TRANSPLANT
International

Supplement 1 to Volume 5, 1992

Proceedings of the
5th Congress of the European Society
for Organ Transplantation
Maastricht, October 7–10, 1991

Editor-in-Chief: Gauke Kootstra

Guest Editors: G. Opelz, W. A. Buurman,
J. P. van Hooff, P. MacMaster, J. Wallwork

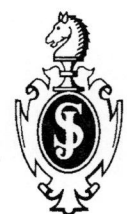

Springer-Verlag Berlin Heidelberg GmbH

TRANSPLANT
International

Official Journal of the European Society for Organ Transplantation

Editor-in-Chief

G. Kootstra
Department of Surgery, University Hospital, P. O. Box 5800,
6202 AZ Maastricht, The Netherlands

Guest Editors

Professor Dr. Gerhard Opelz
Institute of Immunology, University of Heidelberg,
Im Neuenheimer Feld 305,
W-6900 Heidelberg, FRG

Dr. W. A. Buurman
Department of Surgery, University of Limburg,
(B. M. C.) Beeldsnijderdreef 101,
NL-6216 EA Maastricht

Professor Dr. J. P. van Hooff
Department of Nephrology, University Hospital Maastricht,
P. Debyelaan 25,
NL-6202 AZ Maastricht

Mr. P. MacMaster
The Liver Unit, Queen Elizabeth Hospital, Edgbaston,
UK-Birmingham B15 2TH

Dr. J. Wallwork
Papworth Hospital, Papworth Everard,
UK-Cambridgeshire CB3 8RE

Editorial Board

H. Brynger, Göteborg
W. A. Buurman, Maastricht
P. Häyry, Helsinki
R. A. P. Koene, Nijmegen
W. Land, Munich
P. McMaster, Birmingham
M. J. Mihatsch, Basel
G. Opelz, Heidelberg
B. Ringe, Hannover
R. van Schilfgaarde, Groningen
G. Sirchia, Milan
J. P. Soulillou, Nantes
J. P. Squifflet, Brussels
J. Wallwork, Cambridge

International Advisory Board

R. Y. Calne, Cambridge
J. M. Dubernard, Lyon
J. Fabre, East Grinstead, Sussex
L. Fernández-Cruz, Barcelona
A. Flatmark, Oslo
F. Frey, Bern
D. Fries, Paris
C. G. Groth, Stockholm
R. Margreiter, Innsbruck
C. Mawas, Marseille
P. Michielsen, Leuven
E. Möller, Stockholm
P. Morris, Oxford
J. A. Myburgh, Johannesburg
W. L. Olszewski, Warsaw
K. Ota, Tokyo
R. H. Rubin, Boston, Mass.
A. G. R. Sheil, Sydney
S. Slavin, Jerusalem
H. W. Sollinger, Madison, Wis.
T. E. Starzl, Pittsburgh, Pa.
C. R. Stiller, London, Ont.
F. Valderrábano, Madrid

Assistant to the Editor

Pamela Falger

Preface

This supplement to Transplant International contains the Proceedings of the successful 5th Congress of the European Society for Organ Transplantation held in Maastricht from 7–10 October 1991.

Of 827 abstracts submitted to the congress, 548 were selected by the Scientific Committee for either oral or poster presentation. Of these 548 presentations, the guest editors selected 212 full papers for publication in this book.

Two aspects are important where proceedings are concerned – the quality of the papers and the speed of publication. I thank our authors and guest editors, whose combined expertise has given us a guarantee of quality. I also thank our editorial and production teams for their tremendous efforts to hasten editing, proofreading, printing, and publication. In particular, I would like to express my gratitude to Maurits Booster, M. D., and Sylvia van Roosmalen for their assistance and support in seeing this supplement through to completion.

As a concession to time, we have waived some of our stringent rules of style and limited our correspondence with authors by, for example, page proofs being reviewed and corrected in house only. This enables us to publish two months earlier but has the disadvantage that, given the allotted time, we have not been able to ensure that each and every article has an abstract, nor that every "i" has been dotted in the reference lists or in the addresses/institute affiliations of all the authors.

Although contributions to the congress came from every corner of the globe, the core of publications is of European origin, so that this book provides the reader with an update of the state of transplantation in Europe.

May the reader enjoy this book as much as I enjoyed the final editing of it.

Gauke Kootstra, M. D., Ph. D.　　　　　　　　　　　　　　　Maastricht,
Editor-in-chief, Transplant International　　　　　　　　　January 1992

ISBN 978-3-540-55342-7   ISBN 978-3-642-77423-2 (eBook)
DOI 10.1007/978-3-642-77423-2
Published also as Supplement 1 to Volume 5, 1992   ISSN 0934-0874

This work is subject to copyright. All rights are reserved, whether the whole or part of the material is concerned, specifically the rights of translation, reprinting, reuse of illustrations, recitation, broadcasting, reproduction on microfilms or in other ways, and storage in data banks. Duplication of this publication or parts thereof is only permitted under the provisions of the German Copyright Law of September 9, 1965, in its current version, and a copyright fee must always be paid. Violations fall under the prosecution act of the German Copyright Law.

© Springer-Verlag Berlin Heidelberg 1992
Originally published by Springer-Verlag Berlin Heidelberg in 1992

The use of registered names, trademarks, etc. in this publication does not imply, even in the absence of a specific statement, that such names are exempt from the relevant protective laws and regulations and therefore free for general use.

Product Liability: The publisher can give no guarantee for information about drug dosage and application thereof contained on this book. In every individual case the respective user must check its accuracy by consulting other pharmaceutical literature.

23/3020-5 4 3 2 1 0 – Printed on acid-free paper.

TRANSPLANT International

Official Journal of the European Society for Organ Transplantation

Kidney

Liver

Heart, Lung, Heart-Lung

Pancreas, Islets, Small Bowel

Graft Monitoring

Xenografting

Preservation

Immunosuppression

Immunology

Cytokines

Quality of Life

The Donor Problem

Kidney

Transplant Int (1992) 5 [Suppl 1]: S3–S5·

TRANSPLANT
International
© Springer-Verlag 1992

CSA/AZA, in the absence of prednisone, improves linear growth in renal transplanted children

E. David-Neto, W. Nahas, E. C. Sampaio, L. E. Ianhez, E. Sabbaga, and S. Arap

Unidade de Transplante Renal, Servico de Urologia, Hospital das Clinicas da Faculdade de Medicina da Universidade de Sao Paulo, Brazil

Abstract. We compared the results of 44 renal transplants in children, of whom 24 were treated with CSA/AZA and 20 with prednisone in combination with AZA and/or CSA. There were no differences in age distribution or mean ages at transplant between the two treatment groups. The CSA/AZA group had a longer follow-up (29 ± 33 vs 17 ± 18 months). At the last follow-up, five children in the CSA/AZA and none in the prednisone group had lost their grafts. Serum creatinine increased in both groups from 0.7 ± 0.1 mg/dl and 0.9 ± 0.1 mg/dl at the end of the first month to 1.1 ± 0.2 mg/dl in the 36th month (CSA/AZA group) ($P < 0.0001$) and to 1.5 ± 0.6 mg/dl in the 18th month (prednisone group) ($P < 0.05$), respectively. Total cholesterol level was 189 ± 52 mg/dl and 178 ± 60 mg/dl and LDL level was 117 ± 48 mg/dl and 115 ± 51 mg/dl for the prednisone and CSA/AZA groups, respectively. HDL was greater in the CSA/AZA group (50 ± 10 vs 41 ± 10 mg/dl) ($P < 0.03$), and VLDL was greater in the prednisone group (31 ± 13 vs 22 ± 8 mg/dl) ($P < 0.05$). Serum triglyceride was greater in the prednisone group (174 ± 93 vs 112 ± 50 mg/dl) ($P < 0.03$). The standard deviation score for height of the children in the prednisone group did not change (-2.4 ± 1.4 vs -2.1 ± 1.4 SDS), whereas the SDS height score for the CSA/AZA children increased from -3.1 ± 1.7 to -2.6 ± 1.5, -1.9 ± 1.4 and -1.7 ± 1.4, at 12, 24 and 36 months, respectively ($P < 0.001$). CSA/AZA is a good immunosuppressive regime for the first renal transplant in children, but only 75 % tolerated AZA/CSA without same damage to their grafts.

Key words: Renal transplantation – Pediatric – Growth – Cyclosporin A – Prednisone

---

Steroids used for chronic immunosuppression in renal transplantation (RTx) inhibit linear growth in paediatric

Offprint requests to: Dr. E. David-Neto, R. Ferdinando Laboriau, 263, CEP: 01250, Sao Paulo-Brazil

recipients. Since December 1986 we have performed RTx in children followed by triple therapy (CSA/AZA/PRED), stopping the prednisone (PRED) after 6 months in order to improve linear growth. The results of this treatment regime are described here.

Material and methods

A total of 44 children weren enrolled in this study, 24 of them in the CSA/AZA group and 20 in the PRED group, associated with either AZA or CSA or both. The CSA/AZA group comprised 12 children on triple therapy who had PRED withdrawn at 6 months after RTx and 12 who were transplanted a few years before the study started. These children had been maintained on AZA/PRED which was switched to CSA/AZA.

The PRED group comprised children who for various reasons could not have PRED removed from their immunosuppressive regime. The reasons for not stopping PRED were: retransplants (5), CSA nephrotoxicity (2), adequate growth while on PRED (2), nephrotic syndrome (1), haemolytic-uraemic syndrome (1), chronic hepatic disease (1), urinary disorder (1), frequent rejection (2) and parental decision (2). Of these 20 children, four were on AZA/PRED, one on CSA/PRED and 15 on CSA/AZA/PRED.

PRED was started in both groups at 1 mg/kg per day and progressively tapered to 0.12–0.15 mg/kg per day (PRED group) or completely withdrawn by 6 months (CSA/AZA group). CSA was started at 10 mg/kg per day. The dosage was then adjusted to keep the whole-blood trough level (RIA monoclonal specific) around 100–150 ng/ml. AZA was started and kept at 2 mg/kg per day whenever possible.

Table 1. Ages at the start of the study

Age (years)	PRED group	AZA/CSA	Significance of difference
1– 6	6	2	NS
6–12	7	12	NS
12–16	3	7	NS
>16	4	3	NS
Mean + SD	10 ± 5 years	11 ± 4 years	NS
Follow-up (months)			
Mean $\pm$ SEM	17 ± 18	29 ± 33	
Range	3–52	3–55	

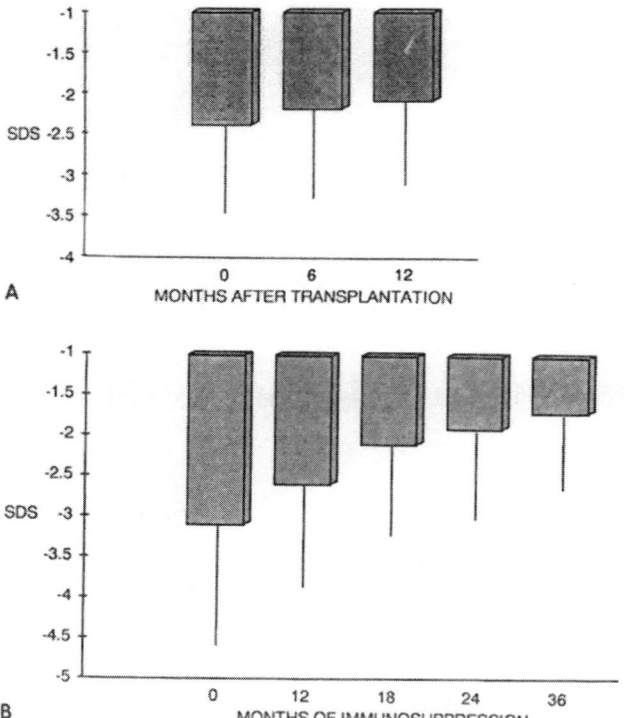

Fig. 1 a, b. Change in standard deviation scores for height after transplantation. **a** PRED group ($P < 0.118$); **b** CSA/AZA group ($P = 0.000$)

The children in both groups had the same age distribution, as seen in Table 1. Mean follow-up was longer in the CSA/AZA than in the PRED group. For this reason we compared data between both groups up to the 18th month.

All results are expressed as mean ± SEM. For continuous variables, analysis of variance was used. Analysis of data between groups was done using, the two-tailed t-test for independent samples with the help of the STATS software.

Results

Serum creatinine (SCr) increased slightly but steadily in both groups. It increased from 0.7 ± 0.1 mg/dl and 0.9 ± 0.1 mg/dl at the end of the first month to 1.1 ± 0.2 mg/dl in the 36th month ($P < 0.0001$) and 1.5 ± 0.6 mg/dl in the 18th month ($P < 0.05$) for the CSA/AZA and PRED group, respectively. There was no difference between the SCr curves up to the 18th month.

In the CSA/AZA group, at the final follow-up, three children had to switch to AZA/PRED because of CSA nephrotoxicity. Two of them are currently well with a mean SCr of 1.2 ± 0.2 mg/dl. The third child lost her graft 1 year later. Four other children in this group lost their grafts, one because of non-compliance, one because of a mistreat acute rejection, one because of haemolytic-uraemic syndrome and one because of arterial thrombosis attributed to CSA toxicity. None of the children in the PRED group lost their graft.

There was no difference in the total and LDL cholesterol levels between the groups. Total cholesterol level was 189 ± 52 mg/dl and 178 ± 60 mg/dl and LDL level was 117 ± 48 and 115 ± 51 mg/dl for the PRED and

CSA/AZA groups, respectively. On the other hand, HDL in the CSA/AZA was greater than in the PRED group (50 ± 10 vs 41 ± 10 mg/dl) ($P < 0.03$), and VLDL was greater in the PRED group than in the CSA/AZA group (31 ± 13 vs 22 ± 8 mg/dl) ($P < 0.05$). Serum triglyceride was greater in the PRED group than in the CSA/AZA group (174 ± 93 vs 112 ± 50 mg/dl) ($P < 0.03$).

AT RTx the children in the PRED group were -2.4 ± 1.4 standard deviation score (SDS) for height. One year later the score had not changed significantly (-2.1 ± 1.4 SDS). In contrast, in the CSA/AZA group, SDS increased from -3.1 ± 1.7 to -2.6 ± 1.5, -1.9 ± 1.4 and -1.7 ± 1.4, at 12, 24 and 36 months ($P < 0.001$).

Discussion

This study illustrates that PRED added to the immunosuppressive regimes for children undergoing RTx leads to some adverse effects that deserve a review of its real need in such recipients, at least on first RTx and in low-risk cases.

We were able to discontinue PRED in 75 % of our first RTx paediatric recipients. In the remaining 25 %, there was either a rejection episode or CSA nephrotoxicity that forced us to reintroduce PRED. These children are currently being treated with another kind of steroid supposed not to have the same adverse effects on growth.

In our group of children, we observed five graft losses in the CSA/AZA group and none in the PRED group. However, all graft losses occurred after a mean of 15 months of CSA/AZA treatment (16 ± 8 months), except for one which occurred in the fourth month (mistreat rejection). As the mean follow-up of the PRED group was currently only 17 months, it is possible that the difference between the two groups in terms of graft loss may disappear with a longer follow-up.

In both groups we observed a steady deterioration of renal function. It was not clear whether this was due to CSA nephrotoxicity or chronic ongoing rejection.

The CSA/AZA group had lower levels of triglyceride and VLDL and higher levels of HDL. Serum lipids have been reported to be higher in patients on CSA/PRED than in patients on AZA/PRED [2]. In our PRED group, 80 % of the patients were also on CSA, and this combination of drugs proved to be more deleterious to serum lipids than the CSA/AZA combination. This raises the possibility that the threat of hyperlipidaemia is not from the CSA, but from the steroids associated with CSA in most protocols. On the other hand, we should note that, al-

Table 2. Linear growth of children in the AZA/CSA group

SDS	Number of children in each category		Significance of difference
	Start	Last follow-up	
$-1 - 0$	0	7	$P < 0.002$
$-1 - -2$	7	5	NS
$-2.1 - -3$	9	3	NS
< -3	8	3	NS
Total	24	18	

SDS, standard deviation score

though higher than in CSA/AZA group, the serum lipids in the PRED group remained within the normal range.

The most striking difference between the two groups was seen in linear growth. We have already demonstrated that PRED in high doses blocks nocturnal GH secretion and in lower doses blocks somatomedin-C activity [3]. In our PRED group the use of 0.12–0.15 mg/kg per day impaired growth. One year after RTx, the children remained -2 SDS below the mean for the height they had been at the time of RTx (Fig. 1 a) and probably will attain adulthood still -2 SDS below mean height, as extensively demonstrated in the literature.

In contrast, the CSA/AZA group demonstrated a catch-up growth of $+0.6$ SDS per year (Fig. 1 b). At the final follow-up, seven of the CSA/AZA children were less than 1 SDS below the mean height for their age (Table 2). If the $+0.6$ SDS per year catch-up growth continues in the years to come we except that all children will be of normal height.

In summary, CSA/AZA was shown to be an excellent immunosuppressive regime for first RTx in paediatric recipients. However, only 75 % of the children tolerated such a regime. The other 25 % still await a new approach which will allow an improvement in their linear growth.

The use of human recombinant GH in very high doses has not been tried by us because the published results on this subject demonstrate an increase in growth rate but do not show a true catch-up growth as evidenced by either the maintenance or a decrease in the SDS for height [1].

References

1. Kamil ES, Yadin O, Ettenger RB, Boechat MI, Pyke-Grimm K, Nelson PA, Lippe BM, Fine RN (1991) Growth after renal transplantation – a potential role for growth hormone therapy. Clin Transplant 5: 208–213
2. Schorn TF, Kliem V, Bojanovski M, Bojanovski D, Repp H, Bunzendahl H, Frei Ulrich (1991) Impact of long-term immunosuppression with cyclosporin A on serum lipids in stable renal transplant recipients. Transplant Int 4: 92–95
3. David-Neto E, Vilares S, Lando V, Nicolau E, Ianhez LE, Sabbaga E, Wajchemberg BL, Arap S (1990) Conversion from azathioprine/prednisone to azathioprine/cyclosporin improves catch-up growth in pediatric renal transplant recipients. Clin Transplant 4: 229–234

TRANSPLANT
International
© Springer-Verlag 1992

Late histopathological findings in renal allografts with four immunosuppressive regimens*

H. Isoniemi[1], **E. v. Willebrand**[2], **J. Ahonen**[1], **B. Eklund**[1], **K. Höckerstedt**[1], **L. Krogerus**[2], **L. Kyllönen**[1], **K. Salmela**[1], and **P. Häyry**[2]

[1] Fourth Department of Surgery and [2] Transplantation Laboratory, Helsinki University, Kasarmikatu 11–13, SF-00130 Helsinki, Finland

The histological changes in renal allografts are usually studied when graft function has already deteriorated. The early results of renal allografts have improved dramatically during the last two decades, but the half-life of renal cadaveric allografts has remained unchanged at approximately 7 years [1]. The mechanism of chronic rejection, and how to prevent it, is not known. We studied the histology of renal allografts under four different immunosuppressive regimens 2 years after transplantation. The aim of this study was to investigate whether histopathological changes exist in the renal allografts with relatively good and stable graft function. We also investigated whether there were differences in allograft histology between four immunosuppressive treatment groups 2 years after transplantation.

Key words: Renal transplantation – Immunosuppression – Histopathology

Patients and methods

Originally 128 consecutive patients with a first cadaveric graft entered a prospective randomized trial. Two-year graft survival was 80% (102 patients). At 2 years all patients with a functioning graft were biopsied. This study group consisted of 89 patients who had an adequate biopsy out of the group of 102 patients. A representative biopsy of 13 grafts was not available because of contraindications to biopsy, patient refusal or inadequate biopsy.

Originally the patients were randomly allocated to four different immunosuppressive groups. One group received triple-drug therapy consisting of cyclosporine (CyA), azathioprine (Aza) and methylprednisolone (MP). Three other groups received all possible combinations of the three immunosuppressive drugs, i.e. CyA + Aza, Aza + MP and CyA + MP [2]. The initial dose of CyA was 10 mg/kg per

* This work was supported by a grant from the Sigrid Juselius Foundation

Offprint requests to: Dr. H. Isoniemi, IV Department of Surgery, Helsinki University Central Hospital, Kasarmikatu 11–13, SF 00130 Helsinki 13, Finland

day, at 1 year the dose was 4 mg/kg per day and at 2 years the mean dose was 3.2 mg/kg per day.

At 2 years 69/89 (78%) patients had normal or near-normal serum creatinine (< 200 μmol/l): mean 148 μmol/l, median 120 μmol/l. Mean and median serum urea were 9.8 mmol/l and 8.0 mmol/l, respectively.

All biopsies were taken two years after transplantation. An automated punch device (Biopty-Cut, Radiplast Bromma, Sweden) was used with ultrasound guidance for percutaneous needle core biopsy. Transplant specimens were obtained with an 18G needle (outer diameter 1.2 mm) which yielded biopsies of 0.9×20 mm. There were no biopsy-related complications using this technique except microscopic haematuria in some cases. Five different stainings were used for light microscopic examination. The specimens were coded and examined by two independent observers. The biopsy was considered representative if it contained at least five glomeruli. Every biopsy was scored separately for histopathological changes in the interstitium (focal and diffuse), glomeruli, vessels (arterioles, arteries and veins) and tubuli (proximal and distal). Altogether 34 different parameters were scored [3]. The histopathological changes were scored semiquantitatively from 0–3 (0 = no change, 1 = mild, 2 = moderate, 3 = severe change).

For testing the correlation between graft function and histological findings the Spearman's rank correlation test was used. For absolute numbers of the four groups, a contigency table was used. For the differences in the intensity of histological changes between the four treatment groups, the Kruskall-Wallis nonparametric test was used. P values > 0.05 were considered significant.

Results

Most of the 34 histological parameters examined showed no changes. Any changes that did occur were usually mild; severe changes were seldom seen. The following score changes were found: diffuse interstitial fibrosis (in 6% of biopsied grafts) diffuse interstitial inflammation (in 2%), glomerular sclerosis (in 3%) and tubular atrophy (in 2%). Diffuse interstitial fibrosis and tubular atrophy were the most common findings, in 2/3 of the grafts, but mostly scored as mild. The other histopathological changes were: diffuse inflammation in interstitium (in 30% of grafts); mesangial matrix increase (37%) and sclerosis (43%) in glomeruli; intimal proliferation (36%) and sclerosis (27%) in vessels; epithelial swelling (36%); basement membrane thickening (25%); anisometric vacuolation (50%); isometric vacuolation (12%); and tubular dilatation (15%). The differences in the frequency of histopathological changes between the four immunosuppressive groups were marginal. The only significant differences in the frequency of changes were in mesangial matrix increase of glomeruli ($P = 0.01$) and in vascular sclerosis ($P = 0.03$), with less frequent changes in the triple therapy group.

Decreased graft function correlated with six histological parameters. These were increasing diffuse fibrosis ($r = 0.40, P = 0.0002$) and diffuse inflammation in interstitium ($r = 0.30, P = 0.005$), sclerosis ($r = 0.33, P = 0.002$) and mesangial matrix increase ($r = 0.34, P = 0.002$) in glomeruli, intimal proliferation in vessels ($r = 0.21, P = 0.05$) and atrophy in tubuli ($r = 0.48, P = 0.0001$).

The histopathological changes were mostly of equal intensity in the four immunosuppressive groups. The only significant differences were seen in diffuse fibrosis in interstitium ($P = 0.05$), mesangial matrix increase in glomeruli ($P = 0.02$), intimal proliferation ($P = 0.03$) and sclerosis ($P = 0.03$) in vessels with fewer changes in the triple-therapy group than in the double-drug regimens. However, other histopathological changes such as diffuse inflammation, glomerular sclerosis and tubular atrophy, were less prominent in the triple-therapy group than in others although the difference was not significant.

A chronic allograft damage index was created for comparison of the four immunosuppressive treatment groups. The index consisted of those six histological parameters which correlated with decreasing graft function. These parameters were diffuse inflammation and fibrosis in interstitium, mesangial matrix increase and sclerosis in glomeruli, intimal proliferation in vessels and atrophy in tubuli. The index was significantly lower in the triple therapy group ($P = 0.009$) (Table 1).

Discussion and conclusion

Two years after transplantation most of the patients (78%) had normal or only slightly increased serum creatinine. Our results demonstrate that even renal allografts with a good and stable graft function exhibit mild histopathological changes, similar to those changes seen in chronic rejection.

Most of the histopathological changes were distributed similarly in the four immunosuppressive groups. There were significant differences only in diffuse interstitial fibrosis, mesangial matrix increase, and vascular intimal proliferation with fewer changes in the triple-therapy group than in any group receiving double-drug treatment.

Table 1. Chronic allograft damage index[a] in the four immunosuppressive groups. Histological biopsy was performed two years after transplantation

Triple ($n = 19$)	Aza + CyA ($n = 23$)	Aza + MP ($n = 25$)	CyA + MP ($n = 22$)	P (Kruskal-Wallis)
1.5	3.2	3.2	4.3	0.009

[a] Sum of diffuse inflammation and fibrosis in interstitium, mesangial matrix increase and sclerosis in glomeruli, intimal proliferation in vessels and tubular atrophy
Mean score per patient per group is presented

However, there was a tendency to less-prominent histopathological changes in the triple-therapy group than in any group receiving a double-drug regimen, and to quantitate this tendency more precisely a new parameter, the chronic allograft damage index was created. The index consisted of those six parameters which were shown to correlate with decreasing graft function, i.e. diffuse interstitial inflammation and fibrosis, glomerular sclerosis and mesangial matrix increase, vascular intimal proliferation and tubuluar atrophy. These are the same histological features which have previously been reported to be associated with chronic rejection [4], which is clinically defined as a gradual but progressive decline in graft function. The chronic allograft damage index was significantly lower in the group receiving triple therapy than in the double-drug treatment groups, thus indicating fewer histopathological changes in the triple-therapy group. The changes in the Aza + MP group, were at the same level as in the other two groups receiving a double-drug regimen. We conclude that triple therapy is more efficacious than any one of the double drug regimens in the prevention of chronic histological changes in renal allografts.

References

1. Cook DJ (1987) Long term survival of kidney allografts. In: Terasaki PI (ed) Clinical transplants 1987. UCLA Tissue Typing Laboratory; Los Angeles, p 277
2. Isoniemi H, Ahonen J, Eklund B, Höckerstedt K, Salmela K, von Willebrand E, Häyry P (1990) Renal allograft immunosuppression. II. A randomized trial of withdrawal of one drug in triple drug immunosuppression. Transplant Int 3: 121–127
3. Isoniemi H, Krogerus L, Willebrand v E, Taskinen E, Grönhagen-Riska C, Ahonen J, Häyry P (1991) Renal allograft immunosuppression. VI. Triple drug therapy versus immunosuppressive double drug combinations: histopathological findings in renal allografts. Transplant Int 4: 151–156
4. Sanfilippo F (1990) Renal transplantation. In: Sale GE (ed) The pathology of organ transplantation. Butterworth, Stoneham, pp 51–101

TRANSPLANT
International
© Springer-Verlag 1992

Flow cytometry evaluation of urinary sediment in renal transplantation

A. Nanni-Costa, S. Iannelli, A. Vangelista, A. Buscaroli, G. Liviano, C. Raimondi, P. Todeschini, G. Lamanna, S. Stefoni, and V. Bonomini

Institute of Nephrology, University of Bologna, Italy

Abstract. The value of exfoliative urinary cytology for the diagnosis of different pathological conditions in renal transplantation is widely recognized. The method, however, has not yet gained full acceptance, mainly because identification of the different cells is not always possible by means of standard staining techniques. In view of its characteristics, flow cytometry (FC) seems to represent a consistently reliable, rapid and innovative approach for differentiating the various cells present in the urinary sediment and assessing their number. This study gives the examination result of 223 urinary specimens from 127 transplanted patients selected according to pathology. Sediment cells, collected from fresh urine samples, were washed, treated with a lysing solution, resuspended in saline solution and directly analysed in a FACSCAN cytometer. Morphological evaluation showed: a small number of cells in patients with stable renal function; a larger number of cells, with predominance of lymphocytes, during acute rejection episodes; an absolute predominance of neutrophils during bacterial infection; large-sized cellular debris in cases of post-transplant tubular necrosis; and small cell debris in cases of cyclosporine cytotoxicity. Lymphocyte surface-marker evaluation made it possible to differentiate lymphocyte populations observed during acute rejection episodes (cytotoxic T-cell, CD8 and HLA class II and NK cells) from those detected during bacterial infection (T-cell CD4 positive). These results suggest that urinary FC may be a reliable diagnostic tool in clinical renal transplantation.

Key words: Renal transplantation – Urinary sediment – Flow cytometry – Lymphocytes

---

The value of exfoliative urinary cytology for the diagnosis of various pathological conditions in renal transplantation

Offprint requests to: Alessandro Nanni-Costa, M.D., Institute of Nephrology, St. Orsola University Hospital, Via Massarenti 9, 40138 Bologna, Italy

has been suggested by various investigators [1, 2, 4, 9]. In particular the detection of lymphocyturia has been indicated as a sign of acute rejection [10].

The main features of standard urinary cytology are its non-invasive nature, ease of execution (usually by Giemsa staining) and the possibility it affords to realize a simple serial monitoring of the patient's condition. Preparing the urinary sediment may, however, give rise to methodological difficulties connected with the quality of material used. At least in some cases identification and quantification of the cells examined may not be possible.

This considerable drawback may be overcome by the use, in this case on urinary sediment, of flow cytometry (FC [6], an up-to-date technique which combines light microscopy examination characteristics, such as multiparametric analysis, with high precision for rapid analysis of individual cells. FC represents a rapid, objective and reliable approach to differentiating and assessing the number of any kind of cell population on the basis of the scatter of a laser beam focused on the cells running through a microscopic capillary called a flow chamber. The light impulses are later processed by a computer which gives a quantitative evalution and a visual picture of the cells examined.

Analysing the results of applying cytometry to urinary sediment diagnosis in renal transplantation may yield interesting results both from the clinical point of view and as regards graft pathophysiology. In clinical terms, it may be possible to identify and quantify sediment cell populations and correlate findings with the varying clinical conditions of the transplant patient, and on an immunological level, it may be possible to identify the profile of the main lymphocyte subpopulations present in the sediment, to compare this with the peripheral circulating subpopulations and to correlate these observations with the immunopathological mechanisms acting in the allograft and/or in the urinary tract.

In this study, a wide range of FC urinary tests were carried out on patients with a clear-cut clinical picture. The aim was to establish whether a correlation exists between urine cytometric results and individual pathology, in which case FC of the urinary sediment would indeed become a valuable diagnostic tool in transplantation.

Patients and methods

The study included 223 urine sediments from 127 transplant patients. All were examined by FC and by normal light microscopy techniques. Samples were divided into five categories selected according to clinical conditions:

1. normal renal function with no clinical or laboratory signs of bacterial infection (41 samples);
2. acute rejection diagnosed from clinical, laboratory, instrument and immunological signs (93 samples);
3. acute infection of the urinary tract diagnosed from clinical signs and culture isolation (57 samples);
4. acute post-transplant tubular necrosis diagnosed via clinical signs (oliguria) and/or laboratory investigations (creatinine clearance < 10 ml/min) (32 samples); and
5. tubular toxicity from cyclosporine (increase in serum creatinine with no sign of rejection, serum cyclosporine > 600 ng/ml (18 samples).

Urinary sediment from 25 normal subjects was examined as a negative control for reference purposes.

Urinary sediment preparation

Fresh urine (10 ml) from the first micturition of the morning was centrifuged at 200 g for 10 min. After removal of the supernatant, the sediment was treated at 22 °C for 10 min with a hypertonic solution (8.3 % NH_4Cl, 1 % $KHCO_3$ and 0.037 % EDTA tetrasodic) in order to lyse out any erythrocytes, after which it was twice washed in phosphate buffer and resuspended in a final volume of 1 ml.

Morphological assessment

Cytomorphometric evaluation of samples was performed using a FACSCAN cytofluorograph (Becton Dickinson, Mountain View, USA). For each sample a cytogram was obtained based on the size and density of each individual cell element, calculated according to the spread of rays emitted by a laser source at a wavelength of 488 nm. From this computerized picture, identification was made of the various cell populations present in the sediment, and for each of these the percentage distribution and overall number was computed.

Analysis of surface markers

In 52 patients suffering from acute rejection (31 cases) or bacterial infection (21 cases) showing a lymphocyturia higher than 500 per ml, determination was made of lymphocyte surface markers on urinary sediment. Peripheral venous blood samples were taken simultaneously. The technique used was that of double immunofluorescence, employing mouse monoclonal antibodies conjugated with fluorescein and phycoerythrin (Table 1), which, because of the

Table 1. Membrane markers and lymphocyte subpopulations

Membrane markers	Monoclonal antibodies	Lymphocyte population
CD3 + TCR	Leu 4 + alpha-beta TCR	T cell
CD3 + HLA class II	Leu 4 + HLA-DR	T-activated cell
CD3 + CD4	Leu 4 + Leu 3	T-helper cell
CD3 + CD8	Leu 4 + Leu 2	T-cytotoxic, T-suppressor (?)
CD16 + CD56	Leu 11 + Leu 19	NK cells

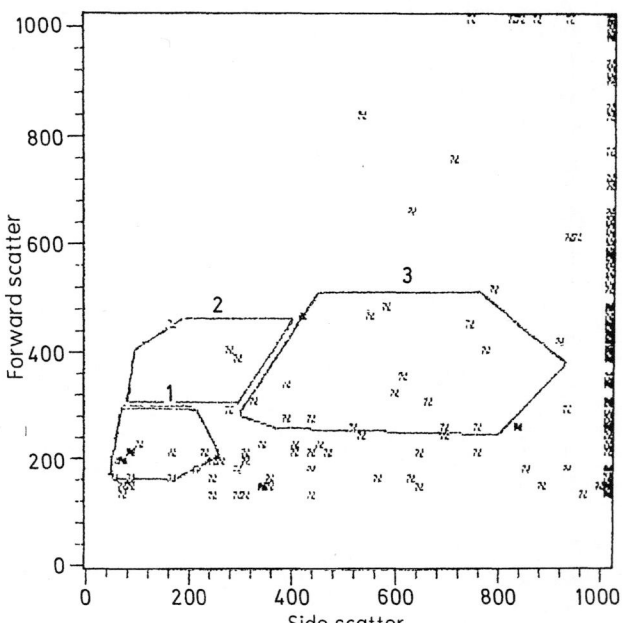

Fig. 1. Cytogram of urinary sediment in a normal subject. The sediment is poor in cells and debris

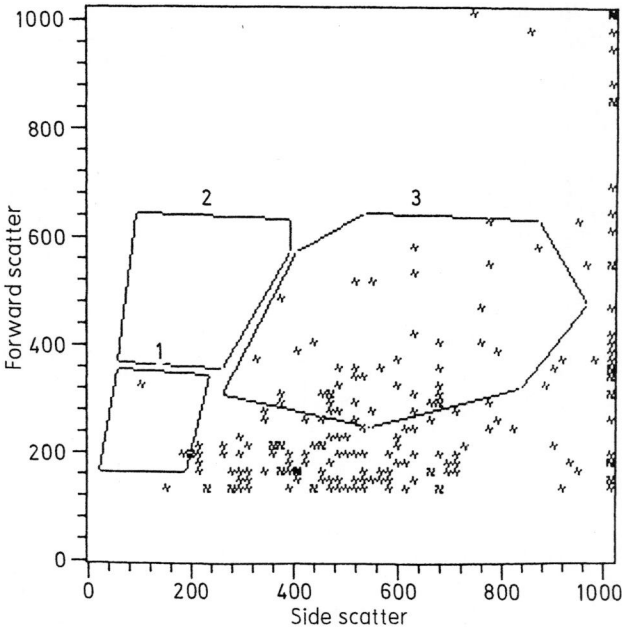

Fig. 2. Cytogram of urinary sediment in transplant patient with stable clinical condition. Cell count appears low

simultaneous use of the two fluorochromes allows simultaneous identification of two different markers on the same cells [3].

To determine lymphocyte surface markers, 0.1 ml of urinary sediment suspension was incubated with 20 µl monoclonal antibody at 22 °C for 15 min, lysed with hypertonic solution and washed twice in buffer solution (PBS) before being brought to a final volume of 0.5 ml.

The same procedure was repeated on samples of venous blood treated with EDTA in order to identify lymphocyte subpopulations in the peripheral blood. Samples were analysed by FACSCAN, obtaining fluorescence cytograms of the antibody-reacting lymphocyte populations. The percentage of positive lymphocytes was calculated for each membrane marker. Lymphocyte viability was assessed, after staining with ethidium bromide, immediately before cytometric analysis. The percentage of viable cells ranged from 55 % to 90 %.

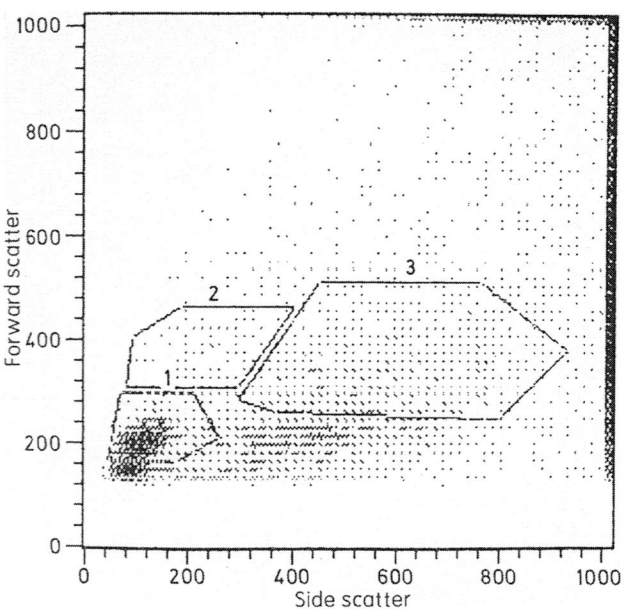

Fig. 3. Cytogram of urinary sediment in transplant patient during an acute rejection episode. Lymphocytes *(bottom right)* clearly predominate

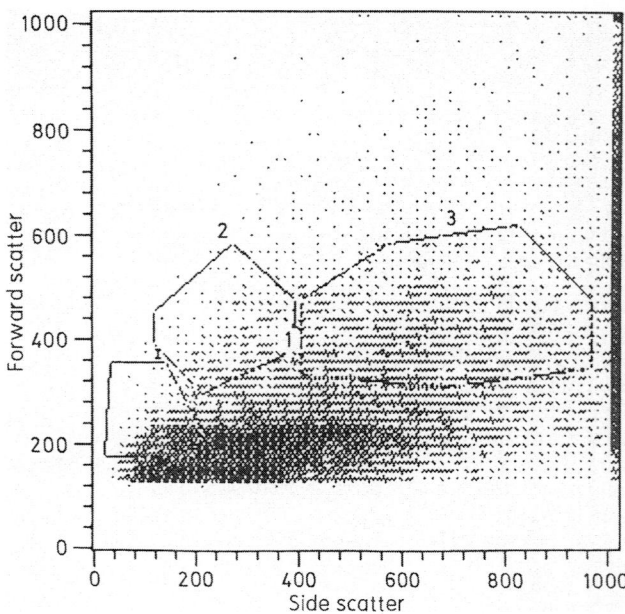

Fig. 5. Cytogram of urinary sediment in patient with post-transplant tubular necrosis. The debris *(right)* has a 'high scatter pattern', i.e. high density and large particles

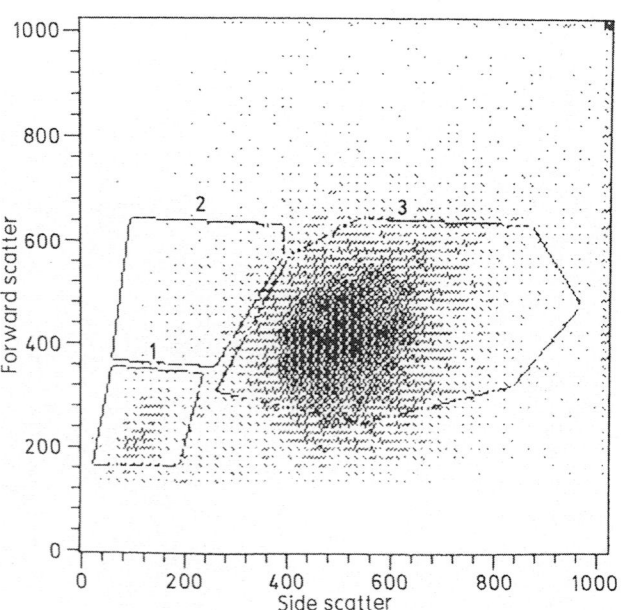

Fig. 4. Cytogram of urinary sediment in transplant patient with urinary infection. Clear prevalence of neutrophils *(middle of picture)*

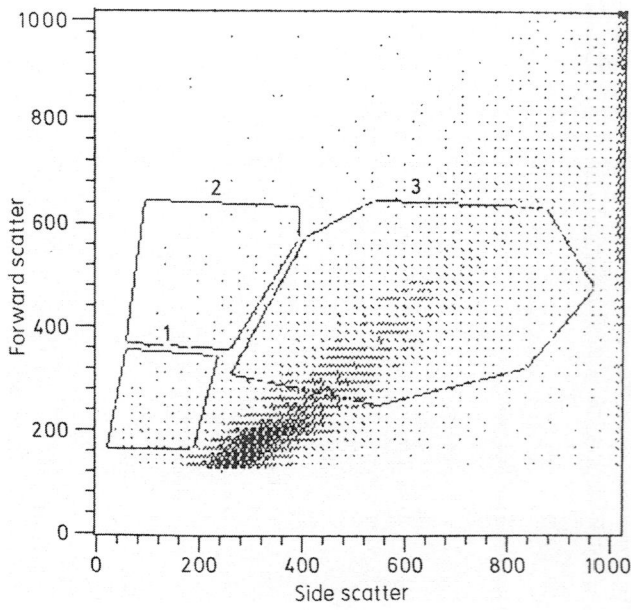

Fig. 6. Cytogram of urinary sediment in transplant patient suffering from cyclosporine toxicity. Debris *(bottom)* has a 'low scatter pattern', i.e. low density and small particles

Statistical analysis

Statistical analysis was performed according to Student's *t*-test for unpaired data.

Results

Figure 1 shows the graphic representation (cytogram), of the urinary sediment in a normal subject as a negative control: the sediment appears extremely poor both in cells and in debris.

Transplant patient cytograms showed a specific morphological pattern according to the clinical condition. Particularly evident are: low cell count in patients with stable renal function (Fig. 2), higher cell count (with lymphocytes clearly predominating) during acute rejection (Fig. 3), and clear prevalence of neutrophils during bacterial infection (Fig. 4). Tubular pathology showed a morphological picture marked by the presence of cell debris. In acute post-transplant necrosis the debris had a high scatter pattern, i. e. high density and large particles (Fig. 5), while in cyclosporine toxicity (Fig. 6) debris had a low scatter pattern, i. e. low density and small particles.

Table 2 shows the number and percentage distribution of identified cell populations in certain of the patient groups (stable clinical condition, acute rejection, bacterial infection and acute tubular necrosis). Patients in a stable

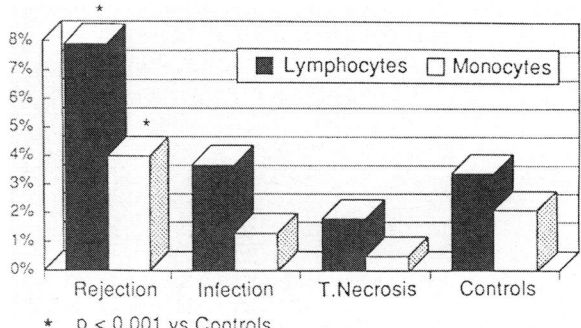

Fig. 7. Lymphocyte and monocyte percent distribution in the various patient groups

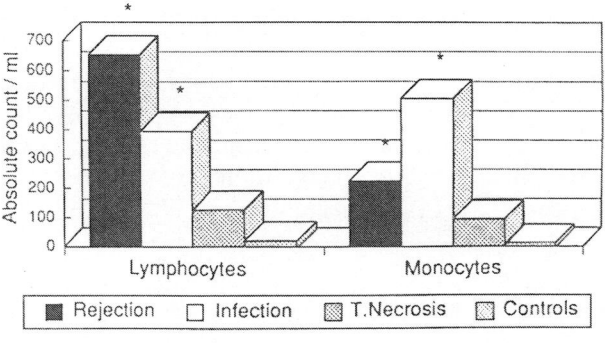

Fig. 8. Lymphocyte and monocyte counts in the various patient groups

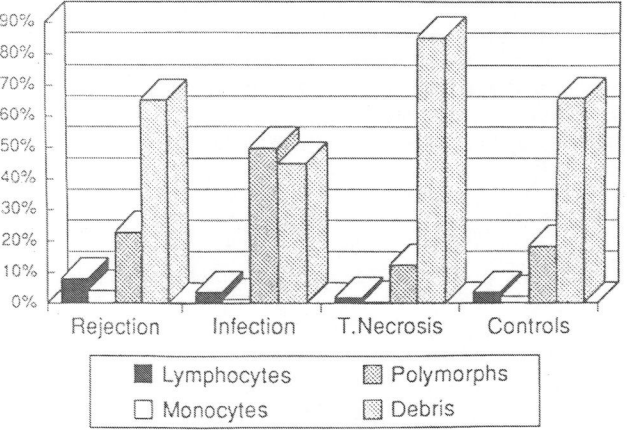

Fig. 9. Percent distribution of lymphocytes, monocytes, polymorphs and debris in the various patient groups

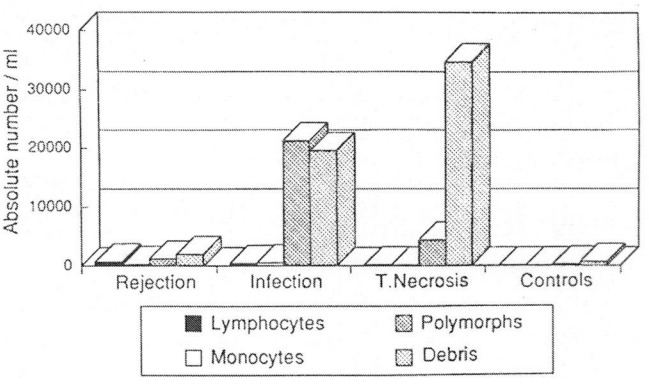

Fig. 10. Cell-count distribution of lymphocytes, monocytes, polymorphs and debris in the various patient groups

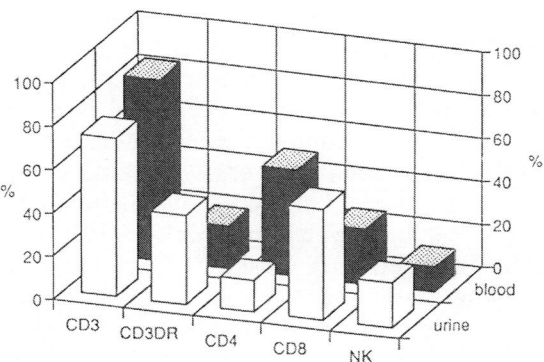

Fig. 11. Lymphocyte subpopulation profile in blood and urine during rejection

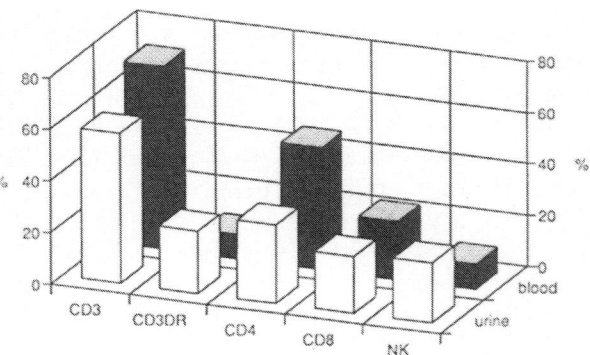

Fig. 12. Lymphocyte subpopulation profile in blood and urine during bacterial infection

clinical condition showed a significantly lower cell count than the other groups ($P < 0.001$).

With regard to the lymphocyte and monocyte percent distribution and absolute count (Figs. 7 and 8), the acute rejection group showed the highest value ($P < 0.001$ vs other groups. Similarly, polymorphs and debris (Figs. 9 and 10) were typical of the bacterial infection and the tubular necrosis groups, respectively.

The distribution of the main lymphocyte subpopulations during acute rejection and bacterial infection is shown in Figs. 11 and 12. During rejection the subpopulation profile differed between the urine and the peripheral blood. The main populations in the sediment were T cells (CD3 and TCR), positive for both CD8 and HLA class II antigens, combined with populations with NK markers and a CD4/CD8 ratio less than 1. In bacterial infection the subpopulation profile in the urine seemed similar to that of the peripheral blood. T populations were predominant, yet the percentage of CD4-positive lymphocytes seemed higher than in rejection, while T-DR-positive, CD8 and NK populations were significantly lower.

Discussion

Despite the noticeable increase in technical equipment currently used in clinical practice, an early and accurate diagnosis of the differing pathological conditions which

Table 2. Number and percent distribution of cellular elements in urinary sediments of renal transplanted patients

	Rejection (n = 93)		Infection (n = 57)		ATN (n = 32)		Controls (n = 41)	
	n	%	n	%	n	%	n	%
Lymphocytes	654* ±267	7.9	394* ±122	3.7	127* ±43	1.8	21 ±25	3.4
Monocytes	225* ±48	4.0	506* ±171	1.3	94* ±63	0.5	11 ±6	2.1
Polymorphs	1143* ±365	22.7	21276* ±5780	49.9	4351* ±794	12.4	184 ±37	18.3
Debris	1954* ±515	65.4	19591* ±6443	45.1	34788* ±13648	85.3	628 ±207	66.2

* p < 0.001 vs Controls
ATN, acute tubular necrosis

may affect a transplanted kidney is problematic for the physician, who sometimes needs time-consuming diagnostic protocols or invasive techniques in order to pinpoint the specific allograft pathology.

FC of the urinary sediment seems to be of real assistance. First of all, the advantage of urine over blood as the medium for patient cytological and immunological monitoring derives from the consideration that, as a product of the transplant organ, urine composition reflects actual intragraft events and is unlikely to be affected by irrelevant systemic events, which may condition blood cell populations. Furthermore, because of its peculiar technical features, urine cytomorphometric analysis offers various advantages over 'classical' cytology: first and foremost, greater simplicity in preparing samples, together with rapidity of execution; second, objectivity, reproducibility and reliability of measurement; third, the ability to obtain a graphic representation and statistical elaboration of the parameters observed [8].

Our results confirm that the diagnostic potential of urine FC is certainly interesting. It allows one to define lymphocyturia during rejection, to identify the morphological profile of urinary sediment in acute tubular necrosis and bacterial infection, to distinguish between a diagnosis of rejection or ischaemic damage in post-transplant oliguria, and to detect tubular damage during cyclosporine administration [7, 11].

In addition, by providing a serial, easily repeatable, non-invasive analysis of the cellular infiltrate of kidney transplants [5], FC may provide further insights for patient clinical monitoring. Our findings on lymphocyte surface markers (Table 1) lead to the identification of the various different lymphocyte subpopulations present in urinary sediment during rejection. The main populations are T cells (CD3 and TCR positive) showing both CD8 and HLA class II antigens, combined with populations with NK markers and a CD4/CD8 ratio less than 1. The antigen pattern of these lymphocytes, probably consisting of active cytotoxic cells, suggests that they come from cytotoxic clones placed in the allograft. These subpopulations also appear significantly different in profile from those circulating in the patient's peripheral blood.

During urinary infections CD4-positive T lymphocytes appear in the urine, probably expressing an immune response against bacterial antigens. Interestingly, the profile

of these populations differs only slightly from that of the peripheral blood.

The results we have reported in this study suggest that monitoring of urinary cytology by means of FC may be a simple, reliable diagnostic tool offering the clinician rapid information on the allograft condition.

Acknowledgment. Supported in part by the Dott. Carlo Fornasini Foundation, Bologna.

References

1. Dooper MM, Bogman MJ, Maas CN, Vooys GP, Koene RA (1989) Immunocytology of urinary sediments in renal transplant patients with deteriorating graft function. Transplant Proc 21: 3596–3597
2. Eggensperger D, Dowd GO, Schweitzer S, Light J (1987) The clinical efficacy of cytodiagnostic urinalysis in the diagnosis of acute allograft rejection: clinico-pathological correlation of 122 specimens. Transplant Proc 19: 1787–1789
3. Fleischer TA, Hagengruber C, Marti GE (1988) Immunophenotyping of normal lymphocytes. Pathol Immunol Res 7: 305–318
4. Krishna GG, Fellner SK (1982) Lymphocyturia: an important diagnostic marker in renal allograft rejection. Am J Nephrol 2: 185–191
5. McWhinnie DL, Thompson JF, Taylor HM, Chapman JR, Bolton EM, Carter NP, Wodd RF, Morris PJ (1986) Morphometric analysis of cellular infiltration assessed by monoclonal antibody labeling in sequential human renal allograft biopsies. Transplantation 42: 353–359
6. Muirhead KA, Horan PK, Poste G (1985) Flow cytometry present and future. Biotechnology 3: 337–355
7. Nanni-Costa A, Stefoni S, Buscaroli A, Iannelli S, Borgnino LC, Stagni B, Raimondi C, Cotti P, Bonomini V (1989) Urinary cytology in renal transplantation. Flow cytometry evaluations. Third European Cytometry User's Meeting, Ghent 1989, pp 123–137
8. Shapiro HM (1988) Practical flow cytometry, 2nd edn. Alan R Liss, New York
9. Simpson MA, Madras PN, Cornaby AJ, Etienne T, Dempsey R, Clowes GH, Monaco AP (1989) Sequential determination of urinary cytology and plasma and urinary lymphokines in the management of renal allograft recipients. Transplantation 47: 218–223
10. Spohn B, Bauer H, Stoetter H, Guth R, Franz HE (1983) Comparison of urine cytology versus fine needle aspiration cytology in monitoring renal allograft disfunction. In: Touraine JL, Traeger J, Betuel H, Brochier J, Dubernard JM, Revillard JP, Triau R (eds) Transplantation and clinical immunology. Excerpta Medica, Amsterdam, pp 218–222
11. Vangelista A, Nanni-Costa A, Fatone F, Buscaroli A, D'Atena T, Bonomini V (1987) Flow cytometry analysis of urinary cytology in renal transplantation. Transplant Proc 19: 1665–1669

Transplant Int (1992) 5 [Suppl 1]: S 13–S 16

TRANSPLANT
International
© Springer-Verlag 1992

Early diagnosis of kidney transplant rejection and cyclosporin nephrotoxicity by urine cytology

M. Kyo[1], F. Gudat[2], P. Dalquen[2], B. Huser[3], G. Thiel[3], N. Fujimoto[1], Y. Ichikawa[1], T. Fukunishi[1], S. Nagano[1], and M. J. Mihatsch[2]

[1] Department of Urology and Renal Transplantation Center, Hyogo Prefectural Nishinomiya Hospital, Japan
[2] Institute of Pathology, University of Basel, Switzerland
[3] Department of Internal Medicine, Cantonal Hospital, Basel University, Switzerland

Abstract. A total of 2000 urine samples from 53 kidney transplant recipients were studied to develop a routine method for the early diagnosis of rejection and cyclosporin (CSA) nephrotoxicity in urine. New-Sternheimer staining and an immunocytochemical technique were used together with classical Papanicolaou staining to differentiate cells in the urine. After cell count and differentiation of second morning urine samples with New-Sternheimer and Papanicolaou stains, immunocytochemistry was performed using antibodies against the following antigens: CD2, CD4, CD8, CD25, CD71 (transferrin receptor), HLA-DR and cytokeratin (Lu-5). Cell counts were obtained for the positively-reacting cells per millilitre of urine. By New-Sternheimer and Papanicolaou staining, CSA nephrotoxicity was characterized by the predominance of proximal tubular cells. During rejection episodes, increased numbers of mononuclear cells and renal epithelial cells were found. Immunocytochemical analysis showed a significant increase in CD2-, CD4-, CD8-, CD25-, CD71-, and HLA-DR-positive epithelial cells and in the ratio HLA-DR/cytokeratin-positive epithelial cells in rejection. CD25-positive cells had the highest sensitivity and specificity for the diagnosis of rejection. Our urine cytology technique proved to be a useful and non-invasive method for the early diagnosis of rejection and CSA nephrotoxicity.

Key words: Urine cytology – Rejection – Cyclosporin nephrotoxicity – Immunocytochemistry – New-Sternheimer staining

The introduction of cyclosporine (CSA) has significantly improved the graft survival rate in renal transplantation [2]. The clinical diagnosis of rejection, however, has become more difficult due to nephrotoxic side-effects of the drug. A non-invasive method is thus needed for daily graft monitoring to complement renal biopsy.

This study was conducted to develop a routine method for the early differential diagnosis of kidney transplant rejection and CSA nephrotoxicity.

Materials and methods

From June 1988 to March 1991, 53 renal transplant patients (19 males, 34 females) with a mean age of 41.8 years (range 9–69) were studied in Basel ($n = 37$) and Nishinomiya ($n = 16$). All patients received CSA and steroids as basic immunosuppression. During the study, 23 rejection episodes in 20 patients and 21 episodes of CSA nephrotoxicity in 18 patients were observed. Rejection was diagnosed by biopsy ($n = 20$) or clinically ($n = 3$). CSA nephrotoxicity cases were also diagnosed by biopsy ($n = 9$) or improvement of renal function after CSA dose reduction ($n = 12$). Two biopsy-proven rejection cases also showed tubular CSA nephrotoxic patterns.

Fresh second-morning urine samples were studied every second day during hospitalization, and after discharge at each medical examination until day 60. Urine samples (25–50 ml) were centrifuged for 10 min at 2000 rpm (700 g), washed in Hank's solution, and counted in a Neubauer's chamber. The cell number was adjusted to about 10000 cells/ml Hank's solution. A cytospin preparation was made in 2 min (for Papanicolaou staining) or 6 min (for immunocytochemistry) at 600 rpm (55 g). For Papanicolaou staining, preparations were fixed immediately with fixspray, Cytostat 400 (Simat AG, Switzerland). The total number of monoclear cells, i.e. lymphocytes and monocytes, and renal epithelial cells (tubular cells and collecting duct cells) was counted.

New-Sternheimer staining was performed for 16 patients in Nishinomiya. After centrifugation for 5 min at 1500 rpm (500 g), lymphocytes/monocytes and renal tubular cells were counted using a simple cell-counting chamber, Kova-System (Miles-Sankyo, Japan). Finally, cell concentration per millilitre of urine of these cells was calculated for each patient.

Immunocytochemical staining was performed by a three-layer alkaline phosphatase anti-alkaline phosphatase (APAAP) method. The monoclonal antibodies used were directed against CD2, CD4, CD8, CD25, CD71, HLA-DR and cytokeratin (Lu-5).

Acetone-fixed cytospin preparations were incubated with the first monoclonal antibody for 30 min at room temperature. After washing with 0.05 M Tris-NaCl buffer, the second incubation with rabbit anti-mouse globulin and the third incubation with the APAAP-complex were performed. After washing, reaction with New-Fuchsin was carried out. Hemalaun was used as counterstain,

Offprint requests to: Masahiro Kyo, M.D., Department of Urology, Hyogo Prefectural Nishinomiya Hospital, 13-9 Rokutanjicho Nishinomiya, 662, Japan

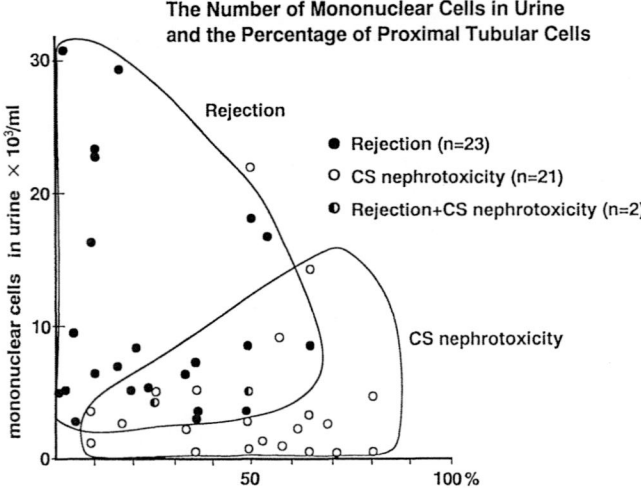

Fig. 1. The number of mononuclear cells in urine and the percentage of proximal tubular cells in all mononuclear cells are shown. Rejection cases showed more mononuclear cells than CSA nephrotoxicity, and in CSA nephrotoxicity proximal tubular cells predominated

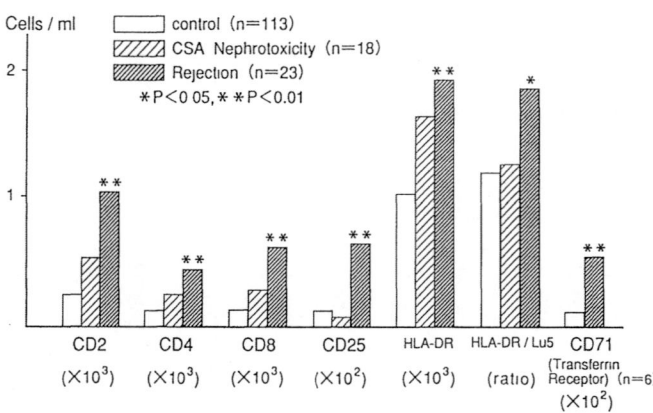

Fig. 2. Immunocytochemical study shows increased numbers of CD2-, CD4-, CD8-, CD25-, CD71-, and HLA-DR-positive cells and the increased ratio of HLA-DR/Lu-5 in rejection. Patients with CSA-nephrotoxicity did not differ from the control group

then 400 mononuclear cells were counted and the cell concentration of positive cells per millilitre of urine was calculated.

Results

Papanicolaou staining

Because of the considerable variation in the number of cells from day to day in the early postoperative days, the first 12 days were not considered in the analysis. Patients with rejections and CSA nephrotoxicity showed increased excretion of mononuclear cells before the clinical diagnosis. All rejection episodes were characterized by an increase in mononuclear cells (mean +/− SD): 1.8 +/− 1.5 to 8.4 +/− 7.5 × 10³/ml). CSA nephrotoxicity cases also showed a slight increase in monocuclear cells (1.7 +/− 2.4 to 6.1 +/− 9.1 × 10³/ml). In cases of CSA nephrotox-

icity proximal tubular cells predominated. These were characterized by size, indistinct cell border, micro- and macro-vacuolization, granular cytoplasm with intracytoplasmic inclusion bodies and eccentric and pyknotic nuclei [14]. The number of mononuclear cells in urine and the percentage of proximal tubular cells among all mononuclear cells at diagnosis of rejection of CSA nephrotoxicity are shown in Fig. 1. Rejection cases showed more mononuclear cells than CSA nephrotoxicity cases ($P < 0.01$), and in CSA nephrotoxicity significantly more proximal tubular cells were found than in rejection ($P < 0.01$).

Immunocytochemical staining

Immunocytochemical staining was performed on 23 urine samples at the time of diagnosis of rejection and 18 urine samples at diagnosis of CSA nephrotoxicity. As control group, 113 urine samples not associated with rejection or CSA nephrotoxicity were used. The mean cell count in rejection cases was significantly higher than in the control group for cells expressing CD2, CD4, CD8, CD25, CD71, HLA-DR and there was also an increased HLA-DR/Lu-5 ratio in rejection (Fig. 2). The CSA nephrotoxicity group showed no significant differences from the control group. Differentiation between rejection and CSA nephrotoxicity cases was possible with the help of CD2*, CD4*; CD8*, CD25** and the ratio HLA-DR/Lu-5* (* $P < 0.05$; ** $P < 0.01$).

For the calculation of sensitivity and specificity, the 75% value of all patients was considered as the upper limit of the normal cell count in urine. The best results for sensitivity and specificity were found in CD25 (Table 1).

New-Sternheimer staining

For screening purposes, New-Sternheimer stain was used. Since 1990, cell counting has been performed on 1500 urine samples at Nishinomiya Hospital. In 10 rejection episodes, 10³ lymphocytes per millilitre of urine on two consecutive days, or more than 2×10^3 lymphocytes per millilitre of urine were observed 3.8 days, on average, before clinical or pathological diagnosis (Fig. 3). Three CSA nephrotoxicity patients excreted proximal tubular cells in the urine at a mean of 4 days before clinical diagnosis.

Table 1. Sensitivity, specificity and predictive value of different antigens for the diagnosis of rejection ($n = 23$)

	CD2	CD4	CD8	CD25	HLA-DR	HLA-DR/Lu5
SE	0.52	0.34	0.52	0.65	0.41	0.58
SP	0.85	0.85	0.86	0.93	0.86	0.76
PVp	0.34	0.24	0.35	0.60	0.20	0.17
PVn	0.92	0.90	0.92	0.95	0.94	0.95

SE, sensitivity; SP, specificity; PV, predictive value of positive (p) or negative (n) cases

S15 top right

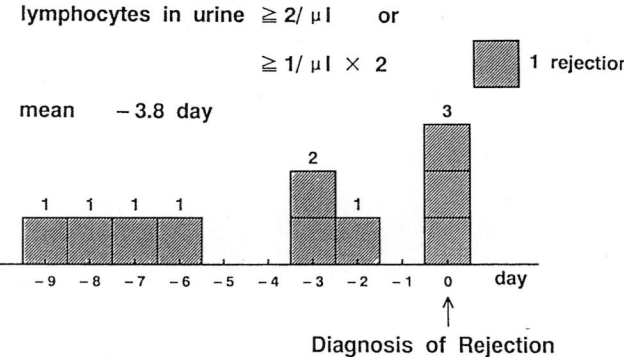

Early Diagnosis of Acute Rejection by New–Sternheimer Stain

lymphocytes in urine ≧ 2/ µl or

≧ 1/ µl × 2

mean – 3.8 day

Fig.3. Results of New-Sternheimer stain in patients with rejection. Rejection episodes were diagnosed on average 3.8 days before the clinical or biopsy diagnosis

Discussion

Objective and if possible non-invasive methods are necessary for the differentiation of rejection and CSA nephrotoxicity. Thick needle biopsy is the standard which allows evaluation of all renal compartments. Fine needle aspiration biopsy permits an analysis of tubulo-interstitial lesions, mainly infiltrating cells and tubular cells [3]. One problem of this technique is the uncertainty of the origin of the aspirated cells, which may come from blood vessels. Despite the use of a thin needle, it is still an invasive method and uncomfortable for the patients. The third method, urine cytology, is the least invasive method for monitoring cellular reacton in the graft. Urine is the easiest material to obtain, and it is the best routine method for graft monitoring, even though urine cytology has the same limitations as fine needle aspiration biopsy in that only tubulo-interstitial lesions can be evaluated.

Several studies on urine cytology have reported the value of lymphocytes [15] or collecting duct cells [4] for diagnosis of rejection. In CSA nephrotoxicity, damaged proximal tubular cells have been found in the urine [13, 14]. A percentage of more than 50 % of proximal tubular cells is highly indicative of CSA nephrotoxicity. Of our CSA nephrotoxicity cases, 65 % showed this predominance of proximal tubular cells, especially those with less than 2000 cells/ml. In cases of more than 2000 cells/ml a gradual increase in lymphocytes and monocytes was also found. In the latter cases, it was difficult to differentiate between CSA toxicity and rejection on the basis of Papanicolaou staining alone. In such cases immunocytochemical studies should also be performed.

Immunotyping of mononuclear cells using monoclonal antibodies has been widely used in recent studies on infiltrating cells in kidney graft biopsies [1]. However, only a few studies have been made in urine cytology. Vangelista et al. [17] found an increase in CD2- and CD8-positive cells in urine during acute rejection. This was confirmed by our study. However, in our study, the highest sensitivity and specificity for rejection was found for CD25-positive cells. Simpson et al. [12] showed that so-

luble urinary IL-2 and IL-2-receptor levels increased in acute rejection, whereas in CSA nephrotoxicity, they were not detected. T-cell activation markers are most helpful for the differential diagnosis of rejection and CSA nephrotoxicity. Another marker indicating T-cell activation is the demonstration of HLA-DR. In normal tissue, HLA-DR antigen is confined to macrophages, dendritic cells, B cells and vascular endothelium [7]. In rejection, however, the expression of HLA-DR antigens increases on renal tubular cells [8]. The ratio HLA-DR/Lu-5 gave better results in the diagnosis of rejection than the absolute number of HLA-DR-positive cells. Lu-5 is a marker of pancytokeratin [5], and in the case of renal damage, the antigen was strongly expressed in tubular cells, but additional HLA-DR expression only occurred in rejection, and not in CSA nephrotoxicity. A positive correlation between the total number of infiltrating cells and anti-transferrin receptor-positive cells in rejection has been reported [8]. Metabolically active cells express transferrin receptor [6]. We found that in all six rejection episodes studied up to now, transferring receptor-positive cells were increased to a similar extent to CD25-positive cells.

In summary, urine cytology is reliable method after the first 2 weeks when urine and cell excretion are less variable than immediately after renal transplantation. The use of New-Sternheimer, Papanicolaou and immunocytochemical stains in combination makes it possible to diagnose rejection and CSA nephrotoxicity earlier than by other clinical means and to differentiate between them.

References

1. Bishop GA, Hall BM, Duggin GG, Horvath JS, Sheil AGR, Tiller DJ (1986) Immunopathology of renal allograft rejection analyzed with monoclonal antibodies to mononuclear cell markers. Kidney Int 29: 708–717
2. Calne RY, Wood AI (1985) Cyclosporin in cadaveric renal transplantation: 3 year follow-up of a European multicentre trial. Lancet 8454: 549
3. Droz D, Campos H, Noel LH, Adafer E, Kreis H (1984) Renal transplant fine needle aspiration cytology: Correlations to renal histology. In: Renal transplant cytology. Proceedings of the Second International Worskhop. Paris Milan Italy Wichitg, pp 59–65
4. Eggensperger D, Schweitzer S, Ferriol E, O'Dowd G, Light JA (1988) The utility of cytodiagnostic urine analysis for monitoring renal allograft injury. Am J Nephrol 8: 27–34
5. Franke WW, Winter S, von Overbeck J, Gudat F, Heitz PU, Staehli C (1987) Identification of the conserved, conformation-dependent cytokeratin epitope recognized by monoclonal antibodies (Lu-5). Virchows Arch A 411: 137–147
6. Gatter K, Brown G, Trowbridge IS, Woolston RE, Mason DY (1983) Transferrin receptors in human tissue: their distribution and possible clinical relevance. J Clin Pathol 36: 539–544
7. Hall BM, Bishop GA, Duggin GG, Horvath JS, Philips J, Tiller DJ (1984) Increased expression of HLA-DR antigens on renal tubular cells in renal transplants: relevance to the rejection response. Lancet 8397: 247–251
8. Henny FC, Weening JJ, Baldwin WM, Oljans PJ, Tanke HJ, Van ES LA, Paul LC (1986) Expression of HLA-DR antigens on peripheral blood T lymphocytes and renal tubular epithelial cells in association with rejection. Transplantation 42: 479–483

9. Mihatsch MJ, Thiel G, Basler U, Ryffel B, Landmann J, Overbeck J, Zollinger HU (1985) Morphological patterns in cyclosporine-treated renal transplant recipients. Transplant Proc 17: 101–116

10. Sanfilippo F, Kolbeck PC, Vaughn WK, Bollinger RR (1985) Renal allograft cell infiltrates associated with irreversible rejection. Transplantation 40: 679–685

11. Seron D, Alexopoulos E, Raftery MJ, Hartey RB, Cameron JS (1989) Diagnosis of rejection in renal allograft biopsies using the presence of activated and proliferating cells. Transplantation 47: 811–816

12. Simpson M, Madras P, Cornaby AJ, Etienne T, Dempsey RA, Clowes GHA, Monako P (1989) Sequential determination of urinary cytology and plasma and urinary cytokines in the management of renal allograft recipients. Transplantation 47: 218–223

13. Simpson M, Madras P, Monaco A (1989) Cytologic examination of urinary sediment in renal allograft recipients. Transplant Proc 21: 3578–3580

14. Stella F, Stella C, Battistelli S, Alfani D, Famulari A, Berloco E, Molajoni ER, Pretagostini R, Rossi M (1986) Monitoring of ciclosporin toxicity by exfoliative urinary cytology in renal transplantation. Contrib Nephrol 51: 152–155

15. Taft PD, Flax MH (1966) Urinary cytology in renal transplantation: association of renal tubular cells and graft rejection. Transplantation 4: 194–204

16. Uchiyama T, Broder S, Waldmann TA (1981) A monoclonal antibody (anti-Tac) reactive with activated and functionally mature human T cells. J Immunol 126: 1393–1397

17. Vangelista A, Nanni-Costa A, Fatone F, Buscaroli A, D'Atena T, Bonomini V (1987) Flow cytometry analysis of urinary cytology in renal transplantation. Transplant Proc 19: 1665–1666

Transplant Int (1992) 5 [Suppl 1]: S17–S20

TRANSPLANT
International
© Springer-Verlag 1992

Haemodynamic changes in human kidney allografts following administration of nifedipine: assessment with doppler spectrum analysis

J. W. S. Merkus[1], L. B. Hilbrands[2], A. J. Hoitsma[2], W. N. J. C. van Asten[1], R. A. P. Koene[2], and S. H. Skotnicki[1]

[1] Clinical Vascular Laboratory, and [2] Department of Nephrology, University Hospital St Radboud Nijmegen, P. O. Box 9101, 6500 HB Nijmegen, The Netherlands

Abstract. Cyclosporin (CyA) has been demonstrated to increase the vascular resistance of renal allografts (RVR), whereas calcium channel blocking agents like nifedipine may counteract this effect. In this study RVR was calculated from renal blood flow (RBF), measured by the clearance of para-aminohippurate (PAH), and mean arterial pressure (MAP). Analysis of Doppler spectra obtained under ultrasonographic guidance was used as a non-invasive method of assessing renal haemodynamics. A comparison was made between these two methods to detect changes in renal haemodynamics which were caused by the administration of 10 mg nifedipine orally to 11 renal transplant recipients treated with CyA. RBF increased significantly (444 ± 176 vs 559 ± 192 ml/min per 1.73 m^2; $P < 0.05$) despite a decrease in MAP (116 ± 10 vs 101 ± 11 mm Hg; $P < 0.05$) after administration of nifedipine. Calculated RVR decreased from 0.31 ± 0.17 to 0.20 ± 0.07 mm Hg $\times$ min/ml ($P < 0.05$). Results of Doppler spectrum analysis were in concordance with these observations. Resistance index (RI) in interlobar arteries decreased from 0.60 ± 0.04 to 0.56 ± 0.06 ($P < 0.05$) and acceleration time (T_{max}) of the Doppler spectrum decreased from 133 ± 32 to 98 ± 32 ms ($P < 0.05$). Theoretically, a lower RI and decreased T_{max} indicate a reduced vascular resistance and changes in vascular wall compliance, respectively. Analysis of Doppler spectra may thus become a useful device for non-invasive assessment of acute changes in RVR.

Key words: Doppler spectrum analysis – Nifedipine – Renal vascular resistance

Analysis of Doppler spectra can be used to assess haemodynamic properties of vascular beds. In human kidney transplantation the analysis of Doppler spectra has been used to estimate haemodynamic changes in kidney allografts. Several reports have been published on the merits of Doppler spectrum analysis in the differential diagnosis of renal dysfunction after transplantation [3, 15]. Parameters derived from Doppler spectra were used to discriminate between different causes of renal dysfunction. The accuracy of this technique, however, is still a matter of debate [13]. More specifically its value in the detection of the nephrotoxic effects of the immunosuppressive drug cyclosporine (CyA) is a matter of controversy [7]. CyA has been shown to increase renal vascular resistance [5], and we have previously shown that intravenous administration of CyA has an impact on renal haemodynamics that can be detected with analysis of Doppler spectra [11]. Calcium channel blockers have been used to ameliorate CyA-mediated renal side-effects, vasodilation most probably being responsible for their beneficial effect [6, 12].

In this study we investigated whether analysis of Doppler spectra enables detection of acute changes in allograft haemodynamics following administration of a calcium channel blocker to patients on CyA treatment. We compared the results of Doppler spectrum analysis before and after administration of nifedipine to CyA-treated kidney allograft recipients undergoing conventional measurements of renal haemodynamics. These observations may contribute to a better understanding of the physiological interpretation of Doppler spectrum-derived information.

Patients and methods

Eleven recipients of a cadaveric renal allograft (9 males, 2 females; mean age 39 ± 12 years) with stable graft function approximately 12 weeks after transplantation were included in the study. The transplantation procedure and post-transplantation care were as described previously [10]. All patients received CyA immunosuppression and low-dose prednisone. None of them were treated with a calcium channel blocker. All patients gave informed consent. Measurements were performed in the out-patient clinic and were started between 8 and 9 a.m. Measurements of renal haemodynamics and echo-Doppler examinations were performed before and after the oral administration of 10 mg nifedipine.

Offprint requests to: J. W. S. Merkus

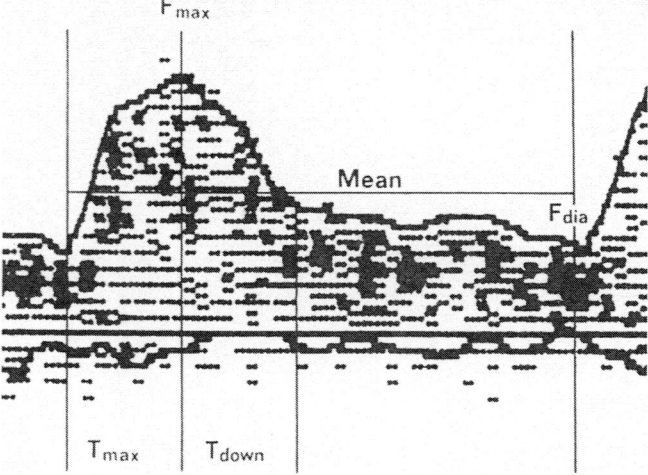

Fig. 1. Doppler spectrum from an interlobar artery with maximum frequency curve and descriptive parameters. F_{max}, maximum systolic frequency shift; F_{dia}, diastolic frequency shift; T_{max}, acceleration time of the systolic deflection; T_{down}, deceleration time of the systolic deflection; Mean, mean frequency shift during one heart cycle

Measurements of renal haemodynamics

During the study patients were in a supine position except during voiding. Blood pressure and heart rate were measured every 3 min with an automatic device (Dinamap, Critikon). Renal clearance of para-aminohippurate (PAH) was used as a marker of effective renal plasma flow (ERPF). After a priming dose, PAH was given by continuous intravenous infusion in a dose adjusted to renal function. After an equilibration period of at least 75 min, urine was collected during three consecutive 30 min intervals. Blood samples were drawn at the midpoint of each interval. A sufficient diuresis was established by an oral water load of 10 ml/kg upon arrival in the ward, followed by IV infusion of a solution of NaCl 0.25 % and glucose 3.3 % at a rate of 400 ml/h, and replacement of excess urinary loss by giving water orally. PAH was measured in serum and urine samples and haematocrit (Ht) in blood samples using standard semi-automated techniques. PAH clearance (ERPF) was calculated using the standard formula UV/P. Renal blood flow (RBF) was calculated as ERPF/1-Ht) and corrected for a standard body surface area of 1.73 m^2. The mean values of five consecutive 3-min interval readings of blood pressure and heart rate around the midpoint of each clearance period were used for analysis. Renovascular resistance (RVR) was defined as mean arterial pressure (MAP) divided by RBF.

Echo-Doppler examinations

Non-invasive examinations were performed with an echo-Doppler scanner (Toshiba SSA-270A), using the B-mode image for guidance of the pulsed wave Doppler sample volume. Doppler spectra were obtained from segmental arteries in the medulla of the allograft and from interlobar arteries near the cortico-medullary junction with a 3.75 MHz sector probe. The angle between the Doppler beam and the artery under investigation was kept below 50° and in the same range in consecutive examinations. With each examination a Doppler spectrum from the common femoral artery on the side of the allograft was also obtained using the 5.0 MHz linear array probe. Doppler spectra were stored on a personal computer for off-line analysis by a user-written program. The program determined a Doppler waveform from the Doppler spectrum representing the instantaneous maximum frequency for every time moment. Subsequently several parameters describing the Doppler waveform were calculated. Figure 1 shows a Doppler spectrum from a segmental artery

and the derived parameters as produced by the computer program. Restistance index (RI) and Pulsatility index (PI) were calculated according the methods of Planiol and Pourcelot [14] and Gosling et al. [9].

The means of blood pressure, heart rate, RBF and RVR of the first three consecutive 30-min periods were used as base-line values. The accompanying first ech-Doppler examination was performed during the third period. Immediately after the end of this period the patient received 10 mg nifedipine orally. Repeated measurements of renal haemodynamics took place from 30 to 60 min after administration of nifedipine. During this period the second echo-Doppler examination was performed.

Statistics

All values are expressed as means ± SD. For comparison of measurements before and after administration of nifedipine, the *t*-test for matched pairs was used. Spearman correlation coefficients (r) were calculated to quantify the correlation between the results of renal function measurements and Doppler parameters. Probability values below 0.05 were considered significant.

Results

The effects of the administration of nifedipine on blood pressure and renal haemodynamics are given in Table 1. Systolic and diastolic blood pressures decreased significantly after nifedipine administration. Mean arterial pressure fell from 116.3 ± 10.0 to 101.1 ± 11.1 ($P < 0.01$). The increase in RBF, despite this fall in MAP, is reflected in a significant reduction in calculated RVR.

Significant changes were also observed in Doppler parameters derived from spectra obtained from the segmental and interlobar arteries of the renal allograft. The acceleration time of the systolic peak of the Doppler waveform (T_{max}) became shorter in both arteries. In the interlobar arteries a significant decrease was found in RI and PI. When renal vascular resistance was correlated with RI obtained from segmental and interlobar arteries, only weak, non-significant, correlations were found ($r = 0.45$ ($P = 0.16$) and $r = 0.57$ ($P = 0.07$), respectively) before administration of nifedipine. After administration of nifedipine, however, RI showed a significant correlation with RVR ($r = 0.66$ ($P = 0.03$) and $r = 0.76$ ($P = 0.007$) in segmental and interlobar arteries, respectively). Figure 2 shows this relationship between RVR and RI from interlobar arteries before and after the administration of nifedipine.

Table 1. Effects of administration of nifedipine on blood pressure and renal haemodynamics

	Nifedipine administration		
	Before	After	P value
Systolic BP (mmHg)	163.0 ± 16.2	142.5 ± 16.6	< 0.01
Diastolic BP (mmHg)	90.6 ± 10.8	77.0 ± 9.6	< 0.01
MAP (mmHg)	116.3 ± 10.5	101.1 ± 11.7	< 0.01
Heart rate (bpm)	63.5 ± 8.6	75.0 ± 14.5	< 0.01
RBF (ml/min per 1.73 m^2)	445 ± 168	559 ± 184	< 0.01
RVR (mmHg × min/ml)	0.32 ± 0.17	0.20 ± 0.07	< 0.01

BP, blood pressure; MAP, mean arterial pressure; RBF, renal blood flow; RVR, renal vascular resistance

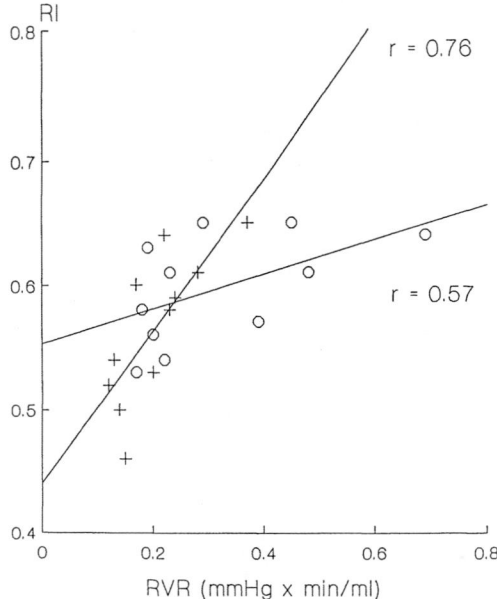

Fig. 2. Correlation of renal vascular resistance (RVR) and resistance index (RI) from interlobar arteries before and after administration of nifedipine. O, Before administration of nifedipine ($r = 0.57$; $P = 0.07$); +, after administration of nifedipine ($r = 0.76$; $P = 0.007$)

In Doppler spectra obtained from the common femoral artery, just distal to the end-to-side anastomosis of the renal artery with the iliac artery, no significant changes were noted after administration of nifedipine.

Discussion

The primary goal of this study was to assess whether Doppler spectrum analysis can detect haemodynamic changes in human kidney allografts after drug-induced haemodynamic interference. We compared changes in Doppler parameters to nifedipine-induced changes in RVR, which was calculated from PAH clearance, haematocrit and MAP. Although the latter calculation only provides a rough estimate, it is commonly used to gain information on global renal vascular resistance [5].

Doppler parameters indicated changes in the haemodynamic properties of the renal allograft. The RI and PI decreased significantly in the interlobar arteries. Also T_{max} decreased in segmental and in interlobar arteries. There were no changes in the Doppler spectra obtained from the femoral artery distal to the renal allograft. Thus it is most likely that the changes observed in the arteries of the allograft are indicative of changes located in the allograft itself, and are not merely the result of a decrease in systemic mean arterial pressure. Moreover, when systemic pressure decreases, no change in RI is expected when renal resistance remains unchanged [2]. The decrease in RI and PI indicates a decrease in vascular resistance. The changed impedance of the renal allograft was confirmed with the measurements of renal haemodynamics, which showed a decrease in RVR.

Correlation of RI and RVR improved markedly after administration of nifedipine. This suggests that one of the two methods of estimation of vascular resistance is more influenced than the other by a variable that has less impact after administration of nifedipine. A possible explanation for this observation is that, after administration of nifedipine, RVR becomes more dependent on the resistance of arteries from which RI was obtained.

RI and PI are generally considered reliable parameters for the estimation of resistance of the distal part of a vascular bed. We found a significant decrease in these parameters in interlobar arteries, which are closest to the probable site of the vasoconstrictive action of CyA [1, 8]. Nifedipine may be expected to have the largest influence on haemodynamics at that site. T_{max} is a parameter which is more difficult to interpret. In clinical renal transplantation, T_{max} has been indicated by Arima et al. [4] as a parameter that is correlated with renal function. In their study a shorter T_{max} was found in renal allografts with stable function, whereas T_{max} was longer in allografts with poor function. In the mathematical model for Doppler waveform analysis introduced by Skidmore and Woodcock [16], T_{max} was regarded as indicative of the elastic properties of the vascular wall: changes in T_{max} reflect changes in vascular wall compliance. Apparently, the vasodilatory effect of nifedipine on the vascular wall of renal arteries that are preconstricted by CyA is reflected in shortening of T_{max} in the Doppler spectrum waveform.

In summary, the changes in renal vascular resistance due to vasodilatory effects of nifedipine are reflected in the Doppler spectrum waveform, in changes in RI, indicating decreased distal resistance to flow, and in changes in T_{max}, reflecting changes in vascular wall compliance. From these observations we conclude that haemodynamic changes in human kidney grafts due to drug interventions can be detected with Doppler spectrum analysis. This may make this non-invasive technique suitable for monitoring acute haemodynamic changes due to drug interventions in human kidney allografts.

Table 2. Results of analysis of Doppler spectra before and after administration of nifedipine

	Nifedipine administration		
	Before	After	P value
Segmental artery:			
F_{max} (Hz)	1612 ± 663	1842 ± 411	0.241
F_{dia} (Hz)	635 ± 328	712 ± 203	0.441
T_{max} (ms)	130 ± 41	79 ± 34	0.014*
RI	0.61 ± 0.05	0.62 ± 0.07	0.874
PI	1.07 ± 0.15	1.08 ± 0.21	0.899
Interlobar artery:			
F_{max} (Hz)	932 ± 209	1037 ± 285	0.261
F_{dia} (Hz)	374 ± 92	448 ± 122	0.070
T_{max} (ms)	133 ± 32	98 ± 32	0.008*
RI	0.60 ± 0.04	0.56 ± 0.06	0.025*
PI	1.07 ± 0.15	0.93 ± 0.17	0.048*
Femoral artery:			
F_{max} (Hz)	2655 ± 783	2927 ± 778	0.056
F_{dia} (Hz)	− 833 ± 233	− 773 ± 222	0.468
T_{max} (ms)	105 ± 14	104 ± 17	0.932
PI	6.1 ± 0.9	5.6 ± 1.5	0.395

* $P < 0.05$; for explanation of parameters see legend to Fig. 1

Acknowledgement. This study was supported by a grant from the Dutch Kidney Foundation (Grant no. C90.1023).

References

1. Abrahams JS, Bentley FR, Garrison RN, Cryer HM (1991) Cyclosporine A directly constricts intrarenal arterioles. Transplant Proc 23: 356–359
2. Adamson SL, Morrow RJ, Bascon PAJ, Mo LYL, Ritchie JWK (1989) Effect of placental resistance arterial diameter, and blood pressure on the uterine arterial velocity waveform: a computer modeling approach. Ultrasound Med Biol 15: 437–442
3. Allen KS, Jorkasky DK, Arger PH, Velchik MG, Grumbach K, Coleman BF, Mintz MC, Betsch SE, Perloff LJ (1988) Renal allografts: prospective analysis of Doppler sonography. Radiology 169: 371–376
4. Arima M, Ishibashi M, Usami M, Sagawa S, Mizutani S, Sonoda T, Ichikawa S, Ihara H, Nagano S (1979) Analysis of the arterial blood flow patterns of normal and allografted kidneys by the directional ultrasonic Doppler technique. J Urol 122: 587–591
5. Curtis JJ, Dubovsky E, Whelchel JD, Luke RG, Diethelm AG, Jones P (1986) Cyclosporin in therapeutic doses increases renal allograft vascular resistance. Lancet i: 477–479
6. Dawidson I, Rooth P, Fry WR, Sandor Z, Willms C, Coorpender L, Alway C, Reisch J (1989) Prevention of acute cyclosporine induced renal blood flow inhibition and improved immunosuppression with verapamil. Transplantation 48: 575–580
7. Don S, Kopecky KK, Fili RS, Leapman SB, Thomalla JV, Jones JA, Klatte EC (1989) Duplex Doppler US of renal allografts: causes of elevated resistive index. Radiology 171: 709–712
8. English J, Evan A, Houghton DC, Bennett WM (1987) Cyclosporine induced acute renal dysfunction in the rat. Evidence of arteriolar vasoconstriction with preservation of tubular function. Transplantation 44: 135–141
9. Gosling RC, Dunbar G, King DH (1971) The quantitative analysis of occlusive peripheral arterial disease by a non-intrusive ultrasonic technique. Angiology 22: 52–55
10. Hoitsma AJ, Wetzels JFM, Van Lier HJJ, Berden JHM, Koene RAP (1987) Cyclosporin treatment with conversion after three months versus conventional immunosuppression in renal allograft recipients. Lancet i: 584–586
11. Merkus JWS, Asten van WNJC, Hoitsma AJ, Koene RAP, Skotnicki SH (1991) Doppler spectrum analysis can detect immediate haemodynamic effects of cyclosporine infusion on human kidney grafts. Transplant Proc 23: 972–973
12. Morales JM, Andres A, Preto C, Ortuno B, Ortuno T, Patermina ER, Hernandez Pablete G, Praga M, Ruilope LM, Rodicio JL (1989) Calcium antagonist treatment of recipients minimizes cyclosporine nephrotoxicity in renal transplantation. A prospective randomized trial. Transplant Proc 21: 1537–1539
13. Perella RR, Duerinckx AJ, Tessler FN, Danovitch GM, Wilkinson A, Gonzalex S, Cohen A, Grant EG (1990) Evaluation of renal transplant dysfunction by duplex Doppler sonography: a prospective study and review of the literature. Am J Kidney Dis 15: 544–550
14. Planiol T, Pourcelot L (1974) Doppler effect study of the carotid circulation, in: White D, McCready V, Vlieger M (eds) Ultrasonics in medicine. Excerpta Medica, Amsterdam, pp 104–111
15. Rigsby CM, Burns PM, Weltin GG, Chen B, Bia M, Taylor KJW (1987) Doppler signal quantitation in renal allografts: Comparison in normal and rejecting transplants with pathologic correlation. Radiology 162: 39–42
16. Skidmore R, Woodcock JP (1980) Physiological interpretation of Doppler shift waveforms-I. Theoretical considerations. Ultrasound Med Biol 6: 7–10

Transplant Int (1992) 5 [Suppl 1]: S 21–S 22

TRANSPLANT
International
© Springer-Verlag 1992

Cyclosporine renal cortical vasoconstriction measured by colour doppler imaging in kidney transplantation

F. Quarto Di Palo[1], **D. Castagnone**[3], **R. Rivolta**[3], **F. Ceccherelli**[2], **A. Elli**[1], **M. Parenti**[1], **P. Palazzi**[1], and **C. Zanussi**[1]

[1] Clinica Medica 1°, and [2] Laboratory Analisi Cattedra 4 Igiene, Università di Milano, Milano, Italy,
[3] Servizio di Radiologia Medica Ospedale Maggiore Milano, Milano, Italy

Important side-effects limit the use of cyclosporine A (CSA), the most insidious of which is nephrotoxicity, which manifests as a preglomerular arteriolar vasoconstriction causing a reduction in glomerular filtration rate (GFR) and renal plasma flow (RPF). This condition is initially purely functional, but with time can become anatomic and irreversible [4].

In clinical practice we lack suitable methods for evaluating CSA vasoconstriction. Our present knowledge is based on indirect information obtained from repeated measurements of plasma creatinine levels and from blood concentrations of the drug. Sometimes more complex and non-routine tests, such as the evaluation of GFR and RPF, or invasive methods, such as renal biopsy, are also employed.

In this study we used the colour-Doppler technique to measure directly the vascular effects of CSA in patients with transplanted kidneys, evaluating changes in blood flow at the hilus and on the cortex of the kidney when the drug was at trough or peak levels.

Key words: Renal transplantation – Cyclosporine – Vasoconstriction – Doppler imaging

Materials and methods

We studied 14 patients with cadaveric renal transplants (seven men and seven women) with a mean age of 34.5 ± 8.5 years. The transplants were well established (34.6 ± 27 months), with good renal function (plasma creatinine < 140 mM/l). None of the patients was taking antihypertensive drugs. All were under triple immunosuppressive therapy, with identical doses of steroids and azathioprine. CSA was taken in two equal daily doses at a mean dose of 4.5 ± 0.5 mg/kg per day. Whole-blood levels of the drug, measured by FPIA (Abbott polyclonal antibody), ranged between 350 and 700 ng/ml. Before the trial, patients took no medications for 12 h.

At 9 a.m. blood samples for the measurement of CSA trough levels and plasma creatinine were taken, mean arterial blood press-

Offprint requests to: F. Quarto Di Palo

ure (MAP) was determined and colour-Doppler spectra obtained. At the end of the procedure, patients took their doses of CSA and 3 h later (peak time) the same determinations were repeated.

To evaluate the effect of the drug on the chronically damaged kidney, the same parameters were repeated on a group of 13 cadaveric renal transplant patients with reduced, but stable, renal function (plasma creatinine 140–350 mM/l).

The ATL Ultramark-9 apparatus with a 3.5 or 5 MHz probe was used to obtain the hilar and cortical colour-Doppler spectra. We used the indices RI (resistive index = peak systolic velocity minus the lowest diastolic velocity divided by peak systolic velocity) and PI (pulsatility index = peak systolic velocity minus the lowest diastolic velocity divided by mean velocity) to eliminate the bias associated with the angle of determination of the velocity in the vessel. With this system it is possible to compare the data obtained at different times with a large margin of specificity, sensitivity and accuracy [1, 3, 6, 7]. All the colour-Doppler values presented are the mean of five successive measurements.

The values are presented as means ± SE. The significance of the differences between the values obtained at trough and peak levels was determined by the t-test for paired data. Linear regression analysis was used to look for relationship between blood cyclosporine and colour-Doppler parameters.

Results

In our patients, the mean CSA blood levels increased from 338 ± 36 ng/ml (trough) to 801 ± 106 ng/ml (peak) ($P < 0.002$). Mean blood pressure (MAP) did not change significantly, being 107.5 ± 5 mm Hg at the trough time and 114 ± 3 mm Hg at the peak time.

The PI and RI measured at the hilus of the kidney did not vary significantly (PI, trough 1.01 ± 0.05 vs peak 1.17 ± 0.10; RI, trough 0.62 ± 0.02 vs peak 0.64 ± 0.03.

The changes in the Doppler spectra of the renal cortex after CSA were more striking. The PI increased from a trough value of 0.82 ± 0.02 to a peak value of 1.11 ± 0.03 ($P < 0.0001$). The change in the RI was analogous, going from a trough value of 0.54 ± 0.009 to a peak value of 0.64 ± 0.007 ($P < 0.0001$).

In the cortex, a positive linear correlation between CSA level and PI value (r, 0.60; $P < 0.02$; $n = 28$) was found. The higher the level of the drug, the more the pe-

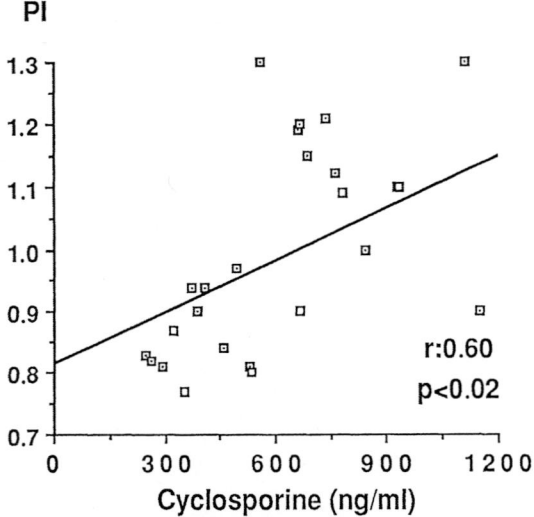

Fig. 1. Relationship between CSA levels in whole blood and pulsatility index (PI) measured on the renal cortex at the same time (*n* = 28)

ripheral resistance increased and the diastolic flow decreased (Fig. 1).

The effect of CSA on colour-Doppler spectra of the kidney in the group of patients with chronically impaired renal function was identical to that observed in well-functioning grafts, except for higher trough values. At the hilus of the kidney PI was 1.32 ± 0.12 at trough vs 1.41 ± 0.15 at peak (NS) and RI was 0.68 ± 0.03 at trough vs 0.70 ± 0.03 at peak (NS). On the renal cortex PI was 1.07 ± 0.09 at trough vs 1.43 ± 0.016 at peak ($P < 0.02$) and RI was 0.62 ± 0.03 at trough vs 0.71 ± 0.03 at peak ($P < 0.03$).

Discussion

Cyclosporine dose-dependently decreased cortical blood flow in the transplanted kidney. The effect was specific and agreed with other reports that show a vasoconstrictive action of the drug on afferent arterioles [5].

Orally administered CSA causes continuous cyclic changes in renal cortical blood flow and in renal vascular resistance related to the varying blood levels of the drug during the daytime. In the patients with good graft function, these variations did not appear to have produced any clinically relevant renal damage. However, the greater nephrotoxicity related to the higher peaks obtained when CSA was given once a day [2] indicates that these vascular changes are not entirely risk free.

The vasoconstrictive effect of CSA is not modified by the presence of impaired renal function. In these cases, an identical level of the drug will produce a greater reduction in blood flow than in the well-functioning kidneys.

It is therefore reasonable to believe that at higher doses of CSA, or in the presence of other concomitant disease states that reduce renal function, these variations in cortical blood flow might play a part in the production of the complex physiopathological phenomenon that leads to nephrotoxicity. If this hypothesis is true, then colour-Doppler imaging which is sensitive, repeatable and non-invasive, may be a new tool for monitoring renal blood flow over time and for evaluating the risk of nephrotoxicity associated with CSA therapy.

References

1. Allen KS, Jorkasky DK, Arger PH, Velchik MG, Grumbach K, Coleman BG, Mintz MC, Betsch SE, Perloff LJ (1988) Renal allografts: prospective analysis of doppler sonography. Radiology 169: 371–376
2. Dieperink H, Leyssac PP, Starklint H, Kemp E (1988) Cyclosporine A administration: once a day or in fractional doses? Transplant Proc 20 [supp 2]: 703–706
3. Leichtman AB, Sorrell KS, Wombolt DG, Hurwitz RL, Glickman MH (1989) Duplex imaging of the renal transplant. Transplant Proc 21: 3607–3610
4. Mason J (1990) Renal side-effects of cyclosporine. Transplant Proc 22: 1280–1283
5. Myers BD (1989) What is cyclosporine nephrotoxicity? Transplant Proc 21: 1430–1432
6. Rifkin MD, Needleman L, Pasto ME, Kurtz AB, Foy PM, McGlynn E, Canino C, Baltarowich OH, Pennel RG, Goldberg BB (1987) Evaluation of renal transplant rejection by duplex doppler examination: value of the Resistive Index. AJR 148: 759–762
7. Skotnicki SH, van Asten WNJC, Beijneveld WJ, van Roosmalen R, Hoitsma AJ, Wijn PFF (1989) Evaluation of renal allografts function by doppler spectrum analysis. Transplant Int 2: 16–22

Transplant Int (1992) 5 [Suppl 1]: S 23–S 25

TRANSPLANT
International
© Springer-Verlag 1992

Monoclonal immunoglobulins in patients with renal transplants: characterization, evolution and risk factors

C. Chakalarovski, Ph. Lang, Cl. Buisson, B. Bourgeon, L. Intrator, L. Deforge, A. Benmaadi, G. Fruchaud, G. Rostoker, Ph. Remy, D. Belghiti and B. Weil

Department of Nephrology and INSERM U 139, Hopital Henri Mondor, Créteil 94010, France

Abstract. Gammopathies were found to be present in 25 (13%) of 192 HIV-negative renal transplant recipients with more than 30 months follow-up prospectively investigated for monoclonal or oligoclonal immunoglobulins (mIg) by agarose gel electrophoresis and immunofixation. Eleven patients had only one monoclonal band, whereas 14 had two or more bands. Of these bands, 60% were IgG kappa, 29% IgG lambda and 11% IgM lambda or kappa, and 90% did not exceed 2 g/l. Most gammopathies occurred early post-transplant (median 5 months) and they were always transient. Some predisposing factors for mIg emergence could be identified: 1. age, but only in women, 2. duration of dialysis, 3. occurrence of prior cytomegalovirus infection, and 4. immunosuppressive regimen including cyclosporine. Serological evidence for active EBV infection was obtained in ten patients, but in six cases infection occurred subsequent to the finding of mIg. In eight patients, the clinical course was characterised by severe infection or tumours (one Kaposi's sarcoma, one B-cell brain lymphoma). The present findings and experimental studies support the view that the development of mIg in renal transplant patients is associated with a failure of regulatory T-cell function. This T-B-cell imbalance requires a careful follow-up in these patients.

Key words: Renal transplantation – Gammopathies

Organ transplantation is associated with an increased risk of developing monoclonal or oligoclonal B-cell lymphomas [2, 10], and a high incidence of monoclonal immunoglobulins (mIg) has recently been described in renal transplant patients [7, 18, 22]. It is unclear whether these mIg are predisposing factors for the development of B-cell malignancies, and they are classifed by Kyle as monoclonal gammopathies of undetermined significance [14, 15]. The present study was performed to evaluate the incidence,

the characteristics and the natural history of these gammopathies. We also tried to determine the risk factors for the occurrence of these mIg.

Patients and methods

HIV-negative renal transplant recipients ($n = 192$) with a functional kidney at 3 months were prospectively investigated for monoclonal or oligoclonal immunoglobulins by agarose gel electrophoresis and by the immunofixation method of Ritchie and Smith [20]. The tests were performed every 3–6 months. All the patients had a follow-up of at least 30 months since transplantation. They received anti-lymphocyte globulins (Mérieux) prophylactically for 2 weeks in association with steroids and azathioprine. Thereafter, patients with low panel reactive antibodies were randomized to receive or not to receive a triple-drug therapy including cyclosporine (CsA). The dose of CsA never exceeded 8 mg/kg per day. Secondary transplant patients and highly sensitized patients were systematically treated with a triple-drug therapy. Finally, the present study included 116 patients treated with a triple-drug therapy and 76 patients treated without CsA.

Statistical analysis was carried out using the chi-squared test or Mann-Whitney U test where appropriate.

Results

Of the study group, 25 (13%) had a monoclonal or multiclonal gammopathy. Of these, 14 (56%) had multiple bands: 12 had two bands, one had three bands and one had four bands. The classification of these mIg showed 22 IgG kappa (60%), 11 IgG lambda (29%) three IgM lambda (9%) and one IgM kappa. The concentration of the mIg was always below 2 g/l except for four bands (3 g/l, 6 g/l, 7 g/l, 15 g/l).

The gammopathies appeared within 2–27 months after transplantation (median, 5 months; mean, 8 ± 6.4 months). In 24 patients there was a period exceeding 2 years since the first detection of the mIg. The bands were always transient. Resolution occured within 12 months in 15 patients, within 12–18 months in five patients and after 18 months in four patients, the longest time being 42 months.

Offprint requests to: Dr. Ph. Lang, Department of Nephrology, Hopital Henri Mondor, Créteil 94010, France

There was no direct correlation between the development of mIg and the sex of the patient. Males represented 64% of the patients with mIg and 68% of those without mIg. Age had an effect on the development of gammopathy, but the higher frequency of mIg in older patients was only observed in women (48.5 ± 7.4 vs 39 ± 10.5 years, $P = 0.006$). No significant difference was observed in men with or without mIg (40 ± 10.2 vs 39.4 ± 9.5 years, respectively).

The duration of haemodialysis prior to transplant was a risk factor for the occurrence of mIg. The mean duration of haemodialysis was 45.7 ± 43 months in patients with mIg compared with 23.7 ± 2 months in patients without mIg ($P < 0.05$).

Continuous prospective virological surveillance of these patients showed that cytomegalovirus (CMV) infection occurred more frequently in patients with mIg than in patients without ($22/25$ vs $98/167$, respectively; $P = 0.01$). Although it was not a significant risk factor, primary CMV infection was more frequent in patients with mIg ($10/22$, 45%) than in patients without ($28/98$, 29%). In six patients the switch from IgM to IgG anti-CMV antibodies was unusually delayed, occurring after 18 months. HBs antigen was detected in only $2/25$ patients and hepatitis-C virus antibodies were confirmed by a recombinant immunoblot assay (RIBA) in $5/20$ (25%) patients. This high percentage is identical to the prevalence found in our transplant population. Significant modification of the serological response to EBV-specific antigens was observed in ten renal transplant recipients. It must be noted that in six patients, these modifications occurred subsequent to the finding of mIg.

The immunosuppresive regimen seemed to have an effect on the development of gammopathy. In the triple-drug therapy group, 16% of the patients had a mIg compared to 8% in those treated without CsA. However, this difference did not reach statistical significance. We found no correlation between the number of rejection episodes per patient and the presence or absence of serum mIg (1.2 ± 0.8 and 1.0 ± 0.7 rejection episodes, respectively).

The number of circulating CD4$^+$ lymphocytes was determined in six patients in parallel with the finding of mIg. The number of CD4$^+$ cells was either less than $150 \, \text{mm}^3$ or, if higher, the CD4$^+$/CD8$^+$ ratio was less than 0.5.

In eight patients, the mIg were associated with the development of severe infections (major wound infection, severe CMV colitis, HSV hepatitis, listeriosis septicaemia, pulmonary aspergillosis, visceral leishmaniasis), or tumours (Kaposis' sarcoma, brain lymphoma).

Discussion

In our study, the incidence of monoclonal and multiclonal gammopathies was 13%. In previous reports using the same sensitive detection method, a similar incidence of mIg has been found after renal transplantation [19, 22].

Gammopathies belonged to either the IgG or the IgM class. IgA was not detected. In B-cell malignancies and in B-cell benign neoplasias, the distribution of mIgG, mIgA and mIgM approximates the frequency of plasma cells producing these heavy chains in bone marrow of healthy adults, i.e. 10% IgM-, 50% IgG-, and 40% IgA-containing cells. The absence or low frequency of mIgA seems to be typical for this category of gammopathy. With respect to the light chain distribution, the kappa/lambda ratio was not altered, in agreement with some reports [18, 19] but not all [22].

The detection of multiple bands has been described in all the categories of gammopathies, but they are found with an unusually high incidence in organ and bone marrow tranplantation [14]. Monoclonal and multiclonal gammopathies had the same outcome, most of them disappearing within 12 months. In the absence of idiotypic study, and although most of the multiple bands had a different light chain, it remains uncertain whether they are produced by a single or by several B-cell clones. The finding of multiple bands or high mIg concentrations did not influence the clinical outcome.

The triggering mechanisms for mIg development remain largely unknown. It is likely that the association of immunosuppressive therapy, chronic antigenic stimulation (the allograft itself) and infection, particularly viral episodes, influence their appearance in genetically susceptible individuals. The depressed humoral and cellular immunity observed in chronic renal failure [1, 13] might also be a risk factor for the emergence of mIg after transplantation, as suggested by this study which shows a high incidence of mIg in patients who have been on dialysis for many years.

It is well known that there is an age-related increase in mIg ascribed to decreased T-cell control of B-cell function [4], but conflicting data have been reported in transplant patients [17, 18, 19, 22]. In the present study, age also had an effect on the development of gammopathies, but this age-related increase was only observed in the women. In other words, the development of mIg in renal transplantation was more frequent in young men than in young women. This observation remains unexplained, but in the general population, B-cell lymphoid proliferations are more frequent in men than in women, possibly indicating that women require the age-cofactor for the emergence of mIg.

Patients treated with the triple-drug therapy had an increased incidence of mIg compared with recipients treated with azathioprine and steroids alone. This may reflect the influence of the intensity of immunosuppressive therapy, but a specific effect of CsA cannot be excluded. This drug can induce autoimmunity [21], increases serum immunoglobulins [11], and promotes B-cell lymphomas experimentally and in humans [11]. Alteration of the cytokine network by CsA might be involved in the pathogenesis of these gammopathies. CsA enhances IL-1 receptor expression [6] and IL-6 gene transcription [24]. However, the link between these in vitro finding and in vivo B-cell stimulation still remains unclear [12].

Other factors may have contributed to the emergence of mIg such as infections, especially from cytomegalovirus which is known to be able to activate B cells and to depress cell-mediated immunity [23]. A recent CMV infection was found in almost 90% of patients developing mIg. Experimentally, CMV-induced immunosuppression is related to genetic factors [8] and this might explain in part why only a relatively small proportion of CMV-infected patients developed mIg.

Reflecting the alteration of cell-mediated immunity, the serological profile of CMV infection in patients who developed mIg was often characterized by the long-term persistence of IgM anti-CMV antibodies. B-cell lymphomas observed in transplant patients are generally associated with EBV infection [16], but the triggering role of EBV infection for mIg development remains uncertain. Because of its inherent ability to transform the host cell, EBV infection might appear as the main triggering factor for mIg emergence, but in the present study, evidence for EBV infection was found only in 40 % of the patients with mIg. However, serological determination of EBV infection is not very reliable in immunosuppressed patients and it remains possible that most mIg in transplant patients are due to an inefficient elimination of EBV-infected cells by cytotoxic T lymphocytes [3]. In our transplant population, only one patient developed a B-cell lymphoma. This patient had two mIg 1 month after a CMV infection, but frequent EBV serological surveys showed that EBV infection occurred only 4 months later in association with the brain lymphoma. This observation suggests that EBV infection was the triggering event for the development of lymphoma, but not for the emergence of the mIg.

Whatever is the triggering event for mIg, their presence imply an insufficient control of B-cell proliferation by relevant T cells. Their detection should be associated with a regular follow-up of the EBV serological profile. The occurrence of an EBV infection in association with a mIg should probably lead to a decrease in immunosuppressive therapy and it could be useful to initiate treatment with acyclovir [9].

Acknowledgements. This study was supported by grants from AURA.

References

1. Cappel R, Van Beers D, Liesnard C, Dratwa M (1983) Impaired humoral and cell mediated immune response in dialysed patients after influenza vaccination. Nephro 33: 21–25
2. Cleary ML, Sklar J (1984) Lympho-proliferative disorders in cardiac transplant recipients are multiclonal lymphomas. Lancet 2: 489–493
3. Crawford DH, Edwards JM Sweny P, Hoffbrand AV, Janossy G (1981) Studies on long term T-cell mediated immunity to Epstein-Barr virus in immunosuppressed renal allograft recipients. Int J Cancer 28: 705–709
4. Crawford J, Eye MK, Cohen HJ (1987) Evaluation of monoclonal gammapathies in the 'well' elderly. Am J Med 82: 39–45
5. Creyssel R, Gibaud A, Cordier JF, Boissel JP (1975) The frequency distribution of heavy chain classes and light chain types of 1000 monoclonal immunoglobulins. Biomedicine 22: 41–48
6. Degiannis D, Stein S, Czarnecki M, Raskova J, Raska K (1990) Cyclosporine induced enhancement of interleukin 1 receptor expression by PHA-stimulated lymphocytes. Transplantation 50: 1074–1076
7. Deteix P, Chapuis-Cellier C, Ghais Z, Lefrançois N, Brusa M, Touraine JL, Traeger J (1985) Systematic survey of immunoglobulin abnormalities; frequency and evolution in organ transplant recipients. Transplant Proc 17: 2651–2654
8. Grundy JE, Mackenzie JS, Stanley NF (1981) Influence of H2 and non-H2 genes on resistance to murine-cytomegalovirus infection. Infect Immun 32: 277–286
9. Hanto DW, Frizzera G, Gajl-Peczalska KJ, Sakamoto K, Purtilo D, Balfour H, Simmons R, Najarian JS (1982) Epstein Barr virus-induced B-cell lymphoma after renal transplantation. Acyclovir therapy and transition from polyclonal to monoclonal B-cell proliferation. N Engl J Med 306: 913–918
10. Hanto DW, Simmons RL (1984) Lymphoproliferative diseases in immunosuppressed patients. In: Morris PJ, Tilney N (eds) Progress in transplantation, vol 1. Churchill Livingstone, Edinburgh, pp 186–208
11. Hattori A, Kunz H, Gill TJ, Shinozuka (1987) Thymic and lymphoid changes and serum immunoglobulin abnormalities in mice receiving cyclosporine. Am J Pathol 128: 111–120
12. Kunzendorf U, Brockmöller J, Bickel U, Jochimsen F, Walz G, Roots I, Offermann G (1991) Promotion of B-cell stimulation in graft recipients through a mechanism distinct from interleukin-6 gene superinduction. Transplantation 51: 1312–1315
13. Kurtz P, Kohler H, Meuer S, Hutteroth T, Meyer Z, Buschenfelde KH (1986) Impaired cellular immune response in chronic renal failure: Evidence for a T cell defect. Kidney Int 29: 1209–1214
14. Kyle RA (1978) Monoclonal gammapathy of undetermined significance – Natural history in 241 cases. Am J Med 64: 814–826
15. Kyle RA (1984) 'Benign' monoclonal gammapathy – misnomer? JAMA 251: 1849–1854
16. List A, Greco A, Vogler L (1987) Lymphoproliferative diseases in immunocompromised hosts: the role of Epstein-Barr virus. J Clin Oncol 5: 1673–1689
17. Peest D, Schaper B, Nashan B, Wonigeit K, Raude E, Pichlmayr R, Haverich A, Deicher H (1988) High incidence of monoclonal immunoglobulins in patients after liver or heart transplantation. Transplantation 46: 389–393
18. Radl J, Valentijn RM, Haaijman JJ, Paul LC (1985) Monoclonal gammapathies in patients undergoin immunosuppressive treatment after renal transplantation. Clin Immunol Immunopathol 37: 98–102
19. Renoux E, Bertrand F, Kessler M (1988) Monoclonal gammapathies in HBs Ag positive patients with renal transplants (letter). N Engl J Med 318: 1205
20. Ritchie RF, Smith R (1976) Immunofixation. III. Application to the study of monoclonal proteins. Clin Chem 22: 1982–1985
21. Sorokin R, Kimura K, Schroder D, Wilson DH, Wilson DB (1986) Cyclosporin-induced autoimmunity. Conditions for expressing disease, requirement for intact thymus and potency estimates of autoimmune lymphocytes in drug-treated rats. J Exp Med 164: 1615–1623
22. Stanko CK, Jeffery JR, Rush DN (1989) Monoclonal and multiclonal gammapathies after renal transplantation. Transplant Proc 21: 3330–3332
23. Van Son WJ, The TH (1989) Cytomegalovirus infection after organ transplantation: an update with special emphasis on renal transplantation. Transplant Int 2: 147–164
24. Walz G, Zanker B, Melton LB, Suthanthiran M, Strom TB (1991) Possible association of immunosuppressive and B-cell lymphoma-promoting properties of cyclosporine. Transplantation 49: 191–194

Transplant Int (1992) 5 [Suppl 1]: S 26–S 29

TRANSPLANT
International
© Springer-Verlag 1992

Cytomegalovirus (CMV) excretion as a factor in the severity of CMV disease in kidney and simultaneous kidney and pancreas transplantation

C. Pouteil-Noble[1], R. Ecochard[2], S. Bosshard[3], B. Lacavalerie[1], A. Donia[1], G. Landrivon[2], J. C. Tardy[3], J. M. Dubernard[1], M. Aymard[3] and J. L. Touraine[1]

[1] Transplantation Unit, Pavillon P, E. Herriot Hospital, Lyon, France
[2] Medical Information Centre, Hotel-Dieu Hospital, Lyon, France
[3] Virology Laboratory, Rockefeller Faculty, Lyon, France

Abstract. The aim of the study was to evaluate the virological parameters associated with the severity of cytomegalovirus (CMV) disease in renal and simultaneous renal and pancreatic transplantation. The association of the viral profile and the severity of the viral disease was analysed taking into account different confounding variables susceptible to linkage with the severity of the CMV infection and the viral parameters. All the patients transplanted between 1 January 1989 and 31 December 1990, a total of 242, were prospectively followed by viral cultures in blood and urine and by serological methods using the detection of CMV-specific IgM and the complement fixation (CF) test. The samples were taken systematically each week for the first month and then at day 90, 180 and every 6 months and also in cases of clinical manifestations related to viral disease. CMV infection was diagnosed virologically by the presence of viraemia, viruria, IgM, or a significant rise in CMV antibody titre in CF. CMV disease was classified as asymptomatic, mild (fever and/or leukopenia), moderate (fever, leukopenia and liver abnormalities), severe (CMV pneumopathy and/or gastrointestinal disease) or fatal. The incidence of CMV infection was 65 % (157/242): 32 % asymptomatic, 36 % mild, 30 % moderate and 2 % severe. The presence of IgM was associated with the severity of CMV disease: 51.4 % of moderate and severe CMV infections in the group with IgM versus only 16 % in the group without IgM ($P < 0.0001$). The risk of having severe or moderate CMV disease was 3.28 times higher in patients with positive IgM. However the serological changes in CF were not significantly associated with the severity of the viral disease since 34.6 % of the patients with CF changes had a severe form versus 20.8 % in the group without CF modification. Viruria was significantly associated with moderate or severe infection: 43.6 % of the patients with viruria had severe infection versus only 12.5 % in the patients without viruria

($P < 0.0002$). The risk of having moderate or severe CMV disease was 3.48 times higher in the patients with viruria. Viraemia was also associated with more severe CMV infection: 48.6 % of moderate or severe CMV infection in the group of patients with viraemia versus 19 % in the group without viraemia ($P < 0.0001$). The risk of having severe or moderate CMV infection was 2.58 times higher in the patients with viraemia. Viraemia was not more associated with severe CMV infection than viruria. Using the maximum likelihood ratio method and the logistic regression model, CMV-specific IgM, viruria and viraemia were each shown to be associated with the severity of CMV disease and the addition of one parameter to the other(s), whatever the type (except the CF changes) and whatever the order of this addition, did not remove the link between the severity and IgM, viruria and viremia. The incidence of severe and moderate CMV disease increased with the number of positive viral parameters (PVP) from 2 % of moderate and severe infections in the group with one PVP, to 28 % in the group with two PVP, to 39 % in the group with three PVP and 68 % in the group with four PVP (trend, 35.95; $P < 0.0001$). Taking the absolute risk of the group of patients without IgM, viruria or viraemia as the basal level, the observed relative risk of severe CMV infection varied from 6.45 in the group with positive IgM without viruria or viraemia, to 10.74 in the group with positive IgM and viruria without viraemia and to 22.5 in the group with the three positive parameters IgM, viruria and viraemia. The different potential confounding factors (recipient and donor serology, renal or renal and pancreatic transplantation, DR compatibility, rejection before CMV infection) did not modify the link between the viral profile and the severity of CMV disease. This study suggests that the severity of CMV disease might be linked to the overspread of the virus as well as to the consequences of a CMV-specific humoral immune response.

Key words: Cytomegalovirus – Kidney transplantation – IgM – Viraemia – Viruria

Offprint requests to: C. Pouteil-Noble, Transplantation Unit, Pavillon P, Hôpital E. Herriot, 5 Place d'Arsonval, 69437 Lyon, Cedex 03, France

Cytomegalovirus (CMV) infection remains the most frequent viral infection in bone-marrow transplantation and in organ transplantation and is responsible for a high morbidity and mortality. Some patients will develop asymptomatic infection detected by systematic viral monitoring and others will develop clinical signs ranging from a self-limited syndrome to severe CMV disease with pneumonia or gastrointestinal disease. However, it is not known whether the viral profile is different in asymptomatic infection than in severe CMV disease, and whether the different clinical forms depend on the viral charge, on the intensity of the viral replication or on the immune status of the recipient.

In bone-marrow transplantation, viraemia is associated with the severity of CMV disease [4, 8] and would be predictive of CMV disease [5]. This marker could be used to determine the initiation of antiviral chemotherapy and to prevent the progression from mild infection to severe CMV disease. In organ transplantation, the association of the clinical signs of CMV disease with the recovery of CMV from sources other than blood, such as urine, remains to be determined. Moreover the use of serological methods such as detection of CMV-specific IgM antibodies by enzyme-linked immunosorbent assay (ELISA) and the significant rise in CMV antibodies using a complement fixation (CF) test need to be assessed in the context of the association with the severity of CMV disease. The aim of the study was to evaluate the virological parameters associated with the severity of CMV disease in renal transplantation and renal and pancreatic transplantation in order to understand the physiopathology of the viral infection better. The viral profile associated with serious disease was determined taking into account the different confounding factors susceptible to linkage with the severity of CMV disease and with the viral parameters. The factors studied were the presence of CMV-specific IgM, the significant increase in CMV antibodies in CF, viraemia and viruria.

Material and methods

Patients

All the patients attending our Transplantation Unit transplanted between 1 January 1989 and 31 December 1990 were included in the study. A total of 242 patients, 191 renal transplant and 51 renal and pancreatic transplant, were thus enrolled.

Virological diagnostic methods and viral monitoring

The serological methods used were the CF test and ELISA. The CF test was performed in microplates with two units of antigen and two units of complement. The detection of CMV-specific IgM was done with the cytomegalovirus IgM EIA (Wellcome) according to the manufacturer's instructions [6].

Cultures were prepared from blood and urine. Specimens were inoculated to human embryonic fibroblasts (MRC5) and cultures were maintained for at least four weeks to detect the CMV isolation because of the slow cytopathogenic effect. A rapid identification was performed by low speed centrifugation of the samples onto MRC5-grown cells followed by detection after 48 h of CMV immediate early antigen by the immunoperoxidase technique with monoclonal antibody E13 (Clonotec).

The viral monitoring was systematic and prospective. Viraemia, viruria and serology were performed weekly from the day of transplantation for the first month and then at day 90, day 180 and then every 6 months. Viral cultures and serology were also performed when clinical symptoms of viral infection occurred.

Definition of CMV infection

The definition of CMV infection was virological and was based on any number of the following signs: viraemia, viruria, seroconversion, the presence of CMV-specific IgM antibodies and significant four-fold rise in the anti-CMV antibody titres by CF.

Classification of CMV disease

Clinical CMV disease was classified in five grades as follows:

– asymptomatic;
– mild (fever and/or leukopenia);
– moderate (fever, leukopenia and liver abnormalities);
– severe (CMV pneumopathy or gastrointestinal disease);
– fatal.

Parameters studied

All the 157 patients included in the study group had at least one positive viral parameter since being infected. The parameters studied were CMV specific IgM antibodies, a significant rise in the CMV antibodies in CF, viraemia and viruria.

Confounding factors

The confounding factors were the factors susceptible, from the literature and from our study, to linkage with the severity of the CMV infection and the viral parameters. They were: recipient age (≤ 55 or > 55 years), donor age (≤ 55 or > 55 years), recipient CMV serology before transplantation, donor serology at the time of organ procurement, the type of transplantation (kidney alone or simultaneous kidney – pancreas transplantation), the degree of HLA A, B, DR compatibility, the degree of anti-HLA immunization before transplantation, the number of transplantations, the type of immunosuppressive therapy, the occurrence of rejection before CMV infection (from the day of the transplantation to 4 days before the diagnosis of CMV infection).

Statistical analysis

The association of severe and moderate CMV infection with viral parameters was compared by means of a two-by-two table for univariate analysis. The Mantel Haenszel test was used to take into account only one confounding variable. Logistic regression was used to take into account more than one confounding variable and to model the relation between the viral profile and the severity of CMV disease.

Results

The incidence of CMV infection was 63%, 157 patients having a CMV infection proved virologically. Of these infections, 32% were asymptomatic, 36% mild, 30% moderate and 2% severe. The presence of CMV IgM was associated with the severity of CMV disease, since 38 patients of the 74 with IgM (51.4%) developed a moderate

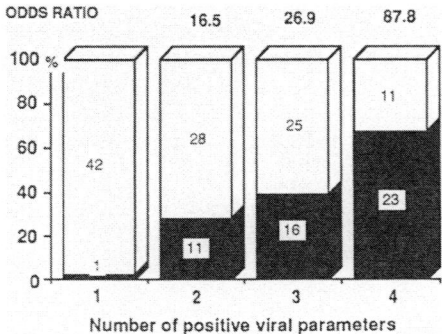

Fig. 1. Severity of CMV infection and the number of positive viral parameters. The incidence of severe and moderate CMV infection increased with the number of positive viral parameters (trend = 35.95; $P < 0.0001$). □, Asymptomatic/mild; ■, moderate/severe

Table 1. Test of significance of the gain when a viral parameter was added. The method used was the maximum likelihood ratio and the model used was logistic regression. The presence of IgM was significantly associated with the severity of CMV disease. The introduction of viruria to IgM in the model did not remove the link between the viral profile and the severity (chi^2 = 7.8; $P < 0.006$). The introduction of viraemia did not modify the association between the severity of the CMV disease and viruria and IgM (chi^2 = 7.9; $P < 0.006$). However, the addition of the CF changes did not add anything to the model (chi^2 = 1.54; $P < 0.22$). Thus, the variables IgM, viruria and viraemia were kept in the logistic regression model to model the risk of having a severe infection according to the viral parameters

Number of positive viral parameters	Parameter	Chi squared	P value
1	IgM	23.4	< 0.0001
2	IgM and viruria	7.8	$P < 0.006$
3	IgM, viruria and viremia	7.9	< 0.006
4	IgM, viruria, viremia and CF changes	1.54	< 0.22 NS

or severe CMV infection versus only 13 out of the 83 patients without IgM (16%). The odds ratio was 5.68 (95% confidence interval, 2.78–11.61) ($P < 0.0001$). The risk of having severe or moderate CMV disease was 3.28 times higher in patients with positive IgM than in patients free of CMV-specific IgM antibodies. However, the serological changes in CF were not significantly associated with the severity of the viral disease, since 34.6% of the patients with CF changes (46/133) had a severe or moderate form versus 20.8% (5/24) in the group without CF modification (odds ratio = 2.01; 95% confidence interval, 0.72–5.64) ($P = 0.3$). Viruria was significantly associated with moderate or severe infection since 44 of the 101 patients (43.6%) with viruria had a severe infection versus 7 of the 56 patients (12%) without only viruria. The odds ratio was 5.40 (95% confidence interval, 2.36–12.4) ($P < 0.0002$). The risk of having moderate or severe CMV disease was 3.48 times higher in patients with viruria than in patients without viruria.

Viraemia was also associated with more severe CMV infection: 48.6% of the patients (35/72) with viraemia developed moderate or severe CMV infection versus 19% (16/85) in the group of patients without viraemia

($P < 0.0001$). The odds ratio was 4.08 (2.04–8.16) and the risk of having a severe or moderate CMV infection was 2.58 times higher in patients with viraemia than in patients free of viraemia. Viraemia was not more associated with a severe CMV infection than viruria since the absolute risk of severe CMV disease was 29% in cases of viruria and 26% in cases of viraemia in the patients having only one positive viral culture, either viraemia or viruria (chi squared = 0.01).

The incidence of severe and moderate CMV disease in increased with the number of positive viral parameters from 2% in the group with one positive parameter, to 28% in the group with two positive parameters, to 39% in the group with three positive parameters and 68% in the group with four positive parameters (trend = 35.95; $P < 0.0001$) (Fig. 1). Specific anti-CMV IgM, viruria and viraemia were each associated with the severity of CMV disease and the addition of one parameter to the other(s) whatever the type (except the CF changes) and whatever the order of this addition, did not remove the link between the severity and IgM, viruria and viraemia, using the method of maximum likelihood ratio and the logistic regression model (Table 1).

The observed absolute risk of severe or moderate CMV infection was 3.1% in patients without IgM, viraemia or viruria, 20% in patients with IgM only, without viraemia or viruria, 33.3% in patients with IgM, with viruria and without viraemia, and 68% in patients with the three parameters positive. Taking the absolute risk of the group of patients without IgM, viruria or viraemia as the basal level, the observed relative risk of severe CMV infection according to the number and the type of viral parameters is shown Fig. 2. The analysis of the different potential confounding factors (recipient serology, donor serology, renal or renal and pancreatic transplantation, DR compatibility, rejection before CMV infection) did not show any modification of the link between the viral profile and the severity of CMV disease (Table 2).

Discussion

The presence of CMV-specific IgM antibodies was associated with the severity of CMV disease whatever the donor and recipient serology and whatever the other confound-

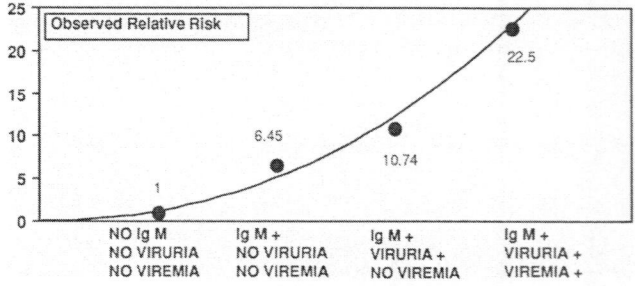

Fig. 2. Observed relative risk of having severe CMV disease and viral parameters in the 157 infected patients. Taking the absolute risk of the group of patients without IgM, viruria or viraemia as the basal level, the observed relative risk of severe CMV infection varied from 6.45 in the group with positive IgM only, without viruria or viraemia, to 10.74 in the group with positive IgM and viruria, without viraemia, and to 22.5 in the group with the three parameters positive

Table 2. Analysis of the confounding factors in the model of the association of the severity of CMV disease with the viral parameters. The method used was the maximum likelihood ratio and the model used was logistic regression. The recipient and donor serology are known from the literature to be linked with the incidence and the severity of CMV infection. In this model, no modification was observed in the link between the severity of CMV disease and the viral parameters (IgM, viruria, viraemia) after taking into account the recipient and donor serology ($P < 0.0001$). CMV infection was more severe in kidney and pancreas transplantation. After taking into account the type of transplantation, the association between the severity of CMV disease and the viral parameters was not modified ($P < 0.0001$). The degree of DR compatibility from 0 to 2 was associated with the severity of CMV disease, a good compatibility protected from serious CMV infection. After taking into account this parameter, the association remained significant ($P < 0.0001$). The occurrence of rejection before CMV infection increased the risk of severe CMV infection. However, this factor was not a confounding factor. Thus, the different potential confounding factors tested did not modify the link between the viral profile and the severity of CMV disease

Confounding variable	Chi^2	P value
None	39.06	< 0.0001
Recipient serology	33.63	< 0.0001
Donor serology	32.51	< 0.0001
Type of transplantation (kidney or kdiney – pancreas)	33.26	< 0.0001
DR compatibility	37.01	< 0.0001
Rejection before CMV infection	38.63	< 0.0001

ing factors. The detection of IgM has previously been found to be associated with a poor prognosis in renal transplantation [7], mainly because it was associated with primary infections. IgM could be the witness of severe infection, but could also play an active role in the aggravation of CMV disease by the formation of immune complexes. The presence of IgM immune complexes (IgM – CIC) using a C1q solid-phase assay has been detected in kidney graft recipients during the second month in infected patients only and as early as the urinary excretion [2]. The dissociation of IgM immune complexes and the characterization of the antibody specificity allowed the CMV specificity of the IgM-CIC to be demonstrated, including IgM antibodies and a 45–47 kDa viral polypeptide [3]. This anti-p 45–47 IgM detected by immunoblotting was always present before the anti-CMV IgM was detected with ELISA and was present in primary infections as well as in recurrent infections [1]. This 45–47 kDa polypeptide could be the main viral target for the CMV-specific IgM antibody response in the early phase of CMV infection, since anti-p 45–47 IgM was detected as early as or before urinary viral excretion. However, the physiopatho-

logical meaning of the production of CMV-specific IgM, not only during primary infections but also during recurrent CMV infection, remains to be elucidated. Complement fixation changes were not associated with severe CMV disease and the significant increase in the titres could reflect the recovery of a normal immune status, when the immunosuppressive therapy is decreased, or be the consequence of an increased immune reactivity concomitant with a mild CMV infection.

Viruria and viraemia were associated with the severity of CMV infection in renal transplantation and this result would be important to confirm in bone-marrow transplantation with the same methodology, since viruria is easier to determine than viraemia, especially in aplastic patients. IgM, viraemia and viruria were each associated with severe or moderate CMV infection. The addition of one factor to the other(s) not only did not remove the link with the severity of CMV infection, but increased the severity of the disease. The striking increased risk of severe or moderate CMV infections with the number of positive viral parameters suggests that the severity of CMV disease might partly be due to the overspread of the virus as well as to the consequences of a CMV-specific IgM immune response.

References

1. Basson J, Tardy JC, Aymard M (1989) Pattern of anti-cytomegalovirus IgM antibodies determined by immunoblotting. A study of kidney graft recipients developing a primary or recurrent CMV infection. Arch Virol 108: 259–270
2. Basson J, Tardy JC, Aymard M (1990) A new C1q solid phase assay for the detection of IgM immune complexes: application to the follow up of kidney graft recipients with recurrent cytomegalovirus infection. J Clin Lab Immunol 31: 43–49
3. Basson J, Tardy JC, Aymard M (1991) Characterisation of immune complexes containing cytomegalovirus-specific IgM antibodies following a kidney graft. J Med Virol 33: 205–210
4. Meyers JD, Flournoy N, Thomas ED (1986) Risk factors for cytomegalovirus infection after human marrow transplantation. J Infect Dis 153: 478–488
5. Meyers JD, Ljungman P, Fisher LD (1990) Cytomegalovirus excretion as a predictor of cytomegalovirus disease after marrow transplantation: importance of cytomegalovirus viremia. J Infect Dis 162: 373–380
6. Schmitz M, von Deimling U, Fleming B (1980) Detection of IgM antibodies to cytomegalovirus (CMV) using an enzyme-labelled antigen (ELA). J Gen Virol 50: 59–68
7. Tardy JC, Pouteil-Noble C, Touraine JL, Aymard M (1987) Prognostic value of anti cytomegalovirus IgM in kidney graft recipients. Transplant Proc 195: 4066–4067
8. Vilmer E, Mazeron MC, Rabian AC, Azogui O, Devergie A, Perol Y, Gluckman E (1985) Clinical significance of cytomegalovirus viremia in bone marrow transplantation. Transplantation 40: 30–35

Transplant Int (1992) 5 [Suppl 1]: S 30–S 31

TRANSPLANT
International
© Springer-Verlag 1992

Prophylaxis of CMV disease by ganciclovir (DHPG) in seronegative recipients of renal allograft from seropositive donors

E. Rondeau[1], B. Bourgeon[2], M. N. Peraldi[1], Ph. Lang[2], C. Buisson[2], K. M. Schulte[2], B. Weill[2] and J. D. Sraer[1]

[1] Service de Néphrologie, Hôpital Tenon, Paris, France
[2] Service de Néphrologie, Hôpital Henri Mondor, Créteil, France

Abstract. In an open-label randomized study of prophylactic treatment by ganciclovir, 23 seronegative recipients of kidney allograft from seropositive donors were randomized to receive from day 14 to day 28 after transplantation either no treatment ($n = 11$) or ganciclovir, 5 mg/kg twice daily ($n = 12$). Both groups were similar in age, immunosuppressive therapy, number of acute rejections and in steroid bolus. Seroconversion occurred in ten patients of the control group (91 %) and in ten of the ganciclovir group (84 %). CMV disease occurred in ten patients of the control group (91 %) and in eight patients of the ganciclovir group (66 %), three of whom had asymptomatic viraemia. The delay between transplantation and onset of CMV disease was significantly increased by ganciclovir prophylaxis (78.5 ± 7.7 vs 46.5 ± 7.5 days, $P < 0.05$). We conclude that in renal transplant recipients at risk of CMV disease, ganciclovir prophylaxis delays the onset of the disease and seems to decrease its incidence and its severity.

Key words: Cytomegalovirus – Ganciclovir – Prophylaxis – Renal Transplantation.

Cytomegalovirus infection is the most frequent infectious complication observed in renal transplant recipients and may cause disease in up to 30 % of patients [8]. A high mortality rate has been reported in patients with CMV pneumonitis [9]. Therefore various methods to prevent CMV infection or disease have been proposed, for example selection of kidney graft from seronegative donors to seronegative recipients [2], prophylactic passive immunization by CMV-immune globulins [6] or prophylactic treatment by oral acyclovir [1]. Although compliance was difficult to obtain, high doses of oral acyclovir have been shown to prevent significantly CMV disease in renal transplant recipients [1]. The most evident effect was obtained in seronegative recipients of kidney from seropositive donors. Ganciclovir, an acyclic guanine analogue, is much more effective in vitro on the inhibition of CMV replication than acyclovir [7], and we [4] and others [3] have shown that ganciclovir is an effective treatment for CMV disease in transplanted patients. Therefore we decided to test the efficacy of prophylactic ganciclovir in renal transplant recipients at particular risk of CMV disease, i.e. seronegative recipients of kidney grafts from seropositive donors.

Patients and methods

Patients and study design

From January 1990 to August 1991, 210 renal transplantations were performed in our two centres (Hôpital Tenon, Paris and Hôpital Henri Mondor, Créteil, France). A total of 23 patients who were seronegative and who had received a kidney from a seropositive donor were included in the study after they had given informed consent. On day 14 after transplantation, patients were randomized to receive either no treatment or ganciclovir, 5 mg/kg twice daily for 14 days. Doses were adapted to the renal function according to the instructions of the manufacturer. As shown in Table 1, the patients in the control group ($n = 11$) and the ganciclovir group ($n = 12$) were similar in mean age, immunosuppressive therapy, steroid pulses, number of rejection episodes, and tune between transplantation and the first rejection crisis. The male/female ratio was opposite in the two groups.

Patients of the control group and ganciclovir group were monitored once a week until the third month post-transplantation for clinical signs, viraemia, viruria, and serological status (ELISA or Latex agglutination). According to the clinical status, bronchioloalveolar lavage and/or gastrointestinal biopsies were performed. CMV antigens were detected by indirect immunofluorescence, and light microscopy was used for determination of the cytopathic effect. CMF infection was detected by serological methods. CMV disease was diagnosed on the association of clinical signs and virus isolation.

Results

As determined by serology, ten patients of the control group (91 %) and ten of the ganciclovir group (84 %) had CMV primary infection after transplantation. However,

---

Offprint requests to: Dr. E. Rondeau, Service de Néphrologie, Hôpital Tenon, 4 rue de la Chine, 75020 Paris, France

Table 1. Patient population

	Control group	Ganciclovir group
Number	11	12
Sex (M/F)	2/9	11/1
Age	39.2 ± 4.4	46.2 ± 4.0
Sequential treatment	11	12
Steroid pulses	3.5 ± 0.9	3.0 ± 1.2
Rejection episodes	1.2 ± 0.3	1.1 ± 0.4
Time to first rejection (days)	20.8 ± 6.3	32.6 ± 11.3

symptomatic CMV disease was observed in the ten patients of the control group but in eight patients of the treated group (91 % versus 66 %, NS). The delay between transplantation and the occurrence of CMV disease was significantly longer in the treated group than in the control group (78.5 ± 7.7 versus 46.5 ± 7.5 days, $P < 0.05$). The severity of the CMV disease was also reduced by ganciclovir prophylaxis, since three patients of this group had asymptomatic disease with positive viraemia, compared with only one patient of the control group. The clinical symptoms were similar in both groups: generalized signs with asthenia, fever, leukopenia, thrombocytopenia (seven cases in the control group and five in the ganciclovir group), pneumonitis (one case in both groups) and gastrointestinal disease (three and one case, respectively); viraemia occurred in six cases in the control group and seven cases in the treated group; CMV was detected by bronchioloalveolar lavage in both groups (three and six cases, respectively). The ten patients of the control group and the eight patients of the prophylactic group who had CMV disease received a therapeutic course of ganciclovir for 14 days and all the patients recovered. No side-effects were observed during prophylaxis or curative treatments by ganciclovir.

Only one graft was lost after an irreversible vascular acute rejection in a patient of the control group. The mean plasma creatinine levels of the patients with a functioning graft was 148 ± 15 and 137 ± 19 µmol/l in the control and the treated group, respectively, after 2 to 23 months of follow-up. The patient survival levels of the rate is 100 % in both groups.

Discussion

Our study demonstrates that prophylactic administration of ganciclovir for 14 days during the 3rd and 4th week after transplantation slightly decreases the incidence of CMV disease in seronegative patients who received a kidney allograft from a seropositive donor. It significantly increases the delay between transplantation and the beginning of CMV disease and seems to decrease the severity of the disease.

Recently it has been shown in allogenic bone marrow recipients that asymptomatic CMV infection of the lung is a major risk factor for subsequent CMV interstitial pneumonia [5], and that prophylactic ganciclovir is effective in preventing the development of CMV interstitial pneumonia in patients with asymptomatic infection. However, these authors reported that a unique 14-day course of ganciclovir was not effective, and that maintenance therapy (5 mg/kg each day intravenously for 5 days per week) until day 120 was required. Although the number of patients included in our study was low, it seems that prophylactic administration of ganciclovir can decrease the incidence and the severity of CMV disease in renal transplant recipients. It significantly delays the onset of the disease. It is likely that a lower rate of CMV disease would have been observed if combined with maintenance therapy. Maintenance therapy, however, will not be easy to administer until oral forms of ganciclovir become available. At the present time, the mortaility from CMV disease in renal transplant recipients, at least in our centres, has disappeared since the systematic screening for CMV infection and the use of ganciclovir in earlier stages of CMV disease. Conversely, the morbidity from CMV disease is increasing, since immunosuppressive treatments are more powerful. One hopes that, in the near future, patients with a high risk of CMV disease will be able to receive prophylactic treatment with oral forms of ganciclovir or its derivatives.

References

1. Balfour HH Jr, Chace BA, Stapleton JT, Simmons RL, Fryd DS (1989) A randomized, placebo-controlled trial of oral acyclovir for the prevention of cytomegalovirus disease in recipients of renal allografts. N Engl J Med 320: 1381–1387
2. Bowden RA, Sayers, M, Flournoy N, Newton B, Banaji M, Thomas D, Meyers JD (1986) Cytomegalovirus immune globulin and seronegative blood products to prevent primary cytomegalovirus infection after marrow transplantation. N Engl J Med 314: 1006–1010
3. Keay S, Petersen E, Icenogle T, Zeluff BJ, Samo T, Busch D, New Man CL, Buhles WC, Merigan TC (1988) Ganciclovir treatment of serious cytomegalovirus infection in heart and heart-lung transplant recipients. Rev Infect Dis 10: S563–S572
4. Rondeau E, Farquet C, Ruedin P, Fries D, Sraer JD (1990) Efficacy of early treatment of cytomegalovirus infection by ganciclovir in renal transplant recipients. Transplant Proc 22: 1813–1814
5. Schmidt GM, Horak DA, Niland JC, Duncan SR, Forman SJ, Zaia JA (1991) A randomized, controlled trial of prophylactic ganciclovir for cytomegalovirus pulmonary infection in recipients of allogeneic bone marrow transplants. N Engl J Med 324: 1005–1011
6. Snydman DR, Werner BG, Heinze-Lacey B, Berardi VP, Tilney NL, Kirkman RL, Milford EL, Cho SI, Bush HL, Levey AS, Strom TB, Carpenter CB, Levey RH, Harmon WE, Zimmerman CE, Shapiro ME, Steinman T, Logerfo F, Idelson B, Schroter GPJ, Levin MJ, McIver J, Leszczynski J, Grady GF (1987) Use of cytomegalovirus immune globulin to prevent cytomegalovirus disease in renal-transplant recipients. N Engl J Med 317: 1049–1054
7. Tyms AS, Davis JM, Jeffries DJ, Meyers JD (1984) BWB759U, an analogue of acyclovir, inhibits human cytomegalovirus in vitro. Lancet ii: 924–925
8. Weir MR, Irwin BC, Maters AW, Genemans G, Shen SY, Charache P, Williams GM (1987) Incidence of cytomegalovirus disease in cyclosporine-treated renal transplant recipients based on donor/recipient pretransplant immunity. Transplantation 43: 187–193
9. Weir MR, Henry ML, Blackmore M, Smith J, First MR, Irwin B, Shen S, Genemans G, Alexander JW, Corry RJ (1988) Incidence and morbidity of cytomegalovirus disease associated with a seronegative recipient receiving seropositive donor-specific transfusion and living-related donor transplantation. Transplantation 45: 111–116

Transplant Int (1992) 5 [Suppl 1]: S 32–S 34

TRANSPLANT
International
© Springer-Verlag 1992

Renal retransplantation in patients with HLA-antibodies

L. Mjörnstedt[1], J. Konar[2], G. Nyberg[1], M. Olausson[1], L. Sandberg[2], and I. Karlberg[1]

[1] Transplant Unit and [2] Blood Centre, Sahlgrenska Hospital, University of Göteborg, Sweden

Abstract. The results of 92 consecutive renal retransplantations, performed during a 5-year period in recipients with HLA-antibodies, were retrospectively analysed. The actuarial 1-year graft survival (1-y GS) was 65% for all retransplantations, as compared with 63% for first grafts in sensitized recipients. For the second ($n = 56$), third ($n = 24$) and fourth-fifth ($n = 12$) grafts 1-y GS was 64%, 71% and 58%, respectively. Acute rejection was the major cause of graft loss (45%). Recipients with > 3 years GS of the preceding transplant had significantly better GS at retransplantation. Also, grafts with no HLA mismatches had significantly prolonged GS. One-y GS was 78% when PRA (panel reacting antibody) was less than 50%, and 60% when PRA was more than 50%. A benefit of repeated mismatches was demonstrated in the subgroup with PRA < 50%, in contrast to recipients with PRA > 50%, suggesting that, in some patients, an absence of antibody response against certain antigens might be used as a basis for future deliberate mismatching.

Key words: Renal retransplantation – HLA antibodies – Graft survival

Regrafting and the presence of HLA-antibodies are factors, which alone or taken together have been reported to impair kidney graft survival [1, 5]. The purpose of the present study was to analyse consecutive renal retransplantations, performed in recipients with preformed HLA-antibodies in our centre during a 5-year period.

Materials and methods

During 1985–89, 92 renal retransplantations were performed in Göteborg in patients with preformed HLA-antibodies. Of these patients, 56 (61%), were second grafts, 24 (26%) third, 10 (11%) fourth

Offprint requests to: Lars Mjörnstedt, M. D, Ph. D., Transplant Unit, Department of Surgery, Sahlgrenska Hospital, S-413 45 Göteborg, Sweden

and 2 (2%) fifth grafts. All grafts but one were cadaveric (CD). Cross matches (CM) with the lymphocytotoxicity test against T and B cells were negative in historical and current symples. Mean cold ischaemia time was 22.1 ± 0.6 h in a range of 9–39 h (CD only). Triple-drug basal immunosuppression with cyclosporine A (CyA) + azathioprine (Aza) + Prednisolone (Pred) was used in 87 (95%) transplantations, Cya + Pred in four cases, and Aza + Pred in one case. ATG induction therapy was given in 47 (51%) transplantations. A group of 38 primary transplantations, also performed in presensitized recipients during this period, was in certain instances used for comparison. The follow-up time was 1–6 years.

Patients

A majority of the recipients were male (67%) and on haemodialysis (69%). The causes of uraemia were: glomerulonephritis (38%), diabetes (14%), chronic pyelonephritis (13%) and polycystic kidney disease (13%). More than 50% panel reacting antibodies (PRA) in current sera were found in 71% of the patients and less than 50% in 25%. Reactivity only against B cells was found in 4% of patients, while 36% of the recipients had a remaining previous graft at the time of transplantation.

Statistical methods

Actuarial graft and patient survival probabilities were estimated by the Kaplan-Meier method. A log-rank test (Mantel-Haenszel) was used to test the equality of survival curves.

Results

For all retransplantations in PRA plus patients taken together, 1-, 2- and 3-year graft survival (1-, 2- and 3-y GS) was 65%, 56% and 45%. No statistically significant difference in GS was seen between second, third or fourth-fifth grafts and the survival curves of regrafts were similar to those of primary grafts in presensitized recipients (Fig. 1a). The causes of regraft loss within the follow-up time were: acute rejection ($n = 22$, 45%); 'chronic rejection' ($n = 13$, 27%); patient death ($n = 8$, 16%); or technical, infectious or other reasons ($n = 6$, 12%). The patient

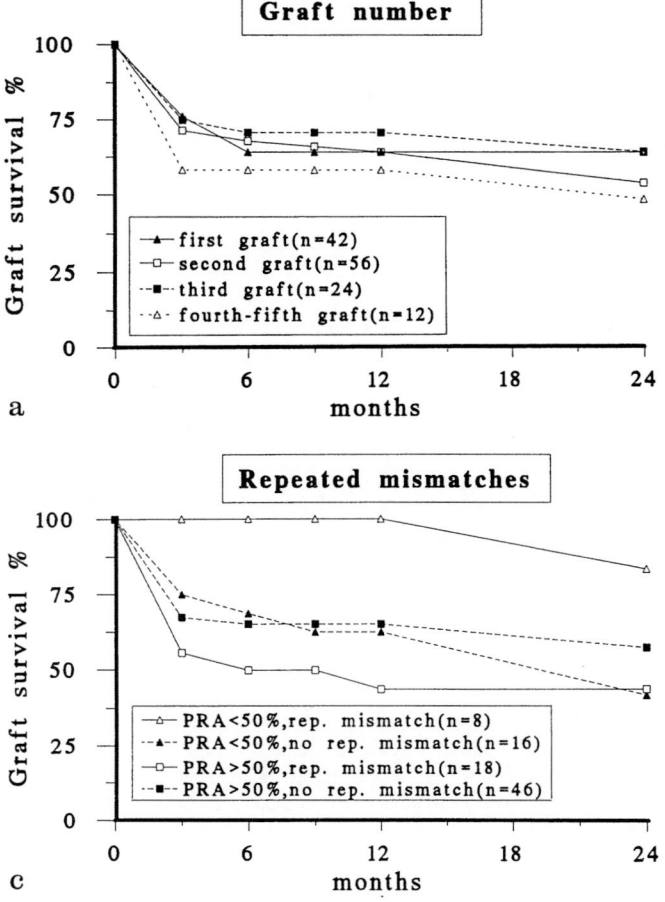

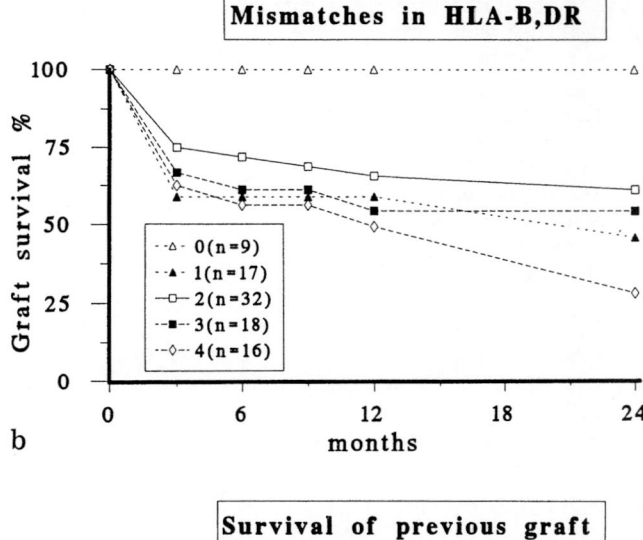

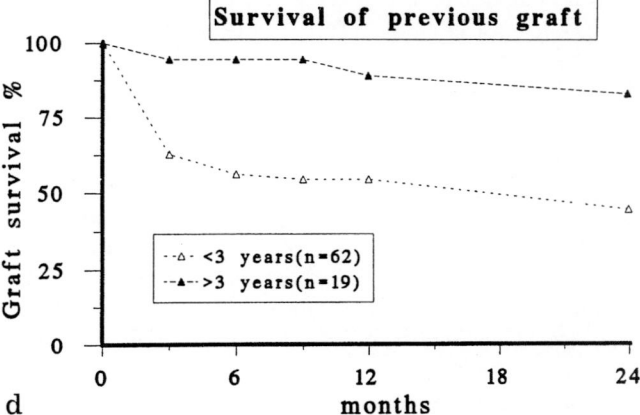

Fig. 1a–d. Survival of renal grafts, in patients with preformed HLA antibodies, transplanted in Göteborg 1985–89. Graft survival is shown in relation to: **a** the graft number; **b** the number of mismatches in HLA-B, DR loci (0 vs 1–4 mismatches; $P < 0.05$); **c** the presence or absence of repeated HLA-A, B or DR mismatches in recipients with more than or less than 50% PRA (repeat mismatch vs no repeat mismatch; $P < 0.05$ for PRA $< 50\%$; n.s. for PRA $> 50\%$); **d** the survival time (less than or more than 3 years) of the previous graft ($P < 0.01$)

survival after retransplantation was 92%, 86% and 81% after 1, 2 and 3 years.

The proportion of highly sensitized ($> 50\%$ PRA) recipients increased after regrafting (Table 1). Patients given their fourth-fifth grafts had the largest proportion of grafts with more than 24 h ischaemia time, grafts lost due to acute rejection and well matched grafts, and were more often male than female (Table 1).

In the regrafted group the influence of various parameters on GS was analysed. In recipients with $< 50\%$ PRA ($n = 26$), 1-, 2- and 3-y GS was 78%, 78% and 60%, as compared with 60%, 54% and 41% in those with $> 50\%$ PRA ($n = 62$). There was a better GS when no mismatches were present in the HLA-B, DR loci (Fig. 1b). A similar, but not statistically significant, benefit of 0 vs > 0 mismatches was seen with matching for the HLA-A + B + DR or HLA-DR. In highly sensitized patients repeat mismatch gave a 1-y GS of 43%, whereas a beneficial effect of repeat mismatch was seen in eight patients with PRA $< 50\%$ (Fig. 1c). A significant difference in GS was observed between recipients who had lost their previous graft in rejection after less than 3 years, compared with those with more than 3 years function (Fig. 1d). Other factors, such as ATG induction therapy, cold ischaemia time more than 24 h, and remaining previous graft at the time of transplantation, did not influence GS significantly.

Discussion

In the present report the survival rate of second and subsequent grafts was similar to first grafts in presensitized recipients, consistent with other reports [1]. This was true despite the fact that the group of regrafted recipients had a higher proportion of highly sensitized recipients and a tendency for longer graft ischaemia as compared with primary grafts. However, in the fourth-fifth grafted group better HLA-matching was obtained, possibly compensating for the other risk factors. A benefit of zero mismatches was demonstrated, particularly when matching for the HLA-B, DR loci. This finding is supported by previous studies [3], whereas others have reported conflicting results [1]. It has been suggested that transplantation across previous mismatches should be avoided, since it increases the risk of early graft loss [2]. In the present report the small subgroup of patients with PRA $< 50\%$ showed significantly better survival of kidneys bearing prevous mismatches, as compared with organs without such antigens. Other centres have reported successful retransplantations with the policy

Table 1. Proportions (%) of various parameters in groups of first or repeated renal transplantations in recipients with performed HLA-antibodies

	First graft (n = 38)	Second graft (n = 56)	Third graft (n = 24)	Fourth-fifth graft (n = 12)
PRA > 50%	45	69	67	83
Cold ischemia time > 24 h	35	37	35	56
Graft loss due to acute rejection	47	42	40	63
0–1 mismatches in HLA-B, DR	24	25	21	58
Male recipients	47	55	75	92

of allowing repeated mismatches, provided no antibody response against these antigens had previously been detected [6]. As also shown, but not concluded, in the latter report, a majority of the recipients with successful transplantations had no or < 50% PRA. The lack of antibody responses against previously-presented foreign HLA antigens could perhaps therefore be used as a basis for 'intelligent mismatching' in the subsequent transplantations. The duration of the previous graft survival was another factor, which in this and earlier [4] reports was found prognostic for the survival of retransplants.

We conclude that in many cases retransplantation of CM-negative kidneys to presensitized patients could be justified. For this group of patients the international programs for kidney exchange are probably even more important, making it possible to obtain HLA-compatible, or in the future perhaps 'intelligently mismatched', organs.

Acknowledgement. This study was supported by grants from The Professor L-E. Gelin Memorial Foundation, Föreningen för njursjuka i Väst-Sverige och Riksförbundet för njursjuka.

References

1. Albrechtsen D, Flatmark A, Lundgren G, Brynger H, Frödin L, Groth CG, Gäbel H (1987) Retransplantation of renal grafts: prognostic influence of previous transplantation. Transplant Proc 19: 3619–3621
2. Barger BO, Shroyer TW, Hudson SL, Deierhoi MH, Barber WH, Curtis JJ, Julien BA, Luke RG, Diethelm AG (1988) Early graft loss in cyclosporin A treated cadaveric renal allograft recipients receiving retransplants against previous mismatched HLA-A, B-, DR-donor antigens. Transplant Proc 20: 170–172
3. Opelz G for the Collaboratory Transplant Study. (1987) Transplant Proc 19: 641
4. Persson H, Frisk B, Smith L, Brynger H (1984) A positive prognostic factor in renal transplantation: Long-term function of previous graft. Transplant Proc 16: 1174
5. Sanfilippo F, Vaughn WK, Bollinger RR, Spees EK (1982) Comparative effects of pregnancy, transfusion, and prior grafts rejection on sensitization and renal transplant results. Transplantation 34: 360–364
6. Welsh KI, van Dam M, Bewick ME, Koffman GK, Taube DH, Raftery MJ, Rigden S (1988) Successful transplantation of kidneys bearing previously mismatched HLA A and B locus antigens. Transplant Int 1: 190–195

Transplant Int (1992) 5 [Suppl 1]: S 35–S 37

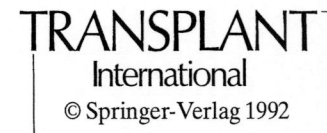

© Springer-Verlag 1992

Bilateral nephrectomy of the native kidneys reduces the incidence of arterial hypertension and erythrocytosis in kidney graft recipients treated with cyclosporin

Y. Vanrenterghem, M. Waer, M. R. Christiaens, and P. Michielsen (for the Leuven Collaborative Group for Transplantation)

Department of Nephrology and Kidney Transplantation, University Hospital Gasthuisberg, B3000, Leuven, Belgium

Abstract. Since the use of cyclosporin (CsA) the incidence of post-transplant arterial hypertension and erythrocytosis has increased sharply. In a retrospective analysis of 707 consecutive first cadaveric kidney graft recipients treated with CsA as basic immunosuppression, the effect of bilateral native nephrectomy on arterial hypertension and erythrocytosis was studied. Patient and graft survival as well as kidney function of the 264 nephrectomized patients were identical to those of the 443 non-nephrectomized patients. In the nephrectomized patients the mean number of rejections during the first year was 0.62 ± 0.88 versus 0.78 ± 1.02 in the non-nephrectomized patients ($P = 0.0285$). At 1 year after transplantation, 65.8% of the non-nephrectomized patients needed hypotensive drugs versus 45.3% of the nephrectomized patients ($P < 0.0001$). Notwithstanding the use of more antihypertensive drugs, diastolic blood pressure in the former group was significantly higher than in the latter group (87 ± 25 versus 83 ± 10 mm Hg; $P < 0.02$). During the first year 44 (9.9%) of the non-nephrectomized patients had haemoglobin levels higher than 17 g/dl versus only six (2.3%) of the nephrectomized patients ($P < 0.0001$). Comparable differences were also found up to 5 years after transplantation. These findings indicate that native nephrectomy is helpful in controlling arterial hypertension and erythrocytosis.

Key words: Renal transplantation – Arterial hypertension – Erythrocytosis – Bilateral nephrectomy – Cyclosporin

Although pretransplant bilateral nephrectomy was routine in the early years of transplantation, most transplant centres now consider that the risks of the procedure do not outweigh the benefits and therefore have abandoned routine native nephrectomy in favour of a more selective approach, such as in cases of chronically infected kidneys [4]. Since the availability of potent antihypertensive agents, even arterial hypertension refractory to haemodialysis alone is often not considered as an indication for removal of the native kidneys. Because the use of CsA has resulted in a sharp increase in the incidence of arterial hypertension, the potential benefits of pretransplant native nephrectomy should be reassessed.

Overproduction of erythropoietin by the native kidneys has been considered as one of the possible causes of post-transplant erythrocytosis, the occurrence of which is often masked by a concomitant bone marrow suppression by azathioprine [13]. As CsA is not a bone marrow suppressant, an increased incidence of erythrocytosis has been reported [7].

The present retrospective study analyses the effect of bilateral native nephrectomy on the incidence of arterial hypertension and erythrocytosis in renal graft recipients treated with CsA as basic immunosuppression.

Patients and methods

Between February 1983 and February 1991, 707 consecutive patients received a first cadaver kidney transplant with CsA as basic immunosuppression. Starting doses of CsA have decreased over the past years from 15 to 10 mg/kg per day. During the last 3 years CsA dose has been adjusted to maintain CsA whole blood levels (specific RIA method) between 200 and 250 ng/ml during the first 3 months. Corticosteroids have been started at a dose ranging between 16 and 24 mg/day tapered every month by 2 mg to 8 mg/day. First rejection crises have been treated with corticosteroids. Corticoresistant rejections have been treated with ATG (Fresenius) or OKT$_3$ (Ortho).

Of the 707 patients, 264 (37.3%) had received a bilateral nephrectomy. In most cases one kidney was removed before transplantation, the other at the time of transplantation. In the remaining 443 patients (66.7%), one or both native kidneys remained in place. Reasons for bilateral nephrectomy were persistent hypertension after starting haemodialysis, chronic pyelonephritis, grade 3 and 4 vesico-ureteral reflux, analgesic nephropathy, bleeding or infected polycystic kidneys and renal malignancies. Demographic data of the nephrectomized and the non-nephrectomized patients are compared in Table 1.

Offprint requests to: Y. Vanrenterghem, Department of Nephrology, University Hospital Gasthuisberg, Herestraat 49, B3000, Leuven, Belgium

Table 1. Demographic data in nephrectomized and non-nephrectomized patients

	Nephrectomized	Non-nephrectomized	Significance of difference
Age at transplant (years)	44 ± 13	43 ± 12	n.s.
Number of pretransplant blood transfusions	17 ± 21	10 ± 15	$P < 0.0001$
Number of B-DR mismatches	1.3 ± 0.8	1.33 ± 0.8	n.s.
Number of HLA-A matches	0.9 ± 0.6	0.9 ± 0.6	n.s.
Number of HLA-B matches	1.0 ± 0.5	1.0 ± 0.6	n.s.

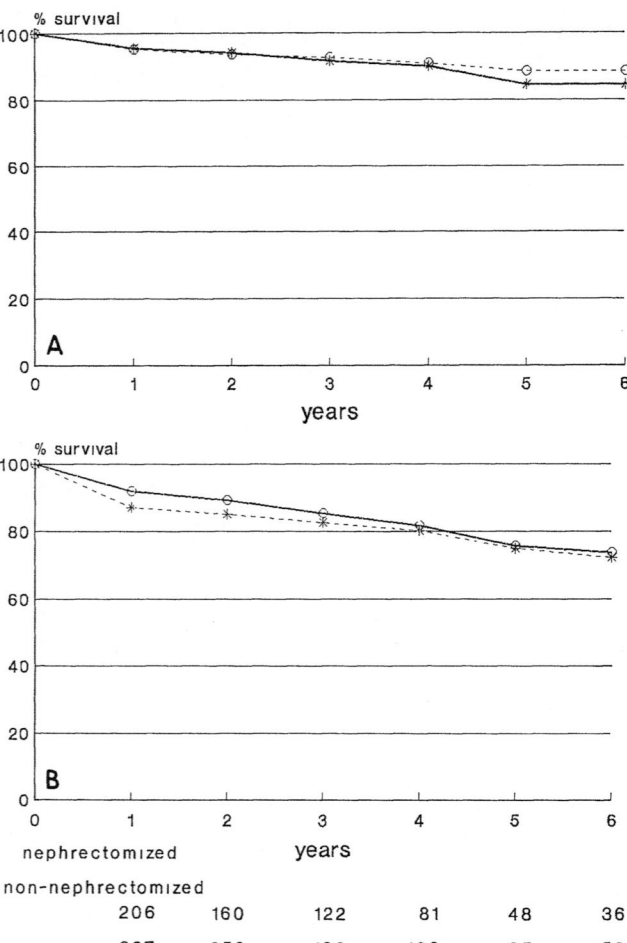

Fig. 1 A, B. Actuarial patient survival (**A**) and graft survival (**B**) in nephrectomized and non-nephrectomized patients. (*Solid line,* nephrectomized patients; *dotted line,* non-nephrectomized patients). At the bottom of the figure the number of patients at risk is given

Patient and graft survival was analysed by the actuarial method. Student's t-test and chi-squared or Fischer's exact probability tests were used where appropriate. Data are presented as mean ± SD.

Results

Although patient and graft survival of the nephrectomized and non-nephrectomized patients were comparable (Fig. 1), acute rejections were more frequently seen in the non-nephrectomized patients. The mean number of rejections per patient during the first post-transplant year was 0.78 ± 1.02 in the non-nephrectomized patients versus 0.62 ± 0.88 in the nephrectomized group

($P = 0.0285$). Serum creatinine and creatinine clearance were, however, not different (Table 2).

Up to 5 years after transplantation a significantly higher percentage of non-nephrectomized patients needed antihypertensive drugs to control arterial hypertension. Notwithstanding the use of more hypotensive agents, diastolic blood pressure was higher in the non-nephrectomized patients (Table 3). Mean haemoglobin and haematocrit levels were significantly lower in the nephrectomized patients (Table 4). During the first year after transplantation 44 (9.9%) of the non-nephrectomized patients had haemoglobin levels higher than 17 g/dl versus only six (2.3%) in the nephrectomized group. Up to 5 years after transplantation, all patients with erythrocytosis necessitating phlebotomy were from the non-nephrectomized group.

Discussion

The potential benefits of bilateral nephrectomy of the native kidneys in renal transplant recipients have mostly been studied in patients treated with conventional immunosuppression. Several authors have found an improved graft survival in the patients with bilateral native nephrectomy [1, 8], while others have not confirmed this finding [2]. In a large study of the SEOPF a lower incidence of renal graft rejection was found in nephrectomized patients [11]. More recently native nephrectomy after transplantation was also shown to improve renal plasma flow in hypertensive transplant recipients, a finding that was also confirmed in animals [3]. In our study no effect on patient and graft survival nor on renal function could be found. In

Table 2. Kidney function in nephrectomized and non-nephrectomized patients

	Nephrectomized	Non-nephrectomized
Serum creatinine (mg/dl)		
at 1 year	1.70 ± 0.67	1.81 ± 0.85
at 2 years	1.78 ± 0.82	1.90 ± 1.33
at 3 years	1.77 ± 1.81	1.81 ± 0.86
at 4 years	1.78 ± 0.89	1.78 ± 0.82
at 5 years	1.67 ± 0.86	1.79 ± 0.87
Creatinine clearance (ml/min)		
at 1 year	56 ± 23	55 ± 23
at 2 years	57 ± 26	54 ± 22
at 3 years	57 ± 29	54 ± 24
at 4 years	58 ± 28	57 ± 29
at 5 years	60 ± 28	56 ± 22

None of the differences between nephrectomized and non-nephrectomized patients are significant

Table 3. Blood pressure in nephrectomized and non-nephrectomized patients

	Nephrectomized	Non-nephrectomized	Significance of difference
Patients treated with hypotensive drugs			
at 1 year	66%	45%	$P < 0.0001$
at 2 years	65%	52%	$P = 0.01$
at 3 years	72%	55%	$P = 0.002$
at 4 years	70%	50%	$P = 0.003$
at 5 years	65%	44%	$P = 0.01$
Systolic blood pressure			
at 1 year	142 ± 20	147 ± 20	n.s.
at 2 years	144 ± 20	145 ± 21	n.s.
at 3 years	143 ± 18	145 ± 19	n.s.
at 4 years	140 ± 18	145 ± 18	$P = 0.05$
at 5 years	138 ± 17	143 ± 17	n.s.
Diastolic blood pressure			
at 1 year	83 ± 10	87 ± 25	$P = 0.02$
at 2 years	84 ± 11	86 ± 11	n.s.
at 3 years	84 ± 10	86 ± 10	n.s.
at 4 years	84 ± 10	86 ± 10	n.s.
at 5 years	81 ± 9	85 ± 9	$P = 0.03$

Table 4. Haemoglobin and haematocrit levels in nephrectomized and non-nephrectomized patients

	Nephrectomized	Non-nephrectomized	Significance of difference
Haemoglobin (g/dl)			
at 1 year	12.3 ± 1.4	13.3 ± 2.1	$P = 0.0001$
at 2 years	12.5 ± 1.3	13.3 ± 1.3	$P = 0.0001$
at 3 years	12.4 ± 1.6	13.1 ± 2.0	$P = 0.001$
at 4 years	12.5 ± 1.5	13.0 ± 2.0	$P = 0.04$
at 5 years	12.5 ± 1.6	13.1 ± 2.1	$P = 0.06$
Haematocrit (%)			
at 1 year	37.6 ± 4.3	40.4 ± 7.0	$P = 0.0001$
at 2 years	38.5 ± 4.4	40.9 ± 6.5	$P = 0.0001$
at 3 years	38.0 ± 4.8	40.4 ± 6.3	$P = 0.0004$
at 4 years	38.7 ± 4.6	40.4 ± 6.6	$P = 0.038$
at 5 years	38.4 ± 4.1	40.2 ± 6.3	$P = 0.06$

agreement with the data of the SEOPF study, the incidence of acute rejection crises was also lower in the nephrectomized group. It may be that the lower incidence of rejections in nephrectomized patients is due to the higher number of pretransplant blood transfusions in these patients.

Several studies have shown that the incidence of hypertension is significantly higher in patients with their native kidneys in place, and that post-transplant hypertension can be controlled by post-transplant nephrectomy [9, 10]. This beneficial effect on blood pressure could, however, not be confirmed by others [2]. Our study indicates that in patients treated with CsA, in which the incidence of hypertension is significantly higher than in patients treated with conventional immunosuppression, native nephrectomy also allows significantly better control of post-transplant hypertension.

Since the use of CsA as basic immunosuppression, a higher incidence of erythrocytosis has been reported [7]. This may be due to the fact that CsA is not a bone-marrow suppressant in contrast to azathioprine, which can mask the true incidence of post-transplant erythrocytosis. Others have suggested a direct stimulating effect of CsA on bone marrow stem cells [12]. Post-transplant erythrocytosis is probably of multifactorial origin. Inappropriate production of erythropoietin by the native kidneys has been suggested as one of the possible factors [13]. In our study haemoglobin and haematocrit levels were significantly lower in the nephrectomized patients. All patients with erythrocytosis necessitating phlebotomy were from the non-nephrectomized group. The lower haemoglobin cannot be explained by a worse kidney function as serum creatinine and creatinine clearance were identical in both groups.

In the past, bilateral native nephrectomy was considered a risky procedure with a substantial morbidity and mortality. Native nephrectomy can now be performed through bilateral vertical lumbotomy incisions with minimal morbidity and no mortality, even in patients under immunosuppression after transplantation [6]. Anaemia in anephric patients, either when waiting for a renal graft or after failure of the graft, can now easily be treated by recombinant erythropoietin. The benefits of the procedure outweigh the risks.

References

1. Advisory Committee to the Renal Transplant Registry (1977) The 13th Report of the Human Renal Transplant Registry. Transplant Proc 9: 9–26
2. Bennett WM (1976) Cost-benefit ratio of pretransplant bilateral nephrectomy. JAMA 235: 1703–1704
3. Coffman TM, Sanfilippo F, Brazy PC, Yarger WE, Klotman PE (1986) Bilateral native nephrectomy improves renal isograft function in rats. Kidney Int 30: 20–26
4. Crosnier J (1981) Indications for kidney transplantation. In: Hamburger J, Crosnier J, Bach JF, Kreis H (eds) Renal transplantation. Theory and practice. Williams and Wilkins, Baltimore, pp 146–176
5. Curtis JJ, Luke RG, Diethelm AG, Whelchel JD, Jones P (1985) Benefits of removal of native kidneys in hypertension after renal transplantation. Lancet II: 739–742
6. Darby CR, Cranston D, Raine AE, Morris PJ (1991) Bilateral nephrectomy before transplantation: indications, surgical approach, morbidity and mortality. Br J Surg 78: 305–307
7. Fang GX, Chan PC, Cheng IK, Li MK (1990) Haematological changes after renal transplantation: differences between cyclosporin-A and azathioprine therapy. Int Urol Nephrol 22: 181–187
8. Krakauer H, Spees EK, Vaughn WK, Grauman JS, Summe JP, Bailey RC (1983) Assessment of prognostic factors and projection of outcomes in renal transplantation. Transplantation 36: 372–378
9. McHugh MI, Tanboga H, Marcen R, Liano F, Robson V, Wilkinson R (1980) Hypertension following renal transplantation: role of the host's own kidneys. Quart J Med 49: 395–403
10. Pollini J, Guttman RD, Beaudoin JG, Morehouse DD, Klasen J, Knaack J (1979) Late hypertension following renal transplantation. Clin Nephrol 11: 202–212
11. Sanfilippo F, Vaughn W, Spees EK (1984) The association of pretransplant native nephrectomy with decreased renal allograft rejection. Transplantation 37: 256–260
12. Stockenhuber F, Geissler K, Sunder-Plassmann G, Kurz RW, Steininger R, Muehlbacher F, Hinterberger W, Balcke P (1989) Erythrocytosis in renal graft recipients due to a direct effect of cyclosporine. Transplant Proc 21: 1560–1562
13. Wolff M, Jelkmann W (1991) Erythropoiesis and erythropoietin levels in renal transplant recipients. Klin Wochenschr 69: 53–58

Transplant Int (1992) 5 [Suppl 1]: S 38–S 39

TRANSPLANT
International
© Springer-Verlag 1992

A logical basis for age matching in organ transplantation: studies of recipient renal function in relation to donor age

P. K. Donnelly, G. Mobb, A. R. Simpson, P. S. Veitch, P. R. F. Bell

Department of Surgery, Leicester University, UK

The ever rising demand for renal transplantation has led to an increased use of older (> 50 years) organ donors [9]. Previous studies have shown that donor-to-recipient age difference is an independent risk factor for allograft survival [3]. A recent multicentre study of 6397 first cadaver renal transplants showed that, where donors are more than 5 years older than the recipient, there is significantly impaired graft survival [11]. The mechanism of this effect is unclear, but it has been suggested that age-related donor factors may influence subsequent graft function.

Pathological studies have shown that native kidneys acquire specific histological (i.e. glomerulosclerosis, interstitial fibrosis) and functional defects in a linear fashion related to increasing age [1, 5]. Whilst graft loss may be seen as the worst outcome from using older donors, impaired function leading to shortened half-life may also occur. Recipients of kidneys from donors > 50 years of age also have a significantly higher creatinine than those from donors < 50 years of age [3]. A study was therefore undertaken to investigate in greater detail the effect of age on the function of donor kidneys in their respective recipients.

Key words: Renal transplantation – Donor age – Kidney function

Patients and methods

Cadaver kidneys were harvested from 48 donors of mean age 36.4 (range 13–67) years. All donors had normal serum creatinine at the time of harvesting. The kidneys were transplanted to 48 recipients of mean age 43.4 (range 19–72) years. Immunosuppressive therapy for all patients consisted of cyclosporin at a starting dose of 17 mg/kg and prednisolone 2.0 mg/kg both tailed as previously described [10]. The patients had been previously transfused and dialysed. All patients had attained a stable level of renal function (serum creatinine below 300 µmol/l) between 6 weeks and 2 years

Offprint requests to: Mr. P. K. Donnelly, Department of Surgery, Leicester General Hospital, Gwendolen Road, Leicester LE5 4PW, UK

post-transplantation. Further assessment of renal function was made by measuring creatinine clearance and glomerular filtration rate (GFR). Serum and urea concentrations of creatinine were measured on automated laboratory analysers which utilized the Jaffe reaction. GFR was measured using a single-injection isotope technique using ethylene diamine tetra-acetic acid (EDTA) labelled with ^{51}Cr [4].

Results

Serum creatinine was found to be positively correlated ($r = 0.371; P < 0.01$) with donor age, whilst there was no correlation with recipient age or time post-transplantation. Creatinine clearance was significantly worse for kidneys taken from older donors ($r = -0.48; P < 0.001$) (Fig. 1 a) whilst there was no significant correlation with recipient age or time post-transplant. GFR was highly significant ($P = 0.0001$) and inversely correlated ($r = -0.527$) with donor age (Fig. 1 b). Recipient age was weakly correlated with GFR ($P < 0.05$) consistent with some matching of older donors to recipients (i.e. within 5 years of age for 13% of the recipients).

Discussion

Previous physiological studies have established that native kidneys show decreasing functional reserve with increasing age [1]. GFR has been shown to decrease linearly from 130 to 80 ml/min in the age range 30–80 years, equivalent to 13 ml/min per decade. Assuming both kidneys contribute equally to the GFR a single normal kidney (not allowing for hyperfiltration) would expect a loss of GFR of 6.5 ml/kidney per decade. The actual loss of GFR in the transplant kidneys was equivalent to 5.7 ml/kidney per decade. It would appear that the transplant kidney has less function for a particular age of donor than would be expected in the native kidney. For example, a 40-year-old patient with a single native kidney would on average expect a GFR of at least 60 ml/min whereas a transplant patient with a kidney from a 40-year-old donor would expect a GFR of only 45 ml/min.

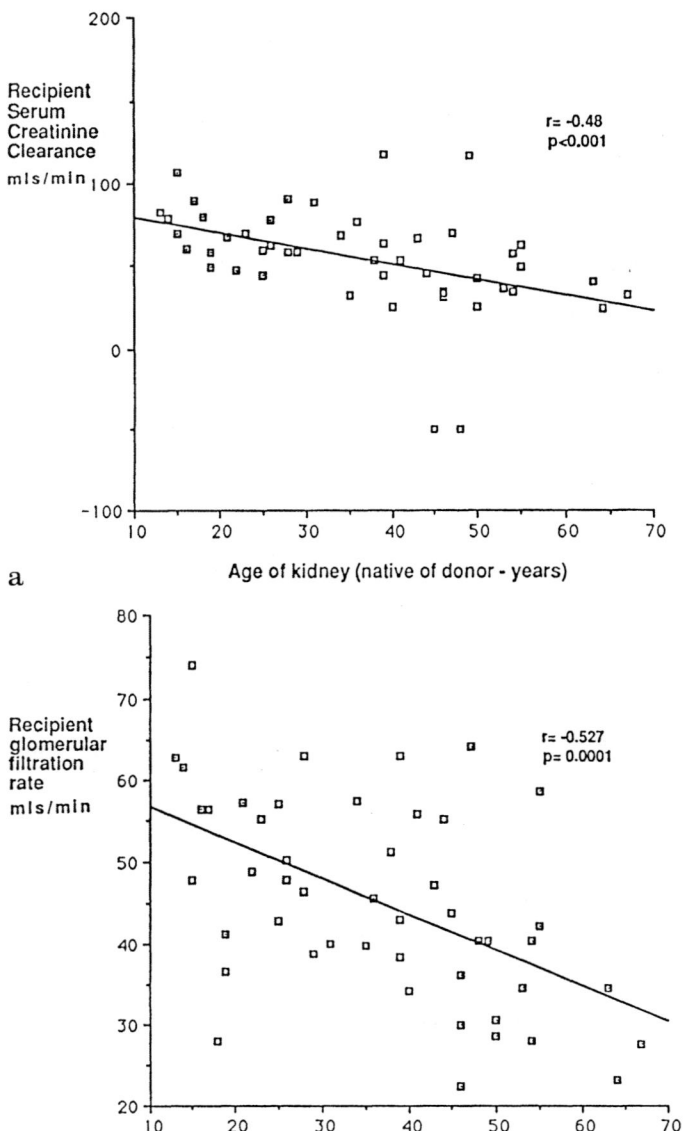

Fig. 1. a Recipient creatinine clearance and age of donor kidney. **b** Recipient glomerular filtration rate and age of donor kidney

tor of functional reserve [8]. At present donor age is not implicated in long-term graft loss which is largely attributed to chronic rejection. This is despite the fact that the half-life of kidneys from donors of 55–69 years of age is only 4.7 years compared with 8 years for donors of 11–24 years of age [6]. Since the histological differentiation of the two processes is by no means precise it would seem wise not to transplant old donor organs to young patients [3, 9]. Multicentre data suggest that a recipient's immune response decreases with advancing age [12], and it would seem logical to take advantage of the favourable immune environment of an older recipient to place an older kidney, which would potentially require less toxic immunosuppressive therapy [2] and possibly be less prone to damaging rejection. Given the rising transplant waiting lists older donor organs should perhaps be offered more frequently to recipients of comparable age.

References

1. Anderson S, Benner BM (1986) Effects of ageing on the renal glomerulus. Am J Med 80: 435–442
2. Cooper JL, Wahlstrom E, Anderson J, Schwerman L, Poterucha J, Krom RAF (1991) Use of cyclosporine with poor initial renal function results in severely diminished renal clearance up to three years following liver transplantation. Transplant Proc 23: 1489–1491
3. Donnelly PK, Simpson AR, Milner AD, Nicholson ML, Horsburgh T, Veitch PS, Bell PRF (1990) Age matching improves the results of renal transplantation with older donors. Nephrol Dial Transplant 5: 808–811
4. Duarte CG, Elveback LR, Liedtke RR (1980) Glomerular filtration rate and renal plasma flow. In: Duarte GCG (ed) Renal function tests. Little Brown and Co, Boston, pp 29–47
5. Kaplan C, Pasternack B, Shah H, Gallo G (1975) Age-related incidence of sclerotic glomeruli in human kidneys. Am J Physiol 80: 227–234
6. Land W, Schneeberger H, Schlieibner S, Illner W-D, Abendroth D, Hillebrand G, Gokel JM, Albert E, Fornara P (1991) Long-term results in cadaveric renal transplantation under cyclosporin therapy. Transplant Proc 23: 1244–1246
7. Leunissen KML, Bosman FT, Nieman FHM, Kootstra G, Vromen MAM, Noordzij TC, van Hooff JP (1989) Amplification of the nephrotoxic effect of cyclosporine by preexistent chronic histological lesions in the kidney. Transplantation 48: 590–593
8. Rao KV, Kasiske BL, Odlund MD, Ney AL, Anderson RC (1990) Influence of cadaver donor age on post transplant renal function and graft outcome. Transplantation 49: 91–95
9. Roels L, Vanrenterghem Y, Waer M, Christiaens M, Grawez J, Michielsen P (1990) The ageing kidney donor: Another answer to organ shortage? Transplant Proc 22: 368–370
10. Taylor J, Horsburgh T, Veitch PS, Bell PRF (1986) The benefit of immediate function to cyclosporin A treated renal allografts. Proc XVIII Int Course on Transplantation. Excerpta Medica, Lyon 19: 3–8
11. Thorogood J, Persijn GG, Zantvoort FA, van Houwelingen JC, van Rood JJ (1990) Matching for age in renal transplantation. N Engl J Med 322: 852–853
12. Yuge J, Cicciarell J (1987) Kidney transplantation and donor-recipient ages. In: Terasaki P (ed) Clinical transplantation. UCLA Tissue Typing Laboratory, Los Angeles

At present kidneys are shared almost exclusively on the basis of 'ageless' HLA matching in which kidneys are assumed to be functionally equivalent provided serum creatinine is normal at the time of retrieval. This study confirms the view that if native kidneys conceal a significant age-related defect of function the same will apply to cadaveric organ recipients. The whole process of retrieval and transplantation seems to further reduce the reserve of the kidney [7]. Whilst the live donor situation provides an opportunity to select the donor organ on the basis of functional studies the same is not true of cadaver organs. Clearly the donor creatinine may mask significant defects and, although there is a large individual range of GFR results, the donor age would seem to be a reasonable predic-

Transplant Int (1992) 5 [Suppl 1]: S 40–S 43

TRANSPLANT
International
© Springer-Verlag 1992

Multicentre trial of ABO-incompatible kidney transplantation

K. Ota*, K. Takahashi, T. Agishi, T. Sonda, T. Oka, S. Ueda, H. Amemiya, T. Shiramizu, H. Okazaki, N. Akiyama, A. Hasegawa, T. Kawamura, H. Takagi, and A. Ueno

Japanese Biosynsorb ABO-incompatible kidney transplant study group

Abstract. A multicentre study of ABO incompatible kidney transplantation using Biosynsorb was started in Japan in November 1989. A total of 51 cases were registered comprising 23 cases of A incompatibility, 26 cases of B incompatibility and two cases of AB incompatibility. The removal of antibodies (IgG and IgM) was carried out using Biosynsorb in 16 cases, plasmapheresis in four cases and use of both combined in 31 cases. The treatment using Biosynsorb was repeated 3.4 times on average. Serum titres of anti-A (IgG and IgM) antibodies decreased to 4.9 ± 5.0 and 2.7 ± 1.7 and for anti-B titres decreased to 2.8 ± 3.5 and 2.4 ± 3.2. Rejection was found in 33 cases: hyperacute one, accelerated acute five, and acute 27. In two cases rejection was developed concomitantly with a steep elevation in antibody titres. Three patients died, two with functioning grafts. Eight grafts were lost. Patient and graft survivals at 2 years were 94.1% and 84.3%, respectively. From these results it is concluded that: 1. Biosynsorb and plasmapheresis are effective in removing anti-A and anti-B antibodies; 2. graft and patient survivals are similar to those in ABO compatible cases; 3. anti-A and anti-B titres less than 16 are recommended at the time of transplantation; 4. anti-A and anti-B titres higher than 128 may be considered as a risk factor for rejection in the early stages after transplantation.

Key words: ABO-incompatible kidney transplantation – Anti-A and anti-B antibodies – Plasmapheresis – Adsorption of antibodies – Biosynsorb

By the end of 1990, 7740 kidneys had been transplanted in Japan. Living donors were used in 28.2% of these cases. Despite our efforts to promote organ donation, the number of transplantations using cadaveric kidneys has not increased to satisfy the demand of 15000 patients on the waiting list. In such a situation we are obliged to use family donors. Accordingly, we often encounter ABO-incompatible potential donor-recipient combinations with no other choice.

Since the introduction of plasmapheresis and the Biosynsorb adsorbent column (Chembiomed, Kawasmi Laboratories) [4] to remove anti-A, and anti-B antibodies, kidney transplantation across the ABO barrier, which hither to was considered very risky, has become a feasible operation.

A multicentre trial including 12 centres was started in Japan in November 1987 and, by the end of December 1990, 51 cases had been registered. This paper describes data obtained from these 51 cases along with the effects and side-effects of Biosynsorb.

Materials and methods

Patients

Patients enrolled in this study were 36 males and 15 females and their average age was 32.6 ± 2.6 years. They were divided into three categories: A-incompatible 23 cases (A to O, 13; A to B, 5; AB to B,

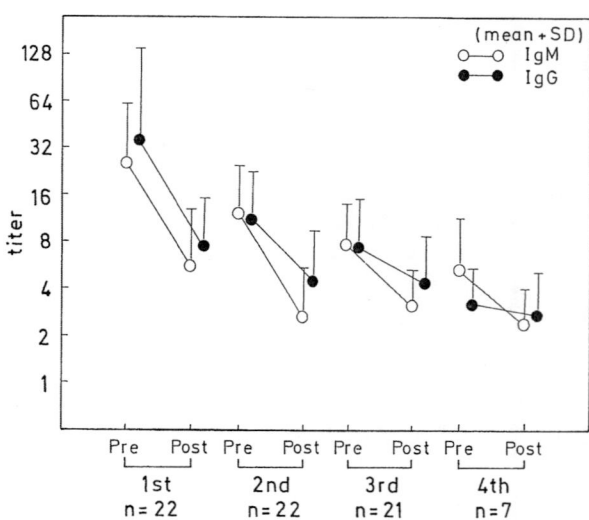

Fig. 1. Average reduction in anti-A antibody for each treatment

Offprint requests to: K. Ota, Kidney Center, Tokyo Women's Medical College, 8-1 Kawada-cho, Shinjuku-ku, Tokyo 162, Japan

5); B-incompatible 26 cases (B to O, 17; B to A, 3; AB to A, 6); and AB-incompatible, two cases. Nine grafts were donated from fathers, 29 from mothers, five from siblings, two from husbands and six from wives. The average mumber of HLA mismatches was 2.4 ± 1.3 and the number of one-way MLR stimulation indices was 19.5 ± 20.1.

Removal of anti-A and anti-B antibodies

All patients were treated with either Biosynsorb and/or double filtration plasmapheresis (DFPP) [1], a method using double filters specially designed to retrieve albumin. Biosynsorb-A was used to remove anti-A and Biosynsorb-B to remove anti-B antibody. The treatment was started 7 days prior to transplantation and repeated three or four times finishing on the day of, or one day before, the operation.

Blood flow and total volume of plasma treated were measured. Titres of anti-A (IgG and IgM) and anti-B (IgG and IgM) antibodies were examined using indirect Coombs, Bromelin and saline test methods along with complement (CH50, C3, C4, C3a and C5a), blood cell count and blood chemistry before, during and after the procedure.

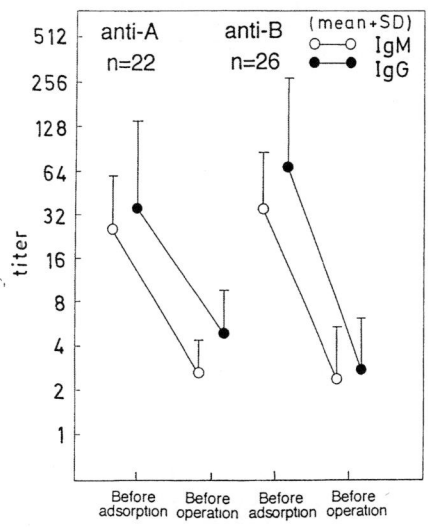

Total plasma treated (ml)   22011 ± 5013   23924 ± 6289   (mean ± SD)

Fig. 2. Reduction in anti-A and anti-B antibody titres before adsorption and before surgery

Immunosuppression

Cyclosporine (CsA), azathioprine (Az) and steroid, were used as the basic immunosuppressive drugs and antilymphocyte globulin and deoxyspergualin were added in the majority of cases. Pulse therapy with methylprednisolone (500 mg/day) for 2–3 days and 5 mg/day of muromonab CD3 for 10 days were used during rejection.

Operation

Kidney transplantation was done using the standard method described by Merrill et al. [7], and the spleen was removed in all except two cases.

Patient and graft survivals

Survivals of patient and graft were evaluated using the Kaplan-Meier method and compared with those obtained from the contemporaneous Japanese kidney transplant registry.

Results

Removal of anti-A and anti-B antibodies

Out of 51 cases, 16 were treated exclusively with Biosynsorb, and 31 with combined Biosynsorb and DFPP. In four cases the treatment with Biosynsorb was stopped within 10 min because of hypersensitivity reactions manifested as chest pain and a fall in blood pressure. These patients were switched to DFPP thereafter.

For the removal of anti-A antibody, 72 sessions of adsorption were carried out for 22 cases. The average volume of plasma processed was 6725 ml. Titres of IgG and IgM antibodies decreased from 17.4 ± 60.3 to 5.3 ± 5.9 (reduction, 43.8%), and 15.1 ± 22.8 to 4.0 ± 4.5 (reduction, 59.0%), respectively.

For the removal of anti-B antibody, 89 sessions of adsorption were carried out for 26 cases. The average vol-

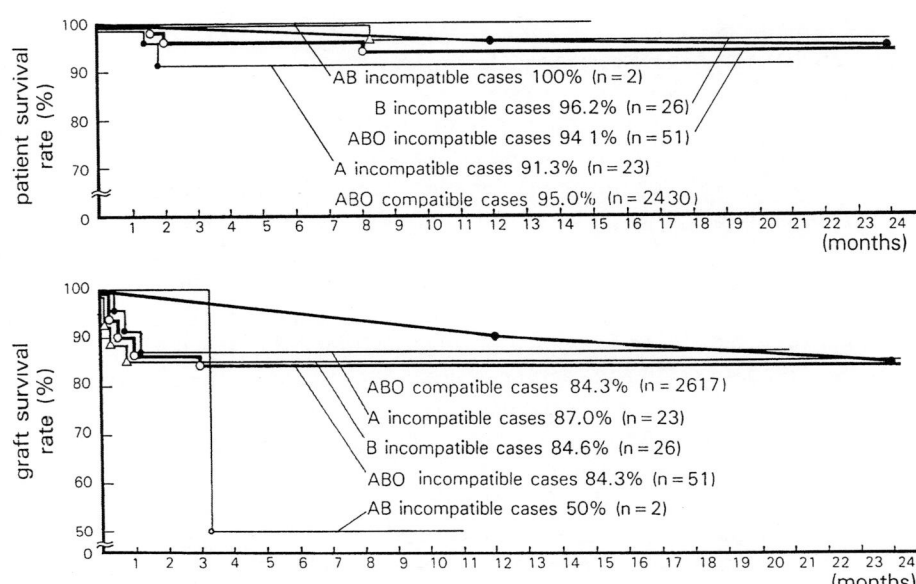

Fig. 3. Patient and graft survival rates (Kaplan-Meier method). ABO incompatible cases were obtained from the Japanese kidney transplant registry

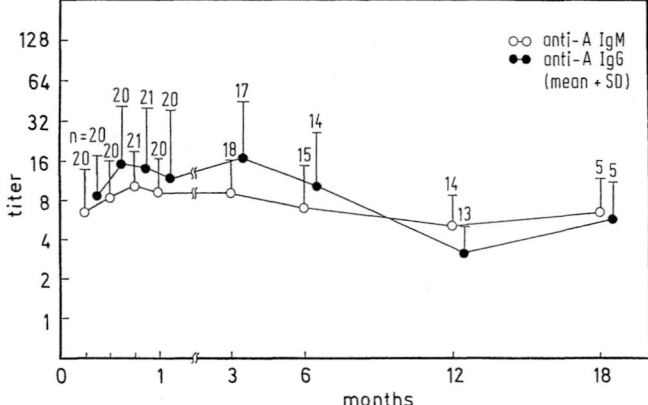

Fig. 4. Levels of anti-A antibody titres after transplantation

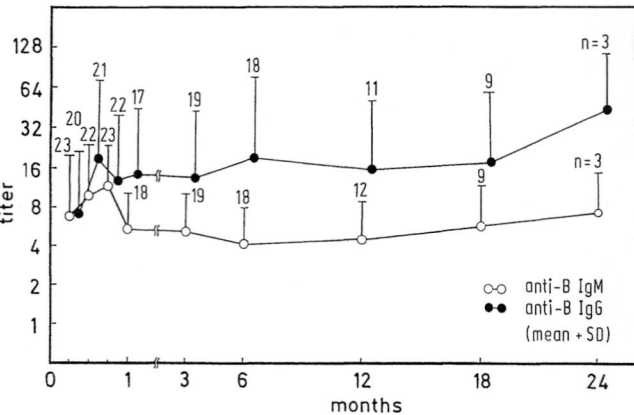

Fig. 5. Levels of anti-B antibody titres after transplantation

ume of plasma processed was 6952 ml. Titres of IgG and IgM antibodies decreased from 33.1 ± 115.9 to 7.5 ± 28.3 (reduction, 66.4%) and 17.6 ± 32.7 to 3.3 ± 4.1 (reduction, 73.3%).

The average preoperative adsorption was 3.4 times and total volume of plasma processed was 23 029 ml for each patient. By repeating the treatment, titres of anti-A IgG and IgM antibodies decreased from 37.0 ± 107.1 to 4.9 ± 5.0 and 26.7 ± 35.8 to 2.7 ± 1.7, respectively, and the titres of anti-B IgG and IgM antibodies decreased from 69.0 ± 202.1 to 2.8 ± 3.5 and 36.2 ± 54.3 to 2.4 ± 3.2, respectively, by the time of transplantation (Figs. 1 and 2).

There were no significant changes in erythrocyte count and level of albumin. A significant change ($P < 0.05$) was observed in the levels of IgG, IgA, IgM, C3a and C5a.

Transplantation and postoperative course

In all cases transplantation surgery was successful. In two cases splenectomy was not performed. Hyperacute and accelerated acute rejection developed in one and five cases, respectively, and in two of the latter, the graft was rejected. Acute rejection developed in 27 cases and in six of these, the graft was rejected. Two of the latter were not splenectomized. In the remaining 21 cases no rejection was found.

Blood type incompatibilities of those 8 cases who had their graft rejected were: A-incompatible, three; B-incompatible, four; and AB incompatible one. No chronic rejection was found in any of the 51 cases.

Three patients died on the 48th, 55th and 244th postoperative day from pancreatitis, brain haemorrhage, and malignant lymphoma, respectively. In two cases, patients died with functioning grafts, while the patient who died of brain hemorrhage was on dialysis after having his graft removed on the 29th postoperative day. Other postoperative complications observed were: cytomegalovirus infection and peritonitis, four cases each; pancreatitis, three cases; urinary tract infection, two cases; and haemorrhagic cystitis, leukopenia, atelectasis, malignant lymphoma, and brain haemorrhage, one case each.

During the observation period of two years, average serum creatinine levels remained around 1.5 mg/dl in both A-incompatible and B-incompatible cases.

As shown in Fig. 3, patient survivals for total cases, and A-, B-, and AB-incompatible cases were 94.1%, 91.3%, 96.2% and 100%, respectively, and graft survivals were 84.3%, 87.0%, 84.6% and 50%, respectively.

Serum levels of anti-A and anti-B antibody

The anti-A and anti-B antibody titres were followed for 2 years. As shown in Fig. 4 the average levels of IgG and IgM anti-A antibody titres fluctuated between 4 and 16, and anti-B titres showed similar fluctuation between 4 and 32 during the observation period. Among five patients who had their grafts rejected within 1 month after transplantation, two showed extremely high antibody titres (IgG, 1024 and 2048; IgM, 1024 and 512), while two patients who had their kidney rejected after 1 month showed no change in antibody titres. The adsorption using Biosynsorb after transplantation was performed 32 times for 11 cases to treat rejection and/or to lower the level of antibodies.

Discussion

There are several measures to remove anti-A and anti-B antibodies. Adsorption using Biosynsorb and plasmapheresis are most commonly used. In this study both of the methods proved to be safe and effective as described by Alexandre et al. [2] and Bannet et al. [3]. The advantage of the former is that no special substitution fluid is necessary. However, the column is very expensive and there is also the risk of hypersensitivity reactions. Plasmapheresis has the potential risk of viral transmission by infused plasma. DFPP, which was introduced to minimize the volume of substitution fluid, proved to be safe and effective. While globulin removed in one session is equivalent to that contained in 5 l of plasma, only 1 l of 7.5% albumin solution was necessary to compensate for the deficiency. There is no difference between A- and B-incompatible cases with regard to the effectiveness of antibody removal.

Since our study had no control group, graft and patient survivals were compared with those obtained from the Japanese registry of kidney transplantation. As shown in Fig. 3, the results obtained in ABO-incompatible cases were similar to those of ABO compatible cases.

There were two cases transplanted without splenectomy. The fact that both of the grafts were rejected within 2 weeks suggests the importance of splenectomy in ABO-incompatible transplantation.

Based on the fact that, in this study, no kidney was rejected in a hyperacute manner, serum levels of IgG and IgM antibodies less than 16 could be considered acceptable to perform ABO-incompatible transplantation. There is controversy as to whether elevation of anti-A and anti-B antibody plays of role in the process of rejection [5, 6]. In our series there were two kidneys rapidly rejected within a week after transplantation concomitant with elevation in IgG and IgM antibody titres. This finding suggests that elevated anti-A and anti-B antibodies triggers and/or enhances rejection crises, particularly in the early stages of transplantation.

It can be concluded that ABO-incompatible transplantation is acceptable if no other donor is available. Graft and patient survivals are nearly equal to those of ABO-compatible cases. For a successful outcome, preparation including splenectomy and reduction of anti-A and anti-B antibody titres below 16 at the time of transplantation is recommended, along with careful monitoring of antibodies and kidney function.

References

1. Agishi T, Kaneko I, Hasuo Y, Hayasaka Y, Sanaka T, Ota K (1980) Double filtration plasmapheresis. Trans Am Soc Artif Intern Organs 26: 406–411
2. Alexandre GPJ, Squifflet JP, Bruyere MD, Latinne R, Reding R, Gianello P, Carlier M, Pirson Y (1987) Present experiences in a series of 26 ABO-incompatible living donor renal allografts. Transplant Proc 19: 4538–4542
3. Bannett AD, McAlack RF, Raja R, Baquero A, Morris M (1987) Experiences with known ABO-mismatched renal transplants. Transplant Proc 19: 4543–4546
4. Bensinger WI, Baker DA, Buckner CD, Clift RA, Thomas ED (1981) Immunoadsorption for removal of A and B blood-group antibodies. N Engl J Med 304: 160–162
5. Chopek MW, Simmons RL, Platt JL (1987) ABO-incompatible kidney transplantation: initial immunopathologic evaluation. Transplant Proc 19: 4553–4557
6. McAlack RF, Bannett AD, Raja R, Kim P, Romano E, Lauzon G (1987) Delayed hyperacute rejection in an ABO-incompatible renal transplant. Transplant Proc 19: 4558–4560
7. Merrill JP, Murray JE, Harrison JH, Guild WG (1956) Successful homotransplantation of the human kidney between identical twins. JAMA 160: 277–282

Transplant Int (1992) 5 [Suppl 1]: S 44–S 46

TRANSPLANT
International
© Springer-Verlag 1992

Should hepatitits-C virus antibody-positive donors be excluded from kidney donation?

C. Pouteil-Noble[1], J. C. Tardy[2], P. Chossegros[3], C. Trepo[3], M. Aymard[2], and J. L. Touraine[1]

[1] Transplantation Unit, Pavillon P, E. Herriot Hospital, Lyon, France
[2] Virology Laboratory, Rockefeller Faculty, Lyon, France
[3] Hepatology Unit, Hotel Dieu Hospital, Lyon, France

Abstract. In organ transplantation, virus transmitted by the donor is associated with a higher risk of severe primary infection after transplantation in the seronegative recipient. In this study, the risk of hepatitis-C virus (HCV) transmission by the kidney was determined, and the morbidity in the recipient assessed. Serum samples from all kidney donors of our Transplantation Unit between 1983 and 1988 were screened for antibodies to anti-HCV by first enzyme-linked immunosorbent assay (Ortho ELISA) and positive samples were confirmed by a second-generation ELISA and the CHIRON RIBA HCV test. Of the 164 kidney donors whose sera were available, five were positive (3%) and all of them were positive with the RIBA test. Liver function was normal in the five donors. Seven recipients received a renal transplant from the anti-HCV-positive donors. Two patients had a follow-up too short to draw any conclusions. Two patients remained anti-HCV-negative up to 36 and 48 months, respectively, but one of them had chronic hepatitis. One patient was anti-HCV-positive before transplantation and remained positive over the 4-year follow-up. The two last patients seroconverted and acute hepatitis occurred at 16 and 101 days after transplantation, respectively. In both cases, no peroperative or postoperative transfusion was given and no other cause of hepatitis could be determined. A cirrhotic evolution was observed within 15 and 36 months in both cases. Thus HCV can be transmitted by a kidney transplant and cadaveric donors positive for anti-HCV antibodies should be excluded from kidney donation.

Key words: Hepatitis C virus – Kidney transplantation – Transmission

Many viruses transmitted by transplanted organs such as cytomegalovirus, herpes simplex virus, Epstein-Barr virus, human immunodeficiency virus, human T cell lymphotropic virus type 1, hepatitis A, hepatitis B, and delta agent can be responsible for severe primary infections in the seronegative recipient [5]. The evolution of the transmitted viral disease in the recipient under immunosuppressive therapy is different from the clinical presentation in the immunocompetent host, going from a fulminant to a chronic persistent infection depending on the type of virus, on the viral charge, on the immune status of the recipient and on the type and (HCV) intensity of the immunosuppressive therapy. In organ transplantation the possible transmission of hepatitis C virus (HCV) has just been reported [7]. In 1989 the possible detection of anti-HCV antibodies against a recombinant viral antigen, C 100-3 [1, 6], then the use of the second-generation ELISA allowing the detection of antibodies against structural and non-structural recombinant antigens and the use of the CHIRON RIBA test as a confirmation test, have improved considerably the diagnosis of HCV infection. If the transmission by blood product transfusion has been proved, other ways of contamination are possible, such as sexual and fetomaternal transmission, as occurs for hepatitis B virus [3, 4, 10].

To assess the risk of HCV transmission by the transplanted kidney we analysed the prevalence of anti-HCV antibodies in 164 organ donors from 1983 to 1988. The serological, biological and clinical follow-up of the respective kidney recipients were analysed in order to determine whether anti-HCV-positive donors should be excluded from organ donation.

Patients and methods

Kidney donors and serological methods

All the stored serum samples from the organ donors from 1 January 1983 to 31 December 1988 in the Virology Department were screened for anti-HCV antibodies and HBs antigen. A first-generation enzyme-linked immunosorbent assay (ELISA) (Ortho HCV ELISA Test system, Ortho Diagnostic Systems, Raritan, N.J.) de-

Offprint requests to: C. Pouteil-Noble, Transplantation Unit, Pavillon P, E. Herriot-Hospital, Place d'Arsonval, 69437 Lyon Cedex 03, France

tecting antibodies against the non-structural proteins, C 100-3 and 5-1-1, was first used. Then, when it became available, the second-generation ELISA which detects antibodies directed against both non-structural proteins, C 200 including C 100-3 and C 33 c., and a structural protein (core), C 22-3, was performed in the donors positive for anti-HCV antibodies with the first generation ELISA. The confirmation test was the CHIRON RIBA second-generation assay, which is an immunoblot assay using the five recombinant antigens, 5-1-1, C 100-3, C 33 c, C 22-3 and superoxide dismutase.

Recipients

All the sera available from the renal transplant recipients receiving a kidney from a positive anti-HCV donor were tested for anti-HCV antibodies from the day of transplantation to the last serum available. The follow-up ranged from one week to 60 months. First- and second-generation ELISA were performed and, in cases of seropositivity, the CHIRON RIBA second-generation assay was used.

Biological parameters including the determination of alanine aminotransferase (ALAT), gamma-glutamyltranspeptidase (γ GT), alkaline phosphatases and serum protein electrophoresis, were evaluated at the time of transplantation and then at 1, 3, 6 and 12 months, and every 6 months, to detect the occurrence of liver dysfunction. Acute hepatitis was defined by an elevation of the transaminase level on two or more determinations at least 2 weeks apart and a normalization of the biology within 6 months. Chronic hepatitis was defined by a persistent elevation of the serum alanine aminotransferase level for more than 6 months. Liver biopsy was performed in cases of chronic hepatitis. All the recipients were followed by the same medical team of the Transplantation Unit and were under the same type of immunosuppressive therapy.

Results

Prevalence of anti-HCV antibodies in kidney donors

The stored serum samples from five of the 164 kidney donors were positive for anti-HCV antibodies. All the patients positive with the first-generation test were reactive with the second-generation assay. The CHIRON RIBA second-generation test confirmed the positivity in the five cases.

No significant difference was observed in the prevalence of anti-HCV antibodies in organ donors whatever the year from 1983 to 1988. All the donors had a normal aminotransferase level at the time of organ procurement, and they were all negative for hepatitis-B surface antigen.

Transmission of HCV infection in the recipients

Seven patients underwent a renal transplant from anti-HCV-positive donors in our Transplantation Department. In two patients, the follow-up was too short to allow any conclusion since one patient died at 7 days from a myocardial infarction and the other patient did not come back to the department after 1 month. Among the five other renal transplant patients, two remained anti-HCV negative on all the sera tested with a follow-up of 48 months and 36 months, respectively. However, one of them had a rise in alanine aminotransferase (ALAT) concentration 30 days after transplantation and then the liver parameters became normal. Then a rise of ALAT and of the γ GT

level occurred from April 1989 to June 1990 without any blood transfusion since transplantation. A liver biopsy was performed for chronic hepatitis and showed hepatosiderosis without signs of acute hepatitis or fibrosis.

One recipient was anti-HCV positive at the time of transplantation and remained positive over a follow-up of 48 months. Anti-HBc antibodies were positive at the time of transplantation. Liver function tests remained normal from the day of transplantation to the last evaluation.

Two patients seroconverted to become anti-HCV positive at 3 and 2 months respectively. The first case was an 18-year-old boy who underwent a second renal transplant on 1 June 1984 and was HBs-antigen-positive. He did not receive any transfusion at the time of transplantation or after transplantation. Two rejection episodes occurred at 18 and 24 days after transplantation. The clinical presentation included a persistent fever from the eighth day, splenomegaly and a persistent leukopenia without active CMV infection. Poor general condition and poor renal function led to transplantectomy 82 days after transplantation. Acute hepatitis occurred from the 101st day while the liver parameters were previously normal. Anti-HCV antibodies were detected at day 101. A liver biopsy was performed 3 years later for chronic hepatitis and showed cirrhosis. He received a third transplant in July 1989 and the last biopsy performed in July 1990 showed the persistence of the cirrhosis but no hepatocellular failure occurred under low-dose azathioprine (25 mg/day).

The second case was a 42-year-old man who underwent a renal transplant on 11 August 1986. He was HBs-antigen-negative and liver function was normal at the time of transplantation. He developed cholestasis 16 days after transplantation and chronic hepatitis was evident. HBs antigen remained negative as well as DNA polymerase and HBV DNA in the serum. Anti-HCV antibodies appeared at 60 days. He did not receive any blood transfusion during or after transplantation. A liver biopsy was performed on 16 May 1987 showing acute hepatitis with minimal agressivity without cirrhosis. Six months later the patient was hospitalized for ascites and oedema of the lower limbs. Electrophoresis showed a rise in gamma globulins and a hypoalbuminaemia and the prothrombin rate was at 60%. All the other causes of chronic hepatitis had been excluded. Although liver biopsy was not repeated, a cirrhotic evolution could be suspected in the absence of cardiac failure and nephrotic syndrome. The patient has not come back to the hospital since October 1987 and a fatal outcome cannot be ruled out.

Thus HCV infection was implicated as the cause of acute hepatitis in both cases with a cirrhotic evolution. To summarise, HCV transmission by the kidney has been proved serologically in two patients of four seronegative patients who received a kidney from an anti-HCV-positive donor. Three patients of the four seronegative recipients had acute hepatitis and all of them developed chronic hepatitis. Two patients out of the three had a rapid cirrhotic evolution. The immunological characteristics and the immunosuppressive therapy of the patients who developed HCV infection were not different from those who did not.

Discussion

The prevalence of anti-HCV antibodies among cadaver donors was 3% from 1983 to 1988 and this rate did not decrease with time although cadaver donors are less transfused nowadays than previously. This high prevalence as compared to the prevalence of 0.6% in the population of blood donors from France or from the United States has also been found by Pereira et al. [7]. This could be due to the blood product transfusions given to the cadaveric donors and to a prolonged stay in intensive care units or in other wards with a risk of transmission. The meaning of the presence of anti-HCV antibodies is certainly not unequivocal since some donors will be able to transmit the anti-HCV antibodies and some not. The passive acquisition of anti-HCV antibodies through plasma or other blood product transfusions in cadaveric donors could not be ruled out, and the real infectivity of the organ is therefore difficult to assess depending on the viral charge and on the replication level. In organ transplantation it is difficult to discriminate between the role of the characteristics of the virus itself as it is in the donor and the role of the immunological status of the recipient in the triggering of overt hepatitis after transplantation. Two patients seroconverted 2 and 3 months after contamination without other cause of HCV transmission, especially without per- or post-operative transfusions and without other cause of hepatitis. In both cases this seroconversion was associated with biological and clinical acute hepatitis 16 and 101 days after transplantation and a rapid evolution to cirrhosis. Three patients acquired chronic hepatitis. The rapid progression of the liver disease in the recipients who became anti-HCV positive after transplantation was comparable to the evolution of HBV hepatitis acquired after transplantation under an immunosuppressive therapy [8].

The rate of seroconversion might be underestimated if a sequential follow-up of the sera of the recipients is not performed for at least 6 months after transplantation. Moreover recipients can be considered as falsely seronegative if the first-generation ELISA is the only test performed. Indeed, it has been shown that patients can have antibodies against structural proteins without antibodies detectable against non-structural proteins. These patients would be positive with the second-generation assay but seronegative with the first generation assay [9]. In the course of HCV infection some patients loose their antibodies [9, 11] against non-structural proteins and keep their antibodies against the structural proteins. This profile has been associated with normalization of the transaminase level and possibly with a decrease or a reversal of HCV replication [9]. In this study all the patients initially anti-HCV positive remained positive with the first- and the second-generation tests, suggesting a persistent viral replication. Amplification techniques should be more sensitive to detect the presence of HCV in the serum before the appearance of IgG directed against anti-C 100-3 [2, 11]. The disappearance of HCV RNA appears to correlate with the resolution of non-A, non-B hepatitis whereas viraemia persists in patients whose disease progresses to chronic hepatitis [2]. No data are available yet on the correlation between the presence or the disappearance of HCV RNA and the persistence or the disappearance of non-structural proteins.

In regard to these results anti-HCV antibody-positive donors should be excluded from organ donation, and this is the policy that we have adopted since 1 January 1990. The ELISA used for screening should be the second-generation ELISA, since antibodies against structural proteins cannot be detected with the first-generation assay, and a better evaluation of the infectivity of the anti-HCV-positive donor will be possible in the future using the HCV RNA amplification technique and the detection of direct markers of HCV replication.

References

1. Choo QL, Kuo G, Weiner AJ, Overby LR, Bradley DW, Houghton M (1989) Isolation of a cDNA clone derived from a blood borne non-A, non-B viral hepatitis genome. Science 244: 359–362
2. Farci P, Alter HJ, Wong D, Miller RH, Shih JW, Jett B, Purcell RH (1991) A long term study of hepatitis C virus replication in non A, non B hepatitis. N Engl J Med 325: 98–104
3. Giovannini M, Tagger A, Ribero ML et al. (1990) Maternal-infant transmission of hepatitis C virus and HIV infections: a possible interaction? Lancet 335: 1166
4. Hess G, Massing A, Rossol S, Schütt H, Clemens R, Meyer zum Büschenfelde KH (1989) Hepatitis C virus and sexual transmission. Lancet II: 987
5. Ho M (1991) Hepatitis C virus. Another agent transmitted by transplanted organs. N Engl J Med 325: 507–509
6. Kuo G, Choo QL, Alter HJ et al. (1989) An assay for circulating antibodies to a major etiologic virus of human non A, non B hepatitis. Science 244: 362–364
7. Pereira BJG, Milford EL, Kirkman RL, Levey AS (1991) Transmission of hepatitis C virus by organ transplantation. N Engl J Med 325: 454–460
8. Pouteil-Noble C, Chossegros P, Caillette A, Raffaele P, Bosshard S, Betuel H, Aymard M, Touraine JL (1990) Influence of chronic cytomegalovirus and hepatitis B virus infections on the outcome of renal transplant. Transplant Proc 22: 1820–1821
9. Pouteil-Noble C, Tardy JC, Chossegros P et al. (1991) Antihepatitis C virus antibodies: prevalence and morbidity in renal transplantation. Transplant Clin Immunol 23: (in press)
10. Riestra S, Suarez A, Rodrigo L (1990) Transmission of hepatitis C virus. Ann Intern Med 113: 411–412
11. Weiner AJ, Kuo G, Bradley DW et al. (1990) Detection of hepatitis C viral sequences in non A, non B hepatitis. Lancet 335: 1–3

Transplant Int (1992) 5 [Suppl 1]: S 47–S 50

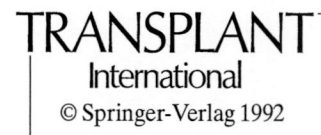

TRANSPLANT
International
© Springer-Verlag 1992

Cadaveric kidney donation beyond the age of 60 years – a comparative analysis of 1180 grafts from different donor age groups

Th. Sautner, M. Gnant, P. Götzinger, P. Wamser, R. Steininger, and F. Mühlbacher

I. Chirurgische Universitätsklinik, Wien, Austria

Abstract. The impact of high donor age on transplantation outcome was analysed in 1180 consecutive cadaveric grafts transplanted in adult recipients. Grafts were divided into three groups acording to donor age (<55 years ($n = 1073$, group 1), 55–59 years ($n = 51$, group 2), ≥ 60 years ($n = 56$, group 3)) and transplantation outcome was compared for these groups. Criteria investigated were the incidence of primary non-function (PNF), initial function (IF) (urine production first 24 h) and long-term function (LTF). The impact of donor age on LTF was analysed among other potential donor, graft and recipient risk factors by the multivariate proportional hazardous model analysis (Cox model). The incidence of PNF was 5.8% (group 1), 11.8% (group 2), and 16.1% (group 3) ($P = 0.002$). Analysis of paired kidneys of PNF grafts in group 2 and group 3 revealed good function for all paired grafts except for one in each group. IF was anuria in 19.7% of group 1, 29.4% group 2 and 21.5% of group 3, oliguria in 18.2% of group 1, 23.5% of group 2 and 32% of group 3. Normal diuresis was found in 62.1% of group, 47.1% of group 2 and 47.3% of group 3 ($P = 0.05$). Independent risk factors for graft survival were year of transplantation, recipient age, panel reactive antibodies, donor age group and number of transplantation. After the exclusion of PNF grafts from the analysis, recipient age, year of transplantation and level of panel reactive antibodies remained as independent risk factors.

Key words: Kidney transplantation – High donor age – Multivariate analysis – Risk factors

---

The growing gap between organs available for transplantation and patients on the waiting lists has led to the consideration of new borderline donor pools such as non-heart-beating donors and donors in extreme age groups [1] during recent years. The use of grafts retrieved from older donors has been discussed widely [3, 6–8]. The objections to the use of such organs, reported as proven signs of kidney aging [2, 4], have been confirmed as well as disproved by analysis of clinical data [3, 8, 9]. Different cut-off points for the subdivision of younger and older donors have been used in reported studies [8, 9]. In the recent past the importance of age-matching between donor and recipient has been discussed [5]. Since 1982, a growing number of recipients have been transplanted with grafts from aged donors at the Vienna Transplant Unit when parameters of donor kidney function were within the normal range. We investigated whether grafts retrieved from older donors or certain donor-recipient age combinations bear a higher risk of graft loss after transplantation. Different higher age groups were introduced to reveal any potential increase of risk over a greater span of increasing donor age.

Patients and methods

Of 1222 consecutive renal transplantations carried out between 1982 and 1991, all cadaveric grafts transplanted to adult recipients (16-years-old and over) were included in the study ($n = 1180$). To investigate the relevance of different cut-off points for donor age, patients were divided into three groups according to donor age: under 55 years (group 1), 55–59 years (group 2), and 60 years and over (group 3).

Variables investigated were donor criteria (sex, cause of death, circulatory condition before explantation, vasopressor therapy, and donor procurement centre), and graft criteria (warm ischaemic time (WIT) and cold ischaemic time (CIT) (Table 1). Recipient criteria were sex, age, primary disease, number of transplantation, panel reactive antibodies (PRA), HLA match, blood units transfused while on dialysis, pregnancies and year of transplantation (Table 2). Potentially interacting variables analysed were age match (donor age = recipient age ± 5 years; donor age = recipient age ± 10 years; or outside these categories) and the simple interaction of donor and recipient age as continuous variables.

Criteria of transplantation outcome were incidence of primary non-function (PNF), urine production during the first 24 h (anuria, <200 ml; oliguria, 200–1500 ml; sufficient function, >1500 ml) and long-term function at 1, 3, and 5 years. Graft function was specified in percent ± SE. Function according to groups was estimated univariately by the Kaplan-Meier method and statistically analysed by

Table 1. Donor and graft variables investigated

Variable	Donor < 55 years	Donor 55–59 years	Donor ≥ 60 years	Significance of difference
Donor:				
Sex (male/female) (%)	68/32	49/51	55/45	$P = 0.02$
Cause of death (%)				
Brain trauma	57	39	40	
Intracereb. bleeding	32	49	53	$P = 0.002$
Other	11	12	7	
Circulatory condition (%)				
Stable	68	53	69	n.s.
Instable	25	39	25	n.s.
Critical	7	8	6	n.s.
Cardiac arrest (yes/no) (%)	8/92	7/93	8/92	n.s.
Donor centre (own/other) (%)	48/52	43/57	44/56	n.s.
Graft:				
WIT (mean) (min)	0.61	0.64	0.60	n.s.
CIT (mean) (h)	21.9	24.6	24.6	n.s.

WIT, warm ischaemic time; CIT, cold ischaemic time

Table 2. Recipient variables investigated

Variable	Donor < 55 years	Donor 55–59 years	Donor ≥ 60 years	Significance of difference
Age (years)	43.7	49.2	48.2	n.s.
Sex (male/female) (%)	61/39	59/41	60/40	n.s.
Primary disease (%)				
Diabetes	8	5	12	n.s.
Other	92	95	88	
PRA (%)				
0%	70	70	85	
1–20%	13	20	7	n.s.
21–60%	10	8	4	
> 60%	7	2	4	
Nr. of transplantation (%)				
1	83	88	89	
2	13	10	7	n.s.
> 2	4	2	4	
A + B + DR mismatch (%)				
1–2	55	57	61	
3–4	43	43	37	n.s.
5–6	2	0	2	
Fullhouse (yes/no) (%)	6/94	8/92	5/95	n.s.
Blood units (%)				
0	13	8	18	
1–5	45	42	46	
6–10	17	14	10	n.s.
> 10	25	36	26	
Pregnancies (%)				
0	74	70	71	
1–2	16	18	18	n.s.
> 2	10	12	11	

the Breslow and Mantel-Cox tests. Distribution of donor, graft and recipient variables in group 3 was compared by the chi-squared test and t-test where appropriate.

All donor, graft and patient criteria were entered in a multivariate proportional hazardous model analysis (Cox model). The impact of factors with an independent significant influence is given as relative risk (RR), indicating the increase or decrease in the risk of graft loss in an arbitrary small interval of time. In addition, to avoid misinterpretation of donor-related factors concerning transplantation outcome, grafts of group 2 and group 3 that showed PNF were compared with their paired kidneys retrieved from the same donor. Cox model analysis was also carried out after exclusion of PNF grafts.

Results

Group 1 contained 1073 grafts, group 2 51 grafts and group 3 56 donor organs. Distribution of the variables was equal in all three groups, except cause of death (brain trauma, 58.3% group 1, 39.2% group 2 and 40% group 3;

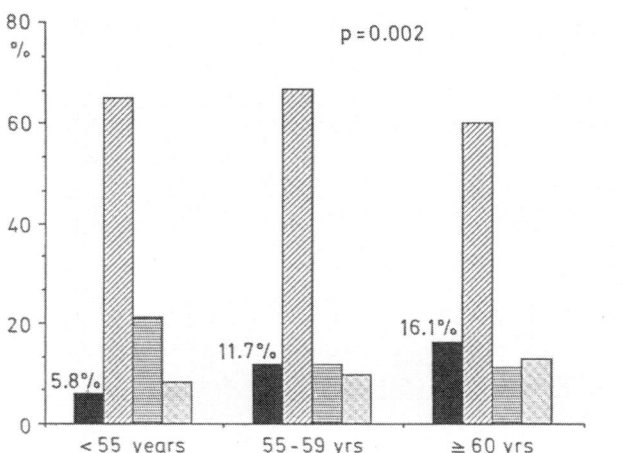

Fig. 1. Incidence of PNF (■), functioning grafts (▨), function loss (▤) and recipient death with functioning graft (▦) (P = 0.002)

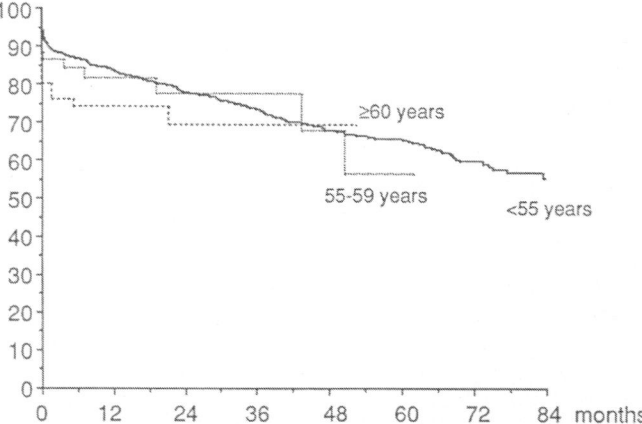

Fig. 2. Graft survival by donor age (Kaplan-Meier estimates); all patients

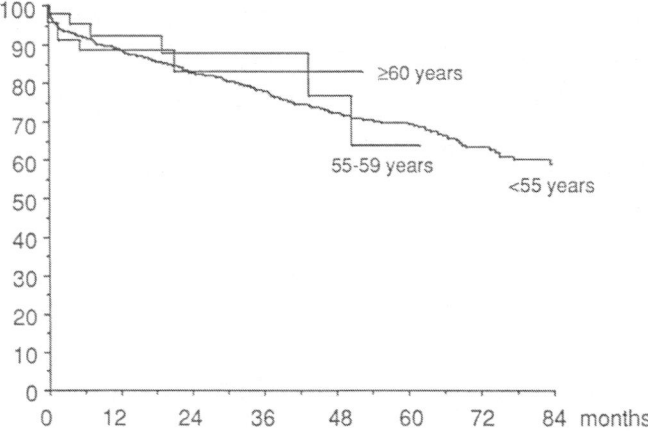

Fig. 3. Graft survival by donor age (Kaplan-Meier estimates); PNF grafts excluded

cerebral bleeding, 30.3% group 1, 49% group 2 and 52.7% group 3; other, 11.4% group 1, 11.8% group 2 and 7.3% group 3; $P = 0.001$). The proportion of grafts from aged donors differed from 1982 to 1990 from 0 to 6.5% (group 2) and 0 to 7.7% (group 3) ($P = 0.004$, 1982–1985 vs 1986–1990).

The incidence of PNF was 5.8% (group 1), 11.7% (group 2) and 16.1 (group 3) ($P = 0.002$) (Fig. 1). Initial diuresis was anuria in 19.7% of group 1, 29.4% of group 2 and 21.5% of group 3, oliguria in 18.2% of group 1, 23.5% of group 2 and 32% of group 3. Normal diuresis was found in 62.1% of group 1, 47.1% of group 2 and 47.3% of group 3 ($P = 0.05$). LTF at 1, 3 and 5 years in univariate analysis (Kaplan-Meier estimates) was $83.7 \pm 1\%$, $73.4 \pm 4\%$ and $65.8 \pm 2\%$ for group 1, $81.5 \pm 5\%$, $77.5 \pm 6\%$ and $56.5 \pm 13\%$ for group 2 and $74.1 \pm 6\%$ and $69.5 \pm 7\%$ for group 3 (observations of group 3 were not made for as long as 5 years) (NS) (Figs. 2 and 3).

Independent factors increasing or decreasing the risk of graft loss revealed by the multivariate proportional hazardous model analysis were: year of transplantation ($RR = 0.86$ for 1 year, $RR = 0.32$ for 1990 vs 1982, $P < 0.0001$); recipient panel-reactive antibodies ($RR = 1.3$ (0% vs 1–40%), $RR = 1.7$ (0% vs > 40%), $P < 0.0001$); recipient age (0.98 (step of 1 year), RR 0.87 (step of 10 years), $P = 0.001$); donor age group ($RR = 1.5$ (group 2 vs group 1), $RR = 2.2$ (group 3 vs group 1), $P = 0.004$); and number of transplantation ($RR = 1.3$ (first vs second), $RR = 1.75$ (first vs third and subsequent), $P = 0.017$) (Table 3). Six grafts in group 2 and nine grafts in group 3 showed PNF.

In group 2 one pair of grafts showed PNF in both recipients, but four of the paired grafts had good function at 6, 14, 15 and 31 months (CIT 23 h (PNF) vs 19 h (paired grafts)). In group 3 also one pair of transplants never showed function, and of the remaining seven paired grafts, six functioned at 6, 8, 13, 14, 21 and 45 months, one recipient died with a functioning graft after 1 month and one graft lost function after 4 months (CIT 28 h (PNF) vs 22 h (paired grafts)).

After exclusion of PNF grafts the Cox model analysis for the remaining transplants revealed an independent influence on graft survival of the following factors: recipient age ($RR = 0.97$ (1 year step), $RR = 0.81$ (10 year step), $P < 0.0001$); year of transplantation ($RR = 0.89$ (1 year step), $RR = 0.40$ (1990 vs 1982), $P = 0.001$); and level of panel reactive antibodies ($RR = 1.2$ (0% vs 1–40%), $RR = 1.57$ (0% vs > 40%), $P = 0.021$).

Age-matching by donor age ± 5 years of recipient age and ± 10 years of recipient age, and the interaction of donor and recipient age entered as continuous variables in the Cox model analysis did not show any effect on transplantation outcome.

Discussion

Grafting of organs retrieved from older donors has increased steadily at the Vienna Transplant Unit during the past 8 years according to the loosening of donor age criteria. In a general comparison with grafts harvested from younger donors the higher incidence of immediate graft loss and early function disorders in aged transplants is noticed.

Donor age above both defined cut-off points ranked among the strongest factors affecting long-term graft function. Yet when grafts suffering PNF were compared

Table 3. Results of Cox model analysis. All grafts vs PNF grafts excluded

Variable	Relative risk (all grafts)	Relative risk (PNF grafts excluded)
Year of transplant		
Single step	0.86 ($P = 0.0001$)	0.89 ($P = 0.001$)
1982–1990	0.32 ($P = 0.0001$)	0.40 ($P = 0.001$)
Number of transplant (first, second, third +)		
Single step	1.30 ($P = 0.017$)	not in the model
First vs third +	1.75 ($P = 0.017$)	
Recipient age (increasing)		
Single year	0.98 ($P = 0.007$)	0.98 ($P = 0.001$)
Ten years	0.87 ($P = 0.007$)	0.81 ($P = 0.001$)
Panel reactive antibodies (0–20%, 21–60%, >60%)		
Single step	1.30 ($P = 0.001$)	1.20 ($P = 0.021$)
0% vs >60%	1.70 ($P = 0.001$)	1.57 ($P = 0.021$)
Donor age (<55, 55–59, ≥60)		
–55 vs 55–59	1.50 ($P = 0.004$)	not in the model
–55 vs ≥60	2.20 ($P = 0.004$)	

with their paired kidneys it appeared that the occurrence of PNF could not solely be accounted for by poor donor quality but had to be interpreted as mainly recipient- and maybe CIT-dependent and might be attributable to immunologically-related failure [10]. A second finding that supports this suspicion is the fact that repeated transplantation, known as a strong risk factor for recipient sensitization and thus poor transplantation outcome, did not show as a significant influence on transplantation outcome in the Cox model when PNF grafts were excluded from the analysis. General factors influencing graft survival were recipient sensitization and recipient age. The positive influence of increasing recipient age on graft survival may be caused by a decrease in immunological response [11]. The improvement in transplantation outcome during recent years, as documented by the decreasing risk of graft loss, can be interpreted as a result of growing technical and immunological management experience of transplantation.

There was no evidence of a favourable effect of age-matching in our data as has been reported recently [5]. Neither could interactions between recipient age and donor age be demonstrated in this cohort of patients as has been shown by the Eurotransplant Group [5]. Nevertheless a possible effect may have been masked by the strong influence of other factors.

High donor age in itself is no obstacle to succesful transplantation. The acceptance of aged donors can increase the number of organs procured substantially. Hence, greater consideration should be given to this reservoir of potential donors.

References

1. Alexander JW, Vaughn WK, Carey MA (1991) The use of marginal donors for organ transplantation: the older and the younger donors. Transplant Proc 23: 905–909
2. Anderson S, Brenner B (1986) Effects of aging on the renal glomerulus. Am J Med 80: 435–442
3. Darmandy EM (1974) Transplantation and the aging kidney. Lancet 2: 1046–1047
4. Davies DF, Shock NW (1950) Age changes in glomerular rate, effective renal plasma flow and tubular excretory capacity in adult males. J Clin Invest 29: 496–507
5. Donelly PK, Henderson R (1990) Matching for age in renal transplantation. N Engl J Med 12: 851–852
6. Matas AJ, Simmons RL, Kjellstrand CM, Buselmeier TJ, Najarian JS (1976) Transplantation of the aging kidney. Transplantation 21: 160–161
7. O'Connor KJ, Bradley JW, Cho SI (1988) Extreme donor age in kidney transplantation. Transplant Proc 20: 770–771
8. Rao KV, Käsiske BL, Odlund MD, Ney AL, Andersen S (1990) Influence of cadaver donor age on posttransplant renal function and graft outcome. Transplantation 49: 91–95
9. Schareck WD, Hopt UT, Gaertner HV, Buesing M, Koeveker G, Smit H (1990) Risk evaluation in the use of kidneys from elder organ donors for transplantation. Transplant Proc 22: 371–372
10. van Speybroeck J, Feduska N, Amend W, Vincenti F, Cochrum K, Salvatierra O (1979) The influence of donor age on transplantation outcome. Am J Surg 137: 374–377
11. Zhou YC, Cecka JM (1989) Clinical transplants. Ed. UCLA Tissue Typing Laboratory, Los Angeles

Transplant Int (1992) 5 [Suppl 1]: S 51–S 53

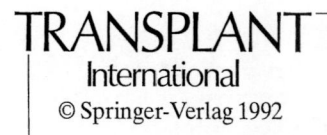

TRANSPLANT
International
© Springer-Verlag 1992

Antibodies against hepatitis C virus among renal transplant patients in Greece

J. Boletis, Ch. Stathakis, H. Papastathi, I. Vafiadi, D. Goumenos, B. Miriagou, A. Hatzakis, A. Kostakis, and Gr. Vosnides

Division of Nephrology and Transplantation, Laiko General Hospital, Athens, Greece

Abstract. To evaluate the prevalence of hepatitis C virus (HCV) infection in Greek renal transplant (RT) patients and its association with abnormal liver function tests (LFTs), serum anti-HCV was determined (Ortho-ELISA test system) in 206 RT and 245 haemodialysis patients (HD) as controls. The prevalence (10.2%) of anti-HCV in RT patients was significantly higher ($P < 0.0001$) than in the Greek general population (0.7%) and lower ($P < 0.0001$) than in the HD patients (23.8%), and was not related to the patients' age, post-transplant time or pre-transplant HD time. None of the anti-HCV RT patients was HBsAg +, whereas 13 (62%) and 12 (57%) of them were anti-HBsAg + and anti-HBc +, respectively. The incidence of abnormal LFTs in anti-HCV + HBsAg – and anti-HCV – HBsAg + RT patients was similar. Our findings indicate that: (a) the prevalence of serum anti-HCV in the Greek RT population is high, although considerably lower than in HD pts; (b) anti-HCV + RT patients have a high incidence of abnormal LFTs, comparable to that seen in HBsAg + RT patients; and (c) in a substantial proportion of anti-HCV + RT patients there is evidence of previous HBV infection.

Key words: Hepatitis C viral infection – Renal transplantation – Abnormal liver function tests

Liver disease is a serious complication of renal transplantation, since death due to liver failure occurs in 8–28% of renal transplant (RT) patients [3, 13]. Although viral hepatitis is one of the most common causes of liver disease complicating renal transplantation [5], until 1989 most cases of acute and chronic HBsAG – viral hepatitis in RT recipients were very loosely attributed to an unidentified hepatitis virus, designated as non-A, non-B virus [1]. In 1989, when an assay for the detection of an antibody against a recombinant viral agent (c100-3) was introduced

[4], a diagnostic tool for hepatitis C viral (HCV) infection became available, and the significance of HCV as a major cause of non-A, non-B hepatitis has since emerged [2]. However, the prevalence and clinical implications of HCV infection in RT patients has not been adequately studied. This, as well as the fact that the frequency of infection with HCV has a considerable geographical distribution [9, 11, 14, 17, 18], motivated us to carry out the present study, the purpose of which was to evaluate the prevalence of HCV infection in a number of patients representative of the Greek RT population and its association with abnormal liver function tests (LFTs).

Materials and methods

Included in the study were 206 RT recipients (49 male, 57 female; aged 43.3 ± 13.6 (17–73) years) who visited the outpatient clinic of Laiko General Hospital, Athens, between July and September 1990. Their pre-transplant haemodialysis (HD) time was 2.4 ± 2.1 (0.2–10) years and their post-transplant time was 3.1 ± 2.8 (0.3–17.5) years. Of the study group, 112 had received a cadaveric graft and 49 a graft from a living related donor. The immunosuppressive regimens consisted of: azathioprine (AZA) + cyclosporin (CsA) + methylprednisolone (MP) (151 patients), AZA + MP (27 patients), CsA + MP (27 patients) and MP only (1 patient). The control group comprised 245 HD patients (137 male, 108 female; aged 56.1 ± 15.1 (19–73) years) who had undergone HD for 4.2 ± 4.4 (0.3–18) years.

Offprint requests to: John Boletis, Fidiou 25, Holargos, 15562, Athens, Greece

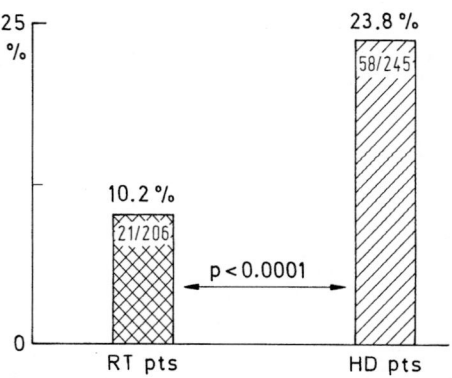

Fig. 1. Prevalence of HCV antibodies in RT and HD patients

Serum antibody against HCV (anti-HCV) was determined with a first generation enzyme-linked immunosorbent assay (Ortho HCV ELISA Test System, Ortho Diagnostic Systems) which detects antibody to a recombinant antigen of HCV (c100-3). Initially reactive samples were retested twice more, and only samples that were repeatedly reactive were considered as positive. Hepatitis B markers were determined with commercially available kits of ELISA-ORGANON (HBsAg, anti-HBs) and E.I.A.-SORIN (HBeAg, anti-HBe, anti-HBc, anti-HBcIgM). Serial LFT measurements (SGOT/SGPT, alkaline phosphatase, γGT and bilirubin) were routinely performed in all patients. LFT results were arbitrarily defined as abnormal when the mean level of two sequential measurements was 1.5 times above the upper limit of the normal range. This definition was chosen because, in RT patients with liver disease, the LFT results are usually not increased [3, 13].

Statistical analyses were performed with the use of the chi-squared test and Student's t-test where applicable.

Table 1. Relation between prevalence of anti-HCV and age in RT patients

Age groups (years)	No. of patients	No. anti-HCV +	%
0–29	29	3	10.3
30–39	49	2	4.1
40–49	57	6	10.5
50–59	58	9	15.5
60–69	12	1	8.3
≥ 70	1	0	0

$P = 0.54$

Table 2. Relation between prevalence of anti-HCV and post-transplant time

Post-transplant time (years)	No. of patients	No. anti-HCV +	%
0–3	131	16	12.2
4–7	61	3	4.9
>8	14	2	14.2

$P = 0.24$

Table 3. Relation between prevalence of anti-HCV and pre-transplant HD time

Time on HD (years)	No. of patients	No. anti-HCV +	%
0–3	136	13	9.5
4–7	22	3	13.6
>8	11	0	0

$P = 0.45$

Table 4. HBV markers in the anti-HCV + RT patients

	No. of patients	%
HBsAg +	0	0
anti-HBc + /anti-HBs +	8	39
anti-HBc + /anti-HBs –	4	19
anti-HBc – /anti-HBs +	5	23
All markers –	4	19
Totals	21	100

Results

Antibody against HCV was repeatedly found to be present in the serum of a significantly higher proportion of RT (21/206, 10.2%) than HD (58/245, 23.8%) patients ($P < 0.0001$) (Fig. 1). The prevalence of anti-HCV in the RT population was not significantly affected by sex (M, 14/149; F, 7/57; $P = 0.70$), age ($P = 0.54$, Table 1), post-transplant time ($P = 0.24$, Table 2) or pre-transplant HD time ($P = 0.45$, Table 3). None of the anti-HCV + RT patients were HBsAG + whereas 13 (62%) of them were anti-HBs + and 12 (57%) were anti-HBc + (Table 4). A similar incidence ($P = 0.26$) of abnormal LFT results was noted in anti-HCV + /HBsAG – and HBsAG + /anti-HCV – RT patients and both anti-HCV + and HBsAG + RT patients, had similar serum creatinine levels ($P = 0.30$) and post-transplant time ($P = 0.94$) (Table 5).

Discussion

The prevalence of anti-HCV + RT patients found in the present study (10.2%) was significantly higher than the very low prevalence (0.7%) found in the Greek general population [15] and significantly lower than the prevalence observed in the HD patients (23.8%). This probably reflects the limitation of test sensitivity, especially in immunosuppressed patients [20]. Regarding the relation between the presence of serum anti-HCV and post-transplantation time or time on HD, the available data are restricted and conflicting [10, 16]. In the present study, no relation was observed between the presence of serum anti-HCV and sex, age, post-transplant time or pre-transplant HD time. It must be noted, however, that in the present study no precise data are available regarding the pre- and post-transplant transfusion history of the patients. None of the 21 anti-HCV + RT patients was found to be HBsAG +, whereas 57% had evidence of previous HBV infection (anti-HBc +) and 62% were immune against HBV (anti-HBs +). This finding is in agreement with the proposal that anti-HBc can be regarded as a 'surrogate assay' for HCV [12, 19] and that, in the majority of anti-HCV + HD patients, there is serological evidence of previous HBV infection [8].

Table 5. Abnormal LFT results, post-transplant time and serum creatinine in anti-HCV + and HBsAg + RT patients

	n	Post-transplant time (years)	Serum creatinine (mg%)	Abnormal LFT	
				n	%
anti-HCV +	21	2.9 ± 2.6	2.7 ± 2.4	14	66
HBsAg +	19	2.9 ± 2.8	2.0 ± 1.4	14	73
P value		0.94	0.30		0.26

In contrast to the infection with HBV [6, 7], data concerning the clinical implications of HCV infection in RT patients are not yet available and this is mainly due to: the very recent availability of the first diagnostic test for hepatitis C [4]; the varying incidence of hepatitis C viral infection in renal transplant units, depending on the geographical origin of the population studied [10, 14, 16, 18]; and the fact that the definition of the hepatic status of RT patients necessitates histological examination, since their liver disease often has a latent course, both clinically and biologically [6]. As a very approximate approach to this matter, the incidence of abnormal LFT results in anti-HCV + and HBsAg + /anti-HCV − RT patients was compared. We found that anti-HCV + patients had a high incidence of persistently abnormal LFT results comparable to that found in HBsAg + patients. This finding suggests that, regarding liver disease, anti-HCV + RT patients probably have an unfavourable course, similar to that seen in HBsAg + RT patients [6, 7]. We also observed that both groups of patients have similar serum creatinine levels and post-transplant time.

In conclusion, the results of the present study indicate that: (a) in Greek RT patients the incidence of HCV infections is significantly higher than in the general population and lower than in HD patients; (b) anti-HCV + RT patients have a high incidence of abnormal LFT results, comparable to that seen in HBsAg + RT patients; and (c) in a substantial proportion of anti-HCV + RT patients there is evidence of previous infection with HBV.

References

1. Alter HJ, Hoofnagle JH (1984) Non-A, non-B: observation on the first decade. In: Vyas GN, Dienstag JL, Hoofnagle JH (eds) Viral hepatitis and liver disease. Grune and Stratton, Orlando, pp 345–354
2. Alter HJ, Purcell RH, Shih JW, Melpolder JC, Houghton M, Choo QL, Kuo G (1989) Detection of antibody to hepatitis C virus in prospectively followed transfusion recipients with acute and chronic non-A, non-B hepatitis. N Engl J Med 22: 1494–1500
3. Braun WE (1990) Long-term complications of renal transplantation. Kidney Int 37: 1363–1378
4. Choo QL, Kuo G, Weiner AJ, Overby LR, Bradley DW, Houghton M (1989) Isolation of a DNA clone derived from a blood-borne non-A, non-B viral hepatitis genome. Science 24: 359–362
5. Debure A, Degos F, Pol S, Degott C, Carnot F, Lugassy C et al. (1988) Liver disease and hepatic complications in renal transplant patients. Adv Nephrol 17: 375–400
6. Dega F, Degott C (1989) Hepatitis in renal transplant recipients. J Hepatol 9: 114–123
7. Dienstag JL (1988) Renal transplantation ahd hepatitis B. Gastroenterology 94: 235–238
8. Elisaf M, Tsianos E, Mavridis A, Dardamanis M, Pappas M, Siamopoulos KC (1991) Antibodies against hepatitis C virus in haemodialysis patients: Association with hepatitis B serological markers. Nephrol Dial Transplant 6: 476–479
9. Esteban JI, Esteban R, Viladomiou L, Lopez-Talavera CJ, Gonzalez A, Hernandez MJ et al. (1989) Hepatitis C virus antibodies among risk groups in Spain. Lancet I: 294–295
10. Gomez E, Aquado S, de Ona M, Martinez A, Gimadevilla R, Sanchez L et al. (1990) Hepatitis C virus antibodies in renal transplant patients. XVII EDTA-ERA Congress, Vienna, Abstract 206
11. Jeffers LJ, Perez GO, De Medina MD, Ortiz-Interian CJ, Schiff ER, Reddy RK et al. (1990) Hepatitis C infection in two urban hemodialysis units. Kidney Int 38: 320–322
12. Koziol DE, Holland PV, Alling DW et al. (1986) Antibody to hepatitis B core antigen as a paradoxical marker for non-A, non-B hepatitis agents in donated blood. Ann Intern Med 104: 488–495
13. Mahony JF (1989) Long term results and complications of transplantation. Kidney Transplant Proc 21: 1433–1434
14. Pol S, Legendre C, Saltiel C et al. (1991) Hepatitis C virus in kidney recipients: Epidemiology and impact on renal transplantation. In: Hollinger FB, Lemon SM, Margolis HS (eds) Viral hepatitis and liver disease. Williams and Wilkins, Baltimore (in press)
15. Politi K, Papathogiannakis N, Richardson SC (1990) Prevalence of antibody to hepatitis C virus in thalassemic patients, in renal patients on hemodialysis and in blood donors. Iatriki 58: 359–364
16. Ponz E, Campistol JM, Barrera JM, Gil C, Andreu J, Bruguera M (1990) Incidence and role of hepatitis C virus in liver disease of renal transplant recipients. XVII EDTA-ERA Congress, Vienna, Abstract 220
17. Roggendorf M, Deinhardt F, Rasshofer R, Eberle J, Hopf U, Moller B et al. (1989) Antibodies to hepatitis C virus. Lancet I: 324–325
18. Roth D, Fernandez JA, Burke GW, Esquenazi V, Miller J (1991) Detection of antibody to hepatitis C virus in renal transplant recipients. Transplantation 51: 396–400
19. Stevens CE, Aach RD, Hollinger FB et al. (1984) Hepatitis B virus antibody in blood donors and the occurrence of non-A, non-B hepatitis in transfusion recipients: An analysis of the transfusion transmitted viruses study. Ann Intern Med 101: 733–738
20. Weiner AJ, Kuo G, Bradley DW, Bonino F, Saracco G, Lee C et al. (1990) Detection of hepatitis C viral sequences in non-A, non-B hepatitis. Lancet 335: 1–3

Transplant Int (1992) 5 [Suppl 1]: S 54–S 57

TRANSPLANT
International
© Springer-Verlag 1992

Value of panel reactive antibodies (PRA) as a guide to the treatment of hyperimmunized patients in renal transplantation

A. Buscaroli, A. Nanni Costa, S. Iannelli, G. Cianciolo, L. De Santis, G. La Manna, S. Stefoni, A. Vangelista, and V. Bonomini

Institute of Nephrology, St. Orsola University Hospital, Bologna, Italy

Abstract. Patient presensitization represents a considerable problem in candidacy for renal transplantation. While it is well known that hyperimmunized patients – panel reactive antibody (PRA) higher than 60% – create difficulties in donor matching and have a worse outcome than non-hyperimmunized patients, less information is available on patients with an intermediate degree of sensitization (30–60%). In order to evaluate how graft outcome relates to such degrees of sensitization, 241 consecutive transplanted patients were divided into two groups on the basis of their previous year's PRA peak: group A, PRA 0–29%; group B, PRA 30–60%. Group A showed a significantly better survival both in the first year (90% vs 79%, $P < 0.05$) and in the third year (82% vs 64%, $P < 0.01$). However, detailed analysis of group B demonstrated that some parameters may significantly influence graft outcome: (1) better compatibility on locus DR; (2) a primary kidney transplant; (3) a dialysis duration of less than 6 months; and (4) the prophylactic use of anti-lymphocyte globulin (ALG).

Key words: Panel reactive antibodies – Locus DR – Dialytic age – Primary kidney transplant – Anti-lymphocyte globulin

The presence of the hyperimmunized patient is a growing problem for kidney transplantation centres where the number of donors is always on the decline while the list of uraemic patients waiting for a graft dramatically increases. Hyperimmunized patients represent a considerable percentage of the waiting list (20–40%) and create a real dilemma in decision making. While it is well known that more than 60% of panel reactive antibodies (PRA) create difficulties both in donor matching and in graft outcome, less information is available on patients with an in-

termediate degree of sensitization [2, 6, 7]. The aim of this study was to analyse the influence of an intermediate degree of sensitization (30–60%) on graft outcome and to assess the best therapeutic strategy for such patients.

Materials and methods

The present study draws on data from 241 kidney transplant patients transplanted in the Nephrology Department of the St. Orsola University Hospital of Bologna from 1985 to 1990 from cadaver donors.

In all patients an accurate pre-transplant study was carried out determining the percentage of antibodies in the serum against a panel of frozen lymphocytes from normal subjects (PRA). The technique used to detect cytotoxicity was complement-dependent NIH standard. Fresh sera were collected from waiting-list patients every 2 months and tested. For this study evaluation was made only on the basis of the PRA peak value in the previons 12 months. Patients were divided into two groups: group A (174 patients, 72%), PRA 0–29%; group B (63 patients, 26%), PRA 30–60%. Over 60% of our case material was confined to isolated episodes (4/241, 1.6%). The distribution of PRA in the patients studied is shown in Fig. 1.

Patients with less than 1 year of follow-up and those with graft failure caused by a primary surgical problem or an accident were excluded from the study. In all cases, steroids plus cyclosporine was the standard initial immunosuppressive therapy. Transplantation in all patients was performed only after a negative donor–recipient crossmatch.

The study was developed in two steps. The first step consisted of comparing groups A and B and determining if there were any dif-

Offprint requests to: Dr. Andrea Buscaroli, Institute of Nephrology, St. Orsola University Hospital, Bologna, Via Massarenti 9, 40138, Bologna, Italy

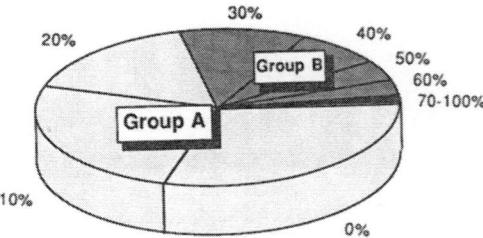

Fig. 1. Distribution of PRA peak values in the 241 patients studied. Group A (PRA <30%) included 174 patients and group B (PRA 30–60%) 63 patients. Four patients with PRA >60% were excluded from the study as being non-evaluable

ferences between the two groups, apart from the PRA peak value, potentially influencing the graft outcome. The second step, and main aim of the study, was to analyse group B alone, in an attempt to define what pre- and post-transplant factors influence graft outcome.

The choice of parameters to be examined for graft outcome related to the following 27 items: (1) *individual characteristics:* sex, age, primary renal disease, blood group, duration of dialysis treatment (months), previous pregnancy, polytransfused or not; (2) *donor characteristics:* provenance of donor (local, shipped), multiorgan graft or not, age difference between donor and recipient; (3) *transplant characteristics:* HLA mismatches on locus A, locus B and locus DR, first or second graft, PRA (latest and highest serum level), cold ischaemia time (h); (4) *clinical characteristics:* time for renal functional recovery after transplantation (days), patient current status (graft functioning, graft failure, death), date of graft failure or death, cause of graft failure or death, survival of graft if failed (months), survival of graft if functioning (months), renal function after 1 year (serum creatinine mg/dl), number of rejection episodes in the first year, number of steroid pulses in the first year, enhancing immunosuppressive therapy (ATG/ALG, OKT3, etc.) in the first 6 weeks, any prophylactic use of antilymphocyte globulin (ALG) in the first weeks [3, 9, 11].

Two kinds of tests were used to evaluate patient outcome after the transplantation: actuarial survival rates using error standard and Z tests to compare two or more groups, and the relative risk (of graft failure in the first year) evaluated for a single field by the odds-ratio test [1].

Results

Comparison of the two groups showed a significantly better survival in group A: 90.4% vs 79.3% in the first year ($P < 0.05$); 87.8% vs 71.1% in the second year ($P < 0.01$); 82.5% vs 64.1% in the third year ($P < 0.01$) (Fig. 2). The relative risk of graft failure in the first year (odds ratio) was also significantly different between groups A and B (0.4 vs 2.3, $P < 0.05$).

Individual, donor, transplant and clinical characteristics did not differ significantly between the two groups (Table 1). Serum creatinine after 1 year was

Table 1. Detailed results of the most significant parameters considered

	Group A – PRA < 30% (n = 174)		Group B – PRA 30–60% (n = 63)		1-year survival (%) (group B)
	No.	%	No.	%	
Sex					
Male	140	80.6	47	74.6	79.5
Female	34	19.4	16	25.4	78.6
Previous pregnancy	4	11.7	3	18.6	–
Age					
0–14 years	2	0.9	0	0.0	–
15–35 years	40	23.1	18	28.6	76.5
35–56 years	116	66.7	39	61.9	80.6
> 55 years	16	9.3	6	9.5	81.8
Dialysis duration					
0–6 months	19	11.0	9	14.3	88.2
7–24 months	64	36.8	25	39.7	78.3
> 24 months	91	52.2	29	46.0	77.4
Polytransfused					
> 5 transfusion	67	38.5	22	34.9	76.2
< 5 transfusion	107	61.5	41	65.1	81.3
HLA-A mismatches					
0	11	6.5	4	6.3	71.4
1	70	40.2	24	38.1	76.7
2	93	53.3	35	55.5	78.1
HLA-B mismatches					
0	2	1.1	0	0.0	–
1	41	23.6	20	31.7	83.3
2	131	75.3	43	68.3	77.5
HLA-DR mismatches					
0	14	8.1	6	9.5	100
1	86	49.4	32	50.8	83.1
2	74	42.5	25	39.7	68.9
Transplant number					
1st graft	168	96.3	55	87.5	82.2
2nd graft	6	3.7	8	12.5	60.0
First 6 weeks enhancement immunosuppression					
Antilymphocyte globulin	75	43.1	32	50.8	a
Plasma exchange	21	12.1	8	12.7	a
OKT3	5	2.9	3	4.8	a
Not treated	83	47.7	35	55.6	72.3

[a] 20 patients were submitted to more than one treatment

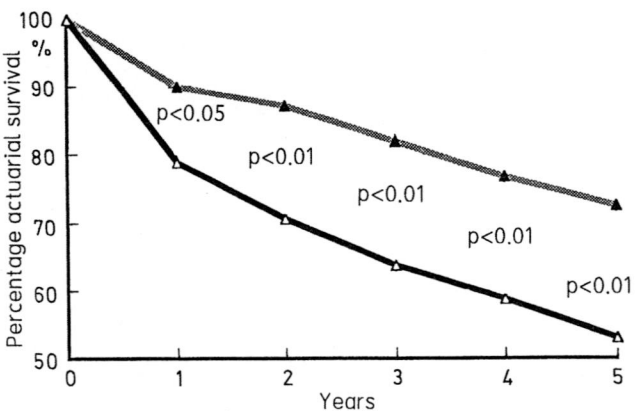

Fig. 2. Actuarial graft survival of group A (PRA < 30%, 174 patients) and group B (PRA 30–60%, 63 patients). ▲, PRA < 30%; △, PRA 30–60%

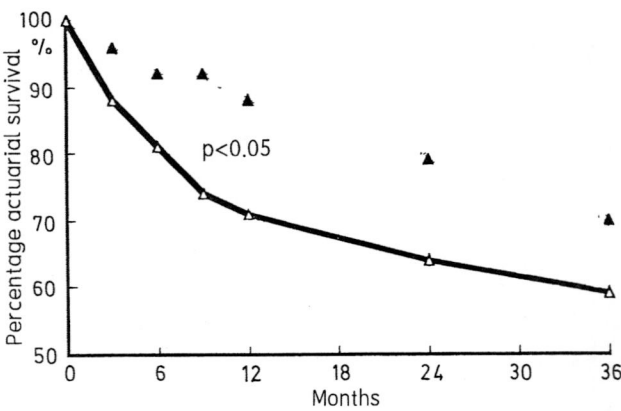

Fig. 3. Effect of the prophylactic use of antilymphocyte globulin (ALG, 28 patients) (not treated, 35 patients) on graft outcome in hyperimmunized patients (PRA 30–60%). ▲, ALG; △, not treated

1.44 ± 0.38 mg/dl in group A and 1.53 ± 0.32 mg/dl in group B, the number of rejection episodes in the first year was 0.70 ± 0.85 vs 1.17 ± 0.94 ($P < 0.001$), respectively, and the number of steroid pulses in the first year 1.27 ± 1.89 vs 2.63 ± 2.98 ($P < 0.001$).

Detailed analysis of group B suggested that some parameters may influence graft outcome:

1. *Compatibility on locus DR:* With no mismatches ($n = 6$) the actuarial survival after 3 years was still 100%; with one mismatch ($n = 32$) it was 83.1% in the first year ($P < 0.01$), 74.9% in the second year ($P < 0.001$) and 65.6% in the third year ($P < 0.001$); and with two mismatches ($n = 25$) it was 68.9%, 57.4% and 50.7% respectively (all $P < 0.001$).
2. *Primary transplant vs retransplant:* Survival for first graft ($n = 55$) was 82.2% in the first year, and 75.1% in the second year while for regrafted patients ($n = 8$) it was 60.0% and 42.9%, respectively. Relative risk for first transplant was 0.3 vs 2.9.
3. *Dialysis time:* Patients who were transplanted without dialysis or with a dialysis duration < 6 months ($n = 9$) showed a better survival (88.2% in the first year) than those with a dialysis duration of 6–24 months (78.3%) ($n = 25$) and those with a dialysis duration > 24 months (77.4%) ($n = 29$), while the difference became less significant at 3 years (74.7%, 61.9% and 62.4%, respectively). The relative risk of the group with a short dialysis duration was 0.5 vs 1.9 in the two latter groups.

Details of the most important items considered are summarized in Table 1.

The prophylactic use of immunosuppressive enhancement therapy – in this case antilymphocyte globulin (ALG) employed in the first weeks from surgery, and usually at the beginning of the second week, before the onset of a rejection crisis – improved graft outcome: 1 year survival was 84.6% in patients treated with prophylactic ALG ($n = 28$), but only 75.0% in untreated patients ($n = 35$). At 3 years, survival still differed but was less significant: 70.0% vs 59.5% in untreated patients (Fig. 3). Serum creatinine after 1 year was 1.51 ± 0.41 mg/dl in the group treated with prophylactic ALG and

1.55 ± 0.15 mg/dl in those not treated. The number of rejection episodes in the first year was 1.01 ± 0.67 for the ALG group vs 1.35 ± 1.15, respectively. Finally the number of steroid pulses in the first year was 1.40 ± 1.34 in the ALG treated patients vs 3.68 ± 3.62 ($P < 0.01$). The relative risk was 0.3 vs 2.9.

Conclusions

This study confirmed that presensitization represents a considerable problem in candidacy for renal transplantation. Based on restricted yet homogeneous case material, the data reported highlight the importance of transplanting as soon as possible. This is, perhaps, the easiest factor on which to work: prolonging dialysis time tends to make the patient more immunologically reactive owing both to repeated contact with artificial material [10] and to the likely clinical need for more transfusions – though our data do not show any significant differences in survival for polytransfused patients, in agreement with previous reports [5]. In this connection the use of erythropoietin is to be welcomed [4]. However, hyperimmunization may also be seen as evidence of a different, more pronounced, immunological reactivity towards the graft. It may thus be helpful to indicate how to manage such patients.

Our data suggest that it is with these patients that greater accuracy in the search for optimum compatibility on the DR locus seems useful, and this can only come about through coordination of transplant centres in organ or recipient exchange. In addition, this study indicates that, once the previous suggestions have been followed, another card can be played to improve the hyperimmunized patient's destiny. By using treatment such as a cycle of ALG to boost immunosuppression in the first weeks after surgery, one both improves late graft outcome and decreases the number of rejection episodes (and consequently the amount of steroids), thus achieving two goals: first, bringing the survival probability of hyperimmunized patients as close as possible to that of non-immunized patients, and second, probably avoiding more infection and steroid-induced complications.

Acknowledgements. This study was supported in part by the Dott. Carlo Fornasini Foundation, Bologna.

References

1. Appleton DR (1988) Analysis of data in nephrology I. Choosing the correct statistical test: dichotomous variables. Nephrol Dial Transplant 3: 91–94
2. Claas FHJ, de Waal LP, Beelen J, Reekers P, Berg-Loonen PVD, de Gast E, D'Amaro J, Persijn GG, Zantvoort F, van Rood JJ (1990) Transplantation of highly sensitized patients on the basis of acceptable HLA-A and B mismatches. In: Terasaki P (ed) Clinical transplant 1989. UCLA Tissue Typing Laboratory, Los Angeles, pp 185–190
3. Gore SM (1983) Graft survival after renal transplantation: agenda for analysis. Kidney Int 24: 516–525
4. Grimm PC, Sinai Trieman L, Sekiya NM (1990) Effect of recombinant human erythropoietin on HLA sensitization and cell mediated immunity. Kidney Int 38: 12–15
5. Iwachi Y, Cecka JM, Terasaki PI (1989) The transfusion effect. In: Terasaki P (ed) Clinical Transplant 1988. UCLA Tissue Typing Laboratory, Los Angeles, pp 283–292
6. Lundgren G, Groth CG, Albrechtsen D (1986) HLA-matching and pretransplant blood transfusion in cadaveric renal transplantation – a changing picture with cyclosporine. Lancet II: 66–69
7. Opelz G (1987) Improved kidney graft survival in non-transfused recipients. Transplant Proc 19: 149–152
8. Rankin GW, Wang X, Terasaki P (1991) Sensitization to kidney transplant. In: Terasaki P (ed), Clinical Transplant 1990. UCLA Tissue Typing Laboratory, Los Angeles, pp 417–424
9. Sanfilippo F, Vaughn WK, LeFor WM, Spees EK (1986) Multivariate analysis of risk factors in cadaver donor kidney transplantation. Transplantation 42: 28–34
10. Stefoni S, Nanni Costa A, Buscaroli A, Colì L, Feliciangeli G, Mosconi G, Scolari MP, Iannelli S, Borgnino LC, Bonomini V (1991) Cellular immunology in regular dialysis: a biological model for biocompatibility evaluation. Nephrol Dial Transplant 6 [Suppl 2]: 4–9
11. Tufveson G, Geerlings W, Brunner FP, Brynger H, Dykes SR, Ehrich JHH, Fassbinder W, Rizzoni G, Selwood NH, Wing AJ (1990) Combined report on regular dialysis and transplantation in Europe, XIX, 1988. Nephrol Dial Transplant 4 [Suppl 2]: 5–32

Transplant Int (1992) 5 [Suppl 1]: S 58–S 59

TRANSPLANT
International
© Springer-Verlag 1992

Cyclosporin A (CsA) and azathioprine (AZA) combination in renal allografts with CsA nephrotoxicity

A. M. Castelao, J. M. Griño, I. Sabate, D. Seron, E. Andres, S. Gilvernet, J. Bover, C. Gonzalez, and J. Alsina

Nephrology Department, Hospital de Bellvitge Princeps d' Espanya, University of Barcelona, Barcelona, Spain

Cyclosporin A (CsA) is a potent immunosuppressive drug whose effect is well known in the organ transplantation field. Treatment with CsA reduces the incidence of rejection and improves graft survival after renal transplantation (RT). However, to set against the clear advantages of CsA, a most important problem is nephrotoxicity [1, 3]. Scientists are therefore seeking new non-nephrotoxic Cs derivatives, but the search has not yet borne fruit.

Teams working in organ transplantation attempt to avoid nephrotoxicity by switching to conventional treatment with azathioprine (AZA), starting 1, 3 or 6 months after transplantation [8, 11]. Conversion from CsA to AZA has not always been successful due to the high incidence of rejection [4]. AZA has also been started immediately after transplantation in combination with CsA at low doses [5], and in some instances no CsA is administered when oliguric acute tubular necrosis is present [10].

In a previous report [2], we presented the short-term results of the treatment with a CsA–AZA combination, reducing the CsA dose and giving a moderate dose of AZA in 21 transplanted patients not achieving acceptable graft function. In the present study we analysed the long-term results in a group of patients whose kidney biopsy examination results were compatible with CsA nephrotoxicity.

Key words: Renal transplantation – Nephrotoxicity – Cyclosporin toxicity

Material and methods

Between March 1984 and March 1990, 377 patients who had received a RT in our hospital were treated with CsA–prednisone (PNS) or CsA–antilymphocyte globulin–PNS (CsA–ALG–PNS). The first group of patients received oral CsA 14 mg/kg per day,

Offprint requests to: Dr. A. M. Castelao. Nephrology Department, Hospital de Bellvitge, C/ Feixa Llarga s/n. 08907, Hospitalet Llobregat, Barcelona, Spain

tapered according to whole blood levels (polyclonal RIA, $n = 300$–800 ng/ml) and PNS 0.25 mg/kg per day. The second group of patients received oral CsA 8 mg/kg per day, tapered according to blood levels, a maximum of six alternate-day doses of 10 mg/kg per day horse ALG, or less if CsA levels were higher than 400 ng/ml, and PNS 0.25 mg/kg per day. Acute rejection (AR) episodes were treated in the first group with three boluses of endovenous methyl-PNS, 0.5 g/day, and with oral PNS, 3 mg/kg per day tapered to 1 mg/kg per day in 1 week and to 0.25 mg/kg per day in 1 month, in the second group.

In 44 of these 377 patients (11.6%), graft function did not achieve an optimal level, with plasma creatinine remaining over 250 µmol/l in a period of 1 to 24 months after RT, in spite of normal CsA blood levels. Because of this, we decreased the CsA dose and added azathioprine (1.01 ± 0.18 mg/kg per day). All the patients received oral co-trimoxazole (one tablet 480 mg every 12 h) when AZA was started, maintaining this treatment during a 3 month period.

Renal percutaneous biopsies were examined by optic, electronic and immunofluorescence microscopy, according to usual techniques. Statistical analyses were performed using the Wilcoxon test.

Results

We studied 44 patients, 28 male and 26 female, mean age 34 ± 12 years. All but one received a cadaver kidney, and two patients underwent a second transplantation. There were no significant differences in age, cold and warm ischaemia time or HLA matching (AB matches 1.5 ± 1.3, DR matches 1.2 ± 0.5) with respect to a control group of 88 randomly selected patients treated with CsA in the same period.

Five patients presented with AR before the drug combination treatment. The general incidence of AR was 34% with the CsA–PNS treatment protocol and 16% with the CsA–ALG–PNS treatment protocol. Biopsy-proven chronic rejection occurred in 16 patients and recurrent or transplant glomerulopathies in another five. *In this study we consider the remaining* **23 patients,** in whom the results of renal biopsy examination were compatible with CsA nephrotoxicity. In all of them we reduced the CsA dose and started AZA (1.01 mg/kg per day), 10.2 ± 16 months after RT.

Table 1. CsA blood levels[a] before and after CsA–AZA combination treatment

	Blood level (ng/ml ± SD)	P value
Before AZA association	396 ± 169	
After 6 months	187 ± 67	0.0001
After 12 months	187 ± 75	0.0001
After 24 months	212 ± 76	0.001
After 36 months	140 ± 48	0.0005

[a] polyclonal RIA, n = 300–800 ng/ml

Table 2. CsA dose before and after CsA–AZA combination treatment

	CsA dose (mg/kg per day ± SD)	P value
Before AZA association	5.1 ± 1.5	
After 6 months	2.7 ± 0.9	0.001
After 12 months	2.9 ± 1.2	0.0005
After 24 months	2.5 ± 1.03	0.0005
After 36 months	2.7 ± 1.05	0.001

Table 3. Plasma creatinine (μmol/l) before and after CsA–AZA combination treatment

	Plasma creatinine (μmol/l ± SD)	P value
Before AZA association	468 ± 228	
After 6 months	289 ± 184	0.012
After 12 months	236 ± 297	0.001
After 24 months	211 ± 67	0.0001
After 36 months	231 ± 81	0.008

CsA blood levels before, and at 6, 12, 24 and 36 months after, the combination treatment are shown in Table 1. CsA doses and plasma creatinine are shown in Tables 2 and 3. AR episodes after combination treatment were seen in two patients, one of whom lost the graft. No opportunistic viral, bacterial or other infections were observed in these patients. The number of urinary infection episodes decreased after the combination treatment (before 1.8 ± 1.43, after 1 ± 1.3).

In three patients we stopped AZA due to leucopenia, thrombopenia and a facial epithelioma 6 to 24 months after the combination treatment. Another two patients abandoned AZA treatment. After a 3-year follow-up, two out of the 24 patients (8.3%) had lost their graft due to AR and non-compliance. Five out of the 12 patients with a follow-up period of more than 4 years lost the graft due to chronic rejection (n = 4) and transplant glomerulopathy (n = 1). The remaining 17 patients have functioning grafts 40 ± 10 months after RT with a mean plasma creatinine of 231 ± 81 μmol/l after 34 ± 13 months of combination treatment.

Discussion

The problem of CsA nephrotoxicity has been under discussion for many years. It is not clear whether conversion from CsA to AZA due to poor renal function improves renal allograft outcome [4]. Routine conversion is not always advisable due to the high risk of rejection and loss of graft function.

In order to avoid CsA nephrotoxicity some authors [6, 7, 9] have reported introducing varions induction treatments, such as triple therapy including CsA, AZA and PNS. In our experience the CsA–AZA–PNS combination has given good results, minimizing CsA nephrotoxicity and preserving long-term renal function. On the other hand infections or neoplasms have been suggested as very frequent complications associated with triple immunosuppression. In our patients urinary infections decreased after combination treatment, and other opportunistic infections were not present. Only one patient suffered a facial epithelioma, with a successful outcome after skin surgery and AZA withdrawal.

In conclusion we think that the CsA–AZA–PNS association is a simple alternative that, applied in an individualized and selective fashion, can reduce CsA nephrotoxicity, allowing an improvement in graft function, without increasing the risk of rejection or opportunistic infections.

References

1. Canafax DM, Shuterland DER, Ascher NL, Simmons RL, Najarian JS (1983) Cyclosporine nephrotoxicity in renal allograft recipients: conversion to azathioprine to improve renal function. Transplant Proc 15 [Suppl 1]: 2874–2877
2. Castelao AM, Griño JM, Sabaté I, Gilvernet S, Andrés E, Sabater R, Alsina J (1989) Cyclospirin A (CsA) and azathioprine (AZA) overlap in renal allografts with impaired renal function. Transplant Proc 21: 1540–1541
3. Flechner SM, Van Buren CT, Kerman R, Kahan BD (1983) The effect of conversion from cyclosporine to azathioprine immunosuppression for intractable nephrotoxicity. Transplant Proc 15 [Suppl 1]: 2869–2873
4. Hoistma AJ, Van Lier HJJ, Wetzels JFM, Berden JHM (1987) Cyclosporin treatment with conversion after three months versus conventional immunosuppression in renal allograft recipients. Lancet I: 584–586
5. Illner WD, Land W, Habersetzer R et al. (1985) Cyclosporin in combination with azathioprine and steroid in cadaveric renal transplantation. Transplant Proc 17: 1181–1184
6. Jones RM, Murie JA, Allen RD, Ting A, Morris PJ (1989) Triple therapy in cadaver renal transplantation. Br J Surg 75: 4–8
7. Landsberg DN, Rae A, Chiu A, Werb R, Taylor P, Chan-Yan C, Manson AD (1989) The use of triple therapy to minimize cyclosporin nephrotoxicity in renal transplantation. Transplant Proc 21: 1550–1551
8. Morris PJ, Chapman JR, Allen RD, Thompson JF (1987) Cyclosporin conversion versus conventional immunosuppression: long-term follow-up and histological evaluation. Lancet I: 586–590
9. Restifo AC, Petrei JJB, Rigby RJ, Hardie IR, Jacob CK, Russ GR, Mathew (1989) A comparison of triple with double therapy (cyclosporin-azathioprine) in low-risk, first cadaveric renal allograft recipients. Transplant Proc 21: 1604–1605
10. Rocher LL, Milford EL, Kirkman RL, Carpenter CB, Strom TB, Tilney NL (1984) Conversion from cyclosporine to azathioprine in renal allograft recipients. Transplantation 38: 669–674
11. Vanrenterghem Y, Waer M, Michielsen P (1985) A controlled trial of one versus three months cyclosporin and conversion to azathioprine in renal transplantation. Transplant Proc 17: 1162–1163

Transplant Int (1992) 5 [Suppl 1]: S 60–S 62

TRANSPLANT
International
© Springer-Verlag 1992

Verapamil (VP) improves the outcome after renal transplantation (CRT)

I. Dawidson, C. Lu, B. Palmer, P. Peters, P. Rooth, R. Risser, A. Sagalowsky, and Z. Sandor

U. T. Southwestern Med. Ctr. and Parkland Hospital, Dallas, Texas, USA

Calcium antagonists (CATs) have a role in the management of certain types of renal insufficiency [6, 15]. These include prophylaxis against post-transplant-associated acute renal failure and cyclosporine A (CsA)-induced renal dysfunction. For the transplanted kidney, CATs may be beneficial in several settings. First, a CAT during organ procurement protects the kidney during ischemic periods [9]. Second, CATs given perioperatively protect the kidney during reperfusion and early after transplantation [2]. Third, CATs also offer protection against CsA nephrotoxicity [1].

Key words: Renal transplantation – Verapamil

Methods

Two prospective randomized clinical studies [1, 2] and one retrospective study were performed [10]. Immunosuppression included 375 mg methylprednisolone on day 1, tapered to 20 mg/day by day 10. Azathioprine, initially 100 mg on day 1 decreased to 25 mg/day for 5 days. Antilymphocyte globulin (14 mg/kg) overlapped with CsA on day 6 (7 mg/kg) and day 7 (12 mg/kg). Verapamil (VP) was initiated on day 3 (study 1), or given into the renal artery (study 2) and continued for 14 days as an oral dose of 120 mg twice daily. Doppler ultrasonography was used to determine blood flow velocities in the renal subcapsular parenchyma. Kidney function was assessed from serum creatinine and glomerular filtration rate (GFR) on days 1 and 7, using subcutaneous ^{125}I-iothalamate [5].

Results

Graft survival

Patients in study 2 have been followed for a mean of 18 months with a current GS for VP patients of 90% (27/30), greater than that for the control patients (68%,

(18/29) ($P < 0.01$). These differences were also confirmed in an actuarial graft survival analysis for all patients ($P < 0.0237$) (Fig. 1). The greatest benefits seem to occur with repeat transplants where only one of ten VP treated patiens lost the graft early. In contrast, three of eight control kidneys were still functioning at 1 year ($P < 0.05$). Since July 1990, all CRT recipients at our transplant center have been receiving perioperative treatment with VP. Figure 1 also includes the actuarial survival curve (as of 16 September 1991) for this group of patients ($n = 53$). The tick marks on the lines indicate the follow-up time for each patient with a surviving graft. The 89% actuarial 1-year kidney graft survival estimate in these patients is similar to the 93% rate among the study 2 patients randomized to VP treatment. Eight simultaneous kidney/pancreas transplants were included in this analysis of 53 CRT recipients.

In the retrospective study in which 17 patients received a CAT for treatment of hypertension, graft survival at one year was 93% versus 78% for 23 patients who did not receive a CAT [10].

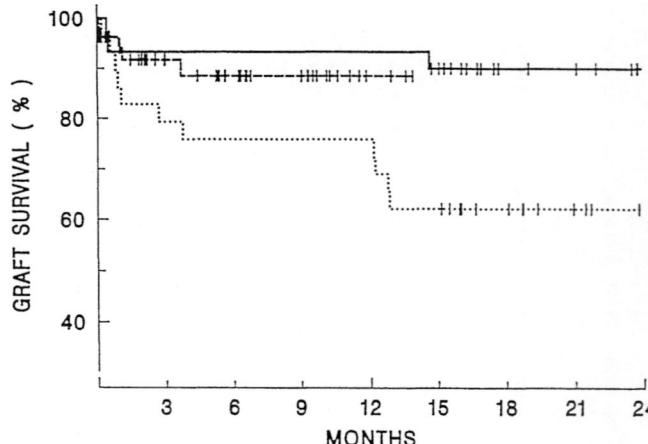

Fig. 1. Actuarial graft survival was significantly improved in 30 patients treated with verapamil *(solid line)* compared with 29 control recipients *(dotted line)* ($P < 0.01$). Currently, 53 kidney recipients receiving perioperative verapamil have an 89% actuarial graft survival *(interrupted line)*

Offprint requests to: I. Davidson, U. T. Southwestern Med. Ctr. and Parkland Hospital, 5323 Harry Hines Blvd. Dallas, Texas, 75235 USA

Rejection episodes

In study 1 of 40 patients, only 3 of 22 patients randomized to VP were treated for a rejection episode within 1 month of transplantation. This was in sharp contrast to 10 of 18 of the control patients treated for rejection ($P < 0.01$) [1]. In the retrospective study, CAT-treated patients had significantly fewer (35 %) first rejection episodes during the 1 year follow-up, in contrast to 83 % in patients who did not receive a CAT ($P < 0.01$) [10].

Rejection episodes

In study 1 of 40 patients, only 3 of 22 patients randomized to VP were treated for a rejection episode within 1 month of transplantation. This was in sharp contrast to 10 of 18 of the control patients treated for rejection ($P < 0.01$) [1]. In the retrospective study, CAT-treated patients had significantly fewer (35 %) first rejection episodes during the 1 year follow-up, in contrast to 83 % in patients who did not receive a CAT ($P < 0.01$) [10].

CsA blood levels and CATs

CsA blood levels were about two times higher in patients reveiving VP compared with controls in both studies [1, 2].

CATs and protection from ischemia

When VP was given intra-arterially during surgery (study 2), serum creatinine values on days 1 and 2 after transplantation were significantly lower compared with control patients. With VP serum creatinine fell by 2.7 mg % between days 1 and 2 in contrast to 1.3 mg % for the control patients. On the second day after transplantation creatinine values were 7.4 and 5.6 mg % for control and VP patients, respectively ($P < 0.01$) [2]. By day 7, the majority of patients (77 %) receiving VP had serum creatinine values below 2.0 mg % versus only 26 % of control patients ($P < 0.01$). Accordingly, on day one GFR was 35 and 19 ml/min for VP and control patients, respectively. By day 7, GFR had increased to 49 and 28 ml/min for VP and control patients ($P < 0.01$).

CATs and CsA nephrotoxicity

Despite the higher CsA blood levels during VP treatment (study 1), serum creatinine levels at 1 week were lower with VP (1.08 ± 0.41 mg %) than those of control patients (1.46 ± 0.46 mg %) ($P < 0.008$). Also the increase in GFR from day 1 to day 7 was greater with VP (32 ± 13 ml/min) compared with 18 ± 13 ml/min in control patients ($P < 0.002$) [1].

Renal blood flow and CATs

CsA-induced blood flow inhibition in animals [13, 14] was later confirmed in CRT recipients where mean diastolic blood flow velocity in ten patients decreased from 10 to 3 cm/s. Despite continued CsA administration, blood flow returned to pre-CsA levels within 3–4 days [14]. Pretreatment with VP prevented this fall in renal blood flow [1]. When VP was given intra-arterially, blood flow was significantly better on the first postoperative day [2]. Only 8 % (2/25) of the VP patients had parenchymal blood flow velocity less than 8 cm/s versus 54 % of the no-CAT patients ($P < 0.01$).

Discussion

These clinical studies demonstrate several significant benefits from perioperative use of VP in CRTs. Most importantly, graft survival and kidney function were improved. This is further supported by the fact that these results have been corroborated by a current 96 % kidney graft survival in CRT recipients with VP given perioperatively (unpublished data). The beneficial effects from CATs may be due to several actions of CATs occurring separately or in combination.

The decreased incidence of acute rejection episodes may be related to the blockage of cellular calcium influx which inhibits lymphocyte activation and macrophage proliferation, both in animal and human in vitro systems [4, 16]. At least part of the beneficial effect of VP on transplant outcome may be due to the increased CsA immunosuppressive effect without accompanying nephrotoxicity because of the increased blood CsA level. Although CATs have complex and incompletely understood interactions with CsA metabolism, both diltiazem and VP compete with CsA for the cytochrome P-450 pathway [9, 12]. In contrast to these two CATs, the dihydropyridine CAT nifedipine does not increase CsA blood concentration [3].

Previously, we demonstrated by in vivo fluorescence microscopy in mice that VP prevents CsA-induced decrease in renal blood flow [13, 14]. Subsequently, these data were confirmed in the clinical setting in CRT recipients [1, 2]. The relative importance of cytoprotection from CATs and their preferential vasodilatation of the afferent arterioles is hard to distinguish. Experimental and clinical data suggest that both mechanisms contribute.

The present studies strongly support routine perioperative use of CATs in CRTs to improve renal function and graft survival. Although VP produces higher CsA blood levels, acute nephrotoxicity is less common and CsA doses are not empirically lowered. Better immunosuppression from increased CsA levels without toxicity probably plays a role in the improved results. Some investigators have steadily reduced the CsA dose to minimize cost [8]. Routine decreases in CsA dose, based on CsA blood levels, may have played a role in the lack of benefits of a CAT in other studies [11]. Based on the results in our two clinical studies the argument could be made not to reduce the CsA dose, but rather accept higher CsA blood levels without nephrotoxicity and gain from increased immunosuppression. Better renal function and graft survival vastly outweigh the small monetary gain from decreased CsA dosing.

In summary, VP restores and maintains renal blood flow and minimizes renal injury associated with organ procurement and cold ischemia. The randomized clinical studies confirm our previous animal research that VP prevents CsA-associated deterioration of renal blood flow. VP-treated patients have improved renal blood flow and improved renal function, despite elevated CsA blood levels. VP given intraoperatively, under adequate blood volume expansion, into the renal artery also reduces the need for postoperative hemodialysis. VP-treated patients have fewer rejection episodes, and most importantly VP is associated with improved graft survival.

The beneficial effect of VP on renal transplant outcome may be related to cytoprotection from ischemia, the preferential vasodilatation of the preglomerular arterioles, elevated blood CsA levels and inherent immunosuppressive properties.

References

1. Dawidson I, Rooth P, Fry W, Sandor Z, Willms C, Coorpender L, Alway C, Reisch J (1989) Prevention of acute cyclosporine-induced renal blood flow inhibition and improved immunosuppression with verapamil. Transplantation 48: 575–580
2. Dawidson I, Rooth P, Lu C, Sagalowsky A, Diller K, Palmer B, Peters P, Risser R, Sandor Z, Seney F (1991) Verapamil improves the outcome after cadaver renal transplantation. JASN (in press)
3. Dy G, Raja R, Mendez M (1991) The clinical and biochemical effect of calcium channel blockers (CCB) in organ transplantation recipients (TR) on cyclosporine (CsA). Transplant Proc (in press)
4. Fry WR, Dawidson I, Alway CC, Rooth P (1988) Cyclosporine A induces decreased blood flow in cadaveric kidney transplant. Transplant Proc 20: 222
5. Israelit A, Long D, White M, Hull A (1973) Measurement of glomerular filtration rate utilizing a single subcutaneous injection of ^{125}I-iothalamate. Kidney Int 4: 346
6. Loutzenhiser R, Epstein M (1990) The renal hemodynamic effects of calcium antagonists. In: Epstein M (ed) Calcium antagonists and the kidney. Hanley & Belfus, Philadelphia, pp 33–73
7. McMillen MA, Lewis T, Jaffe B, Wait R (1985) Verapamil inhibition of lymphocyte proliferation and function in vitro. J Surg Res 39: 76–80
8. Neumayer H, Wagner K (1986) Diltiazem and economic use of cyclosporine. Lancet I: 523
9. Neumayer HH, Wagner K (1987) Prevention of delayed graft function in cadaver kidney transplant by diltiazem: outcome of two prospective, randomized clinical trials. J Cardiovasc Pharacol 10: 170–177
10. Palmer B, Dawidson I, Sagalowsky A, Sandor Z, Lu C (1991) Calcium channel blockers improve the outcome of cadaveric renal transplantation. Transplantation (in press)
11. Prisch JD, Voss BJ, D'Alessandro AM, et al (1990) A controlled, double-blind, randomized trial of verapamil in cyclosporine-treated cadaver renal transplant patients. Abstract presented at the American Society of Transplant Physicians, 9th Annual Meeting, Chicago, May 29–30
12. Renton KW (1985) Inhibition of hepatic microsomal drug metabolism by the calcium channel blockers diltiazem and verapamil. Biochem Pharmacol 34: 2549–2553
13. Rooth P, Dawidson I, Diller K, Taljedal IB (1988) Protection against cyclosporine-induced impairment of renal microcirculation by verapamil in mice. Transplantation 45: 433–437
14. Rooth P, Dawidson I, Clothier N, Diller K (1988) In vivo fluorescence microscopy of kidney subcapsular blood flow in mice; effects of cyclosporine A (CsA), Nva^2) – Cyclosporine (CsG) and isradipine, a new calcium antagonist. Transplantation 46: 566
15. Schrier RW, Arnold ED, Van Putten V, Burke TJ (1987) Cellular calcium in ischemic acute renal failure: role of calcium entry blocker. Kidney Int 32: 313–321
16. Weir MR, Peppler R, Comolka D, Handwerger BS (1988) Additive effects of cyclosporine and verapamil on the inhibition of activation and function of human peripheral blood mononuclear cells. Transplant Proc 20: 240–244

Transplant Int (1992) 5 [Suppl 1]: S 63–S 64

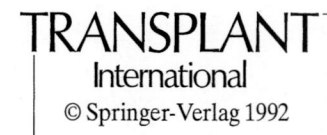
TRANSPLANT
International
© Springer-Verlag 1992

DTPA renal scan assessment of renal allograft dysfunction in rats

D. Dickerson, B. Adams, G. Engelbrecht, G. Boltman, R. Hickman, and D. Kahn

Departments of Surgery and Nuclear Medicine, University of Cape Town and Groote Schuur Hospital, Cape Town, South Africa

The precise cause of allograft dysfunction after renal transplantation often cannot be established by non-invasive means. In clinical practice, radionuclide scans form an integral part of the clinician's armamentarium in the assessment of these patients [1, 2]. Unfortunately, in the clinical setting more than one pathological process may be responsible for the impaired function, making it difficult to correlate the scan appearances with the pathology. In this study in rats we compared the renal DTPA scan appearances of the various pathological processes which may cause renal allograft dysfunction in the immediate post-transplant period.

Key words: Renal transplantation in rats – Kidney dysfunction in rats – DTPA renal scan

Methods

Male Long Evans rats weighing 300–350 g were anaesthetized with ketamine and were assigned to the treatment groups shown below. Animals were subjected to renal transplantation using standard microsurgical techniques to simulate acute rejection. For acute tubular necrosis (ATN) the kidney was rendered ischaemic by clamping the renal artery for 40 min. For cyclosporine toxicity the animals were given a single 10 mg/kg intravenous injection of cyclosporine. Ureteric obstruction and a urine leak involved ligation and division of the ureter, respectively.

The treatment groups were as follows:

Group 1 – Orthotopic transplantation of the left kidney. Normal right kidney ($n = 4$).

Group 2 – Ischaemic injury of the right kidney. Normal left kidney ($n = 4$).

Group 3 – Orthotopic transplantation of the left kidney. Ischaemic injury of the right kidney ($n = 4$).

Group 4 – Cyclosporine toxicity ($n = 4$).

Group 5 – Ureteric obstruction ($n = 2$).

Group 6 – Urine leak ($n = 2$).

Offprint requests to: Dr. D. Kahn, Department of Surgery, Medical School, University of Cape Town, Observatory 7925, Cape Town, South Africa

Renal DTPA scans were performed serially during the first postoperative week. Dynamic acquisitions were obtained on a gamma camera after the intravenous administration of 80–100 MBq of Tc-99m diethylylene triamine pentaacetic acid (DTPA). The renograms were reviewed and the perfusion and function of the kidneys assessed, as indicated by the uptake of the radionuclide and the clearance of the radionuclide, respectively.

Results

The initial renal DTPA scans of the transplanted left kidneys in group 1 showed decreased perfusion and decreased or impaired function when compared with the normal right kidney. Subsequent scans showed further deterioration in the perfusion and function of the left kidney. In group 2 the scans of the ischaemically injured right kidneys demonstrated normal perfusion but impaired function. In the subsequent renograms the perfusion and function reverted to normal. The renal DTPA scans of the animals in group 3, which had a transplanted left kidney and an ischaemically injured right kidney, confirmed the above findings.

The renographic appearances of the kidneys with cyclosporine toxicity in group 4 demonstrated decreased perfusion and impaired function initially. On subsequent scans the perfusion and function were normal. In group 5 the kidneys with ureteric obstruction demonstrated decreased perfusion and impaired function on the initial and subseqeunt renal DTPA scans. The perfusion and function of the kidneys with the urine leak in group 6 were normal according to the DTPA scan. However, extravasation of DTPA was demonstrated.

The renographic findings are summarized in Table 1.

Discussion

The common causes of allograft dysfunction after renal transplantation include acute rejection, ATN, cyclosporine toxicity, and technical complications such as urine leak and ureteric obstruction. Often, invasive methods,

Table 1. Summary of the renal DTPA scan appearances for acute rejection, ATN, Cyclosporine toxicity, ureteric obstruction and urine leak

	Initial scan		Subsequent scan	
	Perfusion	Function	Perfusion	Function
Acute rejection	↓	↓	↓↓	↓↓
ATN	N	↓	N	N
Cyclosporine toxicity	↓	↓	N	N
Urine leak	N	N extravasation	N	N
Ureteric obstruction	↓	↓	↓	↓

N, normal

such as a renal biopsy or angiography, are required to determine the precise cause of the abnormal renal function. The use of radionuclide scans after renal transplantation in patients has been documented previously [1]. Unfortunately, because of the overlap of the various pathological processess which can affect the graft after transplantation, it is difficult to determine the exact scan appearance of the individual pathology so that clinical decisions after renal transplantation are almost never based entirely upon the renal scan appearance. In this study, we created each pathological process which could cause renal dysfunction after renal transplantation and investigated the renal DTPA scan appearances.

In the normal kidney there was rapid uptake of the radionuclide, representing perfusion of the kidney. This was followed by rapid clearance of the radionuclide, representing handling by glomerular filtration and the excretory function of the kidney. Non-functioning kidneys or segmental infarctions did not take up the DTPA and were visualized on the scan as cold lesions.

As demonstrated in this study, the renal scan findings in ATN were good perfusion and poor function with a tendency to revert to normality in subsequent scans. In acute rejection the renal scan showed poor perfusion and poor function which continued to deteriorate in later scans. The initial renal scan appearances of cyclosporine toxicity were similar to acute rejection, but with cyclosporine toxicity there was a trend towards improvement in subsequent scans. Extravasation of contrast on renal scan was indicative of a urine leak. Ureteric obstruction had similar renographic appearances to acute rejection. In the clinical situation an ultrasound would easily distinguish between these two.

We believe that the DTPA renal scan, especially when used serially, is a useful non-invasive investigation in the assessment of allograft dysfunction after renal transplantation. When used in combination with the clinical findings and simple tests, such as ultrasound, the cause of the impaired function can be determined without having to resort to invasive investigations such as a renal biopsy.

References

1. Dubovsky EV, Russell CD (1988) Radionuclide evaluation of renal transplants. Semin Nucl Med 18: 181–198
2. Rutland MD (1985) A comprehensive analysis of renal DTPA studies. 2. Renal transplant evaluation. Nucl Med Commun 6: 21–30

Transplant Int (1992) 5 [Suppl 1]: S 65–S 66

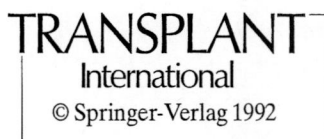

TRANSPLANT
International
© Springer-Verlag 1992

Renal retransplantation in Switzerland: poor HLA matching of first and subsequent allografts does not appear to affect overal graft survival

T. Etienne, C. Goumaz, P. Ruedin, and M. Jeannet

National Reference Laboratory for Histocompatibility, Renal Transplantation Study Group, Swiss Transplant Foundation

Abstract. In Switzerland graft survival after primary renal transplantation can be considered as satisfactory, although our current policy does not favour HLA compatibility except for acute rejectors or sensitized patients. This low level of HLA matching could result in increased sensitization and affect subsequent graft survival. A total of 318 non-primary renal transplants were performed in 293 recipients during the period 1981–1990. Of these, 271 were second transplants, 40 were third transplants and seven were fourth or fifth transplants. Survival rates at 1, 2 and 5 years were 75 %, 68 % and 60 % for second grafts, and 72 %, 60 % and 54 % for third grafts, respectively. Results after multiple grafts were poor, but our experience was limited. The number of sensitized patients (peak PRA > 50 %) awaiting retransplantation slightly increased (51 to 69), but decreased as a proportion (72 % to 66 %). Our policy of relying only marginally on HLA compatibility does not appear to have affected our results adversely.

Key words: Renal retransplantation – Sensitization – HLA compatibility – Organ sharing

In Switzerland graft survival after renal transplantation can be considered as satisfactory (Fig. 1), although our current policy does not favour optimal HLA compatibility except for acute rejectors (< 6 months) and sensitized patients (PRA > 50 %) to whom well-matched kidneys are allocated in priority. Conceivably, this low level of HLA matching (22 % none or one, 41 % two, and 37 % three or four HLA B, DR mismatches, for first transplants) may result in increased sensitization and affect subsequent graft survival. This prompted us to review our data.

Offprint requests to: T. Etienne M.D., Hopital Cantonal Universitaire, 1211 Geneva 4, Switzerland

Materials and methods

A total of 318 non-primary renal transplants were performed in 293 recipients during the period 1981–1990. Of these, 271 were second transplants, 40 were third transplants and seven were fourth and fifth transplants. Among these retransplanted patients, the proportion of sensitized (peak PRA 50–80 %) and highly sensitized (peak PRA > 80 %) patients was 19 % and 29 %, respectively. In cyclosporine-treated patients the proportion of HLA B, DR matching for retransplants was as follows: no mismatches 4.5 %; one, 33 %; two, 38 %; three, 20.5 %; and four 4 %.

Immunosuppressive protocols varied slightly between different centres, and included cyclosporine since approximately 1983, so that 80 % of patients overall were treated with this drug.

Results

Overall second graft survival rates were 75 %, 68 % and 60 % at 1, 2 and 5 years (Fig. 1). The introduction of cyclosporine had a positive impact on second graft survival rates: the 1-, 2- and 5-year survival rates were 80 %, 76 % and 64 % with cyclosporine and 57 %, 48 % and 43 % without cyclosporine. Overall third graft survival rates were 72 %, 60 % and 54 % at 1, 2 and 5 years. In the group of patients who had multiple grafts (four fourth grafts and three fifth grafts), only one patient in each subgroup still had a functioning graft at 1 and 2 years. The other multiple grafts failed within 6 months.

The relatively small number of patients reported in this series did not allow any statistical analysis of the effect of HLA matching. Nevertheless, a trend toward an HLA correlation was gradually emerging, at least for the no-mismatch group: when HLA B, DR antigens were analysed, second grafts with no mismatches had a survival rate of 80 % at 5 years in contrast to a 50 % to 70 % rate with one to four mismatches (in cyclosporine-treated patients).

Overall, the number of sensitized patients (peak PRA > 50 %) awaiting transplantation remained stable and decreased as a proportion (42 % to 32 %) [5]. Considering only patients awaiting retransplantation, we noted a

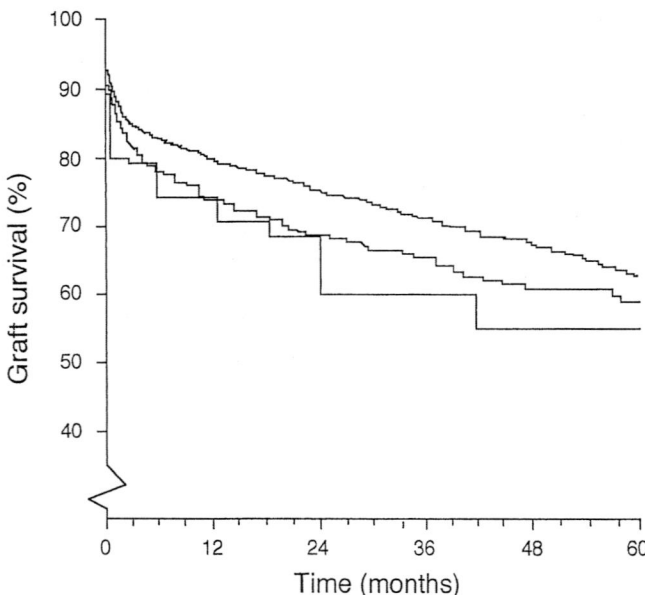

Fig. 1. Actuarial graft survival rates. *Top,* first graft (*n* = 1526); *centre,* second graft (*n* = 271); *bottom,* third graft (*n* = 40)

moderate increase in the number of sensitized candidates: 51 in 1981 and 69 in 1990. However, the proportion of sensitized patients waiting for retransplantation slightly decreased during the period studied (72% to 66%). In the subgroup of highly sensitized patients (peak PRA 80%) this trend was even more obvious (57% to 44%).

Discussion

Despite poor HLA matching of first and subsequent allografts, our regraft survival rates compare favourably with those published by other centres during the same decade [3, 4]. In cyclosporine-treated patients, our overall second graft survival rate was similar to that reported in a European study for one or two HLA A, B, DR mismatches (80% and 76% vs. 80% and 73%, 1- and 2-year graft survival rates). Our overall third graft survival rate is also similar or better than that reported by the same groups [3, 7]. Our experience with fourth and fifth grafts is limited, but not encouraging; however, no definitive conclusion can be drawn. As expected cyclosporine had a positive impact on regraft survival rates at least for second transplants. Our overall patient survival rate is in accordance with that reported elsewhere [1].

A significant influence of HLA matching on graft outcome could not be unequivocally demonstrated in the retransplanted population, although a trend towards an HLA correlation was progressively emerging at least for full matches.

Considering the low level of HLA compatibility achieved for primary grafts, an increased rate of sensitization following rejection of these kidneys could conceivably occur. The impact of HLA matching on sensitization after a failed transplant is still a matter of debate in the literature [2, 6]. Nevertheless, we noted only a modest increase in the number of sensitized and highly sensitized patients awaiting retransplantation. The proportion of sensitized patients even decreased, although it remained relatively high. This relatively high percentage of sensitized candidates is of concern and should be closely monitored. It may partially reflect pretransplant sensitization by blood transfusions in pregnancy (20–30% of patients listed for primary transplantation were sensitized (peak PRA > 50%)).

Our current policy does not favour kidney sharing and HLA compatibility. Nevertheless, our graft survival rates after retransplantation can be considered as good. However, it is our opinion that these data do not provide any argument against an HLA matching effect. We would rather conclude that careful perioperative management of graft recipients and close follow-up of patients may have contributed to these results.

Acknowledgements. We would like to thank Dr. G. Opelz for contributing to the analysis of some of the Swiss data reported here.

References

1. Iwaki Y, Cho RY, Terasaki PI (1987) Regrafts. In: Terasaki P (ed) Clinical transplants. UCLA Tissue Typing Laboratory, Los Angeles, pp 399–407
2. Matas AJ, Frey DJ, Gillingham KJ, Noreen HJ, Reinsmoen NL, Payne WD, Dunn Dl, Sutherland DER, Najarian JS (1990) The impact of HLA matching on graft survival and sensitization after a failed transplant. Evidence that failure of poorly matched renal transplants does not result in increased sensitization. Transplantation 50: 599–607
3. Ogura K, Cecka JM (1990) Cadaver retransplants. In: Terasaki P (ed) Clinical transplants. UCLA Tissue Typing Laboratory Los Angeles, pp 471–483
4. Opelz G (1989) Influence of HLA matching on survival of second kidney transplants in cyclosporine-treated recipients. Transplantation 47: 823–827
5. Pongratz G, Goumaz C, Gore SM, Bradley BA, Jeannet M (1990) Analyse de la fréquence de l'hyperimmunisation anti-HLA chez les patients en attente d'une transplantation rénale. Schweiz Med Wochenschr 120: 1335–1338
6. Sanfilipo F, Goeken N, Niblack G, Scornik J, Vaugn WK (1987) The effect of first cadaver renal transplant HLA A, B match on sensitization levels and retransplant rates following graft failure. Transplantation 43: 240–243
7. Stiller CR, Opelz G (1991) Should cyclosporine be continued indefinitely? Transplant Proc 23: 36–40

Transplant Int (1992) 5 [Suppl 1]: S 67–68

TRANSPLANT
International
© Springer-Verlag 1992

Renal funtional reserve in kidney transplant recipients

R. M. Fagugli[1], **A. Selvi**[1], **L. Fedeli**[2], **R. Brugnano**[1], **M. Cozzari**[1], **U. Buoncristiani**[1]

[1] U. O. Nefrologia e Dialisi-Ospedale Silvestrini, and [2] U. O. Medicina Nucleare Policlinico, Perugia, Italy

In the last few years different authors have observed that kidney transplant recipients with good organ function do not have a renal functional reserve (RFR). This condition is accompained by a high glomerular filtration rate (GFR) [2–6]. We studied RFR in patients with very good organ function under different immunosuppressive therapies, who were divided into groups based on the presence or absence of RFR.

Key words: Renal transplantation – Kidney function

Materials and methods

We studied 18 kidney transplant recipients and eight normal subjects. The patients had a transplant age between 1 and 10 years, were of both sexes, and had a serum creatinine less than 1.4 mg%, and none had diabetes mellitus. In all patients arterial pressure was within normal limits, with or without pharmacological therapy.

Immunosuppressive therapies were cyclosporine ($n = 5$), azathioprine ($n = 6$) and combined ($n = 7$). A pharmacologically-free period was introduced starting 5 days before testing. Patients and controls were on a free diet. RFR was determined by oral protein load (1 g/kg ideal body weight). GFR was determined by ETDA Cr51 and renal blood flow (RBF) by hippuran I^{123} clearance. Statistical analysis was performed with the Student's t-test and the Fischer exact test with a significance level of $P < 0.05$.

Results

There were two groups of kidney transplant recipients: group A, with RFR ($n = 8$), and group B, without RFR ($n = 10$). In group A, basal GFR was 67 ± 28.25 ml/min, significantly lower than in group B (128.6 ± 39.9 ml/min, $P < 0.01$) and in controls (133.6 ± 27.8 ml/min, $P < 0.01$). There was no significant difference between group B and controls. In group A, RFR was similar to normal subjects ($14.1 \pm 11.7\%$ vs $15.1 \pm 10.9\%$; P, NS). RBF was 234.3 ± 65.03 ml/min in group A and 367.7 ± 104.2 ml/min

Offprint requests to: R. M. Fagugli

in group B, both significantly lower than in normal subjects (490 ± 80.7 ml/min; $P < 0.01$) There was no difference in RBF between group A and B. In group A, RBF increment was $18.7 \pm 10.5\%$ and $19.4 \pm 12.1\%$ in the normal subjects.

Filtration fraction (FF) was higher in group B before and after protein load than in group A and normal subjects (0.36 ± 0.09 vs 0.26 ± 0.06 and 0.26 ± 0.09; $P = 0.02$). The transplant age of the two groups was not different (5.7 ± 2.5 in A vs. 4.7 ± 3.1 in B (years)). Cyclosporinaemia was not significantly different (330.5 ± 140 ng/ml in A vs. 447 ± 120.1 ng/ml in B).

In group A, 12.5% were being treated with azathioprine, 37.5% with cyclosporine, and 50% with combined therapy. In group B 50% were being treated with azathioprine, 20% with cyclosporine, and 30% with combined therapy.

There was a total of 11 cases of hypertension, five (45%) in group B and six (55%) in group A. Patients under azathioprine therapy were hypertensive in 66% of cases, and patients under cyclosporine therapy (alone or combined) in 50% of cases. In group B, five patients were being treated with cyclosporine, five were hypertensive, and seven had a transplant age > 5 years (relative risk (Fischer's test), not significant).

Discussion

RFR is currently a matter of debate among nephrologists. Although several studies have been performed on kidney transplant recipients, results are not in agreement. The cause must perhaps be sought in the different types of protocols applied.

We studied kidney transplant recipients with optimal organ function and have noted that these patients consist of two subgroups, the first with RFR comparable with normal subjects, and the second without RFR and a higher GFR. It is important to stress that, whatever the meaning of RFR [1, 7, 8], absence of functional reserve was not due to cyclosporine therapy and that there was no correlation with blood pressure (hypertensive patients were present in both groups). It also seems as though transplantation age has no important effect on RFR. The other point to stress was the presence in the group without RFR of high FF values. This probably indicates the presence of high pressure between afferent and efferent arterioles (high ΔP) or a high ultrafiltration coefficient (k_f).

Next we have to investigate the meaning of RFR absence in prognostic terms and it is necessary to check whether or not hyperfiltration is due to a high protein diet.

References

1. Brenner BM et al. (1982) Dietary protein intake and the progressive nature of kidney disease: the role of hemodynamically mediated glomerular injury in the pathogenesis of glomerular sclerosis in aging, renal ablation, and intrinsic renal disease. N Engl J Med: 307: 652
2. Cairns HS et al. (1988) Failure of cyclosporine treated renal allograft recipients to increase glomerular filtration rate following an aminoacid infusion. Transplantation 46: 79–82
3. Dhaene M et al. (1986) Renal functional reserve of transplanted kidney. Nephron 44: 157–158
4. Fagugli RM et al. (1991) Plasma atrial natriuretic factor and functional reserve in renal transplant reserve. In: Wichtig (ed) Cardionephrology. pp. 507–511
5. Greene ER et al. (1989) Effect of a high-protein meal on blood flow to transplanted human kidney. Transplantation 48: 584–587
6. Magalini SC et al. (1989) Paradoxical effect of short-term protein loading on CsA treated kidney transplant recipients. Transplant Proc 21: 1500–1501
7. Maschio G et al. (1989) Dynamic evaluation of renal function: a chimera for nephrologists? J Nephrol 3: 157–164
8. Zuccala A et al. (1990) Use and misuse of renal functional reserve concepts in clinical nephrology. Nephrol Dial Transpl 5: 410–411

Transplant Int (1992)5 [Suppl 1]: S 69–S 72

TRANSPLANT
International
© Springer-Verlag 1992

Nifedipine improves immediate, and 6- and 12-month graft function in cyclosporin A (CyA) treated renal allograft recipients

S. J. Harper, J. Moorhouse, P. S. Veitch, T. Horsburgh, J. Walls, P. R. F. Bell, P. K. Donnelly, and J. Feehally

Departments of Nephrology and Surgery, Leicester General Hospital, Leicester, UK

Abstract. To investigate the effect of oral nifedipine, a calcium channel blocker known not to modify cyclosporin A (CyA) pharmacokinetics, on immediate transplant function and CyA nephrotoxicity, 68 adult renal transplant recipients were pre-operatively randomized to one of three regimes: A (high-dose CyA, initial dose 17 mg/kg per day, maintenance dose 7 mg/kg per day); B (regime A plus oral nifedipine); C low-dose CyA, initial dose 10 mg/kg per day, maintenance 4 mg/kg per day plus azathioprine 1 mg/kg per day). All three groups received identical steroid regimes. Calcium channel blockers of all types were avoided in groups A and C. Delayed graft function (dialysis dependence by day 4) was seen least frequently in group B ($P < 0.02$). Group B had improved graft function at 6 months compared with group A, identified by differences in serum creatinine ($P < 0.05$), GFR ($P < 0.01$) and ERPF ($P < 0.05$). Similar differences in serum creatinine ($P < 0.05$) and GFR ($P < 0.05$) were also identified at 12 months. Group C also had better 6- and 12-month GFR values than group A ($P < 0.05$ each). The three groups did not differ in donor or recipient age, HLA matching, ischaemic or anastomosis times, frequency of early rejection or whole-blood CyA levels. These results indicate that nifedipine significantly improves immediate and medium-term graft function.

Key words: Renal transplantation – Nifedipine – Calcium channel blockers – Cyclosporin A

The introduction of cyclosporin A (CyA) to solid organ transplantation was associated with significantly improved graft survival rates [1, 5], but its nephrotoxicity remains a major clinical disadvantage.

Although the most common clinical manifestation of CyA nephrotoxicity is an acute reversible impairment of renal function [5], CyA has also been linked with an increase in delayed initial graft function [1], presumably due

to its exacerbation of renal ischaemic injury [16]. In the longer term, a chronic irreversible nephropathy may occur, characterized by a progressive elevation in serum creatinine [13, 14] and diffuse interstitial fibrosis [15]. The pathophysiology of chronic CyA nephropathy is controversial, but there is mounting evidence that vasoconstriction of the afferent glomerular arteriole is the primary abnormality.

There is evidence from retrospective clinical data and experimental studies in animal models that calcium channel blockers may minimize short- and long-term CyA nephrotoxicity [6, 7, 11, 12]. Calcium channel blockers effect a reduction in calcium influx by their action on voltage-dependent slow calcium channels, thereby reducing intracellular calcium ion accumulation, well recognized as a mediator of ischaemic cell injury [2, 18]. Studies in both cardiac and renal ischaemia suggest that calcium channel blockade prior to any ischaemic insult is required for maximum benefit [2, 18]. The capacity of calcium channel blockers to facilitate vascular smooth muscle relaxation, particularly in the afferent glomerular arteriole [9], may be beneficial in chronic CyA nephrotoxicity.

Although the calcium channel blockers verapamil and diltiazem have been shown to be beneficial in CyA-treated renal transplant recipients [3, 20], they are known to modify CyA pharmacokinetics [4], which may cause difficulty in effective control of CyA therapy.

This prospective study was therefore designed using the calcium channel blocker, nifedipine, which does not modify CyA metabolism [4, 10], to investigate whether administration of oral nifedipine could reduce the incidence of delayed graft function and minimize long-term graft deterioration in renal allograft recipients receiving CyA.

Methods

Subjects

Adult cadaver renal allograft recipients ($n = 68$) were randomized pre-operatively to one of three regimes: A, CyA, initial dose of 17 mg/kg per day reduced in a stepwise manner by 2 mg/kg per week

---

Offprint requests to: Dr. J. Feehally, Leicester General Hospital, Gwendolen Road, Leicester LE5 4PW, UK

Table 1. Frequency of delayed initial function in the three study groups

Treatment regime	Number of patients	Incidence (%)
A (High dose CyA)	9/21	43
B (High dose CyA + nifedipine)	2/24	8.3*
C (Triple therapy)	7/23	30.4

* $P < 0.02$

Table 2. Results of serum creatinine, glomerular filtration rate and effective renal plasma flow in the three study groups

	Group A	Group B	Group C
Serum creatinine (μmol/l)			
7 days	394 ± 63	253 ± 58	410 ± 58
28 days	260 ± 40	172 ± 20*	217 ± 34
1 month	206 ± 18	153 ± 11*	166 ± 20
6 months	204 ± 20	155 ± 10*	173 ± 27
12 months	224 ± 23	156 ± 9*	191 ± 28
GFR (ml/min per 1.73 m^2)			
1 month	47 ± 3.9	45 ± 3.3	52 ± 4.1
6 months	32 ± 3.9	45 ± 2.9**	44 ± 3.2*
12 months	28 ± 4.7	43 ± 3.3*	41 ± 4.1*
ERPF (ml/min per 1.73^2)			
1 month	216 ± 13	183 ± 14	191 ± 36
6 months	239 ± 20	237 ± 15*	204 ± 14
12 months	266 ± 23	222 ± 13	184 ± 14

* $P < 0.05$; ** $P < 0.01$ (groups B or C compared with A)

to a maintenance dose of 7 mg/kg per day at 6 weeks; *B,* CyA as in regime A plus oral nifedipine retard 10 mg three times daily for 1 week, then 20 mg twice daily, increasing to 40 mg twice daily if indicated for hypertension; *C,* CyA, initial dose 10 mg/kg per day reducing by 1 mg/kg per week to a maintenance dose of 4 mg/kg per day at 6 weeks. To achieve effective immunosuppression, group C also received azathioprine at a dose of 1 mg/kg per day. All three groups received identical prednisolone regimes. Calcium channel blockers of all types were avoided in groups A and C and other antihypertensive agents were used if clinically indicated.

CyA was given as gelatin capsules in divided doses thrice daily for 2 weeks after transplantation then twice daily. CyA dosage was based on pretransplant dry weight. Half the daily dose was given orally preoperatively, and individuals randomized to group B received the first dose of oral nifedipine at that time.

Highly sensitized individuals (> 50% panel reactive antibodies) or those receiving an HLA-identical live related graft were excluded from randomization. Other factors which may have modified immediate or long-term graft function were documented: donor and recipient age, ischaemic times, anastomosis times, whole-blood CyA levels (days 0–7), antibody status and blood pressure control.

Trough CyA levels were measured in whole blood by high performance liquid chromatography.

Graft function parameters

Delayed initial function was defined as dialysis dependence by the fourth postoperative day in the absence of graft rejection.

Formal investigation of graft function was performed at 1, 6 and 12 months by measurements of serum creatinine concentration and isotopic assessment of glomerular filtration rate (GFR) (^{51}Cr-

EDTA) and effective renal plasma flow (ERPF) (^{131}I-hippuran) using a 'single shot' technique.

Statistics

Statistical analysis was performed with unpaired t-tests, Mann Whitney U and Chi-squared analysis. Data are presented as mean ± standard error of the mean.

Results

Initial graft function

Delayed initial function was seen least frequently in group B in which 2 of 24 patients (8.3%) were dialysis-dependent by day 4, compared with 9 of 21 in group A (43%), and 7 of 23 in group C (30%) ($P < 0.02$, Chisquared) (Table 1).

Graft function up to one year

Serum creatinine. Mean serum creatinine concentrations were significantly lower in group B compared with group A at 1, 6 and 12 months ($P < 0.05$) (Table 2, Fig. 1). *Glomerular filtration rate.* GFR values for group B were higher than for group A at 6 ($P < 0.01$) and 12 months ($P < 0.05$). Group C showed similar improvements in comparison with group A at both 6 and 12 months ($P < 0.05$) (Table 2, Fig. 2). *Effective renal plasma flow.* ERPF was significantly better at 6 months in group B than in group A ($P < 0.05$). There was no significant difference in any graft function parameter at any time point between groups B and C (Table 2, Fig. 3).

There were no significant differences between the three groups in donor or recipient age, HLA mismatches, ischaemic or anastomosis times, mean arterial blood pressure (at any time point), or trough (12-h) whole-blood CyA levels during the first post-transplant week, except at

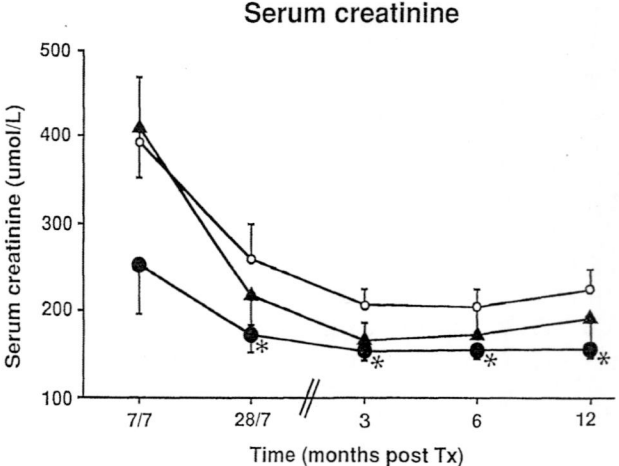

Fig. 1. Serum creatinine concentration during 12 months follow up. ○, group A; ●, group B; ▲, group C

Glomerular filtration rate

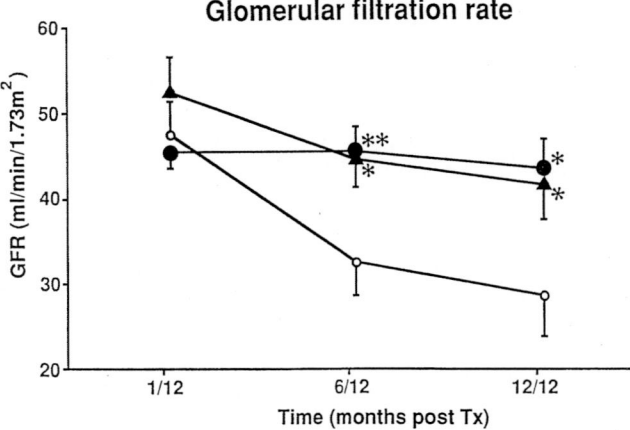

Fig. 2. Glomerular filtration rate during 12 months follow up. ○, group A; ●, group B; ▲, group C

Effective renal plasma flow

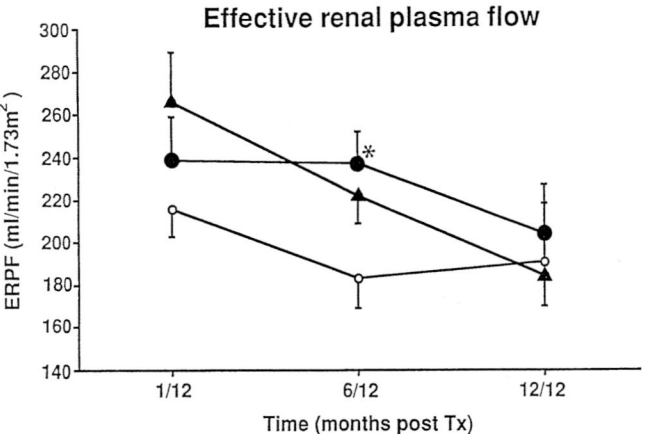

Fig. 3. Effective renal plasma flow during 12 months follow up. ○, group A; ●, group B; ▲, group C

one time point (day 4) when trough levels for group C were significantly lower than those of group A. Documented rejection episodes did not differ in the three groups. However, group B had a significantly higher mean panel reactive antibody status than group A ($P < 0.02$).

Discussion

This study suggests two beneficial effects of nifedipine in renal transplantation using CyA. First, it reduces the incidence of delayed initial function, and second it improves graft function up to 12 months after transplantation. There is a growing body of evidence relating to the beneficial short- and long-term effects of different calcium channel blockers in the context of CyA-treated human renal allograft recipients.

This study supports previous studies of early graft function. The calcium channel blockers diltiazem and verapamil when added to perfusion fluids at organ retrieval and administered to graft recipients have been shown to significantly improve early renal allograft function [3, 20]. Both drugs have the disadvantage of interfering with CyA pharmacokinetics, resulting in unpredictably (30–110 %)

elevated blood levels [4], and high CyA levels have themselves been associated with delayed graft function [7]. We have demonstrated that preoperative oral nifedipine is a simple method of achieving improved initial graft function without the need for uniformity in organ perfusion, which is difficult to achieve while multicentre organ sharing is practised.

The longer-term benefit of calcium channel blockade has previously been suggested by retrospective studies [6, 19]. These reports have presented graft survival data, or relied on serum creatinine concentration or clearance parameters derived from it, to assess graft function. Serum creatinine is a relatively insensitive measurement of graft function and may be particularly unreliable in patients taking CyA [17]. The present randomized study makes a prospective assessment of graft function using proven isotope reference methods for measurement of GFR and ERPF. With a limited follow-up period of 1 year, no significant differences in graft survival were found, but significant benefits in serum creatinine, GFR and ERPF were found if nifedipine was added to CyA.

Delayed initial function has been associated with poor graft outcome so improved function in established grafts may reflect the late consequence of early non-function. However, the benefits of nifedipine are still present if the data are reanalysed using only those with immediate graft function.

This study demonstrates the benefits of nifedipine in patients on a CyA regime which uses larger doses than preferred by some workers. The data thus far do not show any advantage of the nifedipine regime compared with a triple regime using a lower dose of CyA without nifedipine. Further follow-up of this cohort of patients will, however, provide additional evidence of the impact of nifedipine on longer-term graft function and graft survival.

Acknowledgements. The authors would like to thank N. Mistry, H. Hall, A. Sidgwick and S. Weston for their technical expertise in high performance liquid chromatography measurement of cyclosporin A.

References

1. Canadian Multicentre Transplant Study Group (1986) A randomised clinical trial of cyclosporine in cadaveric renal transplantation at three years. N Engl J Med 314: 1219–1225
2. Cheung J Y, Bonventre J V, Malis C D, Leaf A (1986) Calcium and ischaemic injury. New Engl J Med 314: 1670–1676
3. Dawidson I, Rooth P, Alway C et al (1990) Verapamil prevents post transplant delayed function and cyclosporin A nephrotoxicity. Transplant Proc 22: 1379–1380
4. Dy GR, Raja RM, Mendez MM (1991) The clinical and biochemical effect of calcium channel blockers in organ transplant recipients on cyclosporine. Transplant Proc 23: 1258–1259
5. European Multicentre Transplant Trial (1987) Cyclosporine in cadaveric renal transplantation: 5 year follow-up of a multicentre trial. Lancet II: 506–507
6. Feehally J, Walls J, Mistry N et al (1987) Br Med J 295: 310
7. Ferguson CJ, Hillis AN, Williams JD et al (1990) Calcium channel blockers and other factors influencing delayed function in renal allografts. Nephrol Dial Transplant 5: 816–820
8. Kahan BD (1989) Cyclosporine. N Engl J Med 321: 1725–1738

9. Loutzenhiser R, Epstein M (1987) Modification of renal haemodynamic response to vasoconstrictors by calcium antagonists. Am J Nephrol 7 [Suppl 1]: 7–16

10. McNally PG, Mistry N, Idle JR, Walls J, Feehally J (1989) Calcium channel blockers and cyclosporin metabolism. Transplantation 48: 1071

11. McNally PG, Baker F, Mistry N et al (1990) Effect of nifedipine on renal haemodynamics in an animal model of cyclosporin A nephrotoxicity. Clin Sci 79: 259–266

12. McNally PG, Wall J, Feehally J (1990) The effect of nifedipine on renal function in normotensive cyclosporin A-treated renal allograft recipients. Nephrol Dial Transplant 5: 962–968

13. Merion RM, White DJG, Thiru S et al (1984) Cyclosporine: five years experience in cadaveric renal transplantation. N Engl J Med 310: 148–154

14. Morris PJ, French ME, Dunnill MS et al (1983) A controlled trial of cyclosporine in renal transplantation with conversion to azathioprine and prednisolone after three months. Transplantation 36: 273–277

15. Myers BD (1986) Cyclosporine nephrotoxicity. Kidney Int 30: 964–974

16. Parrott NR, Forsythe JLR, Matthews JNS et al (1990) Late perfusion. A simple remedy for renal allograft primary non-function. Transplantation 49: 913–915

17. Ross EA, Wilkinson A, Hawkins RA, Danovitch GM (1987) The plasma creatinine concentration is not an accurate reflection of glomerular filtration rate in stable renal transplant patients receiving cyclosporine. Am J Kidney Dis 10: 113–117

18. Schrier RW, Arnold PE, Van Patten VJ, Burke TJ (1987) Cellular calcium in ischaemic acute renal failure. Kidney Int 32: 313–321

19. Solez K, Racusen LC, Keown PA, Vaughn WK, Burdick JF (1988) The influence of antihypertensive drug therapy on renal transplantation function and outcome. Transplant Proc 20 [Suppl 3]: 618–622

20. Wagner K, Albrecht S, Neumayer HH (1987) Influence of calcium antagonist diltiazem on delayed graft function in cadaveric kidney transplantation: results of a six month follow up. Transplant Proc 19: 1353–1357

Transplant Int (1992) 5 [Suppl 1]: S 73–S 74

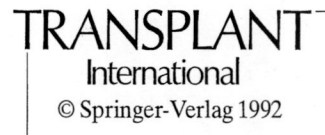

© Springer-Verlag 1992

Post-transplant haemoglobin levels and host kidney status

L. B. Hilbrands, A. J. Hoitsma, and R. A. P. Koene

Department of Internal Medicine, Division of Nephrology, University Hospital Nijmegen, P. O. Box 9101, NL-6500 HB Nijmegen, The Netherlands

Abstract. Erythrocytosis after renal transplantation has been ascribed to inappropriate production of erythropoietin by the recipient's native kidneys. In a retrospective analysis we examined the effect of pre-transplant bilateral nephrectomy on post-transplant haemoglobin level (Hb) and haematocrit (Ht) in 370 renal transplant patients. Hb and Ht were significantly higher in the 341 patients with host kidneys in situ compared with the 29 patients who had undergone bilateral nephrectomy (Hb, 8.5 ± 1.2 mmol/l vs 7.8 ± 1.3 mmol/l, $P = 0.005$; Ht, $41 \pm 6\%$ vs $38 \pm 7\%$, $P = 0.02$). Moreover, a very high Hb and/or Ht (defined as a value above the 80th percentile of the whole group) occurred more frequently in patients with host kidneys in situ (20.5% vs 3.5%, $P = 0.02$). It thus appears that host kidneys significantly contribute to the unexpectedly high haemoglobin levels occurring after renal transplantation.

Key words: Erythrocytosis – Renal transplantation – Nephrectomy

Erythrocytosis is a well-recognized phenomenon in renal transplant recipients. The incidence has been reported to be 6–17% [3, 7, 10], the condition probably being more common in cyclosporine-treated patients than in those treated with azathioprine [5, 8]. Several pathophysiological mechanisms have been proposed, including inappropriate production of erythropoietin (EPO) by the recipient's native kidneys [1, 3, 9]. We investigated retrospectively the effect of pre-transplant bilateral nephrectomy on post-transplant haemoglobin level and haematocrit in a large group of renal transplant patients.

Methods

The study population consisted of all adult patients who had undergone a renal transplantation in our centre from 1 to 10 years previously, and who currently had a functioning graft. Patients with

Offprint requests to: L. B. Hilbrands

polycystic kidney disease, an established cause of erythrocytosis, were excluded. Long-term immunosuppression consisted mostly of azathioprine and prednisone, but a minority of the patients received cyclosporine, usually in combination with prednisone.

The following data were obtained for each patient: sex, age, haemoglobin level (Hb), haematocrit (Ht), serum creatinine concentration, time after transplantation, use of cyclosporine, systolic and diastolic blood pressure, and current number of antihypertensive drugs. The last recorded Hb and Ht were used for analysis. If one or more therapeutic phlebotomies had been performed, the last recorded Hb and Ht preceding the start of phlebotomies were taken. For definition of a very high Hb and/or Ht we arbitrarily chose a limit at the sexspecific 80th percentile (P_{80}) of the whole group.

Statistical analysis was performed with Wilcoxon's test for unpaired data and the chi-squared test where appropriate. A P value smaller than 0.05 was considered statistically significant.

Results

Of the 370 patients who fulfilled the inclusion criteria, 29 had undergone bilateral nephrectomy (BN) for various reasons, and 341 had one or both host kidneys still in situ (HK). The values of the assessed parameters in both groups are summarized in Table 1. Since the use of antihypertensive medication differed significantly in both groups, we reanalysed the data after exclusion of 209 patients who used any kind of antihypertensive drug. Again, both groups did not differ significantly with respect to sex, age, serum creatinine, blood pressure, time after transplantation, and use of cyclosporine (data not shown). Hb, Ht and number of patients with Hb and/or Ht above the P_{80} in this subgroup are given in Table 2.

Discussion

The results clearly show that Hb and Ht were higher in renal transplant patients with host kidneys in situ than in patients who had undergone bilateral nephrectomy before transplantation. In addition, a very high Hb and/or Ht occurred more frequently in HK group.

Since diuretic therapy for hypertension has been associated with higher Hb and Ht levels [6, 7], and patients in

Table 1. Data of patients in the BN (bilateral nephrectomy) and HK (host kidneys in situ) groups

	BN ($n = 29$)	HK ($n = 341$)	P
Males/females	17/12	207/134	NS
Age (years)[a]	42 ± 12	46 ± 13	NS
Time after transplantation (years)[a]	4.8 ± 3.1	4.3 ± 2.6	NS
Serum creatinine (μmol/l)[a]	110 ± 35	129 ± 59	NS
Use of cyclosporine (%)	14	19	NS
Systolic BP (mm Hg)[a]	138 ± 21	144 ± 22	NS
Diastolic BP (mm Hg)[a]	83 ± 10	85 ± 10	NS
Number of antihypertensive drugs[a]	0.4 ± 0.8	1.0 ± 1.1	0.004
Hb (mmol/l)[a]	7.8 ± 1.3	8.5 ± 1.2	0.005
Ht (%)[a]	38 ± 7	41 ± 6	0.02
Hb and/or Ht above P_{80}[b] (%)	3.5	20.5	0.025

[a] Data shown as mean ± SD.

[b] For males Hb > 9.5 mmol/l, Ht > 46%; for females Hb > 8.9 mmol/l, Ht > 45%.

Table 2. Data of patients in the BN (bilateral nephrectomy) and HK (host kidneys in situ) groups after exclusion of patients using antihypertensive medication

	BN ($n = 18$)	HK ($n = 143$)	P
Hb (mmol/l)[a]	8.0 ± 0.9	8.5 ± 1.1	NS
Ht (%)[a]	39 ± 4	41 ± 5	NS
Hb and/or Ht above P_{80}[b] (%)	5.6	27.6	0.05

[a] Data shown as mean ± SD.

[b] For males Hb > 9.4 mmol/l, Ht > 45%; for females Hb > 9.0 mmol/l, Ht > 44%.

the HK group used more antihypertensive drugs, we reanalysed the data after exclusion of all patients who used antihypertensive medication. Although the numbers probably were too small to reach statistical significance for all differences, a trend in the same direction was apparent. Somewhat unexpectedly, no fall in mean Hb and Ht levels was observed after exclusion of patients using antihypertensive medication. It should be stressed however, that the structure of our database did not allow selective exclusion of patients using diuretics instead of all patients using antihypertensive drugs. Other factors that might affect the incidence of post-transplant erythrocytosis were equally distributed between the BN and HK groups.

Our data suggest that host kidneys significantly contribute to the unexpectedly high haemoglobin levels that can occur after renal transplantation. In accordance with our findings, Pollak et al. demonstrated a lower prevalence of bilateral nephrectomy in patients with post-transplant erythrocytosis compared with a control population [7]. It has been postulated that the host kidneys exert their effect on haemoglobin level by inappropriate EPO production. Indeed, selective venous catheterization of transplanted and native kidneys in patients with post-transplant erythrocytosis, revealed that the native kidneys were responsible for the elevated systemic EPO levels occurring in this setting [1, 3, 9].

Because erythrocytosis is associated with an increased risk of thromboembolic events [10], treatment is generally advocated. In addition to repeated phlebotomies, administration of theophylline has recently been shown to be useful by reducing serum EPO levels [2]. Finally, the experience of normalization of haemoglobin levels after bilateral native nephrectomy in 20 out of 22 patients with post-transplant erythrocytosis [4], forms additional evidence for the pathogenetic role of EPO from the host kidneys in this condition.

References

1. Aeberhard JM, Schneider PA, Vallotton MB, Kurtz A, Leski M (1990) Multiple site estimates of erythropoietin and renin in polycythemic kidney transplant patients. Transplantation 50: 613–616
2. Bakris GL, Sauter ER, Hussey JL, Fisher JW, Gaber AO, Winsett R (1990) Effects of theophylline on erythropoietin production in normal subjects and patients with erythrocytosis after renal transplantation. N Engl J Med 323: 86–90
3. Dagher FJ, Ramos E, Erslev AJ, Alongi SV, Karmi SA, Caro J (1979) Are the native kidneys responsible for erythrocytosis in renal allorecipients? Transplantation 28: 496–498
4. Friman S, Nyberg G, Blohmé I (1990) Erythrocytosis after renal transplantation; treatment by removal of the native kidneys. Nephrol Dial Transplant 5: 969–973
5. Gruber SA, Simmons RL, Najarian JS, Vercelotti G, Ascher NL, Dunn DL, Payne WD, Sutherland DER, Fryd DS (1988) Erythrocytosis and thromboembolic complications after renal transplantation: results from a randomized trial of cyclosporine versus azathioprine–antilymphocyte globulin. Transplant Proc 20 [Suppl 3]: 948–950
6. Obermiller LE, Tzamaloukas AH, Avasthi PS, Halpern JA, Sterling WA (1985) Decreased plasma volume in post-transplant erythrocytosis. Clin Nephrol 23: 213–217
7. Pollak R, Maddux MS, Cohan J, Jacobsson PK, Mozes MF (1988) Erythrocythemia following renal transplantation: influence of diuretic therapy. Clin Nephrol 29: 119–123
8. Tatman AJ, Tucker B, Amess JAL, Cattell WR, Baker LRI (1988) Erythraemia in renal transplant recipients treated with cyclosporin. Lancet I: 1279
9. Thevenod F, Radtke HW, Grützmacher P, Vincent E, Koch KM, Schoeppe W, Fassbinder W (1983) Deficient feedback regulation of erythropoiesis in kidney transplant patients with polycythemia. Kidney Int 24: 227–232
10. Wickre CG, Norman DJ, Bennison A, Barry JM, Bennett WM (1983) Postrenal transplant erythrocytosis: A review of 53 patients. Kidney Int 23: 731–737

Transplant Int (1992)5 [Suppl 1]: S 75–S 78

TRANSPLANT
International
© Springer-Verlag 1992

Effect of ATG prophylaxis in sensitized and non-sensitized kidney graft recipients

J. Kaden[2], G. May[1], C. Schönemann[2], P. Müller[1], J. Groth[2], W. Seeger[1], F. Seibt[1], M. Henkert[2], J. Lippert[3]

[1] Kidney Transplant Centre and [2] Department of Immunology, Clinic of Urology, Friedrichshain Hospital, Berlin; and
[3] Humboldt University, Faculty of Medicine, Clinic of Urology, Berlin FRG

Abstract. In our effort to find an optimum immunosuppressive protocol for kidney transplantation we introduced two forms of ATG prophylaxis: 1. high-dose single-bolus prophylaxis (9 mg/kg) in non-sensitized patients (PRA < 5 %); and 2. low-dose 8-day prophylaxis (1.5–3.0 mg/kg) in sensitized patients (PRA > 5 %). A total of 204 kidney graft recipients were included in this study and treated with a triple-drug therapy (TDT). In comparison with TDT-treated controls, in sensitized patients the 8-day ATG prophylaxis resulted in a reduced rate of rejection episodes (25.5 % vs 47 %), an improved 1-year graft survival (82 % vs 71 %) and patient survival (94 % vs 90 %). In non-sensitized patients the high-dose single-bolus ATG prophylaxis induced a T-cell lymphopenia lasting 4 to 5 days and, in comparison with the corresponding controls, resulted in a shortened hospital stay (31.2 days vs 36.7 days), a reduced rate of rejection episodes (25.5 % vs 53 %), an improved 1-year graft survival (92 % vs 86 %) and patient survival (100 % vs 94 %).

Key words: Kidney transplantation – ATG prophylaxis – Rejection episodes – Graft survival – Patient survival

In 1990 Kormos et al. [14] showed that prophylactic rabbit anti-human thymocyte globulin (RATG) achieves a major reduction in early cardiac graft rejection without an increased risk of major opportunistic or bacterial infections, and concluded that RATG would be an important adjunct to contemporary immunosuppressive protocols. Grino et al. [6], using horse ALG, also reported a low incidence of acute rejection episodes after cadaveric renal transplantation. Encouraged by these results we introduced two forms of ATG prophylaxis depending on the sensitization status of the prospective recipient. Sensitized recipients [panel reactive lymphocytotoxic anti-

bodies (PRA) > 5 %] received eight consecutive ATG infusions starting intraoperatively in addition to triple-drug therapy (TDT) consisting of azathioprine (AZA), cyclosporine (CyA) and low-dose prednisolone (PRED). In non-sensitized patients (PRA < 5 %) we inaugurated a new treatment protocol consisting of an intraoperative high-dose single-ATG bolus in addition to TDT.

These treatment protocols were chosen because in our hands the graft survival in sensitized recipients was inferior to that in non-sensitized recipients [3]. The rationale of the protocols was to produce maximal immunosuppression when the recipient was most likely to respond to the new organ.

Materials and methods

Study population

A total of 204 patients who received their cadaveric renal transplant at the Kidney Transplant Centre Berlin-Friedrichshain from April 1987 to November 1990 were included in this study.

Immunosuppressive protocol

All patients received AZA (4 mg/kg) in their dialysis unit immediately before being called to the transplant centre. Methylprednisolone (500 mg intravenously) was given during transplantation, and postoperatively the patients received 40 mg for 7 days, subsequently switching to 35 mg/day PRED for 14 days. A maintenance dose of 10–15 mg/day PRED was then continued for 12 months. Oral CyA was started within 24 h of surgery. The patients received 6 mg/kg divided in two daily doses. During the first postoperative week a maintenance CyA level of 100 ng/ml (RIA, ICN-STAR, SORIN), and thereafter of 200 ng/ml, was the aim. AZA was restarted after surgery at an oral dose of 1 mg/kg and maintained as long as the leucocyte count was greater than 4000/mm³.

Monitoring for rejection and infection

For the diagnosis of rejection the following clinical and laboratory signs were decisive: enlargement and tenderness of the graft, increase in serum creatinine and C-reactive protein, concomitant

Offprint requests to: Dr. J. Kaden, Division of Immunology, Department of Urology, Friedrichshain Hospital, Leninallee 49, O-1017 Berlin, FRG

change in blood urea nitrogen, oliguria, immunoglobulinuria, sonographic changes, immunoactivation in fine-needle aspiration cytology [6], biopsy-proven rejection. Rejection was treated with PRED, 5 mg/kg for 5 days, or with ATG, 1.5–3 mg/kg for 8–10 days depending on the T-cell count ($<200/mm^3$). Infections were classified as either major or minor. Major infections included pneumonia, pyelonephritis, cytomegalovirus (CMV) disease and invasive fungal infection.

CMV infection was diagnosed by the detection of CMV-specific IgM antibodies, a fourfold or greater increase in CMV-specific IgG antibodies (CMV-ELISA, Enzygnost Behring, Marburg, FRG) and/or the fluorescence microscopic detection of CMV antigen-carrying peripheral blood cells or fine-needle-aspirated kidney graft cells [7] by means of monoclonal antibodies (Clonab-CMV, Behring, Marburg, FRG). CMV disease was diagnosed using clinical criteria including leucopenia, spike-like fever, elevation of aminotransferases, thrombocytopenia, deterioration of graft function etc. The treatment of CMV disease depended on the severity of clinical symptoms and included the application of human immunoglobulins with a high content of CMV-specific antibodies (CYTOTECT, Biotest, Dreieich, FRG), the reduction or cessation of AZA for several days and sometimes the prophylactic application of antibiotics.

ATG prophylaxis

We used rabbit anti-human T-lymphocyte globulin (ATG) (Fresenius, Oberursel, FRG) in two different protocols. Non-sensitized patients (PRA $<5\%$) received 9 mg/kg ATG intravenously just before the anastomoses were completed. Sensitized patients (PRA $>5\%$) and patients waiting for a second graft were given 1.5–3.0 mg/kg ATG intravenously for 8 days beginning with the first infusion also intraoperatively before the anastomoses were completed. The daily ATG doses depended on the T-cell count, which needed to be lower than $200/mm^3$.

T-cell count

In order to monitor the ATG effect the cell count was determined three times a week using the spontaneous rosette formation test [11] according to the previously published method [12]. More recently we have been able to confirm and extend our results by FACS analyses (data not published).

Results

Sensitized recipients

In this group, 51 out of 102 sensitized (PRA $>5\%$) or regrafted recipients received an 8-day ATG prophylaxis. The basic immunosuppression in both groups consisted of AZA, PRED and CyA. The results are summarized in Table 1. There was no difference in the postoperative hospital stay (ATG vs non-ATG: 38.9 ± 25.3 days vs 39.6 ± 25.3 days). However, the frequency of rejection crises up to discharge was significantly lower in the prophylaxis group (25.5% vs 47%), and the proportion of functioning grafts was increased by 10%. The improved graft survival was still evident 1 year after transplantation. The 1-year patient survival was also slightly better in the prophylaxis group (94.1% vs 90.2%). In the ATG group three patients did not survive, the causes of death being sepsis (one) and heart failure (two). In the non-ATG group five patients did not survive, the causes of death

being sepsis (one), embolism (one), myocardial infarction (one) and heart failure (two). With respect to CMV infection the proportion of secondary infections was significantly higher in the ATG prophylaxis group, and also in this group the number of patients who experienced oligosymptomatic CMV disease (leucocytopenia $<4000/mm^3$ and fever $\geq 38°$ for at least 2 days) was higher (25/51 vs 14/51). This was also reflected by a higher consumption of Cytotect (Biotest, FRG) in the prophylaxis group (total 4080 ml vs 2760 ml). No difference was seen in the occurrence of polysymptomatic severe CMV disease ($n = 3$ for each group).

Non-sensitized patients

In this group, 51 out of 102 non-sensitized TDT-treated kidney graft recipients received intraoperatively one infusion of 9 mg ATG/kg. No serious side effect was observed. At 24 h post-transplant, the absolute number of T cells (RFC) was decreased from $916 \pm 390/mm^3$ to $187 \pm 121/mm^3$ (Fig.1). This T lymphopenia lasted until the fourth post-transplant day ($284 \pm 173/mm^3$). Thereafter, a slow increase was recorded, reaching the T-cell level of the TDT recipients by day 7. Besides this T lymphopenia, the high-dose single-bolus ATG prophylaxis, in comparison with the controls (Table 2), resulted in a shortened post-transplant hospital stay (31.2 vs 36.7 days), and a reduced rate of rejection episodes (25.5% vs 53%). This is also reflected by the consumption of drugs needed for treatment of rejections (ATG vs non-ATG group: PRED, 19.52 vs 21.96 g; ATG, 2.8 vs 18.8 g; OKT3, 0 vs 45 mg).

With regard to CMV infection diseases there were no differences between the groups, and life-threatening epi-

Table 1. Sensitized kidney graft recipients: triple-drug therapy

	Without 8-day ATG prophylaxis	With 8-day ATG prophylaxis
Patients (n)	51	51
Follow-up time	4.87–1.90	9.89–10.90
Hospital stay (days, mean)	39.6	38.9
Number of recipients with rejection crises	24 (47%)	13 (25.5%)
CMV infections		
primary (n)	5/7	5/7
secondary (n)	17/44	30/44
CMV diseases		
light (n)	19/22	32/35
severe (n)	3/22	3/35
Patient survival (%)		
3 month	94	94
6 month	92	94
12 month	90	94
Transplant survival (%)		
3 month	78	82
6 month	74	82
12 month	71	82

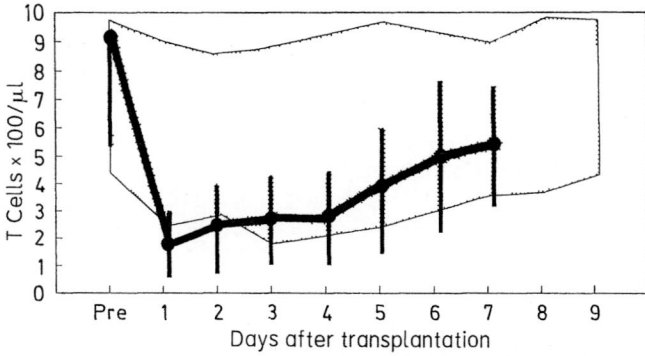

Fig. 1. Absolute number of sheep erythrocyte rosette-forming cells (E-RFC) during in the first week after kidney transplantation. The *black line* represents the mean ± 1 standard deviation of 51 recipients intraoperatively treated with 9 mg/kg ATG-Fresenius in addition to the triple-drug therapy. The *dotted area* represents the absolute number of RFC (mean ± 1 s. d.) in 51 only triple-drug treated recipients.

sodes were not observed. The amount of CMV gamma-globulin infused was almost comparable in the ATG and in the non-ATG groups (7050 vs 6530 ml). With respect to the long-term results, both the 1-year graft survival (92 % vs 86 %) and patient survival (100 % vs 94 %) were clearly improved. It should be noted that three out of four recipients in the prophylaxis group who were on dialysis after 1 year had a primary non-functioning graft. In the non-prophylaxis group, three patients did not survive, the causes of death being sepsis (one), lung embolism (one) and cerebral bleeding (one).

Discussion

In an effort to find an optimum immunosuppressive protocol for organ transplantation many centres are using polyclonal [4–6, 8, 10, 14, 16–18], or monoclonal [1, 2, 9, 15, 16, 19, 20] anti-T-lymphocyte antibodies as prophylaxis in addition to conventional immunosuppressive drugs. The protocols, as well as the antibodies used, are very different. The rationale for using these agents is, first, to reduce the amount of CyA in the early post-transplant period in order to avoid nephrotoxicity, second, to produce maximal immunosuppression when the host is most likely to respond to the new organ, and, third, to reduce the probability of rejections without increasing the risk of infections.

Our data confirm the previously reported excellent overall results with the simultaneous use of ALG, CyA and steroids [4, 6], ALG, AZA and steroids [8, 18] or ALG, AZA, CyA and steroids [10] as induction therapy after kidney transplantation. In contrast to Grundmann et al. [8] and Fries et al. [4], who gave ALG for 14 days and reported a high rate of intolerance and unexplainable fever [8] or an increased rate of clinical CMV infections [4], our protocol included only eight ATG infusions starting intraoperatively.

To demonstrate a beneficial effect of our quadruple-drug induction therapy also in high risk patients, we treated 51 presensitized or regrafted patients according to this protocol. In comparison with TDT-treated sensitized kidney graft recipients (control group) the quadruple-drug induction therapy improved the 1-year graft survival from 71 % to 82 % and the 1-year patient survival from 90 % to 94 %, and reduced the number of patients who experienced rejection crises from 47 % to 25.5 %. This is in contrast to the results of Illner et al. [10] who reported a 55 % frequency of rejection episodes in a comparable group. Thomas et al. [18] reported a shorter hospital stay and a cadaver kidney graft survival rate of 92 % in 40 (but only 38 % presensitized) quadruple-drug-treated recipients. The ATG was also given according to a protocol to reduce the level of total circulating T cells to below 200/mm³.

Thus, the prophylactic use of ATG in addition to the conventional TDT improves the graft survival also in presensitized recipients, seems to be safe because early nephrotoxic side effects were not observed (trough level 100 ng/ml during the first postoperative week) and severe infectious complications did not increase.

In our second series, a newer technique of immunosuppression, high-dose single-bolus ATG and TDT, was used in 51 non-sensitized recipients. The overall patient and graft survival after 12 months (100 % and 94 %, respectively) was excellent. Graft losses occurred in four patients in the study group, but only one due to rejection. Three out of these four grafts were primarily non-functional. However, this situation could still be improved by a better graft survival rate.

Bearing in mind particularly the cost of transplantation, the induction therapy reduced the rate of rejection episodes from 53 % to 25.5 %, shortened the hospital stay on average from 36.7 days to 31.2 days and did not in-

Table 2. Non-sensitized kidney graft recipients: triple-drug therapy

	Without ATG bolus	With ATG bolus
Patients (*n*)	51	51
Follow-up time	3.89–2.90	2.90–11.90
Hospital stay (days, mean)	36.7	31.2
Number of recipients with rejection crises	27 (53 %)	13 (25.5 %)
CMV infections		
primary (*n*)	19/22	17/20
secondary (*n*)	21/29	17/20
CMV diseases		
light	39/40	32/34
severe	1/40	2/34
Patient survival (%)		
3 month	96	100
6 month	94	100
12 month	94	100[a]
Transplant survival (%)		
3 month	92	94
6 month	88	94
12 month	86	92[a]

[a] 8/51 recipients at time of evaluation only 10 month post-transplantation with very well functioning graft

fluence the rate of infectious complications. It should be noted that ATG prophylaxis did reduce the actual rejection rate as opposed to only delaying the onset of rejections. During the first post-transplant week, the CyA trough values were only 100 ng/ml in order to reduce early nephrotoxic side effects. An optimal intraoperative and postoperative immunosuppression was induced by the high-dose single-ATG bolus leading to a T lymphopenia lasting at least 4 days. During this time the first, and may be decisive, contact between host and graft takes place.

Thus, the excellent results of high-dose single-bolus ATG prophylaxis in non-sensitized kidney graft recipients encouraged us to extend this protocol also to sensitized recipients.

References

1. Benvenisty AI, Cohen D, Stegall MD, Hardy MA (1990) Improved results using OKT3 as induction immunosuppression in renal allograft recipients with delayed graft function. Transplantation 49: 321–327
2. Dendorfer U, Hillebrand G, Kasper C, Smely S, Weschka M, Hammer C, Racenberg J, Gurland H-J, Land W (1990) Effective prevention of interstitial rejection crises in immunological high risk patients following renal transplantation: Use of high doses of the new monoclonal antibody BMA 031. Transplant Proc 22: 1789–1790
3. Eichler C, Kaden J, Strobelt V, Oesterwitz H, Scholz D (1989) Cytomegalievirusnachweis mittels monoklonaler Antikörper an Aspirationsmaterial von Nierentransplantaten. Z Urol Nephrol 82: 13–20
4. Fries D, Hiesse C, Charpentier B, Cantarovich M, Lantz O, Benoit G (1989) Optimal results in cadaveric renal transplantation with low-dose cyclosporine and steroids combined with prophylactic anti-lymphocyte globulin. Transplant Proc 20: 23–25
5. Goldman MH, Regester RF, Freeman MB, Tyler B, Tyler JD (1991) Induction therapy with antilymphocyte serum (NATS) increases graft survival and function in kidneys with initial poor function. Transplant Proc 23: 1753–1754
6. Grino JM, Bas J, Gonzalez C, Castelav AM, Seron D, Mestre M, Buendia E, Sabate R, Diaz C, Alsina J (1990) Low incidence of rejection and in vitro donor-specific hyporesponsiveness using pretransplant ALG, low-dose cyclosporine and steroids in kidney cadaveric transplantation. Transplant Proc 22: 1376–1368
7. Groth J, Leverenz S, Koall W, Schmitt E, Kaden J, Schirrow R, Matzanke G, Strobelt V, Barz D, May G, Scholz D (1987) Einfluß immunologischer Faktoren auf die Frühfunktion nach Nierentransplantation. Z Klin Med 42: 2249–2252
8. Grundmann R, Hesse U, Wienand P, Baldamus C, Arns W (1987) Graft survival and long-term renal function after sequential conventional cyclosporin A therapy in cadaver kidney transplantation – a prospective randomized trial. Klin Wochenschr 65: 879–884
9. Hammond Eh, Wittwer CT, Greenwood J, Knape WA, Yowell RL, Menlove RL, Craven C, Renlund DG, Bristow MR, DeWitt CW, O'Connell JB (1990) Relationship of OKT3 sensitization and vascular rejection in cardiac transplant patients receiving OKT3 rejection prophylaxis. Transplantation 50: 776–782
10. Illner W-D, Schleibner S, Abendroth D, Land W (1988) Quadruple-drug induction therapy in highly sensitized patients. Transplant Proc 20 [Suppl 1]: 410–411
11. Jondal M, Holm G, Wigzell H (1972) Surface markers on human B and T lymphocytes. I. A large population of lymphocytes forming non-immune rosettes with sheep red blood cells. J Exp Med 136: 207–215
12. Kaden J, Groth J (1983) Zur Dynamik und diagnostischen Wertigkeit der T-Lymphozytenzahl bei Patienten nach Nierentransplantation. Dtsch Gesundh.-wesen 38: 342–347
13. Kaden J, Strobelt V, Oesterwitz H, Groth J, May G, Eichler C (1987) Monitoring of renal allograft rejection with fine needle aspiration biopsy and serum C-reactive protein determinations. Transplant Proc 19: 1657
14. Kormos RL, Armitage JM, Dummer JS, Miyamoto Y, Griffith BP, Hardesty R (1990) Optimal perioperative immunosuppression in cardiac transplantation using rabbit antilymphocyte globulin. Transplantation 49: 306–311
15. Land W, Hillebrand G, Illner W-D, Abendroth D, Hancke E, Schleibner S, Hammer C, Racenberg J (1988) First clinical experience with a new TCR/CD3-monoclonal antibody (BMY 031) in kidney transplant patients. Transplant Int 1: 116–117
16. Light JA, Khawand N, Ali A, Brems W, Aquino A (1989) Comparison of Minnesota antilymphocyte globulin and OKT3 for induction of immunosuppression in renal transplant patients. Transplant Proc 21: 1738–1740
17. Matas AJ, Tellis VA, Quinn TA, Glicklich D, Soberman R, Veith FJ (1988) Individualization of immediate posttransplant immunosuppression. Transplantation 45: 406–409
18. Thomas F, Cunningham P, Sash C, Gross U, Thomas J (1988) Superior cadaver renal transplantation survival and increased cost-effectiveness using individualized quadruple immunosuppression. Transplant Proc 20 [Suppl 1]: 412–414
19. Weimar W, Baumgartner D, Hendriks GFJ, Hesse CJ, Balk AHHM, Simoons ML, Bos E (1988) The prophylactic use of orthoclone OKT3 in kidney and heart transplantation. Transplant Proc 20 [Suppl 6]: 96–100
20. Wonigkeit K, Nashan B, Schwinzer R, Schlitt HJ, Kurrle R, Racenberg J, Seiler Fr, Ringe B, Pichlmayr R (1989) Use of a monoclonal antibody against the T cell receptor for prophylactic immunosuppressive treatment after liver transplantation. Transplant Proc 21: 2258–2259

Transplant Int (1992) 5 [Suppl 1]: S 79–S 80

TRANSPLANT
International
© Springer-Verlag 1992

Ocular findings in patients with successful renal transplantation

D. Koutsikos[1], B. Agroyannis[1], G. Tserkezis[1], M. Zentelis[2], P. Neamonitis[2], I. Ladas[2], A. Kapetanaki[1], H. Tzanatos-Exarchou[1], P. Founda[1], and A. Katsani[1]

[1] Nephrological Centre, and [2] Ophthalmologic Department, Athens University, Athens, Greece

Successful renal transplantation has a favourable effect on the development of ocular disorders in periodic haemodialysis patients [4]. Certain complications arise in the eyes of the recipients and are attributed mainly to the immunosuppressive medication [2, 3, 6].

The purpose of our study was the recording of the ocular complications in patients with successful renal transplants after long-term stabilization of renal function and immunosuppressive therapy.

Key words: Renal transplantation – Eye disease

Patients and methods

The study included 27 patients, 15 male and 12 female with ages ranging from 26 to 65 years (mean 44.85 ± 10.62), successfully transplanted 9–204 months (mean 85.66 ± 46.76) previously. Haemodialysis periods before transplantation were in the range 1–72 months (mean 26.43 ± 17.46). Serum creatinine ranged between 75 and 380 mol/l (mean 154.62 ± 85.10).

Of the 27 patients, 11 followed a triple and 16 a double immunosuppressive regimen with cortisone doses of 5–15 mg/day (mean 9.17 ± 2.97), azathioprine 50–150 mg/day (mean 95.37 ± 33.45) and cyclosporin A of 100–350 mg/day (mean 184.09 ± 69.99). Other therapy included 17 patients receiving beta-blockers, ten patients diuretics, eight patients Ca channel blockers and eight patients other antihypertensive medication such as clonidine and methyldopa.

The ocular examination consisted of: (1) visual acuity, (2) slit-lamp biomicroscopy, (3) examination of colour vision according to Ischihara, (4) fundus examination under pupil dilatation, (5) exophthalmometry according to Hertel, (6) Coldmann applantation tonometry, (7) Jone's Schirmer test, and (8) fluorescein fundus angiography.

Results

We noted that all renal transplant recipients had pathological ocular findings: five patients had one abnormal ocular finding, seven patients had two, six patients had three and nine patients four or more (Table 1).

Offprint requests to: Dimitris Koutsikos M.D., Aretaieon University Hospital, 76 Vas. Sofias Ave., 115–28 Athens, Greece

Discussion

All patients with successful renal transplants appear to have various pathological conditions of the eyes [4, 7, 8]. The posterior unilateral or bilateral subcapsular cataract that we observed in 74 % of the patients has been atributed to the use of corticosteroids [2, 6]. The same applies for the exophthalmos [4] that we observed in 29 % of the patients. The deposits of Ca^{2+} on the bulbar conjuctiva that occurred in eight patients (29 %) is probably related to secondary hyperparathyroidism [4, 5].

Two findings of this study are most interesting: the high rate of xerophthalmy (60 % of patients) and the uniform microaneurisms of the capillaries in six patients. Xerophthalmy has also been mentioned by other authors at high rates in transplant recipients, and can be attributed to the influence of the chronic use of antihypertensive and immunosuppressive drugs on the secretion of the lacrimal sac [8]. The microaneurisms that were detected by fluoroangiography in six patients have a uniform characteristic presentation in the perifoveal capillary network and retinal pigment epithelium which is different from the presentation in hypertension (Fig. 1). It is the first time that such findings have been described in transplant recipients or other patients and this is a subject of a further study.

Acknowledgements. Special thanks are due to Mrs. Jane Daekidou for secretarial assistance.

Table 1. Incidence of ocular findings in 27 renal transplant patients

Ocular complication	n	Percentage
Xerophthalmy	15/25	60
Calcium deposits in the conjuctival tissue	8/27	29
Posterior subcapsular cataract	20/27	74
Exophthalmos	7/24	29
Hypertensive fundus	9/24	33
Pigment epithelium disorders (drusen)	7/27	26
Findings from fluoroangiography	11/20	55

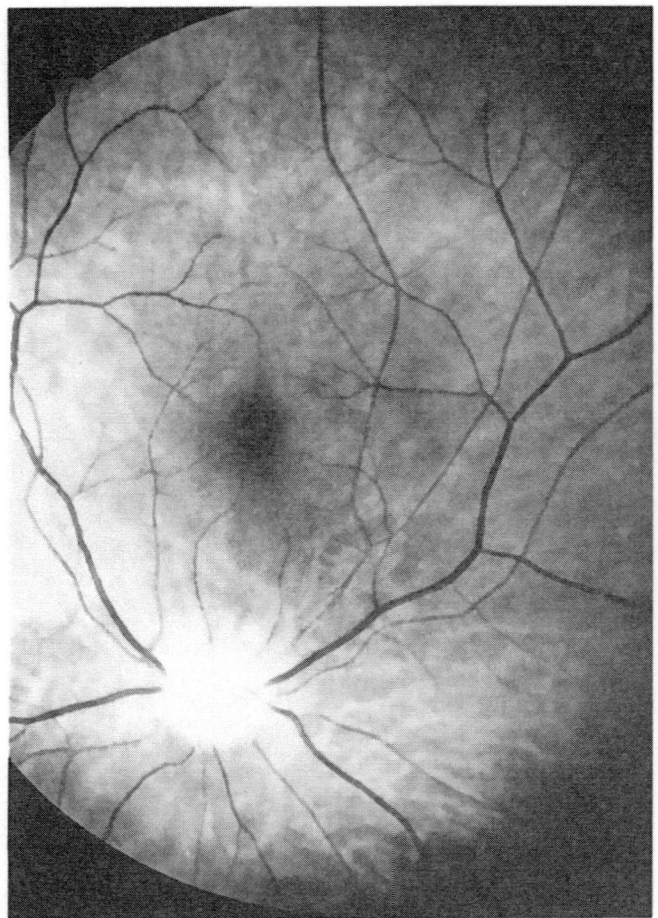

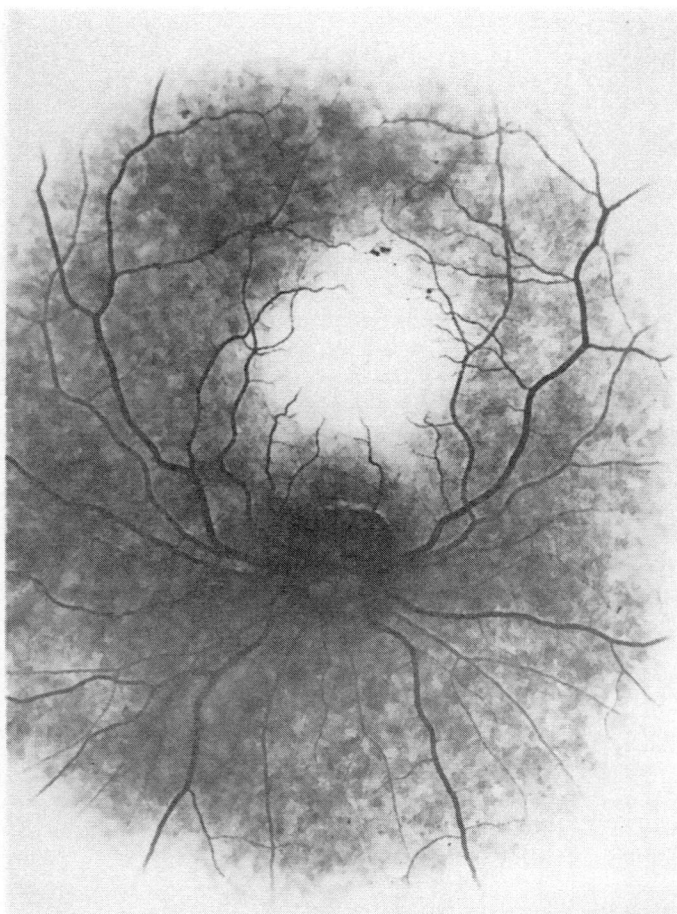

Fig. 1 a–c. Photographs showing the normal fundus (**a**) and microaneurisms in transplant recipients (**b, c**)

References

1. David DS, Berkowitz JS (1969) Lancet II: 149
2. Hovland KR, Ellis PhP (1967) Am J Ophthalmol 63: 283
3. Ker R, Zaruda K, Scheitlin W (1970) Ophthalmol Res 1: 21
4. Kopsa H, Bettelheim H, Gradmer G, Schindt P, Zazgornik J, Balcke P, Pils P (1978) 15th Congress of the EDTA, Proceedings, p 372
5. Perrin D, Vantelon J, Zingraff J (1966) Ann Oculist (Paris) 199: 771
6. Porter R, Crombie AL, Gardner PS, Vldall RP (1972) Br Med J 3: 133
7. Strempel I, Gruber A, Bittner K (1989) Klin Monatsbl Augenheilkd 195: 141
8. Vallino F, Santambrogio S, Elli A et al (1980) Minerva Chir 35: 735

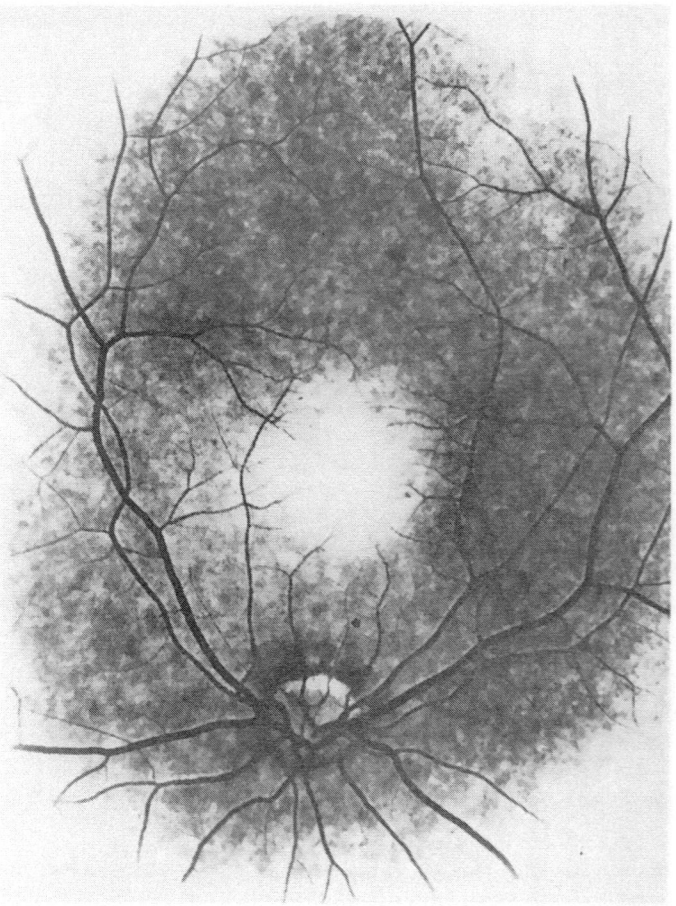

TRANSPLANT
International
© Springer-Verlag 1992

Influence of cyclosporin A (CyA) on renal handling of urate

R. Marcén, N. Gallego, L. Orofino, J. Sabater, J. Pascual, J. L. Teruel, F. Liaño, and J. Ortuño

Department of Nephrology, Hospital Ramón y Cajal, Madrid, Spain

Hyperuricaemia is a frequent side-effect of cyclosporin A (CyA) therapy in renal transplant patients [1, 5–7, 11], and gout arthritis is the cause of considerable morbidity among these patients [5, 7, 8, 10, 11]. However, neither the potential predisposing factors nor the mechanisms of hyperuricaemia have been clearly elucidated. It has been reported that hyperuricaemia in patients on CyA is associated with a lowered glomerular filtration rate, or with a reduced urate clearance [2, 5, 7, 8, 10], due to an increase in the net tubular urate reabsorption or to a decrease in secretion [2, 5]. These conclusions are mostly supported by measurements of the basal clearance rate and fractional excretion of urate, but more precise studies of renal handling of urate by the renal tubule have seldom been performed [2]. The purpose of our study was to investigate the prevalence of hyperuricaemia in our population of renal transplant patients, as well as the risk factors involved. Furthermore, we have evaluated the mechanism of hyperuricaemia by a combined pyrazinamide and probenecid test allowing a better evaluation of urate transport processes than pyrazinamide alone.

Key words: Renal transplantation – Urate excretion – Cyclosporin A

Patients and methods

For the hyperuricemia prevalence study, 169 renal transplant-patients were selected, all of whom had stable graft function and serum creatinine lower than 2 mg/dl. The group comprised 96 males and 73 females, with a mean age of 38 ± 12 years, 80 on azathioprine (Aza) and 89 on CyA. Patient records were reviewed and the following data collected at 12 months: serum and urine urea, creatinine and urate, serum potassium and total CO_2 and the drugs taken at this time. Hyperuricaemia was considered to be present when serum

Offprint requests to: R. Marcén, Servicio de Nefrología, Hospital Ramón y Cajal, Carretera de Colmenar Km. 9.100, 28034 Madrid, Spain

urate level was greater than 8 mg/dl in males and 6.5 mg/dl in females.

The renal handling of urate was studied by a combined pyrazinamide and probenecid test in 31 selected renal transplant patients. All had normal renal function, no clinical evidence of chronic rejection and no history of renal calculi, and none was receiving diuretics or other drugs that alter the synthesis or excretion of urate. The patients were divided into two groups: group 1 comprised ten hyperuricaemic patients on CyA, and group 2 (the control group) comprised 21 normouricaemic patients, (nine on CyA and 12 on Aza.

The combined pyrazinamide and probenecid test consisted of two parts. After two 30-min basal clearances, a single dose of probenecid (2 g) was given orally and four 30-min clearances performed. Pyrazinamide (3 g) was then administered orally, and four additional 30-min clearance studies were performed from 60 to 180 min after pyrazinamide. Maximal uricosuria in the 2 h after probenecid and minimal uricosuria in the 3 h after pyrazinamide were chosen to determine maximal probenecid-induced uricosuria and maximal pyrazinamide inhibition on probenecid-induced uricosuria, respectively. Venous blood samples were obtained at minutes 0, 90, 150, 270 and 330 of the test. Urate, creatinine, sodium and potassium were determined in all blood and urine samples. Adequate urine flow was ensured by the administration of 500 ml tap water 20 min before the test and additional amounts equal to the voided volume after every urine collection. Calculations were performed as previously described [3].

Results

The clinical features of the renal transplant patients at 1 year are shown in Table 1. Hyperuricaemia was more frequent in patients receiving CyA, as was the mean serum urate. Furthermore, there was some degree of graft dysfunction in patients on CyA; serum creatinine was slightly higher and the total CO_2 was lower than in patients on Aza. Ages, sex ratio and percentage of patients on diuretics were similar in both groups. In the hyperuricaemic patients there was no difference in the serum creatinine in relation to immunosuppressive treatment (1.4 ± 0.4 mg/dl) in both groups of patients. However, 16 out of 18 hyperuricaemic patients on Aza (88.9%), and only 31 out of 53 hyperuricaemic patients

Table 1. Clinical features of renal transplant patients according to immunosuppressive treatment

	Aza (n = 80)	CyA (n = 89)	P value
Sex (m/f)	51/29	45/44	NS
Age (yr)	38 ± 10	38 ± 13	NS
Serum urate (mg/dl)	6.1 ± 1.9	7.9 ± 1.9	< 0.001
Serum creatinine (mg/dl)	1.2 ± 0.3	1.4 ± 0.4	< 0.001
Serum total CO_2 (mEq/l)	25.5 ± 2.9	23.7 ± 2.8	< 0.001
No. of patients on diuretic (%)	39 (49)	36 (40)	NS
No. of patients with hyper-uricaemia (%)	18 (24)	59 (60)	< 0.001

Table 2. Results of the combined pyrazinamide–probenecid test

	Group 1 (n = 10)	Group 2 (n = 21)	P value
Sex (m/f)	5/5	14/7	NS
Age (yr)	35 ± 15	42 ± 11	NS
Serum creatinine (mg/dl)	1.3 ± 0.3	1.2 ± 0.2	NS
Serum urate (mg/dl)	8 ± 1.5	5.5 ± 1.3	< 0.001
FE urate (%)[a]	30 ± 13	46 ± 13	< 0.01
Urate secretion (% fl)	21 ± 9.2	32 ± 11.6	< 0.01
Presecretory reabsorption	91 ± 4.7	89 ± 4.9	NS
Postsecretory reabsorption/ secretion	113 ± 27	113 ± 19	NS

[a] During probenecid-induced uricosuria

on CyA (58.4%) were on diuretics ($P < 0.005$). When comparing the hyperuricaemic and normouricaemic patients on CyA, those with high serum urate had increased serum creatinine (1.4 ± 0.3 vs 1.2 ± 0.2 mg/dl, $P < 0.005$).

The pyrazinamide–probenecid test showed a lower fractional urate excretion (FE urate) during the maximal probenecid-induced uricosuria, and a lower urate secretion in hyperuricaemic patients (group 1). However, there were no differences in either the presecretory reabsorption or the postsecretory reabsorption, expressed as postsecretory reabsorption/secretion, between the two groups (Table 2). The lower FE urate in group 1 was associated with a lower urine volume (5.1 ± 2.8 vs 8.2 ± 3.6, $P < 0.05$), despite a similar water balance. Therefore, tubular urate secretion correlated with fractional sodium excretion ($r = 0.46, P < 0.05$).

Discussion

Our study confirms the high prevalence of hyperuricaemia among renal transplant patients on CyA, similar to that reported previously [1, 11]. Differences between our patient series and other series could be attributed to the selection of the patient population, to the definition of hyperuricaemia, or to the time when the study was carried out [6, 7]. We identified two risk factors associated with hyperuricaemia: renal dysfunction and treatment with diuretics. The higher serum creatinine and lower total serum CO_2 levels in patients on CyA would indicate that the existence of graft dysfunction could explain the higher prevalence of hyperuricaemia, as well as the differences in graft function, between normouricaemic and hyperuricaemic patients on CyA. However, a correlation between serum creatinine or creatinine clearance and serum urate levels has not always found, suggesting that renal failure is not the sole determinant of this rise in serum urate [1, 11]. Concerning the influence of diuretics on the development of hyperuricaemia, nearly 90% of patients on either Aza or CyA taking diuretics had high serum urate, but it should be noted that about 40% of hyperuricaemic patients on CyA were not receiving diuretics, and a direct effect of the CyA on urate metabolism could not be proved.

The mechanism causing hyperuricaemia remains uncertain. There is no increased endogenous production of urate [1, 5, 7], and most data support the notion that CyA decreases urate clearance by the kidney [2, 7, 8, 11]. Renal tubular handling of urate has four components: glomerular filtration, proximal tubular reabsorption, proximal tubular secretion and postsecretory reabsorption. CyA could induce hyperuricaemia by modifying several steps in urate excretion. The combined pyrazinamide–probenecid test shows that urate retention is mainly caused by a decrease in urate secretion in the renal tubule, as has been reported previously [2], and no abnormalities on reabsorption were detected. This finding could not be a consequence of renal insufficiency because both groups had the same degree of allograft function, but similar serum creatinine levels do not truly reflect similar renal function [9]. Furthermore, the decline in the glomerular filtration rate produces an adaptive decrease in urate presecretory and postsecretory reabsorption, and a later decrease in urate secretion [4]. The association of lower excretion of urate with a tendency to retain water and sodium by the kidney suggests that the impairment in urate secretion is linked to disorders in renal handling of water and sodium into the proximal tubule, probably mediated by haemodynamic changes induced by CyA.

References

1. Chapman JR, Griffiths D, Harding NGL, Morris PJ (1985) Reversibility of cyclosporine nephrotoxicity after three months treatment. Lancet I: 128–130
2. Chen SL, Boner G, Rosenfeld JB, Scmueli D, Sperling D, Yusim A, Todd-Pokroped A, Shapira Z (1987) The mechanism of hyperuricemia in cyclosporine treated renal transplant recipients. Transplant Proc 19: 1829–1830
3. Colussi G, Rambola G, De Ferrari ME, Rolando P, Surian M, Malberti F, Minetti L (1987) Pharmacological evaluation of urate handling in humans: pyrazinamide test vs combined pyrazinamide and probenecid administration. Nephrol Dial Transplant 2: 10–16

4. Garyfallos A, Magoul I, Tsapas G (1987) Evaluation of the renal mechanism for urate homeostasis in uremic patients by probenecid and pyrazinamide test. Nephron 46: 273–280

5. Hoyer PF, Lee IJ, Oemar BS, Krohn HP, Offner G, Brodehl J (1988) Renal handling of uric acid under cyclosporine A treatment. Pediatr Nephrol 2: 18–21

6. Leunissen KML, Bosman F, van Hooff JP (1985) Cyclosporine, uric acid and the kidney. Lancet I: 708

7. Lyn HY, Rocher LL, McQuillan MA, Schmaltz S, Palella TD, Fox IF (1989) Cyclosporine induced hyperuricemia and gout. New Engl J Med 321: 287–292

8. Noordzy TC, Leunissen KML, van Hoff JF (1990) Cyclosporine induced hyperuricemia and gout. New Engl J Med 322: 335

9. Ross EA, Wilkinson A, Hawkins RA, Danovich GM (1987) The plasma creatinine concentration is not an accurate reflection of the glomerular filtration rate in stable renal transplant patients receiving cyclosporine. Am J Kidney Dis 10: 113–117

10. Tiller DJ, Hall BM, Horvarth JS, Duggin GG, Thompson JF, Sheil AGR (1985) Gout and hyperuricemia in patients on cyclosporine and diuretics. Lancet I: 453

11. West C, Carpenter BJ, Hakale TR (1987) The incidence of gout in renal transplant patients. Am J Kidney Dis 10: 369–371

Transplant Int (1992) 5 [Suppl 1]: S 84–S 86

TRANSPLANT
International
© Springer-Verlag 1992

Erythrocytosis in renal allograft recipients.
Benefit of staggered venous erythropoietin measurements

D. Chevet[1], F. Michel[2], Ch. Mousson[1], Y. Tanter[1], J. M. Rebibou[1], N. Casadeval[3], and G. Rifle[1]

[1] Department of Nephrology-Reanimation, [2] Department of Urology, University Hospital, Dijon, France; and
[3] Hôpital Cochin, Paris, France

Abstract. Two adult renal allograft recipients experienced erythrocytosis – one in acute form – within 3 months of grafting. Involvement of well functioning transplanted kidneys was unlikely whereas staggered erythropoietin measurements detected a high gradient in front of venous remnant kidneys. Because of these results bilateral nephrectomy was performed, which cured polycythaemia. Multiple events leading to polycythaemia after renal transplantation are reviewed and diagnosis and therapeutic schedules are proposed.

Key words: Erythrocytosis – Renal transplantation – Erythropoietin – Erythrapheresis – Bilateral nephrectomy.

The appearance of erythrocytosis after kidney transplantation was first described by Nies et al. in 1965 [15]. It is thought to be a rare and usually temporary post-transplant complication. Nevertheless, recent extensive reviews have indicated an incidence ranging from 8.6 % [11] to 17.3 % [23], with a risk of thromboembolic events in 18 % of cases [23].

It is generally agreed that there are various causes of post-transplant polycythaemia. In 1979, Dagher et al. [7] drew attention to inappropriate production of erythropoietin (EPO) from native kidneys as a major contributing factor. Recently Aeberard et al. [1], Felle et al. [8], Qunibi et al. [18] and Garvin et al. [10] offered strong evidence for this cause–effect relationship in a majority of cases.

The recently-developed sensitive radioimmunoassay for EPO allows the localization of the site of exaggerated EPO production after selective catheterization of native or transplanted kidney veins.

Offprint requests to: Prof. D. Chevet, Service de Néphrologie-Réanimation, Hôpital du Bocage, 2bd de Lattre de Tassigny, 21034, Dijon, France

Case reports

Case 1

A 21-year-old female with Barraquer–Simons syndrome and dense deposits disease had been on maintenance haemodialysis for 1 year. She received rHEPO for 4 months. Then her blood haemoglobin level increased from 5.9 to 11.9 g/100 ml. Before treatment, blood EPO level was 7 mU/ml ($N < 22$ mU/ml). She underwent cadaveric renal transplantation in July 1989. Immunosuppressive therapy included ATG for 20 days, azathioprine and corticosteroids. Vasodilators and α-β blocking drugs were initiated for arterial hypertension (ABP, 170/110 mm Hg). Urine analyses were all normal, creatinine clearance was 77 ml/mn and haemoglobin level (Hb) 10.3 g/100 ml at the end of the first month. Two months later serum creatinine level (SCL) rose from 107 to 220 µmol/l. Transplant biopsy showed acute vascular rejection with interstitial haemorrhages. Cyclosporin A (4 mg/kg per day) was added to the previous regimen and SCL decreased to 164 µmol/l.

Within a 3-week period, facial erythrocytosis, headaches, epistaxis and hypertensive encephalopathy (ABP, 210/120 mm Hg) appeared. Hb was 19.6 g/100 ml and haematocrit value (Hct) 58 %. Leucocyte and thrombocyte counts were in the normal range. No hypoxaemia was detected. Clinical, laboratory and X-ray investigations excluded morphological abnormalities of the transplanted kidney, visceral neoplasm or lymphoproliferative disorder. Bone marrow examination showed 46 % of erythroblasts without cellular abnormality. Two erythrapheresis sessions dramatically improved consciousness state. However, 1 week later, Hb rose again from 12 to 16.5 g/100 ml. Blood EPO level was 94 mU/ml before blood removal. Figs. 1 and 2 show the results of staggered venous EPO measurements.

Because of the severity of the hypertensive crisis, the fast increase in Hb after erythrapheresis sessions and the strong evidence for remnant kidney EPO overproduction, bilateral native nephrectomy was performed. Light microscopic examination of these kidneys showed unidentifiable lesions. BP and Hb returned to normal values within 3 weeks without any antihypertensive drug. Two years later, BP was 130/80 mm Hg, Hb 12.9 g/100 ml, blood EPO level 8 mU/ml and SCL 96 µmol/l. In situ hybridization for human EPO mRNA in patient's kidneys was negative.

Case 2

A 46-year-old male patient underwent maintenance haemodialysis in July 1986 for idiopathic focal glomerulosclerosis. Initially uneventful renal cadaveric transplantation was carried out in January

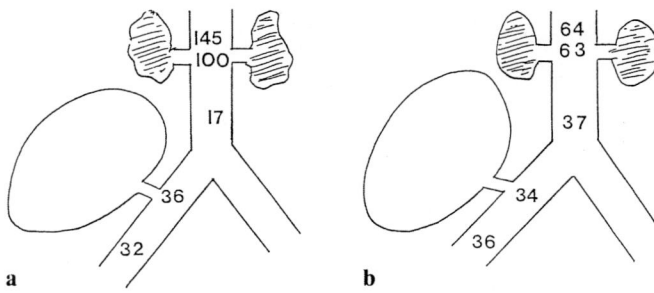

Fig. 1 a, b. Staggered erythropoietin levels (RIA control values 22 mU/ml). **a** case 1, 16 November 1989; **b** case 2, 22 November 1990

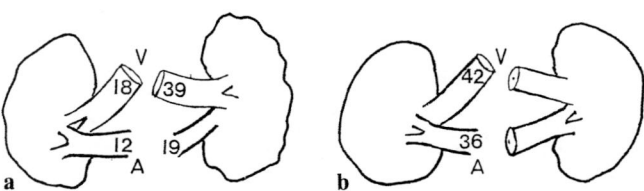

Fig. 2 a, b. EPO levels in arterial and venous samples taken during bilateral renal nephrectomy. Neither renal tumour nor cyst was found. **a** case 1; **b** case 2

1989. The immunosuppressive schedule included ATG (20 days), azathioprine and corticosteroids. Three months later, Hb reached 16.5 g/100 ml when SCL was 145 μmol/l. Chronic polycythaemia slowly progressed to a maximum of 19.1 g/100 ml with Hct 56.3%. The patient experienced mild symptoms such as headaches. Bone marrow aspirate showed 42% erythroblastic reaction and no malignant cells. Markers for haematological proliferative disease were all negative. This non-smoking patient did not have any respiratory disorder or haemoglobinopathy. Complete clinical and laboratory investigations excluded abnormalities of the transplanted kidney or at other sites of visceral neoplasm. Erythrocyte viscosity was 6.5 cP ($N < 4.5$). Blood EPO level was 38 mU/ml ($N < 7$ in matched controls) [20]. Immunosuppressive therapy was unchanged.

The patient was asymptomatic 1 year later except for facial erythrosis. Renal function and BP remained normal. On the other hand, Hb was still 18.8 g/100 ml. Isotopic ^{51}Cr red-cell mass was 53 ml/kg ($N = 42 + 2$). Staggered venous samplings in the iliac vein and vena cava showed an EPO gradient in front of native kidneys (Figs. 1 and 2). Bilateral nephrectomy was performed in November 1990. The weight of both kidneys was 30 g, and only a small cortical cyst was observed in the left one. Hb tapered to 12.6 g/100 ml quickly after surgery and remained in the normal range 1 year later. Post-operative blood EPO level was 14 mU/ml. In situ hybridization for EPO is still in progress.

Discussion

Various aetiological factors have been implicated in post-renal transplant erythrocytosis: acute and chronic rejection [14], transplant arterial stenosis [2], post-transplant hypertension [6], native kidney disease [23]. Other mechanisms have been proposed on theoretical or clinical grounds, including hydronephrosis, hepatic EPO production [13], pancreatic pseudocysts, resolution of hyperparathyroidism [3]. A drug-induced effect has been advocated such as contracted plasma volume by diuretics [16, 17], azathioprine [22] or cyclosporin therapy [5, 9, 21].

Usually, routine clinical and laboratory investigations permit an easy approach to such aetiological factors when the transplant is involved. In addition, the reversibility of the disorder after restoring the renal lesion when possible easily confirms the diagnosis. On the other hand, a successful renal transplantation can allow the appearance of a previously concealed polycythaemic syndrome. Such events can be observed in patients who smoke or in cases of chronic respiratory insufficiency, or sometimes in polycystic kidney disease, when the native kidneys were not removed before grafting. Polycythaemia can also be the first symptom of a myeloproliferative syndrome. Identification of such a syndrome does not pose particular difficulties. From a practical point of view, except in emergency circumstances as illustrated in case 1, measurement of red-cell mass remains, in all cases, an essential procedure before diagnosing a genuine erythrocytosis.

The recently available reliable estimation of EPO by radioimmunoassay or ELISA will certainly make it easier to recognize the cause of polycythaemia after renal transplantation. Indeed, a high level of circulating EPO demonstrates that EPO synthesis is no longer physiologically regulated. In the case of the kidneys, one can postulate that various lesions are able to generate local hypoxia which can stimulate secreting EPO target cells in the interstitium, probably located on peritubular capillary walls [19]. In transplanted erythrocytic patients, one of the main problems, in the absence of other causes, and when the graft is functioning well, is to localize the site of the hypersecretion: are the native kidneys or the grafted one involved? High levels of circulating EPO do not permit such a localization [8, 12, 18]. It was then logical to measure EPO levels in remnant and transplanted kidney veins [1, 7, 10]. We and others have observed a good correlation between the site of overproduction and recovery after surgery. Thus, it seems justified to recommend using this method before making any therapeutic decision. Human EPO mRNA was not identified by in situ hybridization in the removed kidneys (case 1). We have no clear-cut explanation for this failure, but technical reasons (late freezing of the specimens) could be concerned.

Historical and conventional therapy for post-transplant erythrocytosis still remains repeated phlebotomies for many months or years to maintain haematocrit at no more than 45%. Such a procedure avoids disabling symptoms such as headaches or water-induced pruritus, and above all protection from pulmonary embolism or cerebrovascular hazards, whose incidence has been emphasized [23]. This long-term protracted therapy is not always successful, as our case 1 demonstrates. Therefore, aetiological therapies are needed, which allow more constant and predictable results. When endogenous EPO overproduction by remnant kidneys is proved, surgical binephrectomy by a posterior procedure according to Gil-Vernet appears as the definitive therapy choice. Other promising methods include EPO-inhibiting drugs, as advocated for certain converting enzyme inhibitors or well demonstrated for theophylline [4].

References

1. Aeberhard JM, Schneider PA, Vallotton MB, Kurtz A, Leski M (1990) Multiple site estimates of erythropoietin and renin in polycythemic kidney transplant patients. Transplantation 50: 613–616
2. Bacon BR, Rothman SA, Ricanati ES, Rashad FA (1980) Renal artery stenosis with erythrocytosis after renal transplantation. Arch Intern Med 140: 1206–1211
3. Barbour GL (1979) Effect of parathyroidectomy on anemia in chronic renal failure. Arch Intern Med 139: 889–891
4. Barkis GL, Sauter ER, Hussey JL, Fischer JW, Gaber AO, Winsett R (1990) Effects of theophylline or erythropoietin production in normal subjects and in patients with erythrocytosis after renal transplantation. N Engl J Med 323: 86–90
5. Besaras A, Caro J, Jarrell B, Burke J, Francos G, Mallon E, Karsch R (1985) Effect of cyclosporine and delayed graft function on posttransplantation erythropiesis. Transplantation 40: 624–631
6. Curtis JJ (1986) Hypertension and kidney transplantation. Am J Kidney Dis 7: 181–196
7. Dagher JF, Ramos E, Erslev AJ, Alongi SV, Karmi SA, Caro J (1979) Are the native kidneys responsible for erythrocytosis in renal allorecipients? Transplantation 28: 496–498
8. Felle D, Tepavcevid P, Popov J, Vodopivec S, Djisalov M, Curie S, Soltes S, Mitie I, Bozi C, Ilie V (1990) Erythrocytosis following renal transplantation. XIth International Congress of Nephrology, Tokyo, 15–20 July (abstract 525 A)
9. Frassoni F, Bacigapupo A, Piaggio G, Podesta M, Marmont AM (1985) Effect of cyclosporin A on the in vitro growth of hematopoietic progenitors from normal marrow. Exp Hematol 13: 1084–1088
10. Garvin PJ, Reese JC, Lindsey L, Aridge DL, Domoto DT, Ballal S (1991) Bilateral nephrectomy for post-transplant erythrocytosis – Indications and results. Clin Transplant 5: 313–317
11. Heilmann E, Gottschalk D, Gottschalk I, Lison AE (1983) Studies in polycythemia after kidney transplantation. Clin Nephrol 20: 94–97
12. Lamperi S, Carozzi S, Icardi A (1984) Polycythemia is erythropoietin independent after renal transplantation? EDTA-ERA 21: 928–931
13. Meyrier A, Simon P, Boffa P, Brissot P (1981) Uremia and the liver. The liver and erythropoiesis. Nephron 29: 3–6
14. Nellans R, Otis P, Martin DC (1975) Polycythemia following renal transplantation. Urology 6: 158
15. Nies P, Cohn R, Schrier SL (1965) Erythremia after renal transplantation. N Engl J Med 273: 785
16. Obermiller LE, Tzamaloukas AH, Avasthi PS, Halpern JA, Sterling WA (1985) Decreased plasma volume in post transplant erythrocytosis. Clin Nephrol 23: 213–217
17. Pollack R, Maddox NS, Cohan J, Jacobson J (1988) Erythrocythemia following renal transplantation. Influence of diuretic therapy. Clin Nephrol 29: 119–122
18. Qunibi WY, Al Furayh O, Ginn HE, Barri Y, Nichols P, Duffy B, Sheth K, Taher S (1990) Post-transplant erythrocytosis. XIth International Congress of Nephrology, Tokyo, 15–20 July
19. Schuster SJ, Wilson JH, Erslev AJ, Caro J (1987) Physiologic regulation and tissue localization of renal erythropoietin messenger RNA. Blood 70: 316–318
20. Sun CH, Ward HJ, Paul WI, Koyle MA, Yanagawa N, Lee DBN (1989) Serum erythropoietin levels after renal transplantation. N Engl J Med 321: 151–157
21. Tschudi M, Landmann J, Brunner S, Thiel G (1987) Differences in the effect of azathioprine and cyclosporine on erythropoietin after renal transplantation (abstract). Kidney Int 32: 431
22. Webb DB, Price KA, Hutton RD, Newcombe RG, Salaman JR, Orchard J (1987) Polycythemia following renal transplantation: an association with azathioprine dosage? Am J Nephrol 7: 221–225
23. Wickre CG, Norman DJ, Bennison A, Barry JM, Bennett WM (1983) Post renal transplant erythrocytosis: a review of 53 patients. Kidney Int 23: 731–737

Transplant Int (1992)5 [Suppl 1]: S 87–S 92

TRANSPLANT
International
© Springer-Verlag 1992

In vitro FK506 kidney tubular cell toxicity

A. Moutabarrik[1], M. Ishibashi[1], H. Kameoka[1], N. Kawaguchi[1], Y. Takano[1], Y. Kokado[1], S. Onishi[1], T. Sonoda[1], S. Takahara[1], and A. Okuyama[1]

Departments of Urology[1], and Pathology, Osaka University, Osaka, Japan

Abstract. Nephrotoxicity is the most prominent side effect of the new immunosuppressive drug FK506. Some of the histopathological changes associated with cyclosporine (CyA) nephrotoxicity such as tubular vacuolization and glomerular thrombosis have also been reported with FK506 therapy. In this study we used kidney tubular cells in culture to address the issue of FK506- and CyA-induced tubular damage. Exposure of tubular cells to high concentrations of FK506 or CyA (10, 50 and 100 µM) induced a time- and dose-dependent cell injury in vitro characterized by a direct cytotoxic effect on tubular cells as expressed by release of ^{3}H-thymidine from prelabelled cells, N-acetyl-β-D-glucosaminidase (NAG) release and cell detachment. Ultrastructural changes (vacuolization, swelling and mitochondrial enlargement) and inhibition of the growth (DNA and RNA synthesis) of cultured tubular cells were also observed at high concentrations of FK506 and CyA. These concentrations are higher than those reached in clinical situations, but close to the concentrations that may be reached by FK506 or CyA in tissues. Low concentrations of FK506 and CyA (1, 0.1 and 0.01 µM) were not cytotoxic and induced only a minimal inhibitory effect on the growth of tubular cells in vitro. At the same concentration CyA induced more cell detachment, more NAG release and a stronger inhibitory effect on cell growth than FK506 ($P < 0.01$). Since an evident cytotoxic effect was observed only at high concentrations, we can speculate that tubular toxicity is due to the accumulation of drug in the cells inducing cell disruption and death.

Key words: FK506 – Cyclosporine – Kidney tubular cell – Drug toxicity

FK506 is a newly development immunosuppressive drug which has been used successfully in kidney [9] and liver transplantation [7]. Recently, a number of side effects

Offprint requests to: Michio Ishibashi, M. D., Department of Urology, Osaka University Medical School, Fukushima 1-1-50, Fukushima-Ku, Osaka 553, Japan

have been described. Nephrotoxicity appears to be the major adverse effect of this valuable immunosuppressive drug [6]. Some of the features commonly associated with cyclosporine (CyA) nephrotoxicity, such as tubular vacuolization and glomerular thrombosis, have also been observed in patients treated with FK506 [8]. The mechanism by which FK506 and CyA exert their tubular toxicity is not clear, but it has been suggested that the accumulation of the drugs in the cells causes delayed regeneration, morpological changes, and cell death [8]. In the present study, we report an in vitro assessment of kidney tubular cell sensitivity to FK506 compared with CyA, morphological changes induced in tubular cells treated with FK506, and the comparative effect of both these drugs on the growth of tubular cells in vitro.

Materials and methods

Preparation of tubular cells

The LLC-PK1 cell line was used in the present study. This porcine kidney tubular cell line has the characteristics of renal proximal tubular cells [5]. Tubular cells were cultured in medium M199 (Nissui Pharmaceutical Co. Ltd., Tokyo, Japan) supplemented with 10% fetal bovine serum (FBS) (Hyclone Laboratories Inc., Utah. USA). Cell subcultures were obtained by incubating a washed confluent tubular cell culture with a solution of 0.25% trypsin and 0.02% EDTA (Gibco) for 5 min at 37°C.

Drug preparations

FK506 (Fujisawa, Osaka, Japan) was dissolved in absolute methanol. CyA (Sandoz, Basel, Switzerland) was dissolved in absolute ethanol before being added to the media.

Morphometric examination and electron microscopy

Tubular cells were scraped off the culture dish with a rubber spatula and centrifuged at $300 \times g$ for 20 min. The cell pellets were fixed by immersion for 4 h at 4°C in 2.5% glutaraldehyde in 0.1 M cacodylate buffer (pH 7.4). After washing three times in cacodylate buffer, the samples were postfixed for 90 min in 1% osmium at 4°C, dehydrated through ascending grades of alcohol, and embedded in Epon.

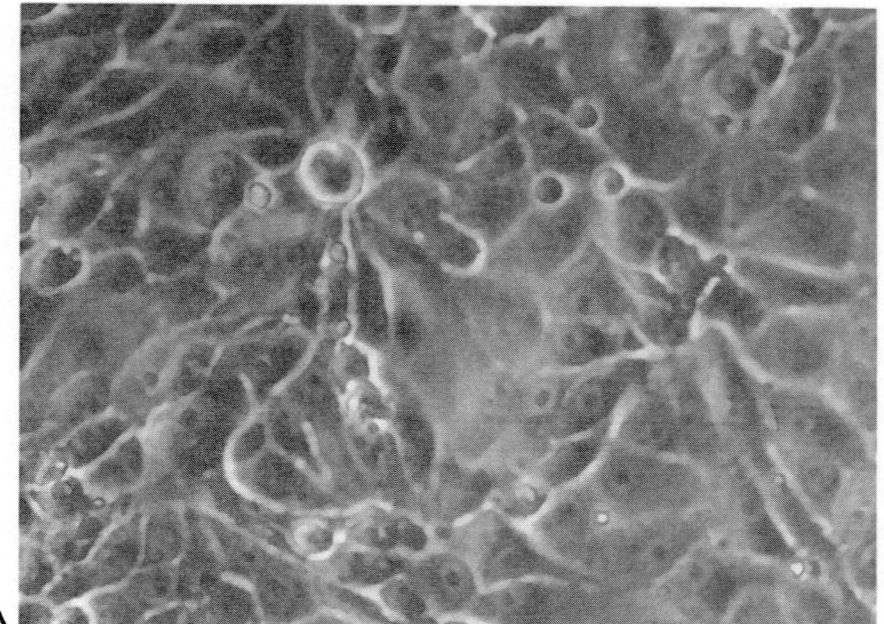

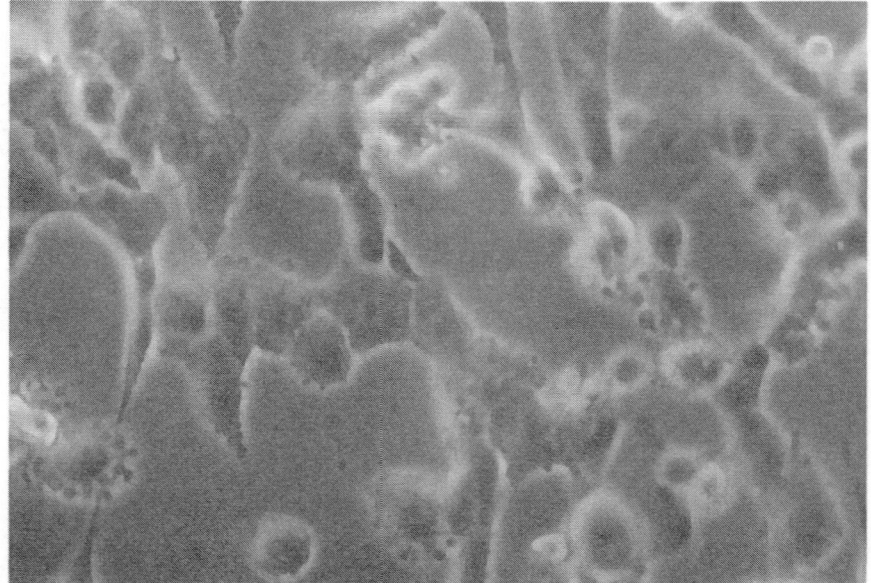

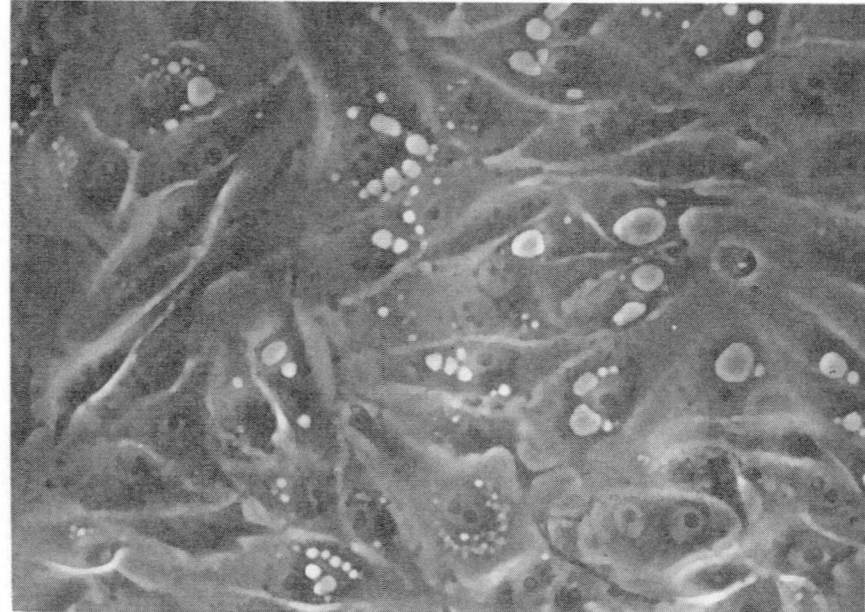

Fig. 1 A–C. FK506-induced cell detachment under light microscopy.
A cultured tubular cells were cultured with medium containing appropriate concentration of vehicle (methanol).
B Tubular cells were cultured with 50 μ*M* FK506 for 5 h. Cell detachment is clearly visible.
C Tubular cells were cultured with 10 μ*M* FK506 for 24 h. Many cells show vacuoles of different sizes

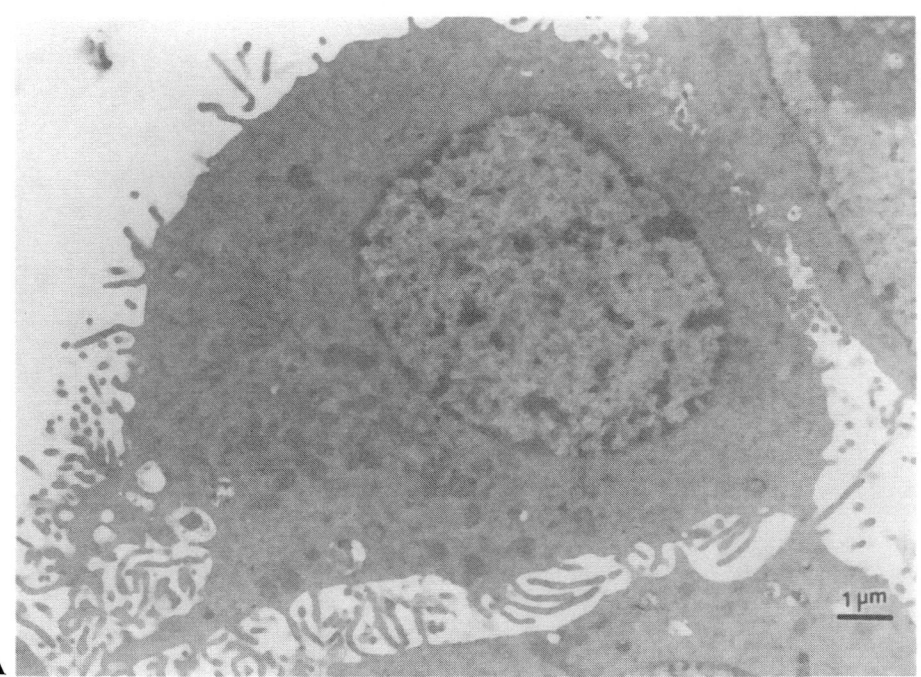

A

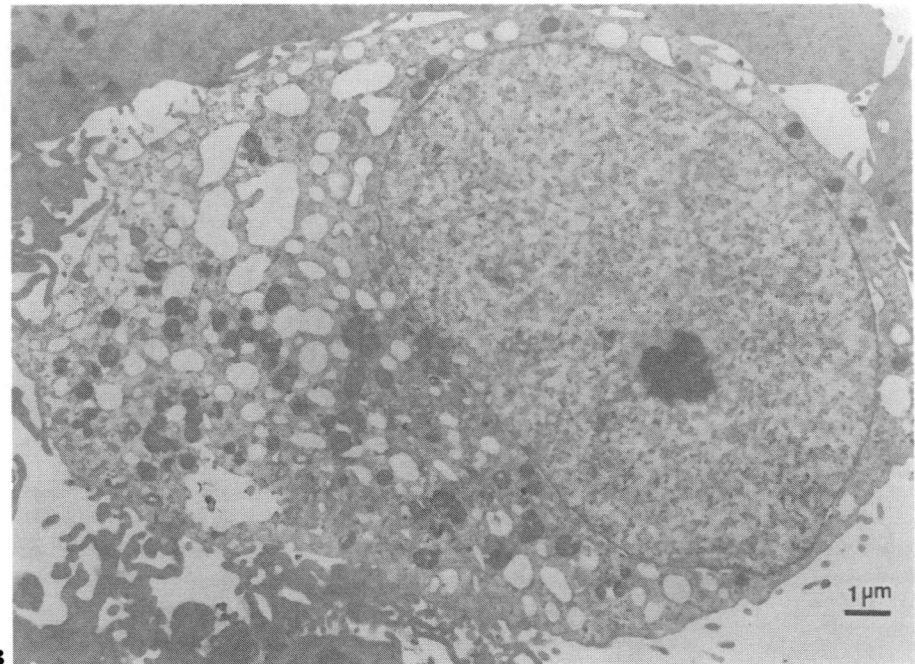

B

Fig. 2 A, B. Ultrastructural changes in tubular cells (LLC-PK1 cell line) exposed to FK506.
A cells incubated with the culture medium containing appropriate concentration of the vehicle.
B cells incubated with 10 μ*M* FK506 for 24 h. Swelling and vacuolization are clearly visible

Semithin (0.5 μm) sections were stained with 1 % toluidine blue. Ultrathin (70–80 nm) sections were examined with uranyl acetate and lead citrate staining in a Hitachi H-7000 electron microscope.

Cell detachment assay

This was determined by direct counting of adherent cells as described previously [10]. Briefly, tubular cells (10^5 cells/cm^2) were plated in 35-mm diameter plastic multiwells in complete medium and were allowed to adhere until confluence was reached. Then the cells were incubated with different concentrations of FK506 or CyA for 4, 10 and 24 h. The vehicle alone served as control. Cell counts were determined by haemocytometer after harvesting the adherent cells with trypsin-EDTA. The data are expressed as percentage of detachment: (number of cells cultured in the presence of appropriate vehicle − number of cells cultured in the presence of test drugs)

× 100/number of cells cultured in the presence of appropriate vehicle).

Drug cytotoxicity assay

This was performed as described previously [4]. Confluent monolayers of tubular cells grown in 24-well plates (Falcon, Oxnard, Calif., USA) were incubated with ^{3}H-thymidine (0.5 μCi/ml of ^{3}H-thymidine) (New England Nuclear, Boston, Mass., USA) in complete medium for 48 h. At the end of the incubation period, radioactive medium was discarded and radiolabelled cells were washed five times with medium. The cells were then incubated for 72 h with different concentrations of FK506 or CyA. ^{3}H-Thymidine-labelled tubular cells incubated with medium alone served as controls. Maximal release was assayed by lysing labelled cells with 0.5 *N* NaOH. After 72 h of incubation, radioactivity of the supernatants was

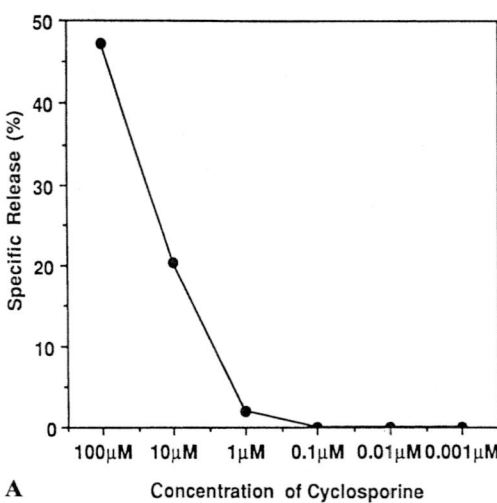

A

CYCLOSPORINE- INDUCED CYTOTOXICITY
IN CULTURED TUBULAR CELLS

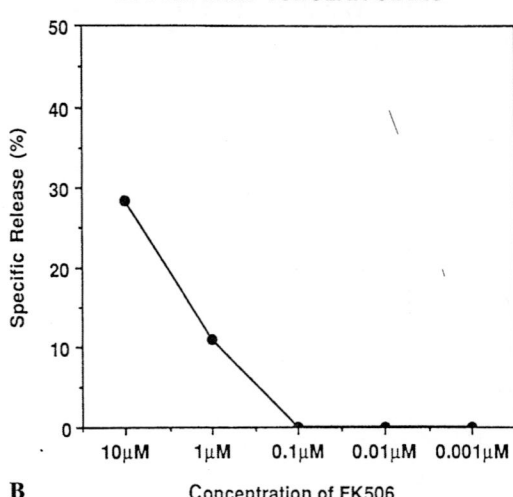

B

FK506 INDUCED CYTOTOXICITY
IN CULTURED TUBULAR CELLS

Fig. 3 A, B. FK506 and CyA induced cytotoxicity. Confluent tubular cells were labelled with ^{3}H-thymidine, thereafter cells were incubated for 72 h with different concentrations of FK506 or CyA. After the end of the period of incubation, radioactivity of the supernatants was measured. Spontaneous release was obtained from the vehicle alone. The maximal release was assayed by lysing cells with 0.5 N NaOH

measured using a liquid scintillation counter (Packard Instruments, Osaka, Japan). The percentage of specific release was calculated as $(E-S) \times 100/(M-S)$, where E is drug-induced release, S is spontaneous release and M is maximal release.

N-Acetyl-β-D-glucosaminidase (NAG) determination

The supernatants from monolayer tubular cells treated with different concentrations of FK506, CyA or appropriate vehicle for 10, 24 and 48 h were assayed for NAG using the *m*-cresolsuphonphthaeinyl-*N*-β-glucosaminidase method (Shionogi NAG assay kit, Shionogi, Osaka, Japan).

DNA and RNA synthesis

Solution (200 µl) containing cells at a concentration of 10^5 cells/ml were grown on a 96-well tissue culture plate (Falcon, Oxnard, Calif., USA) for 24 h in the presence of various concentrations of FK506, CyA or vehicle. The cells were then pulsed with 1 µCi of ^{3}H-thymidine or ^{3}H-uridine (specific activity 25 µCi/mmol and 27 Ci/mmol, respectively) (New England Nuclear, Boston, Mass., USA) for 16 h. Prior to harvesting, the cells were detached using a solution containing 0.05 % trypsin in 0.5 mmol EDTA (Gibco) in PBS and harvested onto filter paper with a plate microharvester (LKB, Wallace Cell Harvester, Pharmacia). The filters were dried and the cells redissolved in 8 ml of scintillation liquid (LKB Scintillation Products, UK) and counted using a beta plate counter (LKB Wallace, Pharmacia, Finland). Results are the mean of three experiments. The data are expressed as percentage of inhibition $= [1 - (\text{cpm B/cpm A})] \times 100$, where cpm A represents the cpm of cells cultured in the presence of appropriate vehicle, and cpm B respresents the cpm of cells cultured in the presence of test drugs.

Results

Cell detachment and ultrastructural changes

Cell detachment was found to be an early marker of FK506- and CyA-mediated tubular toxicity. As early as 5 h after exposure to the highest concentrations of FK506 or CyA (100, 50 and 10 µM), tubular cell detachment was clearly visible under the phase contrast microscope (Fig. 1 B). Table 1 shows the data obtained after 5, 10 and 24 h of incubation of tubular cells with three different concentrations of FK506 or CyA. FK506 or CyA at a concentration of 1 µM did not induce cell detachment independently of the incubation time, but with FK506 or CyA at 10 µM and 50 µM the percentage of cells detached was higher and was increased by prolonging the incubation time. At the same concentration CyA seemed to induce more cell detachment than FK506 ($P < 0.01$).

The most prominent change observed by light microscopy after 24 h treatment with FK506 in non-detached cells was vacuolization. The vacuoles were of different sizes (Fig. 1 C). Profound morphological changes were detectable under the electron microscope after 24 h of tubular cell exposure to FK506 (Fig. 2). These changes included obvious signs of injury with changes in cell shape, membrane cellular irregularity, enlargement of the smooth endoplasmic reticulum, vacuolization and lamellar bodies. Mitochondrial enlargement was observed only at concentrations of 50 and 100 µM of FK506 or CyA (data not shown).

FK506- and cyclosporine-induced cytotoxicity and NAG release

Release of ^{3}H-thymidine by prelabelled cells after exposure to FK506 or CyA was used as a marker of cell disruption. FK506 and CyA induced a dose-dependent release of ^{3}H-thymidine from tubular cells (Fig. 3). After 72 h, cells that were prelabelled with ^{3}H-thymidine and incubated with FK506 doses higher than 0.1 µM released more thymidine than the control monolayer. The specific release induced by 1 µM was 10 %, and 10 µM-induced specific release was around 30 %. FK506 doses less than

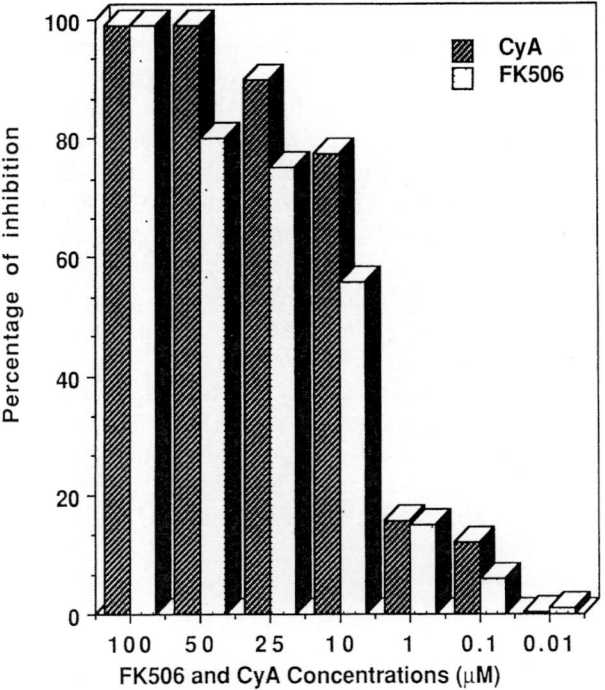

DNA SYNTHESIS INHIBITION BY FK506 AND
CYA IN CULTURED TUBULAR CELLS

Fig. 4. DNA synthesis inhibition by FK506 and CyA in cultured tubular cells. Cells were incubated with FK506, CyA or vehicle for 24 h. At the end of incubation, the cells were pulsed with 1 µC of ^{3}H-thymidine for 16 h

tion CyA had significantly more inhibitory effect on DNA and RNA synthesis than FK506 ($P < 0.01$).

Discussion

Our results show that FK506 and CyA at high doses exert a direct cytotoxic effect on tubular cells, induce ultrastructural changes and strongly inhibit cell growth in vitro. These doses are higher than those reached in plasma in clinical transplantation, but close to the tissue concentrations reached by CyA in the kidney [1]. There is no report available concerning the concentration of FK506 in the tissue but it is not unexpected that FK506, in view of its lipophilic nature, may reach concentrations higher than those in blood and plasma.

An early expression of FK506 and CyA cytotoxic effect seems to be cell detachment. In the first 5 h of exposure of cultured cells to high doses of FK506 or CyA, a high percentage of detached cells was observed. During the same incubation period, at high concentrations of FK506 or CyA, NAG release was very low (data not shown), indicating that the loss of adhesion properties of the cells was not simply a consequence of cell death. These results are consistent with those of Zoja et al. [11] who found that CyA mediated endothelial cell injury by inducing initially cell detachment and subsequently cell lysis. The electron microscope demonstrated non-specific cytoplasmic vacuolations with FK506 treatment. These ultrastructural

0.1 µM (0.01 and 0.001 µM) were not cytotoxic. CyA at 1 µM showed a specific release of 1–5 %, and 10 µM-induced specific release was about 20 %. Doses of CyA less than 0.1 µM) were not cytotoxic. The FK506- and CyA-induced cytotoxicity were not significantly different.

We used NAG release as a specific marker of tubular cell injury. NAG release from tubular cells incubated with FK506 at 10 µM and 1 µM, and CyA at 1 µM for 10, 24 and 48 h was not different from the control (Table 2). In contrast high concentrations of FK506 and CyA (50 µM) induced a significant release of NAG from treated tubular cells at 10, 24 and 48 h ($P < 0.01$), whereas CyA at 10 µM significantly increased NAG release only after 48 h (Table 2). At the same concentration CyA seemed to induce more NAG release than FK506 ($P < 0.01$).

Effect of FK506 and cyclosporine on tubular cell growth

The uptake of ^{3}H-thymidine and ^{3}H-uridine by cultured tubular cells is a marker of cell growth in vitro. A significant dose-related inhibition of DNA synthesis was observed at FK506 or CyA concentrations higher than 1 µM. FK506 and CyA concentrations below 1 µM had only a minimal inhibitory effect (less than 25 %) (Fig. 4).

FK506 and CyA produced a dose-dependent inhibition of RNA synthesis in tubular cells at concentrations higher than 1 µM. Below this concentration the inhibition was modest (less than 20 %) (Fig. 5). At the same concentra-

Table 1. Effect of FK506 and CyA on tubular cell detachment. After reaching confluency the cells were exposed to various concentrations of FK506 and CyA for 4, 10, and 24 h. The remaining cells were then detached with trypsin and counted using a haemocytometer

	cell detachment (%) Incubation time (hours)		
	5	10	24
FK506 50 µM	25	47.5	70
FK506 10 µM	1.2	0.8	20
FK506 1 µM	0.5	0.6	1.0
CyA 50 µM	57.5*	65*	80
CyA 10 µM	0.1	7.5	27.4
CyA 1 µM	0.2	0.0	0.4

* $P < 0.01$ CyA vs. FK506 at the same concentration

Table 2. Kinetics of NAG release from tubular cells treated with FK506 or CyA. Supernatants harvested from cultured tubular cells treated with different concentrations of FK506 or CyA for 10, 24 and 48 h were assayed for NAG

	NAG release Incubation time (h)		
	10	24	48
Control	1.704 ± 0.10	2.41 ± 0.02	4.640 ± 0.19
CyA 50 µM	5.59 ± 0.34*	6.879 ± 0.27*	9.39 ± 0.81*
CyA 10 µM	1.6 ± 0.038	2.403 ± 0.15	5.45 ± 0.09*
CyA 1 µM	1.4 ± 0.002	2.308 ± 0.01	4.28 ± 0.01
FK506 50 µM	4.31 ± 0.36*	4.7826 ± 0.03	6.059 ± 0.4*
FK506 10 µM	1.68 ± 0.09	2.41 ± 0.13	4.27 ± 0.2
FK506 1 µM	1.82 ± 0.02	2.59 ± 0.12	4.69 ± 0.3

* $P < 0.01$ vs. control

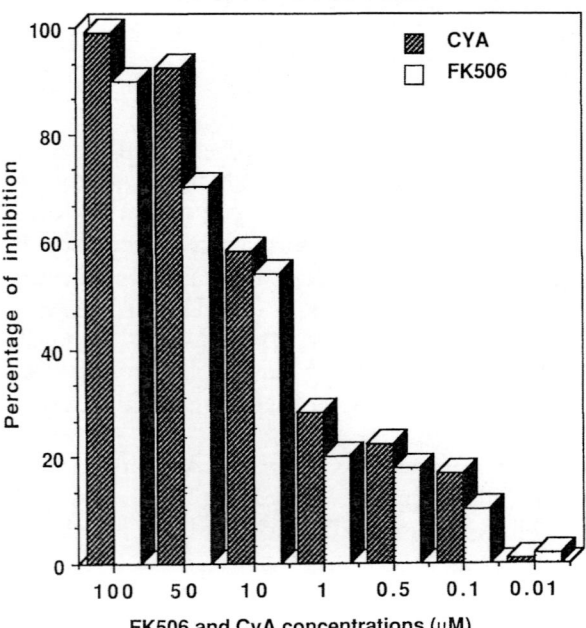

Fig. 5. RNA synthesis inhibition by FK506 and CyA in cultured tubular cells. Cells were incubated with FK506, CyA or vehicle for 24 h. At the end of incubation, the cells were pulsed with 1 µC of ^{3}H-uridine for 16 h

changes corresponded to the cytoplasmic vacuolations visible on light microscopy. The cytoplasmic vacuolization, mitochondrial enlargement and cell swelling induced by FK506 in tubular cells in vitro were similar to the effects reported for CyA treatment [8].

We have assessed the cytolytic effect of FK506 compared with CyA as expressed by ^{3}H-thymidine release from prelabelled cells and NAG release. It appeared that low concentrations of FK506 and CyA (1, 0.1 and 0.01 µM) were without cytotoxic effect. In contrast, high concentrations of FK506 and CyA (100, 50 and 10 µM) were cytotoxic. Zoja et al. [11] also reported that high concentrations of CyA (10 and 50 µM) induced a significant release of ^{51}Cr and lactate dehydrogenase from cultured endothelial cells. The effect of 10 µM and 50 µM seems to be specific to tubular cells since we have observed that cell detachment and cell death in confluent culture of human mesangial cells can be seen only when the concentration of FK506 and CyA is increased to 100 µM (unpublished data).

Our data agree with those of Cole et al. [2], who observed a significant inhibition of DNA and RNA synthesis in both tubular cells and mesangial cells with CyA concentrations higher than 1 µM. The means by which FK506 or CyA exert tubular toxicity remain uncertain. Since significant cytolysis, morphological changes, and delayed growth were observed in vitro only at high concentrations

of FK506, we can speculate as suggested by Mihatsch and Ryffel [8] in CyA toxicity, that at pharmacological doses (below 1 µM) FK506 binds to its binding protein FKBP and inhibits specifically induced gene transcription in lymphoid cells. At these concentrations there is no general inhibition of tubular cell proliferation or protein synthesis. At higher concentrations, the FKBP might be saturated and FK506 may be bound to non-saturable membrane proteins, thus accumulating in the membrane and disrupting membrane function. This accumulation of FK506 may occur not only in the surface membrane but also in the endoplasmic reticulum, mitochondria and Golgi apparatus. Concomitantly, tubular cell proliferation and protein synthesis are inhibited and cellular changes are apparent.

Further studies are required to determine the subcellular basis of FK506 nephrotoxicity and to understand why the kidney is the main target of toxicity. We conclude that, at high concentrations, FK506 and CyA induce cytolysis and morphological changes, and inhibit cell growth. At established therapeutic levels, FK506 and CyA are not cytotoxic in vitro.

References

1. Atkinson K, Biggs JC, Britton K (1982) Distribution and persistence of cyclosporin in human tissues. Lancet II: 1165–1170
2. Cole E, Skorecki K, Cheung F, Wong PY, Fung LS, Levy GA (1988) Cyclosporine A in contrast to cyclosporine metabolite (OL-17) specifically inhibits growth of renal cells in culture. In: Kahan BD (ed) Cyclosporine: therapeutic use in clinical transplantation. Grune & Stratton, London, pp 732–737
3. Demetris AJ, Banner B, Fung J, Shapiro R, Jordan M, Starzl TE (1991) Histopathology of human renal allograft rejection under FK506. Transplant Proc 23: 944–946
4. Hruby ZW, Cybulsky AV, Lowry RP (1990) Effect of tumor necrosis factor on glomerular mesangial cells and epithelial cells. Nephron 56: 410–413
5. Hull RN, Cherry WR, Weaver GW (1976) The origins of a pig kidney cell strain. In Vitro 12: 670–673
6. Ishibashi M (for the Japanese study group) (1991) Japanese study of FK506 in kidney transplantation: Results of early phase II study. Transplant Proc (in press)
7. Jain AB, Fung J, Todo S, Alessiani M, Takaya S, Abu-Elmagd K, Tzakis A, Starzl TE (1991) Incidence and treatment of rejection episodes in primary orthotopic liver transplantation. Transplant Proc 23: 928–930
8. Mihatsch MJ, Ryffel B (1990) Evolution of cyclosporine nephrotoxicity. In: Hatano M (ed) Proceedings of the XIth International Congress of Nephrology. Springer Verlag, Tokyo Berlin Heidelberg New York London Paris Hong Kong Barcelona, pp 576–588
9. Shapiro R, Jordan M, Fung J, McCauly J, Johnston J, Iwaki Y, Tzakis A, Hakala T, Todo S, Starzl TE (1991) Kidney transplantation under FK506. Transplant Proc 23: 920–923
10. Wall RT, Harlan JM, Harker LA, Striker GE (1980) Homocysteine-induced endothelial cell injury in vitro: a model for the study of vascular injury. Thromb Res 18: 113–117
11. Zoja C, Furci L, Ghilardi F, Zilio P, Benigni A, Remuzzi G (1986) Cyclosporin-induced endothelial cell injury. Lab Invest 55: 455–462

Transplant Int (1992)5 [Suppl 1]: S 93–S 97

TRANSPLANT
International
© Springer-Verlag 1992

FK506 mechanism of nephrotoxicity: stimulatory effect on endothelin secretion by cultured kidney cells

A. Moutabarrik[1], M. Ishibashi[1], M. Fukunaga[2], H. Kameoka[1], Y. Takano[1], Y. Kokado[1], T. Sonoda[1], S. Takahara[1], and A. Okuyama[1]

[1] Department of Urology and [2] the First Department of Internal Medicine, Osaka University Hospital, Osaka, Japan

Abstract. The administration of FK506 or cyclosporin A (CyA) to animals and humans induces a decrease in glomerular filtration rate and renal plasma flow and an increase in renal vascular resistance. Endothelins (ET-1), very powerful renal vasoconstrictors, are involved in CyA-related alteration in renal haemodynamics. In this study we sought to determine whether FK506 and CyA had a stimulatory effect on endothelin secretion by cultured kidney cells (tubular and mesangial cells) and whether this stimulatory effect coincided with an increase in ET-1 serum level in FK506- and CyA-treated rats. FK506 concentrations of 1, 0.1, 0.01 and 0.001 μM significantly stimulated ET-1 secretion by cultured tubular and mesangial cells. CyA at 10, 1, 0.1 and 0.01 μM also exerted an enhancing effect on ET-1 secretion in cultured tubular cells whereas CyA only at 10 and 1 μM had a stimulatory effect on ET-1 secretion by human mesangial cells. We observed that the concentrations of CyA that induced the most substantial enhancing effect were 10 or 100 times higher than those required for FK506 to produce the same effect. The concentrations of FK506 or CyA which induced ET-1 secretion by tubular cells and kidney cells were not cytolytic as assessed by N-acetyl-β-D-glucosaminidase (NAG) release and lactic dehydrogenase (LDH) release. FK506 or CyA treatment at toxic doses induced an increase in serum level of ET-1 in treated rats. We conclude that FK506 and CyA induced an increase in the synthesis of endothelin in the kidney which may explain the increase in circulating ET-1. This stimulatory effect may contribute to the genesis of haemodynamic preturbations associated with FK506 and CyA.

Key words: FK506 – Cyclosporine – Endothelin – Mesangial cell – Kidney tubular cell

FK506 is a newly developed immunosuppressive drug which has been used successfully in clinical transplanta-

tion [4, 13]. Among its recognized side effects, nephrotoxicity is the most prominent [3]. Its molecular structure is unrelated to cyclosporin A (CyA), but both agents have similar pharmacological effects and may possibly have the same toxicity. It has been reported that FK506 decreases the glomerular filtration rate (GFR) and renal plasma flow (RFP) and increases renal vascular resistance in humans [19] and in rats [7] treated with FK506. These reversible haemodynamic perturbations that have also been observed in CyA nephrotoxicity, have been linked to the renin angiotensin, adrenergic systems, and thromboxane A2 [8, 11]. Endothelin (ET), a peptide isolated from supernatants of cultured porcine aortic endothelial cells is a very powerful renal vasoconstrictor [20]. ET is ten times more potent than angiotensin II, vasopressin, or neuropeptide Y, making it the most potent endogenous vasoactive substance known [20]. ET appears to have a pivotal role in the pathophysiology of CyA-induced acute renal vasoconstriction and glomerular dysfunction [5]. Renal cell lines and mesangial cells physiologically express mRNA for endothelin and secrete this peptide in the supernatant [14, 21]. In this study we demonstrated that FK506 and CyA have a stimulatory effect on endothelin secretion by kidney cells and this effect coincided with a significant rise in the serum level of ET-1 in FK506- and CyA-treated rats. This finding may contribute to the clarification of the mechanism of FK506- and CyA-induced vasoconstriction and glomerular dysfunction.

Materials and methods

Cell isolation and culture

The LLC-PK1 tubular cell line was used in the present study. This porcine kidney tubular cell line has the characteristics of renal proximal tubular cells [2]. Tubular cells were cultured in medium M199 (Nissui Pharmaceutical Ltd., Tokyo, Japan) with 10% fetal bovine serum (FBS) (Hyclone Laboratories Inc., Utah, USA). Cell subcultures were obtained by incubating a washed confluent tubular cells culture with a solution of 0.25% trypsin and 0.02% EDTA (Gibco) for 5 min at 37 °C.

Offprint requests to: Michio Ishibashi. M.D., Osaka University Hospital, Fukushima 1-1-50, Fukushima-ku, Osaka 553, Japan

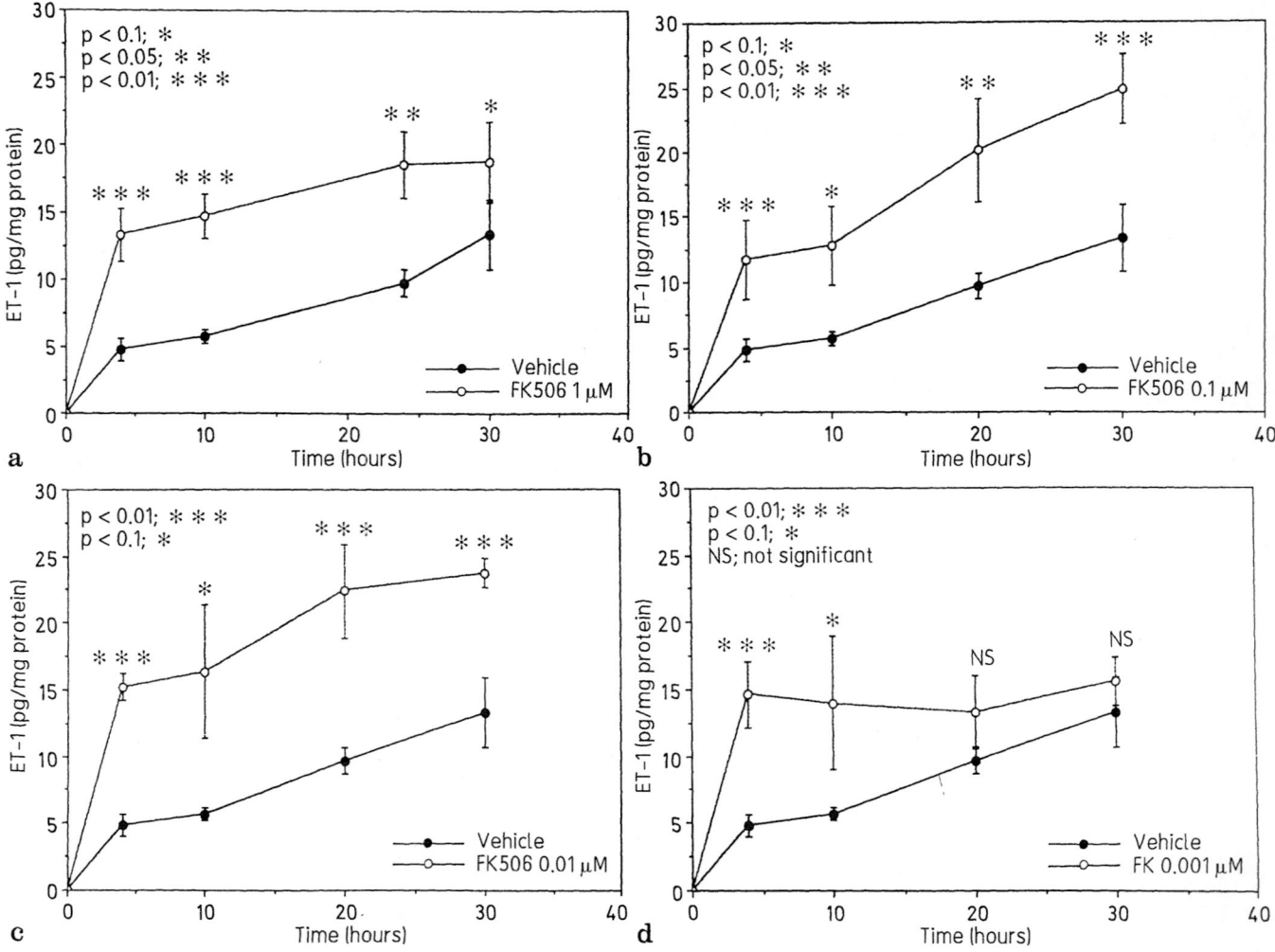

Fig. 1. Kinetics of endothelin production by cultured human tubular cells treated with FK506. Monolayers of tubular cells were incubated with medium containing FK506 at concentrations of 1, 0.1, 0.01 and 0.001 μM. The vehicle alone served as control. The supernatants were harvested at 4, 10, 20 and 30 h and assayed for ET-1

The culture of human mesangial cells (HMC) was performed as previously described [17]. Briefly, glomeruli were isolated from pieces of nephrectomised kidneys and searched for renal cell carcinoma by a consecutive sieving method. Then the glomeruli were seeded onto 10-cm culture dishes (Becton Dickinson, Oxnard, Calif.) and cultured at 37 °C in an atmosphere of 95 % air and 5 % CO_2 using a tissue culture medium RPMI-1640 supplemented with 20 % FBS. HMC between the third passage and the fourth passage were used in this study.

Drug preparations

FK506 (Fujisawa, Osaka, Japan) was dissolved in absolute methanol. CyA (Sandoz, Basel, Switzerland) was dissolved in absolute ethanol before being added to the media.

Animal drug administration

Male Lewis rats weighing 100–120 g were used. FK506 dissolved in 5 % arabic gum solution was administered by gastric gavage at a dose of 5 mg/kg per day. CyA also dissolved in arabic gum was administered by the same procedure at a dose of 20 mg/kg per day. The control rats received the vehicle alone. Each group consisted of five rats. After 12 days administration, the rats' sera were analysed for ET-1.

Sandwich enzyme immunoassay (EIA) for the detection of ET-1

Since human, porcine and rat ET-1 are identical [20], this assay can be used for detection of ET-1 from the three species. After reaching confluence, the tubular cells were fed with M199 10 % FBS and HMC with RPMI 20 % FBS, containing various concentrations of FK506 or CyA. The final methanol or ethanol concentration for all concentrations of FK506 or CyA and vehicle was 0.2 %. The media were collected at 4, 10, 24, 30, 48 and 72 h and analysed for ET-1. The EIA was performed as descibed previously [16]. Briefly, mouse anti-ET-1 monoclonal antibody-coated microtest plates were prepared by adding 100 μl of the monoclonal antibody AwETN40 (20 μg/ml) (kindly provided by Dr. N. Suzuki, Tsukuba Research Laboratory, Takeda Chemical Industries, Japan) to each well, followed by the addition of 300 μl of Block Ace (Snow Brand Milk Product Co., Japan) diluted four times with PBS. ET-1 standards or samples to be tested in 100 μl buffer D (0.02 M phosphate buffer, pH 7, containing 10 % Block Ace, 0.4 M NaCl, and 2 mM EDTA) were added to each well and incubated at 4 °C for 1 day. After being washed with PBS, the plate was reacted with 100 μl anti-endothelin Fab'-horseradish peroxidase (provided by Dr. N. Suzuki) at a dilution of 1/400 in buffer C (buffer containing 50 μM 0.02 M phosphate buffer, pH 7, 1 % bovine serum albumin, with 0.4 M NaCl and 2 mM EDTA) at 4 °C for 1 day. After washing with PBS the bound enzyme activity was measured using o-phenylenediamine as chromogen. The data were analysed by expressing ET-1 production on the basis of total amount of cell protein.

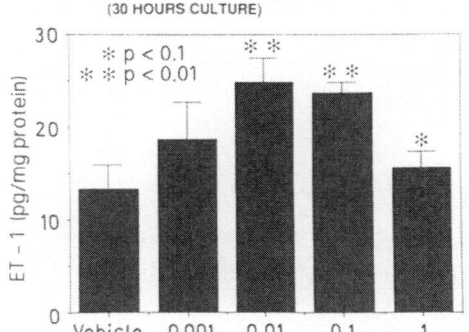

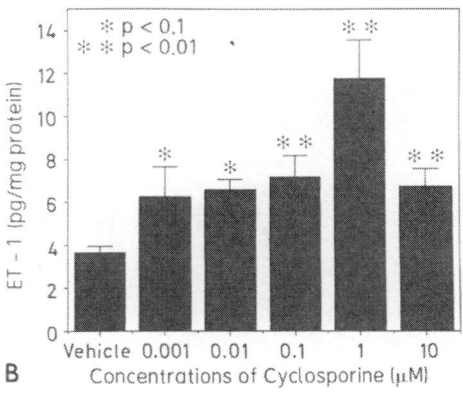

Fig. 2 A. Endothelin production by LLC-PK1 tubular cell line treated with FK506 for 30 h culture. **B** Endothelin production by LLC-PK1 tubular cell line treated with CyA for 10 h

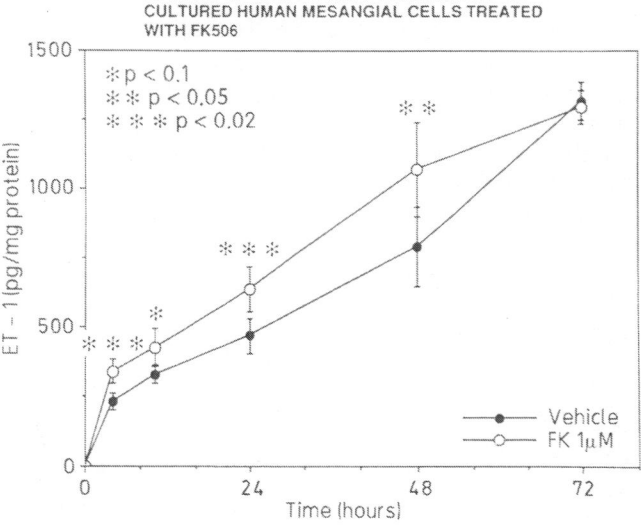

Fig. 3. Kinetics of endothelin secretion by cultured human mesangial cells treated with 1 µM FK506

N-Acetyl-β-D-glucosaminidase (NAG) determination

The supernatants from monolayer of tubular cells treated with different concentrations of FK506, CyA or appropriate concentration of vehicle for 24 h were assayed for NAG. NAG was determined using *m*-cresolsulphonphtaeinyl-N-β-glucosaminidase method (Shionogi NAG assay kit, Shionogi, Osaka, Japan).

Lactate dehydrogenase (LDH) assay

The supernatants harvested from FK506- or CyA-treated HMC at 4, 10, 24 and 48 h were assayed for LDH release by a spectrophotometric assay using commercial kits (Sigma). Maximum release was determined by freezing and thawing the cells three times. Spontaneous release was determined by incubation in medium alone. The results were expressed as percentage of specific release: (LDH test – LDH spontaneous) × 100/(LDH freeze and thaw – LDH spontaneous).

Results

Effect of FK506 and cyclosporine on ET-1 production by LLC-PK1 tubular cell line and human mesangial cells

ET-1 secretion by tubular cells cultured in the absence or presence of FK506 is shown in Fig. 1. Incubation of confluent monolayer tubular cells with culture medium containing vehicle alone resulted in basal production which increased with the duration of incubation. The generation of ET-1 by tubular cells incubated with medium alone was not different from that observed with medium and vehicle (data not shown). FK506 at concentrations of 1, 0.1, 0.01 µM significantly stimulated ET-1 productin in cultured tubular cells. This stimulatory effect was seen at 4, 10, 20 and 30 h incubations. Low concentrations of FK506 (0.001 µM) enhanced ET-1 secretion by tubular cells only with 4 and 10 h incubations. The most substantial enhancing effect of FK506 was observed with concentrations of 0.1 and 0.01 µM (Fig. 1 and 2 A). CyA at concentrations of 10, 1, 0.1 and 0.01 µM also significantly increased ET-1 production by tubular cells (Fig. 2 B). The most marked stimulatory effect was observed with 1 µM CyA. Therefore, it appears that the CyA concentration that induced the maximal enhancing effect was 10 or 100 times higher than the concentration of FK506 that produced the same effect.

As shown in Fig. 3, HMC in vitro secreted more ET-1 than tubular cells (about 50 times). The incubation of HMC with medium and vehicle was not different from that with medium alone. FK506 at 1 µM significantly enhanced ET-1 secretion by cultured HMC with 4, 10, 24 and 48 h of incubation (Fig. 3). FK506 concentrations 0.1, 0.01 and 0.001 also significantly stimulated ET-1 production with a substantial enhancing effect at 0.1 µM FK506 (Fig. 4 A). CyA at 1 and 10 µM had a substantial enhancing effect on ET-1 secretion by HMC whereas concentrations below 1 µM were without significant stimulatory effect (Fig. 4 B). In HMC the maximal stimulatory effect on ET-1 secretion was also obtained with CyA concentrations 10 or 100 times higher than the concentration of FK506 that produced the same effect.

Circulating level of ET-1 in FK506- and cyclosporine-treated rats

After 12 days of oral administration of FK506 or CyA, the rats became sick and lost 30% of their weight. In control rats ET-1 was not detectable in our assay system (less than 1.6 pg/ml). In FK506-treated rats, ET-1 level was 17.7 ± 5.7 pg/ml. In CyA-treated rats, ET-1 level was 18 ± 5.9 pg/ml.

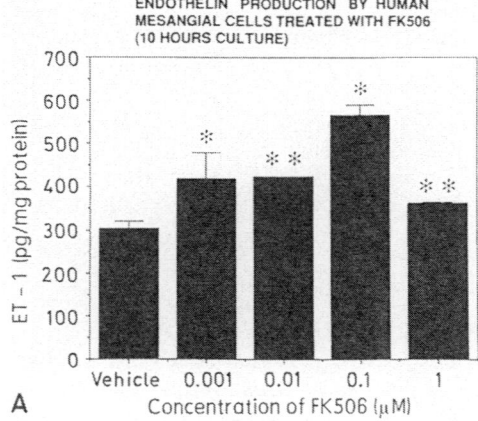

ENDOTHELIN PRODUCTION BY HUMAN
MESANGIAL CELLS TREATED WITH FK506
(10 HOURS CULTURE)

A — Concentration of FK506 (μM)

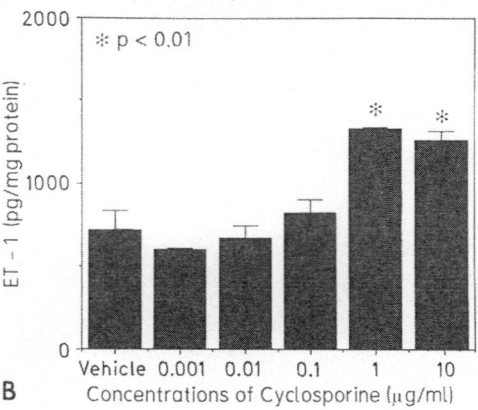

ET-1 PRODUCTION BY HUMAN MESANGIAL
CELLS TREATED WITH CYCLOSPORINE
(48H CULTURE)

B — Concentrations of Cyclosporine (μg/ml)

Fig. 4. A Endothelin production by cultured human mesangial cells treated with FK506 for 10 h culture. **B** Endothelin production by human mesangial cells treated with cyclosporine for 48 h

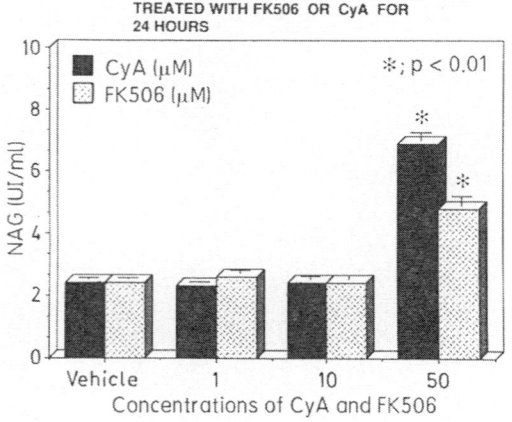

NAG RELEASE FROM TUBULAR CELLS
TREATED WITH FK506 OR CyA FOR
24 HOURS

Concentrations of CyA and FK506

Fig. 5. NAG release from tubular cells treated with FK506 or CyA for 24 h. Supernatants from tubular cells treated with various concentrations of FK506 or CyA were assayed for NAG as descibed in Materials and methods. The vehicle methanol or ethanol served as control

FK506 and cyclosporine NAG release from tubular cells

NAG release was used as a marker of tubular cell injury. NAG release from tubular cells incubated with FK506 doses of 10 μM and 1 μM for 24 h was not different from that of the control (Fig. 5). Furthermore, the kinetics of NAG release (at 4, 10, 24 and 48 h) from tubular cells

treated in vitro with FK506 or 10, 1, 0.1 or 0.01 μM CyA were very similar to those of the vehicle alone (unpublished data). In contrast, high doses of FK506 and CyA (50 μM) induced a significant release of NAG from treated tubular cells ($P < 0.01$).

Effect of FK506 on LDH release from HMC

The cytolytic effect of FK506 and CyA on HMC was assayed using LDH release. HMC treated with FK506 or CyA concentrations 10 and 1 μM for 4, 10, 24 and 48 h showed almost no LDH release (0.1–0.2%). In contrast, with high concentrations of FK506 (50 μM), we observed a relatively high LDH release (Table 1).

Discussion

Extensive investigations have been performed to clarify the mechanism by which CyA and recently FK506 induce tubular and vascular injury which appears to be the primary target in FK506- and CyA-induced damage [5]. In the present study we have demonstrated that FK506 and CyA, at non-cytolytic concentrations, stimulates ET-1 secretion by cultured kidney cells. This effect coincides with an increase in serum level of ET-1 in FK506- and CyA-treated rats.

Renal tubular cell lines synthesise and release ET-1 [14] as is confirmed in this study. ET-1 secretion by tubular cells is stimulated by exposure to a variety of agents such as thrombin, IL-1β, TNF, and TGFβ [10]. FK506 and CyA also stimulated the secretion of ET by tubular cells. Since FK506 and CyA at the range of concentrations tested for ET secretion were not cytolytic (Fig. 6), it is unlikely that the increase in ET secretion in the media could be attributed to cell leakage or release from dying cells. The secretion may therefore be the result of active cellular secretion. The most important enhancing effect on ET-1 secretion by tubular cells was observed with CyA concentrations 10 or 100 times higher than those required for FK506 to produce the same effect. This finding is concordant with the comparative pharmacological effect of both drugs. It has been established that FK506 is 10 or 100 times more immunosuppressive than CyA [18]. Therefore, the present finding lends further support to the relationship between immunosuppressive activity and toxicity.

Human mesangial cells constitutively secrete ET-1 in culture media [21]. The stimulation of HMC by inflammatory mediators such thrombin, thromboxane A2, TGFβ [21] or endotoxin [15] resulted in an increase in ET-1 secretion. HMC, which regulate glomerular filtration, responded to FK506 or CyA treatment in vitro by an increase in their ability to secrete ET-1. This secretion seemed to be an active secretion from cells, since no LDH release (Table 1) was observed at the range of concentration of FK506 or CyA used to induce ET-1 secretion.

The rats' serum levels of endothelin after 12 days oral administration of FK506 or CyA were elevated as compared with values in controls. Kon et al. [5] also reported an elevation in ET-1 serum level 20 min after intravenous administration of CyA in rats. The pathophysiological significance of the stimulatory effect of FK506 and CyA on

Table 1. LDH release from human mesangial cells treated with FK506 or cyclosporine. Supernatants from monolayers of HMC treated with different concentrations of FK506 or CyA were harvested at 4, 10, 24 and 48 h and were assayed for LDH using a spectrophotometric method. The vehicle alone served as control, maximal release was obtained by three cycles of freezing and thawing. The data are expressed as percentage of specific release

	LDH specific release (%) Incubation time (h)			
	4	10	24	48
FK506 1 μM	0.10	0.20	0.10	0.15
FK506 10 μM	0.15	0.10	0.12	0.10
FK506 50 μM	1.80	1.30	9.50	17.00
CyA 1 μM	0.10	0.12	0.10	0.13
CyA 10 μM	0.20	0.1	0.11	0.12
CyA 50 μM	ND	ND	ND	ND

ND, not determined

ET secretion by kidney cells remains to be defined, but as suggested by Kon et al. [5] the increased level of ET-1 following CyA and FK506 may reflect a perturbed ET synthesis and/or metabolism in the kidney after FK506 or CyA treatment, which causes overflow of locally produced ET into the circulation, and changes in tissue and receptor characteristics. Recently, it was demonstrated that CyA-induced glomerular dysfunction involves upregulation of glomerular ET receptors and that this is specific to the kidney [9]. If the effect of ET on glomerular haemodynamics [6] is compared with the effect reported with CyA [1], the two are similar. In isolated perfused kidney exposed to specific anti-endothelin antibody, but not immunized rabbit serum, the CyA-induced fall in RPF and GFR was markedly reduced [12]. The role of endogenous ET in acute CyA nephrotoxicity has been documented in vivo by studies showing that the infusion of specific ET serum partially but significantly prevented the reduction of GFR and RPF induced by intravenous administration of CyA [5]. Since there are only a few reports available concerning the effect of the new drug FK506 on mesangial and tubular cell physiology, this study may provide the experimental background to understanding the glomerular dysfunction which has been reported with FK506 administration [7, 19]. We conclude that the stimulatory effect of FK506 on ET-1 secretion by kidney cells may contribute to the genesis of FK506- and CyA-induced glomerular dysfunction.

References

1. Barros EJG, Boim MA, Ajzen H, Ramos OL, Schor N (1987) Glomerular hemodynamics and hormonal participation in cyclosporine nephrotoxicity. Kidney Int 3: 219–225

2. Hull RN, Cherry WR, Weaver GW (1976) The origin of a pig kidney cell strain. In Vitro 12: 670–674

3. Ishibashi M (for the Japanese study group) (1991) Japanese study of FK506 in kidney transplantation: Results of early phase II study. Transplant Proc (in press)

4. Jain AB, Fung J, Todo S, Alessiani M, Takaya S, Abu-Elmagd K, Tzakis A, Starzl TE (1991) Incidence and treatment of episodes of rejection in primary orthotopic liver transplantation under FK506. Transplant Proc 23: 928–930

5. Kon V, Suguira M, Inagami T, Bradley RH, Ichikawa I, Hoover RL (1990) Role of endothelin in cyclosporin-induced glomerular dysfunction. Kidney Int 37: 1487–1491

6. Kon V, Yoshioka T, Fogo A (1989) Glomerular actions of endothelin in vivo. Clin Invest 83: 1762–1767

7. Kumano K, Wang G, Endo T, Kuwao S (1991) FK506-induced nephrotoxicity in rats. Transplant Proc 23: 512–515

8. Murray BM, Paller MS, Ferris TF (1985) Effect of cyclosporin administration on renal hemodynamics in conscious rats. Kidney Int 28: 767–774

9. Nambi P, Pullen M, Contino LC, Brooks DP (1990) Upregulation of renal endothelin secretion in rats with cyclosporine A-induced nephrotoxicity. Eur J Pharmacol 187: 113–116

10. Ohta K, Hirata Y, Imai T, Kanno K, Emori T, Shichiri M, Marumo F (1990) Cytokine-induced release of endothelin-1 from porcine renal epithelial cell line. Biochem Biophys Res Commun 169: 578–584

11. Perico N, Begnini A, Delaini F, Remuzzi G (1986) Functional significance of exaggerated renal thromboxane A2 synthesis induced by cyclosporine A. Am J Physiol 251: F581–F587

12. Perico N, Dadan J, Remuzzi G (1990) Endothelin mediates the renal vasoconstriction induced by cyclosporine in rat. JASN 1: 76–83

13. Shapiro R, Jordan M, Fung J, Johnston J, Iwaki Y, Tzakis A, Hakala T, Todo S, Starzl TE (1991) Kidney transplantation under FK506. Transplant Proc 23: 920–923

14. Shichiri M, Hirata Y, Emori T, Ohta K, Nakajima T, Sato K, Sato A, Marumo F (1989) Secretion of endothelin and related peptides from renal epithelial cell lines. FEBS Lett 253: 203–206

15. Sugiura M, Inagami T, Kon V (1989) Endotoxin stimulates endothelin release in vivo and in vitro as determined by radioimmunoassay. Biomed Biophys Res Comun 161: 1220–1227

16. Suzuki N, Matsumoto H, Kitada C, Masaki T, Fujino M (1989) A sensitive sandwich-enzyme immunoassay for human endothelin. J Immunol Methods 188: 245–250

17. Tanaka T, Fujiware Y, Orita Y, Sasaki E, Kitamura H, Abe H (1984) The functional characteristics of cultured rat mesangial cells. Jpn Circ J 48: 1017–1029

18. Thomson AW (1989) FK506 how much potential. Immunology Today 10: 6–10

19. Textor S, Wilson D, Weisner R, Porayko M, Dickson E, Krom R (1991) Differences in renal and systemic vasoconstriction during administration of FK506 and cyclosporine. Transplant Proc (in press)

20. Yanigisawa M, Kurihara H, Kimura S, Kobayashi M, Mitsui Y, Yazaki K, Goto Y, Masaki T (1988) A novel vasoconstrictor peptide produced by vascular endothelial cells. Nature 332: 411–415

21. Zoja C, Orisio S, Perico N, Begnini A, Morigi M, Benatti L, Rambaldi A, Remuzzi G (1991) Constitutive expression of endothelin gene in cultured human mesangial cells and its modulation by transforming growth factor β thrombin, and a thromboxane A2 analogue. Lab Invest 64: 16–20

Transplant Int (1992) 5 [Suppl 1]: S 98–99

TRANSPLANT
International
© Springer-Verlag 1992

Early kidney transplantation
may prevent aluminium-related bone disease

K. P. Nordal[1], E. Dahl[2], J. Halse[1], and A. Flatmark[2]

[1] Department of Medicine, and [2] Department of Surgery, The National Hospital, Rikshospitalet, Oslo, Norway

In uraemia patients aluminium (Al) accumulation in bone leads to low turn-over bone disease [4]. Al-related bone disease causes bone pain, non-traumatic fractures and hypercalcaemia, and does not respond to treatment with vitamin D compounds [9]. Al-contaminated dialysate and ingestion of Al-containing phosphate binding agents are the main risk factors for bone Al accumulation [6, 12].

Studies of selected patients have indicated that Al-related bone disease ameliorates after successful kidney transplantation [5, 10], but systematic studies of bone Al have not been reported. In a prospective study we investigated the effect of successful kidney transplantation on bone Al and clinical bone disease.

Key words: Kidney transplantation – Aluminium – Related bone disease

Subjects and methods

Consent to bone biopsy at transplantation was obtained from 84 kidney graft recipients with intact parathyroid glands. Of these patients, 19 (23%) had never been dialysed, and 65 (77%) had been treated by dialysis for 1–44 (median 9) months. After transplantation all were immunosuppressed with a low-dose corticosteroid and high-dose cyclosporin A regimen [7]. Eight recipients died and another 11 returned to dialysis. Of the remaining 65 recipients with a functioning graft, 55 (83%) consented to a second bone biopsy 1 year after transplantation.

Serum creatinine was measured by a standard technique. The transiliac bone biopsies were performed, processed and evaluated as previously described [1]. Aurin–tricarboxylic acid was used to detect stainable Al in bone [8], and Prussian blue to ensure that iron was not responsible for the purple lines.

Results

Seven predialysis (37%) and 50 dialysis (77%) recipients had stainable Al at Tx. In predialysis patients, Al-stained bone surface (AlS) correlated with daily intake of phos-

phate binders ($r = 0.57$, $P < 0.05$). AlS was correlated with dialysis duration ($r = 0.50$, $P < 0.01$) in dialysis patients, and multiple linear regression analysis using a model which comprised daily intake of phosphate binders, dialysis duration, tap-water Al concentration, and serum Al levels confirmed that only dialysis duration could explain the variability in AlS among dialysis patients ($P < 0.01$).

Four patients had symptomatic bone disease with fractures and/or skeletal pain at transplantation. They all had AlS exceeding 45%. All four had been treated with dialysis for more than 24 months, came from areas with high Al content in tap-water, and used phosphate binders. Five asymptomatic patients also had AlS exceeding 45%. All came from areas with high Al content in the water and used phosphate binders, but only one had been on dialysis for more than 12 months.

At follow-up 1 year after transplantation, serum creatinine ranged from 62 to 415 (median 168) µmol/l. AlS had decreased from 13% range 6–23% to 2% (0–3%) ($P < 0.01$), and correlated with AlS at follow-up ($r = 0.58$, $P < 0.0001$). Al had become undetectable in 16 recipients with stainable bone Al at transplantation. No relationship was found between serum creatinine and AlS at 1-year follow-up.

One recipient with symptomatic bone disease and one asymptomatic recipient with AlS > 45% at transplantation had died of infection. Another one with bone pain at transplantation refused a second bone biopsy, but was then without bone pain. In the remaining two with symptomatic bone pain and in the another four with AlS > 45% at transplantation, AlS had decreased (50 to 10%, 51 to 15%, 71 to 0%, 52 to 6%, 75 to 11%, and 60 to 53%, respectively).

Comments

Symptomatic Al-related bone disease is a feared complication of long-term dialysis [11], and increased mortality has been described in severely Al-intoxicated recipients even after transplantation [3]. The present study confirms that successful kidney transplantation cures Al-related

Offprint requests to: K. P. Nordal M. D., Med. Dept. B, The National Hospital, Rikshospitalet, N-0027 Oslo 1, Norway

bone disease [5]. Since Al deposition is related to duration of dialysis [2], the present study underscores the importance of early transplantation.

References

1. Dahl E, Nordal KP, Halse J, Attramadal A (1988) Histomorphometric analysis of normal bone from the iliac crest of Norwegian subjects. Bone Miner 3: 369–377
2. Dahl E, Nordal KP, Halse, Flatmark A (1990) The early effects of aluminium deposition and dialysis on bone in chronic renal failure: a cross-sectional bone-histomorphometric study. Nephrol Dial Transplant 5: 445–456
3. Davenport A, Davison AM, Will EJ, Toothill C, Newton KE, Giles GR (1989) Aluminium accumulation and immunosuppression. Br Med J 298: 458–459
4. Hodsman AB, Sherrard DJ, Alfrey AC, Ott S, Brickman AS, Miller NL, Maloney NA, Coburn JW (1982) Bone aluminum and histomorphometric features of renal osteodystrophy. J Clin Endocrinol Metab 54: 539–545
5. Ihle BU, Buchanan MRC, Stevens B, Becher GJ, Kincaid-Smith P (1982) The efficacy of various treatment modalities on aluminium associated bone disease. Proc Eur Dial Transplant Assoc Eur Ren Assoc 19: 195–202
6. Llack F, Felsenfeld AJ, Coleman MD, Keveney Jr JJ, Pederson JA, Medlock TR (1986) The natural course of dialysis osteomalacia. Kidney Int 29 [Suppl 18]: S 74–S 79
7. Lundgren G, Albrechtsen D, Flatmark A, Gabel H, Klintmalm G, Persson H, Groth CG, Brynger H, Frødin L, Husberg B, Maurer N, Thorsby E (1986) HLA-matching and pretransplant blood transfusions in cadaveric renal transplantation – A changing picture with cyclosporin. Lancet II: 66–69
8. Maloney NA, Ott SM, Alfrey AC, Miller NL, Coburn JW, Sherrard DJ (1982) Histological quantitation of aluminium in iliac bone from patients with renal failure. J Lab Clin Med 99: 206–216
9. Ott SM, Maloney NA, Coburn JW, Alfrey AC, Sherrard DJ (1982) The prevalence of bone aluminum deposition in renal osteodystrophy and its relation to the response to calcitriol therapy. N Engl J Med 307: 709–713
10. Poedenfant J, Salem N, Sypitkowski C, Frame B, Parfitt AM (1985) Reversal of aluminum-related dialysis osteomalacia after transplantation. Bone 6: 405
11. Smith AJ, Faugere M-C, Abreo K, Fanti P, Julian B, Malluche HH (1986) Aluminum-related bone disease in mild and advanced renal failure. Evidence for high prevalence and morbidity and studies on etiology and diagnosis. Am J Nephrol 6: 275–283
12. Ward MK, Feest TG, Ellis HA, Parkinson JS, Kerr DNS (1978) Osteomalacic dialysis osteodystrophy: evidence for a waterborne aetiological agent, probably aluminium. Lancet I: 841–845

Transplant Int (1992) 5 [Suppl 1]: S100–S103

TRANSPLANT
International
© Springer-Verlag 1992

Effect of prostaglandin E₁ on graft function of kidneys from living related donors

S. Ohsaki, S. Teraoka, T. Tojimbara, K. Takahasi, H. Toma, T. Agishi, and K. Ota

Third Department of Surgery, Tokyo Women's Medical College, 8-1 Kawada-cho Sinjuku-ku, Tokyo, Japan

Abstract. Prostaglandin E_1 (PGE_1) was used in renal transplant recipients with living related donors. The drug was given intravenously from day 1 to day 7 after transplantation at a dose of 40 μg/kg twice a day. A total of 45 patients were studied divided into two groups: 25 patients were treated with PGE_1 (group B) and the remaining 20 patients did not receive the drug (group A). In group B, 24-h creatinine clearance (Ccr) was 66 ± 12.8 ml/min compared with 40.3 ± 13.4 ml/min in group A on the fifth postoperative day ($P < 0.05$). Urinary levels of N-acetyl-β-D-glucosaminidase (NAG) and serum levels of platelet factor 4 (PF4) in group B were significantly lower than in group A. On the fourth postoperative day, the urinary excretion of thromboxan B_2 (TxB_2) in group A was higher than in group B, but not significantly (5.1 ± 3.0 ng/day and 2.8 ± 1.1 ng/day, respectively). Acute rejection occurred in four patients in group B and in 10 patients (40%) in group A. The percentage of Leu2a-positive lymphocytes in group B was higher than in group A. We conclude that postoperative administration of PGE_1 improves graft function in kidneys from living related donors.

Key words: Renal transplantation – Prostaglandin E_1 – Doppler ultrasound – Reperfusion injury – Thromboxan B_2 – Lymphocyte subset

Recently, it has been demonstrated that eicosanoids have a beneficial effect on prevention of ischaemic damage and on graft preservation. Current investigations have demonstrated the potent cytoprotective effect of PGE_1 against various types of organ damage. There is, however, little information concerning the effect of this agent in clinical renal transplantation. In a prospective trial conducted in 1990, we gave PGE_1 to renal transplant patients, and also evaluated the effects of PGE_1 on renal allografts from living related donors. We determined graft blood flow, platelet activity, prostaglandin metabolism and immunosuppressive effects.

Offprint requests to: S. Ohsaki, M.D.

Patients and methods

From April 1990 to December 1990, 80 patients were transplanted in our unit for chronic renal failure. To investigate the usefulness of PGE_1, we selected 45 patients randomly and divided them into two groups: 25 patients were treated with PGE_1 (group B) and the remaining 20 patients were not treated with the drug (group A). The proportion of immunological high responders in group A was 54%, and in group B was 57% (Table 1). Transplantation using living related donors was performed in all patients who were then treated with cyclosporin A (CyA), azathioprine (Aza) and methylprednisolone (MP) according to our previously reported protocol. Double filtration plasmapheresis (DFPP) and immunoabsorption methods were performed before transplantation in ABO-incompatible patients.

Administration of PGE_1

During the operation, PGE_1 was administered intravenously at a dose of 20 μg/kg. After the operation PGE_1 was infused intravenously twice daily for 7 postoperative days at a dose of 40 μg/kg.

The parameters studied were peripheral blood count, serum urea, creatinine (Cr), electrolytes, platelet factor 4 (PF4), β-Throm-

Table 1. Comparison between the PGE_1 treatment group and the non-treated control group. There were no significant differences in the donor creatinine clearances, total ischaemic times or graft weights

	PGE_1 group	Control group
Number of cases	20	25
Age (years)	36.7 (25–49)	35.9 (19–52)
Sex (M/F)	12/8	16/9
Type of transplantation		
ABO incompatible	5	4
ABO mismatch	2	2
HLA, AB mismatch		
≥3	3	4
≤2	16	19
MLC stimulation index		
≥20	8	9
≥10	0	6
≤10	8	9
Immunological high responders	11 (57%)	13 (54%)

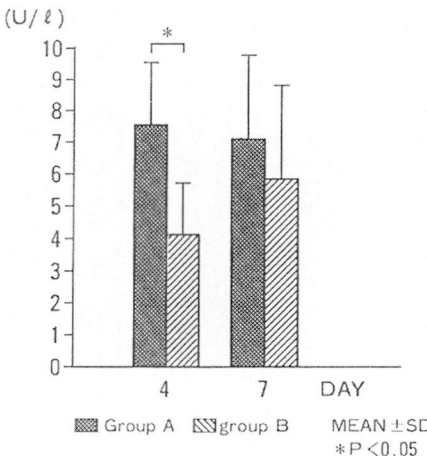

Fig. 1. Urinary NAC levels

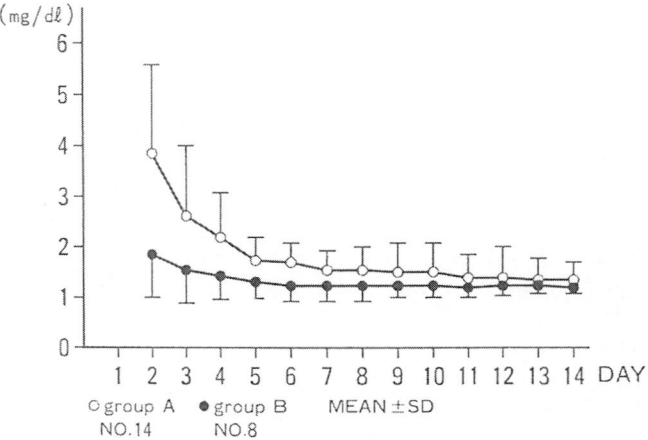

Fig. 2. Changes in the serum creatinine levels. Serum creatinine in group B was decreased more rapidly than in group A, especially in the early postoperative days

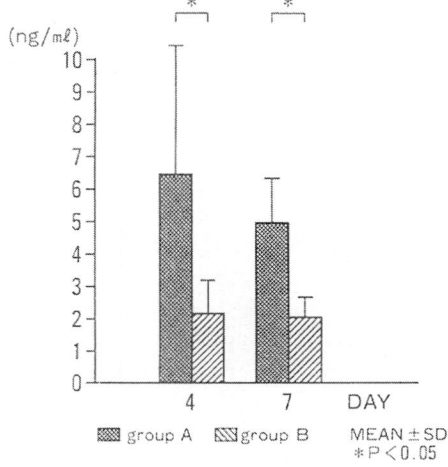

Fig. 3. Serum PF4 levels

boglobuline (β-TG), lymphocyte subset, IgG, IgA, IgM, C3 and C4, and urinary N-acetyl-β-D-glucosaminidase (NAG) and prostaglandin metabolites. The levels of serum PF4, serum β-TG and urinary prostaglandin metabolites were analysed by specific radioimmunoassay. For cases of acute rejection, values were excluded restrospectively from 3 days before the onset of acute rejection.

Doppler ultrasound was used to obtain blood flow velocity curves from the interlobular artery of the transplanted renal allograft. The Doppler flow pattern was observed using a colour Doppler ultrasound scanner SSD680 (Aloka, Japan). The peak systolic velocity (PSV), end diastolic velocity (EDV), average velocity (AGV), pulsatility index (PI) and resistive index (RI) were measured from the interlobular artery of the renal allograft. These parameters were measured at two to four points on the artery and an average was taken.

Statistical analyses

All values are presented as mean ± SD and were analysed by Student's t-test. P-values less than 0.05 were considered to be significant.

Results

The numbers of patients available for study on each postoperative day are shown in Table 2.

Function of renal allograft

The 24-h Ccr values were 42.4 ± 18.9, 40.3 ± 13.5 and 46.1 ± 14.2 ml/min on days 3, 5 and 7, respectively, in group A, and 70.3 ± 20.5, 66.0 ± 12.8 ($P < 0.05$) and 73.2 ± 12.7 ($P < 0.05$) on days 3, 5 and 7 in group B. Urine volume and urine levels of electrolytes were the same in both groups. Levels of urine NAG in group A were 7.6 ± 2.9 U/l on day 4 and 7.1 ± 2.8 U/l on the day-7, and in group B were 4.2 ± 2.2 U/l on day 4 and 6.1 ± 3.7 U/l day 7 (Fig. 1). A dramatic decrease in serum creatinine level was observed in group B after the first 4 days after transplantation, but after 7 days the serum creatinine level was the same as in group A (Fig. 2).

Platelet activity

Serum PF4 level was 6.5 ± 4.9 ng/ml in group A and 2.2 ± 0.87 ng/ml in group B on day 4 ($P < 0.05$) and 5.0 ± 1.4 ng/ml in group A and 2.1 ± 0.7 ng/ml in group B on day 7 ($P < 0.05$) (Fig. 3).

On postoperative day 7, serum β-TG levels were 77.8 ± 26.3 ng/ml in group A and 42.7 ± 4.65 ng/ml in group B ($P < 0.05$).

Urine prostaglandin metabolites

Urinary levels of TxB$_2$ were 5.1 ± 3.0 ng/day in group A and 2.8 ± 1.1 ng/day in group B, and of 6-keto-PGF$_1\alpha$ were 3.8 ± 1.8 ng/day in group A and 3.6 ± 1.4 ng/day in

Table 2. The numbers of patients available for study on each operative day

	Day					
	1	2	3	4	5	7
Group A	19	18	17	16	15	13
Group B	21	20	17	15	13	11

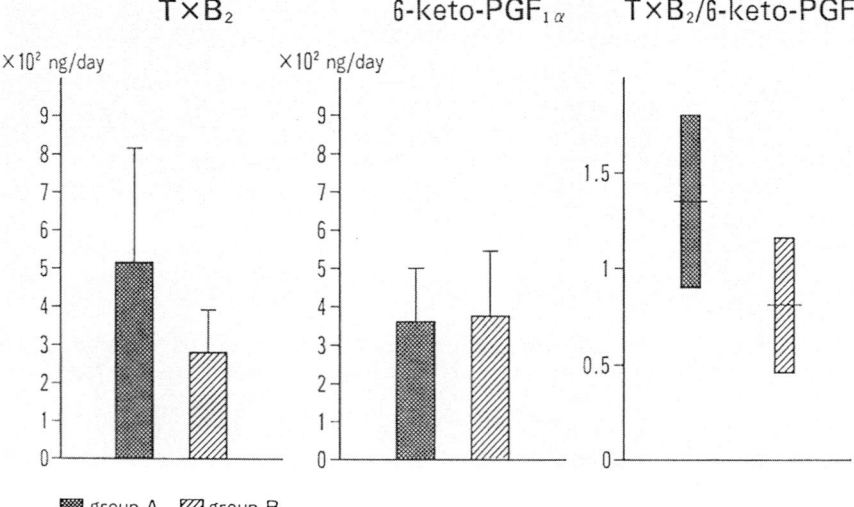

T×B₂ 6-keto-PGF₁α T×B₂/6-keto-PGF₁α

group A group B

Fig. 4. The levels of urine TxB₂, 6-keto-PGF₁α and TxB₂/6-keto-PGF₁α on the fourth postoperative day

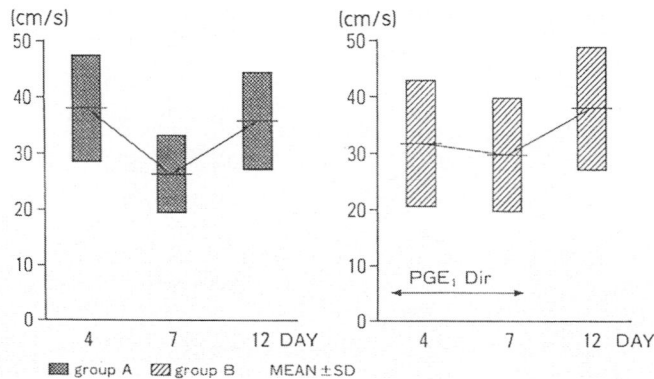

group A group B MEAN ± SD

Fig. 5. Changes in PSV after transplantation. The doppler ultrasound method was used to obtain blood flow velocity curves from the interlobular artery of the transplanted renal allografts. We measured the velocity curve on the same artery of each the renal allograft. The average PSV decreased in the group A but not significantly in the group B

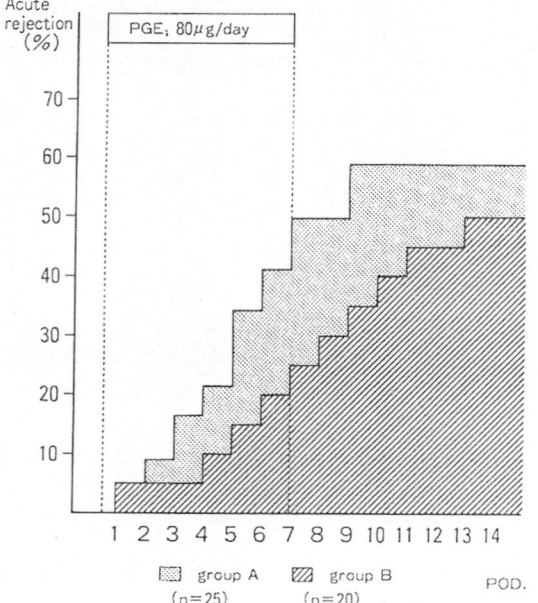

group A (n=25) group B (n=20) POD.

Fig. 6. The proportion of patients with acute rejection on each postoperative day

group B on postoperative day 4. The urinary levels of TxB₂ and TxB₂/6-keto-PGF₁α of group A were higher than those of group B (Fig. 4).

Blood flow in renal allografts

PSV, EDV, RI and PI were measured by Doppler ultrasound methods from the interlobular artery of the renal allograft. RI and PI were increasing at the time of acute rejection in each group, but no difference was observed between the two groups at the time of rejection. Figure 5 shows the changes in PSV that were measured at the time of no rejection following in 2 weeks. PSV measured on day 7 was slightly decreased in group A but showed no change in group B, but the difference between the groups was not significant.

Acute rejection and immunological follow up

The combined rate of acute rejection (AR) from day 1 to day 7 was 40% in group A and 20% in group B. After stopping the infusion of PGE₁ in group B, the number of patients with acute rejection increased and the overall rate of AR was 50% 2 weeks after surgery (Fig. 6). Figure 7 shows the T-cell subsets in the peripheral blood of the patients in whom AR occurred 3 days later. The percentage of Leu2a-positive lymphocytes was $22.2 \pm 3.7\%$ in group A and $34.5 \pm 7.5\%$ in group B ($P < 0.05$). The Leu3a to Leu2a ratio was 2.5 ± 0.4 in group A and 1.4 ± 0.5 in group B. Serum levels of C3, C4, IgG, IgA and IgM were not significantly different between the two groups.

Discussion

PGE₁ possibly protects the renal allograft from ischaemia reperfusion injury by increasing the capillary blood flow and by an immunosupressive effect.

In the PGE₁ group, the 24-h Ccr levels were higher than those in the non-treatment group for 7 postoperative days. Urinary NAG levels in the non-treatment group were

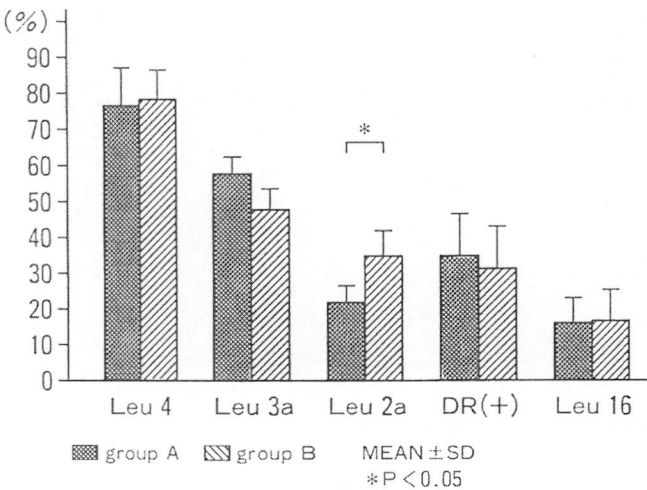

Fig. 7. Lymphocyte subsets on the fourth postoperative day

We studied renal allograft blood flow using a Doppler ultrasound blood perfusion monitor. Flow velocity decreased without rejection on days 5–7 in the non-treated group but did not decrease in the PGE$_1$-treated group. This change in velocity may have been due to tissue oedema or an increase in tissue TxB$_2$ production, but we did not examine this. On the other hand, there were no differences in the early postoperative state (days 1–4). These results suggest that PGE$_1$ improves capillary blood flow, which was not measured by Doppler ultrasound methods in the early postoperative days.

It has been reported that PGE$_1$ induces T-helper cells at low concentrations and T-suppressor cells at high concentrations [7]. The suppression of antigen presentation by macrophages [4, 5, 6], interleukin-1 (IL-1) production by macrophages and IL-2 production by T cells [1] have been demonstrated in an in vivo study. In clinical renal transplantation, there is little information concerning the immunosuppressive effect of PGE$_1$.

Our results demonstrate a low frequency of acute rejection in the PGE$_1$-treated group during PGE$_1$ infusion, and frequent acute rejection after stopping the infusion. During the week after transplantation, the ratio of Leu2a-positive cells in the PGE$_1$-treated group was higher than in the non-treated group. These results suggest that PGE$_1$ may suppress cell immunity and modify T-cell differentiation on renal transplantation.

higher than those of the PGE$_1$ group. It is well known that NAG is included in the lysosome of renal tubular cells. The leakage of hydrolytic enzymes from lysosomes and their activation by acidosis in the ischaemic kidney seem to be critical contributing factors to irreversible change in cells. The marked suppression of urinary NAG activity observed in this study suggests a stabilizing effect of PGE$_1$ on the lysosomal membrane in transplanted kidney injured by ischaemia and reperfusion.

It has been reported that serum TxB$_2$ levels and TxB$_2$/6-keto-PGF$_1\alpha$ increase after reperfusion of a transplanted organ [2, 3]. It is well known that TxA$_2$ activates platelet aggregation and prostaglandin I$_2$ (PGI) inhibits platelet activation. The vasospastic effect of TxA$_2$ together with the increase in TxB$_2$/6-keto-PGF$_1\alpha$ decrease organ blood flow and inhibit the peripheral blood supply. Our results demonstrate that the levels of urinary TxB$_2$, urinary TxB$_2$/6-keto-PGF$_1\alpha$, serum PF4 and serum β-TG in the PGE$_1$ group were lower than in the non-treated group. PF4 and β-TG are released from activated platelets. The suppression of urinary excretion of TxB$_2$ and platelet activation observed in this study suggest that PGE$_1$ suppresses the production of TxA$_2$ from platelets and changes the balance of prostaglandins after reperfusion of the renal allograft. We sugest that PGE$_1$ protects the transplanted kidney from the early ischaemia that occurs immediately after blood reperfusion, and this may be one of the cytoprotective effects of PGE$_1$ in renal transplantation.

References

1. Chouaib S, WelChouaib K, Mertelsmann R, Dupontal B (1985) Prostaglandin e2 acts at two distinct pathways of T lymphocyte activation: Inhibition of interleukin 2 production and down-regulation of transferrin receptor expression. J Immunol 135: 1172
2. Hotter G, Rosello-Catafau J, Bulbena O, Gomwz G, Gelpi E (1990) Prostaglandine E2 and thromboxan B2 levels in rats subjected to pancreas transplantation. Prostaglandins 39: 53–60
3. Klausner JM, Paterson IS, Hechtman HB (1989) Vasodilating prostaglandins attenuate ischemic renal injury only if thromboxan is inhibited. Ann Surg 209: 219–224
4. Scheuer WV, Hobbs MV, Weigle WO (1987) Interference with tolerance induction in vivo by inhibitors of prostaglandin synthesis. Cell Immunol 104: 409
5. Snyder DS, Beller DI, Unanue ER (1982) Prostaglandins modulate macrophage Ia expression. Nature 299: 163
6. Taffet SM, Russel SW (1980) Macrophage-mediated tumor cell killing: regulation of expression of cytolytic activity by prostaglandin E1. J Immunol 126: 424
7. Zimecki M, Webb DR (1976) The regulation of the immune response to T-independent antigens by prostaglandins in B cells. J Immunol 117: 2158

Transplant Int (1992) 5 [Suppl 1]: S104–S106

TRANSPLANT
International
© Springer-Verlag 1992

Renal transplantation in r-HuEPO-treated patients

A. O. Seeberger[1], A. Tibell[2], and G. Tydén[2]

[1] Department of Nephrology and [2] Department of Transplantation Surgery, Karolinska Institute, Stockholm, Sweden

Abstract. After sporadic reports of renal graft artery thromboses, prophylaxis against thrombosis (PAT) was given to all of our r-HuEPO-treated patients ($n = 35$) during a period of 2 years. No thromboembolic events (TEE) occurred in the r-HuEPO-treated group receiving PAT. However, the PAT-protocol (500 ml dextran on days 0, 1, 3 and 5, followed by low doses of aspirin, 160–250 mg daily) resulted in a 54.3 % incidence of bleeding complications, of which 22.9 % were major (i.e., necessitating multiple transfusions or invasive procedures). A group of renal graft recipients ($n = 83$), who were not treated with r-HuEPO and were not given PAT, showed a 10.8 % incidence of bleeding complications of which 2.4 % major. Two cases of TEE were noted in the untreated group. The difference in bleeding complications between the two groups was statistically significant ($0.025 > P > 0.01$). The difference in TEE between the groups was not significant. We found no difference between the groups with regard to early and late graft function and the incidence of acute rejections. In summary, r-HuEPO treatment did not influence the prognosis in renal graft recipients. The use of PAT in the r-HuEPO-treated group resulted in a high incidence of bleeding complications. In consequence, we have abandoned the routine use of PAT in this patient group.

Key words: Renal transplantation – Recombinant human erythropoietin – Prophylaxis against thrombosis

The clinical use of recombinant human erythropoietin (r-HuEPO) has dramatically improved the treatment of uraemic patients. r-HuEPO not only corrects their renal anaemia but also improves their physical condition as reflected by a better appetite and exercise capacity, as well as a reversal of various hormonal and metabolic aberrations, which result in an improvement in their quality of life [1, 5]. However, adverse effects have also been reported, such as hypertension, seizures, diminished dialysis efficiency and clotting of arteriovenous fistulas and grafts [4]. There has also been concern about an increased risk of thromboembolic events (TEE) when performing renal transplantations. After sporadic reports of renal graft artery thromboses, prophylaxis against thrombosis (PAT) was given to all of our r-HuEPO-treated renal graft recipients. The efficiency and side-effects of PAT in this patient group were analysed in the present study.

r-HuEPO treatment has also been shown to influence the immunological response in uraemic patients [3]. We therefore studied the incidence of acute rejections and 1-year graft survival. In addition, early graft function was evaluated, because animal studies have shown that an increase in haematocrit aggravates reperfusion damage during kidney transplantation, thereby worsening early graft function [11].

Materials and methods

A total of 118 adult patients who received a renal transplant during a period of 2 years (June 1988 to June 1990) were studied retrospectively. Of these patients, 35 (group A) had been treated with r-HuEPO, and they were therefore given prophylaxis against thrombosis (PAT) (500 ml dextran on days 0, 1, 3 and 5, followed by low-dose aspirin 160–250 mg daily). The other 83 patients (group B) were not treated with r-HuEPO, and they were therefore not given PAT. The mean haemoglobin value in the r-HuEPO-treated group was 100 ± 15 g/l and in the untreated group 90 ± 20 g/l. The difference in haemoglobin levels between the two groups was statistically significant ($P = 0.005$). Other patient characteristics are shown in Table 1.

Table 1. Patient characteristics

	r-HuEPO + ATP ($n = 35$)	No r-HuEPO + no ATP ($n = 83$)
Mean age (years)	45.7	47.9
Diabetes	11.4 %	14.5 %
HD before transplant	88.6 %	71.1 %
PD before transplant	11.4 %	15.7 %
LD grafts	14.3 %	22.9 %

Offprint requests to: Dr. G. Tydén, Department of Transplantation Surgery, Karolinska Institute, Stockholm, Sweden.

Table 2. Bleeding complications

	GI bleeding	Haematuria	Haematoma
r-HuEPO + PAT (n = 35)	5 (4 major)	8 (4 major)	6 (1 major)
No r-HuEPO, no PAT (n = 83)	2 (2 major)	3	4

Table 3. Serum creatinine levels (μmol/l)

	Day 7	Day 30	6 months	12 months
r-HuEPO + PAT (n = 35)	277 ± 120	208 ± 129	195 ± 122	164 ± 67
No r-HuEPO, no PAT (n = 83)	319 ± 297	184 ± 114	189 ± 144	154 ± 59
P value	0.2473	0.0247	0.0814	0.1884

Table 4. Graft loss during the first year after renal transplantation

	r-HuEPO + PAT (n = 35)	No r-HuEPO, no PAT (n = 83)
Acute vascular rejection	3	8
Chronic rejection	2	2
Non-functioning graft	1	1
Graft artery thrombosis	0	1
Carcinoma in renal graft	0	2
Immunosuppressive treatment removed	1	0

Statistical analyses were performed with the paired Student's t-test and the chi-squared test. Values are given as means ± SD.

Results

No TEE occurred in the r-HuEPO-treated patients receiving PAT (group A). In the untreated group (group B), two cases of TEE were noted (one renal graft artery thrombosis, one deep vein thrombosis). The difference in TEE between the groups was not significant. However, PAT in group A resulted in a 54.3 % incidence of bleeding complications, of which 22.9 % were major, i.e. necessitating multiple transfusions or invasive procedures (see Table 2). No grafts were lost because of these complications. Group B, which was not given PAT, showed a 10.8 % incidence of bleeding complications, of which 2.4 % were major. The difference in bleeding complications was statistically significant both for the total number of complications ($0.025 > P > 0.01$) and for the number of major cases ($0.025 > P > 0.01$). All bleeding complications were observed during the first month after transplantation.

Early graft non-function was defined as an inability to reduce the serum creatinine level on day 1 after transplantation. Early graft non-function was shown by 18 patients in group A (51.4 %) and 37 patients in group B (46.6 %). There was no statistically significant difference between the groups. Eight patients in group A (22.9 %) and 14 patients in group B (16.9 %) required dialysis during the first week after transplantation. There was no statistically significant difference between the creatinine levels in the two groups on day 7 and day 30 and after 6 and 12 months (Table 3).

Ten patients in group A (28.6 %) and 25 patients in group B (30.1 %) did not have a single episode of acute rejection, 14 patients in group A (40.0 %) and 33 patients in group B (39.8 %) had one episode, and 11 patients in group A (31.4 %) and 25 patients in group B (30.1 %) had more than one episode. Three patients in group A (8.6 %) and eight patients in group B (9.6 %) had irreversible rejections. Another four patients in group A (20.0 %) and six patients in group B (16.9 %) lost their grafts during the first year (Table 4). Two patients in group A (5.7 %) and three patients in group B (3.6 %) died during the first year.

Discussion

There has been concern about an increased incidence of TEE in r-HuEPO-treated patients. r-HuEPO increases the haematocrit which results in an increased blood viscosity [8]. Plasma viscosity is not changed by r-HuEPO treatment [10]. Moreover, the platelet count increases significantly during the initial phase of r-HuEPO treatment, but thrombocytosis rarely develops [7]. Platelet adhesion has been shown to increase, while prothrombin, partial thromboplastin time and fibrinogen levels remain unchanged [6]. Bleeding time is shortened by r-HuEPO treatment [6]. Thus r-HuEPO influences several factors which may lead to an increased incidence of TEE.

However, it has yet not been shown that r-HuEPO increases the incidence of coronary, cerebral or peripheral thromboses nor has any study convincingly shown that r-HuEPO treatment is accompanied by an increased risk of vascular access clotting. The reported cases of fistula or shunt thromboses all occurred in patients with 'fistulae-on-risk', such as earlier clotting problems or a technically complicated vascular situation [2, 9].

In 1988 sporadic reports of renal graft artery thrombosis in r-HuEPO-treated patients appeared [12]. In consequence of this, we introduced the use of antithrombotic prophylaxis in all of our r-HuEPO-treated renal graft recipients. Since then, no TEE has occurred in the EPO-treated patients compared with two cases in a group that received neither r-HuEPO nor PAT, but this difference was not statistically significant. However, the protocol resulted in a high incidence of both postoperative and biopsy-related bleeding complications, of which many were major. All the bleeding complications were observed during the first month after transplantation. No graft was lost because of such complications.

Animal studies have shown that a lower haematocrit in rats receiving renal grafts results in better early graft function, independently of preservation time and type of preservation solution [11]. We found a significant difference in haemoglobin levels between our two groups, but no difference with regard to early graft function.

r-HuEPO treatment has been shown to reduce the number of HLA antibodies in some patients [3]. A significant decrease in PRA response and a decrease in T-cell subsets during r-HuEPO treatment has also been reported. We detected no significant difference between our two groups with regard to the incidence of acute rejection and 1-year graft survival.

In summary, no differences between the groups were noted in early and late graft function nor in the incidence of acute rejections. No thromboembolic events occurred in r-HuEPO-treated patients. However, the use of PAT in the r-HuEPO-treated group resulted in a high incidence of bleeding complications. In consequence, we have abandoned the routine use of PAT in this patient group. If PAT is required, the protocol should be less stringent.

References

1. Canadian Erythropoietin Study Group (1990) Association between recombinant human erythropoietin and quality of life and exercise capacity of patients receiving hemodialysis. Br Med J 300: 573–578
2. Eschbach JW, Downing MR, Egrie JC, Browne JK, Adamson JW (1989) USA multicenter clinical trial with recombinant human erythropoietin. In: Baldamus CA, Scigalla P, Wieczorek L, Koch KM (eds) Erythropoietin: from molecular structure to clinical application. (Contributions to Nephrology, vol 76) Karger, Basel, pp 160–165
3. Grimm GC, Sinai-Trieman L, Sekiya NM, Robertson LS, Robinson BJ, Fine RN, Ettenger RB (1990) Effect of recombinant human erythropoietin on HLA sensitization and cell-mediated immunity. Kidney Int 38: 12
4. Gruetzmacher P, Bergmann M, Weinreich T, Nattermann U, Reimers E, Pollok M (1988) Beneficial and adverse effects of correction of anaemia by recombinant human erythropoietin in patients on maintenance haemodialysis. Contrib Nephrol 66: 104
5. Kokot F, Wiecek A, Greszczak W, Klepacka J, Klin M, Lao M (1989) Influence of erythropoietin treatment on endocrine abnormalities in haemodialyzed patients. In: Baldamus CA, Scigalla P, Wieczorek L, Koch KM (eds) Erythropoietin: from molecular structure to clinical application. (Contributions to Nephrology, vol 76) Karger, Basel, pp 257–272
6. Moia M, Mannuci PM, Vizzotto L, Casati S, Cattaneo M, Ponticelli C (1987) Improvement in the haemostatic defect of uraemia after treatment with recombinant human erythropoietin. Lancet I: 1227–1229
7. Samtleben W, Baldamus CA, Bommer J, Gruetzmacher P, Nonnast-Daniel B, Scigalla P, Gurland HJ (1989) Indications and contraindications for recombinant human erythropoietin treatment. In: Baldamus CA, Scigalla P, Wieczorek L, Koch KM (eds) Erythropoietin: from molecular structure to clinical application. (Contributions to Nephrology, vol 76) Karger, Basel, pp 193–200
8. Schäfer RM, Leschke M, Strauer BE, Heidland A (1988) Blood rheology and hypertension in hemodialysis patients treated with erythropoietin. Am J Nephrol 8: 449–453
9. Scigalla P, Bonzel KE, Bulla M, Burghard R, Dippel J, Geisert J, Leumann E, v. Lilien T, Mueller-Wiefel DE, Offner G, Pistor K, Zoellner K (1989) Therapy of renal anemia with recombinant human erythropoietin in children with end-stage renal disease. In: Baldamus CA, Scigalla P, Wieczorek L, Koch KM (eds) Erythropoietin: from molecular structure to clinical application. (Contributions to Nephrology, vol 76) Karger, Basel, pp 227–241
10. Vaziri ND, Ritchie C, Brown P, Kaupke J, Atkins K, Barker S, Hyatt J (1989) Effect of erythropoietin administration on blood and plasma viscosity in hemodialysis patients. Trans Am Soc Artif Intern Organs 35: 505–508
11. Wahlberg J, Jacobsson J, Odlind B, Tufveson G, Wikström B (1988) Haemodilution in renal transplantation in patients on erythropoietin. Lancet II: 1418
12. Zaoui P, Bayle F, Maurizi J, Foret M, Dalsoglio S, Vialtel P (1988) Early thrombosis in kidney grafted into patient treated with erythropoietin. Lancet II: 956

Transplant Int (1992) 5 [Suppl 1]: S 107–S 109

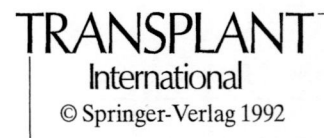

TRANSPLANT
International
© Springer-Verlag 1992

Long-term beneficial effects of azathioprine addition to ongoing cyclosporine-prednisone protocol in renal transplantation

J. Pascual, R. Marcén, L. Orofino, C. Quereda, J. L. Teruel, F. Mampaso, F. Liaño, J. J. Villafruela, and J. Ortuño

Servicio de Nefrología, Hospital Ramón y Cajal, Madrid, Spain

Abstract. Delayed addition of azathioprine (Aza) to an ongoing cyclosporine-prednisone protocol was started 11.3 ± 9.9 months after renal transplantation in 31 patients. Group I ($n = 10$) had chronic renal function deterioration due to chronic rejection, group II ($n = 11$) had repeated or severe acute rejection episodes and group III ($n = 10$) had cyclosporine (Cs) toxicity despite drug tapering. In group I, SCr had risen over the 6 months prior to Aza addition ($P < 0.05$), renal function declining at a rate of -0.13 ± 0.12 SCr^{-1}. In the 6 months post-Aza, renal function improved at a rate of 0.05 ± 0.07 SCr^{-1}, and during the entire follow-up at a rate of 0.05 ± 0.12 SCr^{-1} ($P < 0.01$) with stable Cs levels. In group II the decline in renal function was greater, though the rate of decline was stopped after Aza. In group III, renal function improved in eight patients. After 23 ± 12 months of follow-up, 15 patients had improved graft function, two were stable, 12 had worsened (nine on dialysis) and two had died. Amelioration of chronic graft dysfunction can be achieved by delayed addition of Aza to Cs-prednisone-treated renal allograft patients with chronic rejection or Cs toxicity, with long-term beneficial effects in a high proportion of patients.

Key words: Renal transplantation – Cyclosporine – Azathioprine – Triple therapy – Chronic rejection

The best approach to management of chronic renal allograft dysfunction in cyclosporine (Cs) treated renal transplant (RT) patients has not yet been defined. The current study describes short- and long-term benefits of adding azathioprine (Aza) to Cs-treated RT patients with chronic graft dysfunction due to chronic rejection, repeated or severe acute rejection episodes or Cs toxicity.

Methods

Between March 1986 and March 1991, 200 non-diabetic patients received a cadaveric renal allograft at our hospital. Immunosuppression consisted of Cs (5 mg/kg per day) i. v. for 2 days and then oral Cs (10–12 mg/kg per day) adjusted to give total blood levels (TDx, Abbott, Chicago) in the range 400–800 ng/ml for 1 month and 200–400 ng/ml thereafter. Prednisone was given at a dose of 0.5 mg/kg per day for 1 week and then tapered to 10 mg/day after 1 month. Aza (1–2 mg/kg per day) was added 11.3 ± 9.9 months after RT for 31 of the

Table 1. Renal function and Cs levels before and after addition of Aza to an ongoing Cs-prednisone

	6 months	Aza	6 months	Last visit
Group I				
Number of patients	10	10	10	7
SCr[a]	193 ± 25	255 ± 19	228 ± 22	220 ± 33
1/SCr[b]	0.50 ± 0.05	0.36 ± 0.03	0.41 ± 0.04	0.31 ± 0.08
Cs levels[c]	436 ± 52	286 ± 53	236 ± 54	184 ± 21
Group II				
Number of patients	3	11	8	4
SCr	194 ± 30	290 ± 18	299 ± 43	211 ± 35
1/SCr	0.46 ± 0.07	0.37 ± 0.06	0.23 ± 0.17	0.21 ± 0.08
Cs levels	266 ± 49	332 ± 123	275 ± 33	250 ± 44
Group III				
Number of patients	6	10	10	9
SCr	166 ± 18	210 ± 19	165 ± 14	167 ± 17
1/SCr	0.57 ± 0.08	0.45 ± 0.04	0.57 ± 0.07	0.52 ± 0.09
Cs levels	741 ± 182	469 ± 34	277 ± 40	318 ± 67
All patients				
Number of patients	19	31	28	20
SCr	189 ± 14	253 ± 11	228 ± 18	198 ± 15
1/SCr	0.51 ± 0.04	0.39 ± 0.02	0.40 ± 0.04	0.35 ± 0.05
Cs levels	506 ± 72	361 ± 26	262 ± 25	257 ± 34

Data are mean ± SEM

[a] serum creatinine (μmol/l), excluding graft loss
[b] including 1/SCr = 0 for graft loss (SCr in mg/dl)
[c] in ng/ml
See text for statistical significance

Offprint requests to: Dr. J. Pascual, Department of Nephrology, Hospital Ramón y Cajal, C. Colmenar Km 9,100, 28034 Madrid, Spain

Table 2. Evolution of renal function before and after Aza addition evaluated by the rate of change in 1/SCr

Group	6 months before Aza		Aza start vs. 6 months later	Aza start vs. last follow-up
I	−0.13 ± 0.03	Only functioning grafts	0.05 ± 0.02	0.05 ± 0.02
		1/SCr = 0 for graft loss	0.05 ± 0.02	−0.05 ± 0.06
II	−0.15 ± 0.05	Only functioning grafts	0.04 ± 0.05	0.19 ± 0.07
		1/SCr = 0 for graft loss	−0.03 ± 0.06	−0.11 ± 0.08
III	−0.07 ± 0.04	Only functioning grafts	0.13 ± 0.04	0.13 ± 0.05
		1/SCr = 0 for graft loss	0.13 ± 0.04	0.13 ± 0.05
All	−0.11 ± 0.03	Only functioning grafts	0.08 ± 0.02	0.11 ± 0.03
		1/SCr = 0 for graft loss	0.05 ± 0.03	−0.01 ± 0.04

See text for numbers of grafts in each group and situation and statistical significance

Table 3. Outcome of patient survival and graft function after addition of Aza

	Group (n)			
	I (10)	II (11)	III (10)	All (31)
At 6 months				
Better	7	3	8	18
No change	1	1	1	3
Worse	2	4	1	7
Lost (dialysis)	0	1	0	2
Dead	0	1	0	1
At last follow-up				
Months after Aza	24.9 ± 3.8	16.8 ± 3.8	28.3 ± 2.8	23.1 ± 2.1
Better	3	4	8	15
No change	2	0	0	2
Worse	2	0	1	3
Lost (dialysis)	3	6	0	9
Dead	0	1	1	2

patients. Group I ($n = 10$) had chronic renal allograft dysfunction due to chronic rejection (80% biopsy proven), group II ($n = 11$) had repeated or severe acute renal allograft rejection unresponsive to methylprednisolone boluses, and group III ($n = 10$) had Cs toxicity despite adequate blood levels and drug tapering. The time to initiation of Aza was $19.6 ± 2.8$, $5.9 ± 1.8$ and $8.9 ± 3$ months, respectively. Data are expressed as mean ± SEM and Student's t-test was used for the statistical analysis.

Results

Renal function and Cs levels before and after addition of Aza, rates of renal function changes and outcome of grafts and patients are given in Tables 1–3.

Group I. Three patients lost their grafts 15, 19 and 20 months after Aza addition. Serum creatinine (SCr) had risen over the 6 months prior to Aza addition ($P < 0.05$), renal function declining at a rate of $−0.13 ± 0.03$ SCr^{-1}. In the 6 months post-Aza renal function improved at a rate of $0.05 ± 0.02$ SCr^{-1} ($P < 0.001$) and during the entire follow-up at a rate of $0.05 ± 0.02$ SCr^{-1} excluding the three patients with graft loss ($P < 0.01$). Cs levels did not change significantly.

Group II. Renal function declined at a rate of $−0.15 ± 0.05$ SCr^{-1} before Aza was stopped 6 months after starting ($0.04 ± 0.05$, $n = 8$, $P < 0.025$), when one patient had died of pneumonia and another two had lost their grafts at 4 months. Graft loss also occurred in four patients after 10–19 months after Aza addition. Four patients had improved graft function (rate $0.19 ± 0.07$ SCr^{-1}) $28.2 ± 6.5$ months after Aza. Cs levels were stable.

Group III. Renal function improved 6 months after Aza addition ($−0.07 ± 0.04$ vs. $0.13 ± 0.04$ SCr^{-1}, $P < 0.01$) and this good function was still stable at the last follow-up. One patient died of myocardial infarction 34 months after RT. Only one patient had worse graft function after Aza addition. Cs levels were able to be significantly decreased ($P < 0.005$, basal vs. 6 months; $P < 0.01$, basal vs. last follow-up).

The rate of renal function deterioration for the whole series before Aza addition ($−0.11 ± 0.03$ SCr^{-1}) had been reversed 6 months after Aza ($0.08 ± 0.02$ SCr^{-1}, $n = 28$, $P < 0.001$) and at the last follow-up ($0.11 ± 0.03$ SCr^{-1}, $n = 21$, $P < 0.001$). Considering SCr$^{-1} = 0$ in cases of graft loss, the rates are $0.05 ± 0.03$ SCr^{-1} ($n = 31$, $P < 0.001$) at 6 months and $−0.01 ± 0.04$ SCr^{-1} ($n = 31$, $P < 0.05$) at the end of follow-up. Considering the whole series, Cs levels were decreased after Aza addition ($P < 0.02$).

Discussion

Controlled or routine conversion from Cs to Aza after RT has been attempted to avoid Cs toxicity [3, 4]. However, high rates of acute rejection have been reported [4]. Perioperative triple-drug therapy has given better rejection control, but at the expense of more serious infections and even neoplasms [1] and with unclear advantages regarding patient and graft survival. Our approach of delaying the addition of Aza to an ongoing Cs-prednisone protocol has been of clear benefit for a substantial proportion of patients with dysfunction due to chronic rejection. The reversal in the rate of change in renal function from negative to positive is highly significant in this group, with 70% of functioning grafts after a mean of 2 years of follow-up.

Other groups have reported similar benefits, but with a shorter follow-up [2, 5].

Although advantages of Aza addition in patients with repeated or severe acute rejection episodes are less clear, 36 % had functioning grafts after a mean of 16.8 months of follow-up, a significant proportion if we consider that Aza was really rescue therapy in this group.

Aza addition in patients with Cs toxicity despite normal drug levels allowed a decrease in Cs doses and levels without compromising immunosuppression. After a mean of 28 months, eight out of ten patients had improved renal function and another one had died with a functioning graft: reversal of the rate of graft function deterioration was very evident.

Amelioration of chronic graft dysfunction can be achieved by delayed addition of Aza to Cs-prednisone-treated RT recipients with chronic rejection or Cs toxicity, with long-term beneficial effects in a high proportion.

References

1. De Vecchi A, Tarantino A, Montagnino G, Egidi F, Vegeto A, Berardinelli L, Ponticelli C (1987) A controlled prospective trial of triple therapy with low-dose azathioprine, cyclosporine and methylprednisolone in renal transplantation. Transplant Proc 19: 1933–1934
2. Lorber MI, Flechner SM, Van Buren CT, Sorensen K, Kerman RH, Kahan BD (1987) Cyclosporine toxicity: the effect of combined therapy using cyclosporine, azathioprine and prednisone. Am J Kidney Dis 9: 476–484
3. Morris PJ, French ME, Dunill MS, Hunnisett AGW, Ting A, Thompson JF, Wood RFM (1983) A controlled trial of cyclosporine in renal transplantation with conversion to azathioprine and prednisone after three months. Transplantation 36: 273–277
4. Rocher LL, Milford EL, Kirkman RL, Carpenter CB, Strom T, Tilney NL (1984) Conversion from cyclosporine to azathioprine in renal allograft recipients. Transplantation 38: 669–674
5. Rocher LL, Hodgson RJ, Merion RM, Swartz RD, Keavey S, Turcotte JG, Campbell DA (1989) Amelioration of chronic renal allograft dysfunction in cyclosporine-treated patients by addition of azathioprine. Transplantation 47: 249–254

Transplant Int (1992) 5 [Suppl 1]: S110–S111

TRANSPLANT
International
© Springer-Verlag 1992

Protective effect of vasodilators in donors requiring pressor support

A. R. Pontin, A. Ovnat, J. E. Jacobson, C. R. Swanepoel, D. Kahn

Transplant Unit, Department of Surgery, University of Cape Town and Groote Schuur Hospital, Cape Town, South Africa

Renal dose dopamine given to organ donors improves renal blood flow and therefore should theoretically improve the quality of the renal grafts and increase the incidence of immediate graft function (IGF). Allografts which function immediately have a better long-term survival [1].

Dopamine, in doses of less than 4 µg/kg per min, acts directly on receptors in blood vessel walls in the splanchnic bed causing vasodilation. In contrast, dopamine given at doses of greater than 4 µg/kg per min to hypotensive donors to elevate the systemic blood pressure has a direct adrenergic effect and causes vasoconstriction. This vasoconstriction when combined with the reperfusion injury which occurs after transplantation may jeopardize the chance of the graft functioning immediately. We studied 31 consecutive donors to see if those donors requiring pressor support (dopamine) to maintain systemic blood pressure had a lower incidence of IGF and whether this could be modified by giving the donor vasodilator drugs during procurement of the organs.

Key words: Renal transplantation – Organ donation – Dopamine

Patients and methods

The study group comprised 31 consecutive organ donors. Conventional methods for monitoring and managing the donors were used and, in particular, the donors were given dopamine if the systemic pressure fell below 90 mm Hg despite adequate ventilation and fluid replacement. The dose of dopamine was titrated against its pressor effect on the donor.

The period between the certification of brain death and procurement of the organs was less than 12 h in all donors. The procurement

Offprint requests to: Dr. A. Pontin, Transplant Unit, Department of Surgery, Medical School, Observatory 7925, Cape Town, South Africa

of the kidneys was performed by the same donor team with an *en bloc* removal of the kidneys, aorta and vena cava.

The 31 donors were randomly assigned to receive intravenous vasodilators or not. Phenoxybenzamine 100 mg was given at the start of the operation, and verapamil 5 mg and regitine 10 mg just prior to cross-clamping the aorta. The kidneys were perfused with Euro-Collins solution and stored on ice until transplanted. IGF was defined as adequate renal function such that the patient did not require dialysis in the first postoperative week.

Results

The demographic data of the donors is shown in Table 1. The group of ten donors who received vasodilator drugs had a slightly greater average donor age, a greater male to female ratio, a greater number of grafts perfused in situ, a slightly longer cold ischaemic time, and a greater number of donors requiring dopamine support than the control group not given vasodilators.

The incidence of IGF after transplantation was 81 % in the kidneys procured from donors treated with vasodilators drugs and 52 % in the control group who did not receive vasodilator drugs (Table 2). The survival at 3 months of grafts from donors treated with vasodilator drugs was 94 % and of grafts from the control group was

Table 1. Demographic data of the donors in the vasodilator group and the control group

	Vasodilator group	Control
Number	10	21
Sex (M/F)	9/1	16/5
Perfusion		
in situ	4	3
ex situ	6	18
Organs procured		
kidneys only	6	14
multiple	4	7
Cold ischaemic time (h)	21	18
No. requiring dopamine support	5 (50 %)	8 (39 %)

Table 2. Incidence of immediate graft function (IGF) and 3-month graft survival in the grafts from donors receiving vasodilators and those not receiving vasodilators

	Vasodilator group	Control
Number of grafts	16	25
Immediate function	13 (81%)	13 (52%)
3-month graft survival	15 (94%)	20 (80%)

Table 3. Incidence of immediate graft function in the grafts removed from donors who required dopamine support and were given vasodilators

	Vasodilator group	Control
Donors needing dopamine support	5	8
Number of grafts	6	11
Immediate function	5 (83%)	2 (18%)

80% (Table 2). The beneficial effect of the vasodilator drugs was even more marked in the donors who required dopamine support. Of the grafts removed from donors who required dopamine support, 83% functioned immediately when vasodilator drugs were used compared with 18% when no vasodilator drugs were used ($P < 0.05$) (Table 3).

Discussion

One of the primary goals in renal transplantation is immediate function of the allograft. This can usually be expected in a well-hydrated, well-perfused living donor. However, with brain death, the many pathophysiological changes can effect the microcirculation and reduce the chances of IGF, especially if the donor requires dopamine support [2]. Dopamine is used in excess of 4 µg/kg per min to raise the blood pressure and does so by splanchnic vasoconstriction. The detrimental effects of vasoconstriction in the donor are aggravated by the reperfusion injury which occurs when the organ is transplanted. The reperfusion injury may be reduced by a number of drugs including diuretics, membrane stabilizers, nucleotide savers, scavengers, vasodilators and calcium channel blockers [5]. In this study, a combination of two vasodilators and a calcium channel blocker was used in the donor at the time of organ procurement.

The detrimental effect of dopamine has been shown experimentaly in a brain-dead pig model [3]. Furthermore, this effect could be reduced by pretreatment of the donor with tri-iodothyronine. Similarly, in clinical studies, acute tubular necrosis occurred in 50% of grafts if the donor received dopamine and 28% if they did not [4]. One-year graft survival was 27% for the grafts from dopamine-treated donors and 57% for the grafts from the donors not receiving dopamine [4].

In this study graft function was impaired when the donor had received dopamine. These effects could be reversed by the use of a combination of vasodilators and a calcium channel blocker given at the time of organ procurement. We recommend that all donors who require dopamine for pressor support be given vasodilators and a calcium channel blocker.

References

1. Ferguson RM, Henry ML, Scrimer BG et al (1987) In: Terasaki P (ed) Clinical transplants. UCLA Tissue Typing Laboratory, Los Angeles, p 195
2. Koller J, Wieser C, Kornberger R et al (1990) Influence of the renin-angiotensin system of the organ donor on kidney function after transplantation. Transplant Proc 22: 349–350
3. Pienaar BH, Schwartz I, Roncone A, Lotz Z, Hickman R (1990) Function of kidney grafts from brain dead donor pigs. Transplantation 50: 580–582
4. Schneider A, Toledo-Pereyra LH, Zeichner WD, Allaben R, Whitten J (1983) Effect of dopamine and pitressin on kidneys procured and harvested for transplantation. Transplantation 36: 110–111
5. Scot McDougal W (1988) Renal perfusion/reperfusion injury. J Urol 140: 1325–1331

Transplant Int (1992) 5 [Suppl 1]: S112–S113

TRANSPLANT
International
© Springer-Verlag 1992

The use of OKT3 in steroid-resistant rejections following cadaveric kidney transplantation

B. Rosenkranz, W. Niebel, K. Albrecht, K. Wagner, T. Philipp, and F. W. Eigler

Department for General Surgery, University Hospitals, D-4300 Essen, FRG

OKT3 has been proved to be effective in the treatment of steroid-resistant rejection after renal allograft transplantation [1]. We investigated the clinical course of OKT3 recipients to find out in which cases of steroid resistance OKT3 therapy might be ineffective.

Key words: Renal transplantation – Rejection – OKT3

Material and methods

From December 1986 to October 1990, 380 consecutive cadaveric kidney transplantations were performed. Routine immunosuppression consisted of CsA and prednisone. In cases of high immunological risk, azathioprine was additionally given. If an acute cellular rejection occurred and was confirmed histologically, steroid therapy was administered. Until June 1989 two courses of steroid pulses (3×0.25 g IV) were given, and from then on only one course. In 54 of the 380 patients the rejections were steroid resistant. In all of these cases persisent rejection was confirmed histologically and then treated with OKT3 (5 mg per day for 7–14 days). With regard to age, sex, HLA mismatches and number of transplantations, this group of patients showed no significant differences compared with a group of 326 patients not treated with OKT3. The mean follow-up time was 18 months for the OKT3 recipients and 23 months for the other group. The cases in which rejection was reversed after OKT3 therapy were compared with those with organ loss (Table 1). Patient and graft survival were calculated using the life-table method.

Results

In 54 (17%) of 380 patients, steroid-resistant rejection occurred and was treated with OKT3. In 28 of these patients the graft was rescued (52%) and in 26 cases (48%) the graft was lost. Six patients (11%) of the OKT3 group died within 18 months after transplantation, three of these due to enforced immunosuppression (EBV sepsis; CMV sepsis plus reactivated tuberculosis; enterococcus pneumonia plus peritonitis plus sepsis). One patient died from

aortic dissection developing on top of an iliacal occlusion which occurred under OKT3 therapy. Two other patients died from cardiac failure in generalized sepsis with pre-existent diabetes and from gastrointestinal bleeding subsequent to pre-existing chronic hepatitis plus chronic rejection. In nine cases (17%) OKT3 therapy had to be withdrawn for the following reasons: stomatitis (two), HSV meningitis, somnolence, psychosis and exhaustion (three). Eight of these patients lost their graft, and one graft was rescued later with ATG therapy and showed good function.

In 13 of the cases with organ loss (50%) histological findings showed predominantly perivascular infiltration, endothelial proliferation and/or epithelial necrosis. In the group with good organ function, six biopsies (21%) gave the same result. The number of kidneys preserved in Collins solution was significantly higher in the group with graft loss.

In the OKT3-treated group, 1-year graft survival was 58% ±7% versus 85% ±2% in the patients not treated with OKT3. In the OKT3 group, 1-year patient survival was 90% ±4% versus 95% ±1% in the other patients. The 1-year survival for the patients with restored renal function ($n = 28$) was 100% compared with 81% for the OKT3 recipients ($n = 26$) with graft loss.

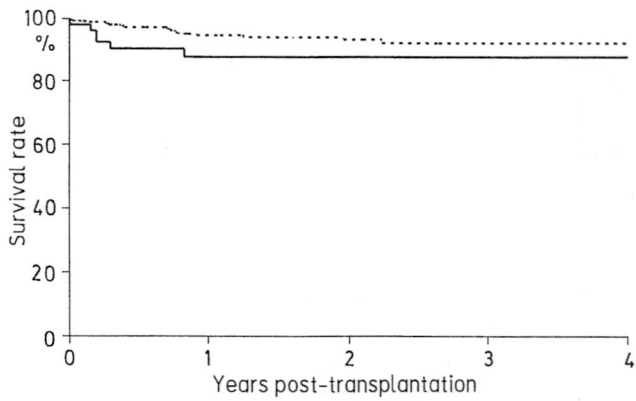

Fig. 1. Actuarial patient survival of OKT3 recipients ($n = 54$) (—) vs. patients not treated with OKT3 ($n = 322$) (----). $P = 0.1$

Offprint requests to: B. Rosenkranz

Table 1. Comparison of OKT3-treated patients: rescued vs. lost grafts

	Good function (> 3 months)	Graft loss (< 3 months)	P
Number of patients	28	26	
Recipient age (years)	41.9 ± 1.9	42.8 ± 2.3	n.s.
Sex (male: female)	17:11	16:10	n.s.
Transplantation number			
First	26 (93%)	23 (88%)	n.s.
Second/third	2 (7%)	3 (12%)	n.s.
Cold preservation (h)	23.14 ± 1.37	22.65 ± 1.35	n.s.
Donor age (years)	37.79 ± 3.42	38.08 ± 4.27	n.s.
Preservation solution			
Collins	13 (46%)	19 (73%)	0.046
UW/HTK	15 (45%)	22 (41%)	
Panel reactive antibodies (%)	3.53 ± 1.9	8.19 ± 4.03	n.s.
Mismatch			
HLA-A	0.82 ± 0.12	0.69 ± 0.12	n.s.
HLA-B	0.78 ± 0.1	0.69 ± 0.12	n.s.
HLA-DR	0.50 ± 0.12	0.53 ± 0.09	n.s.
Withdrawal of OKT3	1 (4%)	8 (31%)	
Start of OKT3 treatment (weeks post-transplantation)	4.6	3.5	
Predominant histological findings			
Perivascular infiltration and/or endothelial proliferation and/or epithelial necrosis	6 (21%)	13 (50%)	0.028
Cellular rejection	22 (79%)	13 (50%)	

Values are means ± SEM

Discussion

The high efficacy of the monoclonal antibody OKT3 for steroid-resistant rejection is well known. On the other hand, during clinical use severe side-effects and even a fatal outcome directly related to OKT3 administration have been observed. The combination of previous high-dose steroid anti-rejection therapy with OKT3 is not recommended because of the high risk of infection [2]. Therefore we reduced steroid treatment to one course. In all cases of steroid resistance the use of OKT3 should be considered carefully, taking into account individual patient risk and histopathological findings. Pre-existent chronic diseases ought not to be underestimated. ATG or triple therapy are alternatives in the treatment of steroid-resistant rejection.

Conclusion

There are alternatives to OKT3 in the treatment of steroid-resistant rejection. In cases of high risk of morbidity and histopathological findings that indicate probable ineffectiveness of OKT3, alternative therapy is used in Essen.

References

1. Cosimi AB (1985) Treatment of rejection: antithymocyte globulin versus monoclonal antibody. Transplant Proc 17: 1526–1529
2. Niebel W, Albrecht KH, Mathers MJ, Feldhoff C, Vögeler U, Eigler FW (1989) Die Therapie der ‚steroid-resistenten' akuten Abstoßung nach allogener Leichennierentransplantation mit ATG und OKT3 – eine retrospektive Studie. In: Lison A, Buchholz B (eds) Spezifische Immunsuppression mit OKT3. Wolfgang Pabst Verlag, pp 75–84

Transplant Int (1992) 5 [Suppl 1]: S114–S115

TRANSPLANT
International
© Springer-Verlag 1992

Aging on the waiting list: should it be a further criterion for cadaver kidney allocation?

M. Salvadori, L. Comparini, E. Bertoni, S. Bandini, G. Mancini, F. Martinelli, P. Tosi, G. Nicita, and R. Lenzi

Department of Transplantation, Careggi Hospital, Florence, Italy

Abstract. Transplant recipients have been selected from our dialysis patients mainly according to the criteria of the best HLA match and the best clinical condition. We have observed that, in using these criteria, most of the patients who receive transplants in the first 2 years on the waiting list. The other patients remain on the waiting list with progressively less chance of transplantation due to a deterioration of their clinical condition and the related increase in risk factors.

Key words: Risk factors – Waiting list – Kidney allocation

Considering that donors are scarce and the chance of receiving a transplant is decreasing [4], the goals in developing an organ allocation system should include fairness (equal opportunity), efficacy and praticality [1]. Many of these goals frequently conflict, so that each transplant center has its own method of allocating kidneys. In this paper we review our experience with criteria for kidney allocation as both a transplant center and a dialysis unit.

Our own transplant program began in 1988. Until then we referred our dialysis patients abroad or to other Italian waiting lists for transplantation. Most of these transplant programs considered HLA-A, -B, -DR matching as the major criterion for kidney allocation. Because of the large size of these waiting lists, two or more equally matched patients were often found. We feel that in such cases the selection of the patient was mainly on a clinical basis.

In order to verify the impact of such a transplant policy on the waiting list, we reviewed the records of our transplant recipients and those of our patients still waiting for a transplant.

Offprint requests to: Maurizio Salvadori, M.D., Department of Transplantation, Villa Monna Tessa, Viale Pieraccini, 18-50100 Florence, Italy

Materials and methods

We reviewed the records of 120 transplant recipients and the records of 58 of our dialysis patients still waiting for a kidney transplant. We also reviewed the records of 180 uraemic patients waiting for a transplant on our waiting list who came from other dialysis units.

After reviewing reports in the literature, we considered the following as risk factors for transplantation:

A. Sensitization [3]. We arbitrarily considered at risk patients with more than 30% panel reactive antibodies.
B. Clinical condition [2].
C. Peripheral vascular disease.
D. Urinary tract disease [6].
E. Age [5]. We considered at risk patients older than fifty years.

According to the presence of one or more of the above risk factors each patient on the waiting list was allocated a 'risk score'.

Results

Figures 1 and 2 show, respectively, the time on the waiting list for our transplant recipients and for our patients still waiting for a transplant. We found that 80% of the transplant recipients received transplants during the initial

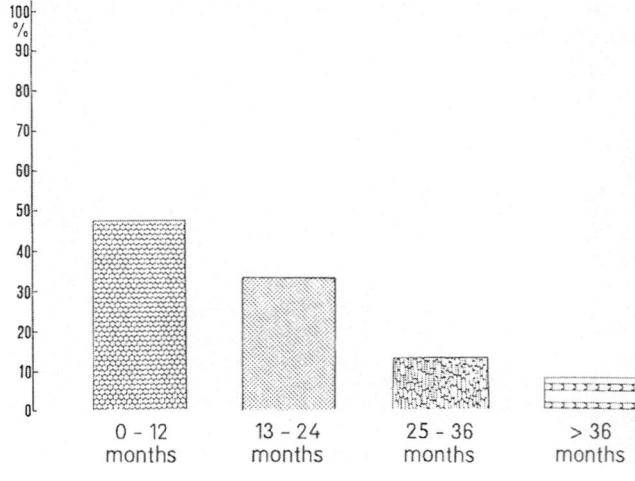

Fig. 1. Time elapsed on waiting list for our 120 transplanted patients

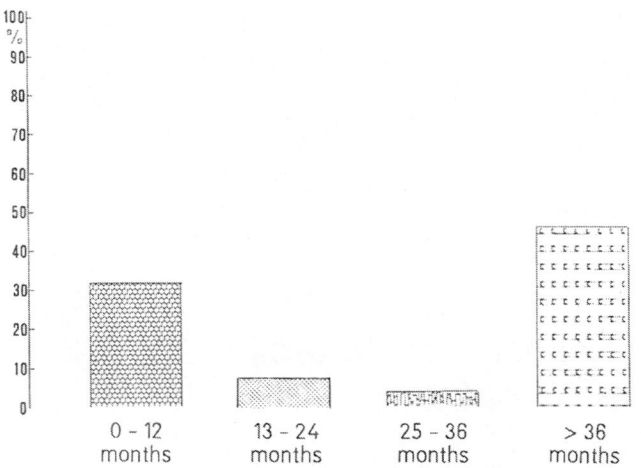

Fig. 2. Time elapsed on waiting list for our 58 dialysis patients still waiting for a transplant

2 years of waiting. In contrast, 47 % of the patients still waiting had been on the list for more than 36 months, and would probably never receive a graft.

The overall prevalence of the risk factors considered were as follows: sensitisation (27 %), poor clinical condition (37 %), vascular disease (21 %), urinary tract disease (23 %) and age (31 %). Of the 180 patients waiting for a transplant on our list, those waiting for 1–2, 3–4, 5–6, 7–8, and more than 8 years had a mean risk score of 0.57, 0.68, 1.54, 2.27 and 1.93, respectively.

Discussion

Most of our dialysis patients who received a transplant did so in the first years of waiting. Only 7 % of the transplant recipients waited longer than 36 months. In contrast, the majority of our patients still waiting for a transplant have been waiting for more than 36 months, and, according to previous reports, these patients have a poor chance of receiving a transplant. We believe that this is a consequence of the selection criteria. Selecting a patient for transplantation relying only on the best match and, secondly, on the best clinical condition, has two consequences:

1. The 'lucky' patients will receive transplants in the first years of waiting with good matches, low risk and good results.
2. For the 'unlucky' patients, the risk factors will increase year by year, and many of them will never be considered for transplantation, particularly in cases of long waiting lists.

Reviewing the records of the uraemic patients waiting for a transplant on our own program, we observed that the incidence of dialysis-related risk factors increases year by year while the patients are on the waiting list. As a consequence, we think that, besides the above-mentioned factors (i.e. good match and good clinical condition), the time on dialysis therapy should also be considered as a criterion in kidney allocation.

References

1. Frey DJ, Matas AJ (1991) Allocation of cadaver kidneys: A survey of the American Society of Transplant Surgeons. Clin Transplant 5: 1–2
2. Hutchinson TA, Duncan C, Thomas JC (1984) Prognostically controlled comparison of dialysis and renal transplantation. Kidney Int 26: 44–48
3. Iwaki Y, Iguro T, Terasaki PI (1985) Effect of sensitization on kidney allografts. In: Terasaki PI (ed) Clinical kidney transplants 1985. UCLA Tissue Typing Laboratory, Los Angeles, pp 139–145
4. Kjellstrand C (1990) The distribution of renal transplants – are physicians just? Transplant Proc 22: 964–965
5. Lee PC, Terasaki PI (1985) Effect of age on kidney transplants. In: Terasaki PI (ed) Clinical kidney transplants 1985. UCLA Tissue Typing Laboratory, Los Angeles, pp 127–134
6. Ramsey DE, Finch WT, Birtch AG (1979) Urinary tract infections in kidney transplant recipients. Arch Surg 114: 1022–1029

Transplant Int (1992) 5 [Suppl 1]: S 116–S 120

TRANSPLANT
International
© Springer-Verlag 1992

Risk factors for development of panel reactive antibodies and their impact on kidney transplantation outcome

Th. Sautner, M. Gnant, C. Banhegyi, P. Wamser, P. Götzinger, R. Steininger, and F. Mühlbacher

I. Chirurgische Universitätsklinik, Wien, Austria

Abstract. The impact of potential risk factors for development of panel reactive antibodies (PRA) in 1078 cadaveric kidney graft recipients was investigated in a multivariate analysis. Multiple transplantation, transfusion of more than five blood units and more than two pregnancies were revealed as factors with a significant independent impact on the formation of high levels of PRA. Multiple transplantation and polytransfusion also affected primary non-function, initial function and long-term graft survival at 1, 3 and 5 years. Incidence of early rejection (within 30 days) was significantly increased with repeated transplantation and decreased with a full-house HLA match. However, these effects on transplantation outcome could only be observed when risk factors lead to the formation of antibodies. In patients with risk factors present, but without subsequent sensitization, the graft survival expectation was the same as in patients in whom risk factors were absent.

Key words: Panel reactive antibodies – Risk factors – Kidney transplantation – Transplantation outcome

High levels of panel reactive antibodies (PRA) are known to be a risk factor for the outcome of renal transplantation. Although some authors have shown that good results can be achieved in patients with elevated PRA [3], and that successful transplantation is possible across the barrier of a positive crossmatch [9], many centres still yield less satisfactory results in sensitized patients [1, 8, 10]. There have been attempts to improve the chances for this group of patients through international exchange programmes which allow the priority transplantation of these patients or even grafting of organs with acceptable HLA compatibility [3, 5]. We investigated which of the factors suspected to have an impact on the development of PRA would prove significant and what their impact was on transplantation outcome. In a subset analysis the independent impact of risk factors on transplantation outcome was investigated.

Offprint requests to: Th. Sautner, I. Chirurgische Universitätsklinik, Alserstr. 4, A-1097 Wien, Austria

Patients and methods

The analysis was carried out on the cohort of cadaveric transplant recipients at our transplant unit in the cyclosporine era. All patients between 1982 and 1991 with available data on preoperative course (duration of kidney disease, waiting time on dialysis, number of blood units transfused prior to transplantation and number of pregnancies) and postoperative follow-up (eventual rejection episodes during the first 30 days, initial function and long-term follow-up) were entered into the study. Grafts lost immediately for technical reasons were excluded ($n = 16$, 1.3 %) with these restrictions, out of a total of 1222 transplants performed, 1078 were able to be analysed.

The cohort was divided into four groups according to PRA level. Group one (GR1) comprised 762 patients with no antibodies, group two (GR2) 142 patients with 1–20 % PRA (low sensitization), group three (GR3) 105 patients with 21–60 % PRA (intermediate sensitization) and group four (GR4) 69 patients with 61–100 % PRA (highly sensitized). The following potential risk factors were investigated:

1. Multiple transplantation (MT) (first, $n = 895$; second, $n = 146$; third or subsequent, ($n = 37$)
2. Blood transfusions (BT) (none, $n = 149$; 1–5, $n = 474$; 5–10, $n = 181$; 10 or more, $n = 274$)
3. Pregnancies (PR) (none, $n = 140$; 1–2, $n = 175$; 3 or more, $n = 104$)
4. Duration of kidney disease (DD) (0–5 years, $n = 510$; over 5 years, $n = 568$)
5. Recipient sex (female, $n = 419$; male, $n = 659$)
6. Recipient age (1–77 years, mean 43.4 ± 14.1 years continuously)

All interactions of the above factors were also investigated. Risk of sensitization was analysed by stepwise polychotomous logistic regression. Factors that revealed a significant impact on the development of PRA were analysed as risk factors for transplantation outcome by their influence on primary non-function (never functioning transplants) (PNF), inital function (IF) (measured by urine output in the first 24 h) [0–200 ml (anuria), 201–1500 ml (oliguria), > 1500 ml (normal diuresis)], incidence of rejection episodes in the first 30 days (ERE) and long-term function (LTF) (at 1, 3 and 5 years). Methods used were the Chi-squared test, Kaplan Meier estimates, stepwise logistic regression and Cox's multivariate proportional hazards model analysis where appropriate. The results of Kaplan Meier estimates are given as percentage of functioning grafts, with standard error (probabilities are given for Breslow and Mantel-Cox tests). The results from stepwise logistic regression and Cox's hazards model analysis are given in relative risks (RR) which indicate the increase in the probability of occurrence of the predicted event.

Transplantation was carried out only after a negative preoperative T-cell cross-match with recent recipient serum (not older than 3 months). The technical details of transplantation and the mode of immunosuppression are described elsewhere [7].

Table 1. Relative risk (RR) and 95 % confidence interval (CI 95 %) of independent risk factors for the development of panel reactive antibodies (PRA). MT, multiple transplantation; BT, blood transfusions; PR, pregnancies

| | PRA | | | | | | |
| | 0 % | 1–20 % | | 21–60 % | | > 60 % | |
	RR	RR	CI 95 %	RR	CI 95 %	RR	CI 95 %
MT							
2nd	1.0	2.2	1.3–3.7	2.2	1.3–4.0	5.7	3.0–11.0
≥ 3rd	1.0	2.0	0.51–7.9	10.0	3.7–29.0	43.0	16–120.0
							P < 0.0001
BT							
1–5	1.0	1.5	0.79–2.8	2.4	0.98–6.1	0.88	0.32–2.4
6–10	1.0	1.5	0.72–3.1	3.9	1.5–10.0	2.1	0.77–5.8
≥ 11	1.0	3.2	1.7–6.2	5.2	2.1–13.0	3.7	1.5–8.9
							P < 0.0001
PR							
1–2	1.0	1.1	0.7–1.9	1.9	1.1–3.3	2.1	0.98–4.3
> 2	1.0	1.2	0.63–2.3	2.9	1.5–5.5	6.4	2.6–14.0
							P < 0.0001
Recipient age							
1 year	1.0	1.0	0.99–1.0	0.99	0.97–1.0	0.98	0.95–1.0
							P = 0.070

Results

Risk factors for PRA formation

Factors with an independent impact on development of PRA were MT with a RR after the second graft of 2.2 for GR2, 2.2 for GR3 and 5.7 for GR4, and after the third graft 2.0 for GR2, 10 for GR3 and 43 for GR4. BT showed a RR of 1.5 (GR2), 2.4 (GR3) and 0.88 (GR4) for 1–5 BT, 1.5 (GR2), 3.9 (GR3) and 2.1 (GR4) for 6–10 BT and 3.2 (GR2), 5.2 (GR3) and 3.7 (GR4) for > 10 BT. PR caused an increase in RR of 1.1 (GR2), 1.9 (GR3) and 2.1 (GR4) for 1–2 PR and 1.2 (GR2), 2.9 (GR3) and 6.4 (GR4) for > 2 PR. Recipient age showed a RR of 1 (GR1), 0.99 (GR2) and 0.98 (GR3) for each 1-year step. Significance levels were $P < 0.0001$ for MT, BT and PR, and $P < 0.07$ for recipient age (Table 1).

In the analysis of interactions among the single variables, none of the interactions revealed an independent impact on development of PRA.

Impact of different PRA levels on waiting time and outcome parameters

Waiting time for transplantation. Waiting time for GR1 was 24.9 months, GR2 31.7 months, GR3 36.1 months and GR4 39.8 months ($P = 0.007$ for GR1 vs. GR2, $P < 0.0001$ for GR1 vs GR3, GR4). The differences between the other groups did not reach significance.

Primary non function. Incidence of PNF (overall 72 patients) was 42 patients (5.5 %) in GR1, nine (6.3 %) in GR2, nine (8.6 %) in GR3 and 12 (17.4 %) in GR4 ($P = 0.002$).

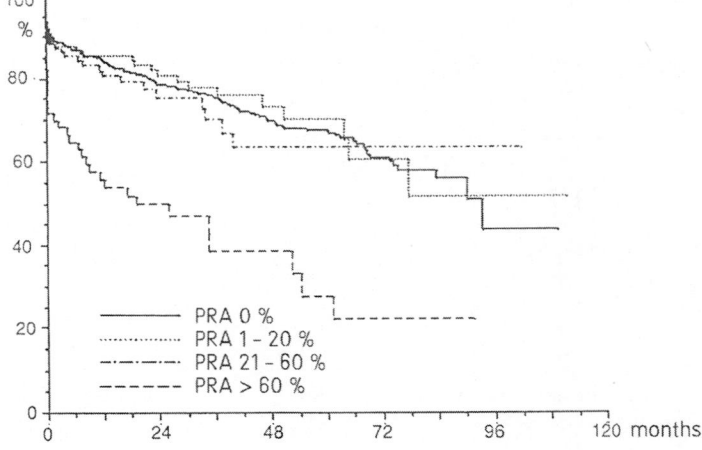

Fig. 1. Percent graft survival for different PRA levels (Kaplan Meier estimates, $P < 0.0001$ Breslow, $P < 0.0001$ Mantel-Cox GR1, 2, 3 vs. GR4)

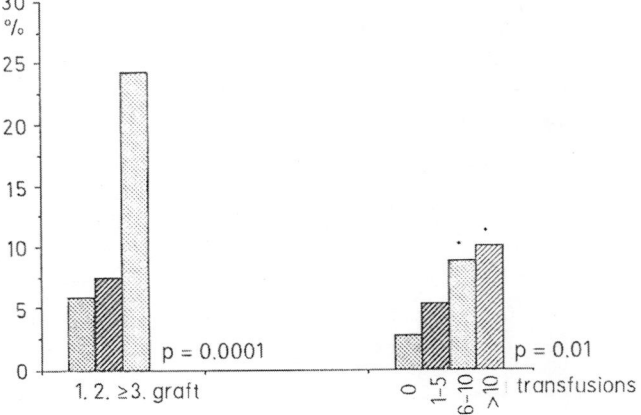

Fig. 2. Differences in incidence of PNF for number of transplantations and number of transfusions

Initial function. IF was anuria for 135 patients (17.7%) in GR1, 35 (24.6%) in GR2, 21 (20%) in GR3 and 20 (29%) in GR4. Grafts showed oliguria in 149 patients (19.5%) in GR1, 14 (9.9%) in GR2, 25 (23.8%) in GR3, and 16 (23.2%) in GR4. Normal diuresis was established in 478 patients (62.8%) in GR1, 93 (65.5%) in GR2, 59 (56.2%) in GR3, and 33 (47.8%) in GR4 ($P = 0.037$).

Early rejection episodes. Total incidence was 518 (48%). Of these, 428 patients (39%) had single episodes (SRE) and 90 (8%) multiple (MRE). SRE occurred in 41.7% in GR1, 37.4% in GR2, 30.7% in GR3 and in 55.7% in GR4. Incidence of MRE within the first 30 days was 6.5% in GR1, 6.1% in GR2, 7.9% in GR3 and 14.8% in GR4 ($P = 0.001$; GR1, 2 and 3 vs GR4).

Long-term function. LTF at 1, 3 and 5 years was $84.5 \pm 1\%$, $75.5 \pm 2\%$ and $67.4 \pm 2\%$ for GR1; $85.3 \pm 3\%$, $77.6 \pm 4\%$ and $69.9 \pm 5\%$ for GR2; $81.8 \pm 4\%$, $69.8 \pm 6\%$ and $63.4 \pm 7\%$ for GR3; and $55.6 \pm 6\%$, $38.4 \pm 7\%$ and $27.4 \pm 8\%$ for GR4 ($P < 0001$; GR1, 2 and 3 vs GR4) (Fig. 1).

Impact of risk factors on outcome parameters

Incidence of PNF.
Multiple transplantation: one graft, $n = 52$ (5.8%); two grafts, $n = 11$ (7.5%); three or more grafts, $n = 9$ (24.3%) ($P < 0.0001$).

Blood transfusions: none, $n = 4$ (2.7%); 1–5 units, $n = 25$ (5.3%); 5–10 units, $n = 16$ (8.8%); >10 units, $n = 27$ (9.8%) ($P = 0.01$).

Pregnancies: none, $n = 53$ (4.9%); one or two, $n = 13$ (7.4%); more than two, $n = 6$ (5.7%) (n.s.).

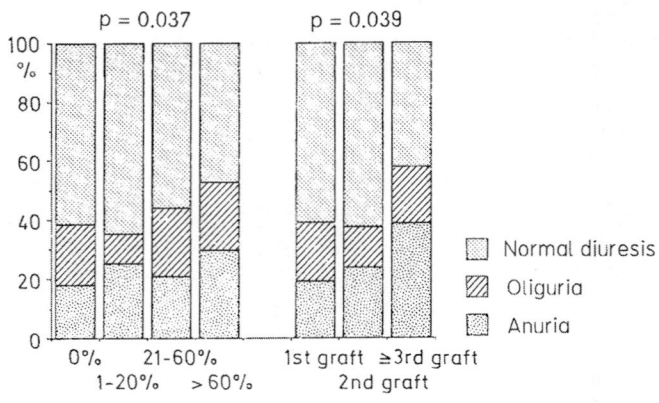

Fig. 3. Differences in initial function (first 24 h) for PRA levels and number of transplantations

Duration of kidney disease: <5 years, $n = 33$ (6.5%); ≥ 5 years, $n = 39$ (6.9%) (n.s.) (Fig. 2).

Initial function. Multiple transplantation: For first grafts, anuria in 163 patients (18.2%), oliguria in 177 (19.8%) and normal diuresis in 555 (62%); for second grafts, anuria in 34 patients (23.3%), oliguria in 20 (13.7%) and normal diuresis in 92 (63%). For third or subsequent grafts, anuria in 14 patients (37.8%), oliguria in 17 (18.9%) and normal diuresis in 16 (43.3%) ($P = 0.039$ (Fig. 3).

Blood transfusions, pregnancies and duration of kidney disease did not significantly affect initial function.

Incidence of rejection episodes. In addition to the suspected risk factors for PRA development, HLA A, B and DR mismatch were included in the stepwise logistic regression analysis for the occurrence of rejection. The following variables revealed a significant independent impact on the occurrence of single (SRE) or multiple (MRE)

Table 2. Relative risk (RR) and 95% confidence interval (CI 95%) of independent risk factors for the occurrence of early rejection episodes (ERE) [single (SRE) or multiple (MRE)] in all patients and in non-sensitized patients only. MT, multiple transplantation; FH, full-house HLA match

	ERE				
	0	1 (SRE)		>1 (MRE)	
	RR	RR	CI 95%	RR	CI 95%
Sensitized patients					
MT					
2nd	1.0	1.2	0.81–1.8	1.5	0.74–3.0
≥3rd	1.0	6.4	2.2–19.0	14.0	4.1–51.0 $P < 0.0001$
Non-sensitized patients					
MT					
2nd	1.0	not in the model		not in the model	
≥3rd	1.0	not in the model		not in the model	
Sensitized patients					
FH					
yes	1.0	0.40	0.21–0.77	0.59	0.18–2.0 $P = 0.012$
Non-sensitized patients					
FH					
yes	1.0	0.38	0.19–0.76	0.68	0.20–2.3 $P = 0.015$

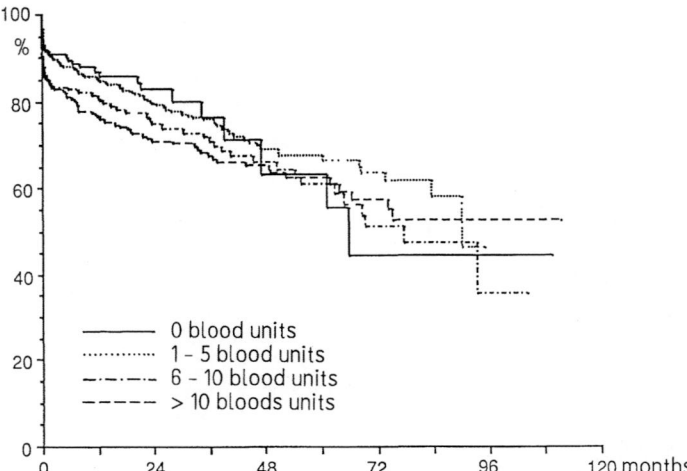

Fig. 4. Percent graft survival by number of blood units transfused (Kaplan Meier estimates, $P < 0.015$ Breslow, $P < 0.002$ Mantel-Cox)

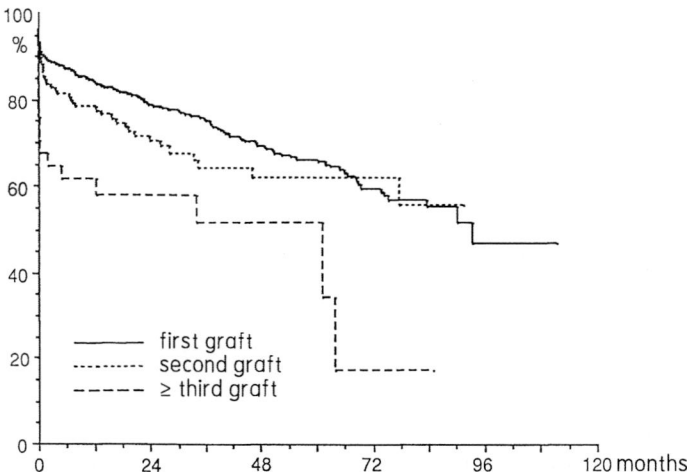

Fig. 5. Percent graft survival by number of transplantations (Kaplan Meier estimates, $P = 0.001$ Breslow, $P < 0.0001$ Mantel-Cox GR1, 2, 3 vs GR4)

rejection episodes. MT showed a RR for SRE of 1.2 for second transplantations and 6.4 for third or subsequent transplantations. The RR for development of MRE was 1.5 for second transplantations and 14 for third or subsequent transplantations ($P < 0.0001$). A six-loci HLA match significantly reduced the risk of SRE and MRE. RR for full-house (FH) match was 0.40 for SRE and 0.59 for MRE ($P = 0.012$).

In the cohort of non-sensitized patients (GR1), the only significant independent risk factor for the occurrence of ERE was a FH match with a RR of 0.38 for SRE and 0.68 for MRE ($P = 0.015$) (Table 2).

The effects of risk factors on LTF were analysed by univariate Kaplan-Meier estimates and Cox's multi-variate proportional hazardous model. Factors having significant impact on LTF in the univariate analysis were BT and MT. Patients who had received no BT had a 1-, 3- and 5-year graft survival of $86.9 \pm 2\%$, $75.5 \pm 5\%$ and $63.7 \pm 9\%$. The graft-function rates for one to five BT were $85.5 \pm 1\%$, $76.3 \pm 2\%$ and $68.7 \pm 2\%$, and with five to ten BT the rates were $80.5 \pm 2\%$, $69.8 \pm 3\%$ and $60.8 \pm 4\%$. For more than ten BT the graft survival was

$76.1 \pm 2\%$, $67.3 \pm 3\%$ and $61.4 \pm 3\%$ ($P = 0.002$ Breslow; $P = 0.015$ Mantel) (Fig. 4).

MT affected graft function at 1, 3 and 5 years as follows: first graft had function rates of $84.5 \pm 1\%$, $75.4 \pm 1\%$ and $66.5 \pm 2\%$, respectively; second grafts $77 \pm 3\%$, $63.6 \pm 4\%$ and $61.6 \pm 5\%$, respectively; and third, fourth and fifth grafts had function rates of $61.1 \pm 7\%$ at 1 year and $52.1 \pm 8\%$ at 3 and 5 years ($P = 0.001$ Breslow; $P < 0.0001$ Mantel) (Fig. 5).

When calculations were carried out for non-sensitized patients only (GR1) no statistically significant effect of the risk factors on graft survival could be demonstrated.

In the multivariate proportional hazards model, in addition to the suspected factors for development of PRA, variables considered as potentially affecting graft survival were entered: donor and recipient age, donor and recipient sex, A, B and DR match, warm and cold ischaemic time and occurrence of early rejection.

Factors increasing the risk of grafts loss were MT [RR 1.37 for second grafts and 1.88 for third and subsequent grafts ($P = 0.008$)], first warm ischaemic time [≤ 5 min, RR 1.3; > 5 min, RR 1.75 ($P = 0.031$)] and incidence of early rejection [RR 1.35 ($P = 0.014$)]. Factors decreasing

Table 3. Relative risk (RR) for graft loss. Variables (RF) with significant influence. Analysis for all patients and for non-sensitized patients only

	RR	P-value
Multiple transplantation:		
PRA > 0		
2nd	1.3	
$\geq$ 3rd	1.8	0.008
PRA $= 0$		
2nd		
$\geq$ 3rd		not in the model
Warm ischaemic time:		
PRA > 0		
1–5	1.3	
6–10	1.7	0.031
PRA $= 0$		
1–5	1.4	
6–10	2.1	0.031
Early rejection episode:		
PRA > 0		
1	1.3	
> 1	1.5	0.014
PRA $= 0$		
1		
> 1		not in the model
Recipient age:		
PRA > 0		
1 year	0.98	
10 years	0.82	< 0.0001
PRA $= 0$		
1 year	0.97	< 0.0001
Disease duration:		
PRA > 0		
> 5 years	0.74	0.024
PRA $= 0$		
> 5 years	0.70	0.011

the risk of graft loss were longer duration of kidney disease [> 5 years, RR 0.74 ($P = 0.024$)] and increasing recipient age [1 year age difference, RR 0.98, and 10 years age difference, RR 0.82 ($P < 0.0001$)].

When calculations were carried out for non-sensitized patients only (GR1) no independent statistically significant effect on graft survival could be demonstrated for the risk factors for PRA formation. The factors remaining significant were warm ischaemic time [1–5 min, RR 1.4 > 5 min, RR 2.1 ($P = 0.006$)], recipient age 1 year age difference, [RR 0.97 ($P < 0.0001$)] and duration of kidney disease $\geq$ 5 years, RR 0.70 ($P = 0.011$)] (Table 3).

Discussion

Almost all of the suspected risk factors seem to affect the development of PRA in a rather complex way. The relative risk for low sensitization (GR1) is hardly influenced by BT and PR as indicated by low RR and confidence intervals. The correlation of few BTs and few PRs with the formation of low PRA levels seems to be loose. Few BTs (0–5) also decreased the risk of high sensitization, a finding that can be partly seen in terms of the transfusion effect [6]. However polytransfusion, multiple pregnancies and multiple transplantation increased the RR for PRA development significantly. MT in particular showed an impressive effect on sensitization. Patients with a history of more than one prior graft have a 40 times higher risk of high sensitization in comparison with first graft recipients.

The impact of increasing recipient age, which lowered the risk for sensitization, was small for the single-year step but decreased the RR by 30% for a recipient age difference of 10 years. This finding is in accordance with the phenomenon of a better transplantation outcome in older recipients because of a decreased immunological response in these individuals [11].

In the presence of PRA, independent factors for single and multiple ERE were MT, which had a strong detrimental effect, and FH HLA match, which reduced the RR of rejection by half. The occurrence of early rejection was not increased by MT in non-sensitized patients. In this cohort only a six-loci HLA match reduced the risk of early rejection significantly. A match of less than six HLA loci did not decrease the risk of early rejection episodes in our cohort of patients.

Early transplantation outcome was affected by multiple transplantations and multiple blood transfusions. These variables showed a detrimental effect in univariate and multivariate analysis. Of all other factors that were entered into the Cox model for graft survival, only increasing warm ischaemic time was found to increase the RR of graft loss, while increasing recipient age and increasing duration of kidney disease decreased the RR of graft failure. The detrimental effect of long-term kidney disease may be an explanation for the finding that a long history of kidney disease has a beneficial impact on graft survival.

HLA matching did not appear to be an isolated factor among the variables entered, which is in contrast to previously published results from multicentre analysis [4].

This finding, documented in a homogeneous cohort of over 1000 grafts followed up at a single centre suggests that the possible benefits of HLA matching are completely masked by stronger effects of several other risk factors.

However, the effects of PRA risk factors on transplantation outcome only show relevance when PRA have been formed. In recipients who have not developed PRA despite risk factors present, MT, BT and PR do not have isolated effects on initial diuresis nor effects on the incidence of PNF or LTF. Here the univariate Kaplan Meier estimates show no significant diversion of the graft function curves. In the Cox model for graft survival in non-sensitized patients, only recipient age, warm ischaemic time and duration of kidney disease revealed an independent influence. PRA act as the mediator and sole effector of risk factor influence on transplantation outcome.

Despite graft exchange programmes for sensitized patients, preoperative crossmatching and aiming for a favourable HLA match, results of transplantation in patients with high PRA levels are still poor. Highly sensitized patients often enter a vicious circle of long waiting times, early graft loss and retransplantation which again increases the risk of further formation of PRA. On the other hand, there seems to be a certain chance of not being sensitized by the risk factors described which gives recipients with risk factors present, but without the subsequent formation of PRA, the same expectation of graft survival as non-sensitized patients.

References

1. Albrechtsen D, Lundgren G, Bratlie A, Brynger H, Fehrmann I, Frödin L, Gäbel H, Lindholm A, Flatmark A (1987) Renal transplantation in presensitized patients treated with cyclosporine. Transplant Proc 29: 1862
2. Claas F (1987) Donor selection for highly immunized patients based on acceptable HLA-A and -B mismatch. Eurotransplant Newsl 44: 6–8
3. Doran M, Coppage M, Ruth J, Fish J, Winsett O, Vaidya S (1987) Renal allograft survival in highly sensitized patients treated with cyclosporine. Transplant Proc 19: 1988
4. Hoof JP, Schippers HMA, van de Steen GJ, van Rood JJ (1972) Efficacy of HLA matching in Eurotransplant. Lancet II: 1385–1387
5. Klouda PT, Ray TC, Gore SM, Bradley BA (1987) Organ sharing for highly sensitized patients. Transplant Proc 19: 731–732
6. Opelz G, Sengar DPS, Mickey MR, Terasaki PI (1973) Effect of blood transfusion on subsequent kidney transplantation. Transplant Proc 5: 249–251
7. Sautner T, Götzinger P, Wamser P, Gnant M, Steininger R, Mühlbacher F (1991) Impact of donor age on graft function in 1180 consecutive kidney recipients. Transplant Proc (in press)
8. Smit JA, Stark JH, Margolius L, Thomson P, Botha JR, Meyers AM, Myburgh JA (1991) Preformed antibodies in predicting clinical renal graft outcome. Transplant Proc 23: 413–414
9. Ting A, Morris PJ (1977) Renal transplantation and B-cell crossmatches with autoantibodies and alloantibodies. Lancet II: 1095–1097
10. Tiwari J, Terasaki PI, Mickey MR (1987) Factors influencing kidney graft survival in the cyclosporine era: a multivariate analysis. Transplant Proc 19: 1839–1841
11. Zhou YC, Cecka JM (1989) Clinical transplants. Ed. UCLA Tissue Typing Laboratory, Los Angeles

Transplant Int (1992) 5 [Suppl 1]: S121–S122

TRANSPLANT
International
© Springer-Verlag 1992

Early or delayed onset of cyclosporine by sequential immunosuppression?

P. Wienand[1], T. Schröder[1], and C. Baldamus[2]

[1] Chirurgische Universitätsklinik Köln-Lindenthal, and [2] Medizinische Universitätsklinik Köln-Lindenthal, Köln, FRG

Abstract. In a prospective randomized trial, 57 renal transplant patients (group A) received a sequential course of 14 days conventional immunosuppression (anti-lymphocyte globulin (ALG), azathioprine and steroids) and cyclosporine and steroids thereafter, while 57 patients (group B) received the conventional immunosuppression for 2 days followed by cyclosporine and steroids. In group A, ALG was tolerated for a mean of 7.8 days while, in group B, conventional therapy had to be changed to cyclosporine therapy after a mean of 2.1 days due to ALG intolerance. Patient survival rates 1 and 2 years after transplantation were 95 % and 92 % in group A and 96 % and 92 % in group B, and graft survival rates were 79 % and 79 % in group A and 89 % and 82 % in group B. In group A, the dialysis frequency in the second, third and fourth weeks after transplantation was significantly higher than in group B. Serum creatinine 1 year post-transplant showed no significant difference between the two groups.

Key words: Renal transplantation – Cyclosporine – Immunosuppressive therapy – Anti-lymphocyte globulin intolerance

It was the purpose of this study to define the most favourable moment for a change from conventional immunosuppression to cyclosporine therapy.

Patients and methods

A total of 114 patients receiving primary cadaver renal transplants were included in a prospective study. The patients were randomly divided into two groups and none was excluded from the study. The patients in group A ($n = 57$) received conventional immunosuppression consisting of azathioprine, steroids and ALG for 14 days after transplantation. Subsequently azathioprine and ALG were replaced with cyclosporine. The patients in group B ($n = 57$) received azathioprine, steroids and ALG for only 2 days post-transplant. Thereafter cyclosporine was given instead of ALG and azathioprine.

When ALG intolerance or fever exceeding 39 °C occurred the conventional treatment was replaced with cyclosporine.

Treatments

ALG therapy. ALG (anti-lymphocyte globulin, Institut Mérieux) was administered at 5 ml/10-kg body weight, maximum 30 ml/day, by a central venous line using continuous mechanical infusion.

Steroid therapy. All patients received 250 mg prednisolone on the first day post-transplant. The dosage was tapered daily in increments of 25 mg to 100 mg, and then every other day in increments of 5 mg, until a permanent dose of 5–10 mg per day was achieved. In cases of graft rejection, a daily dose of 0.5 g methylprednisolone was given 3–5 times.

Azathioprine therapy. A maximum of 3 mg/kg body weight per day was administered while white blood cell counts and platelet counts were monitored. A white blood cell count of less than 3000, and a platelet count of less than 80 000/mm^3 were considered the lower limits.

Cyclosporine therapy. Cyclosporine was initiated at 8–10 mg/kg body weight per day in two doses to achieve whole-blood trough levels of 300 ng/ml assessed by radioimmunoassay (RIA). Cyclosporine was tapered in increments of 1 mg/kg per day when the whole-blood trough levels were exceeded 300 ng/ml.

Perioperative antibiotic prophylaxis. All patients received a perioperative dose of 1.5 g cefuroxime.

Statistical analysis

The cumulative patient and transplant survivals were analysed using the Kaplan-Meier method. Frequencies of dialysis, rejection episodes and kidney function were analysed by linear regression.

Offprint requests to: Priv. Doz. Dr. med. Peter Wienand, Chirurgische Universitätsklinik Köln, Joseph-Stelzmann-Str. 9, D-5000 Köln, FRG

Results:

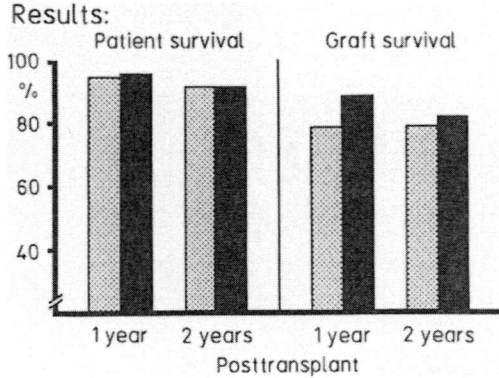

Fig. 1. Patient and transplant survival after early or delayed onset of cyclosporine by sequential immunosuppression. ▨, group A; ■, group B

Results:

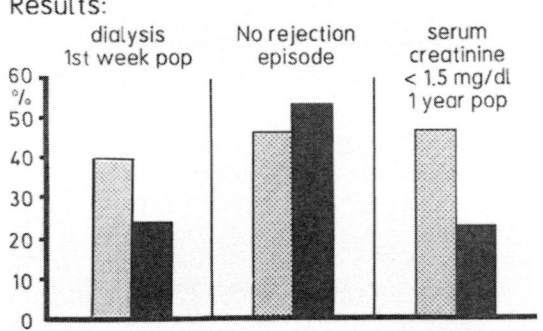

Fig. 2. Frequencies of dialysis, rejection episodes and kidney function in relation to early or delayed onset of cyclosporine by sequential immunosuppression. ▨, group A; ■ group B

Results

Donor data and recipient data did not differ significantly between the two groups with regard to donor age, kidney function and preservation time. All kidneys were stored hypothermicly in Euro-Collins solution. The recipient age and the time between onset of dialysis and transplantation were not significantly different between the two groups, and the HLA-DR histocompatibilities were comparable between the groups.

Patients and transplant survival

Patient survival rates (Fig. 1) 1 and 2 years after transplantation were 95 % and 92 % in group A, and 96 % and 92 % in group B. The graft survival rates in group A were 79 % and 79 %, and in group B 89 % and 82 %. In group A the dialysis frequency (Fig. 2) in the second, third and fourth week postoperatively was significantly higher than in group B.

ALG treatment

The mean time of ALG administration in group B was 2.1 days, but was 7.8 days in group A.

Discussion

In the present study, we sought to determine whether the nephrotoxic side effects of cyclosporine could be avoided by delaying its use in the early post-transplant period. Conventional immunosuppression was applied immediately after transplantation, assuming that in this phase the kidney, having been subjected to cold and warm ischaemia, is especially susceptible to the nephrotoxicity of cyclosporine.

Early conventional immunosuppression and early preceding cyclosporine therapy gave excellent results. Our findings confirm that an early beginning of cyclosporine therapy showed good results.

Conclusion

Patient survival, graft survival, kidney function and rejection episodes showed no significant differences between the two groups. However, the frequency of dialysis was significantly lower in group B. A delayed onset of cyclosporine therapy showed no better results than early cyclosporine therapy.

Transplant Int (1992) 5 [Suppl 1]: S 123–S 128

TRANSPLANT
International
© Springer-Verlag 1992

Application of flow cytometry in clinical renal transplantation

S. Stefoni, A. Nanni-Costa, S. Iannelli, A. Buscaroli, L. C. Borgnino, M. P. Scolari, G. Mosconi, G. Cianciolo, L. B. De Sanctis, and V. Bonomini

Institute of Nephrology, University of Bologna, Bologna, Italy

Abstract. Flow cytometry (FC) may be considered as a fundamental technique in studying cell biology and pathology. It combines the quantitative character of biochemical methods with the multiparametric capacities of microscope analysis in a high-precision process for rapid analysis of individual cell characteristics. Three original FC techniques routinely applied in the field of renal transplantation are reported in the present study. They concern the donor–recipient cross-match test, the morphological analysis of urinary sediment and the modulation of the density of various membrane antigens on the lymphocyte surface. A common factor underlies all these methods: they aim to provide the physician with a reliable diagnostic tool in clinical renal transplantation.

Key words: Flow cytometry – Renal transplant – Lymphocytes

Flow cytometry (FC) today may be considered as a fundamental technique in studying the biology and pathology of cells. Its development and application in biological research and clinical diagnosis respresents a successful example of multidisciplinary 'hybrid technology', based on the confluence of advanced technologies such as radiation physics, computer science, fluorochrome chemistry, cytochemical staining and monoclonal antibody production.

FC has introduced new vistas in the identification and characterization of cell populations [7], combining the quantitative character of biochemical methods with the multiparametric capacities of microscopic analysis in a high-precision technique for rapid analysis of individual cell characteristics [8]. These qualities suggest that FC may be of the greatest use in organ transplantation.

The application of flow cytometry in the field of renal transplantation has hitherto largely consisted of the im-

munological monitoring of patients performed through lymphocyte subset typing by means of fluoresceinated monoclonal antibodies [2, 4]. The technical performance of the last-generation instruments (both analysers and sorters), the increased scientific knowledge and technical experience, and the range of sophisticated diagnostic reagents have progressively extended the scope of flow cytometry techniques to the clinical management of transplanted patients.

This report presents a short review of three FC techniques (designed by us) which are routinely applied at the Nephrology, Dialysis and Transplantation Institute of Bologna University. They concern different areas from among the extremely wide possibilities afforded by FC, but are unified by a common factor: they aim to provide the physician with a diagnostic tool when facing a clinical problem in renal transplantation.

Flow cytometry evaluation of the pretransplant donor–recipient cross-match test in renal transplantation

In renal transplantation the cross-match test (CM) evaluates the existence and degree of presensitization of a potential graft recipient against the kidney donor. It is generally accepted that the presence of preformed antibodies (positive CM) represents an absolute contraindication to transplantation.

The standard optically based method, a complement-dependent cytotoxic assay [12], may sometimes be not completely reliable, even in experienced centres, for purely technical reasons: (1) the difficulty in detecting weak positive reactions (false negative results); (2) a high number of dead or contaminating cells present under light microscopy observation (false positive results); and (3) the possibility of operator errors due to test evaluations not being sufficiently standardized.

In order to optimize pretransplant CM evaluation, we combined the standard light microscopy method with an innovatory FC technique based on cytometrical analysis of the cytotoxic assay itself [13]. Figures 1 and 2 show the

Offprint requests to: Sergio Stefoni, M.D., St. Orsola University Hospital, Via Massarenti 9, 40138 Bologna, Italy

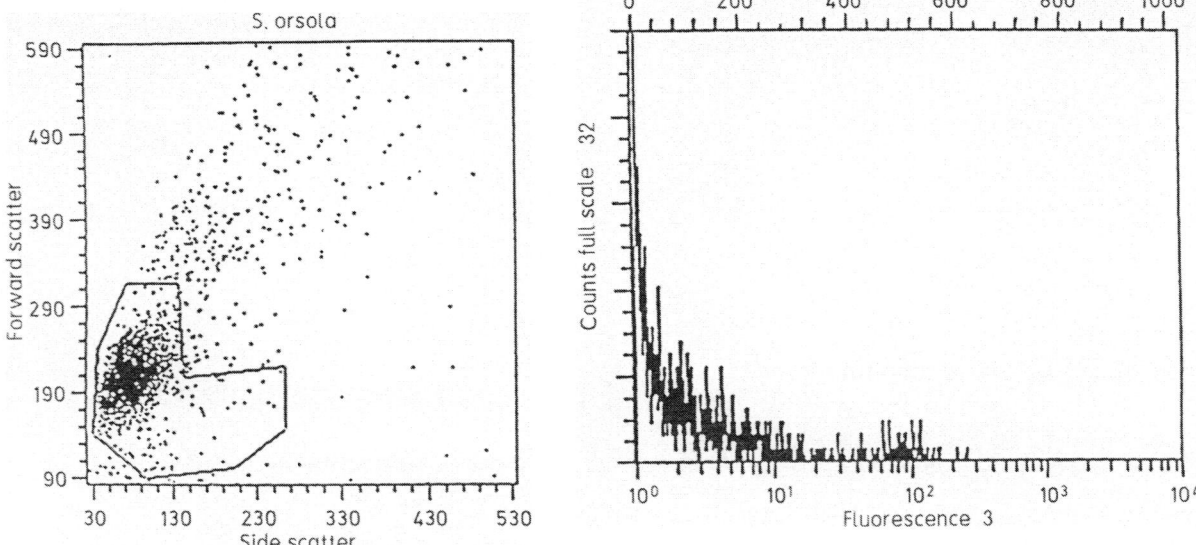

Fig. 1. Cytogram *(left)* and histogram *(right)* of a negative CM test

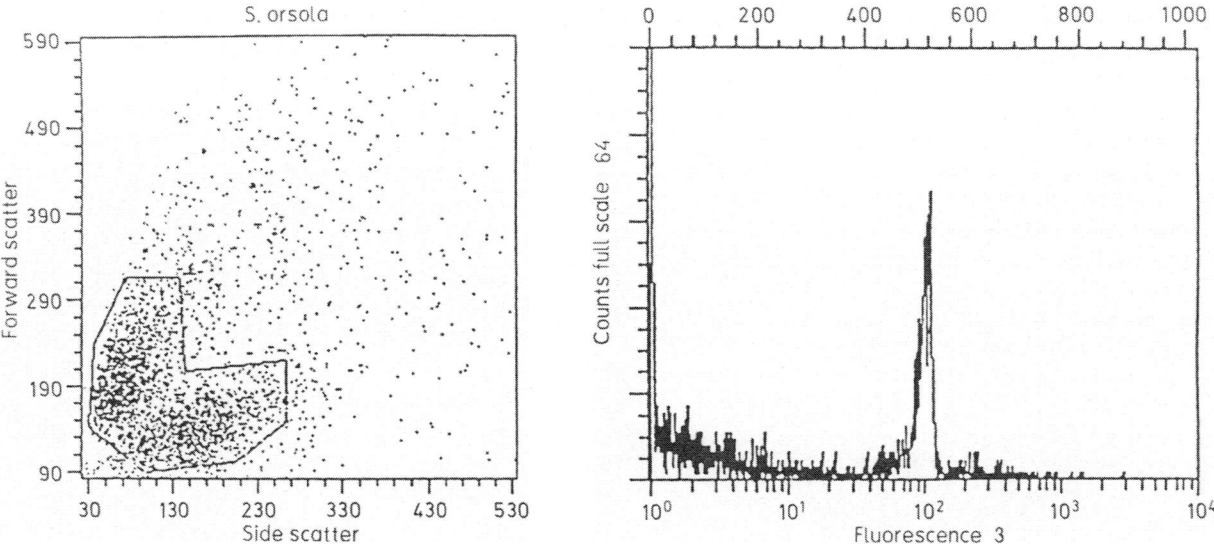

Fig. 2. Cytogram *(left)* and histogram *(right)* of a positive CM test

cytogram and the histogram of negative and positive samples obtained on a FACSCAN Flow Cytometer (Becton-Dickinson). Of note is the unusual shape of the positive dead lymphocytes which fall into the lower right lobe of the established gate window (Fig. 2). The study included 5185 cross-match tests performed over 24 months at the Institute of Nephrology, Bologna University, using lymphocytes from 62 consecutive kidney donors and sera from 431 candidates for transplantation.

Out of the 5185 CM examined by both techniques, 1171 tests (22.6%) proved positive with light microscopy, while 1504 (29.0%) were positive with FC (Fig. 3). The difference is statistically significant ($P < 0.001$). Comparing the two techniques, 719 samples out of the 5185 (13.87%) received different evaluations: 526 CM were positive with FC but negative with light microscopy examination ($P < 0.001$), while 193 proved negative with FC and positive with light microscopy (Fig. 4).

Figure 5 shows the correlation between the results obtained by this technique and graft survival. After 1 month graft survival was significantly higher ($P < 0.02$) in patients for whom CM was evaluated by both techniques, than in a second patient group, in which CM was examined only by light microscopy; after 3 months this difference was reduced and tended to disappear during the first year.

Compared with light microscopy the technical advantages were:

1. Each CM test was assessed on a high number of lymphocytes.
2. Sample evaluation was computerized.
3. The threshold between negative and positive was clearly identified.
4. Detection of weak positive reactions was enhanced.
5. False positive reactions due to insufficient purification of the sample were avoided.

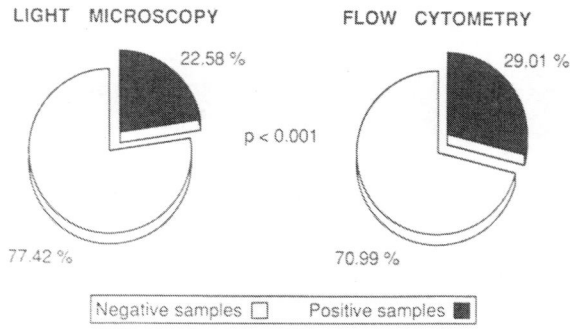

Fig. 3. Percent distribution of positive and negative pattern in 5185 cross-match tests. Light microscopy *(left)* and flow cytometry *(right)*

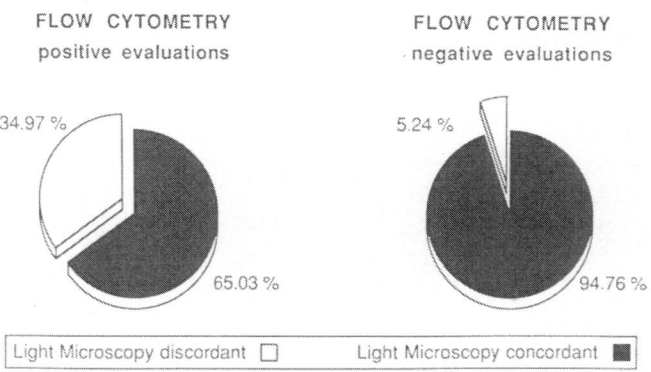

Fig. 4. Comparison of flow cytometry and light microscopy evaluation in 5185 cross-match tests

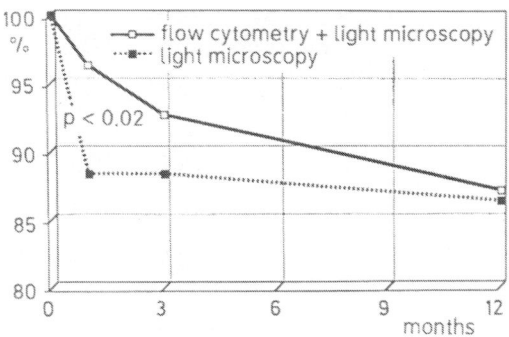

Fig. 5. Graft survival and clinical outcome in patients with negative CM test determined by both flow cytometry and light microscopy evaluation ($n = 51$) or by the standard microscopic technique only ($n = 54$)

6. The risk of selecting candidates with donor presensitization (false negative CM) was reduced.

In short, the cross-match technique we have developed exploits the same biological reaction (i.e. complement-dependent cytotoxicity) as is used in standard light microscopy assays. The advantage of our method over this still-accepted technique for donor–recipient cross-match testing in clinical transplantation is that it increases the sensitivity of the reading, thus reducing the possibility of error.

Clinical results support the validity of this technical improvement, showing that the incidence of primary renal non-function and early graft loss could be reduced. On this basis the new FC technique we have developed seems to be a reliable and helpful assay for pretransplant investigations in renal transplantation, representing an interesting addition or even an alternative to light microscopy cross-match evaluation. A detailed report has been published elsewhere [13].

Urinary cytology

The value of exfoliative urinary cytology for the diagnosis of different pathological conditions in renal transplantation has been suggested by various investigators [11]. In particular, the presence of lymphocytes has been suggested as an indicator of acute rejection episodes [6]. This method, however, has not gained wide acceptance, very likely because of the difficulty in obtaining a reliable identification of the different cells by means of standard staining techniques.

FC may make a significant contribution to this 'pure morphology' approach thanks to its powerful combination of light microscopy examination characteristics, such as multiparametric analysis, and the computerized quantitative evaluation of single cellular elements [10, 15]. The method we designed was aimed at analysing urinary sediment cells in renal transplanted patients in order to define the morphological features of the various populations, i.e. lymphocytes, monocytes/macrophages and granulocytes, involved in the immune response.

We used FC analysis of the urinary sediment in a wide-ranging study involving 233 urine sediment samples from 173 renal transplanted patients, selected on the basis of clinical condition:

A. normal renal function, without clinical or laboratory evidence of bacterial infection
B. acute rejection
C. bacterial infection of the urinary tract
D. post-transplant tubular necrosis diagnosed by clinical signs (oliguria) or laboratory investigation (creatinine clearance lower than 10 ml/min)
E. laboratory signs of cyclosporine cytotoxicity.

Urine sample preparation and instrumental technical details have been reported elsewhere [10].

Results showed that the number and the percentage distribution of the identified cell populations in the patient groups depended on clinical condition. As far as lymphocyte and monocyte numbers were concerned the 'acute rejection' group showed the highest value; similarly polymorphs and debris were typical, respectively, of the 'bacterial infection' and the 'acute tubular necrosis' group.

Figure 6 reproduces urinary sediment cytograms which refer to various clinical conditions: patients with stable renal function had a sediment with a low cell count, acute rejection was characterized by significant lymphocyturia (associated with monocyturia in the case of vascular involvement), while polymorphs and debris predominated in urinary tract infections. During post-transplant tubular necrosis the noteworthy finding concerns the debris which assumes a 'high scatter' pattern, i.e. high density and large size particles, while, interestingly, in patients with clinical or laboratory signs of cyclosporine cytotoxicity the debris

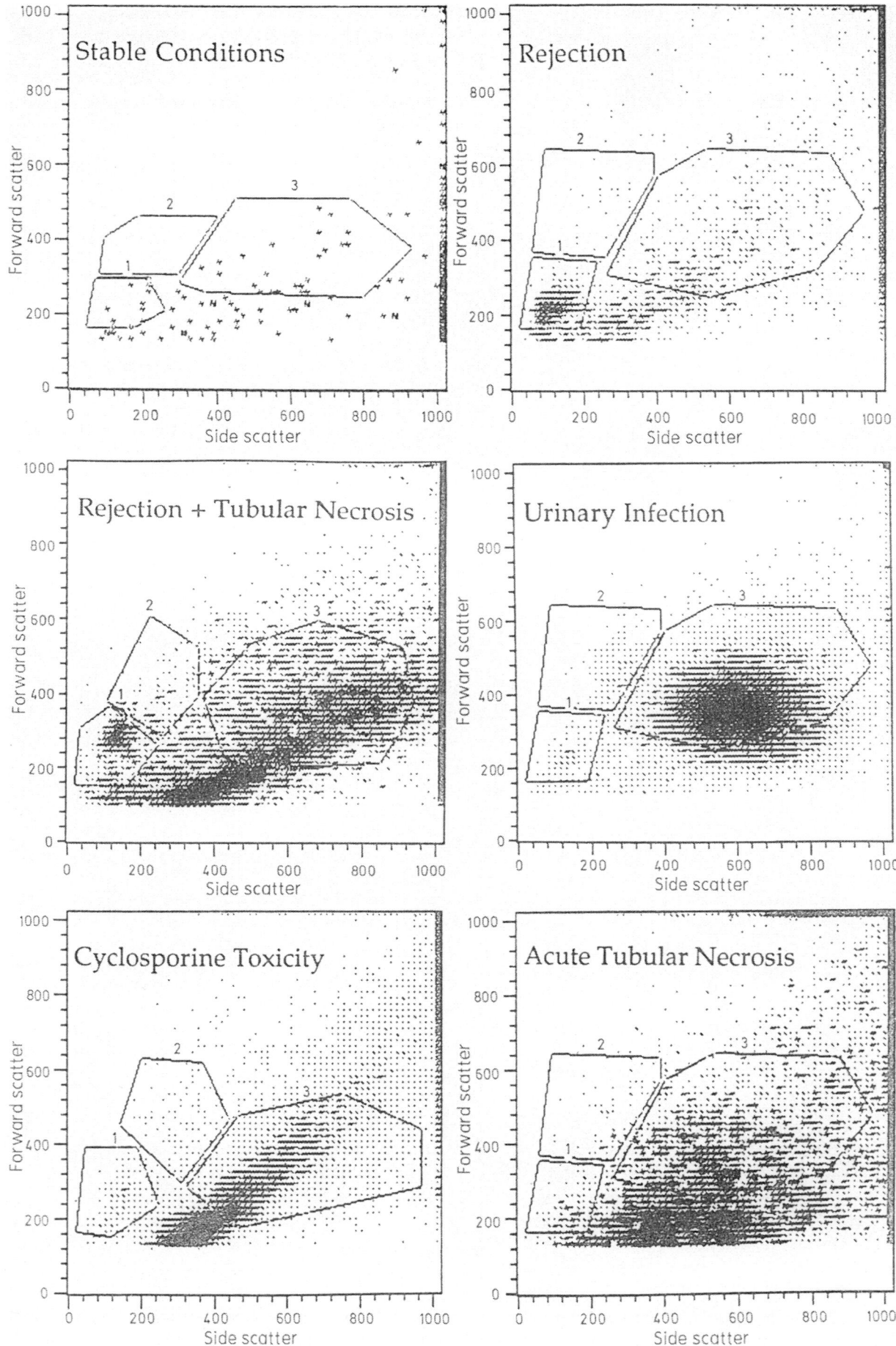

shows a 'low scatter' pattern, i.e. low density and small size particles.

Cytometric urine analysis appears of use as a first-step investigation both in the diagnostic approach to transplant patients and in examining the real morphological situation of the allograft. We hope that in future this test will come to be considered as the morphological equivalent to the creatinine clearance test.

Evaluation of surface antigen expression on lymphocyte membranes

The combined use of FC and monoclonal antibodies enables one to perform a quantitative analysis of the density of the surface antigens expressed on lymphocyte membranes [9]. In order to evaluate whether this determination could be related to the degree of immunological activity, we examined 60 renal transplant patients, chronically treated with cyclosporine and steroids, and 15 normal subjects as a control group.

Isolated peripheral blood lymphocytes were reacted with monoclonal antibodies specific for the antigens of the first and second class of the major histocompatibility complex (MHC), for β2-microglobulin and for the alpha-beta T-cell receptor (TCR) by means of an indirect immunofluorescence technique. A FACSCAN Flow Cytometer (Becton-Dickinson) was used to analyse the mean intensity of fluorescence which is directly related to the number of molecules expressed on the cell surface.

The quantitative expression of MHC antigens (class I and II) and TCR in transplant recipients in a stable clinical condition (quiescence level) was significantly lower (Figs. 7 and 8) than in normal subjects ($P < 0.01$). During episodes of high immunological activity, such as acute rejection episodes and viral infection, TCR (Fig. 8) and MHC class II antigen expression (Fig. 9) showed a significant increase ($P < 0.01$ vs quiescence level). Patients treated with aggressive immunosuppressive therapy (anti-lymphocyte globulin and OKT3 monoclonal antibody intravenously) showed a significant reduction in antigen expression (Figs. 8 and 9) regarding both MHC antigens and TCR ($P < 0.01$ vs quiescence levels).

The main observations emerging from these data are:
1. After renal transplantation the intensity of fluorescence staining of circulating lymphocytes is poor, depending on the reduced density of surface antigens, very likely related to immunosuppressive therapy [5].
2. There is probably a close relationship between clinical phases of high reactivity against the allograft, manifested as acute rejection episodes, and an increased density of TCR and MHC class II antigens [3].
3. The same findings were also observed during CMV infection. In this condition the increased antigen expression reflects an activation phase of T lymphocytes, presumably committed to virus-infected cells [16].

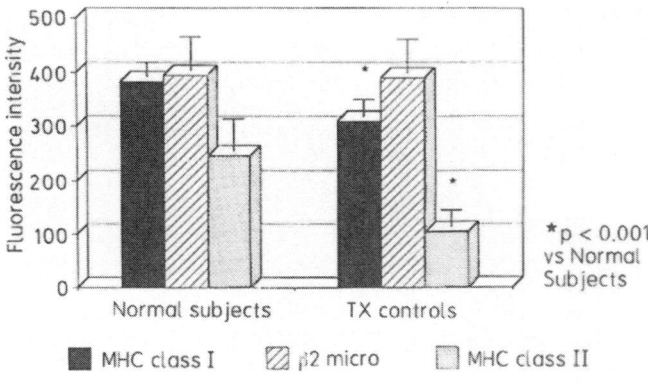

Fig. 7. Quantitative evaluation of MHC antigens (class I and II) and β2 microglobulin expression on peripheral blood lymphocytes in renal transplantation

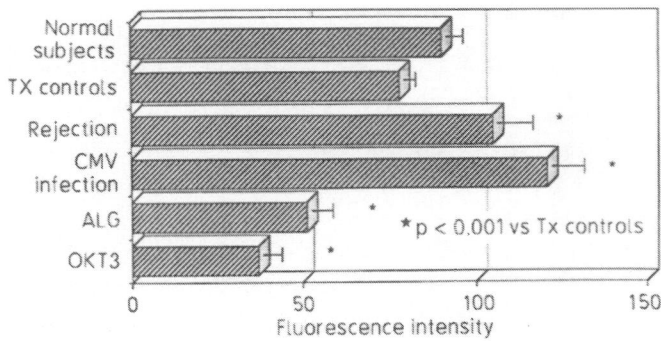

Fig. 8. Quantitative evaluation of TCR expression on peripheral blood lymphocytes in renal transplantation

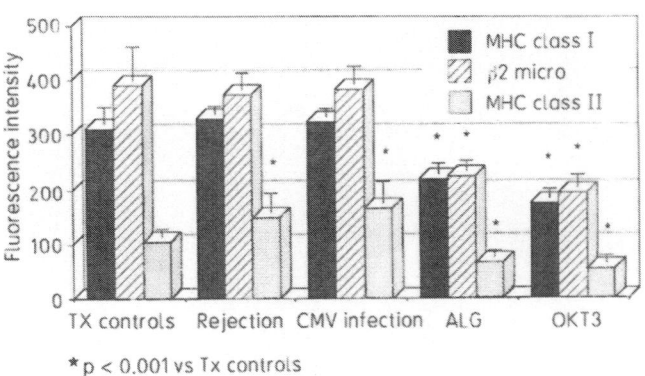

Fig. 9. Up- and down-regulation of MHC antigen expression on peripheral blood lymphocytes in various clinical conditions in renal transplantation

4. The significant reduction in antigen expression in patients treated with ALG is very likely related to the effect of antilymphocyte globulin which unselectively recognizes all lymphocyte structures [11], while the marked alterations which occur during OKT3 treatment depend on rearrangements in the molecular surface structure, such as internalization and modulated re-expression, which take place during treatment [1].

The significant correlations we found between patients with differing clinical conditions and the density of various antigens and receptors expressed on the lymphocyte membrane suggest that the quantitative evaluation of

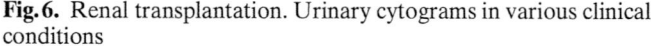

Fig. 6. Renal transplantation. Urinary cytograms in various clinical conditions

these parameters may enable us to go beyond simple lymphocyte subset typing, providing the physician with useful information on lymphocyte functional activity.

Acknowledgment. Supported in part by 'DOTT. CARLO FORNASINI' Foundation, Bologna

References

1. Chatenoud L, Baudrihaye MF, Schindler J, Bach JF (1982) Human in vivo antigenic modulation induced by the anti-T cell OKT3 monoclonal antibody. Eur J Immunol 12: 979–987
2. Colvin RB (1984) Flow cytometry analysis of T cells: Diagnostic applications in transplantation. Ann N Y Acad Sci 428: 5–13
3. Hayry P, von Willebrand E (1986) The influence of the pattern of inflammation and administration of steroids on class II MHC antigen expression in renal transplants. Transplantation 42: 358–363
4. Hoffmann RA, Hansen WP (1981) Immunofluorescent analysis of blood cells by flow cytometry. Int J Immunopharmacol 3: 249–254
5. Koene RP, De Waal RM, Bogman MJ (1986) Variable expression of major histocompatibilitry antigens: role in transplantation immunology. Kidney Int 30: 1–8
6. Krishna GG, Fellner SK (1982) Lymphocyturia: an important diagnostic marker in renal allograft rejection. Am J Nephrol 2: 185–191
7. Loken MR, Stall AM (1982) Flow Cytometry as an analytical and preparative tool in immunology. J Immunol Meth 50: R85–R112
8. Muirhead KA, Horan PK, Poste G (1985) Flow cytometry present and future. Biotechnology 3: 337–355
9. Nanni-Costa A, Vangelista A, Stefoni S, Borgnino LC, Iannelli S, Bonomini V (1987) Quantitative expression of T-cell surface antigens in renal transplantation. Transplant Proc 19: 1600–1602
10. Nanni-Costa A, Stefoni S, Buscaroli A, Iannelli S, Borgnino LC, Stagni B, Raimondi C, Cotti P, Bonomini V (1989) Urinary cytology in renal transplantation. Flow cytometry evaluations. Third European Cytometry User's Meeting, Ghent 1989, pp 123–137
11. Pellet H, Zannier A, Depardon J, Deteix P, Touraine JL (1983) Value of urine cytology for monitoring renal transplantation. In: Touraine JL, Traeger J, Betuel H, Brochier J, Dubernard JM, Revillard JP, Triau R (eds) Transplantation and clinical immunology. Excerpta Medica, Amsterdam, pp 138–143
12. Staff (1974) Transplantation and immunology branch: NIH lymphocyte microtoxicity technique. In: Ray JG, Hare DB, Pedersen PD, Kaynoe DE (eds) Manual of tissue typing techniques. NIH, Bethesda, pp 20–22
13. Stefoni S, Nanni-Costa A, Buscaroli A, Borgnino LC, Iannelli S, Raimondi C, Scolari MP, Bonomini V (1991) Validity of flow cytometry for cross-match evaluation in clinical renal transplantation. Nephron 57: 268–272
14. Ting A (1983) The lymphocytotoxic cross-match test in clinical renal transplantation. Transplantation 35: 403–407
15. Vangelista A, Nanni-Costa A, Fatone F, Buscaroli A, D'Atena T, Bonomini V (1987) Flow cytometry analysis of urinary cytology in renal transplantation. Transplant Proc 19: 1665–1669
16. von Willebrand E, Petterson E, Ahonen J, Hayry P (1986) CMV infection, class II antigen expression, and human kidney allograft rejection. Transplantation 42: 364–367

Transplant Int (1992) 5 [Suppl 1]: S 129–S 132

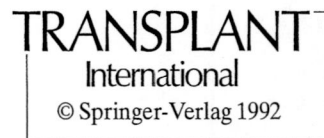

TRANSPLANT
International
© Springer-Verlag 1992

The course of HIV disease in renal allograft recipients

V. Delaney, N. Sumrani, J. Hong, R. Davis, B. Sommer

Department of Surgery, Division of Transplantation, State University of New York Health Science Center at Brooklyn, New York, USA

Abstract. The clinical course of HIV seropositive renal allograft recipients is ill defined. Thus, a retrospective analysis of mortality, morbidity and graft survival was performed in two groups of HIV-positive patients. Group 1 (nine patients), seropositive for an indefinite period of time prior to transplantation (eight IV drug abusers, one homosexual), all lost their grafts after a mean period of 23 ± 11 months from chronic rejection (six), complicated by focal glomerular sclerosis and nephrotic syndrome in three cases, sepsis (two) and death with a functioning graft (one). Four patients died, two from sepsis, one from Kaposi's sarcoma and one from fluid overload. Of the remaining five patients, all on hemodialysis, one had AIDS and four were asymptomatic after a mean period of 44 months following graft failure. Prolonged hospitalizations for both infections and acute rejection were common. Group 2 (six patients) seroconverted in the perioperative period, and two had functioning allografts at 78 and 100 months post-transplant. Causes of allograft loss, patient death and infection-related complications were similar to those of group 1, but acute rejection was rare. In conclusion, HIV infection in renal allograft recipients was associated with poor allograft survival due mainly to rejection, mostly chronic, often complicated by glomerular sclerosis and nephrotic syndrome. Infectious complications requiring hospitalization were also increased.

Key words: HIV – Transplants – Renal – AIDS – Azathioprine – Cyclosporine

More than 70000 people have died of AIDS in the US since its first description in 1981 [2] and it is estimated that an additional 1–2 million are infected with the causative retrovirus, namely HIV [2]. The latter invades, and ultimately destroys, lymphocytes bearing the T4 receptor leading to a relative preponderance of suppressor, or T8, lymphocytes and the production of destructive immunosuppression involving mainly, but not exclusively, cell-mediated immunity [6]. Thus its victims fall prey to a variety of opportunistic infections or unusual B-cell neoplasms and/or a progressive encephalopathy, often accompanied in the terminal stages by severe emaciation [5]. High-risk groups include homosexual males, bisexual men with multiple partners, infants born to infected mothers, and recipients of virus-contaminated blood and tissue products. The frequency of the latter has decreased considerably since 1985 when routine HIV screening of prospective donors became mandatory [15]. The incubation period of HIV is unknown but variable, with some individuals dying of AIDS within 2 years and others remaining asymptomatic for up to 12 years following infection with the virus [2].

Iatrogenic immunosuppression, as used following solid organ transplantation, in patients harboring the virus was thus considered imprudent with the anticipation of earlier death from lethal immunosuppression [1]. By the same token, rejection may be expected to be diminished in both intensity and frequency [2]. Based on the overriding influence of the former consideration, HIV-positive patients are not now (1990) generally considered suitable candidates for transplantation by most centers throughout Europe and the US, although clear-cut data supporting this conclusion are not available in the literature [2]. The uncertainty arises because of both the difficulty in diagnosing AIDS in immunosuppressed patients, the long and variable incubation period, and the usually imprecise timing of infection with the virus. We thus undertook a review of all known HIV-positive renal transplant recipients in a large urban center in the US in an attempt to clarify the clinical course post-transplant.

Materials and methods

A total of 256 patients who received renal transplants between 1976 and 1985 at the State University of New York Health Science Center at Brooklyn consented to HIV testing. Current sera and sera stored at $-70\,°C$ from the time of transplantation were obtained from each

Offprint requests to: Nabil Sumrani, Department of Surgery, Division of Transplantation, State University of New York Health Science Center at Brooklyn, 450 Clarkson Avenue, Box 40, Brooklyn, New York 11203, USA

patient and analyzed for the presence of HIV-1 antibodies by enzyme immunoassay (LAV-EIA; Genetic Systems, Seattle Wash.) and confirmed by Western blot (Immunoblot; Biorad, Richmond, Calif.). Of those tested, 17 were seropositive. Maintenance immunosuppression post-transplant consisted of azathioprine–prednisone until 1983 (four patients) when cyclosporine–low-dose prednisone (13 patients) was employed, both according to standard protocols [14]. Acute rejection was diagnosed by standard clinical and histological criteria [7] and treated with intravenous pulse methylprednisolone (250–500 mg/day) followed by polyclonal anti-lymphocyte globulin (Minnesota: 10–15 mg/kg per day) in biopsy-proven nonresponders.

The following parameters were analyzed: demographics, mortality, graft survival, morbidity, incidence of rejection.

Results

Demographics (Table 1)

A total of 17 patients were HIV positive. Nine of these were positive at the time of transplantation (group 1), six became positive in the perioperative (0–6 months) period (group 2), and two were negative at the time of transplantation, but seroconverted at an unknown time point between 11 and 13 years, respectively, post-transplant (group 3). Mean follow-up periods for groups 1, 2 and 3 were 60 months (range 15–120), 88 months (range 52–94), and 156 months (range 141–168), respectively. Eight of nine patients in group 1 were intravenous drug users, in contrast to group 2 patients in whom the only identifiable risk factor was blood and/or organ donation. Both patients in group 3 were high-risk individuals [IV drug abuser (1) and homosexual (1)].

Table 1. Demographic details of HIV-seropositive renal transplant recipients

	Group 1	Group 2	Group 3
No. of patients	9	6	2
Mean			
Age (years)	31	40	28
Range	20–37	24–56	22–34
Male/female	8/1	5/1	1/1
Cadaveric	6	5	1
Race			
Asian	0 (0%)	1 (16.7%)	0 (0%)
Black	5 (55.6%)	1 (16.7%)	1 (50%)
Caucasian	0 (0%)	1 (16.7%)	0 (0%)
Hispanic	4 (44.4%)	3 (50%)	1 (50%)
Renal disease			
Focal sclerosis	5	2	0
GN	1	1	1
Diabetes	0	1	0
Unknown/others	3	2	1
Risk for HIV			
IVDA	8	0	1
Homosexuality	1	0	1
Blood/organ	0	6	0
CSA/prednisone	7	6	0
AZA/prednisone	2	0	2
Retransplant	1	0	0
Follow-up (months)	60 (15–120)	88 (52–94)	156 (141–168)

Table 2. Causes and times of death (months) in HIV-seropositive renal allograft recipients

Cause of death	N	Group	Survival time post-tx (months)
Gram-negative sepsis	1	1	61
Disseminated mycobacterial avium	1	1	15
Kaposi's sarcoma	1	1	27
Fluid overload, hyperkalemia	1	1	58
Hepatic failure, sepsis	1	2	42
Hepatic failure	1	2	52
Colon cancer	1	2	48
Hepatic failure, sepsis	1	3	144
Hepatic failure, PCP pneumonia	1	3	162

Table 3. Causes of renal allograft loss and graft survival times (months) in HIV-seropositive renal allograft recipients

	Group 1 (n = 9)	Group 2 (n = 6)	Group 3 (n = 2)
No. of surviving allografts	0	2	0
Chronic rejection	(3) 11, 23, 24	(2) 36, 58	(2) 132, 156
Chronic rejection with nephrotic syndrome	(3) 13, 20, 30		
Sepsis	(2) 13, 57	(1) 50	
Death	(1) 27	(1) 57	

Numbers in parentheses are the number of allografts

Mortality (Table 2)

Eight patients died (Table 2) with an overall mortality of 53%. Causes of death in group 1 (four patients) included disseminated *Mycobacterium avium intracellulare* (MAI) infection (1), Gram-negative sepsis (1), cardiorespiratory arrest associated with fluid overload and hyperkalemia (1) and Kaposi's sarcoma (1) at 15, 61, 58 and 27 months post-transplant, respectively. Three patients died in group 2, two of non-A, non-B hepatic failure at 42 and 52 months post-transplant and one of metastatic colon cancer at 48 months. Both patients in group 3 died of liver failure (non-A, non-B), one of whom had concomitant PCP pneumonia, at 162 and 144 months post-transplant, respectively.

Graft survival (Table 3)

All patients in group 1 lost their allografts after a mean period of 23 ± 11 months. Causes of allograft loss included MAI infection of the allograft in association with acute and chronic rejection (1), bacterial sepsis with acute allograft failure superimposed upon chronic rejection as a preterminal event (1), chronic rejection (3), chronic rejection in association with transplant glomerulopathy and/or focal glomerular sclerosis (3, all of whom had nephrotic syndrome) and patient death with a functioning graft (1). Graft survival was 33% in group 2 with a mean follow-up of 89 months (range 78–100). Causes of graft loss included chronic rejection (3) at 36, 50 and 58 months post-transplant, respectively, and patient death with a functioning graft at 57 months. Within this group two patients were alive at the time of writing with functioning allografts, one of whom had biopsy proven chronic rejection with focal glomerular sclerosis and nephrotic syndrome at 80 months post-transplant. The remaining patient had a serum creatinine of 177 μmol/l and minimal proteinuria at 94 months post-transplant. Both patients of group 3 lost their allografts from chronic rejection after 156 and 133 months, respectively.

Morbidity

Infections requiring hospitalization in group 1 included CMV (3), Salmonella (1), recurrent Gram-negative sepsis (2) and MAI (1). Mean hospital stay for allograft-related problems in this group was 11.8 weeks. In group 2 three patients developed unexplained fever in association with pancytopenia with spontaneous evolution 4 to 12 weeks post-transplant. Two patients had transient fever in association with generalized lymphadenopathy (non-specific hyperplasia on biopsy) at 6 and 9 weeks following engraftment. One recipient developed CMV retinitis and one PCP pneumonia. Mean hospital stay for this group was 10.5 weeks. Both patients in group 3 developed AIDS 144 and 162 months post-transplant and within 8 and 11 months following return to dialysis.

At the time of writing a total of six patients were on dialysis, five from group 1 and one from group 2 for a mean period of 44 (range 25–83) months, and two patients had AIDS, but the remaining four were asymptomatic.

Acute rejection was observed in 56% and 17% of group 1 and group 2, respectively.

Discussion

Being a retrospective analysis of a specific sub-group of renal allograft recipients, i.e. those that gave consent for HIV testing, this study has obvious shortcomings. However, since the majority of transplant centers are reluctant to perform renal transplantation in HIV-positive patients and since screening for the virus is now a prerequisite for getting on transplant lists in most countries, this relatively large single-center study presents a possibly unique opportunity to study the natural history of renal transplantation and associated immunosuppression, mainly cyclosporine, in patients with HIV infection.

Patients harboring HIV for unknown periods of time prior to transplantation had a dismal prognosis for allograft survival (Table 3). Surprisingly, from a conceptual stand-point, acute rejection, as diagnosed by standard clinical and histological criteria [7], was common with progression to chronic rejection occurring in the majority, half of whom had glomerular abnormalities in addition. These were suggestive of focal glomerular sclerosis with some features of transplant glomerulopathy [1] and were accompanied by nephrotic range proteinuria. This finding may also represent a recurrence of native glomerular disease, namely focal glomerular sclerosis, the underlying disease in the majority of this particular sub-group

(Table 1) and thought to be more prevalent in blacks [9], intravenous drug abusers [3] and patients with AIDS nephropathy [8]. Even the diagnosis of acute rejection may be called into doubt in this group of patients, since interstitial nephritis can be a manifestation of HIV-associated renal involvement [12] in addition to being one of the hallmarks of acute rejection.

Patients who acquired the virus in the perioperative period while under routine heavy immunosuppression often developed a viral syndrome characterized by fever, pancytopenia and tender lymphadenopathy similar to that reported in previous studies [4, 10, 11], thought to represent the viremic phase of the acute HIV infection. In general, patients in this group and the subgroup which acquired the virus in the later postoperative period (group 3) had better allograft survival when compared with group 1 (Table 3).

Sepsis-related deaths (Table 2) and hospitalizations were more frequent than age- and time-controlled non-HIV renal transplant recipients within the same patient population [13], but whether the concomitant administration of immunosuppression accelerated the time of onset of HIV-related infectious complications is impossible to evaluate from the present data. Liver failure, a prominent pre-morbid clinical feature in the present study, was non-A, non-B, usually associated with sepsis and multiorgan failure, although a concomitant hepatitis C infection was not ruled out.

In summary, renal transplantation in HIV-seropositive patients in the present patient population has a poor prognosis for allograft and patient survival and is associated with substantial morbidity and expense related mainly to infection-related complications. For these reasons, and because dialysis is a readily available alternative treatment modality for end-stage renal disease, the latter is probably the therapeutic modality of choice at the present time.

References

1. Cameron JS (1982) Glomerulonephritis in renal transplants. Transplantation 34: 237–240
2. Feduska NJ (1990) Human immunodeficiency virus, AIDS, and organ transplantation. Transplant Rev 4: 93–107
3. Friedman EA, Rao TKS (1983) Why does uremia in heroin abusers occur predominantly in blacks? J Am Med Assoc 250: 2965–2966
4. L'Age-Stehr J, Schwarz A, Offermann G, Langmaack H, Bennhold I, Niedrig M, Koch MA (1985) HTLV-III infection in kidney transplant recipients. Lancet II: 1361–1362
5. Mills J, Masur H (1990) AIDs related infections. Sci Am 66: 50–57
6. Nabel GJ (1988) Activation of human immunodeficiency virus. J Lab Clin Med 111: 495–500
7. Olsen TS (1986) Pathology of allograft rejection. In: Williams GM, Burdick JE, Solez K (eds) Kidney transplant rejection. Diagnosis and treatment. Marcel Dekker, New York, pp 173–197
8. Prado V, Meneses R, Ossa L, Jaffe DJ, Strauss J, Roth D, Bourgoignie JJ (1987) AIDS-related glomerulopathy: occurrence in specific risk groups. Kidney Int 31: 1167–1173
9. Rao TKS, Friedman EA, Nicastri AD (1987) The types of renal disease in the acquired immunodeficiency syndrome. N Engl J Med 316: 1062–1068

10. Rubin RH, Jenkins RL, Shaw BW, Shaffer D, Pearl RH, Erb S, Monaco A, Van Thiel D (1987) The acquired immunodeficiency syndrome and transplantation. Transplantation 44: 1–4

11. Schwarz A, Hoffmann F, L'Age-Stehr, Tegzess AM, Offermann G (1987) Human immunodeficiency virus transmission by organ donation. Transplantation 44: 21–24

12. Seney FD, Burns DK, Silva FG (1990) Acquired immunodeficiency syndrome and the kidney. 16: 1–16

13. Sumrani NB, Hong JH, Hanson P, Butt KMH (1989) Renal transplantation in blacks: impact of immunosuppressive regimes. Transplant Proc 21: 3943–3946

14. Sumrani N, Delaney V, Ding Z, Butt K, Hong J (1990) HLA-identical renal transplants: Impact of cyclosporine on intermediate-term survival and renal function. Am J Kidney Dis 16: 417–422

15. United Network for Organ Sharing (1987) UNOS Policies, Richmond

Transplant Int (1992) 5 [Suppl 1]: S 133–S 137

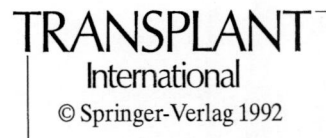

© Springer-Verlag 1992

The Japanese Interferon Study Group (JISG) has established the efficacy of human interferon-β for serious CMV pneumonitis in kidney recipients

K. Takahashi, S. Teraoka, K. Ota, M. Kosaki, H. Okazaki and the JISG

Secretariat of the JISG, Kidney Center, Tokyo Women's Medical College, Tokyo, Japan

The Japanese Interferon Study Group (JISG) is a research organization formed by 30 special hospitals for organ transplantation. A joint multi-centre, double-blind trial was conducted in order to investigate the efficacy of human interferon-β (HuIFN-β) against serious cytomegalovirus pneumonitis in kidney recipients.

Key words: Kidney transplantation – CMV – Pneumonitis – Interferon β

Subjects and methods

Subjects

The subjects were patients diagnosed with cytomegalovirus pneumonitis who received immunosuppressants immediately after kidney transplantations at special kidney transplant facilities. Before the start of the trial, informed consent was obtained from the patients themselves or their relatives.

Test drug

The HuIFN-β reference standard used in the trial was produced from normal human diploid fibroblasts [1] and prepared as a clinical standard drug by Toray Industries. This standard was a freeze-dried preparation that included 2.0×10^6 IU/vial, inert up to 10^7 IU/mg protein. A preparation containing 0.3×10^6 IU/vial was used for the control group. The controller confirmed the indistinguishability of the drug preparations.

Quantitative confirmation of the contents was conducted by Dr. S. Yamazaki of the N.I.H., Japan.

Allocation of the test drug

The test drug was allocated by two controllers (Dr. N. Shimizu, Internal Department, Teikyo University, and Dr. M. Kameyama, Internal Department, Sumitomo Hospital).

Offprint requests to: Kota Takahashi, M.D., Kidney Center, Tokyo Women's Medical College, 8-1 Kawada-cho, Shinjuku-ku, Tokyo, Japan

Dose levels and dosing method

The dose level for both drug preparations was set at a single vial administered three times a day. The administration method involved intravenous drip infusion for 2 h of the contents of a single vial which had been dissolved in 1 ml physiological saline for injection and to which 250 ml saline had been added.

Evaluation method

The improvement in the main clinical symptoms of viral pneumonia was evaluated by separately rating the following factors.

Chest X-ray radiographs. Two radiographs for each case, taken before and after drug administration, were submitted in a blind test by the controller to the Evaluation Committee on Chest X-Ray Radiographs, which conducted the scoring. Standard radiographs shown in Table 1 and Figs. 1–6 were used as references in scoring.

Fever. Improvement rating was assessed from the body temperature (daily maximum) before and after the end of drug administration. A drop below 38 °C was evaluated as 'improved', no drop as 'unchanged', and an increase above 38 °C as 'aggravated'.

Cough. Improvement rating was assessed from the extent of coughing before and after the end of drug administration. Symptoms interfering with sleep were assessed as (+ +), presence of cough as (+),

Table 1. Evaluation criteria for chest X-ray radiographs

Score	Criterion	Figure
0	No abnormal shadow is noted	1
2	Reinforced interstitial shadow is noted, but limited to a portion of lung field of one or both lungs	2
4	Interstitial shadow extends to the periphery of both lung fields	3
6	Manifestation of frosted-glass-type shadow	4
8	Diaphragmatic shadow is noted, but cardiac shadow is unclear; or cardiac shadow is noted, but diaphragmatic shadow is unclear	5
10	Both diaphragmatic and cardiac shadows cannot be seen	6

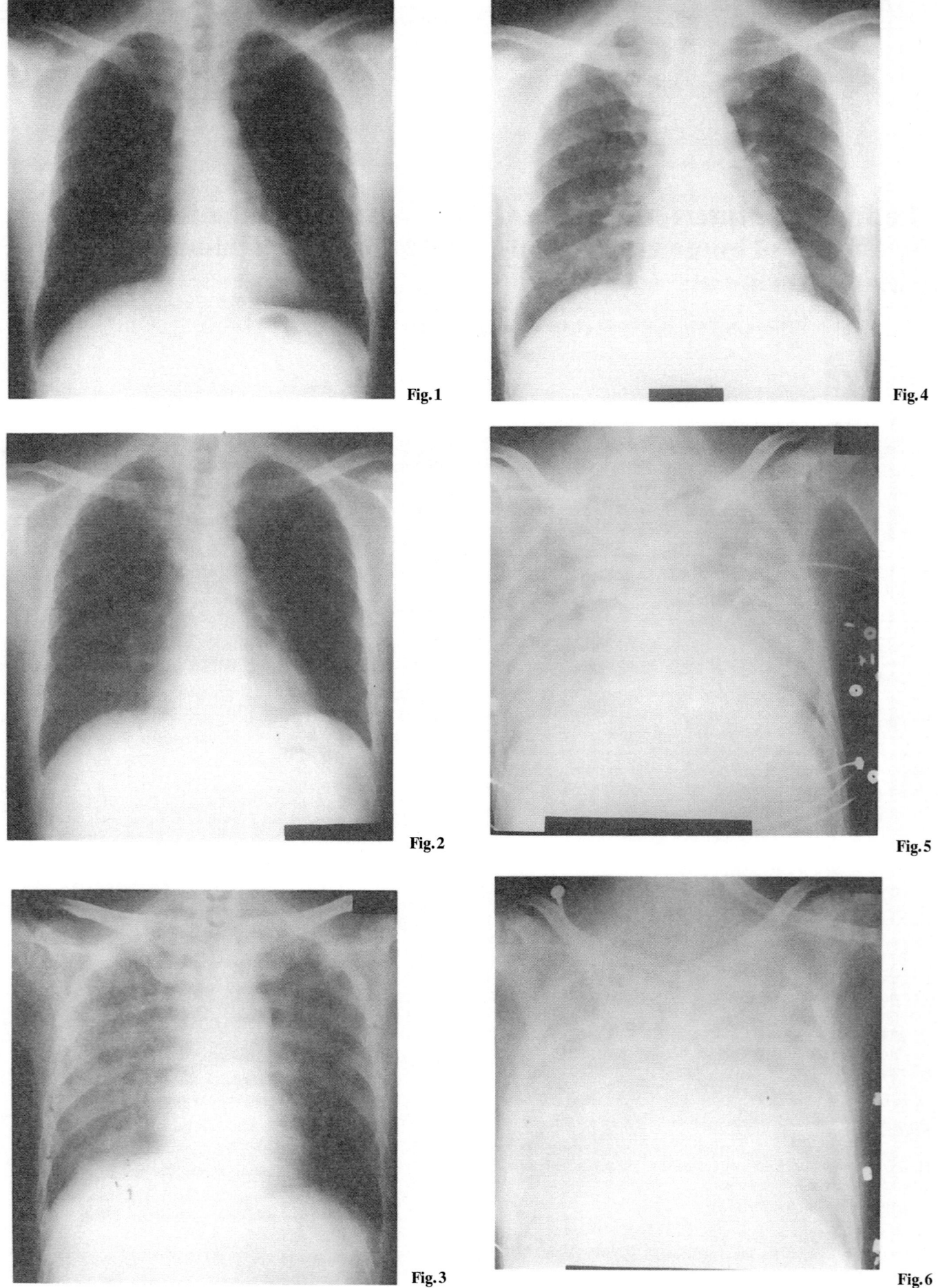

Fig. 1

Fig. 2

Fig. 3

Fig. 4

Fig. 5

Fig. 6

Table 2. Background factors

		6.0 M group ($n = 18$)	0.9 M group ($n = 23$)	Test U	Fisher
Sex	Male	12 (67)	16 (70)	NS	NS
	Female	6 (33)	7 (30)		
Age (years)	~19	2 (11)	2 (9)	NS	NS
	20–29	6 (33)	8 (35)		
	30–39	7 (39)	4 (17)		
	40–49	2 (11)	7 (30)		
	50~	1 (6)	2 (9)		
Severity	Slight	1 (6)	3 (13)	NS	NS
	Moderate	8 (44)	10 (43)		
	Severe	9 (50)	10 (43)		
Weight (kg)	~49	4 (22)	6 (26)	NS	NS
	50–59	9 (50)	13 (57)		
	60~	5 (28)	4 (17)		
Compli-cations	No	10 (56)	17 (74)	NS	NS
	Yes	8 (44)	6 (26)		
Acute rejection	No	15 (83)	22 (96)	NS	NS
	Yes	3 (17)	1 (4)		
Chronic rejection	No	17 (94)	20 (87)	NS	NS
	Yes	1 (6)	3 (13)		
Donor	Living donor	12 (67)	15 (65)	NS	NS
	Cadaveric donor	6 (33)	8 (35)		

Numbers in parentheses are percentages

and no symptoms as (–), and cases with improvement by more than one stage were taken as improved.

Hypoxaemia. Improvement rating was assessed from the PO_2 (room air) before and after the end of drug administration. A PO_2 value below 50 mm Hg was evaluated as (+ +), 50–70 mm Hg as (+), and more than 70 mm Hg as (–), and cases with improvement by more than one stage were taken as improved.

Final global improvement rating. Based on changes in overall clinical symptoms and results of clinical laboratory tests, the global improvement rating was assessed on a six-point rating scale as 'markedly effective', 'effective', 'slightly effective', 'ineffective', 'aggravated', or 'unassessable'.

Results

Number of cases

The total number of cases in the present trial was 43, including 19 in the 6.0 M group and 24 in the 0.9 M group. Two cases were excluded from analysis, including one case where, because of inattention by the physician-in-charge, the patient received the same dose twice and one case where clinical efficacy was evaluated as unassessable because the patient contracted pulmonary tuberculosis either simultaneously with or following CMV pneumonitis. The patient background factors of the 41 evaluated cases are listed in Table 2.

◄――――――――――――――――

Fig. 1–6. Standard radiographs for the radiograph rating described in Table 1

Efficacy

The improvement ratings with regard to chest radiographs, fever, cough and hypoxaemia are listed in Tables 3–6, respectively. Final global improvement rating is listed in Table 7.

The efficacy rate in the 6.0 M group was 50% (9/18 cases), showing a statistically significant tendency compared with the 17% in the 0.9 M group (7/17 cases) (*U*-test: $Z_0 = 1.653$, $P_0 = 0.098$).

Safety

Side effects were noted in 83% (15/18 cases) of the 6.0 M group and in 61% (14/23) of the 0.9 M group. The breakdown is listed in Table 8.

Table 3. Rating of chest X-ray radiographs

Group	Improved	Unchanged	Aggravated	Unassessable	Total[a]	Proportion improved (%)
6.0 M	7	5	6	0	18	39
0.9 M	7	4	9	1	21	33

U test, NS; Fisher, NS
[a] Only 39 cases were analysed because radiographs were missing in two cases

Table 4. Fever rating

Group	Improved	Unchanged	Aggravated	Total[a]	Proportion improved (%)
6.0 M	8	7	1	16	50
0.9 M	4	4	4	12	33

U test, NS; Fisher, NS
[a] Only 28 cases were analysed because in 13 of the 41 cases fever was absent before and after administration of the test drug

Table 5. Cough rating

Group	Improved	Unchanged	Aggravated	Total[a]	Proportion improved (%)
6.0 M	10	3	0	13	77
0.9 M	2	9	1	12	17

U test, $Z_0 = 0.987$, $P_0 = 0.003$; Fisher, $P_0 = 0.008$
[a] Only 25 cases were analysed because in 16 of the 41 cases no coughs occurred before and after administration of the test drug

Table 6. Hypoxaemia rating

Group	Improved	Unchanged	Aggravated	Unassessable	Total[a]	Proportion improved (%)
6.0 M	8	1	3	1	13	62
0.9 M	5	1	4	7	17	29

U test, NS; Fisher, NS
[a] Only 30 cases were analysed because in 11 of the 41 cases no abnormal PO_2 values were noted before and after administration of the test drug

Table 7. Final global rating

	Markedly effective	Effective	Slightly effective	Ineffective	Aggravated	Total	Efficacy rate (%)
6.0 M	6	3	2	4	3	18	50
0.9 M	2	2	8	4	7	23	17

U test, $Z_0 = 1.653$; $P_0 = 0.098$ (+)

Table 8. Side effects

	6.0 M group ($n = 18$)	0.9 M group ($n = 23$)
Fever	15 (83)	14 (61)
Chill	9 (50)	7 (30)
Headache	4 (22)	4 (17)
Fatigue	3 (17)	7 (30)
Anorexia	3 (17)	5 (22)
Nausea, Vomiting	3 (17)	1 (4)
Number of cases	15 (83)	14 (61)

Numbers in parentheses are percentages
None of the differences between the two groups was statistically significant

Table 9. Abnormal laboratory test values

	6.0 M group ($n = 18$)	0.9 M group ($n = 23$)
Decrease in RBC	0 (0)	1 (4)
Drop in Hb	0 (0)	1 (4)
Drop in Ht	0 (0)	1 (4)
Decrease in PLT	2 (11)	5 (22)
Decrease in WBC	2 (11)	8 (35)
Granulcytopenia	0 (0)	1 (4)
Rise in GOT	1 (6)	3 (13)
Rise in GPT	2 (11)	5 (22)
Rise in ALP	1 (6)	1 (4)
Rise in S-Cr	1 (6)	0 (0)
Number of cases	6 (33)	11 (48)

Numbers in parentheses are percentages
None of the differences between the groups was found to be statistically significant

Abnormal laboratory test values were noted in 33% (6/18 cases) of the 6.0 M group and in 48% (11/23) of the 0.9 M group (Table 9).

No difference between the groups was noted in the incidence of side effects and abnormal laboratory test values.

Discussion

The results of kidney transplantation have improved dramatically in recent years with the progress in the development of immunosuppressive drugs. However, infection is still the most common post-transplant complication, often becoming a factor that is decisive in patient survival.

HuIFN-β is a biosubstance with a wide antiviral spectrum, which is marketed as a radical remedy for hepatitis B in Japan, where it is widely used.

The efficacy of interferon on cytomegalovirus infections has been demonstrated by the results of in vitro and in

vivo tests [2]. While interferon administration has been used in an attempt to prevent viral infections immediately after kidney transplantation, there have only been case reports from several open studies on manifest cytomegalovirus pneumonitis, and the degree of therapeutic efficacy in clinical application has not been clarified.

We investigated objectively the efficacy of the drug in a randomized, double-blind, comparative trial. The dose levels used in the present trial were based on the experience from an open study conducted by Takahashi et al. [3]. Since the use of a completely inactive placebo for the control drug poses many ethical problems, and since no approval was obtained from the physicians participating in the trial, a preparation containing less than one-sixth the dose for the treatment group was used for the control group.

While the results showed a clear difference in efficacy between the 6.0 M and the 0.9 M groups, there was no difference in side effects and normal laboratory test values, demonstrating the utility of the drug against cytomegalovirus pneumonitis in the 6.0 M group. Ganciclovir is presently used as the first drug of choice among remedies for cytomegalovirus infections, but based on the results established for HuIFN-β, we wanted to provide with the present study another drug of choice, in addition to ganciclovir, for the therapy of serious cytomegalovirus pneumonitis following kidney transplantation. We are confident that either separate or concomitant use of both drugs can lead to further improvement in therapeutic results following kidney transplantation.

Note
JISG comprises:
1. Participating institutions (in order of number of patients entered): Sapporo City General Hospital; Tachikawa Sogo Hospital; School of Medicine, Chiba University; Kidney Center, Tokyo Women's Medical College (K.T., S.T. and K.O.); Institute of Medical Science, University of Tokyo; Hachioji Medical Center, Tokyo Medical College (M.K.); Hamamatsu University School of Medicine; Nagoya Second Red Cross Hospital; Shiga University of Medical Science; Kyoto Prefectural University of Medicine; Kinki University School of Medicine; Hyogo College of Medicine; Hyogo Prefectural Nishinomiya Hospital; Hiroshima University School of Medicine; Matsuyama Red Cross Hospital; National Nagasaki Chuo Hospital; Fukuoka Red Cross Hospital; and Makiminato Chuo Hospital.
2. Steering committee: K.Ota (Chairman), S.Teraoka, K.Takahashi; H.Okazaki, Sendai Shakaihoken Hospital; M.Kosaki, Hachioji Medical Center, Tokyo Medical College; S.Oshima, Shakaihoken Chukyo Hospital.
3. Evaluation Committee for Chest X-ray Radiographs: K.Simizu, Internal Department, Tokyo Women's Medical College; K.Hara, 3rd Internal Department, Nagasaki University, S.Teraoka, K.Takahashi, K.Ota; T.Tamaki, Hachioji Medical Center, Tokyo Medical College.
4. Participant for Virology: Y.Minamishima, Department of Virology, Miyazaki Medical College.
5. Data Analysis Center: The Controller Committee (N.S., M.K.)

6. Clinical Monitoring Center: Y. Kuwabara, A. Sada, N. Naruse, Toray Industries.

References

1. Kobayashi S, Iizuka M, Hara M, Ozawa H, Nagashima H, Suzuki J (1982) Preparation of human fibroblast interferon for clinical trials. In: Kono R, Vilcek J (eds) The clinical potential of interferons. University of Tokyo Press, Tokyo, pp 55–68
2. Nakamura K, Eizuru Y, Minamishima Y (1988) Effect of natural human interferon-beta on the replication of human cytomegalovirus. J Med Virol 26: 363
3. Takahashi K, Teraoka S, Yagisawa T, Fuchinove S, Honda H, Toma H, Agishi T, Ota K (1987) Effect of human interferon-β on life-threatening viral pneumonitis in kidney transplant recipients. Transplant Proc 19: 4089

Transplant Int (1992) 5 [Suppl 1]: S 138–S 139

TRANSPLANT
International
© Springer-Verlag 1992

Factors affecting the long-term outcome following non-living kidney transplantation

J. Thorogood[1,3], **J. C. van Houwelingen**[3], **J. J. van Rood**[2], **F. A. Zantvoort**[1], **G. M. Th. Schreuder**[2], and **G. G. Persijn**[1]

[1] Eurotransplant Foundation, Leiden, The Netherlands
[2] Department of Immunohaematology and Blood Bank, Leiden University Hospital, Leiden, The Netherlands
[3] University Department of Medical Statistics, Leiden, The Netherlands

The aims of the study were threefold: (1) to analyse the long-term overall kidney graft survival within Eurotransplant for the period 1971–1987; (2) to examine the effect of matching for HLA over the years, with the aid of half-lives after the first post-transplant year; and (3) to take prognostic factors into account for the period 1981–1987, comparing their influence on the long-term outcome of the graft and to predict half-lives for various combinations of factors.

Key words: Kidney transplantation – Long-term-results

Patients and methods

Data on 12 883 first unrelated kidney grafts from non-living donors, transplanted between 1971 and 1987, in 52 renal transplant centres within Austria, Belgium, Germany, Luxembourg and the Netherlands were analysed. Four separate time periods were examined: 1971–1975, 1976–1980, 1981–1984 for patients not treated with cyclosporine (CsA) and 1981–1987 for patients treated with CsA. Estimates of half-lives were obtained from a Weibull model and, for the analysis with prognostic factors, from an exponential model (see Appendix). The half-life estimates the time by which half the grafts would be lost, of those surviving for at least 1 year post-transplant.

Results

Table 1 shows the improvement in graft survival over the years 1971–1987. It can be seen that the half-lives increased by approximately 2 years. The main contribution

Supported in part by the Dutch Foundation for Medical and Health Research (MEDIGON), the J. A. Cohen Institute for Radiopathology and Radiation Protection (IRS) and the Kuratorium für Dialyse und Transplantation.

Offprint requests to: Ms. J. Thorogood, Eurotransplant Foundation, University Hospital, PO Box 2304, 2301 CH Leiden, The Netherlands

to better long-term survival came from improvements in the first post-transplant year. Table 2 shows the changes over the years with respect to number of HLA-B mismatches. The effect of matching for HLA was clearly shown to be important even after the first post-transplant year and in patients receiving CsA. Examining previously identified prognostic factors [1], we observed that donor and recipient age and sex, recipient diagnosis of diabetes and number of HLA-B mismatches all remained of prognostic importance in the longer term. Table 3 shows that the half-lives varied from 14.5 years to 4.9 years, depending on the combination of factors for a given patient.

Discussion

Half-lives increased from 9.7 years for 1971–1975 for patients treated without CsA, to 11.6 years for 1981–1987 for patients treated with CsA. The 30 % gain in overall 5-year graft survival may be largely attributed to improvements in the first post-transplant year, due to such factors as preoperative blood transfusions, prospective HLA-DR matching and use of CsA. The benefits in prolonged renal allograft survival gained by matching for HLA are maintained in the CsA era. Other factors also affect the long-term outcome, namely donor and recipient age and sex and recipient diagnosis of diabetes. Together with number of HLA-B mismatches, these factors in combination lead to large differences in half-lives, estimates ranging from 14.5 to 4.9 years.

Appendix

The Weibull distribution is a generalization of the exponential distribution, allowing for a power dependence of the hazard on time. The survivor function, $S(t)$, for this distribution is $S(t) = \exp(-(\lambda t)^p)$. The hazard function, $\lambda(t)$, is $\lambda(t) = \lambda p (\lambda t)^{p-1}$ and is monotone decreasing for $p < 1$ and monotone increasing for $p > 1$. For $p = 1$ the Weibull model reduces to the exponential model with constant hazard function $\lambda(t) = \lambda$. In the earlier periods, p was significantly smaller than 1, indicating a decreasing hazard rate. In the final

Table 1. Overall graft survival and half-lives

Period	No. of patients	Graft survival (%)		Half-life (years) (95% confidence interval)
		1 year	5 years	
1971–1975	984	57.0	38.8	9.7 (8.4–11.2)
1976–1980	3065	62.2	43.9	10.7 (9.7–11.7)
1981–1984, without CsA	2002	66.0	49.2	10.7 (9.3–12.4)
1981–1987, with CsA	6832	84.5	66.0	11.6 (10.0–13.4)

Table 2. Graft survival and half-lives by number of HLA-B mismatches and period

No. of HLA-B mismatches	No. of patients	Graft survival (%)		Half-life (years) (95% confidence interval)	Standard normal deviate test on half-lives
		1 year	5 years		
1971–1975					
0 HLA-B	320	63.8	45.3	11.1 (8.7–14.3)	$P = 0.042$
1 HLA-B	490	55.1	37.8	9.7 (7.9–12.0)	
2 HLA-B	174	50.0	29.9	7.2 (5.1–10.1)	
1976–1980					
0 HLA-B	992	65.0	50.0	14.5 (12.3–17.2)	$P = 0.001$
1 HLA-B	1741	61.5	41.2	9.3 (8.3–10.4)	
2 HLA-B	332	57.8	39.5	8.7 (6.7–11.3)	
1981–1984, without CsA					
0 HLA-B	550	65.6	51.1	13.0 (10.0–16.7)	$P = 0.005$
1 HLA-B	1193	66.5	49.3	10.8 (9.1–12.8)	
2 HLA-B	259	64.5	44.4	7.5 (5.6–9.9)	
1981–1987, with CsA					
0 HLA-B	1591	87.1	69.7	13.2 (10.6–16.4)	$P = 0.013$
1 HLA-B	3983	84.3	67.0	12.1 (10.2–14.3)	
2 HLA-B	1258	81.7	58.8	9.0 (7.4–11.0)	

Table 3. Half-lives per prognostic group

No. of HLA-B mismatches	Female donor to male recipient	Diabetic recipient	Donor age > 55 years	Recipient < 16 years	Half lives (95% confidence interval)	No. of patients
0	No	No	No	No	14.5 (12.0–17.5)	881
1	No	No	No	No	13.4 (11.8–15.2)	1997
0	Yes	No	No	No	11.1 (8.8–14.1)	210
2	No	No	No	No	10.4 (8.6–12.5)	588
1	Yes	No	No	No	10.3 (8.5–12.4)	496
0	No	Yes	No	No	8.8 (6.2–12.5)	39
1	No	No	No	Yes	8.7 (6.0–12.6)	79
1	No	Yes	No	No	8.1 (5.8–11.2)	101
2	Yes	No	No	No	8.0 (6.3–10.1)	149
0	No	No	Yes	No	6.9 (4.8–9.9)	48
2	No	No	No	Yes	6.7 (4.6–9.8)	51
1	Yes	No	No	Yes	6.6 (4.5–9.8)	22
1	No	No	Yes	No	6.3 (4.5–8.9)	95
2	No	Yes	No	No	6.3 (4.5–8.8)	65
1	Yes	Yes	No	No	6.2 (4.3–8.9)	26
1	Yes	No	Yes	No	4.9 (3.4–7.0)	44
2	No	No	Yes	No	4.9 (3.4–7.2)	24

period (1981–1987, for patients receiving CsA), p was not significantly different from 1 and the exponential model could be used.

Acknowledgement. This work could not have been undertaken without the generous support of all clinicians and their staff from donor hospitals, transplantation centres and tissue typing laboratories, collaborating within Eurotransplant (for a full list, see Thorogood J et al, Transplantation (1989) 48: 231–238).

Reference

1. Thorogood J, van Houwelingen JC, Persijn GG, Zantvoort FA, Schreuder GMTh, and van Rood JJ (1991) Prognostic indices to predict survival of first and second renal allografts. Transplantation (in press)

Transplant Int (1992) 5 [Suppl 1]: S 140–S 142

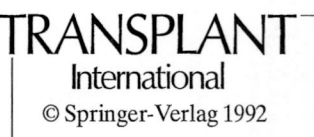
TRANSPLANT
International
© Springer-Verlag 1992

Is repeated mismatching at regrafting deleterious?

G. Tufveson, M. Bengtsson, C. Bergström, L. Frödin, G. Lewén, O. Sjöberg, I. Skarp, T. Tötterman, J. Wahlberg, and B. Wikström

Departments of Surgery (Transplantation Unit), Clinical Immunology and Internal Medicine (Nephrology), University Hospital, Uppsala, Sweden

Abstract. We reviewed our clinical experience of allowing kidney regrafting with a repeated HLA mismatch. We also permitted a weakly positive B-cell cross-match. All patients who received a second or subsequent renal graft ($n = 92$) between January 1985 and June 1990 were analysed for graft survival. The overall 1-year graft survival was 70%. A repeated mismatch occurred in 29 of the patients at at least one HLA locus and their 1-year graft survival was 66%. The balance of the regrafts (63) were performed without a repeated mismatch, and their 1-year graft survival was 70%. Even a weakly positive B-cell cross-match was deleterious; when a grafting with a repeated mismatch was performed only one out of five grafts survived. Our results indicate that retransplantation of renal grafts with a repeated mismatch in the HLA A or B locus can be performed without a negative influence on transplant outcome provided that both the T- and B-cell cross-matches are negative.

Key words: Regrafting – HLA mismatching – B-cell cross-match

In our clinic we had observed an accumulation of patients waiting for regrafting, a phenomenon observed also in many other institutions. Because of this, we decided in January 1985 to give priority to regrafting. Also, we questioned the previous belief that patients previously exposed to HLA antigens should not be grafted with tissue containing the same antigens (repeated mismatch). Contributing to our questioning were two clinical findings: (A) The first Scandinavian multicentre study failed to detect any beneficial effect of DR matching when cyclosporine was used as the main immunosuppressant despite the previously observed beneficial effect of DR matching on graft survival [5]; (B) Taube et al. suggested that it was

possible to remove panel reactive antibodies by means of plasmapheresis and maintain a low level by the use of immunosuppression prior to transplantation and thereafter perform successful grafting [7].

We therefore decided to allow regrafting also with repeated mismatch on locus A, B or DR and perform kidney transplantations against a weakly positive B-cell cross-match. The only mandatory requirement for accepting a regraft was a negative T-cell cross-match.

This paper describes some features of such a policy carried out at a single institution. We have analysed the graft survival of all regrafts performed from January 1985 to June 1990 with regard to graft survival, waiting time, influence of repeated mismatches at any locus and the influence of a current positive B-cell cross-match.

Materials and methods

Patients

All patients who received a second or subsequent renal graft ($n = 92$) between January 1985 and June 1990 were analysed. This patient group represented 23% of the total number of renal graft recipients during the same time period.

Immunosuppression

Base line immunosuppression for these patients generally consisted of conventional triple therapy and in about 50% of the cases ATG (Fresenius AG, Bad Homburg, FRG) or ALG (Horse ALG, Merieux Lyon, France) were given prophylacticly. Anti-rejection therapy consisted of either methylprednisolone, ATG or ALG or OKT-3 (Ortho Pharmaceuticals, Raritan, New Jersey, USA).

Postoperative management

The patients were monitored by daily laboratory parameters. In addition the grafts were frequently biopsied, as described elsewhere [8], as all regrafts were suspected to be of high immunological risk.

Offprint requests to: Gunnar Tufveson, Transplantation Unit, University Hospital, S-751 85 Uppsala, Sweden

Pretransplant immunosuppression

Patients who reacted to more than 50% of a random blood donor panel were also treated with pretransplant plasmapheresis or pretransplant immunoabsorption according to protocols described elsewhere [1, 2]. Nine out of the 29 patients with a repeated mismatch, and 11 out of the 63 patients without a repeated mismatch, received such a treatment.

Cross-match technique

A current cross-match was always performed prior to transplantation. These were carried out using the NIH technique [6] or using the dynal bead technique [9].

Data presentation

The actual results of the procedure were evaluated in terms of 1-year graft survival. The data are expressed as percentage survival of eligible grafts.

Results

The results of this retrospctive study are summarized in Table 1. The overall 1-year graft survival was 70%. The median time on the waiting list was 4.5 months (0–31 months). A repeated mismatch occurred in 29 of the patients at at least one HLA locus and the 1-year graft survival in these patients was 66%. Their median time on the waiting list was 3 months (range 0–19 months). The balance of the regrafts (63) were performed without a repeated mismatch, and their 1-year graft survival was 70%. Their median waiting time was 6 months (0–31 months).

The 29 patients who had a repeated mismatch could be subdivided according to the locus for which they were mismatched. Three of these patients had mismatches in more than one locus and are therefore included more than once in the following discussion, (two of these three patients were doing well at the time of writing). Of 11 patients with a repeated mismatch at the A locus, 82% had a functioning graft after 1 year. Of 15 patients with a repeated mis-

Table 1. Percentage 1-year graft survival and median time on waiting list (range) for regrafts performed at our institution. Influence of repeated mismatch

Regraft group	n	Survival (%)	Waiting time (months)
All	92	70	4.5 (0–31)
With repeated mismatch	29	66	3 (0–19)
Without repeated mismatch	63	71	6 (0–31)
Repeated mismatches			
HLA-A	11	82	
HLA-B	15	60	
HLA-B with negative B-cell cross-match	11	73	
HLA-B with positive B-cell cross-match	4	25	
HLA-DR	6	50	

match at the B locus, only 60% had a functioning graft 1 year later. Amongst these patients, only 11 had a negative B-cell cross-match. The number of patients with repeated DR mismatches was low ($n = 6$), and the graft survival at 1 year was 50%. Only 25% of the grafts (1/4) with a repeated mismatch and a positive B-cell cross-match survived for 1 year.

Discussion

We have shown that regrafts can be performed with a repeated mismatch with approximately the same graft survival as in patients without a repeated mismatch. The advantage of allowing repeated mismatches is that patients waiting for regraft are not unnecessarily denied an otherwise suitable graft. Subanalyses of such a policy shows good graft survival if there is a repeated mismatch at the A or B locus provided that the current B- and T-cell cross-match is negative. In our small experience, even a weakly positive B-cell cross-match should be regarded as a contraindication. The number of observations are too small to allow any firm conclusions regarding DR mismatch. Furthermore, because of a sometimes incomplete DR typing with close to a 20% blank registration of DR genes in the Scandinavian population, that analysis becomes even less meaningful.

Subanalyses of the cause of graft loss of any of the previous grafts as contributing to the outcome of the next graft was not possible in this small patient group. However, theoretically antigen presentation and sensitization may occur within 10 min after revascularization of a graft [4], and therefore the reason for a previous graft loss may only be of academic interest. A somewhat surprisingly good (about 80%) graft survival of repeated mismatched grafts in A and B loci was achieved at 1 year provided that the cross-matches were negative. This could even perhaps suggest that patients without circulating antibodies, despite previous graft exposure, may be tolerant to these antigens.

The ethical implications of our findings for organ allocation seem to fit well into a proposal for future organ allocation within the United States [3] where it was proposed to allocate at least one-quarter of the available kidneys presented to a local harvesting organization to high-risk patients.

In summary, our results indicate that retransplantation of grafts with repeated mismatch in HLA A or B loci can be done without a negative influence on transplant outcome, provided that both the T- and B-cell cross-matches are negative. This procedure makes it more likely for previously grafted patients to receive a graft within a reasonable time.

References

1. Backman U, Fellström B, Frödin L, Sjöberg O, Tufveson G, Wikström B (1989) Successful transplantation in sensitized patients. Transplant Proc 21: 762–763
2. Danielson BG, Wikström B, Backman U, Fellström B, Tufveson G, Sjöberg O (1990) Pretransplant immunoabsorbtion plasma

treatment of HLA-immunized patients – preliminary report. Artif Organs 14 [Suppl 2] 231–232

3. Halasz NA (1991) Medicine and ethics, how to allocate transplantable organs. Transplantation 52: 43–46

4. Haltunen J, Häyry P (1987) Mobile blood-derived components in renal allograft contain significant immunogenic potential. Scand J Immunol 25: 121–126

5. Lundgren G, Groth CG, Albrektsen H, Brynger H, Flatmark A, Frödin L, Gäbel H, Husberg B, Klintmalm G, Maarer W, Persson H, Thorsby E (1986) HLA matching and pretransplant blood transfusions in cadaveric renal transplantation – a changing picture with cyclosporine A. Lancet II: 66–69

6. NIH lymphocyte microcytotoxicity technique (1916) In: Ray JG Jr, Hare DB, Pedersen PD, Mullally DI. NIAID manual of tissue typing techniques 1976–1977. (DHEW publication no. (NIH) 76-545) Government Printing Office, Washington, D. C., pp 22–24

7. Taube DH, Cameron IS, Ogg CS, Welsh KI, Williams DG, Bewick M, Rudge CJ, Kennedy LA, Thick MG (1984) Renal transplantation after removal and prevention of resynthesis of HLA-antibodies. Lancet I: 824–826

8. Tufveson G, Hanås E, Lindgren PG, Larsson E, Andersson T, Fellström B, Wahlberg J, Tötterman T (1989) A review of the Uppsala experience of Biopty-Cut renal transplant biopsies. Transplant Proc 21: 3581–3582

9. Vartdal F, Gaudernack G, Funderud S, Bratlie A, Lea T, Ugelstad J, Thorsby E (1986) HLA class I and II typing using cells positively selected from blood by immunomagnetic isolation – a fast and reliable technique. Tissue Antigens 28: 301–312

Transplant Int (1992) 5 [Suppl 1]: S 143–S 145

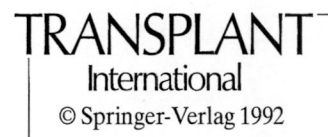
TRANSPLANT
International
© Springer-Verlag 1992

Detrimental role of donor-recipient HLA-DQ$_5$ and -DQ$_6$ disparities on cadaver kidney graft survival

P. Vereerstraeten, M. Andrien, E. Dupont, D. Abramowicz, L. de Pauw, M. Goldman, and P. Kinnaert

Departments of Nephrology and Immunology, CUB Hôpital Erasme, Brussels, Belgium

Abstract. Donor-recipient incompatibility $(D + R -)$ for HLA-DQ$_1$, but not for -DQ$_2$ or -DQ$_3$, is associated with an adverse effect on cadaver kidney graft survival. Until now, however, DQ$_1$ recipients of DQ$_1$-negative kidneys $(D - R +)$ have not been differentiated from DQ$_1$-identical donor–recipient pairs $(D + R +)$ and splits of DQ$_1$, DQ$_5$ and DQ$_6$, have not been studied in that respect. From our data (480 transplantations performed from January 1980 to December 1990), three donor–recipient DQ combinations $(D + R +, D - R +, D + R -)$ were formed for each of four DQ specificities (DQ$_2$, DQ$_3$, DQ$_5$, DQ$_6$). As DR–DQ linkage disequilibrium is well conserved in caucasoid individuals, DQ specificities were inferred from the associated DR specificities. Graft survival rate (%) was significantly lower for the DQ$_5$ $D + R -$ and the DQ$_6$ $D - R +$ combinations when compared with the other corresponding DQ combinations, whereas no significant difference was observed between the DQ$_2$ and DQ$_3$ combinations. In conclusion, if DQ$_1$ plays a prominent role in kidney graft survival, the effects of its splits appear dissociated: DQ$_5$ could be a marker of high antigenicity and DQ$_6$ a marker of high responsiveness.

Key words: Cadaver kidney graft survival – HLA-DQ histocompatibility

In previous retrospective [11] and prospective [12] studies from our centre, donor–recipient HLA-DR disparities characterized by the presence of the antigen in the donor but not in the recipient, or vice-versa, were shown to affect cadaver kidney graft survival differentially. Some of those disparities were beneficial (DR4, DR5 and DR7 in the donor; DR5 in the recipient) whereas others were detrimental (DR1 and DR2 in the donor; DR2, DRW6 and DR7 in the recipient) for graft survival when compared with the other HLA-DR disparities.

More recently, donor–recipient HLA-DQ$_1$-incompatible grafts have been shown to have a poorer 1-year survival (65%) than DQ$_1$-compatible grafts (89%), whereas DQ$_2$ and DQ$_3$ did not influence graft prognosis [7]. In this study, however, DQ$_1$ compatibility involved both identity $(D + R +)$ and DQ$_1$ recipients of DQ$_1$-negative kidneys $(D - R +)$; splits of DQ$_1$, DQ$_5$ and DQ$_6$ were not studied.

The present study was undertaken to investigate the effects of donor–recipient DQ combinations on graft survival, differentiating the $D - R +$ from the $D + R +$ combinations when compared with the incompatible $(D + R -)$ combination, for each of four DQ specificities (DQ$_2$, DQ$_3$, DQ$_5$ and DQ$_6$).

Materials and methods

Patients

From the data collected on 480 cadaver kidney transplantations performed at our centre between January 1980 and December 1990, three groups of donor–recipient DQ combinations $(D + R +, D - R +, D + R -)$ were formed for each of four DQ specificities (DQ$_2$, DQ$_3$, DQ$_5$ and DQ$_6$). As DR–DQ linkage disequilibrium is very well conserved in caucasoid individuals [6], DQ specificities were inferred from their associated DR specificities: DQ$_2$ with DR3 and DR7, DQ$_3$ with DR4 and DR5, DQ$_5$ with DR1 and DRW10, and DQ$_6$ with DR2 and DRW6. This DR–DQ linkage was checked in 114 blood specimens from organ donors in which DR and DQ specificities were simultaneously determined.

Immunosuppressive therapy consisted of cyclosporin, azathioprine and prednisolone as previously described [11]. Prophylactic OKT3 was administered to 193 recipients during the first 2 weeks after transplantation, while the other patients received the triple therapy from the first postoperative day onwards. Rejection episodes were treated with pulses of methylprednisolone in most circumstances and the few corticoresistant episodes with either antilymphocyte globulin or OKT3. All but four recipients had received at least one pretransplant blood transfusion.

Offprint requests to: P. Vereerstraeten, M.D., Department of Nephrology, CUB Hôpital Erasme 808, Route de Lennik, 1070 Brussels, Belgium

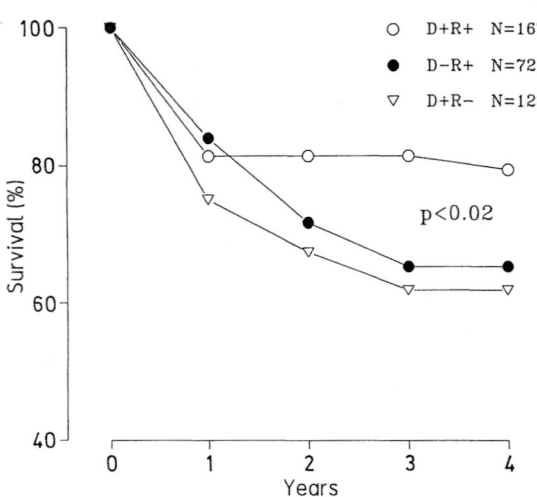

Fig. 1. Donor (D)/recipient (R) HLA-DQ$_1$ combinations and kidney graft survival. D + R + , D positive/R positive; D – R + , D negative/R positive; D + R – : D positive/R negative; NS, not significant; N, numbers of grafts

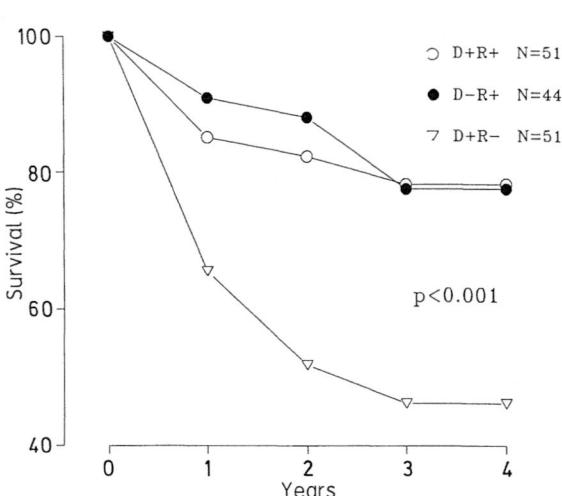

Fig. 2. Donor (D)/recipient (R) HLA-DQ$_5$ combinations and kidney graft survival

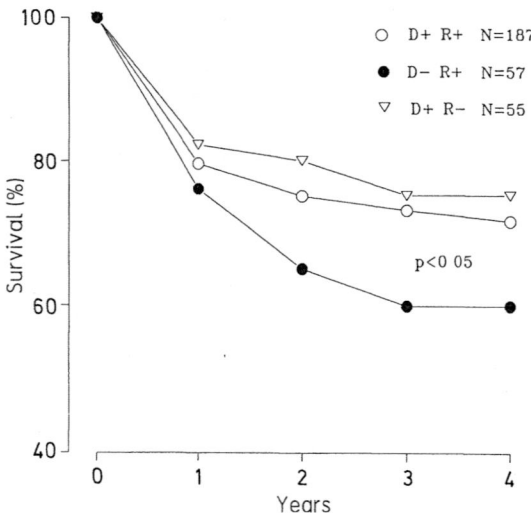

Fig. 3. Donor (D)/recipient (R) HLA-DQ$_6$ combinations and kidney graft survival

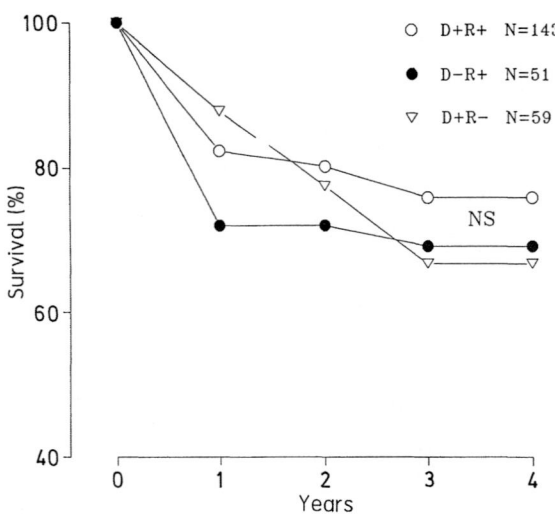

Fig. 4. Donor (D)/recipient (R) HLA-DQ$_2$ combinations and kidney graft survival

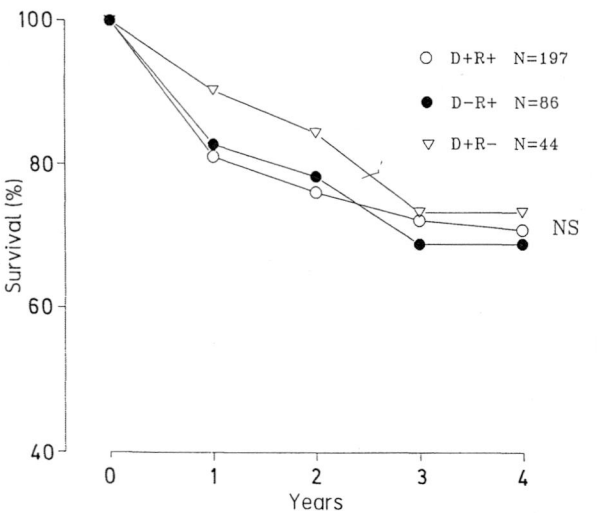

Fig. 5. Donor (D)/recipient (R) HLA-DQ$_3$ combinations and kidney graft survival

HLA typing

HLA-DR and -DQ typing was performed according to the standard NIH microcytotoxicity method [8], using sera obtained in our laboratory and those provided by Eurotransplant.

Statistical analysis

Graft survival was studied according to the actuarial life-table method [5], and differences between survival curves were assessed using the Lee–Desu statistic [4].

Results

The DR–DQ linkage disequilibrium was perfectly conserved between DQ$_5$ and DR1–DRW10 and between DQ$_3$ and DR4–DR5, but somewhat less well between DQ$_6$ and DR2–DRW6 and between DQ$_2$ and DR3–DR7 (Table 1). The overall concordance between the associated DR and DQ specificities was 89% (Table 2), validating the in-

Table 1. Linkage disequilibrium between HLA-DR and -DQ specificities

HLA-DR Specificities	No. of HLA-DQ specificities associated with HLA-DR				
	HLA-DQ$_2$	HLA-DQ$_3$	HLA-DQ$_5$	HLA-DQ$_6$	Total
1			10		10
2			5	25	30
3	24	1			25
4		23			23
5		43			43
W6		3	6	17	26
7	29	8			37
W10			6		6

Table 2. Concordance of associated HLA-DR and -DQ specificities

DQ$_2$ with DR3 and DR7	53/62	85%
DQ$_3$ with DR4 and DR5	66/66	100%
DQ$_5$ with DR1 and DRW10	16/16	100%
DQ$_6$ with DR2 and DRW6	42/56	75%
Overall DQ-DR	177/200	89%

ference of DQ from DR specificities for the total set of our data.

Graft survival was similar for HLA–DQ$_1$ in the D – R + and in the D + R – combinations; it was significantly lower than that observed in the D + R + combination (Fig. 1). When the splits of DQ$_1$ were separately considered, two donor–recipient combinations appeared significantly detrimental for the graft: DQ$_5$ D + R – (Fig. 2) and DQ$_6$ D – R + (Fig. 3). The graft outcome was not significantly different between the DQ$_2$ (Fig. 4) and DQ$_3$ (Fig. 5) donor–recipient combinations.

Discussion

Our results fully confirm the predominant role of DQ$_1$ in cadaver kidney graft survival, but the effects of its splits are dissociated. Whereas DQ$_5$ D + R – grafts behave poorly when compared with either the D – R + or the D + R + combination, survival for the DQ$_6$ D – R + combination is lower than that observed for either the D + R – or the D + R + combination.

The mechanisms underlying these results are still poorly understood as are those involved in alloreactivity. The demonstration of an influence of DQ molecules on kidney graft survival is surprising for, in vitro, the proliferative response observed in mixed lymphocyte reaction depends on DR and DP, but not on DQ molecules [9]. However, the recent demonstration of the prominent role of DQ as immune response molecules in diseases such as type I diabetes mellitus [10] opens the debate for a role of those antigens in transplantation, a hypothesis already put forward by Duquesnoy et al. [3] and more recently by Sengar et al. [7]. Assuming that the model proposed for class II molecules and applied for antigen presentation [2] is valid for alloreactivity, we are currently studying amino acid homologies on the top of the groove formed by the α_1 and β_1 chains of DQ molecules. Interestingly, only one amino acid of exon 2 of the DQ β_1 chain perfectly discriminates DQ$_5$ and DQ$_6$ from the other DQ alleles: glutamine characterizes DQ$_5$ and DQ$_6$ and leucine the other DQ alleles [6]. Whether this difference affects allodeterminant expression remains to be elucidated on a prospective basis.

Alternatively, HLA-DQ molecules produced by immune suppression (IS) genes could be involved in active suppression with respect to a specific antigen, as recently suggested by Altmann et al. [1]. Thus, according to the properties of their DQ molecules, recipients would be responders or nonresponders; DQ$_6$-positive recipients of DQ$_6$-negative kidneys would belong to the first category and recipients bearing other DQ molecules than DQ$_6$ to the second one. Here again, further studies are needed to establish a relationship between the presence of particular DQ molecules and the emergence of suppression mechanisms.

Acknowledgements. This work was supported by the Fonds de la Recherche Scientifique Médicale (grant 1.5.234.87 F) and by the Fondation Universitaire David et Alice van Buuren, Brussels.

References

1. Altmann DM, Sansom D, Marsh SGE (1991) What is the basis for HLA-DQ associations with autoimmune disease? Immunology Today 8: 267–270
2. Brown JH, Jardetsky MA, Saper B, Samraoui P, Bjorkman PJ, Wiley DC (1988) A hypothetical model of the foreign antigen binding site of class II histocompatibility molecules. Nature 332: 845–850
3. Duquesnoy RJ, Annen KB, Marrari MM, Kauffman HM Jr (1980) Association of MB compatibility with successful intrafamilial kidney transplantation. N Engl J Med 302: 821–825
4. Lee E, Desu M (1972) A computer program for comparing K samples with right-censored data. Comput Programs Biomed 2: 315–321
5. Mantel N (1966) Evaluation of survival data and two rank order statistics arising in its considerations. Cancer Chemother Rep 50: 163–170
6. Morel C, Zwahlen F, Jeannet M, Mach B, Tiercy JM (1990) Complete analysis of HLA-DQB1 polymorphism and DR-DQ linkage disequilibrium by oligonucleotide typing. Hum Immunol 29: 64–77
7. Sengar DP, Couture RA, Raman S, Inidal SL (1990) HLA-DQW1 compatibility and cadaveric renal allograft survival. Transplantation 50: 156–158
8. Terasaki PI, Bernoco D, Park MS, Ozturk G, Iwaki Y (1978) Microdroplet testing for HLA-A, -B, -C and -D antigens. Am J Clin Pathol 69: 103–120
9. Termijtelen AM, Erlich HA, Braun LA, Verduyn W, Drabbels JJM, Schroeiers WEM, van Rood JJ, de Koster KS, Giphart MG (1991) Oligonucleotide typing is a perfect tool to identify antigens stimulatory in the mixed lymphocyte culture. Hum Immunol 31: 241–245
10. Todd JA, Bell JI, McDevitt HO (1987) HLA-DQβ gene contributes to susceptibility and resistance to insulin-dependent diabetes mellitus. Nature 329: 599–604
11. Vereerstraeten P, Andrien M, Dupont E, Kinnaert P, Toussaint C (1989) Influence of donor–recipient HLA-DR antigen disparities on cadaver kidney graft survival: an alternative for recipient selection. Transplant Proc 21: 679–681
12. Vereerstraeten P, Andrien M, De Pauw L, Dupont E, Goldman M, Abramowicz D, Kinnaert P (1991) Beneficial effects of some donor–recipient HLA-DR mismatches on cadaveric graft survival: proposal for a new selection policy of recipients. Transplant Proc 23: 385–386

Transplant Int (1992) 5 [Suppl 1]: S146–S147

TRANSPLANT
International
© Springer-Verlag 1992

CMV prophylaxis after renal transplantation with immunoglobulin or CMV-hyperimmunoglobulin – a prospective clinical trial

D. Stippel[1], P. Wienand[1], N. Weißenberg[1], C. Baldamus[2], and U. Kruppenbacher[3]

[1] Department of Surgery, [2] Department of Internal Medicine, and [3] Department of Virology, University of Cologne, Cologne, FRG

Abstract. Three groups of 40 patients each entered this prospective randomized trial. Patients of group A received 2 ml/kg body weight CMV-Polyglobulin, patients of group B 15 g Intraglobin and patients of group C, serving as controls, received no specific anti-CMV prophylaxis. All patients were given the same sequential immunosuppressive therapy. Patient survival and graft function did not show any significant differences at 2 years follow up. The incidence of fever, CMV infections, dialysis and steroid bolus therapy were lower in group A, but without statistical significance. Patients receiving a graft from a CMV–AK-positive donor were at high risk of developing an infection or reactivation of CMV. A study examining this subgroup seems appropriate.

Key words: CMV prophylaxis – Renal transplantation – Immunoglobulin

During the first year post-transplantation CMV infection is a major threat to graft and patient survival. The aim of this study was to examine the effect of prophylactic CMV-hyperimmunoglobulin as compared with immunoglobulin or no CMV prophylaxis.

Materials and methods

During a period of 2 years all recipients of a first or second cadaver renal graft were randomly assigned to one of the three groups (n = 40, each). Patients of group A received a CMV-hyperimmunoglobulin (CMV-Polyglobin, 2 ml/kg body weight) immediately after surgery. Patients of group B received an immunoglobulin (Intraglobin F, 15 g) immediately after surgery. Patients of group C received no specific CMV prophylaxis.

The immunosuppressive regimen was standardized, starting with prophylactic antilymphocyte globulin for 8–10 days, azathioprine

and steroids being switched to long-term immunosuppression with steroids and cyclosporine (whole blood levels of 300 ng/ml).

CMV-KBR titres and CMV-IgM titres (ELISA) were determined prior to surgery and on days 1, 21, 42, 63, 84 and 105 posttransplantation. A rise of four times the initial KBR or an IgM titre > 1:10 was considered a CMV infection/reactivation. Combination with a fever > 38 °C or a rise in serum creatinine, transaminases, leucocytopenia or thrombocytopenia was considered symptomatic of CMV infection. Primary infection was defined as the above together with a preoperative negative CMV-KBR. Reactivation was defined as the above together with a preoperative positive CMV-KBR.

Results

There were no significant differences between the three groups with respect to age, sex, frequency of HLA-A, HLA-B or HLA-DR mismatches, conservation time, anastomotic time, frequency of first versus second transplant or preoperative CMV status. Donor CMV status was known in 71 out of 120 cases. There were no significant irregularities in the distribution of known CMV-negative

Table 1. Frequency of symptoms and complications after renal transplantation depending on the kind of CMV prophylaxis

Results: III

Symptoms	Group A (CMV-IgG) (n = 40) n	Group B (IgG) (n = 40) n	Group C (Control) (n = 40) n
Fever	10	16	14
Pneumonia	1	5	1
Urinary infection	6	6	6
Herpes infection	9	16	6
CMV infection with CMV-immunoglobulintherapy	2	4	3
CMV infection without CMV-immunoglobulintherapy	9	15	12
Dialysis after transpl.	2	7	5
Steroid bolus injection	8	15	14

Offprint requests to: D. Stippel, Department of Surgery, University of Cologne, Joseph-Stelzmann-Straße 9, 5000 Köln 41, FRG

Results I : patient survival

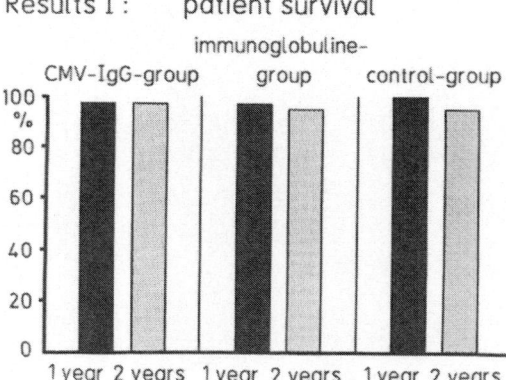

Fig. 1. Patient survival after 1 and 2 years depending on the kind of CMV prophylaxis

Results II : transplant survival

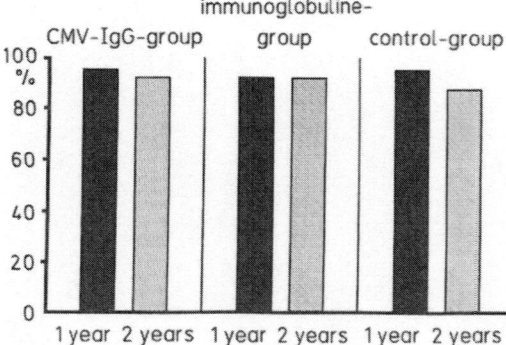

Fig. 2. Graft survival after 1 and 2 years depending on the kind of CMV prophylaxis

donors, but group B was at a slight disadvantage with four negative donors out of 24 with known status compared with 11 out of 23 in group A and 9 out 24 in group C.

There were no significant differences in either patient or transplant survival (Figs. 1 and 2). There were 22 CMV primary infections, and 72 CMV reactivations, the frequency within the three groups being as follows: primary infections: group A 12.5%, group B 27.5%, group C 15%; reactivation: group A 60%, group B 57.5%, group C 62.5% (differences without statistical significance).

Table 1 shows the distribution of various complications between the groups. Group A had the lowest frequency of fever, pneumonia, urinary tract infection, dialysis, and rejection episodes; none of the differences were significant.

Discussion

Administration of CMV-hyperimmunoglobulin or immunoglobulin did not result in a significant improvement in patient or transplant survival. Injection or reactivation developed in 27.5% of patients receiving CMV-hyperimmunoglobulin, 47.5% of patients receiving immunoglobulin and 37.5% of patients of the control group. The number of symptomatic CMV infections leading to therapeutic use of CMV-hyperimmunoglobulin was not significantly different between the groups. There was a tendency towards a lower rate of complications in the CMV-hyperimmunoglobulin group. Considering that there is a subgroup at higher risk (donor CMV-IgG-positive/recipient CMV-IgG-negative) a study examining this subgroup seems appropriate.

Transplant Int (1992) 5 [Suppl 1]: S 148–S 150

TRANSPLANT
International
© Springer-Verlag 1992

Length of time on dialysis prior to renal transplantation is a critical factor affecting patient survival after allografting

J. C. West[1], J. E. Bisordi[2], E. C. Squiers[1], R. Latsha[1], J. Miller[1], and S. E. Kelley[1]

[1] Transplantation Section, Department of Surgery, and [2] Department of Nephrology, Geisinger Medical Center, Danville, USA

Abstract. Within the past year at our transplant center we have had the experience of performing renal allografts in two patients older than 65 years, each of whom had been on hemodialysis more than 10 years. Both resulted in patient mortality within 90 days of transplant (one due to myocardial infarction, the other due to visceral ischemia with infarction). This prompted us to review retrospectively our own data ($n = 204$) and the national (UNOS) data ($n = 10\,971$) regarding transplant outcome, patient age, and length of time on dialysis prior to renal transplantation. This review revealed that patient mortality after transplant increased with the length of end-stage renal disease (dialysis, regardless of type) independent of age, the greatest mortality occurring within the first 6 months of transplant (and not thereafter); graft survival was similar for all age cohorts analyzed. Our review of the literature reveals a paucity of articles pertaining to post-transplant mortality and length of time on dialysis prior to transplant. Our results indicate the following possible conclusions. (1) The length of time of end-stage renal disease therapy prior to renal transplantation is a significant and independent risk factor for post-transplant mortality. (2) Higher priority should be given to this factor when formulating strategies for allocation of scarce resources. (3) Patients on dialysis for extended periods of time who are elderly may be at particularly high risk. (4) Patients being considered for renal transplant should be informed of their individual risk factors for mortality post-transplant based on length of ESRD therapy. (5) Renal transplantation should be considered as early as possible in patients with ESRD (or imminent ESRD).

Key words: Renal transplantation – Dialysis – End-stage renal disease

Within the past year, we have experienced several deaths of renal transplant recipients, each of whom had been on

Offprint requests to: John West, M.D., Department of Surgery Geisinger Medical Center, Danville, PA 17822, USA

hemodialysis for extended periods of time prior to transplantation. This prompted us to review retrospectively our own data ($n = 204$) and the UNOS data ($n = 10\,971$) regarding the effect of length of end-stage renal disease (ESRD) prior to transplantation on patient survival following allografting.

Many factors have been suggested to affect survival following renal transplantation, including recipient age, donor source (cadaver, LRD unrelated) and age, HLA matching, immunosuppressive regimen, and various other pretransplant conditions (e. g. cardiac status, presence or absence of diabetes mellitus, PRA, prior transplant, etc.). To our knowledge, length of time of ESRD prior to transplantation and its impact on patient survival have neither been previously emphasized nor systematically examined.

Materials and methods

Medical records of all adult recipients (> 17-years-old) of cadaver renal transplants performed at our center between 21 April 1981 (inception of program) and 1 September 1990 were reviewed ($n = 204$), revealing the following patient characteristics (see Table 1):

Before 1 February 1984, the standard immunosuppression protocol consisted of azathioprine and prednisolone. After this date all patients were treated with cyclosporine and prednisolone (and frequently triple-drug therapy adding azathioprine). Use of anti-thymocyte globulin (ATG) and OKT3 monoclonal antibody were

Table 1. Patient characteristics ($n = 204$)

Age (years)	
Mean	41.49
SEM	0.89
Range	17.0–70.4
Length of ESRD (months)	
Mean	32.48
SEM	2.4
Range	0–182.9
Immunosuppressive ERA (number of patients)	
Pre-cyclosporin	38
Post-cyclosporin	166

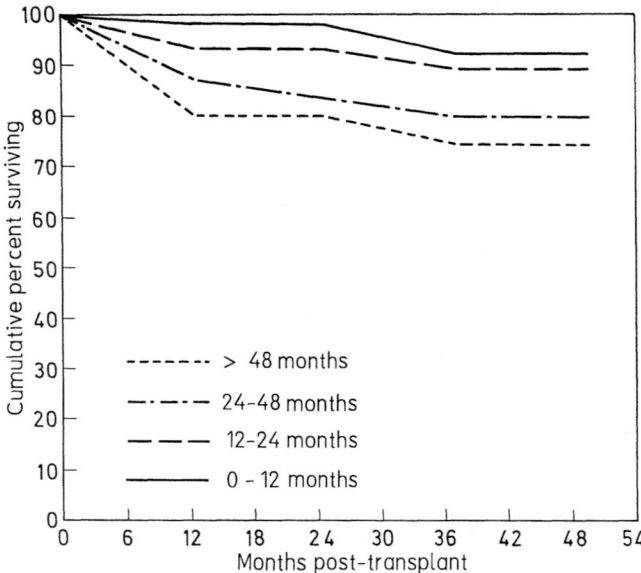

Fig. 1. Patient survival by length of ESRD prior to transplantation

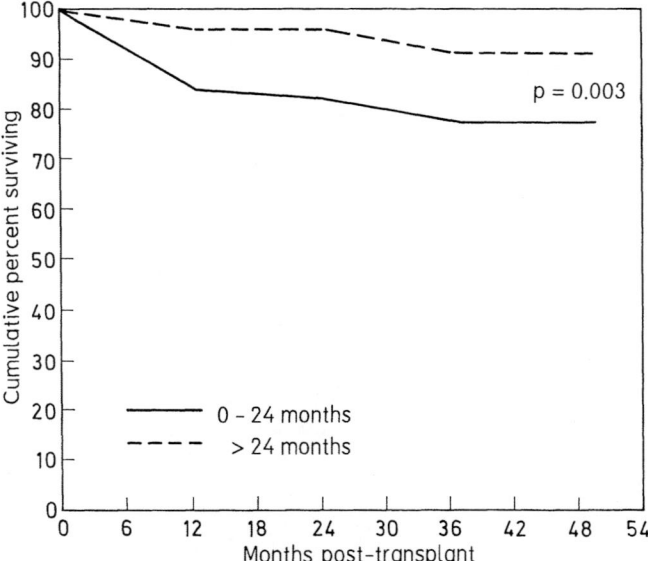

Fig. 2. Patient survival by length of ESRD prior to transplantation

generally reserved for treatment of steroid-resistant or recurrent rejection episodes (and occasionally for induction therapy in the high immunologic risk patient – retransplants, PRA > 75%, etc.).

Also abstracted from the records of each patient were the following: date of transplantation, date of first ESRD treatment (determined as the date of first maintenance dialysis, or date of transplantation if transplanted first without prior dialysis), date of death for those dying with a functioning graft or within 3 months of graft failure and return to dialysis, date of graft failure as defined by date of return to permanent dialysis, date of birth, history of prior transplantation, number of HLA-A,B and HLA-DR loci matches, presence of diabetic nephropathy, immunosuppressive era (see above), and cause of death.

Survival analyses were performed using the Kaplan-Meier product limit method. For purposes of calculating patient survival, any death occurring in a patient with a functioning allograft or within 3 months of return to dialysis following graft failure was considered a graft failure. Patients who returned to dialysis and survived

3 months were censored as to the date of return to dialysis. Patients alive with functioning grafts were censored as of 1 September 1990. No patients were lost to follow-up. Except as noted below, for the purposes of calculating graft survival, return to dialysis and death with a functioning graft were both considered graft losses.

Comparisons of survival between groups were performed with the Gehan's generalized Wilcoxon test. An extension of this test is used for comparing survival in multiple samples. Univariate analysis of the effects of variables on survival was performed using the Wilcoxon rank sum test. The relative contribution of variables to survival was tested with a forward stepwise sequence of chi-squares. The Cox proportional hazards model was also utilized to evaluate the effects of multiple variables on survival. Calculations were performed using CSS.STATISTICA (Stat Soft, Tulsa, Oklahoma) and SAS (SAS Institute, Cary, North Carolina) software on an IBM PS/2.

The United Network of Organ Sharing (UNOS) kindly performed preliminary analysis of their data on adult patients (> 17 years of age) in receipt of cadaver kidney transplants performed between 1 October 1987 and 31 December 1989 ($n = 10\,971$). Patient survival at one year was analyzed by a logistic regression model with consideration of the following variables: age at transplant (> 60-years-old versus < 60-years-old), race, PRA at transplant, status at transplant (home-bound or hospitalized), and length of time on dialysis prior to transplant (> 24 months versus < 24 months).

Results

When patients were assigned to groups based on increasing lengths of ESRD therapy prior to transplantation, a progressive increase in mortality was noted (Fig. 1). Reviewing only those cohorts of patients < 24 months versus > 24 months therapy for ESRD prior to transplantation, the patient survival in the former group post-transplant was significantly better ($P < 0.003$) (Fig. 2, Table 2). Similarly, graft survival was proportionately worse with increasing length of prior ESRD therapy. However, when death as a cause of graft failure was removed from the analysis (e.g. censored) there was no difference in graft survival between the two groups (i.e. the difference in graft survival was completely accounted for by the difference in death rates).

The effects of length of prior ESRD treatment, age, number of prior transplants, and number of HLA-A,B and HLA-DR matches on patient survival were first analyzed by univariate techniques and subsequently by Cox proportionate hazard regression. Only increasing length of prior ESRD treatment and increasing age were independently associated with poorer post-transplant patient survival ($P < 0.003$ and $P < 0.03$, respectively). Age and length of prior ESRD treatment did not correlate with each other. The other variables tested did not significantly influence patient or graft survival.

Table 2. Patient survival (%) by length of prior ESRD ($n = 204$)

Length of prior ESRD (months)	n	Time post-transplant (months)				
		12	24	36	48	60
0–24	115	96.2	96.2	91.4	91.4	91.4
> 24	89	83.3	81.5	77.1	77.1	73.4

Table 3. Relative risk of death at 1 year ($n = 10\,971$)

Variable	Relative risk	n	Percent of total	95 % confidence intervals
Age > 60 years	2.15	1052	9.6	1.77 to 2.61
Black	0.8	2462	22.4	0.67 to 0.96
Homebound	1.44	3146	28.7	1.23 to 1.68
Hospitalized	1.86	777	7.1	1.45 to 2.37
Dialysis > 24 months	1.42	3419	31.2	1.22 to 1.64

Σn 10 971 because these are not mutually-exclusive groups
Σ % of total $\neq 100$ % for the same reason

In order to corroborate our results and to avoid errors inherent in small, single-center analysis, the Scientific Advisory Committee of UNOS agreed to perform a retrospective analysis of their large database. The clinical relationship of length of time of ESRD prior to renal transplantation and its negative effect on patient survival was again confirmed. The effects on 1-year patient survival of age, status at time of transplant, race, PRA, and length of prior ESRD therapy were analyzed. Age > 60 years, status of patients pretransplant (home-bound versus hospitalized), and > 2 years of prior ESRD treatment significantly worsened 1-year patient survival (Table 3).

Cardiovascular disease and infection were the leading causes of death in our patients. There was no difference in the proportion of deaths attributable to cardiovascular disease or to infection in patients with < 24 or > 24 months of prior ESRD therapy.

In summary, increasing the time between institution of ESRD treatment and subsequent transplantation significantly increased the post-transplant mortality in 204 adult cadaveric renal transplant recipients in one center. Preliminary retrospective analysis of a very large database (UNOS) appeared to confirm the significant independent effect of length of prior ESRD treatment on patient survival post-transplant. This effect was independent of age, which was also a significant risk factor for mortality post-transplant. The degree of HLA-A,B and HLA-DR matching and the number of prior transplants did not affect patient survival. The length of prior ESRD treatment worsened graft survival, but only to the extent that it increased mortality.

Discussion

Because of the rapid successes of organ replacement therapy for end-stage organ disease, complex ethical questions have been raised and answers provided regarding equitable allocation of these scarce resources. In the US, the allocation of cadaveric kidneys is based upon a mandatory point system [2], recipients being awarded points based on: (1) time of waiting; (2) quality of antigen match;

and (3) panel reactive antibody (PRA). The 'time of waiting' begins with being activated on the UNOS computer, one point being awarded to the candidate awaiting transplantation for the longest period and fractions of points to those waiting for shorter periods. Additionally, for each year after 1 year of waiting time, 0.5 points are awarded. However, 'time of waiting' is not equivalent to length of time on dialysis – an important distinction. Based upon our results showing that the length of prior ESRD treatment is a significant and independent risk factor for post-transplant mortality, it would seem imperative that strategies for allocating kidneys need to give more weight to this factor rather than the time-honored 'time of waiting'.

Conclusions

Strategies for allocating kidneys need to give more weight to the length of ESRD treatment prior to transplant as this has been shown to be a significant and independent risk factor for post-transplant mortality. Patients on dialysis for extended periods who are elderly may be at particularly high risk. Patients being considered for renal transplantation should be informed of their individual risk of mortality post-transplant based on age and length of ESRD therapy. Finally, renal transplantation should be considered as early as possible in patients with ESRD (or imminent ESRD).

Speculation

Most studies suggest that renal transplantation improves short- and long-term mortality (and rehabilitation) compared with dialysis in similar populations. The present data raises questions as to whether this is true for that subgroup of patients who have survived on dialysis > 2 years. It might be that renal transplantation does not confer a survival advantage to this subgroup and, indeed, may even be associated with a higher mortality rate (at least in the short term). Further studies are necessary to address this question.

Acknowledgements. We are indebted to UNOS (and particularly to Dr. Eric Edwards) for their assistance with this analysis. We are also indebted to Nancy Fetterolf, our own data coordinator, for assistance in our own analysis.

References

1. Matas AJ, Brayman KL, Gillingham KJ (1990) Presentation of renal transplant graft survival data – where should 'death with a functioning graft' be included? Clin Transplant 4: 142–144
2. Phillips MG (ed) (1991) Organ procurement, preservation and distribution in transplantation. The William Byrd Press, Richmond, p 134

Transplant Int (1992) 5 [Suppl 1]: S151–S152

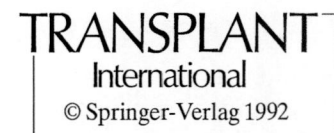

TRANSPLANT
International
© Springer-Verlag 1992

Donor conditions and graft survival – a retrospective study

P. Wienand[1], T. Schröder[1], D. Stippel[1], and C. Baldamus[2]

[1] Department of Surgery, University of Cologne, Cologne, FRG
[2] Department of Internal Medicine, University of Cologne, Cologne, FRG

Abstract. In a retrospective study (one centre) the influence of donor and recipient factors were evaluated ($n = 308$). Head injury as the cause of death and anastomotic time less than 35 min were associated with a significantly better graft survival rate ($P < 0.05$). Although some of the donor factors influence graft survival, a stricter selection of grafts is not advisable, firstly because fewer kidneys would then be offered, and secondly because even comparatively bad graft survival rates are still better than dialysis.

Key words: Renal transplantation – Donor conditions – Graft survival

The analysis of ong-term results after cadaver kidney transplantation evokes the question as to the effects of donor factors. A retrospective study of donor-specific parameters proves their impact on recipient survival, graft survival and renal function 1 year after transplantation.

Materials and methods

From 1981 to 1990, 575 patients received a renal transplant. For 308 of them it was their first graft. The following donor factors were studied: age, cause of death, serum creatinine, diuresis during the last hour before explantation, technique of explantation, multiple organ donor, donor kidney side, renal artery with/without patch, warm ischaemia time, cold ischaemia time, anastomotic time and mode of sharing. Recipient survival and graft survival were calculated by cumulative survival rates by means of the Kaplan–Meier method. Graft function, according to the serum creatinine value 1 year after transplantation, was assessed either by analysing the linear regression, or by defining three different groups of function (good function with serum creatinine below 1.5 mg%, moderate function with serum creatinine between 1.5 and 4 mg%; bad function with serum creatinine higher 4 mg% but without dialysis) and evaluation by cross-tabulation and the chi-squared test.

Results

The 1-year survival rates were 96% for the recipients and 82% for the grafts. Cumulative survival rates after 5 years were 87% for the recipients and 61% for the grafts. None of the investigated parameters had any influence on recipient survival rates, and some of them (technique of explantation, donor kidney side, cold ischaemia time) did not affect graft survival. Donor age between 16 and 55 years, systolic blood pressure lower 140 mmHg, diuresis during last hour about 100 ml and warm ischaemia time up to 5 min resulted in better graft survival rates, though without statistical significance. Head injury was the cause of death in 175 (57%) donors, spontaneous intracranial bleeding in 84 (27.4%), and other causes in 48 (15.6%), such as intoxication, primary brain cancer or suicide. Significantly lower graft survival rates were found for grafts from donors whose deaths were caused by spontaneous intracranial bleeding ($P < 0.02$), as well as for recipients with anastomosing times longer than 35 min ($P < 0.01$). Reduced diuresis during the last hour before explantation correlated with bad graft function, according to higher serum creatinine 1 year after transplantation ($P < 0.02$). However, there was no correlation between recipients' serum creatinine and the donors' diuresis over the last 24 h.

Conclusion

Donor factors and patient survival: no effect

Offprint requests to: Peter Wienand, Priv. Doz. Dr. med., Department of Surgery, University of Cologne, Joseph-Stelzmann-Str. 9, 5000 Köln 41, FRG

Donor factors and kidney survival without effect:
– technique of explantation
– donor kidney side
– cold ischaemia time

Donor factors with effect but not significant:
– donor age between 16 and 55 years
– systolic blood pressure lower 140 mm Hg

– diuresis during last hour 100 ml
– warm ischaemia time up to 5 min

Donor factors with statistical significant effect:
– death caused by spontaneous intracranial bleeding ($P < 0.02$)
– recipients with anastomosing times longer than 35 min ($P < 0.001$)

Transplant Int (1992) 5 [Suppl 1]: S153–S155

TRANSPLANT
International
© Springer-Verlag 1992

Clinical factors which influence the long-term survival of kidney allografts donated from haploidentical donors

T. Yasumura, T. Oka, Y. Ohmori, Y. Nakane, N. Yoshimura, I. Nakai, T. Hamashima

Second Department of Surgery, Kyoto Prefectural University of Medicine, Kawaramachi Hirokoji, Kamigyo-ku, Kyoto, Japan

All patients with renal transplants are very much concerned about their chance of long-term graft function. Chronic rejection is the most common cause of decline in function and graft failure, and after the first post-transplant year, 3–4 % of recipients lose their graft every year [4]. However, the cause, time of onset and mechanism of decline in graft function are not clear. Also unclear is whether clinical and laboratory parameters may predict patients who are at risk of developing chronic rejection. The aim of this study was to find the marker which may determine long-term graft survival in the azathioprine era and in the cyclosporine era.

Key words: Kidney transplantation – Living donors – Long-term survival

Materials and methods

Between April 1990 and March 1982 155 patients were transplanted with one haploidentical renal allograft. Azathioprine (Aza) and prednisolone (PSL) were used for immunosuppressive therapy. Of 155 cases, 133 had been followed up for over 10 years. After excluding 15 cases with grafts rejected within 1 year and 17 cases of death with a functioning graft, the remaining 101 of the 133 cases were subjected to analysis.

Cyclosporine (CsA) was introduced in our institution in April 1982 [2]. The initial immunosuppressive regimen shown in Fig. 1 was applied to 82 cases with a haploidentical renal allograft. At 1 year after transplantation, CsA had been replaced by Aza in 23 cases, and changed to combination therapy with CsA, Aza and PSL in nine cases, mainly due to nephrotoxicity. From January 1987 a new regimen (regimen 2, Fig. 1), in which the dose of CsA was greatly reduced and supplemented with Aza in order to minimize the nephrotoxicity of CsA, was applied in 33 cases. Of a total 115 cases, eight suffered rejection of their graft and six died with a functioning graft within 1 year. No further deaths occurred after the first year. Of the remaining 101 cases, 61, who were followed for over 5 years, were subjected to the analysis. Clinical and laboratory data at 1 year after

Offprint requests to: Tadaki Yasumura, Kawaramachi Kamigyo-ku, Kyoto, 602 Japan

transplantation and the clinical records of every case were reviewed and subjected to multivariate analysis using quantification theory II [3]. Clinical and laboratory factors included in the analysis were episodes of acute rejection and liver dysfunction within 1 year and serum creatine (SCr) level, proteinuria, hypertension and immunosuppressive therapy at 1 year after transplantation.

Results

Marker for predicting 10-year graft function in the Aza era

A variety of factors (Fig. 2) were categorized into groups. These categories were scored by the method of quantification theory II. Each factor score was summed for each case. The distribution of total scores was biphasic and the average total score for the group with 10-year graft function was 0.528 ± 513 (mean $\pm$ SD) and the score for the group with rejected grafts was 0.780 ± 1.023. The discriminating point was located at 0.069 and 85 % of cases with a total score higher than this point had 10-year functioning grafts. SCr level at 1 year after transplantation showed the highest correlation coefficient, followed by hypertension, proteinuria etc.

Curves of actual graft failure rates in four groups categorized according to SCr level are shown in Fig. 3. The two groups with SCr level of less than 1.4 mg/dl had significantly lower failure rates than the other two groups.

Table 1. Correlation coefficients for various factors

Factor	Correlation coefficient
SCr level	0.3547
Immunosuppressive regimen (Aza, CsA, Aza + CsA)	0.3389
Proteinuria	0.1571
Hypertension	0.1517
Liver dysfunction	0.1273
Episodes of acute rejection	0.0999

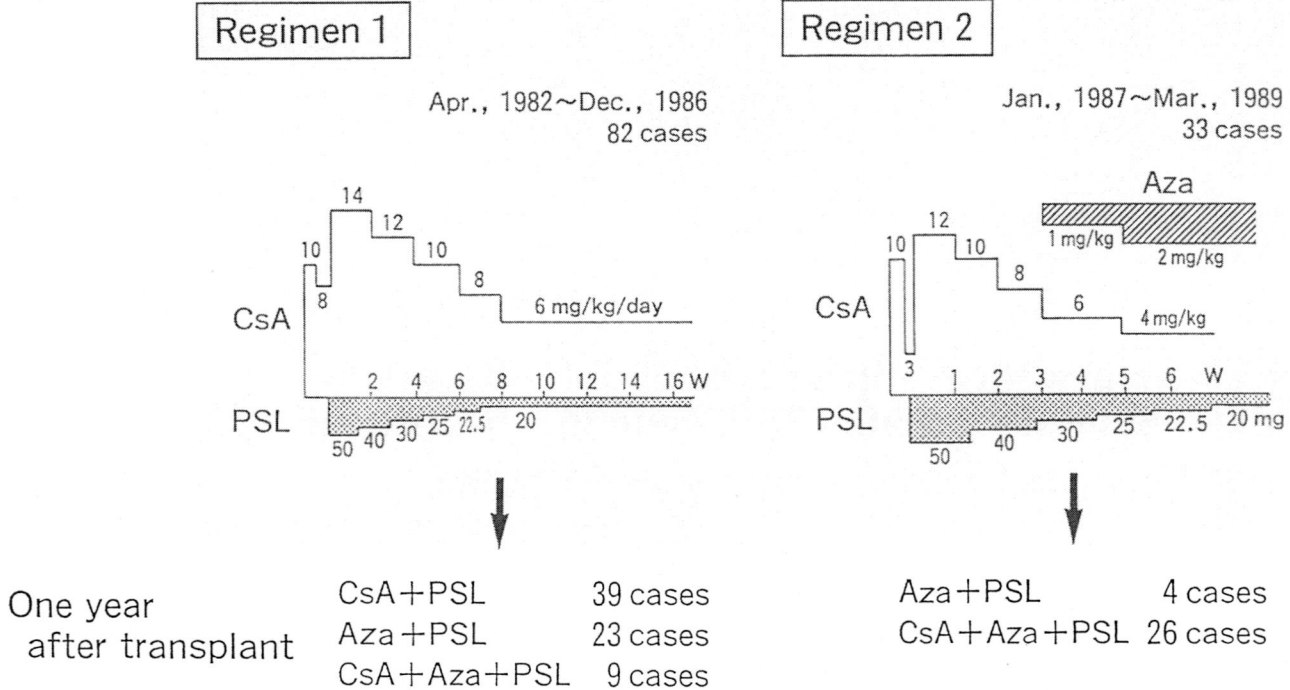

Fig. 1. Initial immunosuppressive regimens and changes of therapy at 1 year after transplantation

Factor	Category	Score
Episode of acute rejection	0 times	0.0938
	1–2 times	0.0775
	3~times	−0.0684
SCr level	~1.0 mg/dl	0.2273
	1.1~1.4 mg/dl	0.3203
	1.5~2.0 mg/dl	−0.3703
	2.1 mg/dl~	−1.1802
Proteinuria	negative	0.1510
	positive	−0.2613
Hypertension	negative	0.3235
	positive	−0.4545
Liver dysfunction	negative	0.1152
	positive	−0.3323
Dose of Aza	≦2.0 mg/kg/day	0.2295
	>2.0 mg/kg/day	−0.1164
Dose of PSL	≦0.2 mg/kg/day	0.1909
	>0.2 mg/kg/day	−0.0628

○ : surviving over 10 years
● : rejected within 10 years
→ : discriminating point

Factor	Correlation coefficients
SCr level	0.2
Hypertension	0.2
Proteinuria	0.16
Liver dysfunction	0.19
Dose of Aza	0.11
Dose of PSL	0.09
Episode of acute rejection	0.06

Fig. 2. Retrospective analysis for factors which may predict 10-year graft function

Correlation between immunosuppressive regimen and long-term graft survival in the CsA era

A variety of clinical and laboratory factors were analysed in 61 cases followed for over 5 years. Calculated correlation coefficients are listed in Table 1. Of six factors, SCr level and immunosuppressive regimen showed significantly higher values. Cumulative graft failure rates were compared between three groups categorized according to immunosuppressive regimen (Fig. 4). The group receiving combination therapy with CsA, Aza and PSL had a significantly lower graft failure rate than the other two groups.

Discussion

In renal transplantation, the most significant factor determining long-term graft function may be HLA matching [1]. Therefore the subjects analysed in this study were restricted to one haploidentical transplant. From the results of this study, it can be concluded that 1-year graft function

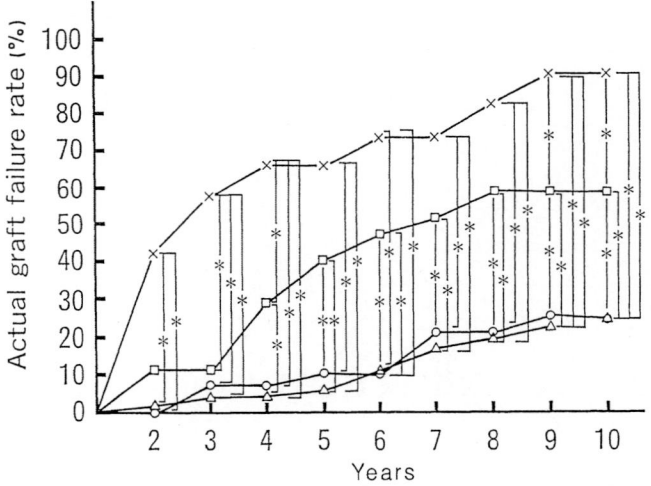

Fig. 3. Curves of actual graft failure rates in four groups categorized by serum creatinine levels at 1 year after transplantation. $\bigcirc$, < 1.0 mg/dl ($n = 28$); $\triangle$, 1.1–1.4 mg/dl ($n = 44$); $\square$, 1.5–2.0 mg/dl ($n = 17$); X, > 2.1 mg/dl ($n = 12$). * $P < 0.05$

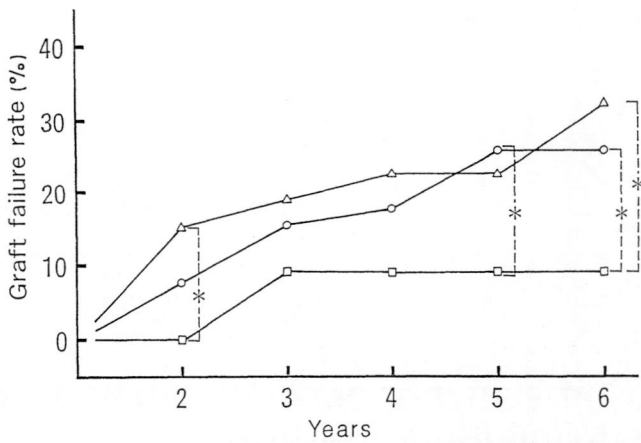

Fig. 4. Curves of cumulative graft failure rates in three groups of recipients treated with CsA + Aza + PSL ($n = 35$), Aza + PSL ($n = 27$) and CsA + PSL ($n = 39$). * $P < 0.05$

is a reasonable parameter for determining long-term graft function in either the Aza or the CsA era, and combination immunosuppressive therapy with CsA, Aza and PSL may be suitable for achieving long-term graft function. However, in this study, three of 133 cases who died with functioning grafts after the first year were excluded. Although exact analysis may not be possible because of these cases, the influence of this exclusion is too small to invalidate the conclusion.

References

1. Cho YW, Terasaki PI (1988) Long-term survival, In: Terasaki PI (ed) Clinical transplants. UCLA Tissue Typing Laboratory, Los Angeles, p 277
2. Oka T, Oinori Y, Aikawa I et al. (1989) Early conversion from cyclosporine to combination therapy with azathioprine in living related kidney transplants. Transplant Proc 21: 1828–1830
3. Tanaka Y, Tarumi T, Wakimoto K et al. (1984) Quantification theory II. In: Tanaka Y (ed) Multivaluate analysis. Kyoritsu, Tokyo, pp 270–295
4. Yasumura T, Aikawa I, Ohmori Y et al. Clinical factors correlated with 10-year graft survival in living related kidney transplantation. III Acute rejection Jpn J Transplant (in press)

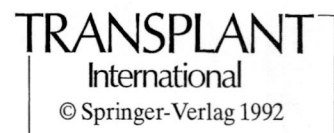

TRANSPLANT
International
© Springer-Verlag 1992

Glomerular hyperfiltration after unilateral nephrectomy in living kidney donors

H. A. Bock, M. Bachofen, J. Landmann, and G. Thiel

Divisions of Nephrology and Organ Transplantation, Departments of Internal Medicine and Surgery, Kantonsspital, Basel, Switzerland

Abstract. Glomerular hyperfiltration, which is expected to occur after uninephrectomy, could potentially damage the non-transplanted donor kidney in living donor transplantation. We therefore prospectively measured renal function (inulin and PAH clearance), albumin excretion and blood pressure in the donors of 30 consecutive living donor kidney transplants before uninephrectomy ($n = 29$) and 1 week ($n = 27$) and 1 year ($n = 16$) after. Hyperfiltration was defined as: (post-nephrectomy inulin clearance)/(0.5 x pre-nephrectomy inulin clearance); hyperperfusion was defined in an analogous way for PAH clearance. Hyperfiltration averaged $128 \pm 5\%$ [SEM] and hyperperfusion $133 \pm 6\%$ 1 week after uninephrectomy. Hyperfiltration was nearly unchanged ($126 \pm 7\%$) 1 year after nephrectomy, whereas hyperperfusion had significantly decreased to $118 \pm 8\%$ ($P < 0.02$). There was no significant change in blood pressure after nephrectomy, and no new cases of hypertension were observed during the 1-year follow-up. The degree of hyperfiltration did not correlate with donor age. Microalbuminuria > 30 mg/24 h was found in two donors 1 week after nephrectomy (one of which normalized at 1 year) and in one additional donor 1 year after nephrectomy. The degree of hyperfiltration did not correlate with albumin excretion rate. In conclusion, no adverse consequences of hyperfiltration were demonstrable during the 1-year observation period, but the prognostic role of occasional microalbuminuria should be further investigated.

Key words: Glomerular hyperfiltration – Living kidney donors – Unilateral nephrectomy

An increased glomerular filtration rate, also termed 'hyperfiltration' is considered an important factor in the pathogenesis of various nephropathies and in the non-immunological progression of chronic renal failure [4]. The paradigmatic example for this is the hyperfiltration which accompanies the early phase of diabetes mellitus [10], and which is considered relevant for the later development of diabetic nephropathy. Since glomerular hyperfiltration is also expected to occur after unilateral nephrectomy for living donor renal transplantation, in 1988 we began a prospective study of hyperfiltration in living kidney donors. The aims of this study were: (1) to determine the degree of hyperfiltration after unilateral nephrectomy; and (2) to determine the incidence of potential consequences of uninephrectomy, such as progressive impairment of renal function, microalbuminuria or arterial hypertension, all of which have been reported to occur with varying frequency after uninephrectomy [2, 3, 7, 9].

Methods

The kidney donors (13 M, 17 F) were studied the day before transplantation ($n = 29$), 1 week after nephrectomy ($n = 27$) and 1 year after nephrectomy ($n = 16$; in one of these, the pre-nephrectomy and the 1-week studies were not carried out for technical reasons). Each study consisted of a hospital admission with overnight urine collection for the determination of albumin excretion and, on the next morning, a combined inulin and PAH clearance with four collections of 40 min each. Blood pressure was measured before the clearance study in the supine position. Urine albumin excretion was measured with an immune-turbidimetric assay, and inulin and PAH using laboratory methods. The hyperfiltration index was computed for each donor as:

$$\frac{\text{Inulin clearance after nephrectomy}}{0.5 \times \text{Inulin clearance before nephrectomy}}$$

An analogous formula was used to calculate hyperperfusion from PAH clearance.

Non-parametric tests (Mann-Whitney U test, paired Wilcoxon test, Spearman's rank correlation) were used for the statistical analysis.

Results

Baseline data

Donor age was between 22 and 68 years (mean 46 ± 2 years); four of the donors were over 60-years-old.

Offprint requests to: Andreas Bock, M. D., Division of Nephrology, Kantonsspital, CH-4031 Basel, Switzerland

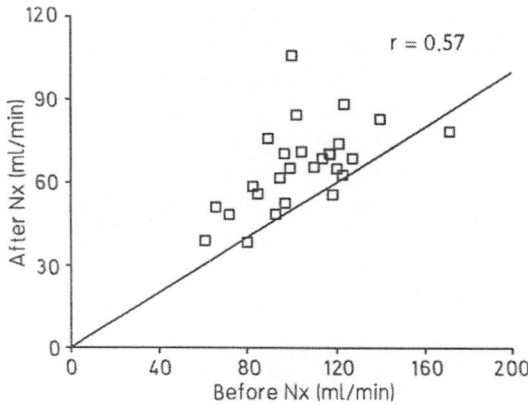

Fig. 1. Inulin clearance of 27 kidney donors before and 1 week after transplantation. The line indicates where the points would be expected if renal function was exactly cut in half by the uninephrectomy. Points above the line indicate hyperfiltration

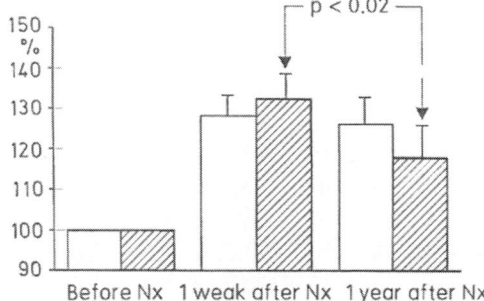

Fig. 2. Hyperfiltration and hyperperfusion after nephrectomy (mean ± SEM). The decrease in hyperperfusion was significant both when all donors were considered (Mann-Whitney U test) or only the ones where follow-up was complete (paired Wilcoxon test). □, hyperfiltration, ▨, hyperperfusion

Of the transplantations, 16 were parent-to-child, 13 were sibling-to-sibling and one was spouse-to-spouse. Weight, the clearances of inulin, PAH and creatinine as well as serum creatinine were normal at baseline (Table 1). The hypertensive maxima of baseline blood pressure (Table 1) are from a 66-year-old and a 58-year-old donor. These two donors were accepted despite known, moderate essential hypertension, because of their urgent wish to donate a

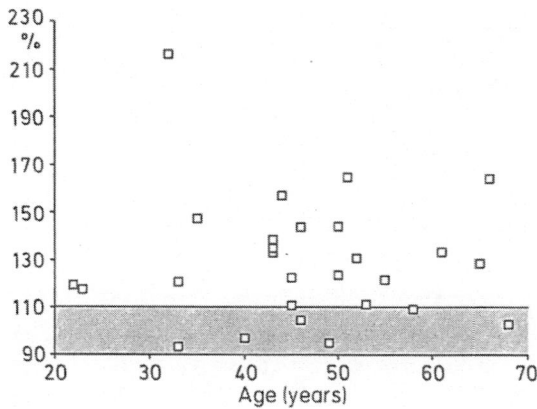

Fig. 3. Donor age versus hyperfiltration after uninephrectomy. No correlation existed

kidney to their child. The remaining 28 donors were normotensive.

Course after nephrectomy

Figure 1 shows inulin clearance before nephrectomy and 1 week after nephrectomy. It is evident that most of the donors' inulin clearance after nephrectomy exceeded 50% of their pre-nephrectomy clearance, i.e. hyperfiltration was present. Mean hyperfiltration (Fig. 2) was $128 \pm 5\%$ (SEM) at 1 week after nephrectomy, mean hyperperfusion $133 \pm 6\%$. Hyperfiltration 1 year after nephrectomy was essentially unchanged $(126 \pm 7\%)$, whereas hyperperfusion had decreased significantly to $118 \pm 8\%$ $(P < 0.02)$. Hyperfiltration exceeding 110% was present in 21 of 27 donors at 1 week after transplantation, and in 12 of 15 donors at 1 year after transplantation. Hyperperfusion of more than 110% was present in 21/27 donors at one week but only in 9/15 donors at one year. The degree of hyperfiltration or hyperperfusion did not correlate with sex, weight, height or donor age (Fig. 3).

Although mean inulin clearance (and, therefore, hyperfiltration) did not change between 1 week and 1 year after nephrectomy, there was a slight, non-significant increase in creatinine clearance which contributed to

Table 1. Weight, blood pressure, and renal function before and after nephrectomy (Nx). Data are given as mean ± SEM [range]

	Before Nx (n = 29)		One week after Nx (n = 27)		One year after Nx (n = 16)	
Weight (kg)	71 ± 2	[47–102]	71 ± 3	[44–100]	69 ± 2	[51–86]
Systolic blood pressure	126 ± 3	[105–170]	126 ± 3	[110–175]	123 ± 3	[110–140]
Diastolic blood pressure	78 ± 2	[60–105]	81 ± 2	[60–100]	82 ± 3	[60–100]
Inulin clearance (ml/')	104 ± 4	[61–171]	66 ± 3	[38–106]	66 ± 4	[43– 97]
PAH clearance (ml/')	548 ± 28	[310–941]	358 ± 20	[213–330]	317 ± 17	[205–326]
Filtration fraction	19 ± 1%	[13– 29]	19 ± 1%	[14– 30]	21 ± 1%	[17– 26]
Creatinine clearance (ml/')	150 ± 8	[88–280]	88 ± 5	[49–196]	101 ± 6	[64–166]
S-creatinine (µmol/l)	64 ± 3	[45– 90]	106 ± 3	[69–169]	90 ± 5	[63–134]

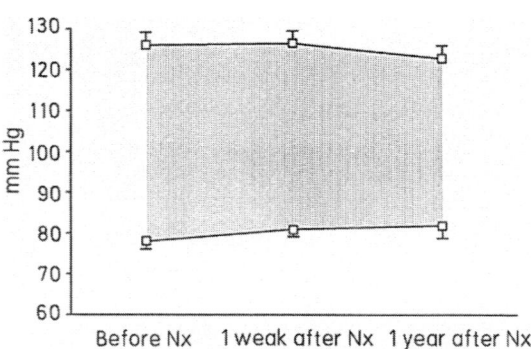

Fig. 4. Mean systolic and diastolic blood pressures (± SEM) before and after nephrectomy

the decrease in serum creatinine between 1 week and 1 year of nephrectomy (Table 1).

Mean systolic and diastolic blood pressure did not change significantly (Fig. 4, Table 1). The two donors with known hypertension remained hypertensive after nephrectomy, but there was no evidence of an increased severity of their hypertension (as judged from blood pressure and antihypertensive therapy). Besides this, a hypertensive blood pressure was only recorded in one 68-year-old donor 1 week after nephrectomy. At that time, this donor was still experiencing considerable pain from his nephrectomy. Although this donor had not yet undergone the 1-year study, he since had several normal outpatient pressure measurements.

Albumin excretion was normal in all donors prior to nephrectomy. After nephrectomy, microalbuminuria of more than 30 mg/24 h was found in a total of three donors, one of which normalized at 1 year after nephrectomy. No risk factors could be identified in these three donors (Table 2). Also, in the entire set of donors, no correlation of albumin excretion with the degree of hyperfiltration or hyperperfusion could be demonstrated.

Discussion

These data confirm that in most living kidney donors, the non-transplanted kidney hyperfilters as soon as 1 week after nephrectomy (Fig. 1). However, in almost one quarter of the donors studied, hyperfiltration was either minimal (< 110 %) or absent. The same 6 out of 27 donors also failed to show hyperperfusion. Thus the entire – presumably endocrine – response to a 50 % reduction in renal mass appeared blunted in these donors. Simple demographic data such as gender, weight, height and age (Fig. 3) were not useful in predicting the hyperfiltration/hyper-

perfusion response. Mean hyperfiltration in this study (+ 128 % and 126 %) was within the range reported by others [1, 6]. Its extent corresponds to the hyperfiltration found in early diabetes mellitus [10], after oral protein loading [5] and after dopamine/amino-acid infusion [8].

Hyperperfusion of approximately the same magnitude accompanied hyperfiltration early after nephrectomy. At 1 year, however, hyperperfusion had significantly decreased despite stable hyperfiltration (Fig. 2). Although PAH extraction was not measured in this study, there is no reason to suspect a decrease in PAH exctraction (which would yield a 'false low' PAH clearance) between 1 week and 1 year after nephrectomy. Rathet, the increase in creatinine clearance from 1 week to 1 year (despite constant inulin clearance, Table 1) suggests that tubular secretory processes are *increased* at 1 year after nephrectomy, perhaps as a consequence of tubular hypertrophy.

The mechanisms mediating this decrease in hyperperfusion are unknown. One may, however, speculate that this increase in renal vascular resistance represents an autoregulatory adaptation of the renal vascular bed. The maintenance of glomerular filtration during the same time (i. e. the trend for filtration fraction to increase, Table 1) could suggest that this resistance increase is predominantly post-glomerular. However, glomerular hypertrophy, such as might occur after uninephrectomy, could also mimic this pattern by increasing the glomerular ultrafiltration coefficient and, therefore, filtration fraction.

No trend to develop arterial hypertension was found in this study (Fig. 4), and there were no *de novo* cases of arterial hypertension. Microalbuminuria > 30 mg/24 h was, however, found in two donors at 1 week after nephrectomy (one of which normalized at 1 year) and in one additional donor at 1 year after nephrectomy. These three donors did not present any obvious risk factors (Table 2). The most likely explanation for this finding is a slight damage to the glomerular filtration barrier, particularly the charge-selective component, perhaps as a consequence of intraglomerular hypertension. Further follow-up of these and future donors is indicated to identify the prognostic significance of this alteration and to determine the specific conditions under which it occurs.

In summary, glomerular hyperfiltration and hyperperfusion after unilateral nephrectomy for living donor renal transplantation occurs early, but only in three-quarters of donors. Although the extent of hyperfiltration is similar to diabetic or protein-induced hyperfiltration, there is stable glomerular filtration during the first year after nephrectomy and no *de novo* hypertension appears to occur during this time. The occasional occurrence of microalbuminuria, albeit unrelated to the degree of hyperfiltration, warrants further study.

Table 2. Data of the three donors who developed microalbuminuria. One-year followup was not yet available (N/A) in the third donor

Age	Sex	Blood press at 1 week	Blood press at 1 year	Hyperfilt. at 1 week	Hyperfilt. at 1 year	Albumin 1 week (mg/24 h)	Albumin 1 year (mg/24 h)
43	f	130/80	110/70	136 %	101 %	94	11
46	m	125/85	140/95	144 %	122 %	10	94
46	m	120/80	N/A	104 %	N/A	38	N/A

References

1. Donadio JV, Farmer CD, Hunt JC et al (1967) Renal function in donors and recipients of renal allotransplantation. Ann Intern Med 66: 106–115
2. Hakim RM, Goldszer RC, Brenner BM (1984) Hypertension and proteinuria: Long-term sequelae of uninephrectomy in humans. Kidney Int 25: 930–936
3. Higashihara E, Horie S, Takeuchi T, Nutahara K, Aso Y (1990) Long-term consequence of nephrectomy. J Urol 143: 239–243
4. Hostetter T, Rennke HG, Brenner BM (1982) The case for intrarenal hypertension in the initiation and progression of diabetic and other nephropathies. Am J Med 72: 375–380
5. Mansy H, Patel D, Tapson JS, Fernandez J, Tapster S, Torrance AD, Wilkinson R (1987) Four methods to recruit renal functional reserve. Nephrol Dial Transplant 2: 228–232
6. Sugino N, Duffy G, Gulyassy PF (1967) Renal function after unilateral nephrectomy in normal man. Clin Res 15: 143
7. Talseth T, Fauchald P, Skrede S et al (1986) Long-term blood pressure and renal function in kidney donors. Kidney Int 29: 1072–1076
8. Ter Wee PM, Rosman JB, van der Geest S, Sluiter WJ, Donker AJ (1986) Renal hemodynamics during separate and combined infusion of amino acids and dopamine. Kidney Int 29: 870–874
9. Watnick TJ, Jenkins RR, Rackoff P, Baumgarten A, Bia MJ (1988) Microalbuminuria and hypertension in long-term renal donors. Transplantation 45: 59–65
10. Wiseman MJ, Saunders AJ, Keen H, Viberti GC (1985) Effect of blood glucose control on increased glomerular filtration rate and kidney size in insulin-dependent diabetics. N Engl J Med 312: 617–621

Liver

Transplant Int (1992) 5 [Suppl 1]: S 163–S 167

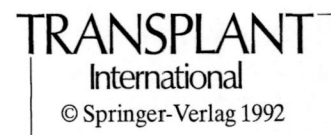

TRANSPLANT International
© Springer-Verlag 1992

The bile acid independent flow is reduced in the transplanted liver

S. Friman, H. Persson, I. Karlberg, J. Svanvik

Department of Surgery, Sahlgrenska Hospital, University of Gothenburg, Göteborg, Sweden

Abstract. Bile secretion is an important indicator of liver graft function. Reports on bile formation by the transplanted liver with stable function some months after operation are scarce. In this study bile flow, bile salt secretion rate (BSSR) and biliary clearance of polyethylene glycol (PEG) 900, a marker of canalicular bile flow, were studied in a group of liver-transplanted (LTX) patients ($n = 8$) 3–6 months after transplantation. A group of cholecystectomized patients with indwelling T-tubes ($n = 6$) served as a control group. Both groups were treated with oral ursodeoxycholic acid (500 mg/day). On the day of the study bile was drained for 6 h by gravity and four-hourly samples were used in the calculations. The relation between bile flow and BSSR analysed with linear regression showed a reduced bile acid independent flow in the liver-transplanted group (0.11 ml/min) compared with the control group (0.20 ml/min). The relation between biliary clearance of PEG 900 and BSSR showed a significantly steeper slope for the cholecystectomized control patients (1.40 ml/μmol) compared with the liver-transplanted patients (0.30 ml/μmol). We conclude, that in spite of stable graft function with normal liver enzmyes, the transplanted liver has a reduced bile acid independent bile flow. The transplanted liver also has a reduced biliary clearance of PEG 900 indicating a reduced canalicular bile flow. The cause of this impaired bile formation could be due to the influence of the immunosuppressive drug cyclosporin, the result of damage to the liver during preservation and reperfusion or the continuous immunological challenge to the graft.

Key words: Bile – Bile secretion – Liver transplantation – Ursodeoxycholic acid – Polyethylene glycol – Cyclosporin

Bile secretion is an important indicator of liver graft function. Bile flow is initially profoundly depressed after or-

thotopic liver transplantation (OLT), but over the following few days the bile volumes and bile acid secretion increase and reach stable levels after 10–14 days, provided that there is a well-functioning liver graft [5, 10, 12, 21].

Bile is an aqueous solution of electrolytes and organic compounds. Bile acids, bilirubin, cholesterol and phospholipds are the major components. Hepatic bile consists of 90% water and the composition is regulated by the canalicular and ductular water fluxes. Sperber, in 1959, postulated that osmotic forces following the active secretion of substances like bile acids generated water flow into the bile canaliculi and numerous studies have since confirmed this assertion [22]. Bile formation is thus initiated at the level of the hepatocytes and is modified by absorption or secretion more distally along the biliary tree. To separate the canalicular from the ductular fraction of the hepatic bile formation, biliary clearances of carbohydrates like erythritol and mannitol have been used for the last 20 years [7, 24]. The validity of these markers has been questioned, and recent studies have shown a higher biliary clearance of polyethylene glycol (PEG) 900, a marker used in studies of kidney physiology, indicating a considerably higher canalicular water influx than previously estimated [8, 9, 11].

Although initial bile formation is an important indicator of graft function, especially during the first postoperative weeks, the reports of bile formation after a few months following liver transplantation when liver graft function is stable, are scarce [1].

The aim of the present study was to investigate the different fractions of the bile formation process in well-functioning liver allografts with no signs of graft dysfunction.

Materials and methods

Drugs, chemicals and solutions

[1,2-³H]-PEG (6.75 mCi/g, range 800–1000 Da with an average molecular weight of 900 Da) and [24-¹⁴C]-taurocholate (46.7 mCi/mmol) were purchased from NEN Boston, Mass., USA.

Offprint requests to: Styrbjörn Friman, M.D., Ph.D., Transplant Unit, Department of Surgery, Sahlgrenska Hospital, S-413 45 Göteborg, Sweden

Table 1. Basal patient data and liver function tests at the time of bile sampling in the liver-transplanted group

Diagnosis	Age	Sex	Time post-transplantation (months)	S-bil (μmol/l)	S-ALP (μcat/l)	S-AST (μcat/l)	S-ALT (μcat/l)
PBC	51	female	3	23	3.7	0.35	0.19
Scl.chol.	26	male	3	48	7.2	0.87	0.93
CAH	43	female	6	45	3.3	0.53	0.56
α-1 anti tryp. def	47	male	4	6	1.9	0.11	0.44
CAH	62	male	3	14	6.9	0.34	0.63
Morbus Osler	40	female	4	9	5.4	0.65	1.00
ALCI	52	male	3	15	5.2	0.16	0.31
Amyloidosis	29	male	3	24	1.9	0.40	0.30
Mean ± SEM	45 ± 5			23 ± 8	4.7 ± 0.9	0.48 ± 0.11	0.63 ± 0.12

ALP, alkaline phosphatase; AST, asparate aminotransferase; ALT, alanine aminotransferase; PBC, primary biliary cirrhosis; CAH, chronic active hepatitis; Scl. chol, sclerosing cholangitis; ALCI, alcohol cirrhosis

Table 2. Basal patient data and liver function tests at the time of bile sampling in the cholecystectomy group

	Age	Sex	Time post-operation (weeks)	S-bil (μmol/l)	S-ALP (μcat/l)	S-AST (μcat/l)	S-ALT (μcat/l)
	58	female	3	18	4.3	0.57	0.62
	44	female	3	20	4.2	0.63	0.68
	38	female	10	17	3.7	0.32	0.53
	73	female	4	14	4.7	0.18	0.34
	50	female	4	7	3.0	0.64	0.63
	79	male	4	17	14	0.67	0.81
Mean ± SEM	57 ± 7			16.3 ± 1.9	5.6 ± 1.7	0.50 ± 0.08	0.65 ± 0.05

ALP, alkaline phosphatase; AST, asparate aminotransferase; ALT, alanine aminotransferase

Sodium glycocholate (grade I, 99 % pure) was obtained from Sigma Chemicals, St. Louis, Mo., USA. Ursodeoxycholic acid (Ursofalk) was manufactured by Falk Co, FRG; Prednisolon by KabiVitrum AB, Stockholm, Sweden; azathioprine (Imural) by Wellcome, London, UK; and cyclosporin (Sandimmun) by Sandoz AG, Basel, Switzerland.

Patients

A group of liver transplanted (LTX) patients ($n = 8$) was studied 3–6 months postoperatively (Table 1). The patients all had stable graft function with normal or only slightly elevated liver enzymes. A choledocho-choledochostomy with insertion of a T-tube had been performed in all cases. The enterohepatic circulation was re-established by clamping the T-tubes within 10 days after transplantation. These patients followed an immunosuppressive protocol of sequential quadruple drug therapy. At the time of investigation their immunosuppression had been reduced to corticosteroids (Prednisolon) 10 mg/day, azathioprine (Imurel) 1–2 mg/kg per day and oral cyclosporin (Sandimmun) 4 mg/kg per day (whole blood levels 150–200 ng/ml). These patients were also given adjuvant treatment with ursodeoxycholic acid (UDCA) starting the first postoperative week at a dose of 500 mg/day.

A group of cholecystectomized patients ($n = 6$), in whom the common duct had been explored at a T-tube inserted, served as a control group. These patients were investigated 3–6 weeks following a cholecystectomy. UDCA at a dose of 500 mg/day was given to these control patients for 14–15 days prior to investigation. All patients had normal or only slightly elevated plasma levels of aminotransferases and bilirubin at the time of the study (Table 2). In this group the T-tubes had been clamped at least 10 days prior to the bile secretion studies.

In a separate group of liver transplanted patients ($n = 8$) the initial bile secretion was followed during the first 7–14 days as long as the T-tube was opened.

All of the patients gave informed consent, and the study was approved by the Ethical Committee of University of Gothenburg for investigations involving human subjects.

Study protocol

Studies of bile formation with stable graft function. The patients fasted during the 12-h period prior to and throughout the test. Fluid loss was compensated by intravenous infusions of Ringer's solution. At the start of the study the T-tube was opened. ^{3}H-labelled PEG 900 (5 μCi) was given intravenously as single bolus injections followed by constant infusions of the marker molecule in saline at a rate of 1.5 μCi/h throughout the study. A period of 2 h was allowed to achieve steady-state plasma concentrations of the two markers. Bile and plasma samples from the following 4 h were used in the calculations. The bile was drained by gravity and collected in pre-weighed vials that were changed every hour. Plasma samples were also collected hourly.

Studies of initial bile formation. In eight patients the initial bile formation was followed. The total bile volume over a 24-h period was collected and from this a sample of bile was analysed as to the bile acid content.

Control experiments. Previous studies have shown that bile volumes drained by gravity correspond well to those obtained when the distal part of the common bile duct is occluded with a balloon [2, 19].

In order to test whether all bile was drained in the described manner, ^{14}C-labelled taurocholic acid was injected intravenously and the recovery in bile over time was measured in one cholecystectomized and one liver-transplanted patient. If bile was lost into the intestines the recovery of the labelled bile acid would be low and the radioactivity would later reappear in bile due to its enterohepatic circulation.

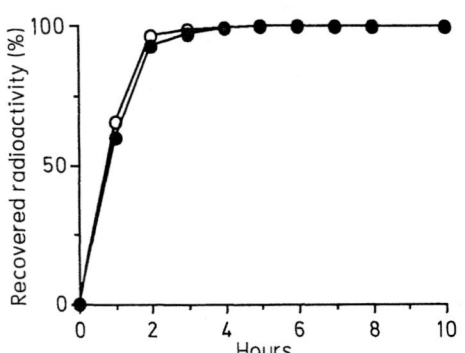

Fig. 1. Time course of recovery of intravenously infused ^{14}C-labelled taurocholic acid in two patients. ●, liver transplanted patient; ○, cholecystectomized patient

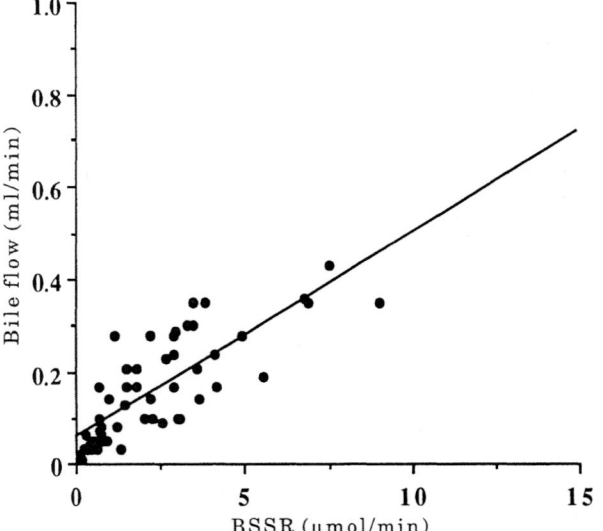

Fig. 2. The relation between bile flow and bile salt secreting rate (BSSR) as expressed with linear regression analysis in eight liver-transplanted patients collected during the first 14 days postoperatively. $Y = 0.06 + 0.044x$; $r = 0.78$; $P < 0.001$. The intercept does not significantly differ from zero

Bile salt assays

The total bile salt concentration in bile was determined by an enzymatic method using 3a-hydroxysteroid dehydrogenase (Sterognost-3a, Nyegaard and Co, Oslo, Norway). Sodium-chenodeoxycholate provided by Nyegaard and Co, was used as a standard. The intra-assay coefficient of variation for determination of sodium-chenodeoxycholate was 2.8% at a concentration of 25 mmol/l and 1.9% at a concentration of 50 mmol/l. The intra-assay coefficient of variation for determination of sodium-glycocholate was 3.8% at a concentration of 25 mmol/l and 2.9% at a concentration of 50 mmol/l [6].

Measurement of radioactivity

To reduce quenching, bile samples were bleached with 10% trichloroacetic acid. To samples of plasma and bile (200 μl) were added 10 ml of Opti-Fluor (Packard Inst., Dovners Grove, Ill., USA). The radioactivity was counted in a TRI-CARB 1500 scintillation counter (Packard). Correction for sample quenching was performed by the spectral index method [17].

Calculations and statistics

Results are presented as means ± SEM. The relationships between bile flow and bile salt secretion rate were analysed by means of linear regression. The calculated intercepts considered to represent the

bile acid independent flow (BAIF) and the slopes were termed the bile acid dependent flow (BADF). Multiple regression analysis with dummy variables was used to compare slopes and intercepts.

The clearance of PEG 900 and mannitol was calculated as the product of bile flow and the ratio between bile and plasma concentrations of the tracers at steady-state conditions.

$$\text{Biliary clearance} = \frac{dpm\ bile}{dpm\ plasma} \times \text{bile flow}$$

The relationships between biliary clearance of PEG 900 and bile salt secretion rate were analysed by means of linear regression. Four-hourly data obtained from each patient were used in these calculations.

Results

Tracer concentrations in plasma

The ^{3}H activity in plasma was stable from the beginning of the first sampling period and throughout the studies.

Recovery in bile of an IV bolus injection of ^{14}C-taurocholic acid

In two separate control experiments the efficiency of the bile drainage procedure was tested by studying the early recovery in bile of an IV bolus injection of a labelled bile acid. During the first 2 h after the injection the majority of the radioactivity was recovered in the hepatic bile outflow (Fig. 1). There was no evident recirculation of labelled bile acids detected by an increased radioactivity in the bile outflow in the following 8 h studied.

Initial bile formation

Bile flow correlated well with the BSSR during the first 7–14 days ($P < 0.01$) (Fig. 2). When the data from the first postoperative days were explored in this manner, the bile acid independent flow of 0.06 ml/min did not differ significantly from zero.

Bile formation with stable graft function

The bile flow, the bile acid concentration and the BSSR were measured during the first hour following the opening of the T tubes. No differences between the control and LTX group were found (Table 3).

Bile flow vs BSSR

Bile flow correlated well with BSSR in both groups of patients (Fig. 3). The slopes of the regression lines did not differ, but the intercept was lower for the LTX group indicating a reduced BAIF (0.11 ml/min) compared with the control group (0.20 ml/min) ($P < 0.05$).

Biliary clearance of PEG 900 vs BSSR

The biliary clearance of PEG 900 correlated well with the BSSR in both groups of patients (Fig. 4). The biliary clearance of PEG 900 was reduced in the LTX group (0.30 ml/μmol) compared with the control group (1.40 ml/μmol) ($P < 0.05$).

Table 3. Bile flow, bile acid concentration and BSSR during the first hour of bile sampling

	Bile flow (ml/min)	Bile acid concentration (mmol/l)	BSSR (μmol/min)
Control ($n=6$)	0.49 ± 0.09	39.2 ± 3.6	19.1 ± 3.6
LTX ($n=8$)	0.55 ± 0.07	45.8 ± 2.0	25.1 ± 3.2

None of the differences between the control and LTX groups was significant

Discussion

In this study the bile formation in liver-transplanted patients with stable graft function was compared with that of a group of cholecystectomized patients. We registered a reduced BAIF as well as reduced biliary clearance of PEG 900 in the liver-transplanted patients.

Previous studies of bile secretion following OLT have mainly been performed during the first 2–3 postoperative weeks and with an interrupted enterohepatic circulation. These studies showed extremely low bile salt secretion rates partly due to continuous drainage of bile and bile acids in combination with low initial bile acid synthesis [5, 10, 12, 21]. The conclusion that can be drawn from these studies, is that bile flow as well as the secretion of bile acids recover gradually during the first 10–14 days. These data are confirmed by our own data (Fig. 2). Our patients received UDCA from the first postoperative day which could account for a slightly higher, but still very low BSSR in our patients. By analysing such initial collections of bile it has been suggested that the BAIF is very low and even absent in the transplanted liver. We feel that this is not a conclusion that should be drawn on bile secretion data from the first postoperative days, since it is obvious that the transplanted liver starts out with no bile secretion at all and that both the BAIF and the BADF increase and stabilize after 2–3 weeks provided that there is no graft dysfunction and that the enterohepatic circulation is restored [1].

The driving force of bile secretion is the active secretion of bile acids into the bile canaliculi [22]. The fraction of hepatic bile generated by the active secretion of bile acids is the BADF. The bile flow is usually linearly related to the BSSR, and the extrapolated bile flow at zero BSSR measures the BAIF [24]. The BADF in our control group was slightly higher (16 μl/μmol) than in previous studies of reference populations [1, 14, 16], probably due to the influence of UDCA. UDCA is known to have high choleretic potency [4, 20] and patients on treatment with UDCA can be expected to have a bile acid pool that consists of 50% UDCA [15]. Our liver-transplanted patients also had a comparable BADF (18 μl/μmol).

The average bile outflow of 0.49 ml/min during the first hour of measurement in the control patients corresponds well to the figure obtained by Prandi et al. [16] and slightly exceeds that reported by Lindblad et al. [14]. Since the present data correspond well to those obtained in earlier studies, where complete biliary drainage was secured by occlusion of the distal common bile duct by a balloon catheter, it is reasonable to assume that all bile was collected also in the present study where drainage by gravity was

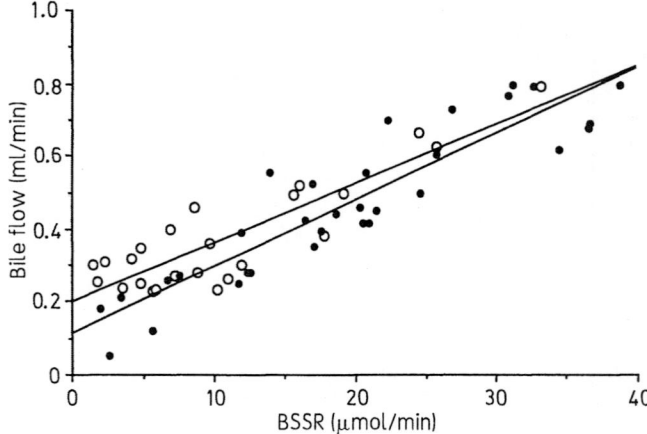

Fig. 3. The relation between bile flow and bile salt secreting rate (BSSR) as expressed with linear regression analysis. LTX *(filled symbols):* $Y = 0.11 + 0.018x$; $r = 0.92$; $P < 0.001$. Control *(unfilled symbols):* $Y = 0.20 + 0.016x$; $r = 0.88$; $P < 0.001$. The intercepts are significantly different ($P < 0.05$)

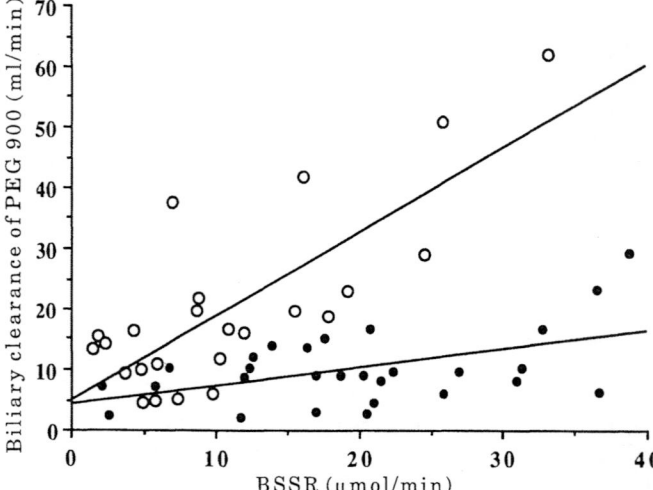

Fig. 4. The relation between biliary clearance of PEG 900 and BSSR as expressed with linear regression analysis. LTX *(filled symbols):* $Y = 4.8 + 0.30x$; $r = 0.55$; $P < 0.01$. Control *(unfilled symbols):* $Y = 4.96 + 1.40x$; $r = 0.78$; $P < 0.001$. The slopes are significantly different ($P < 0.01$)

used. This is further supported by the high biliary recovery within 2 h of intravenously-injected labelled bile acids in the present set-up.

The slightly higher values for bile flow and BSSR seen both in our control patients and even more in our LTX patients are probably due to the bile acid treatment given to these patients. It should be noted that in these observations during the first hour of bile collection no significant differences between the LTX and control patients were found.

The bile acid independent bile flow in man has previously been estimated to be 0.20–0.25 ml/min [1, 14, 16], which is in coherence with our present results in the control group. Our liver-transplanted patients, however, seem to have a reduced bile acid independent bile flow (0.11 ml/min).

Since no method of direct measurement of the canalicular fraction of bile exists, marker molecules like

PEG 900 are used [8, 9, 11]. We found, as a further indication of impaired bile formation in the transplanted liver, a reduced biliary clearance of PEG 900 indicating a reduced canalicular bile flow.

It is well established that cyclosporin in high doses has cholestatic side effects [3], and from animal studies we know that cyclosporin reduces bile formation although no deterioration of liver biochemistry occurs [13, 18, 23]. Our patients were on a low-dose regimen of cyclosporin, but a side effect of this drug must be considered as the cause of the impaired bile formation together with factors like the continuous immunological challenge to the graft and possible permanent injury during preservation and reperfusion.

Acknowledgements. The technical assistance of Ms Monica Wallin, Ms Barbro Berglund and Ms Elisabeth Lundholm is gratefully acknowledged. This work was supported by the Swedish Medical Research Council (grants no. 18x-0494), the Gothenburg Medical Society, the University of Gothenburg and the Swedish Medical Society.

References

1. Bowers BA, Rotolo FS, Watters CR, Cucciaro G, Branum GD, Meyers WC (1989) Regulation of bile secretion following liver transplantation. Transplant Proc 21: 3354
2. Boyer JL, Bloomer JR (1974) Canalicular bile secretion in man. J Clin Invest 54: 773–781
3. Calne RY, White DJG, Thiru S, McMaster P, Craddock GN, Evans DB, Dunn DC, Pentlow BD, Rolles KV (1978) Cyclosporin A in patients receiving renal allografts from cadaver donors. Lancet II: 1323–1327
4. Dumont M, Uchman S, Erlinger S (1980) Hypercholeresis induced by ursodeoxycholic acid and 7-ketolithocholic acid in the rat: possible role of bicarbonate transport. Gastroenterology 79: 82–89
5. Ericzon B-G, Eusufzai S, Kubota K, Einarsson K, Angelin B (1990) Biliary lipid secretion early after liver transplantation. Transplant Proc 22: 1537–1538
6. Fausa O, Skålhegg BA (1974) Quantitative determination of bile acids and their conjugates using thin-layer chromatography and a purified 3a-hydroxysteroid dehydrogenase. Scand J Gastroenterol 9: 249–254
7. Forker EL (1967) Two sites of bile formation as determined by mannitol and erythol clearance in the guinea pig. J Clin Invest 46: 1189–1195
8. Friman S, Rådberg G, Svanvik J (1988) Hepatic clearance of PEG-900 and mannitol in the pig. Digestion 39: 172–180
9. Friman S, Leandersson P, Tagesson C, Svanvik J (1990) Biliary excretion of different sized polyethylene-glycols in the cat. J Hepatol 11: 215–220
10. Haagsma EB, Huizenga JR, Vonk RJ, Albers CJEM, Grond J, Krom RAF, Gips CH (1987) Composition of bile after orthotopic liver transplantation. Scand J Gastroenterol 22: 1049–1055
11. Javitt NB (1982) Hepatic bile formation: assessment of water flow using mannitol and polyethyleneglycol MW 900. In: Bradley SE, Purcell (eds) The paracellular pathway. I Macy Foundation, New York, pp 234–241
12. Javitt NB, Shiu MH, Fortner JG (1971) Bile salt synthesis in the transplanted human liver. Gastroenterology 60: 405–408
13. Le Thai B, Dumont M, Michel A, Erlinger S, Houssin D (1988) Cholestatic effect of cyclosporin in the rat: an inhibition of bile acid secretion. Transplantation 46: 510–512
14. Lindblad L, Scherstén T (1976) Influence of cholic acid and chenodeoxycholic acid on canalicular bile flow in man. Gastroenterology 70: 1121–1124
15. Makino I, Nakagawa S (1978) Changes in biliary lipid and biliary bile acid composition in patients after administration of ursodeoxycholic acid. J Lipid Res 19: 723–728
16. Prandi D, Erlinger S, Glasinovic JC, Dumont M (1975) Canalicular bile production in man. Eur J Clin Invest 5: 1–6
17. Ring JR, Nguyen DC, Everett LJ (1980) The application of spectral analysis in liquid scintillation counting and SIS-spectral index of a sample and SIE spectral index of an external standard. In: Peng CT, Horroks DL, Alpen EC (eds) Liquid scintillation counting: recent application and development. Academic Press, New York
18. Rotolo FS, Branum GD, Bowers BA, Meyers WC (1985) Effect of cyclosporin on bile secretion in rats. 151: 35–40
19. Rundle FF, Cass MH, Robson B, Middleton M (1955) Bile drainage after choledochostomy in man, with some observation on the bile fistula. Surgery 37: 903–910
20. Scherstén T, Linblad L (1979) Biliary cholesterol output during ursodeoxycholic acid secretion in man. In: G Paumgartner, Stiehl A, Gerok W (eds) Biological effects of bile acids. MTP Press, Lancaster
21. Shiffman ML, Carithers Jr RL, Posner M, Moore EW (1991) Recovery of bile secretion following orthotopic liver transplantation. J Hepatol 12: 351–361
22. Sperber I (1959) Secretion of organic anions in the formation of urine and bile. Pharmacol Rev 11: 109
23. Stone BG, Udani M, Sanghvi A, Warty V, Plocki K, Bedetti C, van Thiel DH (1987) Cyclosporin A-induced cholestasis. Gastroenterology 93: 344–351
24. Wheeler HO, Ross ED, Bradley SE (1968) Canalicular bile production in dogs. Am J Physiol 214: 866–874

Transplant Int (1992) 5 [Suppl 1]: S 168–S 169

TRANSPLANT
International
© Springer-Verlag 1992

Quadruple immunosuppression including a new IL-2-receptor antibody and the incidence of infections after liver transplantation

R. Raakow, R. Steffen, M. Knoop, G. Blumhardt, P. Lemmens, M. Wiens, H. Keck, and P. Neuhaus

Department of Surgery, Universitätsklinikum Rudolf Virchow, Berlin, FRG

Immunosuppression is a primary concern after orthotopic liver transplantation (OLT). On the one hand, the graft is at jeopardy through acute or chronic rejection, and on the other, immunosuppression and antirejection therapy increase the risk of infectious complications. Effective immunosuppression therefore should prevent rejections without leading to a high rate of infections, bearing in mind the fact that infections and infection-related complications are the most frequent causes of early death after liver transplantation [1]. With more specific immunosuppression the infectious complications can potentially be minimized. Antithymocyte globulin (ATG) and the first monoclonal antibody OKT3 immunosuppression are non-specific [4]. The replacement of these antibodies in a quadruple immunosuppressive regimen with the new monoclonal IL-2R antibody BT 563 [3] probably reduces the early infection rate. We report on our first experience with BT 563. The incidence of infection was compared with a historical control group with ATG.

Key words: Liver transplantation – Infection – IL-2-receptor antibody – Immunosuppression

Materials and methods

A total of 103 liver transplantations were performed in 98 patients. Between April and September 1990, 33 recipients were treated with BT 563, and compared with 70 consecutive recipients treated with ATG as historical controls. In the BT 563 group no retransplantation was necessary. The median age of the patients was 41 years. In the ATG group there were 65 patients with a median age of 44 years. Five retransplantations were necessary in three patients due to relapsing fulminant hepatitis B (3) and INF (2). Concerning the other indications both groups were comparable.

Offprint requests to: R. Raakow, Department of Surgery, Universitätsklinikum Rudolf Virchow, Augustenburger Platz 1, W-1000 Berlin 65, FRG

Quadruple immunosuppression consisted of steroids, cyclosporin A, azathioprine and rabit antithymocyte globulin (ATG, Fresenius) or the monoclonal IL-2R antibody BT 563 (Biotest). BT 563 was administered as a daily dose of 10 mg IV from day 0 to day 12. In the control group ATG was given from day 0 to day 7 at 5 mg/kg bodyweight IV.

Effects and side effects were diagnosed according to standard procedures. The diagnosis of rejection was established on the basis of pathological changes in liver function tests, clinical signs and histological findings.

Infection prophylaxis remained unchanged in both groups. Knowing that especially Gram-negative bacterial and fungal infections are a major cause of morbidity and mortality following OLT [2], we used selective bowel decontamination (SBD) as described by Stoutenbeek et al. [7]. With SBD we eliminated the endogenous source of Gram-negative bacteria and *Candida* to prevent infections with these pathogens [6]. SBD consisted of the nonabsorbable antibiotics polymyxin B, tobramycin and nystatin as suspension administered via the oropharynx and gastrointestinal tract four times per day. Prophylactic perioperative systemic antibiotic coverage with cefotaxime, tobramycin and metronidazole was added for 48 h. All patients received anti-CMV immunglobulin on day 1 and 14. Acyclovir was given in prophylactic dosage (800 mg/day) for 8 weeks post-transplant. Infections were diagnosed according to criteria proposed by Wiesner et al. [8].

Results

The 1-year survival in both groups was over 90% (ATG 90.8%, BT 563 90.9%). In the ATG group, two patients died from fulminant relapsing hepatitis B after 7 and 8 months, two patients died at 3 and 6 weeks from systemic mycosis, one patient died 11 months after OLT from tumour recurrence and one patient from chronic rejection. In the BT 563 group there were three deaths. One from acute heart failure 11 days after OLT, one from tumour recurrence and one from chronic rejection 6 months after transplantation.

No clinical side effects were noted during the BT 563 treatment period. In the ATG group 24 significant infections were seen in the first 4 weeks after OLT (Table 1). Due to SBD the majority of 21 bacterial infections were related to Gram-positive organisms. Among them were

Table 1. Early infections after OLT under ATG ($n = 70$)

Pathogen	n^a	Site	Organism (n)
Bacteria			
Gram-negative	2	Urinary tract (2)	*Pseudomonas* (1)
Gram-positive	19	Wound infection (4)	*Proteus* (1)
		Urinary tract (3)	*Streptococcus* group D (2)
		Cholangitis (10)	*Nocardien* (1)
		Septicaemia (2)	*Staphylococcus aureus* (1)
			Streptococcus group D (3)
			Streptococcus group D (8)
			Streptococcus viridans (1)
			Staphylococcus coag.-neg. (1)
			Staphylococcus aureus (1)
			Streptococcus viridans (1)
Fungi	3	Septicaemia (2)	*Mucor* (1)
		Pneumonia (1)	*Aspergillus* (1)
			Candida albicans (1)

^a A total of 24 infections were suffered by 19 patients

Table 2. Early infections after OLT under BT 563 ($n = 33$)

Pathogen	n^a	Site	Organism (n)
Bacteria			
Gram-negative	1	Septicaemia (1)	*Escherichia coli* (1)
Gram-positive	4	Cholangitis (2)	*Streptococcus* group D (2)
		Urinary tract (1)	*Streptococcus* group D (1)
		Wound infection (1)	*Staphylococcus aureus* (1)
Virus	1	Pneumonia (1)	CMV

^a A total of six infections were suffered by five patients

Table 3. Incidence of early infections (≤ 28 days)

	ATG	BT 563
Bacterial	21/70 (30%)	5/33 (15.2%)
Viral	0/70 (0%)	1/33 (3.0%)
Fungal	3/70 (4.2%)	0/33 (0%)
Total	24/70 (34.3%)	6/33 (18.2%)

Table 4. Incidence of early rejection (≤ 28 days)

	ATG	BT 563
Incidence	16/70 (22.9%)	3/33 (9.1%)
steroid sensitive	12	2
with response to OKT3	4	1

ten episodes of cholangitis, two bacteraemias, four wound infections and three infections of the urinary tract. There were only two infections of the urinary tract caused by Gram-negative bacteria. In three patients fungal infections were seen. The two patients with fungal septicaemia died 3 and 6 weeks after OLT.

In the BT 563 group, five patients had six infections (Table 2). Five of these infections were caused by bacteria (two cholangitis, one wound infection, one infection of the urinary tract and one septicaemia). One patient de-

veloped severe CMV pneumonia after transplantation. He had to be treated with gancyclovir and anti-CMV immunoglobulin for 39 days and also needed respirator treatment for 14 days. However all infections in the BT 563 group responded to antibiotic therapy.

Observing the incidence of early infections (Table 3) there was a clear difference between the two groups. A higher overall incidence of infection was seen in the ATG group. While two early fatalities due to fungal infections were observed in the ATG group, no infection-related deaths occurred in the BT 563 group.

Discussion

These first results indicate a lower incidence of early infectious complications when ATG is replaced by the new monoclonal IL-2R antibody BT 563 as part of the quadruple immunosuppression after OLT. One possible reason for the observed decrease in early infection was a reduced incidence of early rejection under BT 563 in our experience (Table 4) also described by Otto et al. [5]. Secondly, the monoclonal IL-2R antibody BT 563 inhibits only activated IL-2-dependent T cells, thus resulting in a more specific immunosuppression [4]. In contrast ATG or OKT3 react with all T lymphocytes, thus resulting in a more general immunosuppression, increasing the risk of infection.

Further controlled and prospective studies are necessary to evaluate these observatioans.

References

1. Colonna JO, Winston DJ, Brill JE et al (1988) Infectious complications in liver transplantation. Arch Surg 123: 360–364
2. Cuervas-Mons V, Martinez AJ, Dekker A et al (1986) Adult liver transplantation: an analysis of the early causes of death in 40 consecutive cases. Hepatology 4: 495–500
3. Herve P, Wijdenes J, Bergerat JP et al (1988) Treatment of acute graft-versus-host disease with monoclonal antibody to IL-2 receptor. Lancet II: 1072–1073
4. Herve P, Wijdenes J, Bergerat JP et al (1990) Treatment of corticosteroid resistant acute graft-versus-host disease by in vivo administration of anti-interleukin-2 receptor antibody (B-B10). Blood 75: 1017–1023
5. Otto G, Thies J, Kabelitz D et al (1991) Anti-CD25 monoclonal antibody prevents early rejection in liver transplantation – a pilot study. Transplant Proc 23: 1387–1389
6. Raakow R, Steffen R, Lefebre B et al (1990) Selective bowel decontamination effectively prevents gram-negative bacterial infections after liver transplantation. Transplant Proc 22: 1556–1557
7. Stoutenbeek CP, van Saene HK, Miranda DR et al (1984) The effect of selective decontamination of the digestive tract on colonization and infection rate in multiple trauma patients. Intensive Care Med 10: 185–190
8. Wiesner RH, Hermans P, Rakela J et al (1987) Selective bowel decontamination to prevent gram-neg bacterial and fungal infection following orthotopic liver transplantation. Transplant Proc 14: 2420–2423

TRANSPLANT
International
© Springer-Verlag 1992

Should retransplantation still be considered for primary non-function after liver transplantation?

S. Agnes, A. W. Avolio, S. C. Magalini, M. Foco, and M. Castagneto

Department of Surgery and Division of Organ Transplantation, Catholic University of Rome, Rome, Italy

Abstract. Primary non-function (PNF) of a transplanted liver is a postoperative condition characterized by absence of hepatic recovery due to various insults during harvesting, preservation or revascularization. Until recently early retransplantation (RTx) has been considered the policy of choice. Results of RTx for PNF are unsatisfactory (1-year survival rates ranging from 0 to 34 %). The management of PNF by medical care without RTx with a recovery rate of 80 % and a 1-year actuarial survival rate of 50 % is reported for a series of 33 consecutive liver transplants. The guidelines for the medical care management are given and the results are discussed.

Key words: Liver transplantation – Retransplantation, liver

Primary non-function (PNF) of a transplanted liver is a postoperative condition characterized by absence of hepatic recovery due to various insults during harvesting, preservation or revascularization [3, 10, 16, 20, 22, 28, 30–32, 34]. Its incidence in several series has been shown to range from 7 to 36 %, probably due to different definition criteria employed and great variability of the donor pool [3, 10, 20, 22, 28, 34]. The therapeutic approach to this condition has been the object of discussion. Until recently early RTx has been considered the policy of choice and patient survival has been related to the availability of a suitable organ [21, 26, 30–32].

Unsatisfactory results of RTx for PNF (1-year survival rates ranging from 0 to 34 % [26, 28, 31] and current application of critical care techniques to acute liver failure have changed the approach to PNF, and have lead us to a conservative management without RTx. We report on our series of liver transplants in which PNF was managed by this approach.

Offprint requests to: S. Agnes, M. D., Clinica Chirurgica Universita' Cattolica, Policlinico Gemelli, Largo Gemelli 8, 00168 Roma, Italy

Patients and methods

A total of 33 consecutive liver transplants were performed in 32 patients from 1987 to 1991 at the Catholic University of Rome. Donor acceptance criteria and graft preservation modalities, reported in detail elsewhere [4] are summarized in Table 1. Recipient characteristics have recently been reviewed [2, 7].

Criteria used for the definition of PNF are shown in Table 2, together with those for primary dysfunction (PDF) according to other authors [16, 31].

Supportive management

In the case of PNF, supportive management consisted of both liver function support and extra-liver organ support.

Liver function support consisted of efforts to ensure:
A. optimal perfusion and oxygenation by invasive haemodynamic monitoring, stable haemoglobin level (>10 g/dl), optimization of pulmonary exchanges, pharmacological support with inotropic drugs, when necessary, and prostaglandins PGE_1 (0.5 µg/kg per h) to diminish hepatic vascular resistance;
B. adequate protein supplementation by monitoring and prompt correction of coagulation disorders administering fresh frozen plasma, fibrinogen, antithrombin III and cryoprecipitates, and by maintenance of adequate albumin and vitamin co-factor levels;

Table 1. Donor acceptance criteria and graft preservation modalities

Donor criteria
– age <50 years
– SBP >90 mmHg
– mechanical ventilation <5 days
– serum Na <160 mEq/l
– AST and/or ALT <100 UI/l
– serum bilirubin <2 mg/dl
– PT $>45\%$
– dopamine infusion <10 gamma/kg per min
– no major surgery
– no cardiac arrest
– appearance at laparotomy (color and palpation)

Graft preservation modalities
– use of UW solution (26/33)
– CIT <10 hours
– WIT <70 min

Table 2. Recovery after perioperative injury

Primary dysfunction
- ALT and AST peak 2000–5000 IU/l
- biliary output < 100 ml/day
- low-grade coagulopathy

Primary nonfunction
- ALT and AST peak > 5000 UI/l
- bilirubin peak > 20 mg/dl
- no bile production (at least 5 days)
- severe coagulopathy
- relevant neurological impairment
- lactacidaemia
- ± renal failure
- ± haemodynamic instability

C. artificial nutrition by high glucose and nitrogen content with branched chain amino acids, proscription of aromatic amino acids and low fat supplementation;
D. limitation of intestinal toxic production (lactulose, topically active antibiotics, plasmapheresis).

Extra-liver organ support consisted of:
A. slow withdrawal from mechanical ventilation by pressure support, CPAP;
B. prevention of renal failure by high urinary output using volume, diuretics, dopamine, proscription of nephrotoxic antibiotics and avoidance of high cyclosporin levels;
C. reduction of infectious risk by antibiotic and antimycotic prophylaxis, selective bowel decontamination, aspecific immunoprophylaxis and low grade immunosuppression.

Results

In 32 first transplant patients we observed five cases of PNF (15.6%) and five cases of hepatic liver dysfunction (15.6%) according to the criteria previously defined. In addition, another case of PNF was seen in our only re-transplant carried out because of hepatic artery thrombosis; this case, in which we used unsuccessfully a donor with suboptimal characteristics due to the urgency, was not included in the study.

Early results showed that four of out five patients (80%) recovered in a period ranging from 4 to 9 weeks using critical care procedures. The fifth patient died in the second postoperative week due to evolution towards multiple organ failure. Late results showed that one pa-

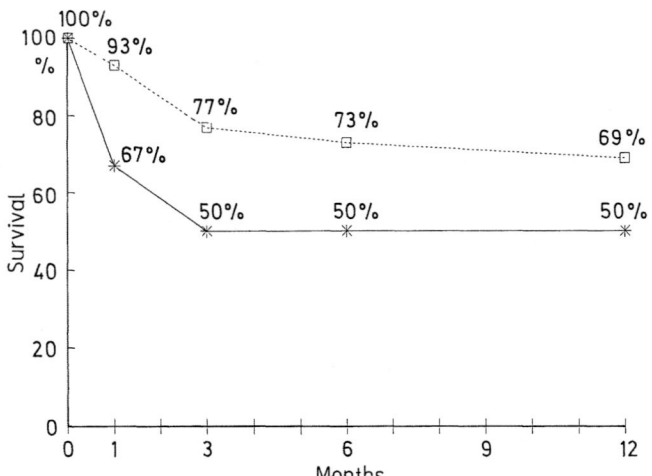

Fig. 1. Actuarial survival trends for livers with PNF and livers without PNF. □, Normal function; *, primary non-function. Liver Transplantation, Catholic University, Rome, Italy

tient of the four died in the second postoperative month from pulmonary aspergillosis, although he was experiencing continuous improvement in liver function. At the time of writing three out of four patients were alive and well at 55, 27, 22 months. Survival trends are represented in Fig. 1, where the group of patients with PNF is compared with the group without PNF (including those with PDF). Actuarial survival rates at 1 year were, respectively, 50 and 69%. In spite of the 19% gap, the difference is not signficant due to the small number of patients (Mantel-Cox, $P = 0.258$; Breslow, $P = 0.143$).

Discussion

In the recent past RTx was the policy of choice for graft failure due to chronic rejection, technical complications and PNF [21, 26, 30–32]. Particularly in the case of PNF, a new liver was usually sought before even attempting an aggressive drug therapy. At present this approach is changing because of the poor results of RTx in this condition, the improving medical management of acute hepatic failure [1, 6, 18] and the lower donor/recipient ratio.

Reasons for failure of the RTx procedure in PNF should be identified in the highly compromised conditions of patients with severe PNF (liver failure and severe extra-hepatic organ compromise) that make a second operation unsuccessful in relation to both intraoperative and postoperative trauma.

Worldwide reconsideration of RTx for PNF is underway [21, 26]. Probably the drive in this direction has been the continuous improvement in critical care procedures for liver failure. Among these we consider of great and probably the greatest importance the clinical introduction of prostaglandins. Prostaglandin PGE₁, initially used for acute hepatic failure [1], has subsequently proved useful for PNF [15, 16]. The close monitoring of the coagulation pattern seems also to be relevant and the recent introduction of measurement and supplementation of antithrombin III may be useful [23]. Monitoring of coagulation has provided a guideline for the selective reintegration of proteins lacking from hepatic synthesis with the effect of avoiding both haemorrhagic complications (cerebral and abdominal) and disseminated intravascular coagulation, which may evolve in multiple organ failure. Fresh frozen plasma administration together with albumin supplementation is also useful to ensure adequate intravascular colloid osmotic pressure by replacing other missing proteins of hepatic synthesis. Parenteral nutrition is fundamental to compensate the great caloric expenditure due to hepatic cell regeneration [19, 27]. It seems especially important to supply high concentrations of branched chain and non-aromatic amino acids [19]. The use of lactulose, intestinal antibiotics and, in selected cases, plasmapheresis are effective in diminishing production and removing toxic substances [9].

In addition other extra-liver organ support procedures that have proved beneficial, are:
A. respiratory care with prolonged mechanical ventilation (pressure support, CPAP) to ensure optimal oxygenation, to diminish respiratory work and to control acid–base equilibrium [23]

B. prevention of renal failure by absolute proscription of potentially nephrotoxic antibiotics and by avoidance of high cyclosporin levels

C. reduction of the infectious hazard by non-specific immunoprophylaxis and by selective bowel decontamination [33]. (In this context it is fundamental to maintain the patient at a low immunosuppressive level.)

From the start of our liver transplant programme we chose to attempt a critical care approach for patients with PNF in consideration of the large experience of our team in the management of liver failure in patients with multiple organ failure, cirrhosis, trauma and sepsis [8, 13, 14]. This policy was also justified by the donor shortage in Italy [29]. We have reported herein our results that show the soundness of this choice as represented by an 80 % recovery rate after PNF and 50 % actuarial survival of this group.

In conclusion, the treatment of PNF is the subject of discussion, but there are two options: retransplantation, which should be done as early as possible, but has been shown to give bad results and to cause organ wastage [26, 28, 31], or supportive management, which, when unsuccessful, precludes late RTx due to multiple organ compromise. Patients are lost also with medical management, but fewer than die as a consequence of surgical trauma added to the critical conditions in RTx, as our small series demonstrates. Various indexes have been proposed to predict the occurrence and severity of PNF from intraoperative or early postoperative parameters [5, 11, 12, 17, 24, 25]; these may be useful to indicate the optimum therapeutic approach.

A wider acceptance of supportive management of PNF would probably lead to a new definition of subgroups that may benefit from medical care and the identification of cases with a worse prognosis in whom supportive management as well as retransplantation would have little success.

References

1. Abecassis M, Falk R, Blendis L et al (1987) Treatment of fulminant hepatic failure with a continuous infusion of Prostin-VR (PGE$_1$). Hepatology 7: 1104
2. Agnes S, Avolio AW, Magalini SC et al (1991) Indicazioni e risultati del programma trapianto di fegato all'Univertita' Cattolica di Roma. Atti XXI Congresso Societa' Italiana Trapianti d'Organo, Milano 25–27 Settembre. 607
3. Asonuma K, Takaya S, Selby R et al (1991) The clinical significance of the arterial ketone body ratio as an early indicator of graft viability in human liver transplantation. Transplantation 51: 164
4. Avolio AW, Agnes S, Magalini SC et al (1991) Importance of donor blood chemistry data (AST, serum sodium) in predicting liver transplant outcome. Transplant Proc (in press)
5. Avolio AW, Agnes S, Pelosi G et al (1991) Intraoperative trends of oxygen consumption and blood lactate as predictors of primary dysfunction after liver transplantation. Transplant Proc 23: 2263
6. Carithers RL, Fairman RP (1989) Critical care of patients with severe liver disease. In: Shoemaker WC (ed) Textbook of critical care, Saunders, p 686
7. Castagneto M, Avolio AW, Agnes S et al (1990) Liver transplantation: Results and personal experience. Proceedings of 5th Postgraduate Course: Recent advances in anaesthesia, pain, intensive care and emergency, Trieste, 21–24 November
8. Chiarla C, Giovannini I, Siegel JH et al (1990) Relationship of plasma cholesterol level to doses of BCCA in sepsis. Crit Care Med 18: 32
9. Conn HO, Lieberthal MM (1979) Mechanism of action of lactulose. In: The hepatic coma syndromes and lactulose. Williams & Wilkins, Baltimore, pp 278
10. Fassati LR, Gridelli B, Rossi G et al (1988) The activity of the liver transplant center in Milan. Transplant Proc 20: 512
11. Forster J, Greig PD, Glynn MF et al (1989) Predictors of graft function following liver transplantation. Transplant Proc 21: 3356
12. Furukawa H, Todo S, Imventarza O et al (1991) Effect of cold ischemia time on the early outcome of human hepatic allografts preserved with UW solution. Transplantation 51: 1000
13. Giovannini I, Boldrini G, Chiarla C et al (1987) Adequacy and support of physiological functions in the acutely ill cirrhotic patient. World J Surg 202: 11
14. Giovannini I, Chiarla C, Boldrini G et al (1988) Calorimetric response to amino acid infusion in sepsis and critical illness. Crit Care Med 16: 7
15. Greig PD, Woolf M, Abecassis SM et al (1989) Prostaglandin E$_1$ for primary non function following liver transplantation. Transplant Proc 21: 3360
16. Greig PD, Woolf GM, Sinclair SB et al (1989) Treatment of primary liver graft nonfunction with prostaglandin E$_1$. Tranplantation 48: 447
17. Gubernatis G, Bornscheuer A, Taki Y et al (1989) Total oxygen consumption, ketone body ratio and a special score as early indicators of irreversible liver allograft dysfunction. Transplant Proc 21: 2279
18. Hasselgren PO (1987) Prevention and treatment of ischemia of the liver. Surg Gynecol Obstet 164: 187
19. Hehir DJ, Jenkins R, Bistrian BR et al (1990) Nutritional in patients undergoing orthotopic liver transplantation. JPEN 9: 695
20. Howard TD, Klintmalm GB, Cofer JB et al (1990) The influence of preservation injury on rejection in the hepatic transplant recipient. Transplantation 49: 103
21. Kamath GS, Plevak DJ, Wiesner RH et al (1991) Primary nonfunction of the liver graft: When should we retransplant? Transplant Proc 23: 1954
22. Makowka L, Gordon RD, Todo S et al (1987) Analysis of donor criteria for the prediction of the outcome in clinical liver transplantation. Transplant Proc 19: 2378
23. Marsh JW, Gordon T, Stieber A et al (1989) Critical care of liver transplant patients. In: Shoemaker WC (ed) Textbook of critical care, Sounders, pp 1329
24. Mimeault R, Grant D, Ghent C et al (1989) Analysis of donor and recipient variables and early graft function after orthotopic liver transplantation. Transplant Proc 21: 2355
25. Miyata T, Yokoyama I, Todo S et al (1989) Endotoxemia, pulmonary complications and thrombocitopenia in liver transplantation. Lancet II: 189
26. Mora NP, Klintmalm GB, Cofer JB et al (1990) Results after liver retransplantation (RETx): a comparative study between "elective" vs "nonelective" RETx. Transplant Proc 22: 1509
27. Reilly J, Mehta R, Teperman L et al (1990) Nutritional support after liver transplantation: a randomized prospective study. JPEN 14: 386
28. Ringe B, Neuhaus P, Lauchart W et al (1989) Experience with hepatic retransplantation. Transplant Proc 21: 2407
29. Scalamogna M, Sirchia G (1990) Transplant organization in Italy. Transplantation 2: 87
30. Shaw BW, Wood R (1989) Improved results with retransplantation of the liver. Transplant Proc 21: 2407
31. Shaw BW, Gordon RD, Iwatsuki S et al (1985) Hepatic retransplantation. Transplant Proc 17: 264
32. Shaw BW, Gordon RD, Iwatsuki S et al (1985) Retransplantation of the liver. Semin Liver Dis 5: 394
33. Weisner RH, Hermans PE, Rakela J et al (1988) Selective bowel decontamination to decrease gram negative aerobic bacterial and Candida colonization and prevent infection after orthotopic liver transplantation. Transplantation 45: 570
34. Williams JW, Vera S, Peters TG et al (1986) Cholestatic jaundice after hepatic transplantation: a nonimmunologically mediated event. Am Surg 151: 65

Transplant Int (1992) 5 [Suppl 1]: S 173–S 174

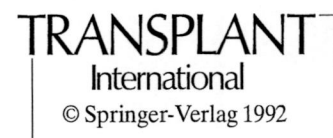

© Springer-Verlag 1992

Increased fibrinolysis in orthotopic but not in heterotopic liver transplantation: the role of the anhepatic phase

C. M. Bakker[1], H. J. Metselaar[1], Th. N. Groenland[2], O. T. Terpstra[3], and J. Stibbe[4]

Departments of [1] Internal Medicine, [2] Anaesthesiology, [3] Surgery and [4] Haematology, University Hospital Rotterdam 'Dijkzigt', Rotterdam, The Netherlands

Abstract. The major cause of increased tissue-type plasminogen activator (t-PA) activity during orthotopic liver transplantation (OLT) is still unclear. Both lack of hepatic clearance of t-PA in the anhepatic period and/or increased endothelial release from the graft upon reperfusion have been suggested. Heterotopic liver transplantation (HLT) avoids resection of the host liver and is therefore a useful model to differentiate these two possibilities. The fibrinolytic system was evaluated in ten patients with OLT and in 18 patients with HLT. A marked increment in t-PA activity was observed during the anhepatic period of OLT, which rapidly normalized after reperfusion. In contrast t-PA activity levels remained normal in HLT. As a reflection of the increased t-PA activity fibrin degradation products were markedly elevated during OLT and plasminogen and α_2-antiplasmin decreased simultaneously during the anhepatic period. In conclusion, the lack of hepatic clearance during the anhepatic period is the most important factor in the evolution of increased t-PA activity during OLT.

Key words: Fibrinolysis – Liver transplantation – t-PA activity – Hepatic clearance

During the past decade, the increase in number of orthotopic liver transplantations (OLT) has led to a better understanding of the coagulation problems encountered during the procedure. Especially during the late anhepatic phase of liver transplantation and soon after reperfusion of the allograft, a dangerous period of hypocoagulation is present in many patients. Increased fibrinolytic activity, found during the anhepatic period in many studies, is an important factor in the origin of massive haemorrhage [3]. The mechanism underlying the increased fribrinolysis is not yet well defined. Lack of hepatic clearance of tissue-type plasminogen activator (t-PA) in the anhepatic phase and/or release of t-PA from either vascular endothelium or hepatocytes upon reperfusion trauma have been suggested as causes of hyperfibrinolysis.

Heterotopic liver transplantation (HLT) avoids the anhepatic period and is therefore a useful model to differentiate the single effect of graft reperfusion on the haemostatic changes from the effect of the anhepatic period. We compared the fibrinolytic activity between OLT and HLT in order to address this question. We also studied the single effect of surgery itself on fibrinolysis in patients undergoing partial hepatic resection (PHR).

Patients and methods

In consecutive series of 10 patients undergoing OLT, 21 patients HLT and 10 patients PHR, arterial blood samples were taken at regular intervals during the whole procedure. OLT was divided into three stages; stage I began with the induction of anaesthesia and ended with the occlusion of blood flow to the patient's own liver, stage II was the anhepatic phase and stage III started at the moment of reperfusion. For the comparison, it was decided that in HLT stage II started 120 min after the beginning of surgery. Blood samples were collected from an unheparinized arterial line in plastic tubes and anticoagulated with trisodium citrate. The samples were immediately placed on melting ice and centrifuged for 30 min at 4°C within 20 min. Plasma was snap-frozen and stored at − 70°C until testing.

Tissue-type plasminogen activator was assayed according to the method of Verheyen et al. [4]. t-PA antigen levels were measured using an ELISA (Biopool IMULYSE t-PA, Umea, Sweden). Tissue plasminogen activator inhibitor (PAI-1) antigen levels were determined by an ELISA (Biopool TINTELIZA, Umea, Sweden). Plasminogen and α_2-antiplasmin levels were assayed according to the method of Friberger et al. [2]. Fibrin degradation products (FbDP) and fibrinogen degradation products (FgDP) were determined by EIA (Organon Technica, Turnhout, Belgium).

The Wilcoxon test for independent samples was used for statistical analysis. Any probability less than 0.05 was considered significant.

Offprint requests to: dr. H. J. Metselaar, Department of Internal Medicine, Room D 420, University Hospital Rotterdam 'Dijkzigt', dr. Molewaterplein 40, 3015 GD Rotterdam, The Netherlands

S174

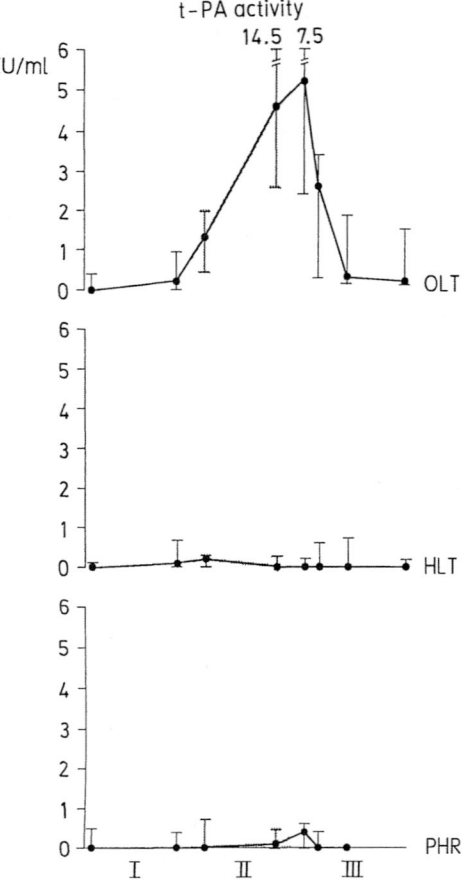

t-PA activity

OLT

HLT

PHR

Fig. 1. t-PA activity (IU/ml, median and quartiles) during stage I, II and III of OLT, HLT and PHR. For explanation of I, II and II see text

Results

The median levels of t-PA activity during OLT, HLT and PHR are shown in Fig. 1. In OLT, t-PA activity increased from 0.2 IU/ml to 5.2 IU/ml at the end of the anhepatic period, and returned to a normal value soon after reperfusion. In contrast, t-PA activity remained within the normal range throughout HLT and PHR. t-PA antigen levels increased significantly from 11.5 ng/ml to 23.7 ng/ml during OLT. In HLT and PHR t-PA antigen levels did not change significantly. Concentrations of FbDP and FgDP rose only during OLT. Levels of PAI-1 antigen, plasminogen and α_2-antiplasmin decreased during OLT until reperfusion and remained virtually unchanged during HLT and PHR.

Discussion

The results obtained in this study clearly show that lack of t-PA clearance during the anhepatic period is essential for the development of a fibrinolytic state during liver trans-

plantation. During the anhepatic period of OLT a marked increase in t-PA activity and t-PA antigen levels was found in contrast to no change in the comparable period of HLT. After reperfusion of the graft, t-PA activity returned to normal values within 15 min. Another proof that lack of clearance, and not reperfusion trauma, causes hyperfibrinolysis comes from the observation that the first venous outflow from the allograft after reperfusion did not contain an increased t-PA activity or antigen level (data not shown). Moreover, as no increase in t-PA activity during PHR was observed, manipulation of the liver per se is not an important factor in the pathogenesis of hyperfibrinolysis.

Another explanation for the enhanced fibrinolytic activity could be an inhibition of PAI-1 by protein C. However, during OLT protein C levels did not change (data not shown).

It has been suggested that the veno–venous bypass used in OLT may induce t-PA release from the vascular endothelium [1]. However no difference in t-PA activity was observed between patients with and without a veno–venous bypass.

The presence of an active fibrinolytic process is also demonstrated by a simultaneous decrease in plasminogen and α_2-antiplasmin during the anhepatic phase. As a reflection of the increased t-PA activity fibrin degradation products were markedly elevated during OLT. Fibrinogenolysis was seen in a limited degree during OLT. Although enhanced fibrinolysis occurred during OLT and not during HLT, no significant difference in blood loss was observed between OLT and HLT. Blood loss, however, is influenced by multiple factors which could have neutralized the single effect of the enhanced fibrinolytic state during OLT.

In conclusion, this study shows that the increased fibrinolytic activity observed during OLT is caused by lack of clearance of t-PA during the anhepatic period.

References

1. Arnoux D, Boutière B, Houvenaegel M, Rousset-Rouvière A, Le Treut P, Sampol J (1989) Intraoperative evolution of coagulation parameters and t-PA/PAI balance in orthotopic liver transplantation. Thromb Res 55: 319–328
2. Friberger P, Knos Gustavsson S, Aurell L, Claeson G (1978) Methods for the determination of plasmin, antiplasmin and plasminogen by means of substrate S-2251. Haemostasis 7: 135–145
3. Porte PJ, Knot EAR, Bontempo FA (1989) Hemostasis in liver transplantation. Gastroenterology 97: 488–501
4. Verheyen JH, Chang GTG, Kluft C, Wijngaards G (1982) A simple sensitive spectophotometric assay for extrinsic (tissue-type) plasminogen activator applicable to measurement in plasma. Thromb Haemost 48: 266–269

Transplant Int (1992) 5 [Suppl 1]: S175–S178

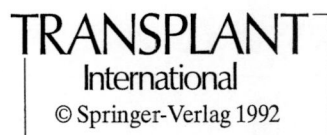

TRANSPLANT
International
© Springer-Verlag 1992

A Pugh score of 8 adequately selects patients with parenchymal cirrhosis for liver transplantation

M. Adler, N. Bourgeois, J. van de Stadt, and M. Gelin

Service Médico-Chirurgical d'Hépato-gastroentérologie, Hôpital Erasme, Brussels, Belgium

Abstract. The aim of our study was to develop simple and highly effective scores to estimate prognosis at 1 year for patients with parenchymal cirrhosis and to define the optimum time for liver transplantation with the same degree of accuracy as the prognosis estimation for primary biliary cirrhosis. The prognostic value of 19 variables was studied retrospectively in 91 patients with parenchymal cirrhosis using multivariate analysis and logistic regression. The best prognostic index was obtained with two independent variables: ascites and aminopyrine breath test. Although the receiver operating characteristic (ROC) curve for these two variables was better than the ROC curve for Pugh score, the percentage of correct prediction was excellent for both indices: 92 % and 87 %, respectively. The critical cut-off value of the Pugh score was 8.8. The prognostic value of a Pugh score ≤ 8 or > 8 was confirmed in a prospective study of 145 cirrhotic patients with 78 % correct prediction. During this period, 21 patients with parenchymal cirrhosis received transplants with a preoperative Pugh score of 9.5 ± 2.0 (mean $\pm$ SEM) and 60 % 1- and 2-year survival. In conclusion in parenchymal cirrhosis, a Pugh score > 8 indicates a poor prognosis at 1 year. This is a simple, easy and highly effective tool to define the optimal time for liver transplantation in this category of patients.

Key words: Liver transplantation – Pugh score – Parenchymal cirrhosis

As emphasized recently by the Hannover group [10] an important issue for defining optimum time for liver transplantation is the estimation of spontaneous prognosis for the following 1 to 2 years. In the field of primary biliary cirrhosis or sclerosing cholangitis, several prognostic

models have been published with certain variables (e. g. age and bilirubin) being consistently included [21]. In the field of parenchymal cirrhosis, however, there is certainly less consistency in the prognostic factors described [2, 4, 5, 7, 9, 14, 16, 17]. The following drawbacks can be emphasized: the high number of variables often kept in the final model, the inclusion of histological features in some studies, the absence of cross-validation, the heterogeneous diagnostic groups and the low predictive value of the model.

The aim of our study was: to construct a powerful prognostic model based on clinical, biological and functional variables in a series of patients with parenchymal cirrhosis; to measure the accuracy of the prediction formula by applying it to another series of cirrhotic patients; to compare the new model with the Pugh score; and finally, to define the cut-off Pugh score value best separating patients with a good prognosis from those who should undergo liver transplantation. In particular, we were interested to know if estimation of quantitative liver function using the aminopyrine breath test could improve the performance of the prediction, as previous investigations showed contradictory results [3, 13, 19].

Patients and methods

Patients

Included in the study were 91 patients with parenchymal cirrhosis (56 % of alcoholic origin). Criteria for defining alcoholism included a daily intake of more than 50 g of alcohol for more than 5 years. Criteria for defining cirrhosis included either a positive laparoscopy and/or liver biopsy (82 patients) or clinico-biochemical features and endoscopic demonstration of oesophageal varices (nine patients) suggesting cirrhosis.

In all the patients, a complete history was obtained and physical examination and laboratory analyses were performed on admission. Abdominal ultrasonography, oesophagogastroduodenoscopy, and a 2-h aminopyrine breath test were performed within 72 h as part of a routine work-up. The status of the patient – living or dead – and the cause of death were established after 1 year.

Offprint requests to: Dr. M. Adler, Service Médico-Chirurgical d' Hépato-gastroentérologie, Hôpital Erasme, Route de Lennik 808, 1070 Brussels, Belgium

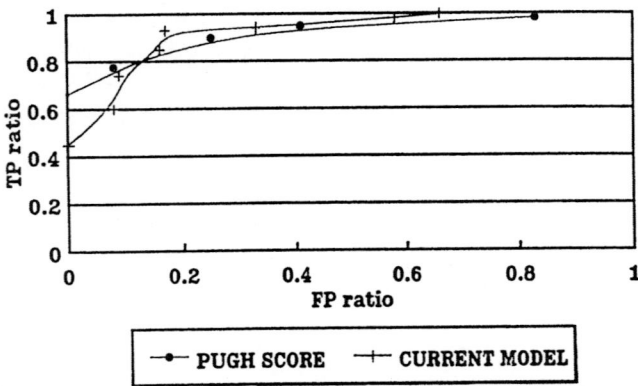

Fig. 1. ROC curves. True positive (TP) ratio (sensitivity) and false positive (FP) ratio (1-specificity) for various cut-off points of the Pugh score (●) and the current model including as variables aminopyrine breath test result and degree of ascites (+)

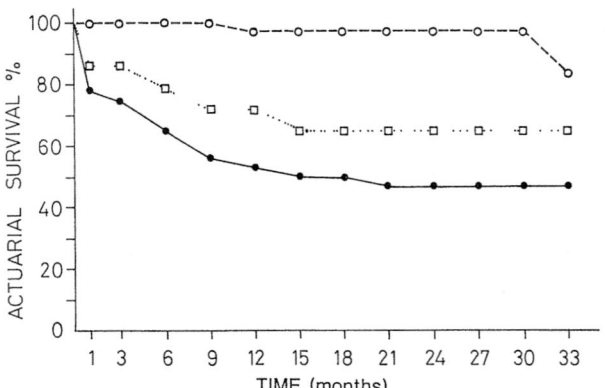

Fig. 2. Actuarial survival of patients with parenchymal cirrhosis ($n = 145$) according to the Pugh classification. ○, Pugh A ($n = 46$); □, Pugh B ($n = 59$); ●, Pugh C ($n = 40$)

In the prospective study, 166 other patients with parenchymal cirrhosis (60% of alcoholic origin) were studied. During the follow-up period, 50 patients with parenchymal cirrhosis were considered for liver transplantation; 21 were transplanted and 29 were turned down.

Statistical methods

In the first series of 91 patients with parenchymal cirrhosis, survival curves were analysed using the actuarial method of Mantel [11]. Variables that achieved statistical significance ($P < 0.01$) in univariate analysis using chi-squared tests were subsequently included in the multivariate analysis. Multivariate analysis of the prognostic variables mentioned above was performed using a stepwise logistic regression procedure [8].

From the regression equation, histograms of predicted probabilities of success were computed for each individual belonging either to the group 'successes' (alive at 1 year) or to the group 'failures' (dead at 1 year). From these histograms, a probability cut-off point could be selected to maximize the proportions of correctly predicted successes and failures. Such studies were carried out for mortality specifically related to liver disease (death due to hepatic failure or severe gastrointestinal bleeding).

Comparison of the discriminative effeciency of the logistic equations including either the best of our 18 variables [2] or the Pugh score was done using the same stepwise logistic regression procedure in terms of probability of correct classification, goodness of fit, accuracy of adjustment of the data to the model and receiver operating characteristic (ROC curves) [12]. The cut-off Pugh score separating patients alive and dead at 1 year was determined.

In the second series of patients, the percentage actuarial survival according to Pugh score (Child-Pugh A = score 5–6; Child-Pugh B = score 7–9; Child-Pugh C = score 10–15) was analysed. The percentage actuarial survival was calculated in this prospective series according to the best cut-off Pugh score and the cut-off point < 0.7 or > 0.7, both obtained in the first series of patients and derived from the logistic equations including as prognostic variables either the Pugh score or aminopyrine breath test result and degree of ascites.

Results

First series of patients with parenchymal cirrhosis

The logistic equation including the Pugh score as predictive parameter was:
$$\ln (p/1-p) = -0.939 (\pm 0.242) \times \text{Pughscore} + 9.332$$
Where ln denotes natural logarithm and p the cut-off point. The number in parentheses is the standard error of regression coefficients and 9.332 is a constant. Taking 0.75 as the cut-off point, the Pugh score obtained from this equation is 8.76, i.e. 9.

Comparison of this last equation with a previously published equation [2], including as predictive variables the aminopyrine breath test result and the degree of ascites, revealed for percentage correct prediction of death and survival at 1 year, goodness of fit and accuracy of adjustment (log likelihood) values of 92% vs 87%, 0.999 vs 0.459, and −34.904 to −17.250 vs −34.904 to −20.206, respectively.

The ROC curve of the two variables (aminopyrine breath test result and degree of ascites) was better than the ROC curve of the Pugh score (Fig. 1). For the same true positive of 90%, false positive would be 17% for the current model and 25% for the Pugh score.

Second series of patients with parenchymal cirrhosis

The percentage actuarial survival according to the Pugh score is depicted in Fig. 2. Actuarial survival at 12 and 24 months was 97% and 97% for Child-Pugh A, 72% and 65% for Child-Pugh B, 52% and 45% for Child-Pugh C. The percentage actuarial survival of patients with a Pugh score of 9 or more (which derives from the first study mentioned above) and equal to or less than 8 in comparison with percentage actuarial survival according to a p value < 0.7 or > 0.7 is represented in Fig. 3. Percentage survival at 12 and 30 months was, respectively, 88% and 84% for a Pugh score ≤ 8, 85% and 79% for a p value > 0.7, 40% and 33% for a Pugh score > 8 and 49% and 41% for a p value < 0.7. The percentage correct prediction of death and survival at 1 year was 77% for a Pugh score ≤ 8 or > 8 and 72% for a p value < 0.7 or > 0.7 in this prospective series of patients.

The Pugh score was calculated retrospectively for the 50 patients considered for liver transplantation. The

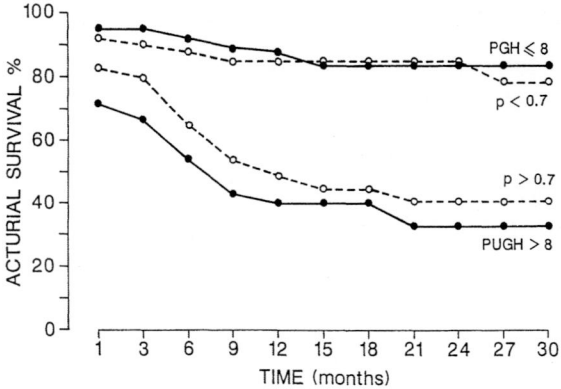

Fig. 3. Actuarial survival of patients with parenchymal cirrhosis (n = 145) according to Pugh score (≤ 8 or > 8) and cut-off point (< 0.7 or > 0.7) from the following equation: ln (p/1-p) = -1.95 ascites + 1.64 aminopyrine breath test $- 0.93$. This equation had a 91 % predictive value in the first series of patients [9]

29 patients turned down and the 21 transplant recipients had, respectively, during their work-up Pugh scores of 9.9 ± 1.6 and 9.5 ± 2.0 (mean $\pm$ standard deviation; $P > 0.05$). These two categories had, respectively, a 24-month actuarial survival of 60 % and 22 %.

Discussion

The prognostic model previously described by us [2], and including at presentation the two variables aminopyrine breath test result and degree of ascites, was compared with the well-establilshed prognostic indicator, the Pugh score.

In the first series of patients, which is in a way a retrospective study, the model with two variables was superior to the model including the Pugh score in terms of percentage correct prediction, goodness of fit, accuracy of adjustment and comparative ROC curves. However, the Pugh score was acceptable as it was correct in 87 % of cases. In the second series of patients studied prospectively, the excellent prognostic value of the Pugh score was validated.

We were mostly interested in trying to define the cut-off value of the Pugh score which best predicts those patients who will die of cirrhosis within 1 year. We propose that a Pugh score of 8 entirely fullfils this requirement. Indeed, this number was obtained from the prognostic equation including the Pugh score in the first series of patients and taking a cut-off point of 0.75 which best separated successes (patients alive at 1 year) and failures (patients dead at 1 year). Moreover the predictive value of a Pugh score of 8 was validated in the prospective study, being here even more efficient than the prognostic model including as variables aminopyrine breath test result and ascites. As emphasized by Wasson et al. [20], the accuracy of the prediction formula can differ in the initial study and in the test sample. This underlines [18] the importance of testing the prediction formula in another group of similar patients.

We conclude from our observations that a Pugh score of more than 8 is adequate for defining optimum time for liver transplantation and is as good as weights generated by a mathematical approach, and can be satisfactory for routine clinical practice. The potential value of a Pugh score of more than 8 as an index of a bad prognosis was further confirmed in a series of 50 patients considered by our group for liver transplantation on the basis of an intuitive combination of clinical and biochemical data suggesting imminent hepatic failure [18]. Retrospective estimation of the Pugh score disclosed that the mean value was more than 8 in both the group receiving transplants and the group turned down.

Estimation of the spontaneous prognosis of cirrhotic patients should improve in the future in terms of sensitivity and predictive value. We suggest that a Pugh score ≤ 8 or > 8 should be used as a reference standard when evaluating new prognostic tests or models. Repeated determination of the measurements, with multivariate analysis utilizing follow-up information to update prognosis, as proposed by Christensen et al. [6], would be a reasonable approach.

References

1. Adams RD, Foley JM (1949) Neurological changes in more common types of severe liver disease. Trans Am Neurol Assoc 74: 217–219
2. Adler M, Van Laethem J, Glibert A et al (1990) Factors influencing survival at one year in patients with nonbiliary hepatic parenchymal cirrhosis. Dig Dis Sci 35: 1–5
3. Albers I, Hartmann H, Bircher J, Creutzfeldt W (1989) Superiority of the Child-Pugh classification to quantitative liver function tests for assessing prognosis of liver cirrhosis. Scand J Gastroenterol 24: 269–276
4. Capone RR, Buhac I, Kohberger RC, Balint JA (1978) Resistant ascites in alcoholic liver cirrhosis. Course and prognosis. Dig Dis Sci 23: 867–871
5. Christensen E, Schlichting P, Fauerholdt L et al (1984) Pronostic value of Child-Turcotte criteria in medically treated cirrhosis. Hepatology 4: 430–435
6. Christensen E, Schlichting P et al (1986) Updating prognosis and therapeutic effect evaluation in cirrhosis with Cox's multiple regression model for time-dependent variables. Scand J Gastroenterol 21: 163–174
7. D'Amico G, Morabito A, Pagliaro L et al (1986) Survival and prognostic indicators in compensated and decompensated cirrhosis. Dig Dis Sci 31: 468–475
8. Dixon WJ (ed) (1983) BMDP statistical software. University of California Press, Berkeley, pp 330–344
9. Gines P, Quintero E, Arroyo V et al (1987) Compensated cirrhosis natural history and prognostic factors. Hepatology 7: 122–128
10. Lautz HU, Pichlmayr R (1989) Special aspects of timing of liver transplantation in patients with liver cirrhosis. Bailliéres Clin Gastroenterol 3: 743–756
11. Mantel N (1966) Evaluation of survival data and two rank order statistics arising in its consideration. Cancer Chemother Rep 50: 163–170
12. McNeil BJ, Keeler E, Adelstein J (1975) Primer on certain elements of medical decision making. New Engl J Med 293: 211–215
13. Merkel C, Bolognesi M et al (1991) Aminopyrine breath test improves prognostic ability of Pugh score in cirrhosis (abstract). J Hepatol 13 [Suppl 2]: 953

14. Poynard T, Zourabichvili O, Hilpert G et al (1984) Prognostic value of total serum bilirubin/glutamyl transpeptidase ratio in cirrhotic patients. Hepatology 4: 324–327

15. Pugh RNH, Murray-Lyon IM, Dawson JL, Pietroni MC, Williams R (1973) Transection of the oesophagus for bleeding varices. Br J Surg 60: 646–649

16. Saunders JB, Walters IRF, Davies P et al (1981) A 20-year prospective study of cirrhosis. Br Med J 282: 263–266

17. Schlichting P, Christensen E, Andersen PK et al (1983) Prognostic factors in cirrhosis identified by Cox's regression model. Hepatology 3: 889–895

18. Sherlock S (1984) Chronic hepatitis and cirrhosis. Hepatology 4: 255–285

19. Villeneuve JP, Infante-Rivard C, Ampelas M, Pornier-Layrag G, Huet PM, Marleau D (1986) Prognostic value of the aminopyrine breath test in cirrhotic patients. Hepatology 6: 928–931

20. Wasson JH, Cox HS, Neff RK (1985) Clinical prediction rules. Applications and methodological standards. New Engl J Med 313: 793–799

21. Wiesner RH (1990) Timing of liver transplantation in primary biliary cirrhosis and primary sclerosing cholangitis. AASLD Postgraduate course 225–245

Transplant Int (1992) 5 [Suppl 1]: S179–S184

TRANSPLANT
International
© Springer-Verlag 1992

Seroprevalence and outcome of hepatitis C in liver transplantation

L. M. Barkholt[1], M. von Sydow[2], L. Magnius[3], B.-G. Ericzon[1], B. Veress[4], and J. P. Andersson[5]

[1] Department of Transplantation Surgery, Huddinge Hospital, Karolinska Institute, Stockholm, Sweden
[2] Department of Virology, Central Microbiological Laboratory of Stockholm County, Stockholm, Sweden
[3] Department of Virology, National Bacteriological Laboratory, Stockholm, Sweden
[4] Department of Pathology, Huddinge Hospital, Karolinska Institute, Stockholm, Sweden
[5] Department of Infectious Diseases, Danderyd Hospital, Karolinska Institute, Stockholm, Sweden

Abstract. A recombinant enzyme-linked immunosorbent assay (ELISA) followed by a neutralization test (NT) and recombinant immunoblot assay (RIBA) were used for the detection of antibody to hepatitis C virus (anti-HCV) in 71 patients receiving 84 orthotopic liver grafts between 1984 and 1990. Before the liver transplantation (LTX) anti-HCV was present in six of the 71 recipients (8.5%) who were accepted for LTX because of acute or chronic liver failure. After LTX anti-HCV could not be detected in one of the patients, but it was continuously present in the others for more than 12 months. Detectable HCV antibodies were not present in the three patients who underwent LTX because of clinical evidence of fulminant NANB hepatitis. Two of 48 (4.2%) previously HCV seronegative recipients, who survived more than 3 months, seroconverted 9 and 16 months, respectively, after transplantation. The postoperative seroconversion was probably due to the transfer of virus via perioperative blood transfusions. Thus, these liver recipients may be able to respond by producing anti-HCV despite immunosuppressive therapy. None of the seven post-transplant HCV-seropositive patients developed symptoms such as icterus or fatigue, which would suggest the presence of liver insufficiency due to HCV infection. However, two of them had increased transaminase levels and histological signs of mild hepatitis. No significant difference was found in 1-year survival, prothrombin complex, albumin levels or the risk for retransplantation in post-transplant anti-HCV-seropositive patients, compared with those without detectable HCV antibodies (71% vs 69%, respectively). Thus, during the study period of 1–5 years, the clinical course of HCV infection was milder than that reported for hepatitis B infection in liver recipients.

Key words: Hepatitis C virus – Liver transplantation

Hepatitis C virus (HCV) is the predominant cause of transfusion-associated non-A, non-B (NANB) hepatitis [3] and may occur concomitantly with hepatitis B virus (HBV) infection [11, 14]. Approximately 50% of NANB virus-infected patients have biochemical evidence of chronic hepatitis and about 20% of these cases develop histological evidence of cirrhosis [1]. In addition, HCV may be involved in the multifactorial genesis of hepatocellular carcinoma [6, 10, 24].

Fulminant or subacute NANB hepatitis may be an indication for performing an acute liver transplantation (LTX) [7]. In the USA chronic NANB hepatitis is the fourth commonest reason for LTX (Starzl, CDC 1989). It is also conceivable that liver recipients may contract an HCV infection after LTX, which has to be taken into account when analysing pathological liver tests after transplantation. In this study recombinant enzyme-linked immunosorbent assays (ELISA) [18] and a neutralization test (NT) as well as a recombinant immuno-blot assay (RIBA) were used to detect antibodies to hepatitis C virus (anti-HCV). The aim of the study was to determine the occurrence of anti-HCV and to explore the role of HCV as a possible cause of the underlying liver disease as well as a cause of postoperative complications.

Materials and methods

Patients

Between November 1984 and July 1990 61 adults (18 to 61 years) and ten children (9 months to 14 years) received a total of 84 liver grafts and were followed for 1–5 years after LTX. The indication for LTX was chronic liver disease in 50 cases, acute and subacute liver failure in eight cases and primary liver malignancy in 13 cases (Table 1). Liver transplantations were performed orthotopically according to the technique described by Starzl et al [25]. The standard immunosuppressive therapy, as previously described [12], consisted of cyclosporin A (Sandoz Ltd, Basel, Switzerland) and prednisolone, until June 1988, when azathioprine (Wellcome, London, UK) was added to the prophylactic regimen. Acute rejection episodes were initially treated with steroids, but if ineffective, rabbit anti-thymocyte globulin (ATG, Fresenius, FRG) or mouse monoclonal antibody (OKT3, Ortho Pharmaceuticals, Raritan, N.J., USA) [12] were given as well.

Offprint requests to: L. M. Barkholt, M. D., Department of Transplantation Surgery, Huddinge Hospital, S-141 86 Huddinge, Sweden

Table 1. Indications for liver transplantation in 71 patients

Indication	Patients (n)
Chronic liver disease	50
Primary biliary cirrhosis	15
Sclerosing cholangitis	10
Posthepatic cirrhosis	6
Autoimmune chronic active hepatitis	5
Cryptogenic cirrhosis	4
Metabolic liver disease	6
Primary biliary atresia	4
Acute and subacute liver failure	8
NANB hepatitis	5
acute	3
subacute	2
Budd-Chiari	2
Toxic hepatic failure	1
Primary liver malignancy	13
Total	71

Serum samples

Serum samples were obtained from each patient before LTX, at 1 week, and 3, 6 and 12 months, and yearly, if possible, after LTX. Additional specimens were analysed if an unexplained elevation of transaminases occurred. Samples from all liver donors to recipients who seroconverted to HCV were available for testing and were kept frozen at $-20\,°C$.

A recombinant enzyme-linked immunosorbent assay (ELISA) (Ortho Diagnostic Systems, Raritan, N.J., USA, or Abbott Laboratories, North Chicago, Ill., USA) was used to detect antibodies to HCV. In addition, reactive samples were tested by a neutralization test, NT (Abbott), and by a recombinant immunoblot assay (RIBA) (Ortho Diagnostic Systems) which utilized four different recombinant HCV antigens (5-1-1, C 100-3, C 22, C 33), representing different structural and non-structural parts of the virus genome. The procedures were carried out according to the manufacturer's instructions. Reactive samples were retested and regarded as positive only if the duplicate test result was above the cut-off value recommended by the manufacturer and if the positive result could be confirmed by NT or RIBA. Information concerning blood transfusions and liver tests were collected from the patients' charts.

Liver biopsies

Liver biopsies were performed when the liver tests were abnormal, but usually to rule out a possible acute rejection. In addition, they were routinely obtained 1 year after LTX. The biopsies were fixed in 4% buffered formaldehyde for 3 h and embedded in paraffin. The sections were stained with haematoxylin-eosin, Ladewig's trichrome, PAS, Russian blue and reticulin.

Results

Prevalence of anti-HCV antibodies prior to liver transplantation

The occurrence of HCV antibodies before LTX and the data about blood transfusions in these liver recipients are shown in Table 2. Before LTX, anti-HCV was present in six of 71 recipients (8.5%). In addition, ELISA reactivity, which could not be confirmed by significant blocking in the neutralization assay, was detected in 10 patients with underlying liver diseases such as autoimmune chronic active hepatitis (CAH) ($n = 3$), primary biliary cirrhosis (PBC) ($n = 3$), post-hepatic cirrhosis (PHC) ($n = 2$), sclerosing cholangitis (SCA) ($n = 1$) or cholangiocarcinoma ($n = 1$). None of the three patients who received transplants because of clinical evidence of acute NANB hepatitis had detectable HCV antibodies.

Incidence of anti-HCV antibodies after liver engraftment

Among the six recipients who were HCV seropositive prior to LTX, two died of septicaemia within the first month. The patients with SCA, primary hyperoxalosis (PHO) and hepatoma (patients no. 2, 3 and 6) were repeatedly HCV seropositive during the follow-up of 1.5–2 years (Table 2). Only one of the six HCV-seropositive recipients had no detectable anti-HCV during the 12-month follow-up. Two liver recipients, one who received a transplant for SCA (no. 7) and the other for toxic liver

Table 2. The occurrence of anti-HCV antibodies in patients undergoing liver transplantation (LTX)

Patient no.	Diagnosis	Transfusions (units)		Anti-HCV antibodies					
		Pre-LTX	During LTX	Pre-LTX	Post-LTX				
					1 week	3 months	6 months	12 month	2 years
1	CAH	No	21	+	+	*			
2	SCA	Yes	12	+	+	+	+	+	+
3	PHO	Yes	9	+	+	+	+	+	+
4	NANB	Yes	I 8	+	+	re-tx			
			II 46	+	+	*			
5	PBC	No	13	+	−	−	−	−	
6	Hepatoma	Yes	12	+	+	+	+	+	
7	SCA	Yes	I 11	−	−	re-tx			
			II 15	−	−	−	−	+[a]	+
8	Tox. hep.	Yes	32	−	−	−	−	−	+[b]

[a, b] Seroconversion 9 and 16 months post-transplant, respectively
CAH, chronic active hepatitis
SCA, sclerosing cholangitis
PHO, primary hyperoxalosis
NANB, NANB hepatitis with cirrhosis

PBC, primary biliary cirrhosis
Tox. hep., toxic hepatic failure
*, patient with fatal outcome
re-tx, liver retransplantation

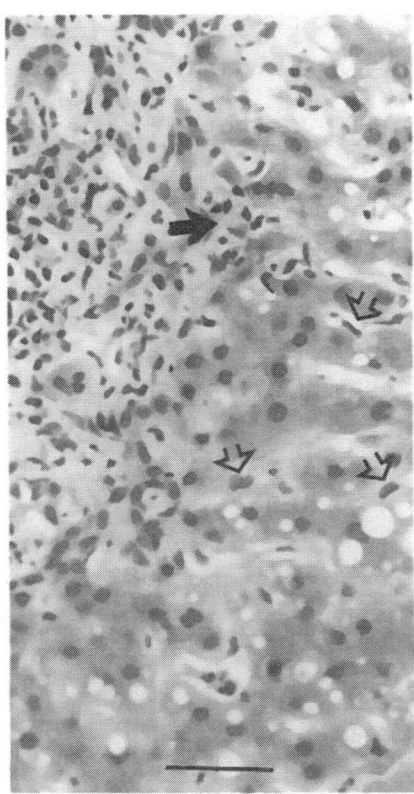

Fig. 1. Inflammatory infiltrate in the portal tract (left) and lymphocyte infiltration in the lobulus *(filled arrow)*. Note fatty changes in hepatocytes and hypertrophic Kupffer cells *(open arrows)*. Haematoxylin–eosin staining. Bar = 50 μm

failure (no. 8) seroconverted to HCV 9 and 16 months after LTX. They continued to be seropositive during the follow-up period of 4.5 and 2.5 years after LTX, respectively.

Clinical outcome in anti-HCV seropositive patients

Long-term follow-up was possible in four of six patients who were anti-HCV positive prior to LTX (Table 3). The patient with a hepatoma (no. 6) suffered from two early

episodes of acute rejection requiring treatment with OKT3. His cholestatic liver tests (total bilirubin 50–70 μmol/l, ALP 6–17 μkat/l) did not normalize, nor did his increased transaminase levels (ALAT 3–6 μkat/l, GGT 3–25 μkat/l). Radiological investigations ruled out vascular or biliary complications. His liver biopsies showed neither rejection nor recurrence of the malignancy after 6 months. Nevertheless, we found a moderate lymphocytic infiltrate within the slightly widened portal tracts. Lymphocytes were also infiltrating the periportal areas of the lobuli, resembling piecemeal necrosis. Furthermore, there was a mild fatty change in the hepatocytes which was accompanied by Kupffer cell hypertrophy (Fig. 1). These changes are consistent with or indicative of NANB hepatitis. Subjectively, he felt well 18 months after LTX. The patients with SCA. PHO and PBC (Nos. 2, 3 and 5) had an uncomplicated postoperative period. They did not receive blood transfusions after the perioperative period. They had normal liver tests and were doing well 1.5–2 years post-transplantation (Table 3).

Clinical outcome in patients with primary HCV infection after transplantation

The two patients who seroconverted to HCV after LTX had been followed at the time of writing for 4.5 and 2.5 years. The patient with SCA (no. 7) received another transplant on day 11 after severe, ATG-resistant rejection and a thrombosed portal vein. His transaminase levels fluctuated (ALAT 2–10 μkat/l, ALP 2.5–4.7 μkat/l) since the time of HCV seroconversion. No signs of rejection were noted in repeated liver biopsies, but mononuclear cells were seen in the sinusoids (Fig. 2 A). Focal cobblestone appearance, mild fatty changes in hepatocytes and single hepatocyte necrosis were also observed, as well as slight cholestasis and multinucleated hepatocytes (Fig. 2 B).

The second patient who received a transplant for toxic liver failure (no. 8) had an uneventful follow-up until 9 months after LTX. Elevated liver tests (ALAT 10 μkat/l, ALP 13 μkat/l) and a low cyclosporin A concentration

Table 3. Influence of HCV on liver function tests in HCV-infected liver transplant patients

Patient no.	Diagnosis	HCV antibodies			Liver test[a]			
		Pre-LTX	Post-LTX		Bil	ALAT	PK	ALB
			6–12 months	> 12 months				
1	CAH	+	*					
2	SCA	+	+	+	21	0.3	99	31
3	PHO	+	+	+	7	0.2	130	22
4	NANB I, II	+	*					
5	PBC	+	–	–	7	0.2	130	39
6	Hepatoma	+	+	+	50	3	130	37
7	SCA I, II	–	+	+	47	10	130	42
8	Tox. hep.	–	–	+	6	20	130	38

[a] At the time of seroconversion or 1 yr post-LTX
Normal values: bil, < 26 μmol/l; ALAT, < 0.7 μkat/l; PK, 70–130 %; ALB 23–42 g/l
CAH, chronic active hepatitis
SCA, sclerosing cholangitis

PHO, primary hyperoxalosis
NANB, non-A, non-B hepatitis
PBC, primary biliary cirrhosis
Tox. hep., toxic hepatic failure
*, patient with fatal outcome

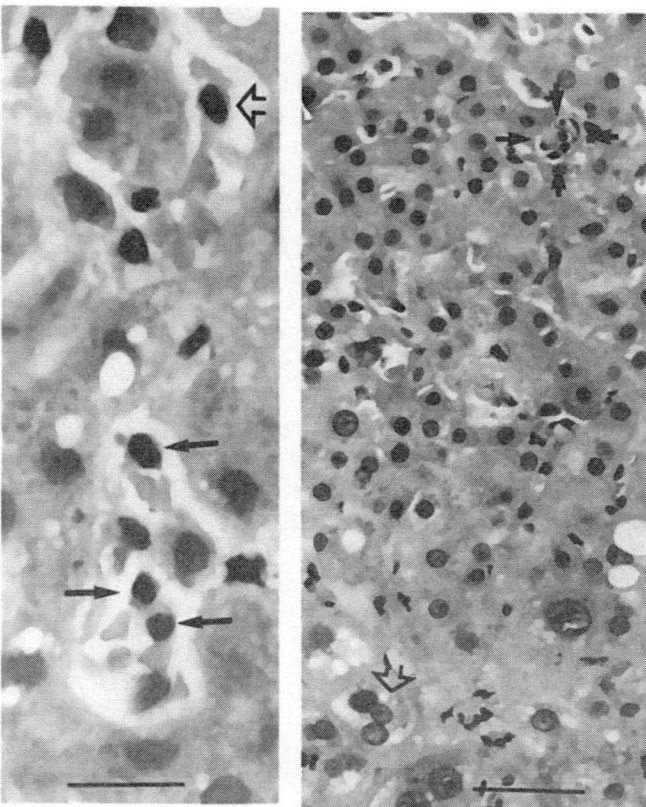

Fig. 2. A Lymphocytes within sinus *(thin arrows)* and hypertrophic Kupffer cell *(open arrow)*. Haematoxylin–eosin staining. Bar = 20 μm. **B** Hepatocyte necrosis *(filled arrows)*, fatty changes and multinucleated hepatocyte *(open arrow)*. Haematoxylin–eosin staining. Bar = 50 μm

were the indications for a liver biopsy which demonstrated signs of low-grade chronic rejection. After the administration of only 1 g of methylprednisolone as anti-rejection treatment the liver tests normalized. HCV seroconversion was detected 16 months after LTX. The patient had a second episode of increased transaminase levels (ALAT 20 μkat/l, ALP 26 μkat/l) 2 months previously. No biopsy was performed, as the ALAT decreased spontaneously within 3 days. His liver biopsy showed multiple foci of malignant changes 2 years after LTX, secondary to a previously diagnosed adenocarcinoma of the rectum, which subsequently led to his death (Table 3).

Patient survival

The blood levels of prothrombin complex (PK) and albumin were used to evaluate graft function. The albumin and PK levels in HCV-seropositive patients 1 year post-transplant, were 34.0 ± 7.8 g/l and 113 ± 27%, respectively. In the anti-HCV-negative patient group, albumin was 34.2 ± 7.9 g/l and PK was 90 ± 39%. Two of the seven patients (29%) with HCV antibodies after LTX received second transplants within the first year. One of them died of multiple organ failure and septicaemia. One additional patient died shortly after surgery because of septicaemia.

Thus, the patient survival for the anti-HCV-seropositive recipients was 71% (five of seven patients) in the first year. In comparison, nine retransplantations (14%) were performed during the first year in 64 post-transplant anti-HCV-seronegative patients, for reasons such as primary non-functioning graft, vascular thrombosis or severe rejection. The 1-year patient survival in this group was 69% (40/64 patients). These differences are not significant.

Epidemiology

Blood transfusions. Six of the eight patients with anti-HCV seropositivity after LTX received blood products before liver replacement (Table 2). One patient worked as a supervisor of drug addicts, and had even been bitten by one of them. In addition to plasma and other coagulation factors, the patients received 8–46 units of packed erythrocytes during the LTX. All of these patients received additional blood transfusions during the first 8 weeks after LTX. The two patients who were found to seroconvert 9 and 16 months after transplantation received no subsequent transfusions. All of the ten patients with a non-specific ELISA anti-HCV reactivity prior to LTX had also received blood transfusions before LTX. All the blood transfusions were given before we began to screen the blood units for anti-HCV.

Donors. Serum samples from three of seven liver donors to the six patients who were anti-HCV positive before LTX and from all three donors to the two recipients who seroconverted were available (two patients had second transplants). They were all anti-HCV negative.

Discussion

The previously obscure condition called NANB hepatitis has now been elucidated, first by the specific cloning of HCV [9] and then by the development of an ELISA to detect antibodies against a major gene product (C100-3) of this virus. In addition, recombinant immunoassays now utilize four antigens [27]. HCV-RNA can also be detected by the polymerase chain reaction [16], a technique not yet routinely available.

SCA, PBC and CAH are chronic liver diseases which are frequently found among candidates for LTX [26]. In these diseases blood transfusions are often required. Patients with SCA and PBC develop gastrointestinal varices which, in the long run, often bleed. The majority of our liver transplant recipients with diagnoses of SCA or PBC had a history of blood transfusions, but HCV antibodies were found in only two of them prior to LTX. Blood transfusions are also assumed to be the primary route of infection for anti-HCV-seropositive patients with CAH, especially when associated with HBV infection [8], but sexual transmission may also occur [2]. In this study, the only one of the six recipients with post-hepatic cirrhosis who was HCV seropositive before LTX had a history of possible blood contact after being bitten by a drug addict.

The patient with subacute NANB hepatitis and a positive anti-HCV prior to LTX had received blood transfusions 20 years before when she delivered a baby. The patient with PHO had also been given several blood transfusions when undergoing haemodialysis 5 years pre-LTX.

The increased incidence of HCV seropositivity in patients with primary liver malignancy has aroused the suspicion that HCV is one of the multifactorial causes [6, 10, 24]. This would be in accordance with the pretransplant HCV seropositivity in our patient with hepatoma.

Fulminant NANB hepatitis is a predominant indication for an acute LTX [7]. Because of the fulminant course (< 8 weeks) these patients may not have had time to produce specific antibodies against HCV prior to LTX. This would accord with the reported mean interval of 15 weeks from the onset of hepatitis to anti-HCV seroconversion [3] which might explain the seronegativity in our three patients with acute liver replacement for clinical evidence of NANB hepatitis. The same authors [7] also noted a mean delay of 22 weeks for seroconversion after blood transfusions and that some patients showed fluctuations in the anti-HCV titre and even became seronegative [3]. Moreover, a liver recipient's NANB hepatitis may have been caused by a second NANB agent [4,20,28] or may have represented a cryptic form of hepatitis B infection in which serological markers are absent [5]. It is also possible that the patient was misdiagnosed as having NANB hepatitis but in fact had a non-viral hepatocellular inflammation.

Seroconversion from HCV negativity prior to LTX to seropositivity may be caused by virus transmission by the transplanted organ or by perioperative blood transfusions. None of the donors to our patients who became seropositive after LTX had detectable HCV antibodies. Therefore, blood transfusions remain the most likely source. In Scandinavia around 0.5 % of blood donors have proved to be anti-HCV seropositive (Dr A. Lindholm, personal communication), which is still a considerable risk. The seroconversion in two patients, 9 and 16 months post-LTX, agrees with reports from other LTX centres [15, 21], but occurs later than in non-immunocompromised patients (12–22 weeks), according to studies of post-transfusion NANB hepatitis [3, 13]. Two patients continued to be seropositive after LTX and had normal liver tests (Tables 2 and 3). Another patient, who was also HCV seropositive before LTX, had a primary HCV infection in the graft as judged by changes in the liver biopsy and by persistent slightly pathological liver tests, at the time of a recurrence of seropositivity (Fig. 1). A similar low-grade effect of an HCV infection in LTX recipients was reported by Read et al [22]. The last pre-LTX seropositive patients who received transplants because of PHC and known NANB hepatitis had been followed for too short a time (1 month) to determine the effect on the graft. The patients who had a primary HCV infection concomitantly had increased transaminase levels at the time of seroconversion.

Unlike HBV infection in the liver graft, HCV infection did not cause severe liver degenerative disease, a finding also reported by others [17, 22]. Furthermore, HCV seemed not to influence graft function in the patients when liver function tests and the frequency of retransplantations were taken into account.

False positive reactivity in anti-HCV ELISA tests was found particularly among samples drawn before LTX. It has previously been shown that patients having autoimmune CAH with high serum immunoglobulin levels may react in a non-specific way in anti-HCV ELISA tests [23], a finding also made in this study. Furthermore, it has been demonstrated that disease activity and immunoglobulin levels in patients with autoimmune CAH are correlated to the reactivity in the anti-C-100-3 region of HCV [19]. Our patients were probably in such a condition when accepted as candidates for LTX.

We conclude that the introduction of anti-HCV testing of blood and organ donors should reduce the risk of hepatitis caused by HCV. In liver tansplant patients such testing should be helpful for distinguishing hepatic inflammation from rejection. In view of the limited size of our sample, seropositivity to HCV does not preclude LTX. However, this point should be re-evaluated by the addition of HCV-RNA assay, which should show the true incidence of HCV in this patient population.

Acknowledgements. Ms. Helene Norder, Berit Hammas, Ulla Magnusson and Pia Andersson are thanked for their skilful technical assistance and Dr. Zoe Walsh and F. P. Walsh for the revision of the language.

References

1. Alter HJ (1989) Chronic consequences of non A-non B hepatitis. In: Seeff LB, Lewis JH (eds) Current perspectives in hepatology. Plenum Medical, New York, pp 83–97
2. Alter MJ, Coleman PJ, Alexander WJ, Kramer E, Miller JK, Mandel E, Hadler SC, Margolis HS (1989) Importance of heterosexual activity in the transmission of hepatitis B and nonA, nonB hepatitis. JAMA 262: 1201–1205
3. Alter HJ, Purcell RH, Shih JW, Melpolder JC, Houghton M, Choo Q-L, Kuo G (1989) Detection of antibody to hepatitis virus in prospectively followed transfusion recipients with acute and chronic nonA-nonB hepatitis. N Engl J Med 321: 1494–1500
4. Bradley DW, Maynard JE, Popper H et al (1983) Posttransfusion non-A, non-B hepatitis: physicochemical properties of two distinct agents. J Infect Dis 148: 254–265
5. Brechot C, Degos F, Lugassy C et al (1985) Hepatitis B virus DNA in patients with chronic liver disease and negative tests for hepatitis B surface antigen. N Engl J Med 312: 270–276
6. Bruix J, Barrera JM, Calvet X, Ercilla G, Costa J, Sanchez-Tapias JM, Ventura M, Vall M, Bruguera M, Bru C, Castillo R, Rodes J (1989) Prevalence of antibodies to hepatitis C virus in Spanish patients with hepatocellular carcinoma and hepatic cirrhosis. Lancet II: 100
7. Chapman RW, Forman D, Peto R, Smallwood (1990) Liver transplantation for acute hepatic failure? Lancet I: 32–35
8. Chiaramonte M, Ngatchu T, Stroffolini T, Rapicetta M, Chionne P, Lantum D Comparison between HBV and HCV infection in a high risk population. The British Society of Gastroenterology A262.
9. Choo Q-L, Kuo G, Weiner AJ, Overby LR, Bradley DW, Houghton M (1989) Isolation of a cDNA clone derived from a blood-borne nonA, nonB viral hepatitis genome. Science 244: 359–362
10. Colombo M, Kuo G, Choo QL (1989) Prevalence of antibodies to hepatitis C virus in Italian patients with hepatocellular carcinoma. Lancet II: 1006–1008

11. Colombo M, Rumi MG, Donato MF, Marcelli R, De Fillippi F, Del Ninno E (1989) Hepatitis C virus infection is frequent in patients with cryptogenic cirrhosis (abstract in topic III). First International Meeting on Hepatitis C, Rome

12. Ericzon B-G, Eusufzai S, Kubota K, Einarsson, Angelin B (1990) Characteristics of biliary lipid metabolism after liver transplantation. Hepatology 5: 1222–1228

13. Farci P, Alter HJ, Wong D, Miller RH, Shis JW, Jett B, Purcell RH (1991) A long-term study of hepatitis C virus replication in non-A, non-B hepatitis. N Engl J Med 325: 98–104

14. Fattovich G, Tagger A, Brollo L, Pontisso P, Realdi G, Ferroni P, Alberti A (1989) Liver disease in anti-HBe positive chronic HBsAg carriers and hepatitis C virus. Lancet II: 797–798

15. Franza A, Miguet JP, Bresson-Hadni S, Coaquette A, Lab M, Njoya O, Vanhems P, Becker MC, Rouget C, Mantion G, Gillet M (1991) Prevalence of hepatitis C virus antibodies in orthotopic liver transplantation: A sequential study of 72 patients. Transplant Proc 23: 1506

16. Garson JA, Tedder RS, Briggs M, Tuke P, Glazebrook JA, Trute A, Parker D, Barbara JAJ, Contreras M, Aloysius S (1990) Detecton of hepatitis C viral sequences in blood donations by 'nested' polymerase chain reaction and prediction of infectivity. Lancet 335: 1419–1422

17. Grendele M, Gridelli B, Colledan M, Rossi G, Fassati LR, Ferla G, Lunghi G, Galmarini D (1989) Hepatitis C virus infection and liver transplantation. Lancet 1221–1222

18. Kuo G, Choo QL, Alter HJ et al (1989) An assay for circulating antibodies to a major etiological virus of human nonA, nonB hepatitis. Science 244: 362–364

19. McFarlane I, Smith H, Johnson P, Bray G, Vergani, Williams R (1990) Hepatitis C virus antibodies in chronic active hepatitis: pathogenetic factor or false-positive result? Lancet 335: 754–757

20. Mosley JW, Redeker AG, Feinstone SM, Purcell RH (1977) Multiple hepatitis virus in multiple attacks of acute viral hepatitis. N Engl J Med 296: 75–78

21. Potterucha JJ, Rakela J, Ludwig J, Taswell HF, Wiesner RH (1991) Hepatitis C antibodies in patients with chronic hepatitis of unknown etiology after orthotopic liver transplantation. Transplant Proc 23: 1495–1497

22. Read AE, Donegan E, Lake J, Ferrell L, Galbraith C, Kuramoto IK, Zeldis JB, Ascher NL, Roberts J, Wright TL (1991) Hepatitis C in liver transplant recipients. Transplant Proc 23: 1504–1505

23. Schwarcz R, von Sydow M, Weiland O (1991) Positive reactivity with anti-HCV ELISA in patients with autoimmune hepatitis – not confirmed with a neutralization test. Scand J Infect Dis 23: 127–128

24. Simonetti RG, Cottone M, Craxi A, Pagliaro L, Rapicetta M, Chionne P, Costantino A (1989) Prevalence of antibodies to hepatitis C virus in hepatocellular carcinoma. Lancet II: 1338

25. Starzl TE, Iwatsuki S, Esquivek CO, Todo S, Kam I, Lynch S, Gordon RD, Shaw BW Jr (1985) Refinements in the surgical technique of liver transplantation. Semin Liver Dis 5: 349–356

26. Starzl TE, Demetris DA, van Thiel D (1989) Liver transplantation. N Engl J Med 1014–1022

27. van der Poel CL, Cuypers HT, Reesink HW, Weiner AJ, Quan S, di Nello R, van Boven JJP, Winkel I, Mulder-Folkerts D, Exel-Oehlers PJ, Schaasberg W, Leentvaar-Kuypers A, Polito A, Houghton M, Lelie P (1991) Confirmation of hepatitis C virus infection by new four-antigen recombinant immunoblot assay. Lancet 337: 317–319

28. Yoshizawa H, Itoh Y, Iwakiri S et al (1981) Demonstration of two different types of non-A, non-B hepatitis by reinjection and cross-challenge studies in chimpanzees. Gastroenterology 81: 107–113

Transplant Int (1992) 5 [Suppl 1]: S 185–S 186

TRANSPLANT
International
© Springer-Verlag 1992

Somatomedin C (IGF I) plasma levels after orthotopic liver transplantation (OLT) in end-stage cirrhotic patients

A. Corti[1], A. De Gasperi[1], G. Oppizzi[2], E. Pannacciulli[1], A. Cristalli[1], G. Fantini[1], E. Mazza[1], M. Prosperi[1], A. Rocchini[1], D. Sabbadini[1], C. Savi[1], A. Scaiola[1], S. Vai[1], F. Romani[3], L. DeCarlis[3], and G. F. Rondinara[3]

Departments of [1] Anaesthesia, [2] Endocrinology and [3] Liver Transplantation, Ospedale Niguarda Ca'Granda, Milano, Italy

Insulin-like growth factors [IGF I and II or somatomedins (SMS)] are polypeptides chemically and biologically correlated with insulin. The main source of synthetic activity and secretion is the liver, although many other tissues have been demonstrated to synthesize SMS [5]. In the circulation, they are not present in a free form, but are mostly bound to a specific carrier protein independently synthesized in the liver. Hepatic or extrahepatic storage organs have not been demonstrated; the half life of the SMS–binding protein complex is between 3 and 4 [1]. Synthesis of SMS is regulated by GH, insulin, thyroxine and nutrition (caloric and protein intake, and nitrogen balance). The role of corticosteroids is still a matter of debate: in patients treated with steroids SMS blood levels have been shown to be within normal limits, while biological activity has been demonstrated to be significantly reduced by SMS inhibitors, probably induced by corticosteroid therapy [2].

The biological properties of SMS are related to their structural homology with insulin, and can be summarized as follows [5]:

A. Insulin-like activity (glucose oxidation, lipogenesis, glycogen synthesis, inhibition of lipolysis and glycogenolysis)
B. Sulphation activity (incorporation of sulphate and leucine into glycosaminglycans of the cartilage)
C. Stimulation of fibroblast multiplication
D. Amplification of other hormone activities (GH)
E. Complementary anabolic activity with insulin.

Low levels of SMS have been demonstrated in hypopituitarism (secondary) or in other diseases independent of GH reduced secretion (primary) such as malnutrition, malabsorption, acute or chronic liver failure and uraemia [2]. Negative nitrogen balance, hypocaloric and/or low protein diets are usually correlated with low levels of SMS. Recently, Schalch et al. reported on the role of or-

thotopic liver transplantation (OLT) in normalizing SMS blood levels in a group of end-stage liver diseased patients [3].

This preliminary paper deals with changes in IGF-I plasma levels (somatomedin C) in a group of patients affected by end-stage liver cirrhosis before and after OLT.

Key words: Liver transplantation – Somatomedin

Patients and methods

Ten patients (eight male, two female) suffering from end-stage post-necrotic cirrhosis and candidates for OLT comprised the study population. Mean age was 42 ± 11 years. Child's classification was B in six and C four patients.

Standard surgical and anaesthetic techniques and a venovenous bypass during the anhepatic phase were used in all the recipients.

Standard immunosuppression included 1 g Solumedrol after reperfusion of the liver and, in the postoperative period, rapidly tapered steroids, RATG (2 mg/kg body weight) for the first 8–10 days, azathioprine (1.5 mg/kg body weight) and cyclosporine.

From day 2 after OLT, nutritional intake included 30 kcal/kg per day and 0.25 g nitrogen/kg body weight. An RIA method (Nichols Institute, San Juan, Calif.) was used to measure IGF-I: normal values in our laboratory are between 0.7 and 2.2 U/ml. Arterial blood samples were drawn from 4 to 6 h before induction of anaesthesia (baseline) and on days 1, 3, 5, 8, 10, 15 and 18 after OLT. The blood samples were stored and retrospectively analysed. Data are reported as mean $\pm$ SD. Student's t-test was used to compare the means. Linear regression analysis was applied to paired data of daily SMS blood levels, daily dosage of steroids, daily caloric intake, daily nitrogen balance, prothrombin time (expressed as percent of normal) and daily bile flow to calculate correlation coefficients. $P \leq 0.05$ was considered significant.

Results

IGF-I plasma levels before OLT were very low $(0.6 \pm 0.4$ U/ml). In six patients mean blood levels were 0.34 ± 0.12 (range 0.22–0.44) U/ml, while in the remaining four patients the levels were within the normal range

---

Offprint requests to: Andrea De Gasperi, II Servizio di Anestesia, Ospedale Niguarda Ca' Granda, Piazza Ospedale Maggiore, 3, Milano, Italy

Table 1. Means ± SD of somatomedin (SMS) blood levels, prothrombin time (PT) and bile flow during the studied period

	SMS (U/ml)	PT (%)	Bile flow (ml/day
baseline	0.6 ± 0.4	50 ± 11	160 ± 189
Day 1	0.9 ± 0.4	61 ± 22	210 ± 166
Day 3	1 ± 0.5'	71 ± 23	180 ± 170
Day 5	1.4 ± 0.9*	71 ± 18*	240 ± 190
Day 7	1.7 ± 0.9**	81 ± 15***	300 ± 175
Day 8	2 ± 0.9**	84 ± 13***	365 ± 100
Day 10	2.2 ± 0.8***	85 ± 25***	430 ± 50
Day 15	1.7 ± 0.8**	81 ± 17***	
Day 18	2.4 ± 1.5***	86 ± 16***	

$^*P \le 0.05$, $^{**}P \le 0.01$, $^{***}P \le 0.001$ vs baseline

(0.8 ± 0.4 U/ml). This profile closely reflected preoperative hepatic function tests which defined Child–Pugh scores for each patient.

Compared with preoperative values (baseline), IGF-I blood levels began to rise significantly 5 days after OLT ($P \le 0.05$ vs baseline), and peaked on the 8th day ($P \le 0.01$ vs baseline). All the patients had normal IGF-I blood levels 15 days after OLT ($P \le 0.01$ vs baseline). At follow-up 1 month later normal SMS blood levels were found in three patients.

The rise in IGF-I blood levels was found to be independent of standard immunosuppressive steroid therapy, dietary intake, insulin supplementation and nitrogen balance. A direct correlation was found between the rate of rise in SMS blood levels and prothrombin time ($r = 0.94$, $P \le 0.001$) from the first day after OLT and bile flow ($r = 0.94$, $P \le 0.005$).

Discussion

Chronic liver diseases are usually associated with decreased levels of SMS, the synthesis of which, is markedly reduced in end-stage hepatic failure. These changes have been demonstrated to be closely correlated with the severity of the liver pathology [4]. In a recent report by Schalch et al. [3], OLT restored normal levels of IGF-I in patients affected by acute or chronic hepatic failure, indicating a possible role of liver transplantation in curing growth retardation in children suffering from chronic hepatic diseases.

In our series of adult patients affected by end-stage postnecrotic cirrhosis admitted to OLT and all with successful transplants, IGF-I blood levels were restored to normal levels within a few days after surgery, giving further confirmation to the data reported by Schalch. Rapid restoration of SMS seems to be related to the very early recovery of synthetic capacity of the newly grafted liver, as

demonstrated by the close correlation with prothrombin time.

Fresh frozen plasma (FFP) has been demonstrated to be virtually IGF-I free (personal, unpublished observation). Since in the early postoperative period FFP is often liberally administered, PT values could be influenced by FFP supplementation, while IGF-I levels should specifically reflect the synthetic capacity of the transplanted liver.

Nutritional intake, exogenous insulin administration and positive nitrogen balance, together with GH and thyroxine, have been demonstrated to promote hepatic synthesis and secretion of IGF-I, while malnutrition, malabsorbtion and negative nitrogen balance have been reported to be accompanied by a reduced level of IGF-I [2]. In our series of patients the increase and normalization in IGF-I blood levels were present in spite of the negative nitrogen balance recorded during the first 5 days after OLT, thus reinforcing the central role played by the restored synthetic capacities of the new liver.

Steroid therapy has been reported to interfere with IGF-I: 66% decreased activity was observed in renal transplanted patients while on steroids [2]. Inhibitors of IGF-I activity were demonstrated to double during steroid therapy, while IGF-I circulating levels were found to be unchanged. The authors stated that steroid therapy was able to induce circulating inhibitors, while IGF-I synthesis was not altered. Since in our study only IGF-I plasma blood levels were measured, the only conclusion we can draw is that the rapidly tapered steroid therapy administered to our patients did not influence either IGF-I synthesis or secretion.

In conclusion IGF-I plasma levels were rapidly restored to normal levels in end-stage cirrhotic patients a few days after OLT. The measurement of IGF-I plasma levels could represent a specific and sensitive indicator of the synthetic capacities of the newly grafted liver. Further studies are needed to define the IGF-I profile during primary non-function and rejection and the possible correlations with the compromised function. In this case retrospective analysis, as performed in this study, is the major drawback.

References

1. Barreca A, Minuto F (1989) J Endocrinol Invest 12
2. Phillips LS, Unterman TG (1984) Clin Endocrinol Metab 13: 145–189
3. Schalch D, Kalayoglu M, Yang H et al (1989) (abstract 1021). Proceedings of 71st Annual Meeting of the Endocrine Society. Seattle
4. Takano K, Hizuka N, Shizume K et al (1977) J Clin Endocrinol Metab 48: 371–376
5. Zapf J, Schmidt CH, Froesh ER (1984) Clin Endocrinol Metab 13: 3–30

Transplant Int (1992) 5 [Suppl 1]: S187–S189

TRANSPLANT
International
© Springer-Verlag 1992

Adjuvant treatment with ursodeoxycholic acid reduces acute rejection after liver transplantation

S. Friman, H. Persson, T. Scherstén, J. Svanvik, I. Karlberg

Transplant Unit, Department of Surgery, Sahlgrenska Hospital, University of Gothenburg, Gothenburg, Sweden

Abstract. Acute rejection, occurring with a reported frequency of 50–70%, is still a dominating problem after liver transplantation. Medication with ursodeoxycholic acid (UDCA) has beneficial effects in different cholestatic conditions and has also been shown to reduce HLA class I antigen expression on hepatocytes in patients with PBC. Since August 1989 we have consecutively treated all patients with primary graft function with UDCA ($n = 41$). Patients transplanted in the first half of 1989 served as a control group ($n = 8$). All patients in this study were given sequential quadruple drug immunosuppression. The treatment group were given oral UDCA 10 mg/kg per day. During the first postoperative month, 17% of the UDCA-treated patients had an episode of acute rejection compared with 75% of the control patients ($P < 0.01$). Liver biochemistry tests 1 month postoperatively were significantly better in patients treated with UDCA. The results suggest that adjuvant treatment with UDCA reduces acute liver graft rejection.

Key words: Ursodeoxycholic acid – Liver – Liver transplantation – Rejection – Immunosuppression

---

Acute rejection is reported to occur in 50–70% of patients receiving liver transplants. Although this is no longer the most frequent cause of death, acute rejection is still a major problem in liver transplant surgery [3, 9, 10, 21]. Ursodeoxycholic acid (UDCA) has been used in the medical treatment of cholesterol gallstone disease, and beneficial effects of treatment with UDCA in different cholestatic liver diseases such as primary biliary cirrhosis, sclerosing cholangitis, chronic hepatitis and biliary atresia have recently been reported [6, 12, 15–18, 22]. The rationale for using UDCA treatment after liver transplantation was to substitute for more toxic bile acids and alter the bile

acid pool to a more atoxic composition, as liver transplantation can be associated with problems due to a number of reasons such as graft dysfunction and drug toxicity.

Materials and methods

Patients

All patients with primary graft function transplanted between August 1989 and June 1991 ($n = 41$) were treated with ursodeoxycholic acid. The mean age was 47 ± 2 years and the distribution of preoperative diagnosis is listed in Table 1. Patients transplanted during the first half of 1989 ($n = 8$) served as a control group. The mean age of the control group was 42 ± 2 years. During this period three patients were lost during or immediately after surgery. These patients did not receive bile acid treatment and are not included in this report.

Operative procedure

All donor livers were harvested in a similar manner using UW solution. No venovenous bypass was used. The median anhepatic time in the control group was 55 min (range 45–75 min) and in the UDCA group, 40 min (range 31–65 min). Perioperative blood loss was comparable, with a median transfusion of 10 units (400 ml) of blood (range 5–80 units) in the control group and a median of 9 units (range 1–41 units) in the UDCA group.

Immunosuppression

Four out of 41 (10%) of the UDCA-treated patients and one out of eight (13%) of the control patients had a positive T-cell cross-match. All patients received blood-group-compatible grafts, eight patients in the UDCA group (19%) received non-blood-group-identical grafts compared with two patients in the control group (25%). All patients received sequential quadruple drug immunosuppression with anti-thymocyte globulin (Mérieux), azathioprine (Imurel, Wellcome) and steroids. Cyclosporine (Sandimmun, Sandoz) was given orally only and was started when the renal function was stable, usually on the 5th to the 7th postoperative day.

UDCA treatment

UDCA treatment was started as soon as possible, usually on the first or second postoperative day and in all cases within the first 5 days. The patients received UDCA (URSOFALK, Falk Co, FRG) orally

---

Offprint requests to: Styrbjörn Friman, M.D., Ph.D., Transplant Unit, Department of Surgery, Sahlgrenska Hospital, S-413 45 Göteborg, Sweden.

Table 1. Preoperative diagnosis in the liver transplanted patients

Diagnosis	Control (n = 8)	UDCA (n = 41)
Advanced chronic liver disease	5	30
Metabolic liver disease		2
Tumour	2	4
Acute fulminant hepatic failure	1	5

Table 2. Liver biochemistry 1 month following orthotopic liver transplantation

	AST (μkat/l)	ALT (μkat/l)	ALP (μkat/l)	Bilirubin (μmol/l)
Control (n = 8)	1.3 ± 0.3	1.9 ± 0.4	12.7 ± 3.0	86 ± 34
UDCA (n = 41)	0.7 ± 0.1**	0.9 ± 0.2*	6.1 ± 0.7**	40 ± 9

* $P < 0.05$; ** $P < 0.01$
AST, asparagine aminotransferase; ALT, alanine aminotransferase; ALP, alkaline phosphatase

at a dose of 10 mg/kg per day. In most cases UDCA was dissolved and given through the patients' nasogastric tube the first postoperative days.

The rejection diagnosis was based on the clinical course and biochemistry in combination with histopathological examination of biopsies in all cases given antirejection treatment.

Results

In the group treated with UDCA, seven patients had a least one episode of acute rejection (17%). In the control group, six out of eight patients (75%) had at least one rejection episode needing treatment during the first postoperative month. The rejection incidence was significantly lower in the UDCA-treated group ($P < 0.01$; Fisher's exact test) (Fig. 1). Biochemistry 1 month after transplantation demonstrated significantly lower average values of aminotransferases and alkaline phosphatases ($P < 0.05$, ANOVA) in patients treated with UDCA than in the control group (Table 2).

At the time of writing the observation time was a median of 12 months (range 4–24) in the treatment group and 24 months (range 3–30 months) in the control group.

In the control group one patient was lost after 9 months due to chronic graft dysfunction and one patient died after 3 months from graft rejection, CMV pneumonitis and fungal septicaemia. In the UDCA-treated group four patients were lost. One patient died after 1 year with infectious complications, one patient died after 5 months due to chronic rejection and one patient due to recurrent hepatocellular carcinoma. The fourth patient died following retransplantation for acute rejection. This patient was early in the series and UDCA treatment was not started until the 5th postoperative day and an acute rejection was diagnosed on the 6th postoperative day.

Discussion

In this study we report a reduced frequency of acute rejection in 41 consecutive liver transplant recipients treated with adjuvant UDCA compared with numbers given in the literature and to a preceding group of eight liver transplant patients. The difference between our groups cannot be explained by improved surgical technique or by differences in immunosuppression protocol since these were not changed during 1989 or later.

UDCA was first discovered in the beginning of this century in bile from a polar bear. This bile acid normally appears in small amounts in the bile acid pool of man. UDCA was first synthesized in Japan in the 1950s and was there used for treatment of different cholestatic conditions, like chronic hepatitis [8]. This atoxic bile acid has also been used to dissolve cholesterol gallstones [14]. In recent years, reports of a beneficial effect of this bile acid on different cholestatic conditions have been frequent [6, 12, 15–18, 22]. UDCA has also been shown to have a direct protective effect on hepatocytes [5, 7]. The rationale for using UDCA after liver transplantation was to substitute for more toxic bile acids and alter the bile acid pool into a more atoxic composition. This would protect the hepatocytes from toxic effects of other bile acids in cases of cholestasis. It has previously been shown that with this treatment, UDCA becomes the dominant bile acid with a proportion of 40–60% [2, 13]. UDCA has also a high choleretic potency, which could be of importance especially during the first weeks postoperatively when bile acid treatment would initiate bile secretion [4, 20].

In a recent retrospective report, however, an Italian group did not see any effect on the rejection frequency following UDCA treatment, but they did not start treatment until the 5th to the 7th postoperative day and since acute rejection probably starts during the first postoperative week, it is important to start treatment on the first postoperative day [19]. This is further supported by treatment failure in one of our patients where treatment was started on the 5th postoperative day.

In a recent study Calmus et al. have shown that treatment with UDCA reduces HLA class I antigen expression on hepatocytes in patients with PBC [1]. Preliminary data from a German group also studying PBC patients confirm the immunomodulating capacity of this bile acid and they found a reduction of HLA class I/II antigen expression on bile duct cells [11]. The ability of this bile acid to alter this antigen expression in these patients may indicate that it also has the potency to alter antigen expression in liver-grafted patients. The reduced rejection frequency seen in the present series may be explained on these grounds. The findings warrant controlled clinical trials as well as studies to analyse the underlying mechanisms.

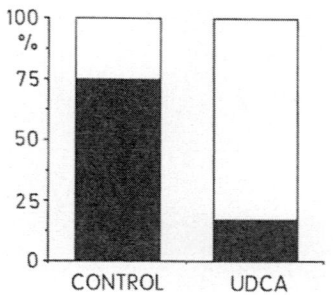

Fig. 1.

Acknowledgements. This study was supported by grants from the Medical Faculty University of Gothenburg, the Swedish Medical Society and Gothenburg Medical Society.

References

1. Calmus Y, Gane P, Rouger P, Poupon R (1990) Hepatic expression of class I and class II major histocompatibility complex molecules in primary biliary cirrhosis: Effect of ursodeoxycholic acid. Hepatology 11: 12–15
2. Chretien Y, Poupon R, Gherardt MF, Chazouilleres O, Labbe D, Myara A, Trivin F (1989) Bile acid glycine and taurine conjugates in serum of patients with primary biliary cirrhosis: effect of ursodeoxycholic acid. Gut 30: 1110–1115
3. Cuervas-Mons V, Martinez AJ, Dekker A et al (1986) Adult liver transplantation: an analysis of the early courses of death in 40 consecutive cases. Hepatology 125: 161–172
4. Dumont M, Uchman S, Erlinger S (1980) Hypercholeresis induced by ursodeoxycholic acid and 7-ketolithocholic acid in the rat: possible role of bicarbonate transport. Gastroenterology 79: 82–89
5. Galle PR, Theilmann L, Raedsch R, Otto G, Stiehl A (1990) Ursodeoxycholate reduces hepatotoxicity of bile salts in primary human hepatocytes. Hepatology 12: 486–491
6. Ghezzi C, Zuin M, Battezzati PM, Podda M (1987) Effects of ursodeoxycholate, taurine and ursodeoxycholate plus taurine on serum enzyme levels in patients with chronic hepatitis. Hepatology 17: 1110
7. Heumann DM, Komito SF, Pandak WM, Hylemon PB, Vlahcevic ZR (1989) Tauroursodeoxycholic acid protects against cholestatic and hepatocytolytic toxicity of more hydrophobic bile salts. Gastroenterology 96: A 607
8. Ichida F (1961) Clinical experience with ursodeoxycholic acid for chronic hepatitis. Diagn Treat 36: 388
9. Kirby RM, McMaster P, Clements D, Hubscher SG, Angrsami L, Sealey M, Gunson BK, Salt PJ, Buckels JAC, Adams DH, Jurewicz WAJ, Jain AB, Elias E (1987) Orthotopic liver transplantation: Postoperative complications and their management. Br J Surg 74: 3–11
10. Klintmalm GBG, Nery JR, Husberg BS, Gonwa TA, Tillery GW (1989) Rejection in liver transplantation. Hepatology 10: 978–985
11. Leuschner U, Dieues HP, Güldütuna S, Birkenfeld G, Leuschner M (1990) Ursodeoxycholic acid (UDCA) influences immune parameters in patients with primary biliary cirrhosis (PBC). Hepatology 12: 957
12. Leuschner U, Fischer H, Kurtz W, Gulduna S, Hubner K, Hellstern A, Gatzen M, Leuschner M Ursodeoxycholic acid in primary biliary cirrhosis, results of a controlled double-blind trial. Gastroenterology 97: 1268–1274
13. Makino I, Nakagawa S (1978) Changes in biliary lipid and biliary bile acid composition in patients after administration of ursodeoxycholic acid. J Lipid Res 19: 723–728
14. Nakagawa S, Makino I, Ishizaki T, Dohi I (1977) Dissolution of cholesterol gallstones by ursodeoxycholic acid. Lancet II: 367–369
15. O'Brien C, Senior JR, Batta AK et al (1989) Ursodeoxycholic acid treatment produces marked clinical and biochemical amelioration of primary sclerosing cholangitis. Gastroenterology 96: 640
16. Podda M, Ghezzi C, Battezzati PM, Bertolini E, Crosignani A, Petroni ML, Zuin M (1989) Effect of different doses of ursodeoxycholic acid in chronic liver disease. Dig Dis Sci 34 [Suppl]: 59–65
17. Poupon R, Chretien Y, Poupon RE, Ballet F, Calmus Y, Darnis F (1987) Is ursodeoxycholic acid an effective treatment for primary biliary cirrhosis? Lancet I: 834–836
18. Poupon RE, Balbou B, Eschwege E, Poupon R (1991) A multicenter controlled trial of ursodiol for the treatment of primary biliary cirrhosis. New Engl J Med 324: 548–554
19. Sama C, Mazziotti A, Grigioni W, Morselli AM, Chianura A, Stefanini GF, Barbara L, Gozetti G (1991) Ursodeoxycholic acid administration does not prevent rejection after OLT. J Hepatol 13 [Suppl 2]: 68
20. Scherstén T, Linblad L (1979) Biliary cholesterol output during ursodeoxycholic acid secretion in man. In: Paumgartner G, Stiehl A, Gerok W (eds) Biological effects of bile acids. MTP Press, Lancaster
21. Starzl TE, Koep LJ, Halgrimson CG, Hord J, Schroter GP, Porter KA, Weil III R (1979) Fifteen years of clinical liver transplantation. Gastroenterology 77: 375–388
22. Ullrich D, Rating D, Schröter W, Hanefeld F, Bircher J (1987) Treatment with ursodeoxycholic acid renders children with biliary atresia suitable for liver transplantation. Lancet II: 1324

Transplant Int (1992) 5 [Suppl 1]: S 190–S 192

TRANSPLANT
International
© Springer-Verlag 1992

Cholestasis and kidney dysfunction in liver transplant patients reduces cyclosporine metabolite excretion

A. Tötterman, M. Lalla, K. Salmela, and K. Höckerstedt

Fourth Department of Surgery, University of Helsinki, Helsinki, Finland

Cyclosporin A (CsA) is metabolized principally by the hepatic cytochrome P 450-dependent microsomal enzyme system and eliminated virtually entirely as metabolites, mainly in the bile [1, 4, 6]. Only less than 1 % of the oral dose is excreted unmetabolized in the urine or bile [5, 7]. Metabolites account for 50–70 % of the total CsA in whole blood [3, 5, 8]. Some of the metabolites have been shown to possess an immunosuppressive and even toxic effect but the role of this effect remains uncertain [2, 9].

In order to evaluate the effect of liver and kidney failure on the metabolism of CsA, we studied twelve patients who had undergone liver transplantation. The samples were collected during the first 4 postoperative weeks.

The aim of the study was threefold: to evaluate (1) whether an impairment of liver function, as measured by standard biochemical liver function tests, decreased the metabolism or excretion of CsA; (2) whether an induction of either the CsA metabolites or the parent compound took place in the first postoperative period; and (3) whether kidney failure, as measured by serum creatinine, correlated with blood levels of CsA or its metabolites.

Key words: Liver transplantation – Cyclosporine – Cholestasis – Kidney dysfunction

Patients and methods

Between August 1989 and January 1991 blood samples from twelve adult patients who had undergone liver transplantation in the Fourth Department of Surgery, University of Helsinki, were studied retrospectively. Samples taken during the first four postoperative weeks were included. The patients comprised eight women (age range 38–65, mean 50 years) and four men (42–62 years, mean 53.5 years). The indications for liver transplantation in the recipients were primary biliary cirrhosis ($n = 6$), sclerosing cholangitis ($n = 2$), liver cancer

Offprint requests to: K. Höckerstedt, M.D., Fourth Department of Surgery, University of Helsinki, Kasarmikatu 11, SF-00130 Helsinki, Finland

($n = 2$), chronic active hepatitis ($n = 1$) and polycystic liver disease ($n = 1$).

Whole-blood CsA was measured with two test, a polyclonal FPIA using polyclonal antibody (polyclonal FPIA, TDx, Abbott) and a radioimmunoassay using a monoclonal specific antibody (SRIA, Sandoz), the latter being more specific for the parent compound. These results (FPIA, $n = 87$; SRIA, $n = 101$) were correlated with standard biochemical liver function tests (s-ASAT, s-ALAT, s-ALP, s-albumin, s-GT, s-bilirubin and plasma thromboplastin time) and with renal function as measured by serum creatinine.

During the follow-up period, nine patients suffered an episode of acute rejection. Five of the patients had a slight rejection, three had a moderate rejection and one had a severe rejection. Rejection was determined by the clinical picture, biochemical parameters and biopsy findings, and treated predominantly with an increase in corticosteroid dose. None of the patients died during the observation period.

In the postoperative period all patients received as immunosuppressive treatment a combination of methylprednisolone, azathioprine and CsA. CsA was administered as a continuous IV dose for 2 weeks postoperatively commencing on the first postoperative day in a dose starting at 1 mg/kg per day and titrated to maintain blood levels at 600 ng/ml measured by RIA. The drug was continued orally when absorption was stabilized. Results are given as the ratio between CsA blood level and CsA dose (mg).

All correlations were calculated with the use of a simple regression analysis, the confidence interval being 95 %.

Results

Neither liver synthesizing capacity, as measured by s-albumin and s-thromboplastin time, nor hepatic cellular injury, as measured by s-ASAT, s-ALAT, and s-GT, showed any significant correlation with blood CsA levels.

With increasing values of s-BIL, blood levels of CsA (FPIA)/CsA input showed a statistically significant rise ($r = 0.631, P = 0.0001$) whereas the change in blood CsA (RIA)/CsA input-levels were not significant ($r = 0.271, P = 0.0477$). There was a positive correlation between s-bilirubin and blood CsA (FPIA)/CsA input ($r = 0.611, P = 0.0001$), a correlation which was not seen with blood CsA (RIA)/CsA input ($r = 0.244, P = 0.084$). S-ALP did not correlate clearly with blood CsA levels.

In the follow-up period there was no statistically significant correlation between blood CsA/CsA input, as

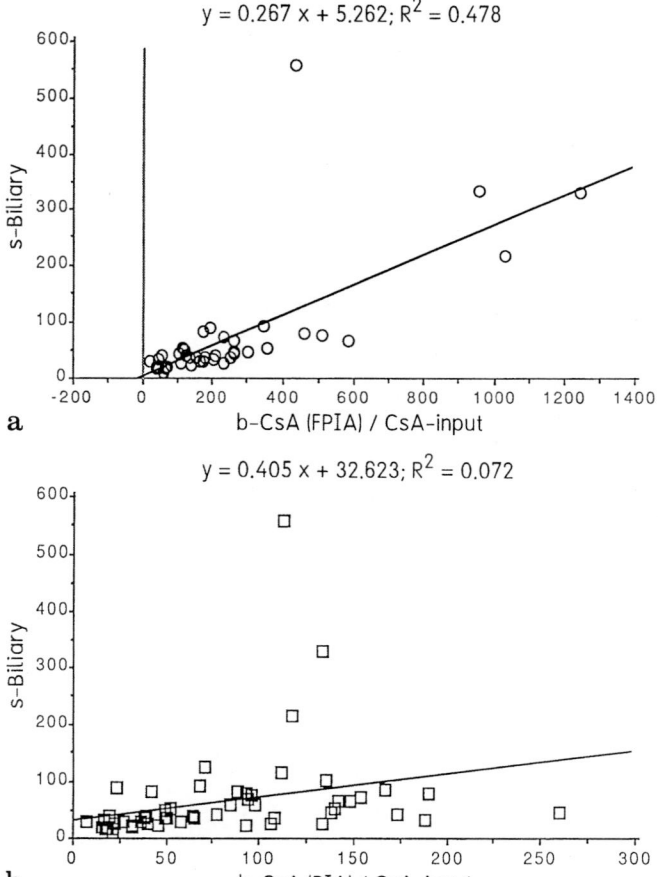

$y = 0.267 x + 5.262; R^2 = 0.478$

$y = 0.405 x + 32.623; R^2 = 0.072$

Fig. 1. a Correlation between serum bilirubin and blood CsA (FPIA)/CsA input. **b** Correlation between serum bilirubin and blood CsA (RIA)/CsA input

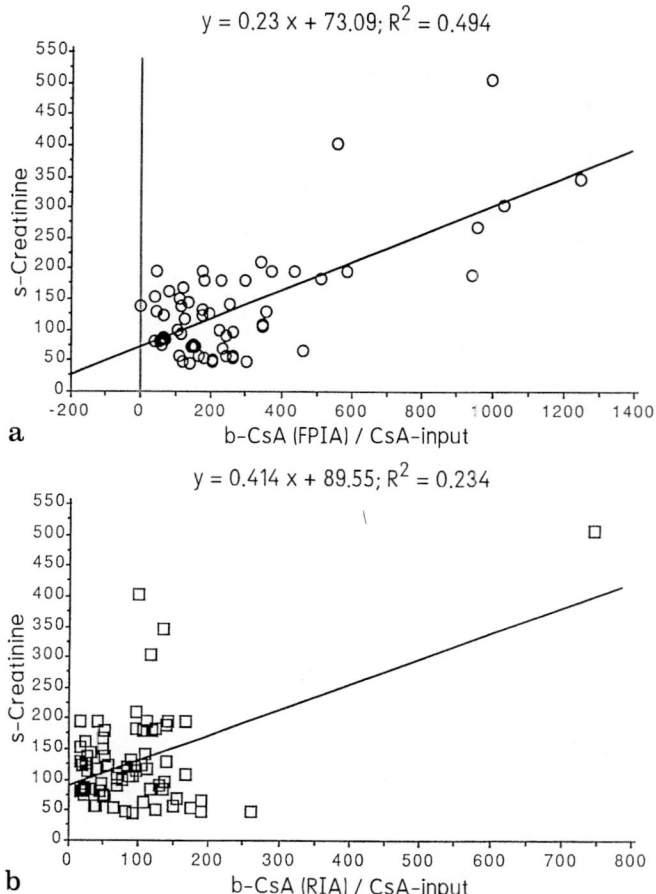

$y = 0.23 x + 73.09; R^2 = 0.494$

$y = 0.414 x + 89.55; R^2 = 0.234$

Fig. 2. a Correlation between serum creatinine and blood CsA (FPIA)/CsA input. **b** Correlation between serum creatinine and blood CsA (FPIA)/CsA-input

measured with either test, and the duration of medication.

With increasing values of serum creatinine, levels of both blood CsA (FPIA)/CsA input and blood CsA (RIA)/CsA input rose significantly, implying a decrease in excretion of both the parent compound and metabolites with renal failure. The correlation was seen both with the FPIA values ($r = 0.7$, $P = 0.0001$) and with the RIA values ($r = 0.48, P = 0.0001$).

Conclusions

The following conclusions were drawn on the assumption that the FPIA test was more specific for measuring whole blood CsA metabolites, whereas the RIA was more specific for blood levels of the parent compound.

This study did not show any correlation with impaired liver cell function and blood levels of CsA or its metabolites. Thus, an impairment in liver function did not decrease the transformation of CsA to its metabolites. Neither was there any reduction in CsA elimination in liver failure, except in cholestasis. With increasing cholestasis we saw a rise in blood levels of especially the CsA metabolites. The concentration of the CsA parent compound was not increased. This implies that cholestasis influences, in particular, the excretion of the CsA metabolites. However, a toxic effect of CsA or its metabolites on the bile

duct system resulting in cholestasis, as seen in cholestasis liver failure, cannot be ruled out.

Short-term administration of CsA did not significantly increase absorption of the drug, in contrast to long-term administration [2].

Despite minor excretion of CsA through the kidneys, we found increasing blood levels of both CsA and its metabolites in kidney dysfunction. CsA is known to be nephrotoxic, thus high blood CsA levels leading to kidney failure cannot be ruled out as an explanation of the correlation.

As further knowledge of the role of the CsA metabolites is gained, the significance of the reduced excretion of CsA in kidney failure and cholestasis will become apparent, and the need for separate blood level monitoring of the metabolites for improved CsA dose adjustment will become necessary.

References

1. Berthallet-Peres P, Bonfils C, Fabre G, Just S, Cano J-P, Maurel P (1987) Metabolism of cyclosporin A. II. Implication of the macrolide antibiotic inductible cytochrome P 45 3c from rabbit liver microsomes. Drug Metab Dispos 15: 391–398
2. Kahan BD (1989) Cyclosporine. N Engl J Med 321: 1725–1738
3. Lensmeyer G, Wiebe D, Carlson I (1988) Deposition of nine metabolites of cyclosporin in human tissues, bile, urine and whole blood. Transplant Proc 20 [Suppl 2]: 614–622

S192

4. Mauer G (1985) Metabolism of cyclosporine. Transplant Proc 17 [Suppl 1]: 19–26
5. Mauer G, Lemaine M (1986) Biotransformation and distribution in blood of cyclosporine and its metabolites. Transplant Proc 18 [Suppl 5]: 25–34
6. Shaw LM (1989) Advances in cyclosporine pharmacology, measurement and therapeutic monitoring. Cl Chemin 85: 1299–1308
7. Venkataramanan R, Starzl TE, Yang S, Burckart GJ, Platchcinski RJ, Shaw BW, Iwatsuki S, van Thiel DH, Sanhui A, Seltman H (1985) Biliary excretion of cyclosporine in liver transplanted patients. Transplant Proc 17: 286–289
8. Wagner O, Scheier E, Heitz F, Maurer G (1987) Tissue distribution, disposition, and metabolism of cyclosporine in rats. Drug Metab Dispos 15: 377–383
9. Yee GC, McGuire TR (1990) Pharmacokinetic drug interactions with cyclosporin (Part I). Clin Pharmacokinet 19: 319–332

Transplant Int (1992) 5 [Suppl 1]: S 193–S 195

TRANSPLANT
International
© Springer-Verlag 1992

Choledochoenterostomy with an anti-reflux mechanism

F. Veiga Fernandes, J. Coutinho, M. P. Henriques, B. da Silva, A. Baptista, A. I. Santos, and F. Godinho

Lisbon Faculty of Medicine, Lisbon, Portugal

Abstract. A new technique of choledochoenterostomy was devised to solve some of the problems of enterobiliary anastomosis with a normal calibre. The distal extremity of the common bile duct is completely surrounded by the bowel mucosa to a length of 3 cm after seromyectomy of a bowel wall rectangle of 4×1 cm. Experimental studies in rats and dogs demonstrated that this procedure prevents the risks of anastomotic disruption and functions like a mechanical unidirectional valve, which has great efficacy in stopping enterobiliary reflux. Studies in ten patients with obstructive jaundice with an extrahepatic biliary dilation less than 1.2 cm diameter submitted to this procedure confirmed the experimental results. All patients were asymptomatic, without jaundice and with normalization of the liver enzymes after 2 months. The permeability of the valvular anastomosis studied by cholangiography, the HIDA ^{99m}Tc test and manometry was quite similar to other classical biliary–enteric anastomosis. In contrast, anti-reflux efficacy was only demonstrated in patients with a valvular anastomosis.

Key words: Choledochoenterostomy – Biliary reconstruction – Liver transplantation

A new technique of choledochoenterostomy was devised in which a unidirectional mechanical valve was created to prevent ascending cholangitis and to protect the anastomosis. This valve was devised to solve the well – known problems of enterobiliary sutures on extrahepatic biliary trees with a normal calibre, as happens in liver transplantation.

Surgical technique

The technique is based on two main steps: a mucomucosal biliary–jejunal anastomosis and complete protection of the distal common bile duct by the external layer of the intestinal mucosa (Fig. 1).

The bowel is prepared by stripping away a 4-cm long rectangle of the seromuscular wall with the width equal to the diameter of the common bile duct (1 cm or less). The separation of the seromuscular layer from the mucosa is facilitated by injecting small amounts of saline solution into the seromuscular plane. The hypervascularized and surplus mucosa bulging through this uncovered rectangle will accept 4–6 cm of the distal biliary tree. The anastomosis between the common bile duct and the bowel is performed 1–2 cm away from the shorter distal side of the rectangle, using three or four interrupted stitches of absorbable material. The longitudinal edges of the seromuscular rectangle are sutured over the common bile duct, which finally remains completely covered by the external layer of the bowel mucosa.

Materials and methods

The surgical technique was first performed on rats which were sacrified 1–2 months after surgery. The morphology of the area involving the biliary enteric anastomosis and the liver was checked and recorded. Samples were collected for microscopic examination.

Surgery was also performed on six dogs which were sacrified between the first and fourth month after surgery. Specimens were collected for histology. Special studies of microcirculation were performed by injecting a blue methylene dye or micropaque material through the common hepatic artery and the superior mesenteric artery. Blood samples were obtained twice a week for bilirubin, alkaline phosphatase, gamma-glutamyl transpeptidase, SGOT, and SGPT, until complete normalization of all parameters was found.

The continent choledochoenterostomy was then performed on ten patients with obstructive jaundice of various causes: five patients with pancreatic adenocarcinoma, one with adenocarcinoma of the Oddi, one with chronic pancreatitis, and three with lithiasis of the main biliary tree. The common bile duct was less than 1.2 cm in diameter in all the patients. A choledochojejunostomy was performed in six of the patients, choledochoduodenostomy in three and cysticjejunostomy in one.

The permeability and functioning of the common bile duct were studied by cholangiography, the HIDA ^{99m}Tc test and manometry, making use of the T tube positioned above the anastomosis. The

---

Offprint requests to: F. Veiga Fernandes, M.D., Lisbon Faculty of Medicine, Avenida do Brasil 200 – 7° Dt°, 1700 Lisbon, Portugal

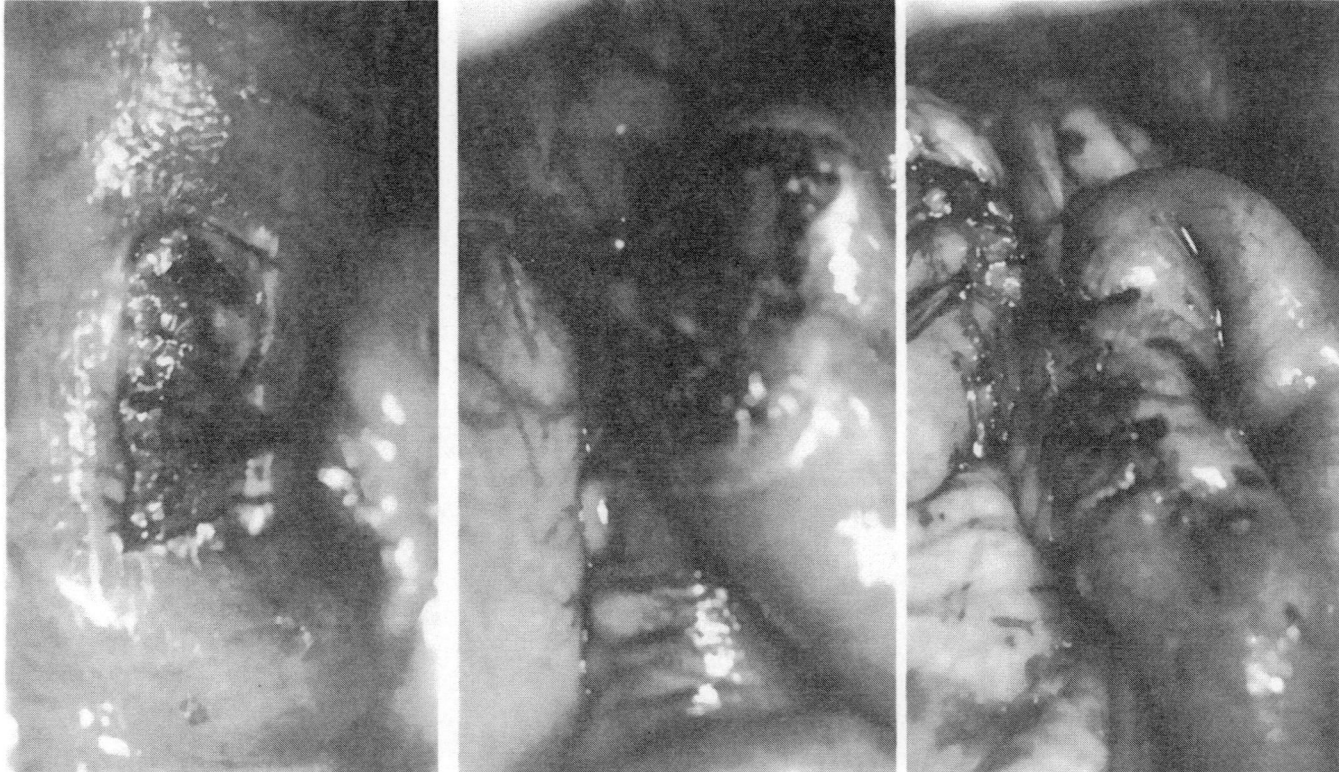

Fig. 1. The main phases of the surgical technique

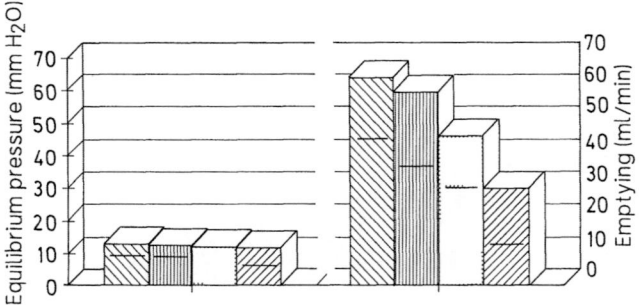

Fig. 2. Values of manometry (equilibrium pressure) and biliary flow of a saline solution in ml/min. Comparison between the valvular anastomosis and other classical types of biliary surgery. ▧ , Valvular anastomosis; ▥ , Choledochojejunostomy; ▦ , Choledochoduodenostomy; ▨ Common duct T tube

anti-reflux capacity of the mechanical valve was tested in the immediate postoperative period using a gamma camera and a sulphur colloid solution of technetium introduced into the Roux-en-Y loop (seven patients) or into the stomach with a liquid meal in three patients with a choledochoduodenostomy. Results were compared with six classical choledochoduodenostomies, six end-to-end choledochojejunostomies and nine cholecystectomized patients with common bile duct exploration (T tube).

Results

Experimental studies

Experimental studies on rats and dogs demonstrated that at 3 months, the common bile duct had adopted a morphology similar to the normal distal choledochus at the intra-duodenal portion, ending in the lumen of the gut with a prominence identical to a normal Vater's papilla. Not one case of choledochoenterostomy disruption was detected. Values of alkaline phosphatase and gamma-glutamyl transpeptidase returned to normal 1–3 weeks after surgery.

Histopathological studies reveal a good parietal vascularization of the common bile duct, with minimum inflammatory cell infiltration, without signs of fibrosis and with a discrete atrophy of the mucosa.

Clinical studies

All patients were asymptomatic, without jaundice and with normalization of liver enzymes (SGOT, SGPT and alkaline phosphatase) 1 month after removal of the T tube.

The basal manometric pressure (equilibrium pressure for the valvular anastomosis, 12.8 ± 2.9 mm) was identical to the values obtained in patients who had undergone different types of biliary surgery (Fig. 2). The emptying of ^{99m}Tc through the common bile duct, and the flow of a saline solution measured in mililiters per minute, with the reservoir positioned 30 cm above the level of the biliary tree $T^{1}/_{2} = 63.4 \pm 19.3$ ml/min), were not significantly different from the same parameters measured after classical choledochoduodenostomy ($T^{1}/_{2} = 44.2 \pm 15.1$ ml/min, $P > 0.1$) or choledochojejunostomy ($T^{1}/_{2} = 56.7 \pm 22.4$ ml/min, $P > 0.1$), but were slightly higher than those obtained in common bile ducts with a T tube $P < 0.05$).

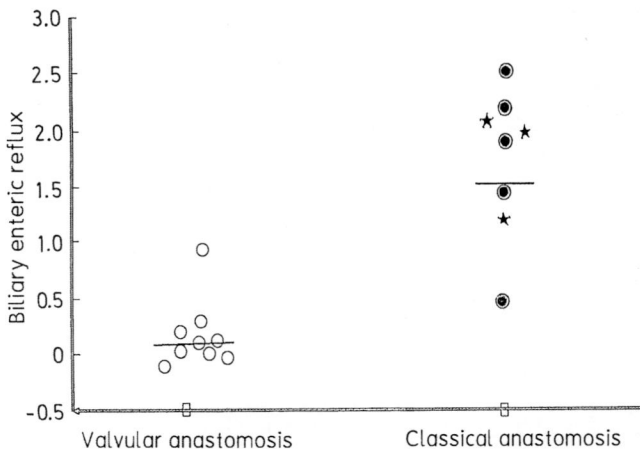

Fig.3. Comparative values of biliary enteric reflux index between the valvular anastomosis (O) and the classical choledochojejunostomy (five patients, ●) and choledochoduodenostomy (three patients, * $P = 0.001$

An anti-reflux efficacy was demonstrated in more than 85 % of the patients, which contrasted with classical biliary-enteric anastomosis patients (Fig.3).

Discussion and conclusions

Direct duct-to-duct biliary anastomosis over a T tube, or Roux-en-Y choledochojejunostomy over an internal stent are the most common types of biliary reconstruction in liver transplantation. A significant percentage of postoperative morbidity and mortality has been related to these types of solution. Biliary tract complications have been considered responsible for technical complications in between 2 % and 35 % of all cases [1–3]. The main causes of biliary reconstruction failures are immediate disruption of the anastomosis and late stenosis of the extrahepatic biliary duct. To obviate some of these problems a new technique of choledochoenterostomy was devised based on the same principles adopted to obtain other kinds of organic mechanical anti-reflux valves.

Experimental studies on rats and dogs demonstrated that the new technique had the following advantages: (1) it prevented the common tendency of biliary anastomotic disruption involving common bile ducts of normal calibre; and (2) the hypervascularized mucosa avoided the risk of fibrotic stricture of the distal choledochus and inhibited the dilation of the proximal biliary tree. The intraluminal passage of the choledochus through the bowel wall caused a very effective enterobiliary anti-reflux effect without biliary obstruction, as was demonstrated in human studies. The choledochoenterostomy surrounded by the mucosa of the bowel functioned as an unobstructed and efficient Nissen fundoplication or a continent ureterocystostomy.

The fundoplication of the mucosa around the common bile duct protected the biliary tree against ascending infection due to the biliary enteric reflux and simultaneously reduced the risk of dehiscence and stricture of the enterobiliary anastomosis. In our opinion, this solution should be recommended in liver transplantation to solve the problems connected with anastomosis performed on common bile ducts of normal calibre.

References

1. Bismuth H, Castaing D, Ericzon BG, Otte JB, Rolles K, Ringe B, Sloof M (1987) Hepatic transplantation in Europe. First report of the European liver transplant registry. Lancet
2. Calne R (1987) Liver transplantation. The Cambridge Kings College Hospital experience. Grune & Stratton
3. Gordon RD, Inatarki S, Esquivel CO, Makowka L, Tzakis A, Todo S, Starzl TE (1988) Liver transplantation. In: Cerilli GJ (ed) Organ transplantation and replacement. JB-Lippincott

Transplant Int (1992) 5 [Suppl 1]: S196–S197

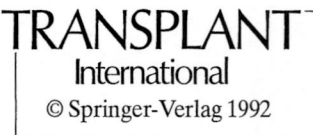

TRANSPLANT
International
© Springer-Verlag 1992

Liver transplantation in hepatocellular carcinoma

E. Jaurrieta, J. Fabregat, J. Figueras, R. Bella, P. Moreno-Llorente, A. Rafecas, J. Torras, T. Casanovas, and L. Casais

Liver Transplant Unit, Hospital de Bellvitge, University of Barcelona, Barcelona, Spain

Abstract. The initial enthusiasm for orthotopic liver transplantation (OLT) in patients with hepatocellular carcinoma (HCC) soon vanished as early recurrences appeared [3, 5, 6]. OLT in HCC remains a controversial issue. We evaluated the efficacy of preoperative studies to select No–Mo patients and determined whether pT stage and histopathological grade (G) have a prognostic significance. A group of 25 patients, all previously thoroughly studied to rule out extrahepatic disease, underwent OLT for HCC. All patients were pNo after pathological study and none of the six patients who died in the postoperative period showed extrahepatic dissemination at necropsy (pMo). The recurrence rate was 43%. The 2 and 5 years actuarial survival was 62% and 43% respectively. The pT and G were not prognostic factors for long-term survival. We think that HCC is still a good indication for OLT because almost 50% of patients have good survival prospects.

Key words: Liver transplantation – Hepatocellular carcinoma – Histopathological staging

Hepatocellular carcinoma (HCC) is one of the liver diseases for which orthotopic liver transplantation (OLT) is indicated. The results reported until now show that the long-term survival is very poor because of a high recurrence rate of the tumour. In order to diminish the recurrence rate after OLT the selection of patients with HCC must be very strict.

The aim of our study was to evaluate the efficacy of pretransplant screening to select patients without locoregional lymph nodes or distant metastases (No-Mo) and to determine whether the T stage and histopathological grade (G) have prognostic significance in long-term survival.

Offprint requests to: E. Jaurrieta, Liver Transplant Unit, Hospital de Bellvitge, University of Barcelona, Feixa Llarga s/n 08907 L'Hospitalet de Llobregat, Barcelona, Spain

Materials and methods

Between February 1984 and December 1990 a total of 25 patients with HCC underwent OLT. The patients' ages ranged from 28 to 64 years (mean, 51.5 years). There were 17 males and 8 females. In screening for extrahepatic spread, ultrasonographic examination of the upper abdomen, CT scan of the thorax, abdomen and cranium and radioisotope bone scanning were carried out routinely. In addition, 22 patients had an exploratory mini-laparotomy. All specimens taken from excised livers were evaluated microscopically to obtain a pathological classification in accordance with the (p)TNM. There were no incidental malignancies.

Results

All the 25 patients were No after pathological study. Six patients died during the postoperative pariod (five of them before 1987) and there was no evidence of tumour at necropsy (Mo). The 2- and 5-year actuarial survival of the 19 patients surviving the postoperative period was 62% and 46%, respectively (Fig. 1), and the recurrence rate was 43%. Of these 19 patients, 13 received transplants more than 24 months previously and were therefore a suitable group for the determination of long-term prognosis. The other six patients with a follow-up between 10 and 16 months were alive without recurrence at the time of writing.

Seven of the group of 13 patients died within 14 months (range 3–14) of OLT; all with tumour recurrence (group I). The other six patients lived for more than 24 months, one of whom died without tumour recurrence at 30 months and the others being alive between 25 and 85 months, with a mean of 48 months (group II).

The pT and histopathological grade (G) were similar in both groups. Group I ($n = 7$): five T4, one T3 and one T2, and five G2 and two G1. Group II ($n = 6$): five T4 and one T3, and two G3, two G2 and 2 G1.

Discussion

The effort to perform liver transplantation for HCC has generally met with failure. However, occasional patients have had long-term survival and perhaps cure [3, 5, 6]. A

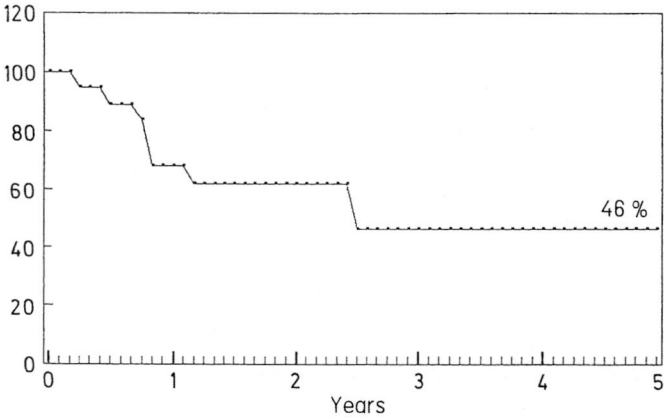

Fig. 1. Actuarial survival curve excluding operative mortality

thorough screening to detect locoregional or distant metastases is necessary. In agreement with Krom et al. [4] and Calne et al. [2], we even perform a laparotomy before liver transplantation to rule out extrahepatic tumour spread. Our pretransplant screening seems to be adequate to select pNo-Mo patients. The recurrence rate was 43%, below that reported by other groups [3, 5]. However, Bis-

muth et al. [1] have reported a very low recurrence rate (10%), probably due to preoperative chemoembolization and the fact that in their series there were smaller and incidental tumours. In our series, pT was not a significant prognostic factor for long-term survival; more cases may be necessary to obtain conclusive results.

In our experience the HCC No-Mo and 'any T' is a good indication for OLT because almost 50% of these patients were long-term survivors.

References

1. Bismuth H, Adam R, Castaign D, Chiche L, Ceriello A (1989) Results of liver transplantation in hepatocellular carcinoma. Proceedings of the Meeting of the E. S. O. T, Barcelona
2. Calne R, Williams R, Rolles K (1986) Liver transplantation in the adult. World J Surg 10: 422–431
3. Iwatsuki S, Gordon R, Shaw B, Starzl TE (1985) Role of liver transplantation in cancer therapy. Ann Surg 202: 401–407
4. Krom RAF, Gips GH, Houthoff HJ (1984) Orthotopic liver transplantation in Groningen, The Netherlands (1979–1983). Hepatology 4: 61S–65S
5. O'Grady J, Polson R, Rolles K, Calne R, Williams R (1988) Liver transplantation for malignant disease. Ann Surg 207: 373–379
6. Ringe B, Wittekind C, Bechstein W, Bunzendahl H, Pichlmayr R (1989) The role of liver transplantation in hepatobiliary malignancy. Ann Surg 209: 88–98

Transplant Int (1992) 5 [Suppl 1]: S 198

TRANSPLANT
International
© Springer-Verlag 1992

Technique of arterial anastomosis in liver transplantation, surgical management in routine situations and anatomical variations

H. P. Lemmens[1], G. Blumhardt[1], P. Neuhaus[1], H. Keck[1], N. Tsiblakis[1], R. Rossaint[2], R. Langer[3], and R. Steffen[1]

[1] Surgical Clinic, [2] Department of Anaesthesiology and
[3] Department of Radiology, Universitätsklinikum Rudolf Virchow, Freie Universität Berlin, Berlin, FRG

Abstract. With a careful donor hepatectomy in order to preserve and, if necessary, to reconstruct accessory liver arteries and a microsurgical technique for the arterial anastomosis the rate of arterial complications after liver transplantation can be kept at a low level.

Key words: Liver transplantation – Arterial anastomosis

Arterial thrombosis is a major factor in morbidity in liver transplantation as it may contribute to graft failure or complications of the biliary tract. It is important to preserve and to reconstruct, if necessary, accessory hepatic arteries of the graft to ensure adequate arterial perfusion after transplantation.

Materials and methods

Between September 1988 and January 1991 144 liver transplantations were performed in 131 adult patients. The indications for transplantation are shown in Table 1.

During donor hepatectomy the coeliac axis was taken including an aortic patch. Accessory arteries were preserved. For eventual vascular reconstruction the iliac vessels (artery + vein) were also routinely taken. The arterial anastomoses were performed with a 7.0 prolene running suture using microsurgical techniques. The patency of the arterial anastomoses was examined routinely every 3 months by Doppler ultrasound, angio-CT scan and, if indicated, by angiography. The follow-up period included a period of 8–35 months (median, 18 months).

Donor organs had regular anatomy in 75 % of cases with variations occurring in 25 %. These variations included accessory left hepatic artery from left gastric artery (11.1 %), accessory right hepatic artery from superior mesenteric artery (7.6 %), combination of both (3.5 %) and others (2.8 %). All accessory right hepatic arteries were reconstructed by end-to-end anastomosis to the donor splenic artery or gastroduodenal artery.

At transplantation anastomosis was performed in general with 7-0 prolene running sutures using an end-to-side technique between the coeliac axis of the graft and the common hepatic artery at the

Table 1. Indications for liver transplantations

	n	%
Posthepatic cirrhosis	69	47.9
Alcoholic cirrhosis	15	10.4
Acute liver failure	12	8.3
PSC	9	6.3
PBC	8	5.6
HCC in cirrhosis	4	2.8
Budd–Chiari	4	2.8
Others	10	6.9
Retransplantations	13	9.0

offspring of the gastroduodenal artery (74.3 %), or splenic artery (13.2 %). In 5.6 % the bifurcation of the hepatic artery was chosen as the site of the anastomosis. An end-to-end technique between the common hepatic artery and the coeliac axis was performed in 2.1 %. In 2.8 % the interposition of a graft (a segment of the donor iliac artery) was necessary for reconstruction.

Results

Table 2. Results

	n
Transplantations	144[a]
Retransplantations	13
Retransplantation for arterial thrombosis	1
Died[b]	13
Arterial stenosis[c]	1
Splenic artery steal syndrome[d]	5
Follow up	18 months (median)

[a] In 131 patients
[b] Upon autopsy no arterial thrombosis or haemodynamically significant stenosis was found to be responsible for death in any case.
[c] In one patient a 70 % stenosis of the common hepatic artery could be identified at the site of the anastomosis three months after transplantation. Since the liver function was excellent no further therapy was considered.
[d] During follow up a moderate increase in the aminotransferase levels and slight liver function impairment was observed in five patients. This was shown to be caused by a splenic artery steal syndrome with splenomegaly. Therefore an embolization of the splenic artery and/or splenectomy was performed. Thereafter the aminotransferase levels as well as the liver function tests normalized in all patients.

Offprint requests to: H. P. Lemmens, Department of Surgery, Free University Berlin, Klinik Rudolf Virchow, Augustenburgerplatz 1, 1000 Berlin 65, FRG

Transplant Int (1992) 5 [Suppl 1]: S199–S200

TRANSPLANT
International
© Springer-Verlag 1992

Biliary neopterin for differentiation between liver allograft rejection and viral graft infection

R. Margreiter[1], C. Aichberger[1], A. Königsrainer[1], G. Reibnegger[2], G. Weiss[2], and H. Wachter[2]

[1] Department of Transplant Surgery and [2] Institute of Medical Chemistry and Biochemistry, University Hospital, Innsbruck, Austria

Differential diagnosis between rejection and infection of a liver graft still represents a major problem. Rising concentrations of neopterin in serum or urine sensitively indicate rejection or infectious complications after renal, cardiac or bone marrow transplantation [3]. Neopterin has been shown to be even more sensitive when measured locally, e.g. in the pancreatic juice of patients after pancreas allotransplantation [1]. In the present study, we measured urinary and, for the first time, biliary neopterin concentrations in nine liver allograft recipients during the early post-transplant period.

Key words: Liver transplantation – Rejection – Infection – Biliary neopterin

Materials and methods

Urine and T-tube bile samples were collected from two female and seven male patients after orthotopic liver transplantation over a period of 25 days on average. The underlying liver disease was chronic active hepatitis in five patients, alcohol-toxic cirrhosis in one and haemochromatosis in one. Prophylactic immunosuppression consisted of cyclosporin A, steroids and azathioprine. Rejection was diagnosed on the basis of clinical symptoms, impaired liver function, reduced bile production, and urinary neopterin excretion as well as graft histology. Acute graft rejection episodes were treated with boluses of methylprednisone as described elsewhere [2]. The urinary neopterin/creatinine ratio was measured in first-morning urine by high-performance liquid chromatography (HPLC). Biliary concentrations were determined according to a method previously described for assessment of neopterin in serum [4]. This technique uses solid-phase extraction combined with on-line elution from the solid phase onto the HPLC column. The method is also applicable for biliary specimens. Samples (50 µl) were diluted with aqueous sodium chloride (450 µl, 0.015 mol/l) and centrifuged at 10000 g for 5 min. The supernatant (100 µl) was mixed with 10 µl 0.1 mol/l Fe^3P + EDTA solution and incubated for 20 min at room tempera-

ture. To 100 µl of this mixture, 10 µl phosphoric acid (5 mol/l) was added and 100 µl of the resulting mixture transferred to the solid-phase cartridge and processed further as described previously [4]. The biliary neopterin concentrations measured by HPLC were compared with results obtained with a commercially available radioimmunoassay (Henning-Berlin, Berlin FRG).

Results

Increased urinary neopterin concentrations were seen to be associated with immunological and infectious complications such as acute rejection ($n = 6$), cytomegalovirus (CMV) infection ($n = 2$), hepatitis B ($n = 1$), hepatitis C ($n = 1$) and herpes infection ($n = 1$). During every rejection episode, rising biliary neopterin concentrations were found. The elevation in bile fluid and particularly the decrease in neopterin concentration subsequent to successful anti-rejection therapy were more pronounced and rapid than in urine. However, biliary neopterin concentrations began to increase about 24 h after urinary values started to rise. In contrast to their effect on urinary neopterin, CMV infection and hepatitis and herpetic infections were not associated with rising biliary neopterin concentrations.

In a patient with repeated rejection episodes resistant to various therapeutic attempts, biliary and urinary neopterin concentrations were invariably higher than in patients who responded well to anti-rejection treatment.

Discussion

The preliminary results of this study suggest that the determination of biliary neopterin concentrations facilitates differentiation of acute allograft rejection from viral infections after liver transplantation. Biliary neopterin appears not to increase in various forms of viral infections such as CMV, herpes and hepatitis. Since rejection can often not be distinguished from viral graft infection, even by histomorphology, measurement of biliary neopterin

Offprint requests to: Prof. R. Margreiter, M.D., Department of Transplant Surgery, University Hospital, Anichstraße 35, A-6020 Innsbruck, Austria

may provide important information in addition to histology, clinical data and urinary neopterin.

The rise in urinary neopterin concentration preceded that in biliary neopterin concentration by 24 h. Elevated urinary neopterin seems to reflect the systemic activation of cellular immunity. It is remarkable, however, that viral infections, particularly viral hepatitis, did not cause a rise in biliary neopterin concentration.

Although not proven, it is very likely that hepatic neopterin is produced by Kupffer cells. It could be speculated that the delayed rise in neopterin levels in the bile fluid when compared with urinary neopterin is caused by a defective reticulo-endothelial system (RES). Its impaired function can be due to ischaemic damage and/or the fact that donor Kupffer cells are gradually replaced by recipient cells. Since hepatitis viruses are known to block the RES, no neopterin is produced during this type of infection.

If these results can be confirmed in a larger number of patients, biliary neopterin would be a very useful tool for diagnosing liver allograft rejection.

References

1. Königsrainer A, Reibnegger G, Öfner D, Klima G, Tauscher T, Margreiter R (1989) Transplant Proc 22. 671–672
2. Tilg H, Vogel W, Aulitzky WE, et al. (1989) Transplantation 48: 594–599
3. Wachter H, Fuchs D, Hausen A, Reibnegger G, Werner ER (1989) Clin Chem 27: 81–141
4. Werner ER, Fuchs D, Hausen A, Reibnegger G, Wachter H (1987) Clin Chem 33: 2028–2033

Transplant Int (1992) 5 [Suppl 1]: S 201–S 205

TRANSPLANT
International
© Springer-Verlag 1992

Total hepatectomy and liver transplant for hepatocellular adenomatosis and focal nodular hyperplasia*

I. R. Marino, V. P. Scantlebury, O. Bronsther, S. Iwatsuki, and T. E. Starzl

Department of Surgery, University of Pittsburgh, School of Medicine and the Veterans Administration Medical Center, Pittsburgh, Pa., USA

Abstract. Extensive hepatocellular adenomatosis (HA) and focal nodular hyperplasia (FNH) represent a proliferation of hepatic cells that occurs most frequently in women. These lesions are uncommon in the pediatric age group, accounting for 2 % of pediatric hepatic tumors, and are extremely rare in males. The etiology of HA and FNH has been correlated with the use of oral contraceptives. We report to the best of our knowledge the first series of patients treated with OLTx for HA and FNH (five cases). All these patients had lesions involving at least 90 % of the hepatic parenchyma and all underwent major hepatic surgery before OLTx because of life threatening complications. One patient died in the immediate postoperative period following retransplantation for primary non-function of the first OLTx. Four out of five patients are currently alive from 4.1 to 9.6 years after OLTx. Our results justify the use of OLTx for symptomatic patients with HA and FNH who cannot be treated with conventional hepatic resections.

Key words: Hepatocellular adenomatosis – Focal nodular hyperplasia – Liver transplantation

Indications for orthotopic liver transplantation (OLTx) have been continuously expanding. Hepatic replacement for primary and metastatic malignancy of the liver has been the subject of numerous reports [7, 14, 17, 18, 21, 23, 30]. Nevertheless, the indication for such aggressive therapy for benign neoplasms of the liver has yet to be defined. The role of OLTx for extensive hepatic adenomatosis (HA) and focal nodular hyperplasia (FNH) is analyzed in this study.

HA is a disease seen mainly in women. Before the use of oral contraceptives, HA was amongst the rarest of tumors. In two large pathological reviews of material collected between 1907 and 1954, only six patients with HA were found [2, 9]. Since the use of oral contraceptives from 1960, more examples of liver cell adenomas have been published [1]. It is also possible to observe lesions of this type even in the pediatric age group [29]. The term FNH was introduced in 1958 by Edmondson [4]. It occurs most often in women and can be associated with oral contraceptives [16]. This pathological process has also been described as occurring in pediatric patients [27].

Because of the characteristics of these two liver lesions, treatment of symptomatic patients usually consists of surgical resection. In fact the majority of these tumors may be resected with conventional subtotal hepatectomies.

This study describes our experience in patients treated with OLTx for multiple HA, with one patient having associated extensive FNH. In all five patients, more than 90 % of the liver parenchyma was involved with the lesions, thus preventing a curative hepatic resection.

This report represents, to the best of our knowledge, the first series of OLTx for multiple HA and for FNH with long-term follow-up.

Case reports

Case 1

Patient 1, a white female born in 1965, was referred for OLTx evaluation in January 1982 because of end-stage liver disease secondary to type I glycogen storage disease and HA. She had undergone an end-to-side portacaval shunt 9 years previously to improve her growth and the metabolic abnormalities associated with glycogen storage disease [8, 24].

During this period the child was followed with serial sonographic examinations of the liver which began to reveal intrahepatic masses. Until 1981, no symptoms were referable to these masses. However, a liver biopsy of one lesion was obtained and this proved to be an adenoma.

In September 1981 the patient had the onset of severe abdominal pain and tenderness with enlargement of her liver. This was thought

* Aided by Research Grants from the Veterans Administration and Project Grant No. DK 29 961 from the National Institutes of Health, Bethesda, Maryland

Offprint requests to: Thomas E. Starzl, M. D., Ph. D., Department of Surgery, 3601 Fifth Avenue, Falk Clinic 5C, Pittsburgh, Pennsylvania 15213, USA

to be due to intrahepatic hemorrhage resulting in obstruction of the biliary tree and subsequent hepatic failure. The patient's condition deteriorated further 3 months later. Abdominal CT scan confirmed that hepatomegaly was secondary to multiple intrahepatic masses (Fig. 1). She was placed on the transplant list due to progressive liver failure, the potential risk of malignant transformation of the HA, and because the lesions appeared to be unresectable by a conventional approach. At OLTx her native liver was found to be enlarged with the parenchyma almost completely replaced by multiple nodules, which histologically proved to be adenomas (Fig. 2).

The patient developed portal vein thrombosis 1 year after OLTx with hepatopetal collateral circulation adequately perfusing the liver. Because of repeated episodes of gastrointestinal tract bleeding, she underwent a distal spleno-renal shunt for control of portal hypertension [19]. Over the past 9 years, her liver function has been excellent, and the most recent liver enzyme levels performed in August 1991 were normal.

Case 2

Patient 2, a white female born in 1948, presented in November 1980 with abdominal tightness, anorexia and weight loss. An abdominal CT scan demonstrated multiple defects within the liver. There was no history of birth-control pill ingestion, although in May 1980 she presented with menorrhagia which was successfully treated for an 11-day period with hormone replacement.

In December 1980, because of dyspnea secondary to ascites and liver enlargement, a laparotomy was performed. She was found to have multiple masses in both lobes of the liver, and a large amount of hemorrhagic ascites. Liver biopsy was consistent with multiple HA. The patient was referred to our institution for further evaluation. A right hepatic trisegmentectomy was performed. The remaining portion of the left lobe still had some residual nodules. The histologic diagnosis on the removed parenchyma was multiple HA with no evidence of malignancy. Tamoxifen was started in an attempt to prevent further growth of the residual adenomas.

In January 1982 the patient presented with increasing abdominal girth and a palpable abdominal mass. Abdominal CT scan demonstrated massive enlargement of the residual lateral left segment due to multiple large masses, which occupied most of the parenchyma. The patient was activated as a liver transplant candidate, and a suitable donor became available on 5 March 1982. At surgery the residual left lobe of the liver was markedly enlarged. The hepatectomy specimen weighed 4250 g. Histological examination demonstrated multiple HA replacing almost the entire liver parenchyma, with signs of focal necrosis and cholestasis. The postoperative course was uneventful and she was discharged.

In August 1991 she was found to have multiple lesions in the lungs. These lesions proved to be metastases possibly of hepatocellular carcinoma. However, pathology failed to reveal any malignant lesion in the native liver at the time of OLTx, and no lesions were found at CT scan of the transplanted liver in August 1991. The most recent liver function tests performed in August, 1991, more than 9 years following OLTx, were normal.

Case 3

Patient 3, a black female born in 1965, had a history of oral contraceptive use since age 13 years. She presented with moderate pruritus and hepatomegaly 2 years later. A diagnosis of possible multiple HA was entertained, based on ultrasound and CT examinations showing multiple low density lesions involving both lobes of the liver. In May 1981, she had an episode of intraabdominal hemorrhage (from one of the adenomas) requiring emergency operation and left lateral segmentectomy. Examination of the surgical specimen confirmed the diagnosis of HA. Subsequently the patient has several episodes of intrahepatic bleeding which led to the resection of a segment of the right lobe 18 months later. In March 1983 the patient was referred to our institution for possible OLTx. Abdominal CT showed recur-

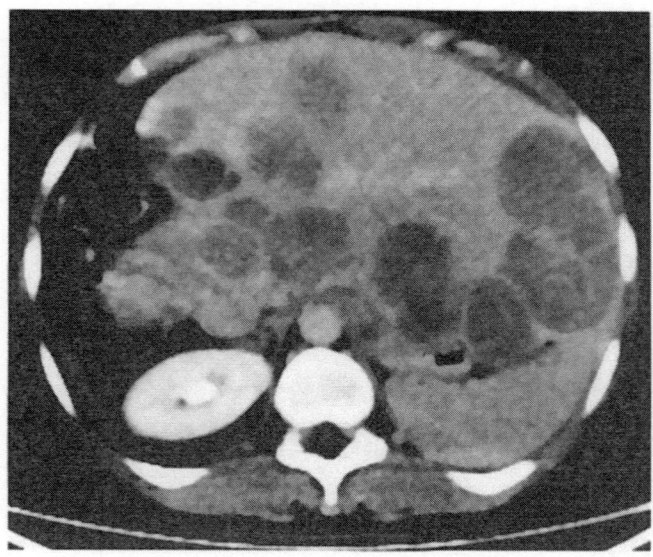

Fig. 1. Pre OLTx CT scan, case no. 1. Multiple hepatic masses occupying almost all the liver parenchyma

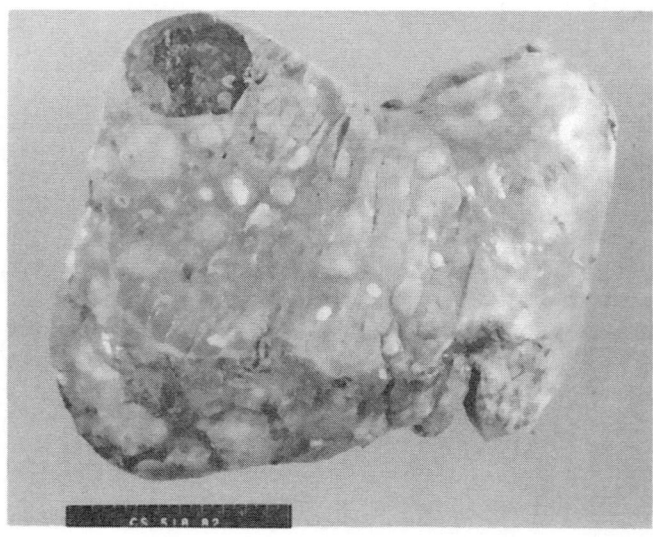

Fig. 2. Case no. 1, recipient liver (a portion has been removed for biochemical study). Multiple nodules distorting the surface are clearly discernible

rence of the lesions with involvement of the entire liver (Fig. 3). The patient was felt to be a suitable candidate for OLTx. An OLTx was performed on 25 September 1984. The native liver weighed 2600 g with distortion of the parenchyma by numerous soft lobulations. Histologic examination confirmed the diagnosis of multiple HA.

The patient's quality of life in the last seven years has been excellent. She graduated from college Nursing School and is working full time. The most recent liver function tests performed in September 1991 were normal.

Case 4

Patient 4, a white female born in 1977, had a familial history of liver adenomatosis. Her mother underwent a liver resection for HA in 1981 and presently was four new HA. Her 8-year-old brother also has multiple HA. Since age 7 years the patient has had multiple recurrent episodes of abdominal pain. In May 1987 an ultrasound and CT scan of the liver revealed the presence of multiple masses, the

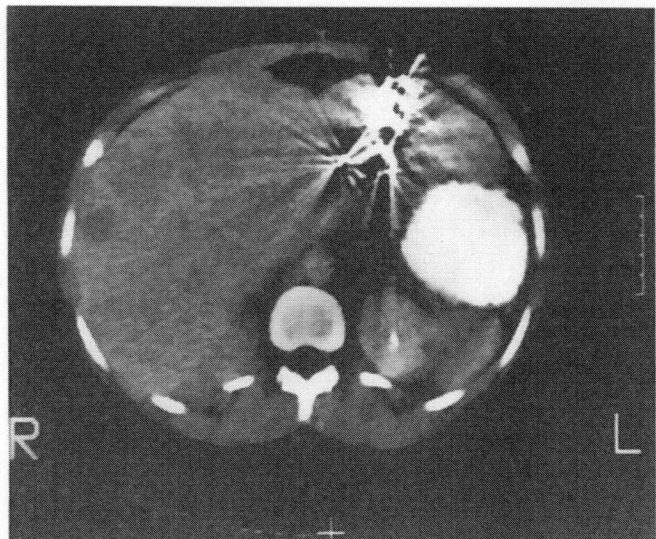

Fig. 3. Pre OLTx CT scan, case no. 3. Surgical clips (related to previous left and right segmental resection) can be noted in the liver. Inhomogenicity with multiple low density areas can be noted throughout all lobes of the liver

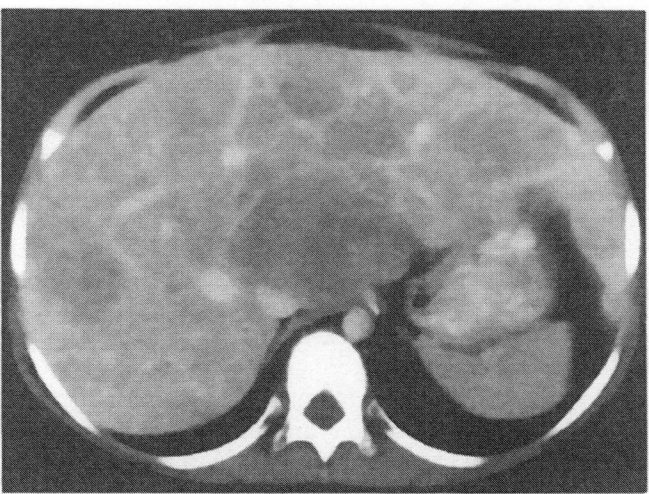

Fig. 4. Pre OLTx CT scan, case no. 4. Multiple hepatic mass lesions of various sizes are spread throughout the entire liver

largest of these being 10 cm in diameter (Fig. 4). In June 1987 she developed fever and abdominal pain. Repeat ultrasound and CT scan of the abdomen revealed a mass with an air fluid level in the right lobe of the liver consistent with an abscess. The remaining hepatic parenchyma was replaced by tumor. At laparotomy the abscess including a portion of the tumor and normal appearing liver were excised for histology. Material was also sent for cultures. Histology confirmed the presence of a HA with associated hemorrhage and necrosis; cultures were positive for Salmonella. The pathological characteristics of the patient's tumor resembled those of her mother.

She was referred to our institution 2 months later for transplant evaluation. Abdominal CT showed inhomogeneity with multiple low-density areas throughout all lobes of the liver (Fig. 4). She was found to be a good candidate of OLTx because of her progressive clinical deterioration and the unresectability of her lesions. The hepatectomy specimen showed multiple tumor masses measuring from 0.5 to 7.0 cm in diameter and replacing 90 % of the liver parenchyma (Fig. 5). In addition to adenomas, histology revealed multiple lesions of FNH.

She is presently in excellent condition, attending school full time, and the last liver function tests performed in August 1991 were normal.

Case 5

Patient 5, a white female born in 1944, had a long history of diarrhea which had been ascribed to irritable colon syndrome. In April 1987 an abdominal CT scan showed multiple masses in the liver. She then underwent a laparoscopy with liver biopsy and a diagnosis of adenoma was made. The patient had been taking daily 17-alfa-estradiol therapy for 2 years up until she was discovered to have hepatic ademonas.

In October 1987 she presented to another institution with acute onset of dull right upper abdominal quadrant pain. A new CT scan performed at that time revealed two small areas suspected of blood collections inside of the right lobe of the liver. The patient was transferred in stable condition to our institution for further evaluation. The other parameters were unremarkable. CT scan of the abdomen showed hepatic adenomas involving the entire left lobe with extension into the anterior segment of the right lobe (Fig. 6). She was considered to be probably not treatable with conventional hepatic resection and she was activated as a liver transplant candidate with the idea to attempt a left trisegmentectomy when a liver became available. A suitable donor was identified on 24 December 1987, and the patient was explored. The liver seemed almost completely replaced by multiple adenomas, except for the anterior segment of the right lobe which appeared free of disease. A left trisegmentectomy was attempted. However, residual adenomas were encountered in the intersegmental plane between the anterior and the posterior segments of the right lobe. Consequently, a decision was taken to perform an OLTx. The patient required 129 units of packed red blood cells during the procedure, and this was probably partially related to her high presensitization and the presence of cytotoxic antibodies (PRA 50 %) [20]. Histological examination of the native liver showed multiple HA replacing almost the entire liver parenchyma with both small and large cell dysplasia of a mild to moderate degree, but no definite evidence of malignancy. The transplanted liver underwent primary non-function and the patient developed renal failure. On 27 December 1987, she underwent a second OLTx. The second liver functioned, but she developed severe necrotizing pancreatitis and died on 4 January 1988.

Discussion

Hepatic adenomas and FNH represent a proliferation of hepatic cells that occurs most frequently in women [5]. These lesions are very rare in the pediatric age group accounting for 2 % of hepatic tumors [3], and extremely rare in males [5]. A strong relationship has been postulated between HA and the use of oral contraceptives [1, 5, 15]. Even FNH may be hormone dependent [15], and is often associated with use of birth-control pills [5, 16]. Hepatic adenomas have also been reported as a frequent complication of metabolic diseases, including type I glycogen storage disease, galactosemia, and tyrosinemia [5, 10].

These aspects of HA and FNH are represented in the patients of our series of whom all were female. Two of them were in the pediatric age. One had used oral contraceptives for several years. One had received short-term hormone therapy for menhorragia, while another had 2 years of estrogen administration before the clinical onset of the liver disease. The background for the multiple HA in one patient was type I glycogen storage disease.

Both HA and FNH are benign tumors but their definitive diagnosis can only be made on the basis of the micro-

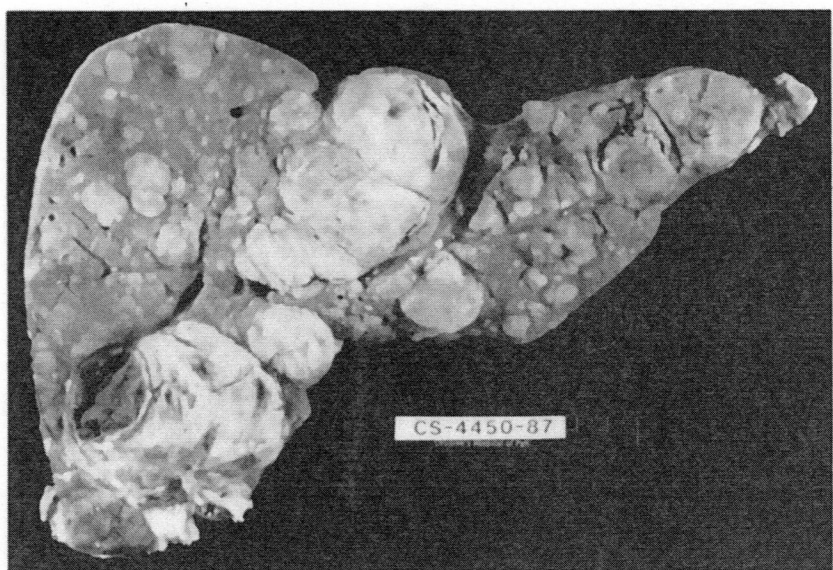

Fig. 5. Case no. 4. Cross-section of the recipient liver. The parenchyma is in most part replaced by circumscribed, irregular nodules ranging from 0.2 to 7.0 cm

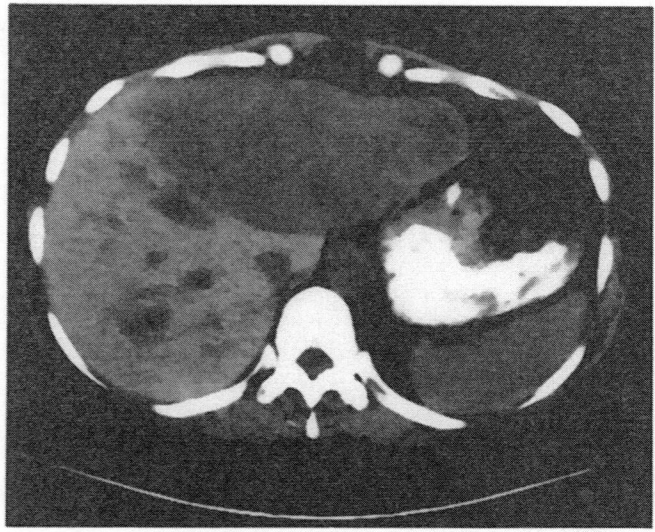

Fig. 6. Pre OLTx CT scan, case no. 5. A large hypodense lesion is demonstrated involving the entire left hepatic lobe with extension into the anterior segment of the right lobe. There is an additional smaller round lesion in the posterior segment of the right lobe

scopic examination of the biopsy material. Radiological examinations including ultrasound, radionuclide scintigraphy, CT and angiography are helpful in studying, grading and following the patient, but they cannot offer absolute diagnostic parameters. The histological differential diagnosis for HA includes hepatocellular carcinoma and hepatoblastoma in the pediatric population [11, 28]. HA can be differentiated from FNH because the former does not contain bile ductules, which are always present in FNH [4].

The clinical history in our patients suggested relatively fast-growing hepatic lesions. The median interval from the first diagnosis to OLTx was 20 months (range: 7 months to 4 years).

The usual clinical presentation of HA is different from that of FNH. Generally adenomas result in bleeding and necrosis, as occurred in all four of our HA cases. Emergency surgery is required for intraabdominal hemorrhage in one third of the patients [5], and this had been the case in patients no. 2 and no. 3. In contrast FNH is usually asymptomatic and commonly is an incidental clinical or autopsy diagnosis [5, 15]. In patient no. 4 who had mixed HA and FNH, symptoms were from a liver abscess.

The development of hepatocellular carcinoma within a HA have been reported in a few patients taking oral contraceptives [15] and in patients with type I glycogen storage disease [31]. Reports have described regression of HA after discontinuation of birth control pills [6, 26] and of cases of regression with dietary therapy in patients whose HA was associated with type I glycogen storage disease [22].

Both for HA and FNH, the approach to therapy should be conservative. If there are single or few lesions, exploratory laparotomy and resection should be recommended for HA and FNH if conventional extirpation techniques are feasible. In extensive cases of asymptomatic FNH, a biopsy to confirm the diagnosis and a long-term radiological non-invasive follow-up may be preferable to a dangerous extensive resection. Even large lesions may be stable for a lifetime. However, the diagnosis must be certain, and it must be recognized that in expert hands, even hepatic trisegmentectomies can be done safely [12–14, 25].

Watching and waiting is a less attractive option for HA because the natural history is unpredictable and the possible risks of bleeding and malignant transformation are higher. In our patient no. 2, lung metastases of hepatocellular carcinoma were found 9.5 years after OLTx without evidence of tumor recurrence in here native liver which was removed in two stages separated by more than a year, or in the transplanted liver.

In the cases reported here, drastic treatment was indicated. The lesions which occupied 80% or more of the liver, were symptomatic, multiple and non-resectable short of fatal hepatectomy. The 80% long-term survival (mean 7.5 years) provides retrospective justification as well as encouragement for further trials in similar highly selected patients.

Acknowledgements. The authors thank Donna Ross for her invaluable help with manuscript editing.

References

1. Baum JK, Holtz F, Bookstein JJ, Klein EW (1973) Possible association between benign hepatomas and oral contraceptives. Lancet II: 926–929
2. Benz EJ, Baggenstoss AH (1953) Focal cirrhosis of the liver: its relation to the so-called hamartoma (adenoma, benign hepatoma). Cancer 6: 743–755
3. Dehner LP (1978) Hepatic tumors in the pediatric age group:- A distinctive clinicopathologic spectrum. In: Rosenberg HS, Boland RP (eds) Perspectives in pediatric pathology, vol 4. Yearbook Medical Publishers, Chicago, pp 217
4. Edmondson HA (1958) Tumors of the liver and intrahepatic bile ducts. In: Atlas of tumor pathology Sect. 7, fasc. 25, Armed Forces Institute of Pathology, Washington DC
5. Edmondson HA, Craig JR (1987) Neoplasms of the liver. In: Schiff L, Schiff ER (eds) Diseases of the liver, 6th edn. J.B. Lippincott Company, Philadelphia, pp 1109-1158
6. Edmondson HA, Reynolds TB, Henderson B, Benton B (1977) Regression of liver cell adenomas associated with oral contraceptives. Ann Intern Med 86: 180–182
7. Esquivel CO, Iwatsuki S, Marino IR, Markus BH, Van Thiel DH, Starzl TE (1987) Liver transplantation for hepatocellular carcinoma and other primary hepatic malignancies. In: Sugahara K (ed) New trends in gastroenterology. Printed in Shinkoshuppan, Kyoto, pp 323–332
8. Greene HLT, Slonim AE, Burr IM (1979) Type I glycogen storage disease: a metabolic basis for advances in treatment. In: Barness LA (ed) Advances in pediatrics, vol 26: 63–92
9. Henson SW, Gray HK, Dockerty MB (1956) Benign tumors of the liver. 1 Adenomas. Surg Gynecol Obstet 103: 23–30
10. Howell RR, Stevenson RE, Ben-Menachem Y, Phyliky RL, Berry DH (1976) Hepatic adenomata with Type I glycogen storage disease. JAMA 236: 1481–1484
11. Ishak GG, Glunz PR (1967) Hepatoblastoma and hepatocarcinoma in infancy and childhood: report of 47 cases. Cancer 20: 396–422
12. Iwatsuki S, Starzl TE (1988) Personal experience with 411 hepatic resections. Ann Surg 208: 421–434
13. Iwatsuki S, Todo S, Starzl TE (1990) Excisional therapy for benign hepatic lesions. Surg Gynecol Obstet 171: 240–246
14. Iwatsuki S, Starzl TE, Sheahan DG, Yokoyama I, Demetris AJ, Todo S, Tzakis AG, Van Thiel DH, Carr B, Selby R, Madariaga J (in press) Hepatic resection versus transplantation for hepatocellular carcinoma. Ann Surg
15. Kerlim P, Davis GL, McGill DB, Weiland LH, Adson MA, Sheedy PF II (1983) Hepatic adenoma and focal nodular hyperplasia: Clinical, pathologic, and radiologic features. Gastroenterology 84: 994–1002
16. Kinch R, Lough J (1978) Focal nodules hyperplasia of the liver and oral contraceptives. Am J Obstet Gynecol 132: 717–727
17. Margreiter R (1986) Indications for liver transplantation for primary and secondary liver tumors. Transplant Proc 18 [Suppl 3]: 74–77
18. Marino IR, Todo S, Tzakis AG, Klintlmalm G, Kelleher M, Iwatsuki S, Starzl TE, Esquivel CO (1988) Treatment of hepatic epithelioid hemangioendothelioma with liver transplantation. Cancer 62: 2079–2084
19. Marino IR, Esquivel CO, Zajko A, Malatack J, Scantlebury VP, Shaw BW, Starzl TE (1989) Distal splenorenal shunt for portal vein thrombosis after liver transplantation. Am J Gastroenterol 84: 67–70
20. Marino IR, Weber T, Kang YG, Esquivel CO, Starzl TE, Duquesnoy RJ (1989) HLA alloimmunization and blood requirements in orthotopic liver transplantation. Transplant Proc 21 [Suppl 1]: 789–791
21. Neuhaus P, Brolsch CE, Ringe B, Pichlmayr R (1986) Liver transplantation for liver tumors. Recent Results Cancer Res 100: 221–228
22. Parker P, Burr L, Slonim A, Ghisham FK, Greene H (1981) Regression of hepatic adenomas in Type Ia glycogen storage disease with dietary therapy. Gastroenterology 81: 534–546
23. Rolles K (1987) Liver transplantation for hepatocellular malignancy in Europe: In: Sugahara K (ed) New trends in gastroenterology. Printed in Shinkoshuppan, Kyoto, pp 333–338
24. Starzl TE, Putnam CW, Porter KA, Halgrimson CG, Corman J, Brown BI, Gotlin RW, Rodgerson DO, Greene HL (1973) Portal diversion for the treatment of glycogen storage disease in humans. Ann Surg 178: 525–539
25. Starzl TE, Koep LJ, Weil R III, Fennell RH, Iwatsuki S, Kano T, Johnson ML (1980) Excisional treatment of cavernous hemangioma of the liver. Ann Surg 19: 25–27
26. Steinbrecher UP, Lisbona R, Hvang SN, Mishkin S (1981) Complete regression of hepatocellular adenoma after withdrawal of oral conctraceptives. Dig Dis Sci 26: 1045–1050
27. Stocker JT, Ishak KG (1981) Focal nodular hyperplasia of the liver: a study of 21 pediatric cases. Cancer 48: 336–345
28. Weinberg AG, Finegold MJ (1983) Primary hepatic tumors of childhood. Hum Pathol 14: 512–537
29. Wheeler DA, Edmondson HA, Reynolds TB (1986) Spontaneous liver cell adenoma in children. Am J Clin Pathol 85: 6–12
30. Yokoyama I, Todo S, Iwatsuki S, Starzl TE (1990) Liver transplantation in the treatment of primary liver cancer. Hepatogastroenterology 37: 188–193
31. Zangeneh F, Limbeck GA, Brown BI, Emch JR, Arcasoy MM, Goldenberg VE, Kelley VC (1969) Hepatorenal glycogenosis (Type I glycogenosis) and carcinoma of the liver. J Pediatr 74: 73–83

Transplant Int (1992) 5 [Suppl 1]: S 206–S 208

TRANSPLANT
International
© Springer-Verlag 1992

Liver transplantation for fulminant liver failure in children

R. Mondragon[1], G. Mieli-Vergani[2], N. D. Heaton[1], A. P. Mowat[2], V. Vougas[1], R. Williams[3], and K. C. Tan[1]

Departments of [1] Surgery and [2] Paediatrics, and
[3] Institute of Liver Studies, King's College Hospital and King's College School of Medicine and Dentistry, London, UK

Abstract. The mortality rate of fulminant hepatic failure (FHF) in childhood has remained between 70 % and 95 % despite recent improvements in medical therapy. Liver transplantation has become an important therapeutic option in adults with this entity, but has been infrequently performed in children. Many children do not receive transplants because of the rapid progression of the illness and the lack of suitable donor livers. We present our experience in liver transplantation in children with FHF. Between March 1988 and December 1989, seven children aged between 15 months and 12 years received eight liver transplants. The aetiology of FHF was viral hepatitis in five and drug hepatotoxicity (carbamazepine) in two. Five of our patients were in grade III–IV coma. Reduced-sized livers were used in six of the eight transplants. The postoperative morbidity included viral and fungal infections, and abdominal bleeding. Two patients died from graft-versus-host disease and one from brain aspergillosis. Four patients (57 %) survived a median follow-up of 15 months. Liver transplantation should be the therapeutic option in children with FHF where the chances of medical recovery are poor.

Key words: Transplantation – Liver transplantation – Fulminant hepatic failure

Fulminant hepatic failure (FHF), an infrequent and catastrophic illness in children, is characterized by widespread necrosis of hepatocytes and is caused by a wide variety of hepatic insults. The condition, first defined by Trey and Davidson, requires the development of hepatic encephalopathy within 8 weeks of the onset of illness in an individual with no evidence of previous liver disease [18]. The mortality rate for this condition has remained between 70 % and 95 % despite recent improvements in medical therapy [6, 10, 15].

Liver transplantation is increasingly accepted as a treatment modality for FHF specially in adults [3, 9, 13, 19]. The experience in children is scarce, mainly because of the rapid evolution of the illness and the lack of paediatric donor livers.

We present our experience in liver transplantation in seven children with FHF.

Material and methods

From March 1988 to March 1991, 148 patients received 161 orthotopic liver transplants at King's College Hospital, of whom seven were children with FHF. There were four males and three females, with a mean age of 6 years (range 1–12 years). The causes of the FHF were acute viral hepatitis in five (four non-A non-B hepatitis, and one hepatitis A) and carbamazepine toxicity in two (Table 1).

Preoperative medical management included the correction of the coagulation disorders by plasma, cryoprecipitate infusion or exchange transfusion. Endotracheal intubation was instituted when patients had difficulty in controlling secretions or in grade IV encephalopathy. Intracranial pressure (ICP) was monitored in children with cerebral oedema. Mannitol and thiopentone infusions were used to reduce the intracranial pressure. The decision for transplantation was made according to 'The King's College Criteria' [11] which includes: age < 10, > 40 years; aetiology (non-A non-B hepatitis, and idiosyncratic drug reactions); jaundice more than 7 days; prothrombin time > 50 s; and serum bilirubin > 300 µmol/l (providing that no absolute contraindication for transplantation such as uncontrolled sepsis, cardiovascular instability or irreversible brain damage is present). Two children met three criteria, and five met four or more criteria for transplantation.

Six of the seven children presented with hyperbilirubinaemia (median 403 mmol/l, range 87–632), and transaminaemia (mean 1470 IU/l, range 144–6000). Hepatic encephalopathy was stage II in two, stage III in three and stage IV in two. All had severe coagulopathy as evidenced by prolongation of prothrombin time, with a mean value of 63 s (range 33–104 s). However, with the correction of the coagulopathy at the time of transplantation the prothrombin time decreased to a mean value of 16 s.

Orthotopic liver transplantation, and reduced-sized liver transplantation were performed according to accepted techniques [5, 17]. Veno-venous bypass was not used. Baseline immunosuppression was achieved with cyclosporin A (CsA), steroids and azathioprine.

Offprint requests to: Mr. K. C. Tan, Department of Surgery, Liver Transplant Surgery, King's College Hospital, Denmark Hill, London SE5 9RS, UK

Table 1. Clinical and biochemical data of the seven children receiving transplants

Sex	Age (months)	Diagnosis	Bilirubin (mmol/l)	AST (IU/l)	Creatinine (mmol/l)	PT (s)	Coma grade	Ascites
F	72	Carbamazepine hepatotoxicity	507	1325	107	63	III	Yes
F	24	Carbamazepine hepatotoxicity	87	6000	91	87	III	Yes
M	48	NANB hepatitis	370	638	51	32	III	No
M	132	NANB hepatitis	632	776	106	104	IV	Yes
M	144	Hepatitis A	507	1325	107	63	III	No
F	84	NANB hepatitis	555	465	81	33	II	No
M	12	NANB hepatitis	389	144	62	48	II	Yes

NANB, non-A non-B hepatitis; AST, aspartate aminotransferase; PT, prothrombin time; Coma grade, encephalopathy grade

The dosage of CsA was adjusted according to daily radioimmuno-assay levels to maintain a trough level of 150–200 ng/ml. Episodes of allograft rejection were treated with pulse doses of steroids.

Results

Liver transplantation was performed from 1 to 5 days (mean 3 days) after the patient was listed in the 'emergency' category with the UK Transplant Service. Eight liver transplants were performed in seven children; one child required retransplantation 6 months later because of severe biliary obstruction. Two patients received a full-sized graft; reduced-sized grafts were used in six, utilizing the left lateral segment in three and the left tobe in three (Table 2).

The operative procedure was technically simple because of the absence of portal hypertension and no previous abdominal operations. The presence of coagulopathy including fibrinolysis, resulted in mean blood losses of 1400 ml (range 515–4000 ml). The histology of the excised livers showed massive or submassive hepatocellular necrosis, bridging between portal tracts and central veins and portal tract inflammatory cell infiltrate.

Postoperative complications developed in five of the children. Acute rejection was diagnosed and treated in three. Abdominal bleeding was a problem in two (one required a laparotomy), fungal infection in two (disseminated candidiasis in one and brain aspergillosis in one), CMV pneumonitis in two, biliary obstruction and subhepatic abscess in one, and portal vein thrombosis in one who required a thrombectomy (Table 3).

Three children died during an observation period of 3 to 22 months. Two children developed graft-versus-host disease (GVHD). They were treated with high doses of steroids, antilymphocyte globulin and thalidomide. In both cases disseminated CMV infection was detected and treated with gancyclovir. Neither of them responded to anti-GVHD therapy, and died with disseminated infection. One patient developed brain aspergillosis and never responded to aggressive medical therapy.

Of the seven patients, four (57%) were alive at the time of writing. The median duration of follow-up was 15 months (3 months to 3 years). Neurological recovery in the survivors was complete.

Discussion

The criteria for selecting children with FHF who are suitable for liver transplantation remain difficult to establish. The decision has to be taken before the development of severe complications, such as cerebral oedema, hypoglycaemia, renal failure and sepsis. The decision for transplantation was taken for our children with the assistance of the King's College Criteria [11]. Using these criteria it has been shown that in patients with more than three factors present mortality without transplantation is up to 95%.

Once the decision for transplantation has been taken, the coagulopathy should be corrected with the administration of fresh frozen plasma, cryoprecipitate, platelets and exchange transfusions. If clinical signs of cerebral oedema are detected, the insertion of an extradural ICP monitor is advisable [14]. Episodes of raised ICP can be successfully managed with hyperventilation, hyperosmolar mannitol and thiopentone infusions.

The lack of suitable paediatric donor livers makes the use of reduced-sized and ABO-incompatible grafts necessary. Four of our children received transplants across ABO blood group barriers. These grafts have previously been associated with an increased incidence of severe rejection, arterial thrombosis and cholangitis [7]. In the present series, no such association was demonstrated. Because of the possible complications, the use of ABO-incompatible grafts can only be recommended in emergency situations. Five of our grafts were reduced-sized grafts. It has been shown by others that graft and patient survival is the same in full-sized or reduced-sized grafts [12].

Table 2. Graft type and surgical complications

Patient		Graft type (segments)[a]	Complications
1		Standard	
2		II, III, IV.	
3		Standard	
4		II, III	Intraabdominal bleeding biliary obstruction
	(R)	II, III	Subhepatic abscess
5		II, III	
6		II, III, IV	Intraabdominal bleeding
7		II, III, IV	Portal vein thrombosis

[a] Hepatic segments according to Couinaud; R, retransplantation

Table 3. Postoperative complications in the children transplanted

		Mortality
Acute rejection	3	
Pneumonia	3	
Intraabdominal bleeding	2	
Graft versus host disease	2	2
CMV infection	2	
Fungaemia	2	1
Biliary obstruction	1	
Portal vein thrombosis	1	
Subhepatic abscess	1	
Retransplantation	1	
		3 (42%)

Several defects in immunological function have been described in patients with FHF [1, 8, 21]. These defects, together with the use of invasive monitoring, immunosuppression, broad spectrum antibiotics, and treatment for graft rejection, render the child highly suceptible to bacterial and fungal infections [16, 20]. This appears to be reduced by the use of selective bowel decontamination. If sepsis is suspected the aggressive use of antibiotics and antifungals is recommended.

GVHD is a complication rarely seen after liver transplantation in adults, and few cases have been reported [2, 4]. Two of our cases developed GVHD, and both had received reduced-sized livers from an adult donor. Several factors may have been involved in the development of GVHD in these children. A relatively large pool of immunologically competent cells is grafted into a small host with defective immunological function which makes them incapable of mounting an effective response against transplanted lymphocytes. The results of treatment with CsA, increased doses of steroids, antilymphocyte globulin and thalidomide proved dissappointing.

The survival rate obtained so far with liver transplantation is encouraging (57%). In our experience, and in other adult centres, the survival rate in patients with FHF is significantly lower than for elective cases. To improve the results early referral of these children to centres with facilities and experience in liver transplantation is desirable. Better criteria for transplantation which identify early those children who will not survive without transplantation need to be developed.

References

1. Altin M, Rajkovic IA, Hughes RD, Williams R (1983) Neutrophil adherence in chronic liver disease and fulminant hepatic failure. Gut 24: 746–750
2. Bhaduri BR, Tan KC, Humphreys S, et al (1990) Graft-versus-host-disease after orthotopic liver transplantation in a child. Transplant Proc 22: 2378–2380
3. Bismuth H, Samuel D, Gugenheim J, Castaing D, Bernuau J, Rueff B, Benhamou JP (1987) Emergency liver transplantation for fulminant hepatitis. Ann Intern Med 107: 337–341
4. Burdick JF, Vogelsang GB, Smith WJ, et al (1988) Severe graft versus host disease in a liver transplant recipient. N Engl J Med 318: 689–691
5. de Hemptinne B, Salizzoni M, Yandza TC, et al (1987) Indications, technique and results of liver graft volume reduction before orthotopic tranplantation in children. Transplant Proc 19: 3549–3551
6. European Association for the Study of the Liver (1979) Randomized trial of steroid therapy in acute liver failure. Gut 20: 20–23
7. Gungenheim J, Samuel D, Reynes M, Bismuth H (1990) Liver transplantation across ABO blood group barriers. Lancet II: 519–523
8. Imawari M, Hughes R, Gove C, Williams R (1985) Fibronectin and Kupffer cell function in fulminant hepatic failure. Dig Dis Sci 30: 746–750
9. O'Grady JG, Williams R, Calne R (1986) Transplantation in fulminant hepatic failure. Lancet II: 1227
10. O'Grady JG, Gimson AES, O'Brien CJ, et al (1988) Controlled trials of charcoal hemoperfusion and prognostic factors in fulminant hepatic failure. Gastroenterology 94: 1186–1192
11. O'Grady J, Alexander GJM, Hayllar KM, et al (1989) Early indicators of prognosis in fulminant hepatic failure. Gastroenterology 97: 439–445
12. Otte JB, de Ville de Goyet J, Sokal E, et al (1990) Size reduction of the donor liver is a safe way to alleviate the shortage of size-matched organs in pediatric liver transplantation. Ann Surg 2211: 146–157
13. Peleman R, Gavaler J, Van Thiel D, Esquivel C, Gordon R, Iwatsuki S, Starzl T (1987) Orthotopic liver transplantation for acute and subacute hepatic failure in adults. Hepatology 7: 484–489
14. Potter D, Peachey T, Eason J, Ginsburg R, O'Grady J (1989) Intracranial pressure monitoring during orthotopic liver transplantation for acute liver failure. Transplant Proc 21: 3528
15. Ring-Larsen H, Palazzo V (1981) Renal failure in fulminant hepatic failure and terminal cirrhosis. Gut 22: 585–591
16. Rolando N, Harvey F, Brahm J, et al (1991) Fungal infection: a common, unrecognised complication of acute liver failure. J Hepatol 12: 1–9
17. Starzl TE, Iwatsuki SI, Esquivel C, et al (1985) Refinements in the surgical technique of liver transplantation. Semin Liver Dis 5: 349
18. Trey C, Davidson LS (1970) In: Popper H, Schaffner F (eds) Progress in liver diseases. Grune and Stratton, New York, p 282
19. Vickers CH, Neuberger J, Buckels J, McMaster P, Elias E (1988) Transplantation of the liver in adults and children with fulminant hepatic failure. J Hepatol 7: 143–150
20. Wajszczuk CP, Dummers S, Ho M, Van Thiel DH, et al (1985) Fungal infections in liver transplant recipients. Transplantation 40: 347–353
21. Wyke RJ, Rajkovic IA, Eddleston ALWF, Williams R (1980) Defective opsonization and complement deficiency in serum from patients with fulminant hepatic failure. Gut 21: 643–649

Transplant Int (1992) 5 [Suppl 1]: S 209–S 210

TRANSPLANT
International
© Springer-Verlag 1992

The impact of the different severe infections on the outcome of liver transplantation. A study of 150 patients

N. P. Mora, B. S. Husberg, T. A. Gonwa, R. Goldstein, and G. B. Klintmalm

Baylor University Medical Center, Transplantation Services, Dallas, Texas, USA

Severe infection (Sev Inf) is still the main cause of morbidity and mortality after liver transplantation (LTx) [2, 3, 4]. The aim of our study was to analyze how each type of infection, bacterial, fungal or viral, influences the rates of morbidity and mortality after LTx.

Key words: Liver transplantation – Infections

Patients and methods

Between March 1988 and December 1989, 180 LTx were performed in 150 adult patients with a follow-up of 5–26 months. Surgery was performed as described by Starzl et al. [6]. Standard immunosuppression with CyA plus prednisolone was administered. Intravenous imipenem was used as antibiotic prophylaxis intraoperatively and for the first 5–7 postoperative days. Selective antifungal prophylaxis was administered with low doses of amphotericin B in high-risk patients (i. e. in need of intensive care before LTx) for 10 days after LTx.

Sef Inf included all episodes of sepsis, meningitis, pneumonia, wound infection, gastrointestinal infection, peritonitis, intra-abdominal abscess, hepatic abscess, cholangitis, and hepatitis. The definition of Sev Inf excluded uncomplicated urinary infection, localized herpes infection, and infection episodes not requiring hospitalization. All fungal infections were included. Patients were divided into four groups according to the presence of the specific type of Sev Inf: bacterial (B), $n = 50$; fungal (F), $n = 19$; viral (V), $n = 44$; and not-infected patients (NI), $n = 72$. Patients with more than one type of Sev Inf entered more than one of the three groups.

The number of days in intensive care after LTx, total hospital stay, 3-month mortality rate and 1-year and 2-year actuarial patient survival in the three infection groups were compared with the NI group as control in order to assess how each type of Sev Inf affects the outcome of LTx.

Results

The results are summarized in Tables 1–4. NI patients demonstrated an optimal survival and outcome after LTx. When viral infection was present there was an increase in

the number of days in intensive care and in the total length of hospital stay, but survival and 3-month mortality rates were not decreased significantly. Bacterial infections significantly affected 3-month mortality rates, and morbidity was also higher than in the NI group. The study presents a very low incidence of fungal infection, which was probably caused by the selective amphotericin protocol that was

Table 1. Patient survival after liver transplantation according to the presence of the different types of severe infections. NI, not infected; B, bacterial infection; F, fungal infection; V, viral infection. * $P = 0.0007$ vs NI; ** $P = 0.027$ vs NI

Group	6 months (%)	12 months (%)	18 months (%)	24 months (%)
NI ($n = 72$)	97.2	97.2	94.4	94.4
B ($n = 50$)	81.9*	71.5*	71.5*	71.5*
F ($n = 19$)	94.7	68.4**	68.4**	68.4**
V ($n = 44$)	93	86.6	86.6	86.6

Table 2. 90-day mortality after liver transplantation according to the presence of the different types of severe infections. NI, not infected; B, bacterial infection; F, fungal infection; V, viral infection. * $P = 0.031$ vs NI

Group	Deaths/patients	Mortality (%)
NI	2/72	2.78
B	7/50	14*
F	0/19	0
V	2/44	4.55

Table 3. Number of days in intensive care after liver transplantation according to the presence of the different types of severe infections. NI, not infected; B, bacterial infection; F, fungal infection; V, viral infection

Group	Mean ± SD	P value (versus NI)
NI ($n = 72$)	3 ± 11	
B ($n = 50$)	12 ± 15	0.0001
F ($n = 19$)	11 ± 14	0.0001
V ($n = 44$)	8 ± 11	0.0001

Offprint requests to: G. B. Klintmalm, M. D., Ph. D., Baylor University Medical Center, Transplantation Services, 3500 Gaston Avenue, Dallas, TX-75246, USA

Table 4. Total hospital stay (days) after liver transplantation according to the presence of the different types of severe infections. NI, not infected; B, bacterial infection; F, fungal infection; V, viral infection

Group	Mean ± SD	P value (versus NI)
NI (n = 72)	20 ± 17	
B (n = 50)	42 ± 31	0.0001
F (n = 19)	48 ± 32	0.0001
V (n = 44)	38 ± 27	0.0001

used. Nevertheless, fungal infection was associated with the lowest survival rate of the four groups, even though all deaths occurred later than the first 3 months after the first LTx.

Conclusions

Infection has been demonstrated to be the primary cause of death after liver transplantation [1]. Invasive fungal infections showed the worst prognosis with a high late mortality [5, 7]. Bacterial infections demonstrated higher morbidity and mortality after LTx compared with the NI group, and viral infections caused higher morbidity without modifying 3-month mortality and patient survival rates. To our knowledge, there are no previous studies focusing on how the three main types of infection affect the outcome and survival after LTx.

References

1. Carithers RL, Fairman P, Méndez-Picon G (1988) Postoperative care. In: Maddrey WC (ed) Transplantation of the liver. Elsevier, New York, pp 111–141
2. Colonna JO, Winston DJ, Brill JE, et al. (1988) Infectious complications in liver transplantation. Arch Surg 123: 360–364
3. Ho M, Wajszczuk CP, Hardy M (1983) Infections in kidney, heart and liver transplant recipients on cyclosporine. Transplant Proc 15 [Suppl. 1]: 2768–2772
4. Kusne S, Dummer JS, Singh N, et al. (1988) Infections after liver transplantation. Medicine 67: 132–143
5. Shahh PM, Just G (1989) Fungal infections in organ transplantation. In: Holmberg K, Meyer RD (eds) Diagnosis and therapy of systemic fungal infections. Raven Press, New York, pp 71–78
6. Starzl TE, Iwatsuki S, Esquivel CO, et al. (1985) Refinements in the surgical technique of liver transplantation. Semin Liver Dis 5: 349–356
7. Wajszczuk CP, Dummer JS, Ho M, et al. (1985) Fungal infections in liver transplant recipients. Transplantation 40: 347–353

Transplant Int (1992) 5 [Suppl 1]: S211–S213

TRANSPLANT
International
© Springer-Verlag 1992

Hepatic support by hepatocyte transplantation in congenitally metabolic diseased rats

M. Nozawa[1], H. Ikebukuro[1], I. Otsu[1], M. Inagaki[2], H. Ebata[2], and M. Mito[2]

[1] Department of Surgery, Meikai University 1-1 Keyakidai, Sakado, Saitama, Japan
[2] Second Department of Surgery, Asahikawa Medical College 4–5 Nishikagura, Asahikawa, Japan

Abstract. Nagase analbuminemic rats (NAR), which lack albumin synthesis in the liver, underwent intrasplenic hepatocyte transplantation (HCTx), and the long-term effects were studied using functional and morphological examinations. Hepatocytes were isolated from congenic F344 rats with collagenase infusion, and 1×10^7 cells were injected into the spleen of 3-month-old NAR ($n = 10$). Serum albumin increased with time, reaching 53.9 mg/dl 14 months after HCTx, which was equivalent to 2.1% (maximum 4%) of serum albumin in normal rats. On the other hand, untreated NAR showed persistently low serum albumin levels (0.99 ± 0.23 mg/dl at 10 months). According to immunostaining with anti-rat albumin antibody at 16 months after HCTx, hepatocyte grafts occupied 27–41% of the spleen area and weighed 120–420 mg, which was equivalent to 0.8–2.9% of a whole liver. Our study demonstrated that grafted hepatocytes can grow in the spleen with the ability to synthesize albumin. HCTx in NAR is a new experimental system to monitor the function and survival of grafted heptocytes without sacrificing the animals by measuring serum albumin levels. Certain manipulations to facilitate the growth of grafted hepatocytes are necessary to achieve sufficient hepatic support in HCTx.

Key words: Intrasplenic hepatocyte transplantation – Nagase analbuminaemic rat

When isolated hepatocytes are grafted into a rat spleen, they can grow gradually until they ocuppy about 40% of the spleen area with preserved liver cell function as has been reported by Mito et al. [2]. The technique could be a useful treatment for metabolic diseases due to liver enzyme deficiencies and acute liver failure. However, it has been difficult to monitor the function of grafted hepatocytes in the spleen and to assess how much they assist the host liver function, because there are few suitable animal models for these studies. We performed intrasplenic hepatocellular transplantation (HCTx) in albumin-deficient rats, and monitored the function of grafted hepatocytes by measuring serum albumin levels in order to evaluate the effects of HCTx on congenital metabolic diseases.

Materials and methods

Male NAR (RT1l) ($n = 10$, 200–250 g body weight, 3 months old, supplied by Sasaki Institute, Tokyo) underwent intrasplenic hepatocyte isotransplantation under ether anaesthesia. Hepatocytes were isolated from congenic F344 rats (RT1l) by collagenase infusion according to the method of Seglen [7], and approximately 1×10^7 hepatocytes in 0.2 ml of Hank's solution were injected into each recipient's spleen. The viability of the hepatocytes at the time of isolation, assessed by trypan blue staining, was 85%. Blood samples were taken from each rat at intervals for 20 months after HCTx, and serum albumin levels were measured by radioimmunoassay (RIA). The specific rabbit antiserum against rat albumin was prepared in the Hormone Assay Center, Institute of Endocrinology, Gunma University (Maebashi, Japan) and used for RIA [4]. Age-matched untreated NAR ($n = 9$) and adult F344 rats ($n = 5$) served as controls.

At 12 months after HCTx, spleens were removed from three HCTx rats, followed by serum albumin measurements at 2 month intervals. At 18 months after HCTx, another three rats were sacrificed for morphometric analysis of grafts in the spleen. The spleen was perfused through the portal vein for fixation with periodate-lysin-paraformaldehyde containing 0.1% glutal aldehyde. Then the spleen was sliced along the long axis and mixed with rabbit anti-rat albumin serum (Capple, USA) for immunostaining. The total area of the hepatocyte graft and graft fraction rate (%) were measured using a CB-Tasper system. The volume of the graft was also estimated from the fraction rate and the spleen weight.

The results were analysed using the Student's t-test or the Cochran-Cox test, and the values are shown as mean $\pm$ SE.

Results

All but two rats which underwent HCTx survived for at least 16 months after HCTx until some of the rats were sacrificed. Serum albumin levels of untreated NAR were very low throughout the observation period

Offprint requests to: Masumi Nozawa M. D., Department of Surgery, Meikai University 1-1 Keyakidai, Sakado, Saitama 350-02, Japan

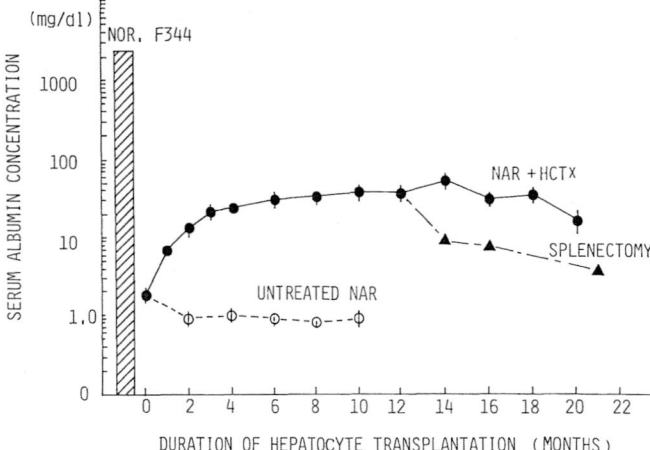

Fig. 1. Serum albumin levels in F344 normal rats ($n = 5$), untreated NAR ($n = 9$), and NAR with intrasplenic hepatocyte isotransplantation (HCTx) ($n = 10$). Some of the NAR with HCTx ($n = 2$) underwent splenectomy 12 months after HCTx

(0.99 ± 0.23 mg/dl at 10 months) compared with the normal F344 rats (2455 ± 62 mg/dl). Serum albumin levels of the transplanted group were 6.9 ± 1.1 mg/dl 1 month after HCTx, which was significantly higher than those of the untreated NAR group (0.92 ± 0.06 mg/dl at 2 months, $P < 0.01$). The levels increased until 14 months (53.9 ± 9.2 mg/dl, maximum 88.3 mg/dl) and declined from 16 to 18 months. Serum albumin dropped considerably after splenectomy in NAR with HCTx (8.8 ± 0.2 mg/dl 2 months after splenectomy), though it never decreased to the level of untreated NAR (Fig. 1).

The graft fraction rates in three rats which were sacrificed 16 months after HCTx were 27.1, 36.1 and 40.9% (Fig. 2, Table 1). There was a clear correlation between serum albumin levels and estimated hepatocyte graft volumes in the spleen (Table 1).

Discussion

Liver transplantation has been performed successfully in humans for the treatment of congenital metabolic diseases [8]. However, many transplant candidates, especially children, do not get the benefits of liver transplantation because of a serious donor shortage. Thus, various alternative methods have been sought clinically as well as experimentally. We have reported short-term and long-term effects of fetal liver transplantation in congenital metabolically diseased rat models [5, 6]. In the present study we transplanted adult hepatocytes in NAR and observed the long-term growth and function of the grafts.

NAR is a rat mutant in which serum albumin levels are very low (0.05% of normal rats) due to an albumin mRNA defect in the liver [3]. This trait is transmitted in an autosomal recessive fashion. Following HCTx, serum albumin increased considerably with time. It reached 88.3 mg/dl in one rat 14 months after HCTx, which was equivalent to 4% of normal rat serum albumin. Morphological study showed that grafted hepatocytes occupied 40.9% of the spleen in the same rat 16 months after HCTx, which was equivalent to 2.9% of a whole liver weight. The volumes of grafted hepatocytes in the spleen parralleled the serum albumin levels in NAR with HCTx. Moreover, serum albumin levels dropped significantly following splenectomy in HCTx rats. All these results suggest that grafted hepatocytes in the spleen grow with time and give the main contribution to albumin production in albumin-deficient rats.

Gupta et al. reported that when hepatocytes from the HBsAg-producing transgenic mouse were isografted into the spleen of normal mice, serum HBsAg was present from 3 days after HCTx, and increased from 20 to 168 ng/ml over a period of 20 weeks [1]. Thus, measuring serum albumin levels in NAR following HCTx or measuring serum HBsAg levels in mice following HCTx of

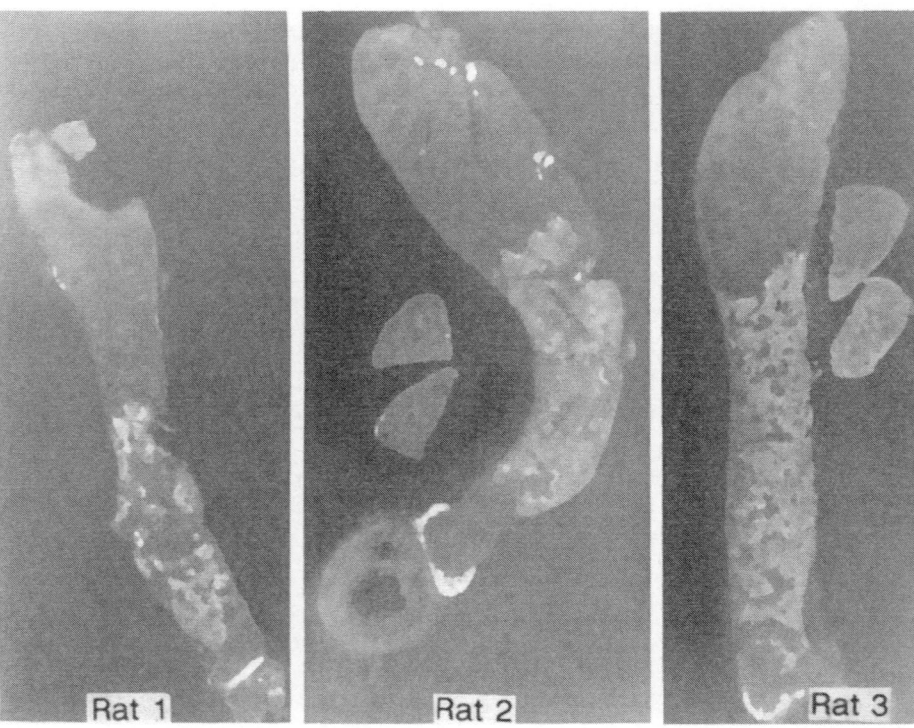

Fig. 2. Rat albumin immunostainings of hepatocyte grafts in the spleen 16 months after HCTx

Table 1. Morphometric analysis of intrasplenic hepatocyte grafts in the rats shown in Fig. 2

Rat no	Serum albumin (mg/dl)	Total area of HC in the spleen (mm²)	Total volume of HC in the spleen (mg)
1	12.3	16.5 (27.1%)	120
2	31.5	29.7 (36.1%)	350
3	42.3	32.7 (40.9%)	420

HC, hepatocytes

HBsAg-producing hepatocytes enabled us to monitor the function, survival and fate of grafted hepatocytes without sacrificing the animals.

We have reported the effects of orthotopic whole liver transplantation (OLTx) in NAR and found that serum albumin increases rapidly to normal range immediately after OLTx [4]. Since the function of grafted hepatocytes is equivalent to only 2% that of OLTx, certain manipulations to facilitate hepatocyte growth are necessary to achieve sufficient function. However, HCTx may be useful as a method for liver enzyme replacement in such conditions as congenital enzyme-deficient disease.

Acknowledgements. We wish to thank Dr. S. Nagase, Sasaki Institute, Tokyo, and Prof. K. Wakabayashi, Institute of Endocrinology, Gunma University, Maebashi, for their contributions to our study.

References

1. Gupta S, Chowdhury NR, Jagutiani R, Gustin K, Aragona E, Shafritz DA, Chowdhury JR, Burk RD (1990) A novel system for transplantation of isolated hepatocytes utilizing HBsAg producing trangenic donor cells. Transplantation 50: 472–475
2. Mito M, Ebata H, Kusano M, Onishi T, Saito T, Sakamoto S (1979) Morphology and function of isolated hepatocytes transplanted into rat spleen. Transplantation 28: 499–505
3. Nagase S, Shimamune K (1979) Albumin-deficient rat mutant. Science 205: 590–591
4. Nozawa M, Jujo H, Masumoto H, Otsu I, Ikebukuro H, Tanaka K, Nagase S, Ozawa K (1987) Effects of liver transplantation in congenitally albumin-deficient rats. Transplant Proc 19: 1091–1094
5. Nozawa M, Otsu I, Ikebukuro H, Makino S (1991) Effects of fetal liver transplantation in rats with congenital metabolic disease. Transplant Proc 23: 889–891
6. Otsu I, Ikebukuro H, Nozawa M (1989) Effects of fetal liver transplantation in congenitally enzyme deficient rats. Transplant Proc 21: 2357–2359
7. Seglen PO (1976) Preparation of isolated rat liver cells. In: Prescott DM (ed) Methods in cell biology, vol 13. Academic Press, New York, pp 29–83
8. Wolf H, Otto G, Giest H (1986) Liver transplantation in Crigler-Najjar syndrome. Transplantation 42: 84

Transplant Int (1992) 5 [Suppl 1]: S 214

TRANSPLANT
International
© Springer-Verlag 1992

Blood transfusion in orthotopic liver transplantation: six-year experience

S. K. Donica, L. C. Roberts, P. K. Duke, S. T. Black, T. H. Swygert, T. C. Gunning, M. A. E. Ramsay, and A. W. Paulsen

Departments of Anesthesiology, Baylor University Medical Center and UT Southwestern Medical Center, Dallas, Texas, USA

Patients undergoing orthotopic liver transplantation (OLT) are susceptible to massive blood loss and require transfusion. Possible reasons for increased transfusion demands include platelet abnormalities, thrombocytopenia secondary to hypersplenism, clotting factor deficiencies, fibrinolysis, increased surgical blood loss associated with portal hypertension and previous surgical procedures, and hypothermia. The purpose of this study was to review trends in blood product usage during our first 6 years of experience performing OLT.

Key words: Liver transplantation – Blood transfusion

Methods

A retrospective review was undertaken of 544 complete data sets generated during 558 procedures in 487 patients between 21 December 1984 and 30 June 1991. Veno-venous bypass was used routinely. A Haemonetics Cell Saver was used beginning in 1987 when not contraindicated by tumor or infection. Frequent thromboelastography and occasional coagulation profiles were obtained. Red blood cells were transfused to maintain a hematocrit of 25–30%. Fresh frozen plasma (FFP), cyroprecipitate (Cryo), and platelets (Plat) were transfused as indicated to maintain hemostasis. Crystalloid and colloid were administered to maintain hemodynamic stability when blood products were not appropriate.

Patients were grouped by academic year. Mean ± standard error of the mean are reported for BPRBC (banked packed red blood cells), CS (cell saver), TRC (total red cells = BPRBC + CS), FFP, Plat, and Cryo. Data were analyzed using t-tests with Bonferroni multiple comparisons and the Kruskall-Wallis one-way analysis of variance. P values < 0.05 were considered significant. Annual intraoperative blood product usage for OLT and total annual institutional blood product usage were analyzed.

Results

When 1989–1991 are compared to earlier years there is a significant decrease in the administration of BPRBC, FFP, Plat, and Cryo (Fig. 1). The percentage of TRC given as CS units increased from 14.5% in 1986 to 34% during 1990–1991. There was no significant difference in TRC

Offprint requests to: L. Clayton Roberts, M. D., 3600 Gaston Avenue, Wadley Tower, Suite 654, Dallas, Texas 75246, USA

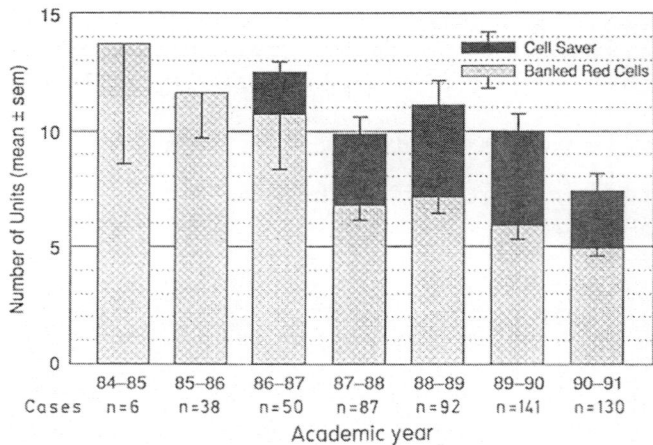

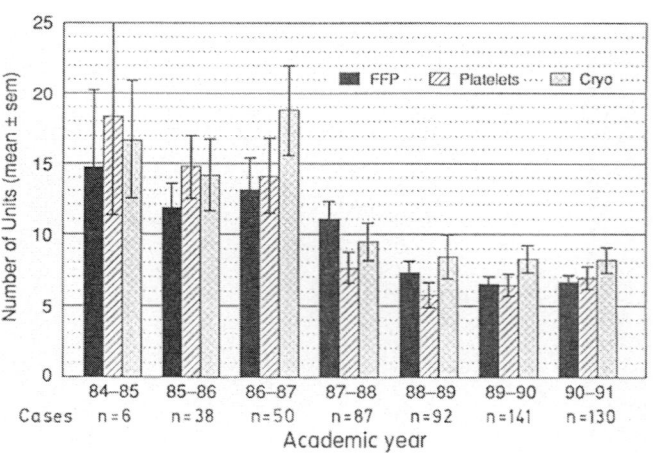

Fig. 1. Blood product usage during OLT

over time. Current annual intraoperative blood product administration during OLT, based on 139 cases, represents 9.1% of the total 46406 units of blood products consumed by the institution.

Discussion

Possible reasons for decreased blood product usage with time include improvements in the management of coagulopathies and refinements in surgical technique. OLT does not place excessive demands on blood bank resources.

Transplant Int (1992) 5 [Suppl 1]: S 215–S 216

TRANSPLANT
International
© Springer-Verlag 1992

Liver transplantation for small HCC in cirrhosis

F. Romani, C. V. Sansalone, P. Rimoldi, G. Rondinara, L. de Carlis, L. S. Belli, F. Riolo, V. Pitotta and L. Belli

Department of Surgery and Transplantation Unit Pizzamiglio II, Niguarda Hospital, Milan, Italy

Segmental liver resection is generally considered the treatment of choice for small HCC in cirrhotic livers. Although in selected patients with small encapsulated nodules and low alpha-fetoprotein levels long-term survival can be expected after resection [4], Western experience is still limited, and follow-up studies too short so that the data presently available cannot be considered satisfactory [3].

The true value of alcoholization as a possible alternative therapy in these patients is still to be ascertained. When using these treatment modalities, the major problem is the high tumour recurrence within the liver [1, 6]. Three main reasons could explain these clinical observations:

1. inadequate resection of the original tumor;
2. unrecognized multifocal HCC;
3. newly generated tumours in the remnant cirrhotic parenchyma.

The rationale for liver transplantation is the oncological accuracy of the ablation of the liver, and the possibility of a simultaneous cure of the associated cirrhosis [2].

In our programme of liver transplantation, begun in 1985, we accepted as an indication small HCC in cirrhotic livers. We present here our initial experience with 19 cases.

Key words: Liver transplantation – Liver cirrhosis

Materials and methods

From January 1985 to September 1991, 121 patients received liver homografts at our centre for various end-stage liver diseases. In 22 cases the indication was small HCC complicating cirrhosis. Here we consider only 19 patients with a follow-up greater than 6 months.

Offprint requests to: Federico Romani, M. D., Department of Surgery Pizzamiglio II, Niguarda Hospital, 20162 Milan, Italy

All patients were asymptomatic and the tumours were occasionally detected by serial US scans and alpha-fetoprotein determinations. The aetiology of the cirrhosis was alcoholic in two patients and post-hepatitic in 17 patients. Six patients were HBV-positive at the time of transplantation.

According to the Child's classification of liver disease, six patients were Child A, ten patients Child B and three patients Child C. High alpha-fetoprotein levels were found only in three cases. A complementary treatment with chemioembolization was carried out in two patients while on the waiting list.

All cases received homografts according to standard techniques and all organs were harvested using UW solution. The characteristics of the cancer involvement were assessed using serial specimens of whole organs.

Results

As a consequence of careful examination of the removed liver 14 patients were found to have a single lesion while five had multiple lesions (ranging from two to four nodules). The extent of cancer involvement was underestimated in nearly 20% of our patients if compared to the preoperative assessment. Tumour sizes were less than 3 cm in diameter in 13 cases and between 3 and 5 cm in six patients (Table 1).

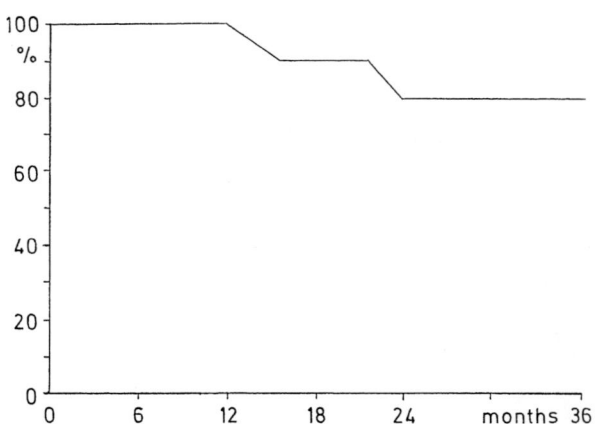

Fig. 1. Actuarial survival curve of 18 cases with small HCC nodules complicating cirrhosis

Table 1. Indications for liver transplantation in 19 patients with small HCC in cirrhosis, with a follow-up period of 6–53 months

	Tumour diameter (cm)		Number of lesions		Child's classification			Alpha-fetoprotein	
	< 3	3–5	Single	Multiple (2–4)	A	B	C	Normal	> 10 mg
Number of patients	13	6	14	5	3	13	3	15	4

One patient died 7 days postoperatively due to PGNF, accounting for an in-hospital mortality rate of 5%. Two patients died of tumour recurrence 12 to 20 months after transplantation. The remaining 16 patients were currently still alive with no overt recurrence during a follow-up between 6 and 53 months. The actuarial survival rate at 3 years was about 80% (Fig. 1).

Discussion

Our promising results in terms of control of tumour recurrence and 3-year survival rates do not match with data from previously reported series [5, 7, 8]. However, this should not be a surprise because at the beginning liver transplantation was performed for large, unresectable tumours, probably in a more advanced stage compared to our cases.

We are convinced that the proper treatment for the patient with a small hepatocellular carcinoma in a cirrhotic liver must be selected from among transplantation, segmental resection and alcoholization. For patients in Child B an C classes, liver transplantation is surely the proper treatment. Still questionable remains the choice for patients with better liver function. Several issues are against liver transplantation: shortage of liver donors; time spent on waiting list; mortality and morbidity still greater than other procedures; and risk of virus recurrence in HBV-positive patients.

Nevertheless, oncological accuracy and the parallel possibility of cure of the cirrhosis strongly recommend liver transplantation. Unfortunately, data collected so far come from diffferent groups of patients not comparable with one another. We therefore consider justified a prospective controlled trial to clearly determine the survival, quality of life and recurrence with all three procedures.

References

1. Belghiti J, Panis Y, Farges O, et al. (1991) Intrahepatic recurrence after resection of hepatocellular carcinoma complicating cirrhosis. Ann Surg 214: 114–117
2. Belli L, Romani F, Belli LS, et al. (1989) Reappraisal of surgical treatment of small hepatocellular carcinoma in cirrhosis: clinico pathological study of resection or transplantation. Dig Dis Sci 34: 1571–1575
3. Bismuth H, Houssin D, Ornowski J, Meriggi F (1986) Liver resection in cirrhotic patients: a Western experience. World J Surg 10 S
4. Franco D, Capusotti L, Smadja C, et al. (1990) Resection of hepatocellular carcinomas: results in 72 European patients with cirrhosis. Gastroenterology 98: 733–738
5. Iwatsuki S, Starzl TE, Todo S, Gordon RD, et al. (1988) Experience in 1000 liver transplants under cyclosporine-steroid therapy: a survival report. Transplant Proc S 1: 498–504
6. Matsumata T, Kanematsu T, Takenaka K (1989) Patterns of intrahepatic recurrence after curative resection of hepatocellular carcinoma. Hepatology 9: 457–460
7. O'Gray JG, Polson RJ, Rolles K, et al. (1988) Liver transplantation for malignant disease. Ann Surg 207: 373–379
8. Ringe B, Wittekind C, Bechstein WO (1989) The role of liver transplantation in hepatobiliary malignancy. Ann Surg 209: 88–89

Heart, Lung,
Heart-Lung

Transplant Int (1992) 5 [Suppl 1]: S 219–S 220

TRANSPLANT
International
© Springer-Verlag 1992

Results of acute heart retransplantation in Eurotransplant

J. de Boer[1], B. Cohen[1], J. Thorogood[1], J. D'Amaro[2], and G. G. Persijn[1]

[1] Eurotransplant Foundation, Leiden, The Netherlands
[2] Department of Immunohaematology, University Hospital, Leiden, The Netherlands

Abstract. In 1988 a special programme for acute retransplantation was introduced in Eurotransplant, giving patients awaiting acute retransplantation priority in the selection procedure. Due to scarcity of donor hearts the question arose whether graft survival after acute retransplantation justified the use of these hearts for this category of patient. A retrospective analysis on the results of transplantations performed in patients who were awaiting acute retransplantation within Eurotransplant was done. In 18 out of 46 cases the patient was treated prior to retransplantation with some kind of mechanical support device. Of the 46 grafts, 28 failed. The actuarial 1-year graft survival in this study group was 36%. In comparison, graft survival for primary cardiac transplantation is approximately 81%. Graft survival after acute heart retransplantation is very poor, especially when the patient has been pretreated with a severe mechanical support system.

Key words: Heart transplantation – Retransplantation – Graft survival – Mechanical support – Bridging

Acute graft failure, especially in heart transplantation, leads to a serious life-threatening situation, which can only be treated with immediate retransplantation. Therefore, a new programme was initiated in Eurotransplant in 1988. This so called 'High Urgency Program' included two rules:

- All donor centres had to offer each available donor heart for this special category.
- Patients on the 'high urgency' list had the highest priority in the selection procedure.

The question was raised if, in the light of the shortage of donor organs, the results justify acute retransplantation.

Patients and methods

As of 1 September 1991, 98 patients were assigned to the 'high urgency' category. A total of 45 patients, 43 male and 2 female, actually received retransplants and one patient returned to the high urgency list another retransplantation. In 18 cases, the patient was treated prior to retransplantation with mechanical support (five

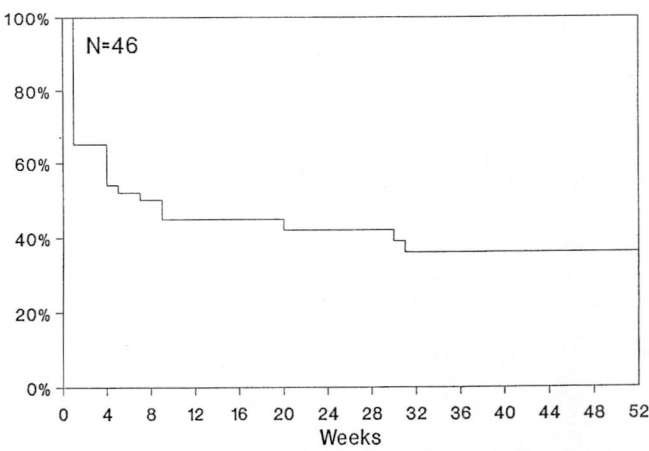

Fig. 1. Graft survival in heart retransplantation, Eurotransplant Jan 1988–Aug 1991

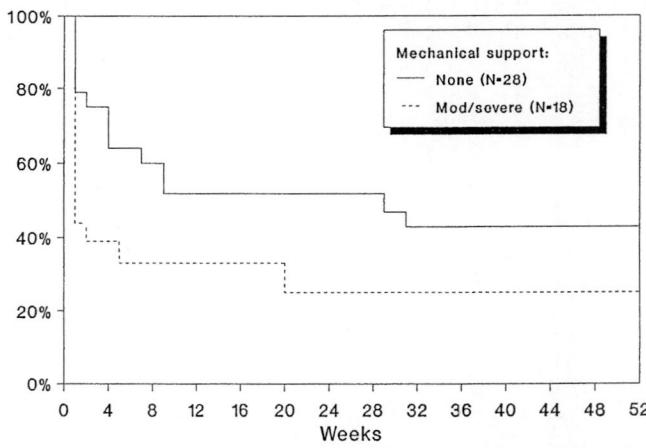

Fig. 2. Graft survival in heart retransplantation, Eurotransplant Jan 1988–Aug 1991

Offprint requests to: J. de Boer, M.D., Eurotransplant Foundation, P.O. Box 2304, 2301 CH Leiden, The Netherlands

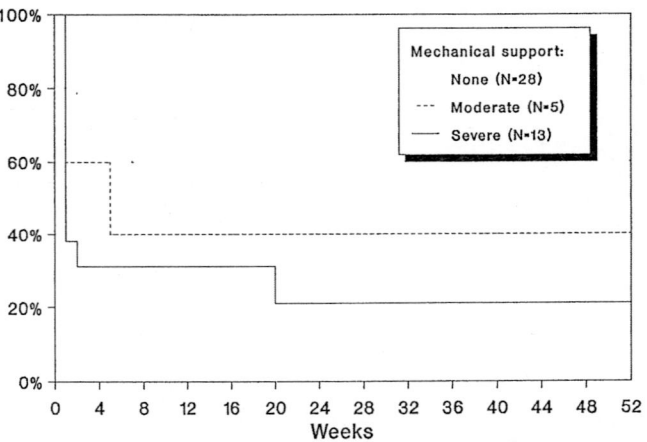

Fig.3. Graft survival in heart retransplantation, Eurotransplant Jan 1988–Aug 1991

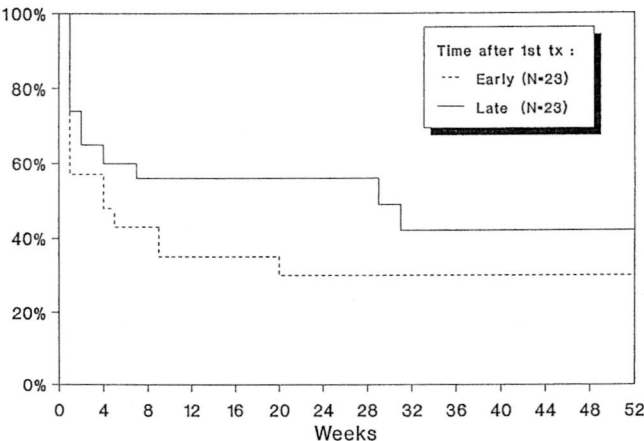

Fig.4. Graft survival in heart retransplantation, Eurotransplant Jan 1988–Aug 1991

patients with intra-aortic counterpulsation and 13 with a ventricular assist device). In 23 cases the patient was retransplanted within 30 days (the early retransplantation group), the others were retransplanted after more than 30 days (the late retransplantation group).

Results

The results of the follow-up analysis of the 46 transplantations are shown in Fig.1. The overall graft survival was 36% at 1 year. Of the 46 transplants, 28 (61%) failed within 1–213 days (median 5 days), 17 of these within 1 week. From the group that received mechanical support prior to retransplantation, 13 grafts failed within 1–319 days (median 3 days), while 15 of the 28 without mechanical support failed within 1–213 days of retransplantation (median 21 days). However, the 1-year survival of grafts in the two groups were not significantly different (Fig.2). Moderate support (i.e. intra-aortic counterpulsation) had no effect on the graft survival (40% at 1 year vs 43% for the group without mechanical support), while the graft survival of the severe support group (i.e. the ventricular assist group) was much lower (21% 1-year graft survival) (Fig.3, P = ns).

The late retransplantation group did somewhat better than the early retransplantation group (42% 1-year graft survival vs 30%) (Fig.4, P = ns).

Discussion

Our results are lower than those of the International Society for Heart and Lung Transplantation, which reported 49% patient survival at 1 year in regrafted cardiac patients [2], compared with 81% 1-year patient survival for primary transplantation [2], as also reported by Cabrol et al. [1]. However, these patients received a cardiac retransplant also after chronic rejection while the patients in our study received their second graft only after acute failure.

The question remains as to whether the poorer graft survival results obtained in patients after acute cardiac retransplantation justifies the use of a higher urgency code for those patients than for those awaiting primary cardiac transplant. The number of acute retransplantations is still too low to draw final conclusions.

Acknowledgements. We are grateful to the medical staff, nurses and administrators of the participating cardiac transplant centres for providing the necessary data for this special analysis.

References

1. Cabrol C, Gandjbakhch I, Pavie A, et al. (1991) Cardiac retransplantation, la Pitie experience. Transplant Clin Immunol 22: 169–175
2. Kriett JM, Kaye MP (1991) The Registry of the International Society for Heart and Lung Transplantation: Eighth Official Report. J Heart Lung Transplant 4: 491–498

Transplant Int (1992) 5 [Suppl 1]: S 221–S 223

TRANSPLANT
International
© Springer-Verlag 1992

Right ventricular failure after heart transplantation: relationship with preoperative haemodynamic parameters

C. Campana[1], A. Gavazzi[1], R. Marioni[1], A. D'Armini[2], N. Pederzolli[2], C. Larizza[3], C. Berzuini[3], L. Martinelli[2], M. Vigano[2], and C. Montemartini[1]

[1] Division of Cardiology and [2] Division of Cardiac Surgery, IRCCS Policlinico S. Matteo
[3] Department of Computer Sciences and Systems, University of Pavia, Pavia, Italy

Abstract. The prevalence of right ventricular failure after orthotopic heart transplantation, evaluated in 196 patients, was 11.7%, as assessed by the presence during the first postoperative month of right atrial pressure > 10 mm Hg. Two deaths, related to refractory right ventricular failure, were observed within the first month, both in subjects with preoperative pulmonary arteriolar resistances > 5 Wood Units. The haemodynamic profile after heart transplantation showed a significant decrease ($P < 0.01$) and an early normalization of pulmonary arterial pressure, pulmonary wedge pressure and pulmonary arteriolar resistances, while right atrial pressure slowly decreased until the third month. In a long-term analysis of survival (death within 1 year) the probability of death was significantly related to the values of right atrial pressure and cardiac index during the first month after heart transplantation. Otherwise, the presence of elevated values of right atrial pressure did not show a significant correlation with the echocardiographic right ventricular end-diastolic diameter nor with the presence of right bundle branch block. The careful selection of patients referred for the cardiac transplantation (mean value of pulmonary arteriolar resistances in the evaluated subjects was 2.5 ± 1.5 Wood Units) improves the probability of avoiding the appearance of severe right ventricular failure in the postoperative period in most cases. The best predictor of right ventricular failure remains to be clearly identified.

Key words: Right ventricular failure – Pulmonary hypertension – Pulmonary vascular resistances – Heart transplantation

---

The development of secondary pulmonary hypertension is a frequent finding in patients with advanced cardiac failure referred for heart transplantation. The evaluation of the degree of pulmonary hypertension and pulmonary vascular resistances is a critical issue in defining the indication for orthotopic cardiac transplantation. Previous experience in transplantation of patients with high pulmonary resistances has resulted in donor right heart failure generally in the early postoperative period.

It is still unclear which among the various preoperative haemodynamic parameters indicative of pulmonary hypertension is a good predictor of the clinical and haemodynamic evolution after cardiac transplantation.

The purposes of this study were to verify the prevalence of right ventricular failure after cardiac transplantation, to characterize the potential predictors of right ventricular failure after cardiac transplantation, and to evaluate the short-term (1 and 3 months) and long-term (1 year) mortality after heart transplantation in relation to the haemodynamic parameters before and after the cardiac transplant.

Methods

Between November 1985 and April 1991, 196 orthotopic cardiac transplants were performed at the IRCCS Policlinico S. Matteo of Pavia, according to the criteria of the clinical programme of heart transplantation.

The patients ranged from 9 to 67 years of age (mean age 43.2); 176 were males and 20 were females. All patients showed advanced cardiac failure and were ascribed to III or IV NYHA functional class. The indications for heart transplantation were dilated cardiomyopathy in 96 patients, ischaemic cardiac disease in 85, valvular heart disease in 13, and hypertrophic cardiomyopathy in 2 cases.

The preoperative cardiac catheterization data were available for all 196 patients. The death of 13 patients occurred within the first month, 6 between the first and the third month and 15 three months later after heart transplantation. The postoperative catheterization data were completely lacking in 13 cases and 6 other cases had only one evaluation after cardiac transplant, because the patients died.

The haemodynamic data were derived from right heart catheterization by the Swan-Ganz thermodilution technique. The systolic, diastolic and mean pulmonary arterial pressures, the mean right atrial and pulmonary capillary wedge pressures, the cardiac output, and pulmonary vascular resistances expressed in Wood Units, were recorded before transplantation and at the first and third month after surgery. If preoperative pulmonary vascular resistances were > 5 Wood Units, the pretransplant haemodynamic evaluation

Offprint requests to: Carlo Campana, M. D., Division of Cardiology, IRCCS Policlinico S. Matteo, I-27100 Pavia, Italy

was also carried out after the administration of vasodilators (nitroprusside graded infusion at a starting dose of 0.2 µg/kg per min).

In the analysis of the post-transplant data, the presence or the absence of right bundle branch disturbances in the 12-lead surface ECG was considered, according to the hypothesis that this finding could be related to right ventricular distension.

In a limited group of patients (64 patients, mean age 42 years) it was possible to analyse the echocardiographic parameters; two-dimensional and Doppler echocardiograms in the parasternal short and long axis, and apical two- and four-chamber views were obtained, respectively, at the first and third month after cardiac transplantation. The echocardiographic images were analysed to assess right ventricular size (right ventricular diastolic diameter).

Statistics

The results are presented as mean ± standard deviation. Means were compared using the non-paired Student's t-test; statistical significance was defined as $P < 0.05$.

A survival analysis was performed using a logic-linear model, considering nine different variables and various associations between them.

Results

Two deaths because of refractory right ventricular failure in the early postoperative period were observed, both in patients with preoperative pulmonary arteriolar resistances > 5 Wood Units.

The prevalence of right ventricular failure in the whole population was 11.7%, considering that 23 patients showed, at the first month evaluation, a right atrial pressure > 10 mmHg (mean 13.17 ± 2.39 mmHg (range 11–20 mmHg).

The haemodynamic profile was characterized by an early normalization of pulmonary artery pressure (PAP) (pretransplant systolic PAP 48.6 ± 18.3 mmHg; mean PAP 33.1 ± 12.9 mmHg; diastolic PAP 23.4 ± 10.9 mmHg; first month systolic PAP 28.3 ± 8.3 mmHg; first month mean PAP 18.1 ± 6.07 mmHg; first month diastolic PAP 10.8 ± 5.3 mmHg; third month systolic PAP 28.3 ± 8.6 mmHg; third month mean PAP 18.2 ± 6.4 mmHg; third month diastolic PAP 11.7 ± 5.8 mmHg), pulmonary wedge pressure (PWP) pretransplant PWP 23.5 ± 11.2 mmHg; first month PWP 9.3 ± 5.3 mmHg; third month PWP 9 ± 5.2 mmHg) and pulmonary arteriolar resistances (PAR) (pretransplant PAR 2.5 ± 1.5 W.U., first month PAR 1.5 ± 0.8 W.U., third month PAR 1.5 ± 0.9 W.U.).

Right atrial pressure (RAP) showed a slow decrease until the third month (pretransplant RAP 7.9 ± 6 mmHg; first month RAP 5.5 ± 3.9 mmHg; third month RAP 4.9 ± 3.3 mmHg).

The values of cardiac output and cardiac index before transplantation were, respectively, 4.0 ± 1.2 l/min and 2.2 ± 0.6 l/min per m^2. After heart transplant surgery, the related values of cardiac output and cardiac index were: first month, 5.7 ± 1.1 l/min and 3.3 ± 0.7 l/min per m^2; third month 5.8 ± 1.2 l/min and 3.3 ± 0.7 l/min per m^2.

In the short-term survival analysis none of the eight pretransplant haemodynamic variables provided a significant predictive capacity. In the long-term evaluation, in contrast, the nine post-transplant variables supplied a predictive survival power, but only considering the values related to the first month, according to the formula:

$$P \text{ (death within one year)} = \frac{e^{3.7 - 0.14 \times AD1 - 1.8 \times CI1}}{1 + e^{3.7 - 0.14 \times AD1 - 1.8 \times CI1}}$$

Then the values of right atrial pressure and cardiac index for first month after cardiac transplantation showed a significant predictive capacity.

On the other hand, the pretransplant and 3 months post-transplant parameters did not supply statistical predictivity. In relation to two different subgroups with right atrial pressure for the first month after heart transplantation > or ≤ 10 mmHg, the preoperative haemodynamic patterns did not show statistically significant differences.

The evaluation of the echocardiographic parameters showed mean values of right ventricular end-diastolic diameter (RVEDD) of 27.9 ± 5.1 mm for the first month and 26.4 ± 5.02 mm for the third month (NS). If they were related to the right atrial pressure, in the presence of right atrial pressure > 10 mmHg, RVEDD was 28.6 ± 5.3 mm for the first month and 25.2 ± 5.8 mm for the third month. In the presence of right atrial pressure < 10 mmHg RVEDD was 27.4 ± 4.9 mm for the first month and 27.1 ± 4.3 mm for the third month, without significant differences among the groups.

The prevalence of right bundle branch disturbances (complete or incomplete block) after cardiac transplantation was 43% (84/196 patients). In the subgroup of patients with right atrial pressure > 10 mmHg, the prevalence of right bundle branch block was 56% (13/23 patients), without significant differences compared with all transplant recipients.

Discussion

Pulmonary hypertension is observed in most patients affected by advanced cardiac failure referred for heart transplantation. Generally the subjects who show pulmonary hypertension and high pulmonary vascular resistances are not good candidates for orthotopic heart transplantation, because of the presence of severe risk of acute perioperative right ventricular failure. The subjects with pulmonary vascular resistances > 5 or 6 Wood Units are usually not admitted to the cardiac transplant programme, even if there has not been a wide agreement on this subject.

The Wood Unit has traditionally been used to measure pulmonary vascular resistance, but according to certain authors [1], the pulmonary vascular resistance index unit (PVRI) identifies better the subjects at higher risk for right ventricular failure after cardiac transplantation.

The transpulmonary pressure gradient (TPG = PAPm-PWP) also seems to be a good marker of level of pulmonary hypertension to define the contraindications to orthotopic heart transplant and to show a different early and late risk of death [3].

According to other studies [2], the increased risk of death imposed by high pulmonary vascular resistances is continuously variable and it is not correct to identify a cut-off level.

An accurate selection of patients referred for cardiac transplantation according to pulmonary hypertension and pulmonary vascular resistances is an important condition to avoid the development of right ventricular failure. According to these criteria, the prevalence of right ventricular failure observed in this study was not remarkable. The mean values of preoperative pulmonary vascular resistances in all transplant recipients were 2.5 ± 1.5 W.U. The evolution of haemodynamic parameters after cardiac transplant confirmed a significant reduction and normalization in pulmonary arterial pressure and pulmonary wedge pressure, a behaviour which can define a good readaptation after surgery. This finding was not evident in right atrial pressure, as an expression of the right ventricular adaptation may be the presence of chronic volume overload.

The findings related to the presence of right bundle branch block and to the degree of right ventricular end diastolic diameter were not significantly different in patients with higher right atrial pressure and in the subjects with first month right atrial pressure within 10 mm Hg.

In a complex statistical evaluation of long-term survival, nevertheless, the haemodynamic data represented a useful parameter because the values of right atrial pressure and cardiac index for the first postoperative month showed a significant relationship with the probability of death.

References

1. Addonizio LJ, Gersony WM, Robbins RC, Drusin RE, Smith CR, Reison DS, Reemtsma K, Rose EA (1987) Elevated pulmonary vascular resistance and cardiac transplantation. Circulation 76 [Suppl V]: V-52
2. Kirklin JK, Naftel DC, Kirklin JW, Blackstone JH, White-Williams C, Bourge RC (1988) Pulmonary vascular resistance and the risk of heart transplantation. J Heart Transplant 7: 331–336
3. Murali S, Kormos RL, Uretsky BF, Schecter D, Reddy PS, Hardesty R, Ruffner RJ, Breisblatt WM, Griffith BP, Armitage JM (1990) Pre-operative pulmonary hypertension and mortality after orthotopic cardiac transplantation. J Heart Transplant 9: 56

Transplant Int (1992) 5 [Suppl 1]: S 224–S 227

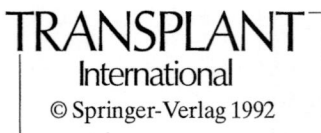

TRANSPLANT
International
© Springer-Verlag 1992

Preoperative prostaglandin E1 treatment to prevent right ventricular failure after orthotopic heart transplantation

A. Wasler[1], F. Iberer[1], K. H. Tscheliessnigg[1], H. Metzler[2], H. Gombotz[2], J. Berger[2], T. Auer[1], and B. Petutschnigg[1]

[1] Department of Surgery and [2] Department of Anesthiology, University of Graz, Graz, Austria

Abstract. Elevated pulmonary vascular resistance (PVR) and pulmonary hypertension (PH) are high risk factors for early graft failure in orthotopic heart transplantation (oHTx). The need for an oversized donor in patients with elevated PVR aggravates the shortage of suitable donor organs. To decrease the elevated PVR to values suitable for orthotopic heart transplantation prostaglandin E1 (PGE1) was administered in 11 patients (11 male, mean age 49.2 years, mean dosage 35 ng/kg per min over 6–8 days). Ten days after the discontinuation of the PGE1 therapy, recatheterization was done. All haemodynamic data were determined by right heart catheterization using a Swan Ganz catheter and thermodilution technique before, and 10 days after, PGE1 treatment. The Wilcoxon signed ranks test was used for statistics. PVR significantly decreased in all patients (5.5 to 2.8 Wood units, $P < 0.005$). All patients were considered to be suitable for oHTX and put on the waiting list. At the time of writing, in eight of these patients (eight male, mean age 49.6 years; four ischemic, four dilatative CMP) oHTX had been successfully performed. No right ventricular failure occurred in the postoperative phase. These results sugest that long-term moderation of elevated PVR by PGE1 therapy weeks or months before transplantation enables oHTX in patients with elevated PVR.

Key words: Pulmonary hypertension – Pulmonary vascular resistance – Orthotopic heart transplantation – Prostaglandin E1

Orthotopic heart transplantation (oHTx) in end-stage congestive heart disease is complicated by secondary pulmonary hypertension (PH) and consecutive elevated pulmonary vascular resistance (PVR). PH and elevated PVR are outstanding risk factors for early postoperative mor-

tality in oHTX [9]. Patients with an elevated PVR of 4 to 6 Wood units (WU) are not generally accepted for oHTX. However, no clear definition of the borderline between orthotopic and heterotopic heart transplantation concerning elevated pulmonary pressure and PVR has yet been found [12]. Moreover, the reversibility of elevated PVR to values tolerated by the unconditioned transplanted right ventricle complicates the definition of the borderline indication.

In cases of PVR values higher than 4–6 WU the use of an oversized donor heart is indicated [19]. Some centres prefer the heterotopic transplantation [15] technique or perform heart lung transplantation which are at higher risk and have inferior long-term results compared with oHTx. To enable oHTx in patients with high PVR and to avoid the unindicated implantation of oversized donor hearts for borderline indications we used the selective pulmonary vasculature dilatator prostaglandin E1 (PGE1) to induce a long-lasting moderation of elevated PVR.

Materials and methods

Patients, indication for PGE1 therapy, pretreatment right heart catheterization

In 1990 33 patients were evaluated for cardiac transplantation at the University of Graz, Department of Transplantation. Eleven patients presenting a PVR higher than 3 WU or a mean pulmonary artery pressure higher than 30 mm Hg were considered to be at risk for postoperative right ventricular failure and were included in this study (Table 1). All patients were on digitalis, ACE inhibitors and diuretics. This therapy was continued until recatheterization was done.

Catheterization technique

A Baxter Eduard Swan-Ganz 7F thermodilution catheter was introduced through the right internal jugular vein and advanced to the pulmonary artery wedge position using radiographic and haemodynamic guidance. Haemodynamic data were recorded with a Hellige

---

Offprint requests to: Wasler Andre, M.D., Universitätsklinik für Chirurgie, Transplantationschirurgie, Fach 65, Auenbruggerplatz, A-8036 Graz, Austria

Table 1. Demographic data

Patients	Sex	Age	Diagnosis
1	m	45	dilative
2	m	46	ischaemic
3	m	32	dilative
4	m	61	ischaemic
5	m	57	dilative
6	m	33	dilative
7	m	51	ischaemic
8	m	54	dilative
9	m	60	ischaemic
10	m	61	ischaemic
11	m	42	dilative

Table 2. Haemodynamic data before PGE1 treatment

Patient number	PAPs (mmHg)	PAPd (mmHg)	PAPm (mmHg)	CO (l/min)	PVR (WU)
1	83	27	47	4.7	4.2
2	70	42	52	3.5	3.4
3	69	47	37	3.8	3.0
4	65	24	38	3.7	3.2
5	45	23	35	2.0	5.2
6	47	22	33	3.0	4.3
7	79	31	53	5.9	3.1
8	135	50	94	3.6	13.9
9	78	36	56	2.1	9.5
10	71	19	36	3.5	6.3
11	79	32	50	3.9	4.9

PAP, pulmonary artery pressure; s, systolic; d, diastolic; m, mean; CO, cardiac output; PVR, pulmonary vascular resistance; WU, Wood units

Table 3. Haemodynamic data after PGE1 treatment

Patient number	PAPs (mmHg)	PAPd (mmHg)	PAPm (mmHg)	CO (l/min)	PVR (WU)	Outcome
1	98	32	55	4.9	3.1	oHTx
2	63	26	36	5.0	3.0	oHTx[a]
3	50	22	36	4.0	0.5	oHTx
4	58	27	38	4.3	1.8	d.w.w.
5	45	19	29	5.7	1.9	d.w.w.
6	30	15	24	3.0	1.8	oHTx
7	71	27	46	5.9	2.8	oHTx
8	80	39	37	3.9	5.7	d.w.w.
9	73	31	42	4.0	3.8	oHTx[b]
10	52	17	28	5.0	2.5	oHTx
11	78	27	45	3.9	3.6	oHTx[c]

d.w.w., died while waiting for oHTx

[a] died 10 months after oHTx: *Pneumocystis carinii* pneumonia

[b] died 3 months after oHTx: ventricular fibrillation

[c] died on day 20 after oHTx: acute rejection

Table 4. Haemodynamic data ($n = 11$)

	Before PGE1	After PGE1	
PAPsys (mmHg)	74.6 (45–135)	63.4 (30–98)	$P < 0.05$
PAPdia (mmHg)	32.3 (19–50)	25.6 (15–39)	$P < 0.05$
PAPm (mmHg)	48.9 (33–94)	37.8 (24–55)	$P < 0.05$
Wedge (mmHg)	30.5 (17–44)	27.5 (15–40)	ns
CO (l/min)	3.6 (2–5.9)	4.5 (3–5.7)	$P < 0.05$
PVR (Wood)	5.5 (3–13.9)	2.8 (0.5–5.7)	$P < 0.005$

Servomed. The cardiac output was calculated with a 9520 cardiac output computer of the American Edwards Laboratories. Oxygen and nitroglycerine tests were performed during right heart catheterization.

PGE1 treatment

PGE1 (Minprog, Upjohn) was initiated at a dosage of 5 ng/kg per min. During the first 24 h a stepwise dosage augmentation was performed until a mean dosage of 35 ng/kg per min (25–60 ng) was reached [16]. The PGE1 dosage was maintained continuously for 6–8 days using a motor syringe pump via a central i.v. line. At the expected end of treatment the dosage was tapered during another 24 h. The amount of the dosage increase was dependent on the occurrence of side effects, such as headache, abdominal pain, systemic hypotension, oedema and joint pain. In all patients the dosage increase was performed until side effects appeared. To induce tolerance to high doses of PGE1 intravenous piritamide, diuretics and catecholamines at dosages up to 8 µg/kg per min were administered. After PGE1 therapy all patients were discharged for 10 days.

Recatheterization, statistics

After 10 days all patients were readmitted to our department. In all patients the PGE1 treatment had been discontinued for a minimum of 8 days before recatheterization was done using identical techniques to the investigation before the PGE1 treatment. Statistical evaluation was performed using the Wilcoxon signed ranks tests. Significance was assumed for $P < 0.05$.

Results

The baseline results of right heart catherization are presented in Table 2. The results of the right heart catherization 1 week after the discontinuation of the PGE1 treatment are summarized in Table 3. In all patients the haemodynamic data improved (Tables 3 and 4). The PVR significantly decreased in all 11 patients treated with PGE1. In eight patients the CO increased, in ten patients a reduction in the systolic PAP occurred, and in nine patients the diastolic and the mean PAP decreased. No correlation could be found between the reduction in PVR during right heart catheterization using oxygen or nitroglycerine and the PGE1-induced long-term moderation of PVR.

At the time of writing eight of the PGE1-treated patients had undergone orthotopic heart transplantation according to the techniques described by the Stanford group [13]. The mean interval between PGE1 treatment and oHTx was 2 months (10–152 days). The donor/recipient body weight relationship indicated no use of oversized donors in this patient cohort (Table 5). In the early postoperative period all patients were prophylactically treated with PGE1 starting from the weaning of the cardiopulmonary bypass. No right heart failure or tricuspid valve insufficiency was observed after transplantation. Three patients died due to *Pneumocystis carinii* pneumonia (10 months after oHTx), ventricular fibrillation (3 months after oHTx) and therapy-resistant acute rejection grade 4 (20 days after oHTx).

Table 5. Donor/recipient body-weight ratio

Patient number	PVR before PGE1	PVR after PGE1	Body-weight ratio
1	4.2	3.1	1.0
2	3.4	3.0	1.2
3	3.0	0.5	1.1
4	4.3	1.8	1.0
5	3.1	2.8	1.3
6	9.5	3.8	0.9
7	6.3	2.5	1.2
8	4.9	3.6	1.0

Discussion

Pulmonary vascular resistance of 6–8 WU is generally accepted to be an absolute contraindication for oHTx [8]. In contrast, right ventricular decompensation and failure has also been observed in patients presenting slightly elevated or near normal values [12]. The exposure of the donor heart to the new haemodynamic conditions of the recipient after weaning from bypass leads, in cases of right ventricular afterload mismatch, to a right ventricular overload pattern [3] which results in hypocontractility [14]. To get used to the new right ventricular afterload conditions about 2 weeks of training and adaptation are required. After that time the upper normal range of right and left ventricular filling pressure is reached [3]. The danger of right ventricular failure increases when primary right ventricular dysfunction induced by prolonged ischaemic time [3], preservation damage or body size mismatch complicates the haemodynamic situation [11]. The use of donor hearts which are larger, have reduced ischaemic time and have not undergone any significant trauma while supporting the donor in patients with marginal PVR has been suggested [19]. However, all these factors affecting the function of the transplanted right ventricle contribute to the imprecise limit of PVR beyond which oHTx is contraindicated.

Most centers accept 6 WU as the borderline for oHTx [1, 2]. To overcome these problems prostaglandins are perioperatively used at many centres. PGE1 is a short-acting, potent pulmonary vasodilator which increases myocardial contractility [4], decreases PVR, increases cardiac output [4] and is an immunosuppressive agent [11].

The effect of PGE1 on elevated PVR and PH after mitral valve replacement [5] and after coronary bypass grafting [6] has been reported. The postoperative effect of prostaglandins on acute right ventricular failure after heart transplantation has been proved [17, 20]. Higgenbottam reported successful bridging to heart-lung transplantation with continous prostacycline therapy in patients with fixed primary pulmonary hypertension [10].

We decided on PGE1 because of its short time of action and its 80–90% metabolism at the first lung passage [7]. Because of the application in the upper vena cava the main effects of PGE1 occur in the lesser circuit. Treatment of severe side effects is a simple dosage reduction.

PGE1 decreased PVR in all patients. The pulmonary vasodilating effect of PGE1 results in an improvement in the left ventricular filling pressure. In addition, the increased contractility of the myocardium results in improved cardiac output and in a long-lasting reduction in the right ventricular afterload. Nevertheless, the persistence of the decreased PVR values for weeks after stopping the PGE1 therapy has to be further investigated. The improvement of the left ventricular performance [18] and the sympathomimetic effect of the applied catecholamines might contribute to the long-lasting effect.

Despite seriouly elevated PVR and PAP values before PGE1 treatment, after treatment all patients were suitable for oHTx according to generally accepted criteria. On the one hand we circumvented heterotopic heart transplantation in highly elevated PVR, and on the other hand the waste of oversized donor organs could be avoided as none of the transplanted right ventricles failed.

The use of oxygen or nitroglycerine enables the demonstration of the reversibility of the elevated PVR during right heart catheterization but their effect is not specific to the pulmonary vasculature and it does not result in long-term moderation of the elevated PVR. The influence of the PGE1 treatment on survival time and life quality while on the waiting list cannot be determined yet, but there is a trend towards better working capacity and life expectancy for patients after PGE1 treatment.

In conclusion, we have proved the reversibility of the vasoconstrictive component of the PVR in a model independent of oxygen or nitroglycerine examination. It can be assumed that patients responding to PGE1 therapy while on the waiting list do not develop right ventricular failure under PGE1 therapy after oHTx. There is a long-term moderation of elevated PVR. Patients also presenting with borderline PVR can be accepted for oHTx. We are able to accept donor organs that are not much oversized and might have longer ischaemic times. This increases the probability of obtaining a suitable donor heart and reduces the risk of wasting organs due to right ventricular failure.

References

1. Addonizio LJ, Gersony WM, Robbins RL, Drusin RE, Smith CR, Reison DS, Reemtsma K, Rose EA (1987) Elevated pulmonary vascular resistance and cardiac transplantation. Circulation 76 [Suppl V]: V–52
2. Armitage JM, Hardesty RL, Griffith BP (1987) Prostaglandin E1. An effective treatment of right heart failure after orthotopic heart transplantation. J Heart Transplant 6: 348–351
3. Bathia JSJ, Kirshenbaum JM, Shemin RJ, Cohn LH, Collins JJ, DiSesa VJ, Young PJ, Mudge GH, St. John Sutton M (1987) Time course of resolution of pulmonary hypertension and right ventricular remodeling after orthotopic cardiac transplantation. Circulation 4: 819–826
4. Clayman CB (1975) The prostaglandins. JAMA 8: 904–906
5. D'Ambra MN, LaRaia PJ, Philbin DM, Watkins D, Hilgenberg AD, Buckley MJ (1985) Prostaglandin E1. A new therapy for refractory right heart failure and pulmonary hypertension after mitral valve replacement. J Thorac Cardiovasc Surg 89: 567–572
6. Dewhirst WE (1988) Prostaglandin E1 for refractory right heart failure after coronary artery bypass grafting. J Cardiothorac Anesth 2: 56–59
7. Ferreira (1967) Prostaglandins: their disappearance from and release into circulation. Nature 216: 868

8. Fonger JD, Borkon AM, Baumgartner WA, Achuff SC, Augustine S, Reitz BA (1986) Acute right ventricular failure following heart transplantation: improvement with prostaglandin E1 and right ventricular assist. J Heart Transplant 5: 317–321

9. Heck CF, Shumway SJ, Kaye MP (1989) The Registry of the International Society for Heart Transplantation: sixth Official Report – 1989. J Heart Transplant 4: 271–276

10. Higgenbottam T, Wheeldon D, Wells F, Wallwork J (1984) Long-term treatment of primary pulmonary hypertension with continuous intravenous epoprosterol (Prostacyclin). Lancet II: 1046–1047

11. Iberer F, Wasler A, Tscheliessnigg KH, Metzler H, Rehak P, Kleinert M, Popper H, Auer T, Gombotz H, Petutschnigg B, Rödl S, Giegerl E (1990) Prostaglandin in der Herztransplantation-Prävention des Rechtsherzversagens und der Abstossung. Z Herz, Thorax, Gefäßchir 14: 33–37

12. Kirklin JK, Naftel D, Kirklin JW, Blackstone E, White-Williams C, Bourge R (1988) Pulmonary vascular resistance and the risk of heart transplantation. J Heart Transplant 7: 331–336

13. Lower RR, Shumway NE (1960) Studies on orthotopic heart transplantation of the canine heart. Surg Forum 11: 18–24

14. Pascual JMS, Fiorelli AI, Bellotti GM, Stolf NAG, Jatene AD (1990) Prostacyclin in the management of pulmonary hypertension after heart transplantation. J Heart Transplant 9: 644–651

15. Shumway SJ, Baughman KL, Traill TA, Cameron DE, Fonger JD, Gardner TJ, Achoff SC, Reitz BA, Baumgartner WA (1989) Persistent pulmonary hypertension after heterotopic heart transplantation: a case report. J Heart Transplant 8: 387–390

16. Swan P, Tibballs J, Duncan A (1986) Prostaglandin E1 in primary pulmonary hypertension. Crit Care Med 1: 72–73

17. Tscheliessnigg KH, Iberer F, Zenker G, Kleinert M, Auer T, Gombotz H, Breinl E, Metzler H, Dacar D, Mächler H, Popper H, Lanzer G, Wasler A, Petutschnigg B, Rödl S (1990) Right ventricular failure and tricuspid regurgitation after orthotopic cardiac transplantation. Diagnosis and treatment. Trasplante 1(3): 113–117

18. Virgolini I, Kaliman J, Fitscha P, O'Grady J, Rogatti W, Sinzinger H (1989) Beneficial effect of long-term PGE1 treatment in left ventricular heart failure. Prostaglandins Leukot Essent Fatty Acids 38: 177–180

19. Wahlers TH, Haverich A, Schäfers HJ, Hermann G, Fieguth HG, Borst HG (1987) Risk factors of right heart failure (RHF) after orthotopic heart transplantation (HTX) (abstract). J Am Coll Cardiol 9: 90A

20. Weiss CI, Park JV, Bolman RM (1989) Prostaglandin E1 for treatment of elevated pulmonary vascular resistance in patients undergoing cardiac transplantation. Transplant Proc 21: 2555–2556

Transplant Int (1992) 5 [Suppl 1]: S 228–S 230

TRANSPLANT
International
© Springer-Verlag 1992

Phenotype of endomyocardial biopsy-derived T-lymphocyte cultures and chronic rejection after heart transplantation

K. Groeneveld[1], **A.H.M.M. Balk**[2], **A.J. Ouwehand**[2], **E.H.M. Loonen**[1], **M. vd Linden**[2], **S. Strikwerda**[2], **B. Mochtar**[2], **N.H.P.M. Jutte**[1], and **W. Weimar**[1]

[1] Department of Internal Medicine I, Erasmus University Rotterdam, Rotterdam, The Netherlands
[2] Thorax Center, University Hospital Rotterdam-Dijkzigt, Rotterdam, The Netherlands

Abstract. Chronic rejection (CR) is a major problem in long-term survival in heart transplantation. We analysed whether the occurrence of CR correlates with the incidence of acute rejections (AR) or with characteristics of endomyocardial biopsy-derived cell cultures. CR was diagnosed by annual angiography and defined as all coronary vascular changes. One year after transplantation 24 of the 63 patients had CR (38%). The incidence of AR in CR + and CR − patients was comparable. The patients in both groups had similar individual median percentages of EMB-yielding cell cultures. During the first year the CR − patients had more cultures in which at least 60% of the cells were CD4 + T cells (50% vs 37%, $P = 0.05$), due to a stronger CD4 predominance in the first 6 months. In the second year the CD4 predominance in the patients diagnosed as CR + after 1 year tended to be higher ($P = 0.08$). The patients had comparable percentages of cultures predominated by CD8 + T cells, $\gamma\delta$ T cells or NK cells, irrespective of the time interval. These results might indicate that CD4 + T lymphocytes play a dual role in the aetiology of CR.

Key words: Chronic rejection – Heart transplantation – CD4 + T cells

Introduction

The long-term survival of heart transplant recipients is limited by the development of accelerated coronary artery disease. Knowledge about the aetiology and treatment of this disease, commonly referred to as chronic rejection (CR), is limited [1]. Libby et al. describe a model in which CR was the result of a cellular immunological reaction in the graft arteries [4]. In this model the major cell type involved was the host CD4 + helper T cell.

After heart transplantation endomyocardial biopsies (EMB) are taken at regular intervals to diagnose acute rejection. We analysed whether the development of CR is related to the occurrence of acute rejection episodes. We also compared patients with and without CR with respect to growth patterns and phenotypic composition of cells grown from EMB [6, 10] to analyse whether the occurrence of CR is correlated with any of these characteristics.

Materials and methods

Patients

We studied 63 consecutive cardiac allograft recipients transplanted between January 1988 and February 1990. The median age of the patients was 50 years, with a range of 19 to 59 years. All patients had received preoperative blood transfusions and all received cyclosporine and low-dose prednisone as maintenance immunosuppression. In the early post-transplantation period serial EMBs were obtained at weekly intervals. Later EMBs were taken less frequently. The rejection grade was assessed according to the criteria of Billingham. Only is cases of infiltrate with myocyte necrosis (grade 2) was antirejection therapy instituted. During the first year pTx we received 12 to 23 EMBs from each patient (median 15 EMBs). In the second year pTx 2–5 EMBs per patient were obtained.

Diagnosis of CR was assessed by annual coronary angiography and defined as the presence of all coronary vascular changes, including minor wall irregularities of the epicardial branches and the intramyocardial branches. All coronary angiographies were scored by consensus of two of us (AHMM B and M vd L).

Culture method and phenotypic analysis

Endomyocardial biopsies were cultured as described by Ouwehand et al. [6]. Surface differentiation antigens of the EMB-derived cultures were analysed as described before [6]. A phenotypic marker was defined as predominant when at least 60% of the cells were positive.

Statistics

Unless stated otherwise data were analysed by the Mann-Whitney U test.

Offprint requests to: Kees Groeneveld, Ph.D., Department of Internal Medicine I, Bd 299, Erasmus University Rotterdam, P.O. Box 1738, 3000 DR Rotterdam, The Netherlands

Table 1. Median individual percentage of CD4 or CD8 predominance ($\geq 60\%$ of the cells) in T-cell cultures from CR + and CR − patients derived from EMBs taken during different time intervals

Time interval	Predominant phenotype	Median % of cultures (number of patients)		
		CR + patients	CR − patients	P-value
First year	CD4	37 (24)	50 (39)	0.05
	CD8	33 (24)	25 (39)	0.60
0–180 days	CD4	44 (24)	59 (39)	0.06
	CD8	27 (24)	20 (39)	0.54
180–360 days	CD4	10 (24)	33 (35)	0.80
	CD8	50 (24)	33 (35)	0.58
Until first	CD4	50 (17)	50 (27)	0.32
acute rejection[a]	CD8	20 (17)	0 (28)	0.10

[a] rejection biopsy included

Results

Patients

One year after transplantation, 24 of the 63 patients studied (38%) were diagnosed as having CR. The median age of these 24 CR + patients (50 years, range 17–59 years) was similar to that of the CR − patients (50 years, range 17–58 years).

During the first year post-transplantation the number of EMBs obtained from CR + and CR − patients were comparable: CR + patients median number of EMBs, 15 (range 13–23); CR − patients, 16 (range 12–23). After 12 months, 17 CR + patients (71%) and 29 CR − patients (74%) had had one or more periods of acute rejection. The number of acute rejection episodes was not related to the development of CR.

Cell cultures

Lymphocyte cultures (to a minimum of 10^6 cells) could be established from at least one EMB from all patients. After 1 year the CR + and CR − patients had comparable median percentages of biopsies yielding T-cell cultures: CR + patients; 43%; CR − patients, 33%; $P = 0.45$. The percentage growth from biopsies of CR + and CR − patients at different time intervals during this first year was also highly comparable.

In the first year the CR − patients had a higher percentage of cultures in which at least 60% of the cells were CD4 + T cells (CR − patients, median percentage 50%; CR + patients, 37%; $P = 0.05$) (Table 1). This difference in CD4 predominance was mainly caused by the EMB obtained in the first half year ($P = 0.06$), since in the second half year CD4 + T cells predominated in CR + and CR − patients in equal percentages ($P = 0.80$). CR + patients tended to have a higher percentage of CD8 + T-cell-dominated cultures from EMBs obtained before the first acute rejection episode ($P = 0.10$). In other time intervals the percentages of cultures dominated by CD8 + T cells in both patient groups were comparable. There were no differences between CR + and CR − patients with respect to the predominance of NK or γδ cells.

Second year

Eleven CR + patients and 15 CR − patients could be studied for a second year. Two of the 15 patients negative for CR after 1 year developed CR during the second year. The 13 CR − patients and the two newly diagnosed CR + patients did not differ with respect to the characteristics of the graft infiltrating cells. This might very well be due to the small number of patients and small number of EMBs obtained in the second year. Five of the 11 patients diagnosed as having CR after 1 year had at least one acute rejection during the second year, compared with only one of the 13 patients who at the end of the second year were still CR − ($P = 0.17$, Fisher test).

The 11 CR + patients were compared with the 13 CR − patients concerning the cultures derived from EMBs obtained during the second year. The patient groups had comparable median percentages of cell growth and predominance of CD8 + T cells. There were no differences in the predomination of either NK cells or γδ T cells. During the second year the 11 CR + patients tended to have a higher percentage of cultures dominated by CD4 + T cells ($P = 0.08$). We, therefore, also analysed the CD4 predominance in these 11 CR + and 13 CR − patients in the first year (Fig. 1). During the first 6 months the CR − patients tended to have a higher median percentage of CD4-dominated cultures ($P = 0.09$). This difference diminished in the second half year ($P = 0.88$).

Discussion

We analysed whether the development of chronic rejection can be related to the occurrence of acute rejection episodes or to characteristics of EMB-derived cultures of graft infiltrating cells.

In our patient group the occurrence of acute rejection episodes was not related to the development of CR. The percentage rejectors in both groups was similar, and a relationship between the number of acute rejection episodes and the development of CR was not found. These results are in agreement with those reported by other groups [2, 5]. However, Uretsky et al. [8] demonstrated a relationship between the occurrence of major acute rejection episodes during the first year after transplantation and the subsequent development of CR. These conflicting results might be explained by differences in the definitions of both acute rejection and CR.

With the exception of predominance of CD4 + T cells, the CR + and CR − patients were highly comparable when data concerning growth patterns and phenotypic composition of graft infiltrating cells for the complete first year after transplantation were analysed. The patient groups had highly similar percentages of lymphocyte growth from EMBs irrespective of the time interval. Kaufman et al. [3] demonstrated an association between lymphocyte growth from EMBs taken during the first 3 months post-transplantation and the subsequent development of CR. In our study the CR + and CR − patients had highly similar percentage growth from EMBs obtained during the first 90 days (data not shown). These

S230

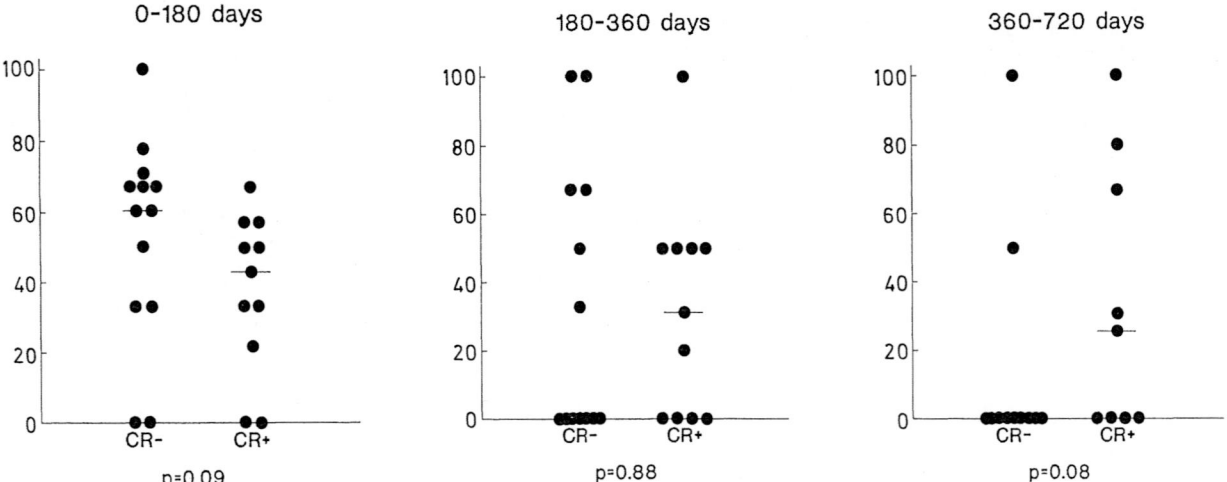

Fig. 1. Individual percentages of T-cell cultures from endomyocardial biopsies (EMB) in which CD4 + T cells predominated (≥ 60% of the cells). EMBs were taken at different time intervals pTx from 11 patients with CR at 1 year after transplantation and 13 patients without CR at 2 years after transplantation. Median percentages are indicated

conflicting results might be caused by differences in the growth medium, or by differences in the definitions of both cell growth and CR.

The CR + and CR − patient groups had comparable percentages of γδ T-cell-dominated cultures from EMBs obtained before the diagnosis of CR. The presence of γδ T cells seems not to be related to CR, since Vaessen et al. [9] showed that in the years after diagnosis of CR the EMB-derived cultures from CR + and CR − patients also yielded γδ T cells in comparable frequencies.

The most pronounced difference between CR + and CR − patients was found in the predominance of CD4 + cells (Table 1). During the first half year the CR − patients had a higher percentage of CD4-dominated cultures, while in the second half year no differences between the two groups were found (Table 1). In the second year post-transplantation the CR + patients showed a higher median percentage of CD4-dominated cultures compared with the patients who remained free from CR during the first 2 years (Fig. 1). The change in time of this difference between CR + and CR − patients was due to a decline in CD4-dominated cultures in the CR − patients.

The higher CD4 predominance in the patients having CR is in agreement with the model described by Libby et al. [4], in which CD4 + helper T cells interacting with foreign HLA class-II antigens are thought to play an important role. Histological evidence for the importance of class-II antigens in relation to CR has come from Salomon et al. [7], who demonstrated high class-II expression on endothelial cells in arteriosclerosis lesions from human cardiac allografts. We do not have an explanation for the stronger CD4 predominance in the cultures from the CR − patients during the first 6 months after transplantation. One might speculate that the patients diagnosed as having CR at the end of the first year developed CR because of the lack of graft infiltrating CD4 + T cells.

In conclusion, analysis of heart allograft infiltrating cells in relation to CR does not lead to the definition of a factor with prognostic value for the development of CR. The differences between CR + and CR − patients in the predominance of CD4 + T cells in EMB-derived cultures and the change with time of this difference might indicate

that CD4 + T cells play a dual role in the aetiology of chronic rejection.

Acknowledgment. This work was supported by grant 89.055 from the Netherlands Heart Foundation.

References

1. Balk AHMM, Weimar W (1992) Chronic heart graft rejection in the clinical setting. In: Paul LC, Solez K (eds) Organ transplantation: long term results. Marcel Dekker Inc, New York
2. Gao SZ, Schroeder JS, Alderman EL, Hunt SA, Silverman JF, Wiederhold V, Stinson EB (1987) Clinical and laboratory correlates of accelerated coronary artery disease in the cardiac transplant recipient. Circulation 76 [Suppl V]: V56–61
3. Kaufman CL, Zeevi A, Kormos RL, Zerbe TR, Keenan RJ, Uretsky BF, Griffith BP, Hardesty RL, Duquesnoy RJ (1990) Propagation of infiltrating lymphocytes and graft coronary disease in cardiac transplant recipients. Hum Immunol 28: 228–236
4. Libby P, Salomon RN, Payne DD, Schoen FJ, Pober JS (1989) Functions of vascular wall cells related to development of transplantation-associated coronary arteriosclerosis. Transplant Proc 4: 3677–3684
5. Narrod J, Kormos R, Armitage J, Hardesty R, Ladowski J, Griffith B (1989) Acute rejection and coronary artery disease in long-term survivors of heart transplantation. J Heart Transplant 8: 418–421
6. Ouwehand AJ, Vaessen LMB, Baan CC, Jutte NHPM, Balk AHMM, Essed CE, Bos E, Claas FHJ, Weimar W (1991) Alloreactive lymphoid infiltrates in human heart transplants: loss of class II directed cytotoxicity more than three months after transplantation. Hum Immunol 30: 50–59
7. Salomon RN, Hughes CCW, Schoen FJ, Payne DD, Pober JS, Libby P (1991) Human coronary transplantation-associated arteriosclerosis: evidence for a chronic immune reaction to activated graft endothelial cells. Am J Pathol 138: 791–798
8. Uretsky BF, Murali S, Reddy PS, Rabin B, Lee A, Griffith BP, Hardesty RL, Trento A, Bahnson HT (1987) Development of coronary artery disease in cardiac transplant patients receiving immunosuppressive therapy with cyclosporine and prednisone. Circulation 4: 827–834
9. Vaessen LMB, Ouwehand AJ, Baan CC, Jutte NHPM, Balk AHMM, Claas FHJ, Weimar W (1991) Phenotypic and functional analysis of T cell receptor γδ-bearing cells isolated from human heart allografts. J Immunol 147: 846–850
10. Zeevi A, Fung JJ, Zerbe TR, Kaufman C, Rabin BS, Griffith BP, Hardesty RL, Duquesnoy RJ (1986) Allospecificity of activated T cells grown from endomyocardial biopsies from heart transplant patients. Transplantation 41: 620–626

Transplant Int (1992) 5 [Suppl 1]: S 231–S 233

TRANSPLANT
International
© Springer-Verlag 1992

The clinical value of ultrasonic tissue characterization in the management of heart transplant patients

E. Lieback, M. Nawrocki, R. Meyer, J. Bellach, H. Warnecke, and T. Cohnert

Germany Heart Institute, Berlin, FRG

Abstract. The purpose of this study was to evaluate the rejection process by ultrasonic tissue characterization. Serial 2D echocardiographic images were obtained within 24 h prior to an endomyocardial biopsy. The end-diastolic echoframes were digitized into a computer matrix. A region of interest was placed into the anteroseptal segment of each scan. Image texture was analysed by four major groups of texture analysis (first-order histogram, co-occurrence matrix, run-length statistic, power spectrum). In 23 patients, 408 biopsies were taken after each examination, so that correlation between the ultrasonic tissue measurements and the histological state of the tissue could be determined. When rejection occurred, heterogeneity, brightness and contrast of texture increased. Of 117 texture parameters originally claculated, three parameters (inverse difference moment, run-length non-uniformity, ring sums of power spectrum) that characterized rejection were determined by means of discriminance analysis. Compared with biopsy findings, echocardiographic sensitivity for moderate rejection was 93.3% and specifity 83.6%. Our study indicates that acute rejection is associated with changes in echocardiographic texture. Serial echocardiographic texture analysis can reliably identify heart transplant rejection.

Key words: Heart transplantation – Rejection – Echocardiography – Tissue characterization

To date echocardiographic diagnosis of rejection has mainly been concerned with the analysis of functional, particularly diastolic, parameters of the heart [1]. We wanted to prove with our study whether morphological, i.e. structural, changes of the myocardium caused by rejection, can be discovered by analysing the grey-level distribution (texture analysis) of echocardiograms. This echocardiographic tissue characterization procedes in the reproducible connection which exists between the structure of tissue and its acoustic properties [2]. The digital processing of echocardiographic images with texture analysis is one possibility to detect acoustic properties of tissue. Echocardiographic texture is defined as spatial distribution of echo amplitudes or grey levels.

Methods

The study group comprised 23 heart transplant recipients. The mean follow-up period was 16.8 ± 9.8 months. A total of 408 endocardiographic examinations were compared with the results of endomyocardial biopsies. The echocardiographic examinations were strictly standardized.

The end-diastolic echocardiographic images were digitized in a $512 \times 512 \times 6$ bit matrix of the image-processing system. In each echocardiogram a region of interest with a standard size of 25×25 pixels was placed in the anteroseptial segment of the left ventricle. In this region of interest the texture parameterization was done. Four main groups of texture analysis [3, 4] were used: (1) first order histogram; (2) co-occurrence matrix; (3) run length analysis; (4) power spectrum.

At each examination 117 texture parameters were calculated and set in relation to the histological results of the biopsies. Then we tried to prove which set of texture parameters were necessary and sufficient to distinguish between the histological conditions of the myocardium after heart transplantation, and we tried to prove as well whether rejection can be discovered by analysing the ultrasound image texture. Step by step we reduced all available parameters using the Friedmann tests and Fischer's analysis of discriminance.

Results

Figures 1 and 2 show the grey-level distribution in the region of interest of a selected patient in a phase without rejection and at the time of rejection. Already visually you can notice a significant difference in grey-level distribution. Additionally, texture analysis can quantify this visual difference.

The reduction of the 117 texture parameters using Friedmann tests and Fischer's analysis of discriminance led us to the result that three texture parameters describe

---

Offprint requests to: Evelin Lieback, Germany Heart Institute, Augustenburger Platz 1, 1000 Berlin 65, FRG

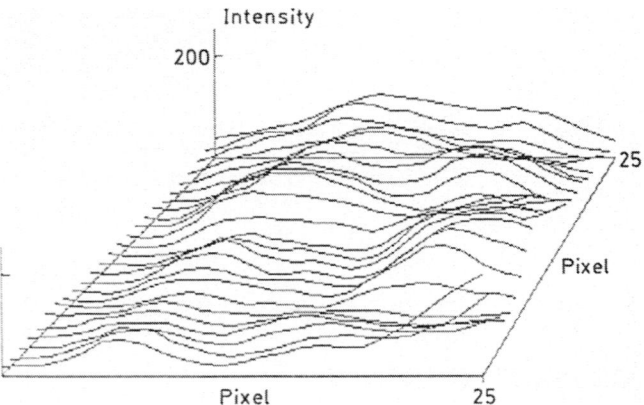

Fig. 1. Pixel map of the region of interest of a patient in a phase without rejection

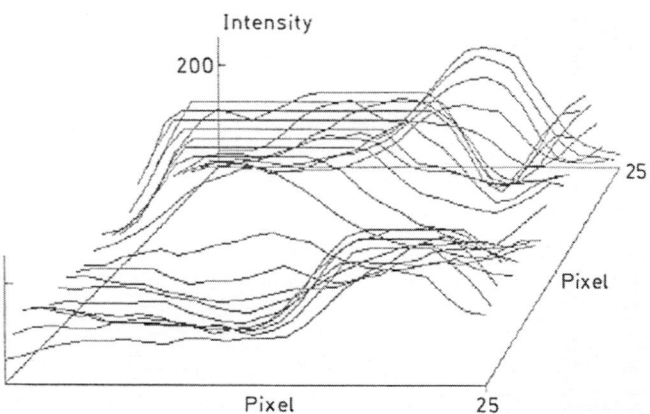

Fig. 2. Pixel map of the region of interest of the same patient at time of rejection

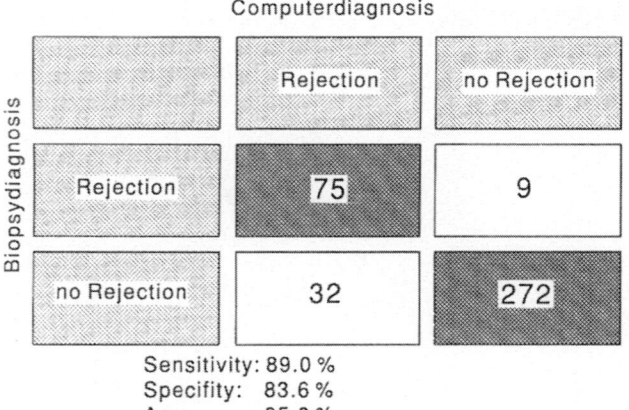

Fig. 3. Computer classification 'rejection' and 'no rejection'

the echocardiographic texture of the myocardium after heart transplantation. These three parameters are: inverse difference moment DX = 2 unjudged, run length non-uniformation vertical and power spectrum sector sum 0–30°.

Figure 3 shows the computer classification of 'rejection' or 'no rejection' using these three texture parameters. The sensitivity of the computer classification compared with biopsy diagnosis was 89% and the specificity 83.6%.

Discussion

We assume that, although there is no direct relationship between image texture and structure of tissue during rejection, with rejection the connected processes of cell infiltration, myocytolysis, interstitial oedemas and perfusion changes can lead to changes in the acoustic properties of the myocardium and therefore, also, to changes in the echocardiographic texture.

In a few cases the results of biopsies were different from those of the texture analysis. Because of artefacts of echocardiographic examination, the results of texture analysis can be wrong positive or wrong negative. Wrong positive texture analysis can also occur when there are other toxic effects on the myocardium (i. e. toxic noxes or myocarditis). On the other hand the biopsies can be wrong negative, because of the so called 'sampling error'. The echocardiographic examination area is many times larger than the histological one. The echocardiographic region of interest with the 25 × 25 image points is equivalent to a myocardial area of about 8 × 8 mm, in comparison with the nm area of histological myocardial samples.

We found limitations which lower the diagnostic value of this method also in the technical/method area. It was not always possible to analyse the 2D echocardiogram quantitatively, although there were no strong adiposities or lung emphysema in heart transplant recipients. It depends mainly on the technical representation of cardial structures and the connected digital image analysis whether a reliable diagnosis of rejection with the texture analysis of echocardiographic images can be done. Early postoperatively, the diagnostic security can be improved with additional examinations by noninvasive processes, for example intramyocardial ECG.

Summary and conclusion

Summarizing our research results, we come to the following conclusions:
1. You can infer the structure of the myocardium using the analysis of grey-level distribution (texture analysis) of echocardiograms.
2. The results of texture analysis correlate with the histomorphological results after heart transplantation.

This opens new possibilities for non-invasive diagnosis of rejection after heart transplantation.

Therefore, postoperatively, transplant recipients should be checked echocardiographically in short time intervals. If texture parameters point to suspicion of rejection, a control biopsy should be taken. The number of necessary biopsies can be decreased by this method. This is recommended particularly in the first 12 postoperative months after transplantation.

References

1. Aende I, Simon R, Seegers A, Daniel W, Heublein, Hetzer R, Haverich A, Hood WP, Lichtlen P, Schützenmeister R, Wenzlaff P (1990) Diastolic dysfunction during acute cardiac allograft rejection. Circulation 81: 66–70
2. Chandrasekaran K, Bansal RC, Greenleaf JF (1986) Evaluation of rejection process by analysis of backscatter from 2D-Echo images in a heterotopic heart transplantation model. Ultrason Imaging 8: 38
3. Galloway MM (1975) Short note – Texture analysis using gray level run lengths. Comput Graphics Imaging Processes 4: 172–175
4. Haralick RM, Shanmugam K, Dinstein I (1973) Textural features of image classification. IEEE Trans Syst Man Cybernet SMC-3: 610–621

Transplant Int (1992) 5 [Suppl 1]: S234–S237

TRANSPLANT
International
© Springer-Verlag 1992

Coronary flow reserve is impaired early after cardiac transplantation

P. Mullins, J. Scott, D. Aravot, C. Dennis, S. Large, J. Wallwork, and P. Schofield

Transplant Unit, Papworth Hospital, Huntingdon, UK

Abstract. The highest mortality rate after cardiac transplantation, at present, occurs within the first year after cardiac transplantation. The state of the coronary microcirculation soon after cardiac transplantation has not been previously assessed. We investigated the hypothesis that coronary flow reserve (CFR) is impaired in the early postoperative period after cardiac transplantation. A 3F intracoronary Doppler flow probe was inserted into the left anterior descending coronary artery and maximal coronary flow was assessed using the non-endothelial-dependent vasodilator papaverine. We compared two groups of patients: group A – 13 patients studied 3 months after operation; and group B – 25 patients studied at a median of 4 years after operation (range 2–8 years) without coronary occlusive disease (COD). CFR was defined as the quotient of maximum hyperaemic to resting velocity (vel). CFR was markedly impaired in group A patients compared with group B (3.3 SEM 0.3 versus 4.2 SEM 0.2, $P < 0.01$). No significant differences between mean resting or peak velocities, original diagnosis, age, active rejection, blood pressure, lipid levels, ischaemic time, cyclosporin levels or cytomegalovirus (CMV) status were noted. Responses to papaverine in resistance coronary vessels are impaired in the early postoperative period after cardiac transplantation. This is caused by a combination of higher resting flow and lower peak flow in the early group. This impairment of function in the coronary microcirculation may contribute to early graft dysfunction and reflect changes in vascular smooth muscle function leading to the development of COD.

Key words: Cardiac transplant – Coronary microcirculation – Impairment of endothelial vasodilation

Cardiac transplantation is established as standard therapy for end-stage heart failure [11]. The main causes of

Offprint requests to: Dr. P. A. Mullins, Transplant Unit, Papworth Hospital, Papworth Everard, Huntingdon, Cambridge CB3 8RE, UK

death within the first year are infection and rejection [11]. These conditions may be accompanied by deterioration in cardiac graft function by mechanisms which are poorly understood. The main cause of late graft failure is COD [11]. This disease is diffuse and often affects smaller coronary vessels in contrast to conventional atherosclerosis [6]. The pathophysiology of COD is still unclear [19].

The coronary microcirculation is an important determinant of the ability of the heart to respond appropriately to physiological stimuli such as exercise, and ischaemia [3, 8]. In the absence of significant epicardial coronary arterial stenoses the ability of the coronary microcirculation to conduct hyperaemic blood flow can be assessed [7]. Experimentally, the ability of the coronary vascular bed to vasodilate in response to pharmacological stimuli, such as papaverine, at a constant perfusion pressure can be measured in humans. The use of small-diameter (3 French) intracoronary Doppler flow catheters allows subselective estimations of coronary blood velocity in individual coronary vessels [8, 24]. This is a simple, reproducible method for evaluating coronary flow reserve [23]. This method has been more extensively evaluated than any other technique currently employed [10].

Perioperative factors may damage the coronary arterial system and damage vascular smooth muscle in patients after cardiac transplantation. We investigated the hypothesis that coronary flow reserve using the non-endothelial-dependent vasodilator papaverine is impaired in patients soon after cardiac transplantation.

Methods

Patients

Studies were performed in a total of 38 cardiac transplant recipients; 33 males and 5 females (Table 1). The mean age of all patients was 46 years (range 21–60 years). Of the 38 patients, 20 had originally undergone transplantation for ischaemic heart disease, and the remainder for dilated cardiomyopathy. Group A (13 patients) was

Table 1. Patient details

	Group A (n = 13)	Group B (n = 25)
Age	52 (range 43–60 years)	45 (range 21–59 years)
Sex	All Male	Male – 20; female – 5
Original diagnosis	IHD – 7; DCM – 6	IHD – 13; DCM – 12
Heart rate	90 (19)	84 (17)
BP	95 (6)	96 (3)
LVEDP	8 (4)	7 (2)
Ischaemic time	160 (50)	154 (43)
Cyclosporin level	504 (351)	259 (150)
HDL cholesterol	1.1 (0.6)	1.0 (0.3)
LDL cholesterol	4.8 (1.2)	4.4 (0.2)
Triglycerides	2.5 (1.3)	1.9 (0.9)
CMV + or mismatch	10	19

All values + standard deviation where appropriate
IHD, ischaemic heart disease; DCM, dilated cardiomyopathy; LVEDP, left ventricular end-diastolic pressure; BP, mean systemic pressure; CMV, cytomegalovirus

assessed 3 months after transplantation. Group B (the remaining patients) consisted of cardiac transplant recipients without evidence of coronary occlusive disease on coronary angiography at a median of 4 years postoperatively (range 2–8 years).

Immunosuppressive regime and drug therapy

In group B, 14 patients were receiving double therapy, i.e. cyclosporin and azathioprine or steroids. The remaining group B patients and all group A transplant recipients received triple immunosuppressive therapy (cyclosporin, azathioprine and steroid therapy). None of the patients received β-antagonist therapy or premedication. All vasoactive medication (e.g. calcium antagonists) was omitted 24 h prior to the procedure.

Biopsy protocol

All patients underwent right ventricular endomyocardial biopsy on the day of coronary angiography. These samples were examined by conventional light microscopy and graded according to standard histological criteria for the presence of acute cellular rejection [1] and evidence of vascular rejection.

Blood analysis

Routine analysis was performed for full blood count, urea and electrolytes, liver function tests, fasting lipids (total cholesterol, HDL and LDL cholesterol) and trough whole-blood cyclosporin level on the day of study.

Catheterization protocol

The patients were fasted prior to cardiac catheterization. Coronary angiography was performed via the right femoral artery in all patients using the Judkins technique. Coronary injections were performed manually using up to 8 ml of intracoronary radio-opaque contrast (Niopam) and ciné film recordings made in multiple projections. After routine angiography the proximal left anterior descending coronary artery was centred for optimal viewing. A period of at least 10 min was allowed to elapse before the study continued to eliminate vasoactive effects from the contrast medium.

Heparin, 10000 units, was given intravenously. A size 8F angioplasty guiding catheter was advanced into the left coronary ostium. A 0.014 inch guidewire was advanced into the distal part of the left anterior descending coronary artery. Using a monorail technique, a

size 3F 20 MHz intracoronary Doppler flow probe (Schneider, UK) was advanced over the guidewire into the proximal segment of the left anterior descending coronary artery. The Doppler flow probe and the range gate of the velocimeter were adjusted to obtain good quality phasic and mean coronary blood flow velocity signals. These signals were recorded with the surface electrocardiogram on a Mingograf recorder (Siemens-Elema, Sweden). A temporary pacing wire was inserted into the apex of the right ventricle, and the pacing rate set at five beats per minute below the resting value for each patient.

Baseline resting and phasic coronary blood flow velocity were taken in each patient. After an initial intracoronary 2 mg test dose of papaverine hydrochloride administerd via the guiding catheter, further injections of up to 14 mg papaverine (2 mg/ml in 0.9% saline) were given until maximum flow was achieved. The hyperaemic response was recorded in the form of maximum blood flow velocity in centimetres per second (cm/s). Velocity profiles were allowed to return to baseline levels between doses of the various drugs. CFR was defined as the ratio of the peak flow velocity (PFV) achieved with papaverine compared to the resting blood flow velocity (RVF).

Coronary angiography

Each coronary angiogram was assessed by two independent observers blinded to the clinical history. The coronary lumen was defined as the effective perfusion channel and measurement was performed in diastolic frames. Quantitative measurements of arterial diameter in coronary vessels were performed using digital electronic calipers (Sandhill Scientific). This method has previously been used in studies examining both coronary occlusive disease progression [17] and coronary flow reserve [9]. Two views were taken and projected onto a sheet of paper using a Tagarno system. The arterial diameter was measured in the left anterior descending coronary artery from tracings of the projected image, at a distance of 2–3 mm from the tip of the Doppler flow probe. The diameters were calculated using the mean of the measurements of these two views. Left ventricular angiography was performed at the end of the study.

Statistical analysis

Results are expressed as means with standard deviations for continuous measurements, and frequencies for categorical variables. The means of the two groups were compared pairwise using the Student's t-test. Statistical validity was accepted for P values < 0.05.

Ethical committee approval

This study was approved by the Huntingdon District Health Authority Ethical Committee.

Results

CFR was impaired in group A patients compared with group B (Table 2) – 3.3 SEM 0.3 versus 4.2 SEM 0.2 ($P = 0.01$). There was an overall increase in both groups in the percentage of LAD diameter compared with baseline (group A – + 20% SD 8%; group B – + 14% SD 4%). The heart rate in group A was higher than group B, but this did not reach statistical significance (Table 1). There was no important difference in mean systemic pressure between the two groups for each drug or drug combination. Other clinical variables did not differ between the two groups either (Table 1). Acute cellular rejection was present in two patients in group A and three Group B patients dur-

Table 2. Coronary blood flow

	CFR	Resting velocity (cm/s)	Peak velocity (cm/s)
Group A $n = 13$	3.3 (0.3)	8.0 (1.0)	25.3 (3.7)
Group B $n = 25$	4.2 (0.2)	6.6 (0.7)	28.3 (3.6)

Values (SEM)
CFR, coronary flow reserve

ing the study. The coronary flow reserve of these patients was 3.2 (SD 1.7) similar to the group A mean value (3.3 SD 1.0). There was no evidence of vascular rejection in any of the patients in either group.

Discussion

This study demonstrates that impairment of coronary flow response to papaverine occurs in patients soon after cardiac transplantation. Since there were no significant differences in proximal coronary arterial diameter between groups after papaverine, these responses must be mediated by differences in coronary microvascular function. Cardiac mortality occurs, at present, predominantly within the first 90 days after cardiac transplantation from infection and rejection [11, 20]. It is possible that this high attrition rate is related in part to coronary vascular dysfunction during this period.

Papaverine is a non-specific vasodilator which acts principally on resistance rather than proximal coronary vessels [25]. This is confirmed by the fact that there were no significant differences in LAD diameter after the drug in the two groups studied here. The causes of abnormal vasodilator response may include donor-related sympathetic endothelial coronary arterial damage [18] followed by smooth muscle responses, cold perfusion injury [21], vascular rejection [2], conventional atherosclerosis risk factors [26] or a combination of these. Experimentally, vascular endothelial damage initially leads to platelet deposition and vasoconstriction [5]. Vascular smooth muscle migration, proliferation and hypertrophy occur within days and persist for several weeks [22]. If the endothelial injury is severe, smooth muscle proliferation continues. Abnormal vasodilatory response to intracoronary nitroglycerine has previously been reported in proximal coronary vessels early after cardiac transplantation [12]. We have demonstrated that the coronary microcirculation non-endothelial function is abnormal soon after cardiac transplantation. Any change in coronary flow reserve in the early group of patients at increasing times from operation are unclear at present.

It is notable that the patients with angiographically normal coronary arteries at least 2 years after operation had a CFR consistent with previously published results in conventional and transplant patients [13]. In these patients, it is likely that any early vascular vasodilatory dysfunction initially improves, except in those patients who subsequently develop coronary occlusive disease [14]. Longitudinal studies are underway at present to evaluate this. The only established treatment of for end-stage coronary occlusive disease at present is cardiac retransplan-

tation [15]. Unfortunately the mortality rates are higher than in first-time cardiac transplant recipients, and there may be a higher recurrence rate of coronary disease. The use of angioplasty for treatment of proximal coronary stenoses in patients with coronary occlusive disease is of some benefit in the short term [16], but longer-term results are not available. Coronary artery bypass grafting has been attempted in a limited number of cases [4]. The diffuse and distal disease limits widespread application of this method of revascularization. This lack of effective treatment for coronary occlusive disease indicates that a better understanding of the pathophysiology of the disease is important. These results suggest that efforts to reduce coronary artery damage at the time of cardiac implantation, and to prevent vascular smooth muscle dysfunction could reduce the high early mortality in cardiac transplant recipients and retard or prevent the development of coronary occlusive disease.

Conclusion

Coronary flow reserve is impaired in patients soon after cardiac transplantation. Non-endothelial-dependent vasodilatory dysfunction occurs in the coronary microcirculation soon after cardiac transplantation. This may contribute to the early mortality in cardiac transplant recipients and be related to the development of coronary occlusive disease.

Acknowledgements. We would like to thank Dr. G.I.Verney, Dr. N.R.B.Cary, and the staff of the Radiography department at Papworth Hospital for their support during this study.

References

1. Billingham ME (1981) Diagnosis of cardiac rejection by endomyocardial biopsy. J Heart Transplant 1: 25–30
2. Billingham ME (1987) Cardiac transplant atherosclerosis. Transplant Proc [Suppl 5]: 19–25
3. Canty JM, Klocke FJ (1985) Reduced myocardial perfusion in the presence of pharmacologic vasodilator reserve. Circulation 71: 370–377
4. Copeland JG, Butman SM, Sethi G (1991) Successful coronary artery bypass grafting for high-risk left main coronary artery stenosis after cardiac transplantation. Ann Thorac Surg 49: 106–110
5. Forstermann U, Mugge A, Alheid U, Bode M, Frolich JC (1989) Endothelium-derived relaxing factor (EDRF): a defence mechanism against platelet aggregation and vasospasm in human coronary arteries. Eur Heart J 10 [Suppl F]: 36–37
6. Gao SZ, Alderman EL, Schroeder JS, Silverman JF, Hunt SA (1988) Accelerated coronary vascualr disease in the heart transplant patient: coronary arteriographic findings. J Am Coll Cardiol 12: 334–340
7. Hoffmann JF (1984) Maximal coronary flow and the concept of coronary vascular reserve. Circulation 70: 153–159
8. Hoffmann JF (1981) A critical view of coronary reserve. Circulation 75 [Suppl I]: I–6
9. Kern MJ, Deligonul U, Vandormael M et al (1989) Impaired coronary vasodilator reserve in the immediate postcoronary angioplasty period: analysis of coronary artery flow velocity indexes and regional cardiac venous efflux. J Am Coll Cardiol 860–872

10. Klocke FJ (1987) Measurements of coronary flow reserve: defining pathophysiology versus making decisions about patient care. Circulation 76: 1183–1189
11. Kriett JM, Kaye MP (1990) The registry of the international society of heart transplantation: Seventh official report – 1990. J Heart Transplant 9: 323–330
12. McGinn AL, Wilson RF, Olivari MT, Homans DC, White CW (1988) Coronary vasodilator reserve after human orthotopic cardiac transplantation. Circulation 78: 1200–1209
13. McGinn AL, Christensen BV, Meyer SM, Simon A, Kubo SH, Laxson DD, Wilson RF (1991) Nitroglycerin-induced coronary dilation is impaired early after cardiac transplantation (abstract). J Am Coll Cardiol 17: 309A
14. Mullins PA, Scott JP, Aravot DJ, Large SR, Cary N, Wallwork J, Schofield PM (1991) Small vessel coronary occlusive disease after cardiac transplantation (abstract). J Am Coll Cardiol 17: 308A
15. Mullins PA, Scott JP, Dunning JJ, Aravot DJ, Large SR, Cary N, Wallwork J, Schofield PM (1991) Cardiac transplant waiting lists, donor shortage and retransplantation: implications for using donor hearts. Am J Cardiology 68: 408–409
16. Mullins PA, Shapiro LM, Aravot DJ, Scott JP, Large SR, Wallwork J, Schofield PM (1991) Experience of PTCA in orthotopic cardiac transplant recipients. Eur Heart J (in press)
17. O'Neill BJ, Pflugfelder PW, Singh NR, Menkis AH, McKenzie FN, Kostuk WJ (1989) Frequency of angiographic detection and quantitative assessment of coronary arterial disease one and three years after cardiac transplantation. Am J Cardiol 63: 1221–1226
18. Rowe SK, Kleiman NS, Cocanougher B, Smart FW, Minor ST, Raizner AE, Henry PD, Roberts R, Pratt CM, Young JB (1991) Effects of intracoronary acetylcholine infusion early versus late after heart transplant. Transplant Proc 23: 1193–1197
19. Schroeder JS, Hunt SA (1991) Chest pain in heart transplant patients. N Eng J Med 324: 1805–1806
20. Sharples LD, Caine N, Mullins P, Scott JP, Solis E, English TAH, Large SR, Schofield PM, Wallwork J (1991) Risk factor analysis for the major hazards following heart transplantation – rejection, infection and coronary occlusive disease. Transplantation (in press)
21. Takahashi A, Hearse DJ, Braimbridge MV, Chambers DJ (1990) Harvesting hearts for long-term preservation. J Thorac Cardiovasc Surg 100: 371–378
22. Weidenger FF, McLenachan JM, Cybulsky MI, Gordon JB, Rennke HG, Hollenberg NK, Fallon JT, Ganz P, Cooke JP (1990) Persistent dysfunction of regenerated endothelium after balloon angioplasty of rabbit iliac artery. Circulation 81: 1667–1669
23. Wilson RF, White CF (1986) Intracoronary papaverine: an ideal vasodilator for studies of the coronary circulation in conscious humans. Circulation 73: 444–451
24. Wilson RF, Laughlin DE, Ackell PH, Chilian WM, Holida MD, Hartley CJ, Armstrong ML, Marcus ML, White CW (1985) Transluminal, subselective measurement of coronary artery blood flow velocity and vasodilator reserve in man. Circulation 72: 82–92
25. Yanagisawa M, Masaki T (1988) Endothelin, a novel endothelium-derived peptide: pharmacological activities, regulation and possible roles in cardiovascular control. Biochem Pharmacol 12: 1877–1883
26. Zeiher AM, Drexler H, Wollschlager H, Just H (1991) Modulation of coronary vasomotor tone in humans. Circulation 83: 391–401

Transplant Int (1992) 5 [Suppl 1]: S 238–S 241

TRANSPLANT
International
© Springer-Verlag 1992

Determinants of graft arteriosclerosis after heart transplantation

C. D. Scott, I. W. Colquhoun, K. Gould, J. Au, and J. H. Dark

Cardiothoracic Centre, Freeman Hospital, Newcastle-upon-Tyne, UK

Abstract. Accelerated graft coronary artery disease (TxCAD) is now the most common complication limiting long-term survival after heart transplantation. This study examines its association with several potentially causative factors. The study population comprised all 73 transplants recipients at this centre between May 1985 and June 1989 who survived at least 2 years. Coronary angiography was performed in every patient at 2 years after transplantation and annually thereafter. All angiograms were retrospectively examined for any evidence of TxCAD. The number of rejection episodes and history of cytomegalovirus (CMV) infection were determined from patient records. Fasting serum triglycerides, and total and HDL cholesterol were measured at between 18 and 60 months after transplantation. Patients with advanced TxCAD ($>70\%$ stenoses) had a mean of 1.4 ± 1.4 rejection episodes in the first year compared with 0.5 ± 0.8 episodes in those without TxCAD ($P < 0.05$). The mean number of episodes in all patients with any evidence of TxCAD was 0.8 ± 1.1 which was not significantly different from those without TxCAD. There were no association between exposure to CMV infection and TxCAD or between hyperlipidaemia and TxCAD. We conclude that frequent episodes of allograft rejection are associated with the development of advanced TxCAD. Hyperlipidaemia is not associated with the development of TxCAD in the first 5 years after transplantation. A history of exposure to CMV is not associated with TxCAD in our patients possibly because of our routine use of anti-CMV hyperimmune globulin in CMV-mismatched patients.

Key words: Heart transplantation – Graft arteriosclerosis

Accelerated coronary artery disease is now the most common complication limiting long-term survival after heart transplantation [2, 4]. Suggested causes of this phenomenon include those common to patients with native coronary artery disease such as hyperlipidaemia, hypertension and diabetes [6, 11] and those peculiar to heart transplant recipients such as allograft rejection and transplant related cytomegalovirus infection or reactivation [10, 11, 15, 16, 19, 20].

The results of previously published studies have been contradictory with regard to the importance of hyperlipidaemia after transplantation [6, 8]. A consensus has emerged that allograft rejection and cytomegalovirus infection are associated with accelerated coronary artery disease [10, 15, 16, 19, 20] although it is not unanimous [1, 8].

This angiographic study of both early and advanced coronary artery disease in transplant recipients re-examines several of these potential associations.

Methods

The study population comprised all 73 adult transplant recipients at this centre between May 1985 and June 1989, who survived at least 2 years after surgery. The operative technique was as described by Lower et al. [14]. All patients were immunosuppressed with cyclosporin, azathioprine and prednisolone. Aspirin was given routinely only to those patients with angiographically demonstrated coronary artery disease. Those recipients who were CMV-antibody-negative at the time of transplantation with a CMV-positive donor (CMV mismatch) were given prophylactic anti-CMV hyperimmune globulin. Full details of the protocol employed have been published previously [7].

Coronary angiography

Coronary angiography was performed in all patients, first at 2 years after transplantation and then annually. All coronary angiograms were reviewed by two of the investigators independently and consensus was then reached. Coronary artery disease was said to be present if any irregularity of coronary vessels was detected. The severity of stenoses was visually estimated. Advanced coronary artery disease was defined as a stenosis of 70% or greater in any major epicardial coronary artery or occlusion of any visible vessels.

Offprint requests to: Dr. C. D. Scott, Cardiothoracic Centre, Freeman Hospital, High Heaton, Newcastle-upon-Tyne, NE7 7DN, UK

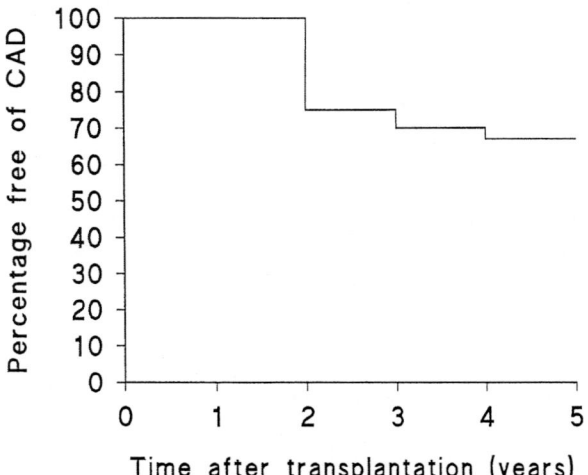

Fig. 1. A survival curve representing those transplant recipients free of proven coronary artery disease at the indicated time after transplantation

Hyperlipidaemia

All transplant patients at this centre are encouraged to eat a low-fat diet with a high polyunsaturated to saturated fat ratio. Blood lipid profiles were obtained at a minimum of 18 months after transplantation. Total cholesterol, HDL cholesterol and triglycerides were measured in each patient after a 16-h fast.

CMV infection

CMV infection was determined by donor-recipient mismatch (defined above) or by the presence of CMV IgM antibody and/or isolation of CMV from the urine from a patient with an otherwise unexplained pyrexial illness.

Allograft rejection

Each patient underwent routine endomyocardial biopsies weekly until 6 weeks after transplantation, fortnightly until 3 months, monthly until 6 months and 3-monthly thereafter. Additional biopsies were performed as clinically indicated. A rejection episode was defined by a biopsy indicating moderate or severe rejection according to the Billingham classification [3].

Statistical analysis

Results are expressed as mean ± 1 standard deviation. Comparative analyses were performed using the Student's t-test, Mann-Whitney U test and Fisher's exact test. A probability $p < 0.05$ was considered significant.

Results

A survival curve was constructed by the Kaplan-Meier technique [13] showing the percentage of transplant patients free of proven coronary artery disease as a function of time after transplantation (Fig. 1). The percentage of patients free from proven coronary artery disease was 75% at 2 years, 70% at 3 years ($n = 42$), 67% at 4 years ($n = 16$) and 67% at 5 years ($n = 8$).

Of a total of 25 patients with coronary artery disease, ten have advanced disease, the majority of the remaining 15 have only minor luminal irregularities.

There have been three deaths in the study population, one due to malignancy in a patient with no coronary disease and two due to coronary disease. One of these patients had advanced disease identified angiographically ante-mortem, the other had only minor disease documented. Post-mortem examination subsequently proved this to be a considerable underestimade of the severity of disease.

Rejection

Patients with coronary disease had a total of 0.8 ± 1.1 episodes of rejection in the first year after transplantation compared with 0.5 ± 0.8 episodes in those without. This difference was not statistically significant. However those with advanced disease had significantly more episodes (1.4 ± 1.4) than those with no disease ($P < 0.05$, Mann-Whitney). No patient had any rejection episode after the first postoperative year.

Hyperlipidaemia

The lipid profiles of the study patients are detailed in Table 1. There were no significant differences in serum levels of triglycerides, or total or non-HDL cholesterol between any of the groups with severe, mild or no coronary disease.

Cytomegalovirus infection

Of 25 patients with coronary artery disease, four (16%) were CMV mismatched or had reactivation/reinfection compared with nine (19%) of 48 patients with no evidence of coronary disease. This difference was not significant ($P = 0.52$).

Discussion

Limitations of the study

Coronary angiography is currently the best method available for studying coronary artery disease in transplant patients but it is less than ideal. It is not able to distinguish

Table 1. Blood lipid profiles of patients with severe, mild or no coronary disease. Values are expressed as mean ± 1 standard deviation

	Coronary disease	No coronary disease	Significance
Total cholesterol (mmol/l)	7.4 ± 1.4	7.3 ± 2.0	NS
Non-HDL cholesterol (mmol/l)	5.9 ± 1.5	6.2 ± 2.1	NS
Triglycerides	2.42 ± 1.23	2.37 ± 1.50	NS

different underlying pathological processes [12] and it also probably underestimates the severity of disease [9].

The serum lipid levels in this study were based on single samples. However they were all performed at least 18 months after transplantation when serum lipids can be expected to be more stable than in the immediate perioperative period [6].

Prevalence of graft arteriosclerosis

The prevalence of graft coronary disease in our patients is comparable with that found in other studies [1, 6, 8, 17, 22]. There were however some differences in diagnostic criteria. In common with most other studies [1, 8, 16, 20], we accepted any luminal irregularity as indicative of coronary disease. Pascoe et al. [17] recorded only lesions causing greater than 30% stenosis of any vessel. Eich et al. [6] identified coronary disease by evidence of perfusion defects or impaired left ventricular function using isotope techniques and confirmatory coronary angiography. The prevalence of disease diagnosed by routine angiography would probably have been higher.

Rejection

We have confirmed, in our patients, previous findings that frequent episodes of allograft rejection [16, 20] are associated with graft arteriosclerosis. This association was limited, however, to those with advanced disease and was not significant for all patients with coronary artery disease. Some previously published studies have also found limited [16] or no such associations [8].

The underlying reason for this variation in the apparent importance of allograft rejection is probably that current techniques only indirectly assess the immune process responsible for coronary disease. The standarad technique of surveillance endomyocardial biopsy assesses only cell-mediated myocardial rejection. Antibodies reactive against vascular endothelium have been shown to be associated with atherosclerosis in non-transplant patients [5]. Several studies have indicated the importance of antibody-mediated rejection in the development of graft coronary disease [11, 18]. Although acute antibody-mediated rejection is often accompanied by cell mediated rejection the processes may differ in severity and response to treatment [21].

Hyperlipidaemia

We have found no association between blood lipids and the development of coronary disease in our patients. Gao et al. [8] reported an association with plasma triglycerides at 1 year after transplantation but it was not consistent over time. Hess et al. [11] reported a clear association between coronary disease and hypercholesterolaemia in combination with cytotoxic B-cell antibodies but there were only 14 patients in the study. In a larger study of 38 patients Eich et al. [6] also found an association with hypercholesterolaemia. However, the frequency of rejec-

tion episodes in each group was not stated. The overall incidence of coronary artery disease may have been abnormally high in this study [6] given that the diagnostic techniques would have missed minor coronary artery disease and that the stated incidence was similar to other series [1, 8, 17, 22].

The lack of association between blood lipids and transplant-related coronary disease may seem surprising in view of the well-known association of hyperlipidaemia and coronary atheroma in the general population. This may be due to the aetiological dominance of relatively rapid immunological processes in the first years after transplantation. The effects of hyperlipidaemia in these patients may only become apparent over a much longer period.

Cytomegalovirus infection

Our finding of no association between CMV infection and coronary disease is in contrast to several large published studies [10, 15, 19]. At this centre routine surveillance of anti-CMV IgG levels amongst asymptomatic seropositive patients is not performed. Thus some patients classified in other studies [10, 15] as having had CMV infection would not be in this analysis. Another centre using routine anti-CMV hyperimmune globulin [1] has reported similar findings to our own although the criteria for CMV infection were not stated in this report. We have found that anti-CMV hyperimmune globulin prevents or greatly ameliorates clinical CMV illness in mismatched patients; it may also prevent CMV-related graft coronary disease in this group.

Conclusion

We have confirmed that frequent allograft rejection is associated with the development of advanced graft coronary disease. In contrast to other studies, we have not demonstrated any effect of CMV exposure, we believe that our use of anti-CMV hyperimmune globulin in all CMV-mismatched recipients may be protective in this respect. In common with many other studies, we have found no association between blood lipids and accelerated coronary disease. The effects of hyperlipidaemia may only become apparent over a much longer period after transplantation.

References

1. Balk AHMM, Linden MVD, Meeter K, et al (1991) Is there a relation between transplant coronary artery disease and the occurrence of CMV infection (abstract). J Heart Lung Transplant 10: 188
2. Bieber CP, Hunt SA, Schwinn DA, et al (1981) Complications in long term survivors of cardiac transplantation. Transplant Proc 13: 207–211
3. Billingham ME (1985) Diagnosis of cardiac rejection by endomyocardial biopsy. J Heart Transplant 1: 25–30
4. Billingham ME (1989) Graft coronary disease: the lesions and the patients. Transplant Proc 21: 3665–3666

5. Cerilli J, Brasile J, Sosa J, et al (1987) The role of autoantibody to vascular endothelial cell antigens in atherosclerosis and vascular disease. Transplant Proc 14 [Suppl V]: 47–49

6. Eich D, Thompson JA, Ko D, et al (1991) Hypercholesterolaemia in long term survivors of heart transplantation: An early marker of accelerated coronary artery disease. J Heart Lung Transplant 10: 45–49

7. Freeman R, Gould FK, McMaster A (1990) Management of CMV antibody negative patients undergoing cardiac transplantation. J Clin Pathol 43: 373–376

8. Gao SZ, Schroeder JS, Alderman EL, et al (1987) Clinical and laboratory correlates of accelerated coronary artery disease in the cardiac transplant patient. Circulation 76 [Suppl V]: 56–61

9. Gao SZ, Johnson D, Schroeder JS, et al (1988) Transplant coronary artery disease: histopathologic correlations with angiographic morphology (abstract). J Am Coll Cardiol 11: 135A

10. Grattan MT, Moreno-Cabral CE, Starnes VA, Oyer PE, Stinson EB, Shumway NE (1989) Cytomegalovirus infection is associated with cardiac allograft rejection and atherosclerosis. JAMA 261: 3561–3566

11. Hess MJ, Hastillo A, Mohanakumar T, et al (1983) Accelerated atherosclerosis in cardiac transplantation: role of cytotoxic B-cell antibodies and hyperlipidaemia. Circulation 68 [Suppl II]: 94–101

12. Johnson DE, Gao SZ, Schroeder JS, DeCampli W, Billingham ME (1989) The spectrum of coronary artery pathologic findings in human cardiac allografts. J Heart Transplant 8: 349–359

13. Kaplan EL, Meier P (1958) Nonparametric estimation for incomplete observations. Am Stat Assoc 10: 457

14. Lower RR, Stofer RC, Shumway NE (1961) Homovital transplantation of the heart. J Thorac Cardiovasc Surg 41: 196–202

15. McDonald K, Rector TS, Braunlin EA, Kubo SH, Olivari MT (1989) Association of coronary artery disease in cardiac transplant recipients with cytomegalovirus infection. Am J Cardiol 64: 359–362

16. Narrod J, Kormos R, Armitage J, et al (1989) Acute rejection and coronary artery disease in long term survivors of heart transplantation. J Heart Transplant 8: 418–421

17. Pascoe EA, Barnhart GR, Carter WH, et al (1987) The prevalence of cardiac allograft arteriosclerosis. Transplantation 44: 838–839

18. Rose EA, Smith CR, Petrossian GA, Barr ML, Reemtsma K (1989) Humoral immune responses after cardiac transplantation: correlation with fatal rejection and graft atherosclerosis. Surgery 106: 203–207

19. Stovin PGI, Sharples L, Hutter JA, Wallwork J, English TAH (1991) Some prognostic factors for the development of transplant related coronary artery disease in human cardiac allografts. J Heart Lung Transplant 10: 38–44

20. Uretsky B, Murali S, Reddy S, et al (1987) Development of coronary artery disease in cardiac transplant patients receiving immunosuppressive therapy with cyclosporine and prednisone. Circulation 76: 827–834

21. Yowell RL, Hammond EH, Bristow MR, Watson FS, Renlund DG, O'Connell JB (1988) Acute vascular rejection involving the major coronary arteries of a cardiac allograft. J Heart Transplant 7: 191–197

22. Zusman DR, Stinson EB, Oyer PE, et al (1985) Determinants of accelerated graft atherosclerosis in conventional and cyclosporin treated heart transplant recipients (abstract). J Heart Transplant 4: 587

Transplant Int (1992) 5 [Suppl 1]: S 242–S 245

TRANSPLANT
International
© Springer-Verlag 1992

Role of CMV pneumonia in the development of obliterative bronchiolitis in heart-lung and double-lung transplant recipients

J. Cerrina[1], F. Le Roy Ladurie[1], P. H. Herve[1], F. Parquin[1], S. Harari[1], A. Chapelier[1], G. Simoneau[2], P. Vouhe[1], and P. H. Dartevelle[1]

[1] Centre Chirurgical Marie Lannelongue, Plessis Robinson, France
[2] Hopital Antoine Beclere, Clamart, France

Abstract. Obliterative bronchiolitis (OB) is the main cause of late mortality after lung transplantation. Cytomegalovirus infection has been associated with late graft failure. The aim of this study was to determine whether the development of OB was related to CMV pretransplant serological status and to CMV infections. The study group comprised 36 lung transplant recipients (27 HLT and 9 DLT) who survived more than 4 months, of whom 47% developed OB (defined by the persistence of an unexplained obstructive disease: FEV1/VC < 0,7). OB occurred more frequently: (1) in seronegative recipients with seropositive donors (8/9) than in seropositive recipients (7/19) or seronegative well-matched recipients (2/8); and (2) in patients who experienced CMV pneumonia (11/16) and CMV recurrence (11/16). Since matching seronegative recipients is the best way to prevent CMV infection, we believe that seronegative grafts must be reserved for seronegative recipients.

Key words: Lung transplantation – CMV infection – CMV pneumonia – Obliterative bronchiolitis

Obliterative bronchiolitis (OB), initially described in 1901 by Lange [11], occurred when injury to small conducting airways is repaired by proliferation of granulation tissue. OB has been described in fume exposure, viral infections, adverse drug reaction and connective tissue diseases [3]. A similar pulmonary disorder was reported in 1984 in heart and lung transplant recipients by the Stanford group: five of their first 14 long-term surviving heart-lung transplant recipients developed progressive obstructive airway disease [1]. Post-mortem material and open-lung biopsies, which were available from three recipients, showed a histological pattern of OB. Since this report OB has been observed by all lung transplant teams in the three

types of lung transplantation (heart-lung, double and single lung). The incidence of OB varies between 24 and 67% in long-term survivors after lung transplantation [10, 14].

OB has been suggested to occur more frequently in cases of poorly controlled lung rejection [14]. The role of CMV infection has also been implicated as a causative factor in OB [10] and the development of coronary artery disease in the transplanted heart and late renal graft failure [4, 12].

Our aim was to analyse if the development of OB in double-lung (DLT) and heart-lung transplant (HLT) recipients was related to CMV pretransplant serological status and to CMV post-transplant infection.

Patients and methods

Of the 39 HLT and 14 DLT performed at Marie Lannelongue Hospital from June 1986 to November 1990, we studied 36 (27 HLT and 9 DLT) who survived more than 4 months and were at risk of OB. There were 18 males and 18 females; their ages ranged from 9 to 53 years (mean: 33 ± 12 years). The mean follow up was 718 ± 69 days. The original diagnoses were: primary pulmonary hypertension ($n = 10$), respiratory insufficiency ($n = 16$), Eisenmenger's syndrome ($n = 7$), chronic pulmonary embolism ($n = 3$). The immunosuppressive regimen consisted of: cyclosporin (CyA) adjusted to achieve whole blood levels of 150–300 ng/ml, azathioprine 1–2.5 mg/kg per day and prednisone 0–1 mg/kg per day beginning at day 7. Rabbit antilymphocytic globulin was administered for the first 7 postoperative days. Acute allograft rejection (AAR) was treated by the administration of 1 g methylprednisolone for 3 consecutive days.

The CMV serological status of donors and recipients were determined using an ELISA method (D + = seropositive donor; D – = seronegative donor; R + = seropositive recipient; R – = seronegative recipient). CMV seronegative blood products were used for all patients. Mismatched recipients (D + /R –) received anti-CMV immunoglobulins 250 mg/kg per week for 6 weeks (Centre Transfusion Sanguine Lille, France). Symptomatic CMV infections were treated with ganciclovir (10 mg/kg per day for 15–21 days). The immunosuppressive regimen was not altered when active CMV infection was diagnosed.

Offprint requests to: Dr. J. Cerrina, Centre Chirurgical Marie Lannelongue, 133 Avenue de la Résistance, 92350 Plessis Robinson, France

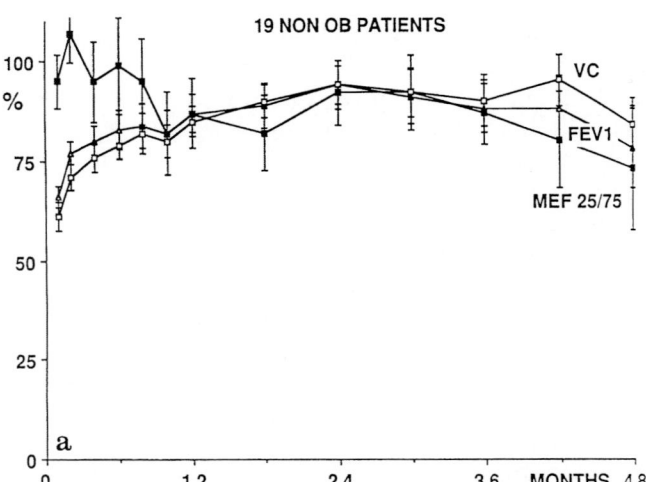

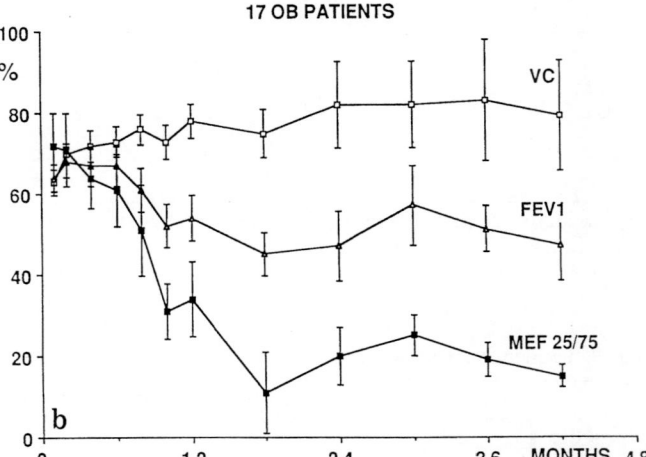

Fig. 1. Evolution of pulmonary function tests ($\square$, VC; $\triangle$, FEV1; $\blacksquare$, MEF 25/75:) expressed as percentage of predicted values in the two groups of patients (mean ± s. e. m.). *Left panel,* non-OB patients; *right panel,* OB patients

Follow-up

Pulmonary functional tests. Spirometry was performed using computerized Gould equipment (2400, Respiratory Function Laboratory; Gould Instruments, Cleveland, Ohio, USA). Vital capacity (VC) was measured as inspiratory vital capacity. Forced expiratory volume in 1 second (FEV1) and expiratory flow between 25 and 75% of forced vital capacity (MEF 25/75) were read from the largest of three flow-volume curves. Data were expressed as percent of the subjects' own predicted values.

Pulmonary functional tests were performed twice a week during the postoperative course. After their discharge, patients were monitored every 2 weeks for 6 months and then monthly.

Bronchoscopy. Fibreoptic bronchoscopy [bronchial aspiration, bronchoalveolar lavage (BAL) and at least five large trans-bronchial biopsies (TBB)] were routinely performed on days 15, 30, 45, 90 or in the event of symptoms such as fever, chest radiographic abnormalities or decrease in pulmonary function. In addition, TBB were performed during the month following treatment of an episode of confirmed histological AAR. TBB samples were studied for histological patterns of allograft rejection using the Lung Rejection Study Group criteria [18] and for the presence of specific viral inclusions and other opportunistic agents. The presence of virus was assessed in BAL fluid by HES staining, indirect immunofluorescent assay and shell vial culture. Viral culture of blood and urine and serological studies were performed weekly throughout the postoperative stay and every time the patients returned to our institution.

Definitions

CMV infection was defined by the presence of CMV in lung, blood and/or seroconversion. Infection was considered as symptomatic disease when clinical, radiological or biological abnormalities compatible with CMV disease were present: fever, gastrointestinal symptoms, interstitial shadows on chest radiographs, elevated liver enzymes, cytopenia or mononucleosis.

CMV pneumonia was defined by the association of
- the presence of CMV in lung specimens (bronchoalveolar lavage or transbronchial biopsies);
- histological patterns of viral alveolitis on TBB [15]; and
- lung infiltrates on chest radiographs.

OB was diagnosed when the FEV1/VC ratio was less than 70% for more than 3 months in the absence of other causes and independent of the presence of a histological pattern of OB on TBB. A severe OB was considered when FEV1 was lower than 40% of predicted values.

Statistical analysis

Results are expressed as mean ± SD (except for pulmonary functional tests expressed as mean ± s.e.m.). Patients were separated into two groups according to the occurrence of OB. The chi-squared test with Yates' correction and non-paired Student's t-test were used to compare the two groups. $P \leq 0.05$ was considered the threshold for significance.

Results

A total of 17 OB occurred in the 36 patients. Their mean age (35 ± 12 years) and sex ratio (8 female, 9 male) did not differ from the non-OB group (37 ± 11 years; 10 female, 9 male). The mean delay to OB occurrence was 271 ± 41 days (range 76–678 days). Ten of the 17 patients with OB became severe and eight of these patients died. OB was confirmed histologically in 13 of the 17 patients (eight post-mortem examinations and five TBB sample examinations). The time-course for the results obtained in the pulmonary function tests are shown in Fig. 1. Initial pulmonary function tests were similar in both groups with a trend for a higher initial MEF_{25-75} in the patients without OB.

Relationships between CMV serological status and OB

The results presented in Table 1 show that among the nine D + /R –, eight developed OB. Only two OB were noted among the eight D – /R –. Six OB occurred in 19 seropositive recipients. OB was more frequently observed in D + /R – patients than in the two other groups D – /R – and R + (Table 1).

Table 1. Incidence of OB related to CMV serological status

	OB	Non-OB	Total
D – /R –	2	6	8
D + /R –	8*	1	9
R +	7	12	19
Total	17	19	36

OB was more frequently observed in D + /R – patients than in D – /R – and R + .

* P < 0.01

Table 2. Incidence of OB related to CMV infection

	OB	Non-OB
Total patients	17	19
No infection	3	6
CMV infection	14	13
Pneumonia	11*	5
Recurrence	11*	5

OB was observed more frequently in patients who experienced CMV pneumonia and CMV recurrence

* P < 0.01

Table 3. Incidence of CMV infection related to CMV serological status

	Patients	Pneumonia	Recurrence
D – /R –	8	0	0
D + /R –	9	7*	5
R +	19	9	11
Total	36	16	16

Pneumonia was more frequently observed in D + /R – patients than in D – /R – and R + patients

* P = 0.05

Relationships between CMV infection and OB

Asymptomatic infection was observed in two cases (Table 2). Symptomatic infection was experienced by 25 patients (69%), 16 of whom (64%) had CMV pneumonia. CMV recurrence was observed in 16 patients (64%). No deaths occurred as a result of CMV infection. OB was detected more often in the 16 patients who experienced CMV pneumonia (11 vs 5; $P < 0.01$) and in the 16 patients with recurrence of CMV infection (11 vs 5; $P < 0.01$).

The results presented in Table 3 show that none of the eight D – /R – patients had CMV infection. CMV pneumonia, but not CMV recurrences, were more frequently observed in the D + /R – patients as compared with R + and D – /R – patients ($P = 0.05$).

Discussion

This study shows that OB is more frequently observed in cases of CMV pneumonia, CMV recurrences and in CMV mismatched recipients (D + /R –). The incidence of OB was 47% in this study while in the literature incidences from 24% to 67% have been reported [16]. This range in

the incidence of OB may be due to several factors: (a) differences in duration of follow-up (the longer the follow-up, the higher the risk of OB); (b) differences in the nature of the immunosuppressive regimen or in the patients' management [16]; and (c) the different criteria which were used for the diagnosis of OB (some studies used histological criteria on TBB [10], while others (reference 15 and this report) used pulmonary function tests). Although tissue diagnosis must be considered the 'gold standard', the use of TBB instead of open-lung biopsy increases the chance of missing the diagnosis, since in TBB samples bronchioles are scarce and sometimes absent. Moreover, the distribution of OB is patchy [16] contributing to a decrease in the sensitivity of TBB for diagnosis of OB. Therefore we suggest that pulmonary function tests could be a more sensitive procedure for detecting OB. In this study a persistent decrease in the FEV1/VC ratio (below 70%) was used. The accuracy of this criterion was confirmed by all the autopsy examinations.

CMV infection and CMV pneumonia (69% and 44% in our patients, respectively) were more frequently noted after lung transplantation than subsequent to other organ transplantations [7]. The high incidence of CMV infection was related to the high proportion of CMV seropositive donors and/or recipients leading to a small number of well-matched D – /R – patients (22%). CMV pneumonia was the main visceral CMV disease after lung transplantation (64% of our patients with CMV infection experienced pneumonia). The infection was more frequently observed in D + /R – patients (77%) reflecting the severity of primary infection. None of the patients with CMV pneumonia died but recurrences were frequent (64%). The absence of death was probably due to early diagnosis and early treatment with ganciclovir. The use of an association of sensitive laboratory tests (shell vial culture, immediate fluorescence assay, immunohistochemical staining) allowed early diagnosis of CMV infection. The high incidence of recurrence may be due to the short duration of ganciclovir treatment.

OB was more frequently noted in our patients with CMV mismatch, CMV pneumonia or CMV infection recurrences. Similar results were reported by Keenan et al. who reported that OB was more often observed in patients who had CMV infection (the three D + /R – and nine of the ten R + developed OB when compared with six of the 14 D – /R –). In addition, seven of the eight patients with CMV pneumonia developed OB. The role of CMV recurrence was not studied. The discrepancies in interpretation of results between Keenan et al. [10] and our results is due to differences in serological status of the two populations [D – /R – patients were 51% (Keenan et al.) vs 22% (this report)]. In contrast, Scott et al. [14] failed to find any association between CMV infection and OB occurrence.

The mechanisms whereby CMV infection favours occurrence of OB remain unclear [2, 5]. We have previously reported that CMV pneumopathy was associated with activation of T lymphocytes and macrophages. Several findings support this notion: (a) serum levels of neopterin (a marker of macrophage activation) and soluble IL2 receptor [9] are increased; and (b) genes coding for IL1β, IL6 and serine esterase B are expressed in BAL cells indicating in situ activation of both macrophages and cytotoxic cells [8]. Substances released by these activated cells (TNFα, IL1β and proteases) may induce lung damage. Furthermore, activated macrophages synthesize growth factors which may account for the fibroblastic proliferation that is observed in OB [6].

CMV infection is obviously not the sole cause of OB since OB was observed in D − /R − patients who remained free of CMV infection. It has been reported that AAR is closely linked to OB [16]. However, CMV infections and AAR may be closely related since: (a) donor-specific alloreactivity assessed by primed lymphocyte testing on BAL cells appeared soon after CMV infection [10] and (b) the expression of MHC class II antigens is increased during CMV infection in infected cells [13, 17].

In conclusion, the prevention of the occurrence of CMV infection after lung transplantation is important. Seronegative donor and recipient matching is the most reliable way to avoid CMV infection in lung transplant recipients. Seronegative grafts must therefore be reserved for seronegative recipients.

References

1. Burke CM, Theodore J, Dawkins KD, et al (1984) Post-transplant obliterative bronchiolitis and other late sequelae in human heart-lung transplantation. Chest 86: 824–829
2. Burke CN, Glanville AR, Theodore J, Robin EU (1987) Lung immunogenicity, rejection and obliterative bronchiolitis. Chest 92: 547–549
3. Epler GR, Colby TV, McLoud TC, Carrington CB, Gaensler EA (1985) Bronchiolitis obliterans organizing pneumonia. N Engl J Med 312: 152–158
4. Fryd DS, Peterson PK, Fergusson RM, et al (1980) Cytomegalovirus as a risk factor in renal transplantation. Transplantation 30: 436–439
5. Grundy JE, Shanley JD, Griffiths PD (1987) Is cytomegalovirus interstitial pneumonitis in transplant recipients an immunopathological condition? Lancet 2: 996–998
6. Hertz M, Henke C, Greenheck J, et al (1991) Pathogenesis of obliterative bronchiolitis after lung and heart-lung transplantation: a possible role for platelet-derived growth factor. Am Rev Resp Dis 143: A468
7. Ho M (1990) Epidemiology of cytomegalovirus infections. Rev Infect Dis 12: S701–S710
8. Humbert M, Cerrina J, Rain B, et al (1991) Interleukin-1β, interleukin-6 and serine esterase B gene expression in bronchoalveolar cells after lung and heart-lung transplantations. Am Rev Resp Dis 143: A600
9. Humbert M, Emilie D, Cerrina J, et al (1991) Soluble interleukin-2 receptor (sIL-2R) and neopterin (N) seric levels after lung and heart-lung transplantations. Am Rev Resp Dis 143: A460
10. Keenan RJ, Lega ME, Dummer JS, et al (1991) Cytomegalovirus serological status and post-operative infection correlated with risk of developing chronic rejection after pulmonary transplantation. Transplantation 51: 433–438
11. Lange W (1901) Ueber eine eigenthümliche Erkrankung der kleinen Bronchien und Bronchiolen. Dtsch Arch Klin Med 70: 324–364
12. Loebe M, Schuler S, Zais O, Warnecke H, Fleck E, Hetzer R (1990) Role of cytomegalovirus infection in the development of coronary artery disease in the transplanted heart. J Heart Transplant 9: 707–711
13. Rubin RH (1990) Impact of cytomegalovirus infection on organ transplant recipients. Rev Infect Dis 12: S754–S766
14. Scott JP, Higenbotham TW, Sharples L, Clelland CA, Smyth RL, Stewart S, Wallwork J (1991) Risk factors for obliterative bronchiolitis in heart-lung transplant recipients. Transplantation 51: 813–817
15. Smith CB (1989) Cytomegalovirus pneumonia: state of the art. Chest 95: 182S–187S
16. Theodore J, Starnes VA, Lewiston NJ (1990) Obliterative bronchiolitis. Clin Chest Med 11: 309–321
17. Von Willebrand E, Petterson E, Ahonen J, Häyry P (1986) CMV infection, class II antigen expression and human kidney allograft rejection. Transplantation 45: 394
18. Yousem SA, Berry GJ, Brunt EM, et al (1990) A working formulation for the standardization of nomenclature in the diagnosis of heart and lung rejection: lung rejection study group. J Heart Transplant 9: 593–601

Transplant Int (1992) 5 [Suppl 1]: S246–S248

TRANSPLANT
International
© Springer-Verlag 1992

The use of allopurinol in the inhibition of obliterative bronchiolitis of the transplanted lung

J. P. Scott[2], **and J. Wallwork**[1]

[1] Transplant Unit, Papworth Hospital, Cambridge, UK, [2] Mayo Clinic, Rochester, Minnesota, USA

Abstract. Long-term survival following lung transplantation has been limited primarily by the development in patients' lungs of a rejection-related obliteration of terminal bronchioles by fibroblasts. It is known to result from frequent and persistent acute lung rejection and its physiological features include a progressive decline in the lung function measurement of forced expiratory volume in 1 s. We report the dramatic effect on this hitherto usually fatal condition of a specific inhibition of purine metabolism at the xanthine oxidase enzyme by the hypoxanthine analogue allopurinol. The effect of this drug in heart-lung transplant patients with deteriorating lung function in reducing the rate of rejection and in stabilizing lung function was apparent over as short a follow-up period as 3 months and in ten patients. Although the follow-up time is short, we believe the effects are so striking as to require reporting although the mechanisms of this phenomenon are not yet well understood.

Key words: Xanthine oxidase – Allopurinol – Lung transplantation – Obliterative bronchiolitis – Rejection

Since the commencement of successful clinical trials of heart-lung transplantation, long-term survival has not been possible as a direct result of obliteration of small airways by fibrous tissue [obliterative bronchiolitis (OB)] [2]. International registry figures indicate survival as poor as 58 % at 2 years [12].

Frequent, persistent and severe acute pulmonary rejection, are the major confirmed risk factors for the development of OB [16]. The frequencies of both acute and persistent acute lung rejection are related to progressive decline in the patients' baseline forced expiratory volume in 1 s (FEV_1), which is in turn characteristic of OB [16].

Pathologically, OB is characterized by progressive destructive occlusion of small airways from a variety of

causes [15, 17]. In lung transplant recipients occlusion of small pulmonary blood vessels may also occur [6, 7]. Fibroblast proliferation in small airways is probably triggered by local immunological injury in parallel with the parenchymal perivascular immature lymphocytic infiltrates described as occurring during pulmonary rejection [3, 6, 7]. The findings of open-lung biopsies and of postmortem studies suggest that the often abrupt fall in FEV_1 characteristic of OB is associated with critical occlusion of numerous small airways by fibrous tissue [16, 17]. At our institute, only four of our first 14 patients survived 1 year following the development of OB.

The role of oxygen free radicals (OFR) in the genesis of lung injury and of fibrosis has previously been reported [5]. The production of OFRs is from several cellular sources, including xanthine-oxidase-catalysed reduction of hypoxanthine or xanthine. The potent stimulation by OFR of fibroblast proliferation has recently been described [14].

Allopurinol, a xanthine oxidase inhibitor, has been used in transplant organ preservation as has mannitol and other drugs with OFR scavenging properties [1, 9, 11]. Allopurinol has slight toxicity by itself, but has a major interaction with the widely used immunosuppressant antimetabolite azathioprine.

Offprint requests to: Dr. J. P. Scott, Division of Thoracic Diseases and Internal Medicine, East 18th Floor, Mayo Clinic, 200 1st Street, Rochester, Minnesota 55905, USA

Table 1. Azathioprine (Aza) dosage (mg/day), cyclosporin (CyA) dosage (mg/day), whole blood monoclonal radioimmune assay of CyA levels (ng/ml), prednisolone (P) dosage (mg/day) and patient weight (kg), prior to therapy with allopurinol

Patient	Aza dose	CyA dose	CyA level	P dose	Weight
1	25	350	281	0	62
2	12.5	325	230	0	55
3	37.5	1175	113	0	56
4	75	150	152	10	50
5	100	400	403	5	74
6	175	900	41	10	57
7	25	225	93	2.5	52
8	25	325	334	10	57
9	150	325	1028	15	63
10	50	1425	325	15	50

Table 2. Number of acute lung rejection (R) and infection (I) episodes in the 3 months prior to commencing allopurinol

Patient	R episodes	I episodes
1	2	0
2	0	0
3	0	1
4	6	0
5	4	1
6	4	0
7	1	0
8	2	1
9	2	0
10	2	0

Table 3. Mean change in percent predicted forced expiratory volume in one second (FEV_1) in the 3 months before and in the 3 months after institution of therapy with allopurinol for each of the ten patients

Patient	Mean change in FEV_1 (% of predicted)	
	3 months before	3 months after
1	− 8.8	− 5.0
2	− 5.0	0.0
3	− 3.1	+ 3.1
4	− 30.9	+ 2.0
5	− 28.5	+ 9.6
6	− 25.6	0.0
7	− 11.0	+ 7.3
8	− 5.3	+ 2.7
9	− 7.6	+ 2.0
10	− 14.0	+ 3.5

Methods

Since April 1984, 101 patients have received HLT at our institute, of whom 66 were alive at the time of writing, 46 of whom more than 1 year after surgery. Of the 66 survivors, ten patients (six male, four female), of average age 32.6 years (range 21–47 years) and average time since transplantation of 982 days (range 267–1665 days), had an irreversible decline in FEV_1 over the 6 months prior to the commencement of this study. All patients were considered at high risk for the development of OB, with frequent and persistent episodes of treated acute lung rejection. Average FEV_1 prior to allopurinol therapy was 53.7% of predicted (range 20.9–91.2%).

These patients were therefore commenced on allopurinol 200–600 mg/day in order to achieve a serum urate less than 0.20 mmol/l. The azathioprine dosage was initially reduced to 25% of the previous dose.

Lung function, blood chemistry, haematology, and whole-blood monoclonal assays for cyclosporine were performed and immunosuppression dosage recorded on a regular basis before and after allopurinol therapy was commenced (Table 1). The frequency of infection and rejection episodes was also recorded (Table 2), as was the rate of hospital admissions.

Results

Mean white blood count in the 3 months prior to commencement of allopurinol was 6.1 (range 4.7–7.9) and was 6.0 (range 4.9–7.0) in 3 subsequent months ($P = NS$). There was also no significant difference in neutrophil count, lymphocyte count, haemoglobin, platelets, cyclosporine dose or levels, nor in oral steroid dosage. All but

one patient had a stable or increased weight over the 3 months following commencement of the drug.

Mean change in FEV_1 over the 3 months prior to the introduction of allopurinol was − 13.9% of predicted FEV_1 (+/− standard error 3.3). The mean change in FEV_1 in the next 3 months was + 2.4% (+/− standard error 1.3). The difference between the mean change in FEV_1 before and after allopurinol was commenced was significant when analysed using the paired Student's t-test ($t = 4.26$; $P = 0.003$. Individual mean changes in FEV_1 are given in Table 3.

Rejection episodes averaged 2.4/patient per 3 months before and 0.3/patient per 3 months after commencement of treatment with allopurinol; using McNemar's test with continuity correction this difference was significant ($z = 2.5$; $P = 0.013$). The frequency of infection was comparable, averaging 1.6 episodes/patient per 3 months before and 1.5 episodes/patient per 3 months after allopurinol was started ($P = NS$).

Discussion

We have demonstrated the short-term effect of high-dose allopurinol in preventing further decline in FEV_1 towards disability and death which has plagued lung transplantation. This prospective study was not randomized, reflecting our level of clinical concern for these patients with deteriorating lung function. The mechanism of this effect is unknown, but the reduction in the frequency of rejection without an overall increase in the frequency of infection suggests its effect is not merely an enhancement in the overall level of immunosuppression.

Since under conditions of ischaemia, and perhaps under those of inflammation, inhibition of xanthine oxidase may result in a reduction in OFR generation [10] and OFR have been implicated in the genesis of fibroblast proliferation [14], it is possible that allopurinol has had this striking effect by way of OFR inhibition [8]. The alternative hypothesis is that the interaction of allopurinol and azathioprine results in a change in the profile of active azathioprine metabolites [4], including 6-mercaptopurine, and this results in an enhancement of anti-inflammatory and/or immunosuppressive activity. Some support for this second hypothesis can be argued from the report of the attenuated decline in FEV_1 in HLT patients following the initial introduction of azathioprine at Stanford [6].

The OFR hypothesis can be assessed by measurement of secondary products of OFR, such as lipid hydroperoxide [13] and the alternative hypothesis can be examined by study of azathioprine metabolites [4].

These results should be cautiously interpreted, since this was not a randomized study and accordingly we have now undertaken a prospectively randomized study in recent HLT recipients prior to initial hospital discharge. The long-term effects are not yet known. However, if further studies confirm this observation, the implications for lung transplantation are potentially profound. The internationally reported prospects of 58% survival at 2 years after undergoing the established combined heart and lung transplant procedure [12] could be significantly improved. The dramatic fall in acute lung rejection without apparent change in the level of immunosuppression, and with no increase in the level of infection, suggests that this approach may well have wider application in the general transplant field. We are aware of the short follow up in these patients, but believe that the possible implications of this preliminary study require us to report these observations for comment and criticism.

References

1. Bonser RS, Fragomeni LS, Edwards BJ, et al (1990) Allopurinol and desferoximine improve canine lung preservation. Transplant Proc 22:557–558
2. Burke CM, Theodore J, Baldwin JC, et al (1986) Twenty-eight cases of human heart-lung transplantation. Lancet I:517–519
3. Clelland CAC, Higenbottam TW, Otulana BA, et al (1990) Histological classification of acute lung rejection in heart-lung transplantation. J Heart Transplant 9:177–186
4. Elion GB, Callahan S, Rundles RW, Hitchings GH (1963) Relationship between metabolic fates and antitumor activities of thiopurines. Cancer Res 23:1207–1217
5. Fogt F, Zilker T (1981) Total exclusion from external respiration protects lungs from the development of fibrosis after paraquat in the immunosuppressed host. Clin Chest Med 2:19–39
6. Glandville AR, Baldwin JC, Burke CM, Theodore J, Robin ED (1987) Obliterative bronchiolitis after heart-lung transplantation: Apparent arrest by augmented immunosuppression. Ann Intern Med 107:300–304
7. Griffith BP, Paradis IL, Zeevi A, et al (1988) Immunologically mediated disease of the airways after pulmonary transplantation. Ann Surg 208:371–378
8. Gruber DF, O'Halloran KP, Farese AM (1989) Xanthine oxidase potentiation of reactive oxygen intermediates in isolated canine peripheral neutrophils. J Biol Response Mod 8:462–467
9. Hajjar GB, Toledo-Pereyra LH, MacKenzie GH (1987) Twenty-four hour heart-lung preservation and oxygen free radical scavengers. Transplant Proc 19:1342–1344
10. Junod AF (1989) Oxygen free radicals and the lungs. Intensive Care Med 15:S21–23
11. Kennedy TP, Rao NV, Hopkins C, Pennington L, Tolley E, Hoidal JR (1990) Role of reactive oxygen molecules in experimental colitis. Gut 31:786–790
12. Kriett JM, Kaye MP (1990) The registry of the international society for heart transplantation: seventh official report–1990. J Heart Transplant 9:323–330
13. Miyazawa T, Fujimoto K, Oikawa S (1990) Determination of lipid hydroperoxides in low density lipoprotein from human plasma using high performance liquid chromatography with chemiluminescence detection. Biomed Chromatogr 4:131–134
14. Murrell GA, Francis MJ, Bromley L (1990) Modulation of fibroblast proliferation by oxygen free radicals. Biochem J 265:659–665
15. Scott JP, Higenbottam TW, Clelland CAC, et al (1989) The natural history of obliterative bronchiolitis and occlusive vascular disease of patients following heart-lung transplantation. Transplant Proc 21:2592–2593
16. Scott JP, Higenbottam TW, Sharples L, et al (1991) Risk factors for obliterative bronchiolitis in heart-lung transplant recipients. Transplantation (in press)
17. Yousem SA, Burke CM, Billingham ME (1985) Pathologic pulmonary alterations in long-term human heart-lung transplantation. Hum Pathol 16:911–923

Transplant Int (1992) 5 [Suppl 1]: S 249–S 251

TRANSPLANT
International
© Springer-Verlag 1992

Evaluation of the International Society for Heart Transplantation (ISHT) grading of pulmonary rejection in 100 consecutive biopsies

J. Hunt[1], **S. Stewart**, **N. Cary**, **T. Wreghitt**, **T. Higenbottam**, **J. Wallwork**[3]

Departments of [1] Pathology, [2] Respiratory Physiology and [3] Surgery, Papworth Hospital, Cambridge, UK; and
[4] Department of Virology Addenbrooke's Hospital, Cambridge, UK

Heart-lung and lung transplantation are accepted treatments for patients with end-stage pulmonary vascular disease or parenchymal lung disease [4, 5, 10]. Survival rates for heart-lung and lung transplantation are lower than those for heart transplantation alone. The 5-year actuarial survival for heart-lung transplantation has been 41 % largely due to rejection and infection remaining as the limiting factors for long-term survival [3].

A standardized nomenclature for the histological grading of pulmonary rejection was formulated by the International Society for Heart Transplantation (ISHT) in July 1990 [12]. Infection, however, is a major problem in the histological assessment of lung recipient biopsies, potentially limiting the usefulnes of such a classification. In this study, 100 consecutive transbronchial biopsies (TBBs) from lung transplant recipients were analysed, together with microbiological and serological data, in order to evaluate the proposed ISHT grading system for pulmonary rejection and the importance of concomitant infections in the histological interpretation of TBBs.

Key words: Pulmonary rejection, ISHT grading – TBBs histology

Materials and methods

Patients

From September 1990 to March 1991, 100 consecutive TBBs were obtained from 43 patients during routine surveillance or clinically indicated procedures. The patients included four single lung and 39 heart-lung recipients and their ages ranged from 18 to 59 years (mean 34.1). The transbronchial procedure has previously been described [1].

Histology

The biopsies were fixed in 10 % neutral buffered formalin and processed in a Shandon Hypercenter. Routine biopsies were processed

overnight and clinically urgent specimens were processed using a short 2-hour cycle. The paraffin-embedded material was serially sectioned and stained with haematoxylin and eosin. Special stains performed on all cases included Perls'/elastic van Gieson for connective tissue, PAS and Grocott's methenamine silver method for fungal hyphae and the cysts of *Pneumocystis carinii*. Additional special stains were performed as appropriate, e. g. Ziel-Neelsen stains for acid fast bacilli in cases with granulomatous inflammation. Accompanying bronchioalveolar lavage (BAL) specimens were fixed in 100 % alcohol and prepared slides stained with haematoxylin and eosin and by Grocott's methenamine silver method. Cytospin preparations were made if required. All the histological material was reviewed by S. S.

Microbiology

Specimens from either the BAL or transbronchial samples were sent for viral culture including cultures for HSV and CMV. In patients who were known CMV mismatches or seropositive, early detection

Table 1. Results of ISHT grading system applied to 76 TBBs

	(a)	(b)	(c)	(d)	Total
Grade A (acute rejection)					
1. Minimal	4	9	0	1	14
2. Mild	14	15	0	1	30
3. Moderate	7	6	0	0	13
4. Severe	0	0	0	0	0
Grade B (airway inflammation)					
B1.	0				
B2.	1				

Grade C (oblit. bronchiolitis)	**Grade D (chronic vascular rejection)** 5
C1a 5	
C1b 2	
C2a 1	
C2b 0	

Grade 0 (no abnormality) 14	Grade E (vasculitis) 0

Grade A, suffixes (a) with bronchiolar inflammation
(b) without bronchiolar inflammation
(c) with bronchial inflammation
(d) no bronchioles present
Grade B1, lymphocytic bronchitis; B2, lymphocytic bronchiolitis
Grade C1, sub total; C2 total; a active, b inactive

Offprint requests to: James Hunt, Department of Pathology, Papworth Hospital, Papworth Everard, Cambridge, CB3 8RE, UK

Table 2. Biopsies in which rejection could not be assessed due to histological evidence of infection

Nature of infection (histological)	Number of biopsies (n = 22)	Confirmed by appropriate culture serology (n = 16)
CMV Pneumonitis	12	11
Bacterial infections (bronchitis/organizing pneumonia)	4	3[a]
Asp – invasive	2	(1)[b]
– bronchocentric/ granulomatous	1	1
– pneumonia	1	1[c]
PCP	2	N/A

Asp, *Aspergillus fumigatus;* PCP, *Pneumocystis carinii pneumonia;* N/A, not applicable
[a] *Pseudomanas aeruginosa,* 2; *Haemophilus influenza,* 1
[b] One biopsy not sent for culture
[c] *Herpes simplex* virus also cultured

Table 3. Results of microbiological investigations in biopsies graded for rejection

Type of infection	Number of isolates (n = 22)
Pseud infections	11
CMV	3
Asp	2
Other bacteria[a]	4
Mixed infections[b]	2
	22

Pseud, *Pseudomanas aeruginosa;* Asp, *Aspergillus fumigatus*
[a] Includes: *Branhamella catarrhalis, Acinetobacter* spp., *Haemophilus influenzae, Staphylococcus aureus*
[b] Includes: Adenovirus/Pseud; CMV/Asp

Table 4. Rejection grades assigned to biopsies with microbiological evidence of concomitant infection

Rejection grade	Number of biopsies (n = 22)
0	2
A1a	2
A1b	4
A2a	5
A2b	4
A2d	1
B2	1
C1a	1
A1b/C1a/D[a]	1
Total	22

[a] Multiple rejection grades assigned on one biopsy

of CMV was performed by the DEAFF (Direct early antigen fluorescent focus) test. Other infectious agents investigated by serological methods and according to clinical suspicion included toxoplasmosis, adenovirus, influenza virus, mycoplasma spp., legionella and Epstein-Barr virus. A review of all microbiological data from specimens that included sputa, blood cultures, throat swabs and BAL was undertaken for specimens taken 2 days prior to, and 2 days following, biopsy procedures.

Results

Gradable rejection was shown by 76 TBBs. The grades assigned at the time of biopsy are shown in Table 1. The majority of TBBs showed acute rejection, predominantly mild acute rejection, grade A2, and there were no cases of severe acute rejection. In six TBBs more than one grade was assigned, e.g. grade A2a (mild acute rejection) together with grade C1b (obliterative bronchiolitis) and grade D (chronic vascular rejection). Rejection could not be assessed in 24 TBBs. In the majority of cases (22), this was due to histological evidence of infection. In all but two biopsies this was confirmed by the appropriate microbiological cultures or serological investigation. The results are shown in Table 2. From only one procedure was the material inadequate for assessment, and in one biopsy the effects of a previous biopsy obscured the histology. In the two TBBs thought to be infective at histology (but 'culture negative'), one showed features suggestive of a viral pneumonitis and one showed a non-specific pneumonitis. In the 76 TBBs assessed as gradable for rejection, in 22 cases the caveat 'exclude infection' was included in the histological report. Analysis of the microbiological data showed eight of these cases to have significant positive cultures in addition to 14 out of the 54 cases graded confidently for rejection. Table 3 shows the patients culture/serological results. The rejection grades assigned to these biopsies at the time of reporting are shown in Table 4.

Discussion

This study validates the use of the TBB for the diagnosis of infection and rejection in heart-lung and single-lung transplant recipients, in keeping with previous reports [2, 8]. In only a single biopsy procedure was the material insufficient for a diagnosis. The number of biopsy specimens required to evaluate significant lung rejection is uncertain but the Lung Rejection Study Group [12] recommend a minimum of five transbronchial specimens containing lung parenchyma to be taken from the donor graft at each biopsy procedure. The ISHT Working Formulation Grading of Rejection can be applied to TBBS and in this study over three-quarters of the biopsies were assigned a grade to aid clinical management, most frequently Grade A, acute rejection. Perivascular infiltrates in TBBs are not specific for rejection, and the major differential diagnosis is infection [9]. Analysis of microbiological results showed evidence of a concomitant respiratory tract infection in 22 out of 76 biopsy procedures where a grade had been assigned, and emphasises the importance of reviewing all the data before assigning a final grade. Examination of the grades assigned in these cases, Table 4, shows no trend towards a particular grade and in particular no evidence of a preponderance of acute rejection with airways inflammation. The respiratory infections were presumably upper airways infections in these cases.

TBBs are useful for the diagnosis of complications in lung transplantation patients. The histological diagnosis of infection in this study was shown to be highly specific and only two false positive histological diagnoses of infection were made on biopsy material when accompanying microbiological data were analysed. CMV is a major problem. Although there are special techniques available that increase the sensitivity of detection [7, 11], the diagnosis of CMV disease in the lung requires the demonstration of CMV inclusions together with an accompanying pneumonitis [6]. Culture and serological evidence of CMV indicates infection as seen in four out of 22 biopsies which had been graded but which also had evidence of a concomitant infection. CMV pneumonitis with inclusions and surrounding inflammation was not confused with rejection in our study.

References

1. Higenbottam T, Stewart S, Penketh A, Wallwork J (1988) Transbronchial lung biopsy for the diagnosis of rejection in heart-lung transplant patients. Transplantation 46:532–539
2. Higenbottam T, Stewart S, Wallwork J (1988) Transbronchial lung biopsy to diagnose lung rejection and infection of heart-lung transplants. Transplant Proc 20:767–769
3. Kriett JM, Kaye MP (1991) The Registry of the International Society for Heart and Lung Transplantation: Eighth Official Report – 1991. J Heart Lung Transplant 10:491–498
4. Penketh ARL, Higenbottam TW, Hakim M, Wallwork J (1987) Heart and lung transplantation in patients with end-stage lung disease. Br Med J 295:311–314
5. Reitz BA, Wallwork J, Hunt SA, Pennock JL, Billingham ME, Oyer PE, Stinson EB, Shumway NE (1982) Heart lung transplantation? Successful therapy for patients with pulmonary vascular disease. N Engl J Med 306:557–564
6. Sissons JGP, Borysiewicz LK (1989) Human cytomegalovirus infection. Thorax 44:241–246
7. Steinhoff G, Behrend M, Wagner TOF, Hoper MH, Haverich A (1991) Early diagnosis and effective treatment of pulmonary CMV infection after lung transplantation. J Heart Lung Transplant 10:9–14
8. Stewart S, Higenbottam TW, Hutter JW, Penketh ARL, Zebro TJ, Wallwork J (1988) Histopathology of transbronchial biopsies in heart-lung transplantation. Transplant Proc 20: 764–766
9. Tazelaar HD (1991) Perivascular inflammation in pulmonary infections: implications for the diagnosis of lung rejection. J Heart Lung Transplant 10: 437–441
10. Theodore J, Levington N (1990) Lung transplantation comes of age. N Engl J Med 332:772–774
11. Weiss LM, Movahed LA, Berry GJ, Billingham ME (1990) In situ hybridization studies for viral nucleic acids in heart and lung allograft biopsies. Am J Clin Pathol 93:675–679
12. Yousem SA, Berry GJ, Brunt EM, Chamberlain D, Hruban RH, Sibley RK, Stewart S, Tazelaar H (1990) A working formulation for the standardisation of nomenclature in the diagnosis of the heart and lung rejection: Lung Rejection Study Group. J Heart Transplant 9:593–601

Transplant Int (1992) 5 [Suppl 1]: S 252–S 254

TRANSPLANT
International
© Springer-Verlag 1992

Coronary flow reserve and coronary occlusive disease

P. A. Mullins, J. P. Scott, D. J. Aravot, C. Dennis, S. R. Large, J. Wallwork, and P. M. Schofield

Transplant Unit, Papworth Hospital, Cambridge, UK

Abstract. The functional effects of coronary occlusive disease (COD) in cardiac transplant patients on small-resistance coronary vessels are unclear. We investigated the changes in coronary flow reserve (CFR) in response to the non-specific smooth muscle vasodilator papaverine. A 3F Doppler probe was inserted into the left anterior descending (LAD) coronary artery in 61 patients following orthotopic heart transplantation. Studies were performed in 57 males and 4 females with a mean age of 46 years (range 20–61 years). The median time from operation was 4 years (range 3 months to 10 years). Coronary blood velocity was measured at rest (RFV) and maximum hyperaemia (PFV) produced by intracoronary papaverine. Coronary flow reserve (CFR) was defined as the ratio of PFV to RFV. Minor lesions in epicardial vessels were found in 23 transplant patients. The mean percentage diameter of the most severe lesion in the coronary tree was 23% SD 3% including 12 lesions in the LAD coronary artery itself (mean 24% SD 4%). Patients with COD had an impaired CFR (2.6 SEM 0.2) compared with normals (3.9 SEM 0.2, $P = 0.0003$), adjusting for year after operation. Mean resting flow velocity was similar in both groups (minor COD, 6.8 cm/s SEM 1.2; normals, 7.1 cm/s SEM 0.6), but mean peak flow velocity response to papaverine was reduced (16.5 cm/s SEM 2.5 versus 27.3 cm/s SEM 2.6; $P = 0.007$). In the presence of minor epicardial disease, coronary flow reserve in resistance vessels was reduced due to impairment of peak flow. This demonstrates that non-endothelial-dependent coronary resistance vessel vasodilatation is abnormal and may be caused by a defect in vascular smooth muscle function.

Key words: Cardiac transplant – Coronary microcirculation – Coronary occlusive disease

---

Coronary occlusive disease is the major long-term problem facing cardiac transplantation [8]. Clinical monitoring of the disease is usually dependent on serial coronary an-

Offprint requests to: Dr. P. A. Mullins, Transplant Unit, Papworth Hospital, Papworth Everard, Huntingdon, Cambridge CB3 8RE, UK

giography. This is insensitive for detecting coronary occlusive disease in heart transplant patients [4, 10] and underestimates its presence compared with post-mortem data [13]. It also affects small- and medium-sized coronary vessels. It is not possible to assess these vessels angiographically. The relationship between coronary structure defined by angiography and prognosis in cardiac transplant patients is therefore not clear.

Coronary angiographic assessment of conventional and transplant-related coronary occlusive disease has other limitations. For example, it is possibility that narrowings of intermediate 'severity' are significant [9]. Coronary flow reserve measurements are increasingly being used as potential methods for estimating the physiological impact of coronary pathology [3], including coronary disease which may affect smaller vessels [11].

Coronary flow reserve is defined as the ratio of the maximum to the resting coronary flow at a given perfusion pressure, when coronary vessels are maximally vasodilated. In the normal coronary circulation, coronary flow reserve is reduced by lesions producing approximately 35–50% stenosis or more in primary coronary arteries [6, 7, 9]. To maintain myocardial blood flow, coronary resistance vessels vasodilate to compensate for the resistance offered by proximal stenoses [7]. The maximal flow at a given coronary perfusion pressure is predominantly determined by the total cross-sectional area of the resistance vessels. A reduction in the number, calibre or impaired function of these coronary resistance vessels could have a marked impact on coronary flow reserve. This may limit their ability to respond to reductions in myocardial flow produced by proximal coronary lesions [5].

The relationship between 'minor' angiographic abnormalities and myocardial perfusion has not previously been assessed in a large number of cardiac transplant patients.

Patients and methods

Patients

This study was approved by the Huntingdon District Health Authority Ethical Committee. A group of 61 patients was investigated after cardiac transplantation; 55 males and 6 females. Of these, 56

Table 1. Patient variables

	Heart rate	MAP (mm Hg)	LVEDP (mm Hg)	Age (years)	Sex	Hct (%)
'Minor' COD	87 (11)	96 (2)	9 (1)	47 (12)	22 M 1 F	40 (3)
Normal	83 (12)	94 (3)	8 (2)	47 (9)	33 M 5 F	38 (2)

All values + standard deviation where appropriate
COD, coronary occlusive disease; MAP, mean arterial pressure; LVEDP, left ventricular end-diastolic pressure; Hct, haematocrit

Table 2.

	Group 1	Group 2
Original diagnosis	IHD 12 DCM 11	IHD 20 DCM 18
Median time post-operation (years)	5 (0.3–10)	4 (0.3–8)
Ischaemic time (min)	160 (45)	157 (40)
CyA level	282 (252)	326 (220)
Cholesterol	6.2 (1.0)	5.65 (1.9)
HDL cholesterol	0.95 (0.5)	1.0 (0.7)
LDL cholesterol	5.3 (1.4)	4.6 (1.2)
Triglyceride	2.2 (1.3)	1.9 (0.6)

All values + standard deviation where appropriate
COD, coronary occlusive disease; CyA, cyclosporin; DCM, dilated cardiomyopathy; IHD, ischaemic heart disease

were receiving cyclosporin and azathioprine immunosuppression with or without steroid therapy. No patients were taking β-antagonist therapy. All vasoactive medication (e. g. calcium antagonists) was omitted 24 h prior to the procedure. None of the patients received premedication. Patients underwent right ventricular endomyocardial biopsy on the day of coronary angiography. These samples were examined by conventional light microscopy and graded according to standard histological criteria for the presence of acute rejection [1].

The patients were fasted prior to cardiac catheterization. Coronary angiography was performed via the right femoral artery in all patients using the Judkins technique. Coronary injections were performed manually using up to 8 ml of intracoronary radiopaque contrast (Niopam) and ciné film recordings made in multiple projections. After routine angiography the proximal left anterior descending coronary artery was centred for optimal viewing. A period of at lest 10 min was allowed to elapse before the study continued to eliminate vasoactive effects from the contrast medium.

Heparin 10000 units was given intravenously. A size 8F angioplasty guiding catheter was advanced into the left coronary ostium. A 0.014-inch guidewire was advanced into the distal part of the left anterior descending coronary artery. Using a monorail technique, a size 3F 20 MHz intracoronary Doppler flow probe (Schneider, UK) was advanced over the guidewire into the proximal segment of the left anterior descending coronary artery. The Doppler flow probe and the range gate of the velocimeter were adjusted to obtain good quality phasic and mean coronary blood flow velocity signals. These signals were recorded with the surface electrocardiogram on a Mingograf recorder (Siemens-Elema, Sweden).

Baseline resting and phasic coronary blood flow velocity were taken in each patient. After an initial intracoronary 2-mg test dose of papaverine hydrochloride via the guiding catheter, further injections of up to 14 mg of papaverine (2 mg/ml in 0.9 % saline) were given until maximum flow was achieved. The hyperaemic response was recorded in the form of maximum blood flow velocity in centimetres per second (cm/s). Velocity profiles were allowed to return to baseline levels between doses of papaverine.

Each coronary angiogram was assessed by two independent observers blinded to the clinical history. Coronary occlusive disease was defined as any evidence of disease in primary or secondary coronary arteries on angiography. The primary coronary arteries were defined as the left anterior descending coronary artery, left circumflex coronary artery and right coronary artery (primary vessels). Their main branches were classified as secondary coronary arteries (diagonal, obtuse marginal, and posterolateral or posterior descending branch of the right coronary).

Coronary disease was graded according to the stenosis diameter of the most severe lesion in primary or secondary coronary vessels compared with an adjacent 'healthy' artery. The coronary lumen was defined as the effective perfusion channel and measurement was performed in diastolic frames. Quantitative measurements of arterial diameter in coronary vessels were performed using digital electronic calipers (Sandhill Scientific). Coronary angiography was performed at rest, at peak hyperaemia and changes in coronary diameter measured. Left ventricular angiography was performed at the end of the study.

Coronary flow reserve and coronary vascular resistance index

Coronary flow reserve, was defined as the ratio of the peak flow velocity (PFV) achieved to the resting blood flow velocity (RFV). To offset any changes in blood pressure during the study, a coronary vascular resistance index (CVRI) was calculated from the following expression:

$$CVRI = \frac{\text{Mean BP at peak flow} \backslash PFV}{\text{Mean BP at rest} \backslash RFV}$$

where BP = aortic blood pressure.

Statistical analysis

Results are expressed as means with standard errors for continuous measurements, and frequencies for categorical variables. Linear regression analysis was performed to adjust coronary flow reserve measurements for the year after operation. Unpaired Student's t-tests were used to assess differences between group means. Statistical significance was assumed for P values < 0.05.

Results

The median time from operation for all cardiac transplant patients was 4.5 years (range 3 months to 10 years). Of the transplant recipients, 32 had originally undergone transplantation for ischaemic heart disease, and the remaining 29 patients for dilated cardiomyopathy. For the groups investigated, relevant patient information, haemodynamic measurements and other variables are shown in Tables 1 and 2. Patients with 'minor COD' were significantly further out from operation compared with normal transplant patients ($P = 0.007$). Several variables which could potentially be related to the development of coronary occlusive disease (Table 2), did not show any association with impaired coronary flow reserve. The mean age of the donor hearts was 26.5 years (SEM 1.5 years). The mean cold ischaemic time was 159 min (range 77–260 min). The donors for 16 (26 %) patients were female and for the remaining 45 were male.

Normal coronary angiograms were found for 38 cardiac transplant patients, and 23 transplant patients had minor lesions in epicardial vessels. The mean percentage diameter of the most severe lesion in the coronary tree was 23 % SD 3 % including 12 lesions in the left anterior descending coronary artery itself (mean 24 % SD 4 %). Nine of these patients had minor coronary disease in one

Table 3. Coronary flow measurements

	CFR	CVRI	RFV	PFV
'Minor' COD	2.5 (0.2)	0.42 (0.04)	6.8 (1.1)	16.5 (2.5)
COD	3.9 (0.2)	0.26 (0.02)	7.1 (0.6)	27.3 (2.6)

Values in parentheses are SEM
CFR, coronary flow reserve; RFV, resting flow velocity (cm/s); PFV, peak flow velocity (cm/s); SEM, standard error of the mean; CVRI, coronary vascular resistance index; COD, coronary occlusive disease

primary or secondary vessel, four patients had disease in two vessels, while the remainder had disease in three or more coronary arteries.

Coronary flow reserve measurements

Adjusting for year from operation, patients with minor COD had a significantly impaired coronary flow reserve and a higher coronary vascular resistance index ($P < 0.0001$) (Table 3). The mean resting coronary blood flow was similar in both groups. Mean peak flow velocity was also impaired compared with normals ($P = 0.007$). There was overall dilation by $+18\%$ (SD 6%) of the left anterior descending coronary artery in both groups in response to papaverine. Reproducibility of the arterial diameter measurements was acceptable with minimal inter-observer ($r = 0.91$) and intra-observer variation ($r = 0.95$).

Discussion

This study demonstrates a reduction in coronary flow reserve and maximum hyperaemic coronary blood flow in cardiac transplant patients with minor proximal coronary occlusive disease. The degree of stenosis in the left anterior descending coronary artery was relatively minor, and affected this vessel in only 52% (12/23) of cases. In addition there were no differences between the groups in the degree of vasodilation produced by papaverine in the proximal left anterior descending coronary artery. This suggests that the dilatory dysfunction occurs in the coronary resistance vessels in these patients.

This reduction in coronary flow reserve and maximum hyperaemic coronary flow could be explained by progressive occlusion of resistance vessels [12]. Occlusion of small tertiary (branches of primary and secondary coronary vessels) coronary branches is commonly seen at postmortem [2], but would have to be extremely widespread to have such a large effect on its own. Aspects of the function of resistance vessel vascular smooth muscle may also be damaged during the development of coronary occlusive disease. Both these factors may operate.

Other alternative explanations for impairment of coronary flow reserve and peak coronary flow in the group with coronary occlusive disease need to be excluded. There were no obvious significant differences in heart rate, myocardial contractility or ventricular dilatation, elevated left ventricular end-diastolic pressure or in haematocrit levels between the three groups. It is known that left ventricular hypertrophy, ventricular wall motion abnormalities and collateral vessels can produce abnor-

mal flow reserve measurements [6]. None of the patients had these features.

Functional assessment of the coronary vasculature in patients with coronary occlusive disease is attractive. However, the clinical importance of these reductions in coronary flow reserve and peak hyperaemic response in individual cardiac transplant patients is unknown. Longitudinal studies are underway to evaluate the relevance of these findings.

Conclusion

Coronary flow reserve and hyperaemic response to the non-endothelial-dependent vasodilator papaverine is significantly impaired in heart transplant recipients when 'minor' coronary occlusive disease is present on coronary angiography. Dysfunction of the coronary microcirculation may contribute to the significant late morbidity and mortality produced by the disease. This may probe an important method of evaluating coronary occlusive disease in patients following cardiac transplantation.

Acknowledgements. We would like to thank Dr. G.I. Verney, and the staff of the radiographic and cardiac technical departments at Papworth Hospital for their support during this study.

References

1. Billingham ME (1981) Diagnosis of cardiac rejection by endomyocardial biopsy. J Heart Transplant 1:25–30
2. Billingham ME (1987) Cardiac transplant atherosclerosis. Transplant Proc 4 [Suppl 5]:19–25
3. Buss PD (1990) The coronary circulation. In: Nichols WM, O'Rourke MF (eds) McDonald's blood flow in arteries. Edward Arnold, Sevenoaks, pp 360–380
4. Gao SZ, Alderman EL, Schroeder JS, Silverman JF, Hunt SA (1988) Accelerated coronary vascular disease in the heart transplant patient: coronary angiographic findings. J Am Coll Cardiol 12:334–340
5. Gould KL, Lipscomb K, Calvert C (1975) Compensatory changes of the distal coronary vascular bed during progressive coronary constriction. Circulation 51:1085–1094
6. Hartley CJ (1989) Review of intracoronary Doppler catheters. Int J Cardiac Imaging 4:159–168
7. Klocke FJ (1987) Measurements of coronary flow reserve: defining pathophysiology versus making decisions about patient care. Circulation 76:1183–1189
8. Kriett JM, Kaye MP (1990) The Registry of the International Society for Heart and Lung Transplantation: Seventh official report–1990. J Heart Lung Transplant 9:323–336
9. Marcus ML, Skorton DJ, Johnson MR, Collins SM, Harrison DG, Kerber RE (1988) Visual estimates of percent diameter coronary stenosis: 'a battered gold standard'. J Am Coll Cardiol 11:882–885
10. O'Neill BJ, Pflugfelder PW, Singh NR, Menkis AH, McKenzie FN, Kostuk WJ (1989) Frequency of angiographic detection and quantitative assessment of coronary arterial disease one and three years after cardiac transplantation. Am J Cardiol 63: 1221–1226
11. Opherk D, Zebe H, Weihe E, et al (1981) Reduced coronary dilatory capacity and ultrastructural changes of the myocardium in patients with angina pectoris but normal coronary angiograms. Circulation 63:817–825
12. Talman CL, Winniford MD, Rossen JD, Simmonetti I, Kienzle MG, Marcus ML (1990) Polymorphous ventricular tachycardia: a side effect of intracoronary papaverine. J Am Coll 15:275–278
13. Uys CJ, Rose AG (1984) Pathologic findings in long-term cardiac transplants. Arch Pathol Lab Med 108:112–116

Transplant Int (1992) 5 [Suppl 1]: S255–S258

TRANSPLANT
International
© Springer-Verlag 1992

Tricuspid valve insufficiency as a complication of endomyocardial biopsy

L. Wiklund[1], K. Caidahl[2], C. Kjellström[3], B. Nilsson[1], G. Svensson[1], and E. Berglin[1]

[1] Department of Cardiothoracic Surgery, [2] Department of Clinical Physiology, and [3] Department of Pathology, Sahlgrenska Hospital, Gothenburg, Sweden

Abstract. The purpose of this study was to investigate the occurrence of major tricuspid insufficiency caused by endomyocardial biopsy in heart transplant recipients. Endomyocardial biopsy was used for the detection of rejection and Doppler echocardiography was performed at regular intervals. Six of 96 heart transplant patients (6.3 %) had sudden appearance of large tricuspid regurgitation, all of which were directly related to a preceding biopsy. Chordal tissue was identified histologically in biopsy samples of all six patients. All patients developed symptoms of right ventricular failure which was confirmed by right heart catheterization. Three patients subsequently underwent valvuloplasty for ruptured chordae tendineae of either of the three leaflets. Two of these three patients were free from symptoms during follow-up, but the third patient developed moderate tricuspid regurgitation and clinical symptoms. It is concluded that endomyocardial biopsy, although it is the most useful tool for detection of rejection, should be used with caution with regard to anatomical structures and the risk of damage to the tricuspid valve must not be neglected. It is also concluded that valvuloplasty of the tricuspid valve can be successfully performed in a transplanted heart.

Key words: Chorda tendineae rupture – Echocardiography – Endomyocardial biopsy – Heart transplantation – Tricuspid insufficiency

---

Percutaneous endomyocardial biopsy was introduced by Caves et al. in 1972 and was an important contribution to the detection of rejection after heart transplantation [4]. The technique is still the preferred method for diagnosis of rejection in the transplanted heart and is regarded as safe with a low morbidity and mortality. Complications such as transient arrhythmias, transient bundle branch block, transient nerve palsies, puncture site bleedings and endocarditis occur in low frequency. Major complications are rare, cardiac perforation, pneumothorax and tamponade

being reported in less than 0.4 % [4, 5]. Henzlova et al. recently reported coronary artery–right ventricular fistulas in four out of 74 patients after endomyocardial biopsies [8].

Rupture of chordae tendineae of the tricuspid valve as a complication of endomyocardial biopsy has recently been reported by Braverman et al. [3] in five heart transplant recipients.

The aim of the present study was to investigate the occurrence of large tricuspid valve insufficiency secondary to chordal destruction caused by the bioptome when obtaining endomyocardial biopsies in heart transplant recipients.

Patients and methods

Between January 1988 and August 1991, 96 orthotopic cardiac transplantations were performed in 78 men and 18 woman at our center. Ages ranged from 16 to 63 (mean 43) years.

To detect rejection episodes, weekly endomyocardial biopsies were used during 6 weeks post-transplantation. Thereafter, biopsies were obtained every fortnight for 6 weeks, monthly for 3 months, and then every 3 months. Biopsies were also occasionally obtained when rejection was clinically suspected.

In the standard technique for right ventricular biopsy a bioptome (Caves–Schultz) is percutaneously introduced into the right internal jugular vein through an introducer, and guided by fluoroscopy. The bioptome is advanced with its jaws closed until it reaches the right ventricular septal endocardium. The bioptome is withdrawn 1 cm, and with its jaws opened, it is readvanced into the septal endocardium. The jaws are then closed, and the bioptome is withdrawn with the biopsy [4]. Wnen the standard approach offered difficulties the right femoral vein was punctured. In rare cases the left subclavian vein was used.

Doppler echocardiography was performed after each biopsy for the first 2 months and then at the yearly follow-up. We used an Acuson-128 or Acuson-128XP (Acuson, Mountain View, Calif., USA) equipped with a 3.5 or 2 MHz phased array transducer to obtain two-dimensional echocardiographic recordings. The three patients who were subjected to tricuspid valvuloplasty were also investigated through the transoesophageal approach using a 5 MHz transducer. The degree of tricuspid regurgitation was semiquantitated by colour-flow Doppler and by continuous-wave Doppler on the basis of the systolic regurgitant flow relative to the area of the right atrium as well as on the basis of the intensity of the regurgitant jet (Table 1) [3, 7, 13].

The sudden occurrence of large (grades 3–4) tricuspid valve regurgitation was regarded as a possible adverse effect of a preceding biopsy. In these patients the biopsy samples were histologically re-

---

Offprint requests to: Dr. Lars Wiklund, Department of Cardiothoracic Surgery, Sahlgrenska Hospital, S-413 45 Gothenburg, Sweden

Table 1. Semiquantitative grading of tricuspid regurgitation by echocardiography

Degree of insufficiency	Grade	Echocardiography findings
Minor	0.5	Weak not holosystolic jet
Mild	1	Weak holosystolic jet detectable
Moderate	2	Syst. jet < 50 % right atrial area
Moderate to severe	3	Jet > 50 % right atrial area
Severe	4	Jet filling right atrium completely

Table 2. Frequency and grading of echocardiographically estimated postoperative tricuspid regurgitation in 96 consecutive patients

	Grading of tricuspid insufficiency				
	< 0.5	1	2	3	4
No. of patients	28	24	27	10	2
%	29.2	25	28.1	10.4	2.1

Echocardiography was not performed in five patients

Table 3. Development and grading of tricuspid insufficiency as estimated by echocardiography and the number of biopsies in three patients who underwent valvuloplasty

Patient number	Tricuspid regurgitation			No. of biopsies[a]
	Before chordal rupture	After chordal rupture	After valvuloplasty	
1	0.5	4	3	17
2	2	3–4	2	16
3	0.5	4	0.5	5

[a] Number of biopsies taken between the last normal echocardiography and the one which first showed a large tricuspid regurgitation

evaluated for the presence of chordal tissue [11, 12]. The biopsies were processed, sectioned and stained as recommended by the International Society for Heart Transplantation [2].

Case reports

A total of 9790 biopsies were obtained during 1780 different procedures. During the first year a mean of 18 biopsies/patient were obtained, with a range of 12 to 27 biopsy procedures for every heart transplant recipient. The following maximum degrees of tricuspid regurgitation were estimated by echocardiography: in 28 patients grade < 0.5, in 24 patients grade 1, in 27 patients grade 2, in 10 patients grade 3, while two patients were judged as having grade 4. Five patients had no echocardiographic evaluation because of early mortality (Table 2). Of nine patients with a large tricuspid regurgitation (grade 3–4), this appeared suddenly in six. In these patients chordal rupture with a prolapse of the tricuspid leaflet into the right atrium was echocardiographically visualized in three cases. In all six patients, chordal tissue, and in three cases papillary muscle, was found histologically. Quite a few samples contained fibrous tissue, which was interpreted as previous biopsy site. This fibrous tissue was not surrounded by endocardium as were the fragments of chordae tendineae when tangenitally sectioned or cross-sectioned. All patients had clinical symptoms of right ventricular failure such as fatigue, dyspnoea, liver tenderness, pitting oedema, and elevated liver enzymes. Right heart catheterization confirmed a moderate right ventricular failure. Pulmonary artery pressures at rest were 31.6 mm Hg ± 6.2 (systolic), 10.6 mm Hg ± 1.3 (diastolic) and 17.0 mm Hg ± 1.0 (mean). Exercise pulmonary artery pressures were 47.8 mm Hg ± 6.2 (systolic), 16.8 mm Hg ± 4.6 (diastolic) and 29.8 mm Hg ± 4.3 (mean). The three patients who subsequently underwent valvuloplasty because of suspected rupture of chordae tendineae are described in detail below.

Case 1

A 51-year-old man who underwent heart transplantation for end-stage ischaemic heart disease had a pulmonary vascular resistance of 4/2 (undilated/dilated) Wood units. One month postoperatively only minimal tricuspid regurgitation was found (grade 0.5) and the patient had no clinical symptoms. Five months later regurgitation grade 4 and prolapse of the septal leaflet of the tricuspid valve were detected. The patient had pitting oedema, dyspnoea, fatigue, liver tenderness and elevated liver enzymes. Chordal tissue and papillary muscle were found histologically from one biopsy taken in the interval between the last normal and the first pathological echocardiographic investigation. During this interval two moderate rejections were treated with high dose methylprednisolone and antithymocyte globulin, respectively. Furthermore, two mild rejections were treated with bolus doses of methylprednisolone. Altogether, the patient was subjected to 17 biopsy procedures between the last normal echocardiography and the one which first showed a large regurgitation. One year after the transplantation, valvuloplasty with a Carpentier's ring no. 32 was performed via a sternotomy. Ruptured septal chordae tendineae were noticed. Postoperatively, echocardiography showed tricuspid regurgitation grade 2, which 6 months later had increased to grade 3 concomitant with appearance of symptoms like fatigue and oedema.

Case 2

A 45-year-old man with end-stage ischaemic heart disease and a pulmonary vascular resistance of 5/2.8 Wood units underwent heart transplantation. One week after transplantation tricuspid regurgitation grade 2 was present. This increased to grade 3 4 months postoperatively with a prolapse of the septal leaflet into the right atrium and clinical symptoms of oedema and fatigue (Fig. 1). Chordal tissue and structures from papillary muscle were found in three biopsies from the same occasion. During that time 16 biopsies were taken and a moderate rejection was treated with antithymocyte-globulin. Two mild rejections were treated with bolus doses of methylprednisolone. The patient subsequently underwent valvuloplasty via sternotomy and received a Carpentier's ring no. 34. Some chordae tendineae of the septal leaflet were ruptured. The tricuspid regurgitation was postoperatively been graded 2, and the patient was currently doing well and free from symptoms.

Case 3

This patient is a 41-year-old man with ischaemic heart disease who received a transplant in 1984, and another 7 years later due to chronic rejection. He had a complicated second postoperative course with renal insufficiency, wound rupture and mediastinitis. Echocardiographically, the tricuspid regurgitation was estimated at grade 0.5. It was technically difficult to perform the endomyocardial biopsy because of a rotation of the heart. The patient developed signs of vascular rejection and was successfully treated with plasmapheresis four times. After a biopsy 4 months postoperatively tricuspid valve regurgitation of grade 4 was suddenly detected and echocardiography showed evidence of chordal rupture of the tricuspid valve with leaflet prolapse into the right atrium. Histologically, connective tissue like chordae tendineae was found in the biopsy taken immediately preceding the echocardiography (Fig. 2). Clinical symptoms such as pitting oedema, dyspnoea, and fatigue occurred. Valvuloplasty was performed via a right thoracotomy and cannulation of the femoral artery and caval veins and a Carpentier's ring no. 32 was inserted. Chordae tendineae from the lateral part of the anterior tricuspid leaflet and the lateral part of the posterior tricuspid leaflet were found to be ruptured. Postoperatively the patient had renal insufficiency and underwent dialysis. One month postoperatively there was no tricuspid regurgitation and the patient was doing well.

Discussion

After heart transplantation tricuspid regurgitation of varying degree is found. Initially this can be caused by in-

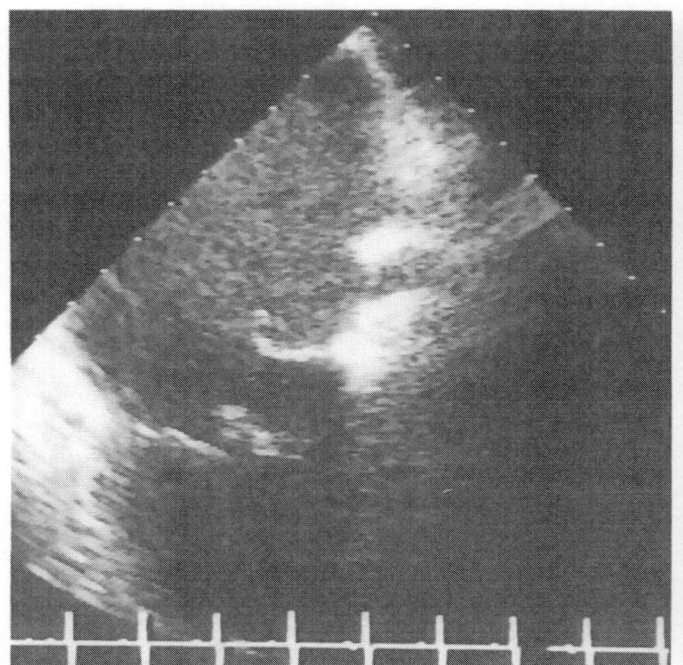
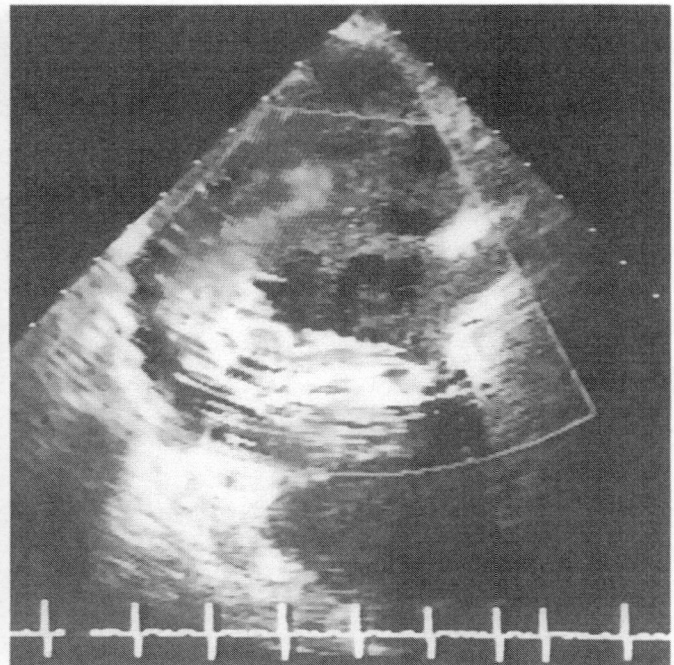

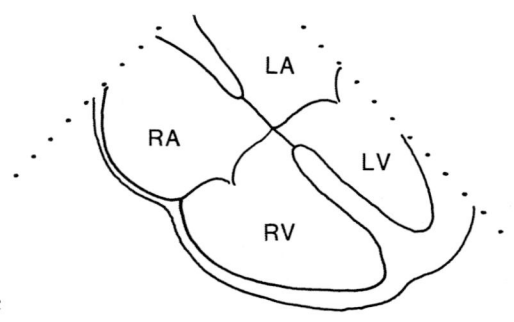

Fig. 1. a Doppler-echocardiographic evaluation of case 2 before valvuloplasty.
b The regurgitant jet filling up the right atrial area.
c Schematic illustration of the echocardiography: RA, right atrium; RV, right ventricle; LA, left atrium; LV, left ventricle

creased pulmonary vascular resistance to which the donor heart is not accustomed. The presence of tricuspid regurgitation in transplant recipients has been discussed in the literature, among others by Herrman et al. [9]. They did, however, not see any correlation in their study between the number of biopsies and tricuspid regurgitation.

Akasaka et al. recently reported a high frequency of tricuspid insufficiency in heart-lung transplant recipients, although these patients did not undergo endomyocardial biopsies. The authors speculated that the reason for atrioventricular valve regurgitation could be undetected rejection of low grade resulting in papillary muscle dysfunction [1].

In our study we found moderate to severe tricuspid regurgitation in 13% of heart transplant patients. Of all patients in our series, 6.3% had tricuspid regurgitation caused by endomyocardial biopsy as determined from the sudden occurrence and histological findings. This is an incidence similar to that reported by Braverman et al. [3] from 1442 biopsies obtained on 440 separate occasions. They did not report any clinically significant consequences from the biopsy damage, whereas in our patients the ruptured chordae tendineae was a severe complication that resulted in valvuloplasty in three patients (3.1%).

There are special anatomical features in the right ventricle to have in mind when considering the risks of endomyocardial biopsy. Thus, there are long chordae tendineae and short papillary muscles anchored at different levels and unevenly spread out in the whole ventricle making it theoretically possible for a bioptome to catch chordae tendineae at any point.

The technique of performing endomyocardial biopsy has been well described [4]. The importance of approaching the right ventricular septum with closed bioptome jaws so as not to catch chordae tendineae has been stressed, but even if these measures are taken, the jaws have to be opened at some point. Since fluoroscopy does not reveal the presence of chordae or papillary muscle, it is impossible to detect if they have been caught in the bioptome. It is not possible to recognize or differentiate the specific tissue that has been caught in the bioptome jaws. The fact that, in our study, chordal tissue or papillary muscle were found in the biopsy samples from all six patients with suspected biopsy damage of the tricuspid valve points to the importance of an immediate echocardio-

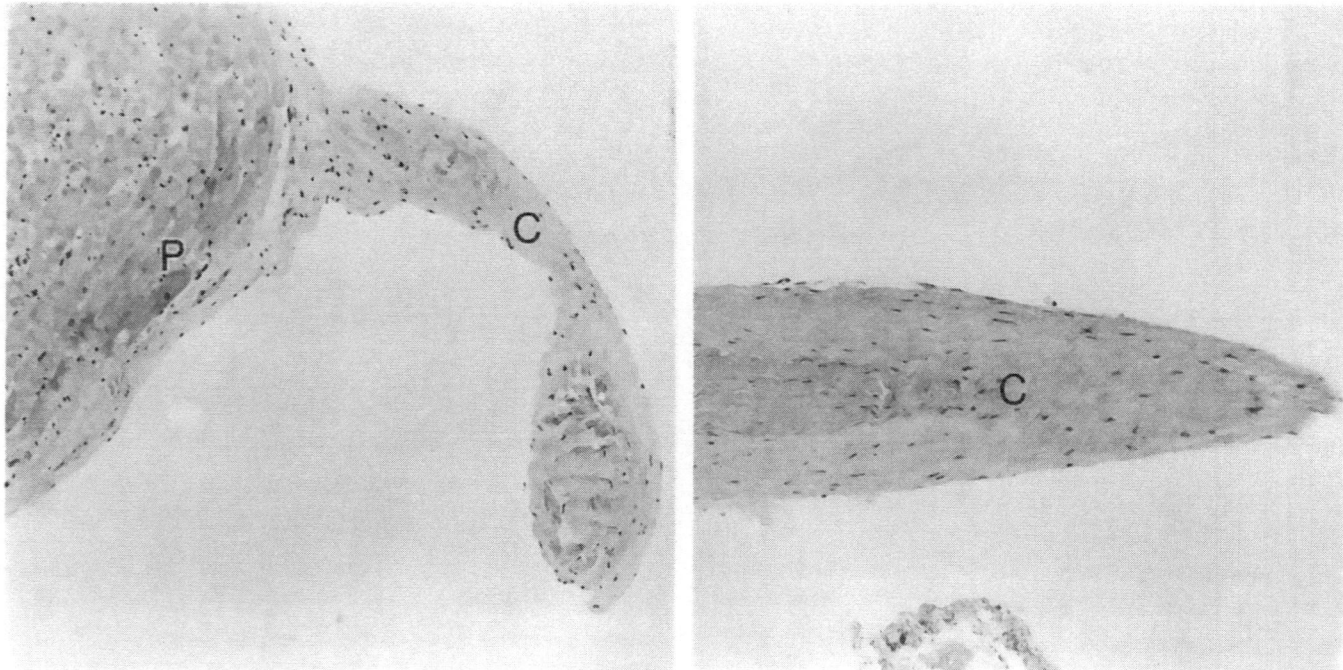

a   b

Fig. 2 a, b. Endomyocardial biopsy samples from a heart transplant patient showing papillary muscle *(P)* and chordal tissue *(C)*

graphical follow-up in patients with either post-biopsy symptoms or histological findings of chordal tissue to avoid severe undetected tricuspid valve regurgitation. Whether there were histological findings of chordal tissue in patients with a lower degree of tricuspid regurgitation was not investigated, but since no patient had clinical symptoms or showed echocardiographical signs of chordal rupture it was not considered necessary.

Miller et al. have proposed transthoracic echocardiography-guided biopsies as an alternative to fluoroscopy guidance. They pointed out several advantages, such as elimination of cumulative radiation exposure for the physician and the patient, a greater amount of information on ventricular function and pericardial effusion, avoidance of the expense and congestion of operating theatres and catheterization laboratories, and, most important, that it allows the physician to obtain endomyocardial biopsies safely from the entire right ventricular surface, including the free wall, apex and septum [10].

Although endomyocardial biopsy is the most useful tool for the detection of rejection it should be used with careful consideration of anatomical features and consciousness of the risk of damage to the tricuspid valve. It is also concluded that valvuloplasty of the tricuspid valve can successfully be performed in a transplanted heart.

References

1. Akasaka T, Lythall DA, Kushwaha SS, Yoshida K, Yoshikawa J, Yacoub MH (1990) Valvular regurgitation in heart-lung transplant recipients: a doppler color flow study. J Am Coll Cardiol 3:576–581
2. Billingham ME, Cary NRB, Hammond ME, Kemnitz J, Marboe C, McCallister HA, Snovar DC, Winters GL, Zerbe A (1990) A working formulation for the standardization of nomenclature in the diagnosis of heart and lung rejection: heart rejection study group. J Heart Transplant 9:587–593
3. Braverman AC, Coplen SH, Mudge GH, Lee R (1990) Ruptured chordae tendineae of the tricuspid valve as a complication of endomyocardial biopsy in heart transplant patients. Am J Cardiol 66:111–113
4. Caves PK, Schultz WP, Dong E Jr, Stinson EB, Shumway NE (1974) New instrument for transvenous cardiac biopsy. Am J Cardiol 33:264–267
5. Fowles RE, Baim DS (1986) Endomyocardial biopsy: In: Grossman W (ed) Cardiac catheterization and angiography. Lea and Febiger, Philadelphia; pp 506–516
6. Fowles RE, Mason JW (1982) Endomyocardial biopsy. Ann Intern Med 97:885–894
7. Haverich A, Albes JM, Fahrenkamp G, Schäfers H-J, Wahlers T, Heublein B (1991) Intraoperative echocardiography to detect and prevent tricuspid valve regurgitation after heart transplantation. Eur J Cardiothorac Surg 5:41–45
8. Henzlova MJ, Nath H, Bucy RP, Bourge RC, Kirklin JK, Rogers WJ (1989) Coronary artery to right ventricle fistula in heart transplant recipients: a complication of endomyocardial biopsy. J Am Coll Cardiol 14:258–261
9. Herrmann G, Simon R, Haverich A, Crener J, Dammenhayn L, Schäfers HJ, Wahlers Th, Borst HG (1989) Left ventricular function tricuspid incompetence, and incidence of coronary artery disease late after orthotopic heart transplantation. Eur J Cardiothorac Surg 3:111–118
10. Miller LW, Labovitz AJ, McBride LA, Pennington DG, Kanter K (1988) Echocardiography-guided endomyocardial biopsy. A 5 year experience. Circulation 5 [Suppl. III]:III99–102
11. Silver MM (1983) Gross examination and structure of the heart. In: Silver DM (ed) Cardiovascular pathology. Churchill Livingstone, Edinburgh, pp 15–19
12. Thideman K-U, Ferraus VJ (1983) Ultrastructure of the heart. In: Silver DM (ed) Cardiovascular pathology. Churchill Livingstone, Edinburgh, pp 70–72
13. Waagstein F, Caidahl K, Wallentin I, Bergh C-H, Hjalmarsson Å (1989) Long-term β-blockade in dilated cardiomyopathy. Effects of short- and long-term metoprolol treatment followed by withdrawal and readministration of metoprolol. Circulation 80: 551–563

Transplant Int (1992) 5 [Suppl 1]: S259–S261

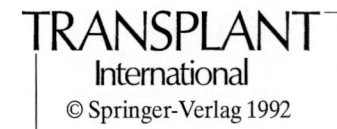
TRANSPLANT
International
© Springer-Verlag 1992

Occurrence of lymphoproliferative disorder after heart transplantation is related to the total immunosuppressive load

R. M. L. Brouwer[1], A. H. M. M. Balk[2], and W. Weimar[1]

Departments of [1] Internal Medicine, and [2] Cardiology, University Hospital Rotterdam 'Dijkzigt', Rotterdam, The Netherlands

Abstract. Heart transplant recipients are at a high risk for the development of post-transplant lymphoproliferative disorders (PTLD). We explored the relationship between the incidence of PTLD and the immunosuppressive therapy in 150 consecutive patients who received a cardiac transplant at our centre. None of our patients treated with cyclosporin A and prednisone only ($n = 41$) developed PTLD. In contrast, 6 of 101 patients who were previously treated with anti-T-cell preparations suffered from PTLD. No relationship was found between the type of anti-T-cell therapy and the incidence of PTLD. We conclude that the high incidence of PTLD in heart transplant recipients is related to the total immunosuppressive load and not related to a single agent like OKT3.

Key words: Heart transplantation – Lymphoproliferative disorders – Immunosuppressive load

The long-term use of immunosuppressive drugs after organ transplantation is associated with an increased incidence of neoplasia. Of great concern is the striking number of lymphoproliferative disorders in heart and heart-lung recipients [4]. These tumours, commonly of B-cell origin, frequently occur at extranodal sites, are associated with Epstein-Barr virus infections, are often fatal, but may undergo regression if immumnosuppressive therapy is reduced [1, 2, 3, 6]. A major factor influencing the development of post-transplant lymphoma appears to be the intensity and type of immunosuppression. Several authors reported an additional increased risk after the administration of OKT3 [5, 7]. The objective of our study was to explore the relationship between the use of anti-T-cell therapy and the incidence of PTLD in heart transplant recipients.

Offprint requests to: W. Weimar, M. D., Department of Internal Medicine, University Hospital Rotterdam 'Dijkzigt', Dr. Molewaterplein 40, 3015 GD Rotterdam, The Netherlands.

Methods

Patients

Between 1 January 1985, the beginning of the cardiac transplantation programme, and 20 December 1990, 150 orthotopic heart transplantations were performed at the University Hospital, Rotterdam. One patient received a second transplant, for whom the data are combined. Six patients who died within 15 days of transplantation and two patients with a follow-up less than 1 month were excluded from the present analysis. We therefore were able to include data on 142 patients in our variables associated with the risk of having post-transplantation lymphoproliferative disorder after cadiac transplantation (PTLD). The mean age of our patients was 44 ± 1 years, and were male. The indications for transplantation were dilated cardiomyopathy (69 patients), ischaemic cardiomyopathy (70) and other severe cardiac diseases (3).

Immunosuppressive regimens

Immunoprophylaxis. Maintenance immunosuppression consisted of the prednisone-cyclosporin A combination in all patients. For immunoprophylaxis in the first week after transplantation several protocols were used. All patients received high-dose steroids in the perioperative phase which was gradually decreased to a maintenance dose of 10 mg prednisone after 3 months. In 62 patients cyclosporin A was given intravenously during the first 5 days after transplantation and oral administration of CsA was started at day 4, in the remaining patients equine antithymocyte globulin (hATG) (Institute Merieux, Lyon, France), 425 lymphocytotoxic units (0.5 ml) per kilogram for 3–7 days ($n = 28$) or anti-T-cell monoclonal antibody OKT3 (Orthoclone OKT3, Ortho Pharmaceutical, Raritan, N.J., USA), 5 mg/day for 7 days ($n = 51$) was given. These 79 patients also received short-term (5 days) azathioprine (100 mg/day) and CsA was started at day 5 (8 mg/kg orally per day).

In all patients, CsA dosage was adjusted to the plasma levels of the drug. Until November 1988, a non-specific assay for CsA (RIA, Sandoz, Basle, Switzerland) was used (target range 100–200 ng/ml). After November 1988, a specific monoclonal antibody (Cyclo-Trac SP, Incstar, Stillwater, Minnesota, USA) was used to measure the plasma concentration of the parent drug (target range 50–125 ng/ml).

Rejection treatment. Rejection episodes were treated in a uniform manner throughout the study period. Endomyocardial biopsies

Table 1. Indication for anti-T-cell therapy

	Number of patients
Prophylaxis only	
hATG	10
OKT3	28
For treatment of rejection	
rATG	17
OKT3 and rATG	5
Both for prophylaxis and treatment of rejection	
hATG and rATG	16
OKT3 and rATG	23
hATG, rATG and OKT3	2
Total	101

rATG, rabbit antithymocyte globulin; hATG, equine antithymocyte globulin

Cumulative dose: OKT3 43 mg (25–100 mg); rATG 1090 mg (299–4200 mg)

were graded using the criteria as proposed by Billingham. In the case of moderate or severe rejection in the first 4 weeks after transplantation, patients were treated with rabbit ATG (rATG, National Institute for Public Health, Bilthoven, The Netherlands) in a dosage to keep the T-cell count $< 150 \text{ mm}^3$ for 3 weeks). First-line treatment for moderate rejection occurring more than 4 weeks after transplantation was 1 g methylprednisolone per day intravenously for 3 days. Refractory rejection episodes were treated with either rATG (see above) or OKT3 (5 mg/day) for 10 days.

Pathological studies

The diagnosis of post-transplantation lymphoproliferative disorder was based on histological examination of excision biopsy or autopsy material.

Results

One and three year survival in our patients was 91% and 89%, respectively. Detailed information on the indication for anti-T-cell therapy is given in Table 1. In six patients treated with anti-T-cell therapy a diagnosis of post-transplantation lymphoproliferative disorder was made. Three of these patients were treated with OKT3 (two patients with OKT3 alone), three patients with polyclonal anti-T-

cell therapy and one patient both with OKT3 and RATG. Detailed information on the characteristics of these patients is given in Table 2.

In contrast, none of the 41 patients treated with CsA and prednisone alone developed PTLD (incidence 0%, 95% CI 0–9%). The difference in incidence between two the groups: 6%, 95% CI of the difference 1–13% ($P < 0.05$).

A number of factors that might be associated with the development of PTLD were examined. No statistically significant differences were found in age, time after transplantation, cumulative CsA dose, plasma levels or cumulative steroid dose.

Four patients died, despite reduction or withdrawal of immunosuppression and treatment with acyclovir i.v.

Discussion

The most striking observation in our study was that none of the patients who was treated with CsA and prednisone alone developed a post-transplantation lymphoproliferative disorder. Of the six patients who developed PTLD, all were treated with anti-T-cell therapy, either as immunoprophylaxis or for treatment of rejection. Of these six patients, only three were treated with OKT3 whereas the remaining three received a polyclonal anti-T-cell preparation. Our findings are in contrast with the observations made by Swinnen et al. [7]. They concluded that a substantial increase in the incidence of post-transplantation lymphoproliferative disorder occurred after the addition of OKT3 to their immunosuppressive regimen. They also found a relationship between the incidence of PTLD and the cumulative dosage of OKT3. How can this discrepancy be explained? One possibility is the type of maintenance immunosuppression. Swinnen et al. used triple drug treatment (CsA, prednisone and azathioprine) whereas at our centre patients are treated with CsA-prednisone only. Furthermore, the cumulative dose of OKT3 given to their patients who subsequently developed PTLD was high (between 70 and 135 mg per patient) and our patients received a median total dose of 35 mg. In view of this difference and our observation that none of our patients treated with CsA and prednisone alone suffered from PTLD, it is more likely that the high incidence of PTLD in their patients was due to a greater total immunosup-

Table 2. Characteristics of the patients with post-transplantation lymphoproliferative disorder

Patient No.	Cumulative OKT3 dose (mg)	Cumulative rATG dose (mg)	Cumulative hATG dose (days)	Time to PTLD (months)	Pathological findings		Clinical status (time from diagnosis)
					Hist	IP	
4	none	4200	5	6	IBL	M	Dead (5 months)
28	none	none	3	30	IBL	P	Dead (1 month)
52	none	920	none	25	PC	M	Dead (1 month)
59	50	960	none	7	IBL	M	Alive in CR (29 months)
79	35	none	none	11			Alive with recurrence (16 months)
84	35	none	none	4	DM	P	Dead (1 month)

rATG, rabbit antithymocyte globulin; hATG, equine antithymocyte globulin; IP, immunophenotype; Hist, histology; IBL, immunoblastic lymphoma; PC, plasma cell tumor; DM, diffuse mixed lymphoma; M, monoclonal; P, polyclonal; CR, complete remission

pressive load, than that a single agent, like OKT3, was responsible.

References

1. Hanto DW, Frizzera G, Gajl-Peczalska KJ, et al (1982) Epstein-Barr-virus induced B-cell lymphoma after renal transplantation. N Eng J Med 306:913–918
2. Hanto DW, Frizzera G, Gajl-Peczalska KJ, Simmons RL (1985) Epstein-Barr virus, immunodeficiency, and B cell proliferation. Transplantation 39:461–472
3. Nalesnik MA, Jaffe R, Starzl TE, et al (1988) The pathology of posttransplant lymphoproliferative disorders occurring in the setting of cyclosporine A-prednisone immunosuppression. Am J Pathol 133:173–192
4. Penn I (1987) Cancers following cyclosporine therapy. Transplantation 43:32–35
5. Ren EC, Chan SH (1988) Possible enhancement of Epstein-Barr virus infections by the use of OKT3 in transplant recipients. Transplantation 45:988–989
6. Starzl TE, Porter KA, Iwatsuki S, et al (1984) Reversibility of lymphomas and lymphoproliferative lesions developing under cyclosporine-steroid therapy. Lancet I:583–587
7. Swinnen LJ, Costanzo-Nordin MR, Fisher SG, et al (1990) Increased incidence of lymphoproliferative disorder after immunosuppression with the monoclonal antibody OKT3 in cardiac-transplant recipients. N Eng J Med 323:1723–1728
8. Weintraub J, Warnke RA (1982) Lymphoma in cardiac allotransplant recipients. Transplantation 33:347–351

Pancreas, Islets, Small Bowel

Transplant Int (1992) 5 [Suppl 1]: S 265–S 267

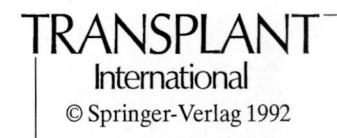

TRANSPLANT
International
© Springer-Verlag 1992

Perfusion imaging of pancreas allografts using technetium-99m hexamethyl propylene amine oxime

M. H. Booster[1], E. A. J. M. Schoenmakers[2], A. J. M. Rijnders[2], G. A. K. Heidendal[2], M. J. P. G. van Kroonenburgh[2], J. P. van Hooff[3], G. Kootstra[1], and H. G. Peltenburg[3]

Departments of [1] Surgery, [2] Nuclear Medicine, and [3] Nephrology, University Hospital Maastricht, P.O. Box 5800, 6202 AZ Maastricht, The Netherlands

Abstract. The vascular integrity and major changes in perfusion can be determined by visual interpretation of radionuclide flow studies. We studied the potential of a new radiopharmaceutical technetium-99m hexamethyl propylene amine oxime (^{99m}Tc-HMPAO) in the particular setting of pancreas transplantation. Perfusion was measured by perfusion indices (PI). Changes in graft perfusion were estimated by three independent observers. A predefined scale from 0 to 4 was used, with 0 representing no visualisation of the graft and 4 denoting sharp countour delineation and distinct demarcation from the background. In order to investigate the relation between perfusion of the pancreas graft and its exocrine function, we measured the amylase excretion rate (AER) in the urine, expressed in units per hour. It is concluded that ^{99m}Tc-HMPAO is a suitable radiopharmaceutical for pancreas allograft imaging. For the assessment of the vascular integrity in the direct postoperative period, the scintigram is very reliable. Although a correlation between exocrine function of the graft and the perfusion score was not established, it is possible to make a clear sorting of AER measurements into different groups.

Key words: Pancreas transplantation – Perfusion – Scintigraphy – HMPAO

The early diagnosis and treatment of graft rejection and graft thrombosis are of major importance in pancreas transplantation since these grafts have little potential for recovery. The vascular integrity and major changes in perfusion can be determined by visual interpretation of radionuclide flow studies. Many different radiopharmaceuticals have been proposed, but each one has certain drawbacks. Background activity, bolus variations and changes in systemic flow often make it impossible to interpret the results. The potential of a new agent, technetium-99m hexamethyl propylene amine oxime (^{99m}Tc-HMPAO), was demonstrated in cerebral perfusion studies. This highly lipophilic complex passively penetrates biological membranes, as shown by a high brain uptake after IV injection. After passing the cell membrane, an intracellular reaction with glutathione takes place, converting the agent into a hydrophilic compound. Due to this intracellular metabolism, the compound remains in the cell and is not cleared from the tissue as easily as, for instance, the widely used perfusion marker in kidney transplantation, diethylene triamine penta-acetic acid (^{99m}Tc-DTPA). It is therefore possible to make static scintigraphic images in which the extraction of HMPAO is proportional to the regional perfusion of the graft. We studied the potential of ^{99m}Tc-HMPAO in the particular setting of pancreas transplantation.

Patients and methods

Pancreas transplantation was carried out in 20 diabetic type 1 patients (13 men, 7 women). Mean age at the moment of transplantation was 36 years. Of these 20 patients, 10 underwent a combined pancreas/kidney transplantation, 7 a pancreas-alone transplantation and 3 a pancreas subsequent to a kidney transplantation. The pancreas graft included a donor duodenal segment, and exocrine drainage was established via an anastomosis between the duodenal segment and the bladder. In case of pancreas-alone grafting, the donor spleen was always included to maintain the normal anatomical vascular interrelation. In those cases, the spleen was ex vivo irradiated with 1200 rad in order to prevent graft-versus-host disease.

The patients were studied in the supine position. After IV administration of 185–370 MBq ^{99m}Tc-HMPAO, images were taken with a large field-of-view gamma-camera (Gemini 700). Thirty frames of 2 s each were immediately followed by 50 frames of 30 s. Perfusion studies were carried out on the first day after transplantation, subsequently within the next 2 weeks and thereafter dependent on the clinical course.

Perfusion was measured by perfusion indices (PI). Changes in graft perfusion were estimated by three independent observers. A predefined scale from 0 to 4 was used, with 0 representing no visualisation of the graft and 4 denoting sharp contour delineation and dis-

Offprint requests to: M. H. Booster, Department of Surgery, University Hospital Maastricht, P. O. Box 5800, 6202 AZ Maastricht, The Netherlands

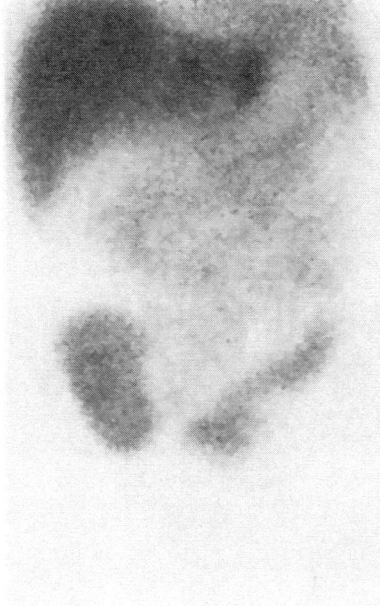

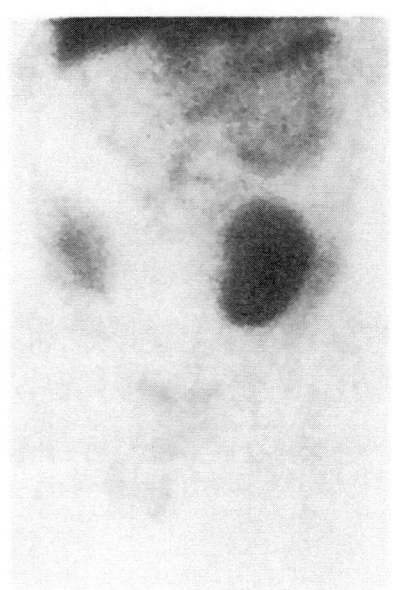

Fig. 1. Technetium-99m hexamethyl propylene amine oxime (^{99m}Tc-HMPAO) perfusion image obtained 20 min after injection. This patient received a combined pancreas/kidney transplantation. Both organs are visualised very well, and there is a high target-to-background ratio. Perfusion indices (PI) score was 4

Fig. 3. Typical scintigraphic image of pancreas graft thrombosis. This patient received a combined pancreas/kidney transplantation. However, no activity is seen in the lower right abdomen and in the area of the aortal bifurcation, where the pancreas was transplanted. The simultaneously transplanted kidney has a good perfusion

Results

Quality of the scintigraphic images

The ^{99m}Tc-HMPAO scintigraphic images had a high target-to-background ratio. Static images with clear definition of the inserted grafts were obtained up to 20 min after administration of the tracer (Fig. 1). Optimally perfused grafts (PI = 4) showed parallel rising configurations of the graft and aorta time-activity curves (Fig. 2). The results were not affected by variation in the bolus injection, systemic flow or organ depth. Uptake of the tracer reflected the regional perfusion of the graft.

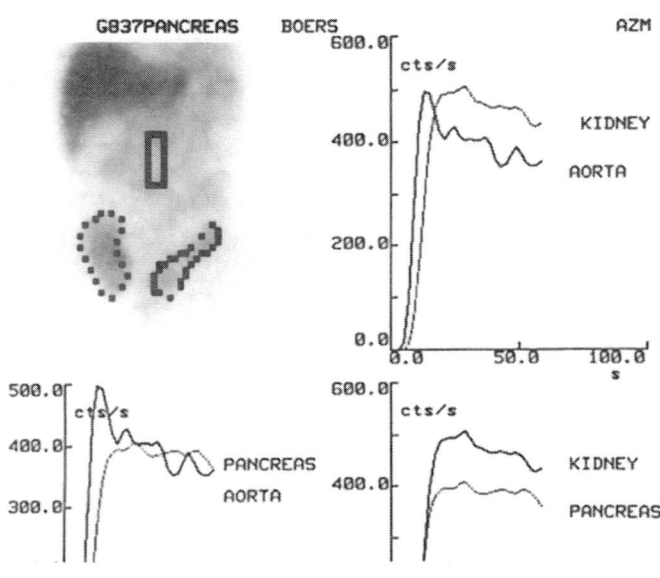

Fig. 2. Optimal perfusion of the graft includes a parallel rising configuration of the graft and aorta time-activity curves

Vascular integrity assessment

In the direct postoperative period (within 24 h after transplantation) HMPAO scintigraphic studies invariably indicated in 4 patients a non-perfused allograft with a PI score of 0 (Fig. 3). The AER was minimal in these patients (less than 400 U/h). Exploration of the grafts showed thrombosis in 3 and accelerated acute rejection in 1 patient. In-

tinct demarcation from the background. Furthermore, a semiquantitative analysis of aorta versus graft time-activity curves was performed.

In order to investigate the relation between perfusion of the pancreas graft and its exocrine function, we measured the amylase excretion rate (AER) in the urine, expressed in units per hour.

Table 1. Relationship between relative amylase excretion rate (AER %) and PI score 3 months after transplantation

	n	Mean AER %	Interval
PI = 0	9	3 %	0.5–14.5
PI = 1	8	9 %	1 –30.5
PI = 2	8	74 %	1.3–97.8
PI = 3	8	82 %	52.3–95.8
PI = 4	1		

itial PI scores from 2 to 4 were found in 16 patients. All these patients had AER above 4000 U/h.

In patients who had received a combined pancreas/spleen transplant, variable persistent reductions in perfusion of the spleen with time were observed up to the point at which there was almost no splenic uptake at all. This reduction in splenic perfusion did not affect the pancreas perfusion. Histological studies of spleens removed 7 months after transplantation revealed extensive fibrosis.

Relation between PI score and AER

There was no relation between the magnitude of the PI score and that of the AER. In order to be able to compare results between recipients, the AER had to be expressed as a percentage of the maximum observed rate (AER%) in each recipient.

In the first 3 months after transplantation, no statistical correlation between AER% and PI score could be established. HMPAO scintigraphic studies failed to detect acute rejection in 6 out of 10 cases.

In 10 of the 20 patients, the follow-up was long enough to evaluate the relationship between AER% and PI score after 3 months (Table 1).

The overall effect of differences in AER% between PI scores was significant ($P < 0.008$; Kruskas-Wallis 1-way ANOVA test). This effect was mainly caused by the significant difference between groups PI = 1 and PI = 3 ($P < 0.011$; Wilcoxon rank sum test). During long-term follow-up, both AER% and PI score exhibited gradually decreasing values. Histological examination of the pancreas graft at 9 months' follow-up in 2 patients with a PI score of 0 revealed chronic rejection with extensive fibrosis.

Discussion

With HMPAO scintigraphic studies it is possible to assess perfusion in pancreas allograft recipients. The quality of the scintigraphic images is high, and extraction of the lipophilic compound is proportional to the regional perfusion of the graft.

Non-perfused allografts were invariably discriminated with a PI score of 0 in our study. This makes ^{99m}Tc-HMPAO scintigraphy a very reliable method for detecting early graft thrombosis.

Acute rejection was not detected in all cases. This is probably due to the fact that the macrovascular changes caused by acute rejection do not appear as rapidly as, for instance, clinical and laboratory findings. If HMPAO is employed as a promising tool for pancreas allograft rejection, the value of monitoring becomes questionable.

Although a clear correlation between PI scores and the AER was not found, PI scores stratified AER measurements 3 months after transplantation. Furthermore, a gradual persistant decline of values was observed in the PI scores as well as in the AER, indicating the relationship between chronic rejection and deteriorating graft perfusion.

In summary, ^{99m}Tc-HMPAO is a suitable radiopharmaceutical for pancreas allograft imaging. For assessment of the vascular integrity in the direct postoperative period, the scintigram is very reliable. Although a correlation between exocrine function of the graft and the PI score was not established, it is possible with the PI score to make a clear sorting of AER measurements into different groups.

References

1. Costa DC, Ell PJ, Cullum ID, et al (1986) The in vivo distribution of ^{99m}Tc-HMPAO in normal man. Nucl Med Commun 7: 647–658
2. Dewanjee MK (1990) The chemistry of ^{99m}Tc-labeled radiopharmaceuticals. Semin Nucl Med 20: 5–27
3. Kung HF (1990) New technetium 99m-labeled brian perfusion imaging agents. Semin Nucl Med 20: 150–158
4. Neirinckx RD, Burk JF, Harrison RC, et al (1988) The retention mechanism of technetium-99m-HMPAO: intracellular reaction with glutathione. J Cereb Blood Flow Metab 8: S4–S12
5. Teule GJJ, Leunissen KML, Halders SGEA, et al (1989) Serial radionuclide determinations of graft perfusion in pancreas spleen transplantation. Transplant Proc 21: 2795–2796
6. Volkert WA, Hoffman TJ, Seger RM, et al (1984) ^{99m}Tc-propylene amine oxime: a potential brain radiopharmaceutical. Eur J Nucl Med 9: 511–516
7. Walovitch RC, Williams SJ, Lafrance ND (1990) Radiolabeled agents for SPECT imaging of brain perfusion. Nucl Med Biol 17 (1): 77–83

Transplant Int (1992) 5 [Suppl 1]: S 268–S 269

TRANSPLANT
International
© Springer-Verlag 1992

Prospective analysis of pancreatic grafts with duplex-Doppler ultrasound: value of resistive index in the diagnosis of rejection

R. Gilabert[1], L. Fernandez-Cruz[2], C. Bru[1], M. J. Ricart[3], A. Saenz[2], and E. Astudillo[2]

Departments of [1] Radiology and [2] Surgery, and [3] Transplant Unit, University of Barcelona, Barcelona, Spain

The diagnosis of rejection and its differentiation from other causes of pancreatic graft dysfunction remain the basic problem in pancreas transplantation. A previous study with pulsed Doppler (PD) done at our institution demonstrated an increase of the resistive index (RI) during pancreatic graft rejection episodes [1]. The aim of the study was to determine prospectively the utility of duplex-Doppler (DD) ultrasound (US) in identifying the cause of pancreatic graft dysfunction. The major clinical categories were graft rejection and graft pancreatitis.

Key words: Duplex-Doppler ultrasound, pancreatic rejection – Pancreatic rejection diagnosis

Patients and methods

The study group included 23 whole pancreas grafts transplanted in to 22 patients (16 male, 6 female; mean age 36 years). Eighteen patients had combined kidney/pancreatic grafts from the same donor, 3 patients had sequential (not simultaneous) kidney and pancreatic grafts, and 2 patients had pancreas-alone grafts. The surgical technique consisted of whole pancreas transplantation with anastomosis of the graft's portal vein and celiac trunk to the recipient vena cava and iliac artery, respectively. The exocrine graft secretions were drained into the urinary bladder. DD examinations were performed with a 3.75-MHz transducer. Pancreatic size, echostructure, perigraft and intra-abdominal fluid were evaluated by US. The PD study was done to assess the permeability of the vascular pedicle at the hilar level. A venous and arterial Doppler spectrum (DS) were also obtained at the graft parenchyma (head, body, tail). The arterial DS was quantified by the RI [RI = (peak systolic velocity – end diastolic velocity)/peak systolic velocity], and the final RI was derived from the average of the 3 parenchymal levels sampled in the study. All patients underwent a baseline study 48–72 h after grafting, during graft dysfunction episodes and in the follow-up investigation.

Offprint requests to: Prof. L. Fernandez-Cruz, Department of Surgery, Hospital Clinic, Villarroel 170, Esc. 6 – 4° Piso, E-08036 Barcelona, Spain

The diagnosis of graft pancreatitis was based on clinical data (abdominal pain), increase of serum amylase and lipase levels (> 800 U/l or > 400 U/l, respectively), improvement after urinary drainage, rise of cytomegalovirus immunoglobulin (IgG)/IgM antibody or pancreatic biopsy (+) revealing inclusion bodies. The rejection status of the graft was based on clinical data (pain, temperature > 38 °C), reduction of urinary amylase levels (> 50 % of normal pre-rejection value), fluctuations of serum amylase level and improvement after rejection treatment.

Results

Normal grafts have a homogenous structure, and the graft size did not exceed the expected dimensions of a normal pancreas. Peripancreatic fluid was found in 22.7 % of these grafts after surgery, but it did not persist more than 6 weeks in uncomplicated cases. On PD examination, the venous spectrum consisted in a continuous flow. The arterial waveform was characterized by a systolic peak followed by a continuous flow throughout diastole. No significant differences were observed between RI on baseline exploration (0.63 ± 0.01) and those obtained in stable grafts (0.62 ± 0.01). Nineteen episodes of graft pancreatitis were diagnosed, being documented at a mean time after transplantation of 246 ± 58 days $(r = 11–850)$. The aetiology of these episodes was bladder dysfunction or urethral stenosis in 13 and infection in 5 (cytomegalovirus infection in 4, urinary tract infection due to *Pseudomonas aeruginosa* in 1). The cause of the remaining episode could not be determined. US results were pathological in 10 of 19 episodes of graft pancreatitis, disclosing perigraft fluid $(n = 10)$, hypoechogenicity $(n = 2)$ and heterogenous echostructure $(n = 1)$. No increase of RI was observed during the episodes of graft pancreatitis: mean RI was 0.61 ± 0.001, which is not significant when compared with RI prior to the episode of graft pancreatitis (0.63 ± 0.006) and with RI in stable grafts.

Some 24 episodes of pancreatic graft rejection were diagnosed; simultaneous kidney/pancreas rejection in 13 and pancreas-alone rejection in 11. Rejection episodes occurred at a mean time after transplantation of

54 + 11 days ($r = 7$–235). Kidney graft rejection preceded the pancreas rejection in 6 episodes. US results were pathological in 14 episodes of graft rejection, disclosing peri-graft fluid ($n = 9$), increase of graft size ($n = 8$), heterogenous echostructure ($n = 8$), hypoechogenicity ($n = 3$) and duodenal wall oedema ($n = 1$). PD showed an increase of RI in 18 episodes of pancreatic graft rejection: mean RI was 0.75 + 0.03 in simultaneous kidney/pancreas rejection. These values were statistically significantly higher, $P < 0.001$, when compared with basal pre-rejection values; the mean increase of RI was also significantly higher in isolated pancreas rejection (38 %) than in cases of simultaneous kidney/pancreas rejection (22 %). Reversal of the rejection was seen in 18 episodes (75 %). Loss of pancreatic function occurred in 6 episodes, with progressive worsening on PD study in spite of rejection therapy.

In conclusion, real-time US abnormalities were more prominent in pancreatic graft rejection than in graft pancreatitis. The RI in graft pancreatitis was not significantly different than that in stable grafts. Rejection was associated with a significant drop of the urinary amylase activity and a marked increase of RI. The mean increase of RI over basal values was 22 % in pancreas grafts with simultaneous kidney rejection and 38 % in isolated pancreas graft rejection.

Reference

1. Gilabert R, Fernández-Cruz L, Bru C, Sans A, Andreu J (1988) Duplex-Doppler ultrasonography in monitoring clinical pancreas transplantation. Transplant Int 1: 172–177

Transplant Int (1992) 5 [Suppl 1]: S270–S271

TRANSPLANT
International
© Springer-Verlag 1992

Reperfusion injury of pancreas allografts: relation to islet cell function

H. G. Peltenburg[1], **B. H. R. Wolffenbuttel**[1], **M. H. Booster**[2], **P. P. C. A. Menheere**[3], **K. M. L. Leunissen**[1], **G. Kootstra**[2], and **J. P. van Hooff**[1]

Departments of [1] Nephrology and Transplantation, [2] General Surgery, and [3] Clinical Chemistry, University Hospital Maastricht, Maastricht, The Netherlands

It is unknown to what extent preservation and/or reperfusion may damage islet cells in pancreas allografts. In this study, the release of insulin after reperfusion was used as a marker of injury to the islet cell and compared with the best insulin secretory response (ISR) after glucagon stimulation over a period of 100 days after pancreas transplantation.

Key words: Pancreas reperfusion injury – Pancreas transplantation

Patients and methods

All recipients suffered from diabetes mellitus type I, with absent C-peptide response after glucagon stimulation, and were treated with insulin 3–4 times daily; the pre-transplant hemoglobin (HbA$_{1C}$) level was 9.2 ± 4.1; average diabetes duration was 12 years; mean age was 36.5 years. The recipients' characteristics are summarized in Table 1. The technique of pancreas allograft transplantation is described in [1]. Briefly, a segment of duodenum and the pancreas are transplanted with bladder deviation. In the procedure with a pancreas transplantation alone, the spleen is included after irradiation ex vivo with 600 rad. All organs are preserved with UW solution. Immunosuppression consisted of cyclosporin A (CyA) 4 mg/kg IV, dosage adjusted after an initial oral dose with trough levels 0.1–0.2 mg/l (high performance liquid chromatography, HPLC, whole blood); PRN 60 mg on day 1, tapered to 10 mg on day 3, ultimately to 5 mg; azido thymidine (AZT) 1.5 mg/kg. The first anti-rejection treatment involved rATG, the second OKT3, the third PRN 100 mg 3 alternate days. Glucagon stimulation was carried out on day 1 after transplantation, then twice a week or more frequently depending on the clinical course. Glucagon 1 mg was given slowly (over 1 min) IV, and samples were drawn 5, 10, 15, and 30 min after injection. The ISR to glucagon was expressed as the incremental area under the curve (iAUC in mU/l per 30 min). The insulin release after reperfusion was measured directly before and every 15 min during the first 2.5 h after reperfusion of the implanted pancreas allograft. The iAUC was

calculated and the release after reperfusion expressed as iAUC in mU/l per 150 min.

The insulin level was determined with a commercially available radioimmunoassay (RIA) (Pharmacia, Uppsala, Sweden) after polyethylene glycol (PEG) precipitation. The C-peptide content was determined with a RIA (Byk-Sangtec, Dietzenbach, FRG). The amylase activity was measured by catalyzing the hydrolysis of p-nitrophenyl-a-d-maltahexaoside at 37°C for 3 min; a bichromatic rate technique (405 and 510 nm) was used to measure the absorbance of the developed p-nitrophenol.

Results and discussion

Table 1 summarizes the recipients' characteristics. No relation was found between either the cold or the warm ischemia time and the release of insulin after reperfusion. Table 2 shows the results of the ISR after glucagon stimulation. The correlation between the ISR and amylase excretion rate (AER; U/h) is also shown. There was no relation between amylase release after reperfusion and the highest AER after pancreas transplantation (data not shown). However, there was an inverse relation between insulin release after reperfusion (U/l per 150 min) and the maximum insulin secretion response after glucagon stimulation (U/l per 30 min) measured within the first

Table 1. Summary of recipient characteristics

Recipient No.	Sex	Age (years)	Pancreas transplant type	Follow-up (months)	Dr-mis-matches	CIT (h)	Rejection episodes
1	M	36	PA	3	2	20	1
2	F	29	PA	6	2	13	3
3	M	32	SPK	18	1	12	1
4	M	36	SPK	6	1	19	1
5	M	48	SPK	12	2	11	0
6	F	23	PA	4	1	11	2
7	M	45	PAK	4	0	20	0
8	M	43	SPK	3	1	19	?

PA, pancreas-alone; PAK, pancreas after kidney transplant; SPK, simultaneous pancreas kidney transplant; CIT, cold ischemia time

Offprint requests to: H. G. Peltenburg, Department of Nephrology and Transplantation, University Hospital Maastricht, P.O. Box 5800, 6202 AZ Maastricht, The Netherlands

Table 2. Quantitative results of insulin secretory response (ISR) after glucagon 1 mg IV in pancreas allograft recipients (mU/l per 30 min); correlation with amylase excretion rate (AER)

Recipient	First ISR	Maximum pre-rejection		During rejection		Maximum post-rejection		Correlation with AER			
		Day	ISR	Day	ISR	Day	ISR	n	r	SEE	P
1	351	9	948	14	434	16	858	9	0.57	3677	0.11
2	323	11	3338	13	2434	20	5037	7	0.91	549	0.004
3	219	6	820	13	58	21	501	7	0.48	3618	0.27
4	125	4	177	7	114	14	800	5	0.55	4030	0.33
5[a]	347	–	–	–	–	–	1370	11	0.92	1313	0.0001
6	905	6	1561	14	141	48	561	9	0.91	1229	0.001
7[a]	493	–	–	–	–	–	1980	9	0.15	8087	0.68
8[a]	85	–	–	–	–	–	111	11	0.37	167	0.26

[a] No rejection in recipients 5 and 7; all responses of recipient 8 were low
SEE, standard error of estimate

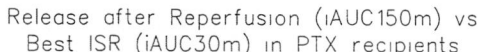

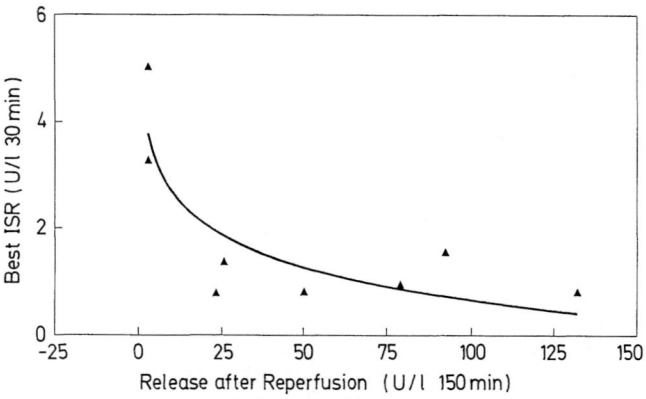

Fig. 1. Release of insulin after reperfusion vs maximum ISR after glucagon stimulation in pancreas transplant recipients

3 months after transplantation (Fig. 1). This relation was significant at the level of $P < 0.01$.

In conclusion, pancreas allografts varied considerably in their output of insulin directly after reperfusion. Furthermore, an inverse relation was shown between insulin release after reperfusion and stimulation, and no relation between amylase release after reperfusion and unstimulated maximum amylase secretion within 100 days after pancreas allograft transplantation.

Reference

1. Kootstra G, Van Hooff JP, Jorning PJG, et al (1987) A new variant for whole pancreas grafting. Early experience. Transplant Proc 19: 2314

TRANSPLANT
International
© Springer-Verlag 1992

Isolation of pig pancreatic islets by a new method with hydraulic shaking: preliminary report*

G. L. Viviani[1], **I. Fontana**[2], **A. Zecchi**[1], **R. Bottino**[2], **R. Sanna**[1], **L. Lione**[1], **G. Sacchi**[1], **G. Falzetti**[1], **U. Valente**[2], and **L. Adezati**[1]

[1] Department of Endocrinology and Metabolism and [2] Transplant Unit, University of Genova, Genova, Italy

The limited availability of human pancreas represents a serious problem in islet transplantation. In the past few years many efforts have been made to isolate pancreatic islets from large mammals in order to achieve valid and reproducible isolation methods [1–4].

For several reasons swine may be considered an ideal source of islet tissue because of the similarity between human and porcine insulin and because of the easy availability of pig pancreata. Some papers have been published recently on this topic with good results [1, 5–7].

However, some problems, such as islet dissociation into single cells after collagenase digestion, are not completely solved. In this article, an automated method involving a hydraulic shaking system is described for islet isolation from the pig pancreas, developed in our laboratory and derived from Ricordi's model.

Key words: Pancreatic islets, pig – Isolation

Materials and methods

Pancreata were obtained from a local slaughterhouse from 6–9-month-old animals weighing on average 120 kg. The warm ischemia time was 24 ± 8.2 min, and the cold ischemia time was 151 ± 39 min. The organs were distended by 2 ml/g pancreatic tissue of collagenase (6 mg/ml) solution (Worthington type IV biochemicals, Freehold, N.J.; 176 U/mg).

Ten splenic pancreatic lobes were processed. After distension, the pancreata were cut into 10-cm^3 pieces and digested in a chamber continuously perfused with HBSS at 37°C. The chamber was derived from Ricordi's digestion chamber with some modifications (material Plexiglas; inner volume 500 ml; peristaltic pump flow rate 100 ml/min). Shaking was performed by a second peristaltic pump providing a recirculation flux (maximum of 520 ml/min) that allowed a controlled and continuous, gentle disruption of pancreatic tissue.

The inlet of the recirculation pump was located at the top of the chamber, and the outlet, on the side. Digestion time was checked by observation every 2 min under a microscope. When free islets were detected, the collagenase solution was diluted and collected in 5 l fresh HBSS supplemented with 2% fetal calf serum (FCS) at 4°C. Mean collecting time was 40 ± 6 min. Islet purification was performed by discontinuous Ficoll gradients as described by other authors [5, 7].

Viability and morphological integrity were evaluated by staining with dithizone and a combination of inclusion and exclusion dyes (acridine orange and ethidium bromide) and by light microscopy demonstrating positive aldehyde-fuchsin staining [8].

For determination of the volume, the islets were counted under a microscope equipped with a calibration grid and were divided into 5 diameter classes (50, 100, 150, 200, > 250 μm), considering the islet spheres. Groups of 5 islets were used for insulin secretion as previously described [9]. All results are expressed as mean ± SEM.

Results

The hydraulic shaking system allowed a complete digestion of the pancreatic tissue. Average digestion time was 18.5 ± 1.4 min. After this time the islets were shunted in fresh HBSS; the mean collecting time was 40 ± 6 min. At the end of the procedure only a fibrous network and little pieces of nondistended parenchyma remained in the digestion chamber.

The isolation yielded 7921 ± 1443 islets/g pancreas expressed as EN/g pancreas with a volume of 913 ± 135 mm^3 islet tissue (13.99 mm^3/g pancreas). After the density gradient purification, 44% of the islet tissue was recovered, corresponding to 3557 ± 556 EN/g pancreas with a volume of islet tissue of 410 ± 53 (6.28 ± 0.9 mm^3/g pancreas).

The insulin secretory response to glucose (300 mg/dl) plus theophylline (5 mmol/l) was 7.3 ± 1.5 times the basal rate.

Discussion

In the past few years, some methods for the isolation of islets of Langerhans from the pig pancreas have been published [1, 5–7, 10–11]. Nevertheless, many aspects need to be solved.

* This work was partly supported by C.N.R. grant no. 89.0344.14

Offprint requests to: G.L. Viviani, Department of Endocrinology and Metabolism, DiSEM, Viale Benedetto XV 6, 16132, Genova, Italy

Ricordi reported a marked fragility of swine islets: This represents a serious problem because of a possible rapid dissociation of the pancreas into single cells during the isolation procedure. To overcome this problem, the automated procedure developed for the human pancreas was largely modified by Ricordi's group, increasing the circuit diameters, lowering the temperature of the heating circuit, and reducing the continuous mechanical shaking.

In our isolation method, only one recirculation circuit was used, and the inner chamber volume was enlarged (500 ml). Moreover, the chamber was made of transparent material that allowed continuous observation of the digestion procedure. A hydraulic shaking system replaced the mechanical one of Ricordi's method and represents the most important difference between the two methods.

Hydraulic shaking allows a more gentle disruption of the tissue and may be more tightly controlled. Moreover, the hydraulic shaking may be calibrated in order to obtain the appropriate continuous agitation.

An average digestion of 19 min was necessary to obtain free islets and to start the collecting phase. This time is shorter than that reported from other authors [6, 8]. Only Ricordi reported a lower digestion time [5]. These different results may be explained either by the type and concentration of collagenase used, which was slightly increased in comparison with other reports, or by the shaking system adopted, as it was continuous but more gentle.

The islets obtained showed morphological integrity and a good viability, and all the exocrine tissue was dissociated into single cells. Moreover, the yield was relatively high and the functional response good. These results let us hypothesize that, at least for the fragile pig pancreas, a continuously hydraulic shaking method may represent an elective way to isolate intact islets.

If alternative sources of islet tissue prove to be useful in reversing diabetes and promoting survival after rejection, isolating islets from large mammals may become very important. This method may be transferable to other animals after introducing some modifications and may represent a valid possibility for obtaining intact and viable islets for xenotransplantation.

References

1. Ricordi C, Finke EH, Lacy PE (1986) A method for the mass isolation of islets from the adult pig pancreas. Diabetes 35: 649–653
2. Calafiore R, Calcinaro F, Basta G, Pietropaolo M, Falorni A, Piermattei M, Brunetti P (1990) A method for the massive separation of highly purified, adult porcine islets of Langerhans. Metabolism 39: 175–181
3. Ricordi C, Socci C, Davalli AM, Staudacher C, Baro P, Bertova A, Sassi I, Gavazzi F, Pozza G, Di Carlo V (1990) Isolation of the elusive pig islet. Surgery 107: 688–694
4. Finke E, Marchetti P, Falqui L, Swanson C, McLear M, Olack B, Scharp D, Lacy P (1991) Large scale isolation, function and transplantation of islets of Langerhans from the adult pig pancreas. Transplant Proc 23: 772–773
5. Olack B, Swanson C, McLear M, Longwith J, Scharp D, Lacy PE (1991) Islet purification using Euro-Ficoll gradients. Transplant Proc 23: 774–776
6. Hesse UJ, Weyer J, Meyer W, Isselhard W, Pichlmeier H (1989) Transplant Proc 21: 2763–2764
7. Mellert J, Hopt UT, Hering BJ, Bretzel RG, Federlin K (1991) Influence of islet mass and purity on reversability of diabetes in pancreatectomized pigs. Transplant Proc 23: 1687–1689
8. Ricordi C, Gray DWR, Hering BJ, Kaufman DB, Warnock GL, Kneteman NM, Lake SP, London NJM, Socci C, Alejandro R, Zeng Y, Scharp DW, Viviani GL, Falqui L, Tzakis A, Bretzel RG, Federlin K, Pozza G, James RFL, Rajotte RV, DiCarlo V, Morris PJ, Sutherland DE, Starzl TE, Mintz DH, Lacy PE (1990) Islet isolation assessment in man and large animals. Acta Diabetol Lat 27: 185–195
9. Liu X, Federlin KF, Bretzel RG, Hering BJ, Brendel MD (1991) Persistent reversal of diabetes by transplantation of fetal pig proislets into nude mice. Diabetes 40: 858–866
10. Viviani GL, Borgoglio MG, Fontana I, Borgoglio A, Nocera A, Leprini A, Comaschi M, Valente U, Adezati L (1989) Azathioprine decreases insulin secretion in human islets. Transplant Proc 21: 2714–2716
11. Ricordi C, Socci C, Davalli AM, Staudacher C, Baro P, Vertova A, Sassi I, Gavazzi F, Bertuzzi F, Pozza G, Di Carlo V (1990) Effects of pancreas retrieval procedure on islet isolation in the swine. Transplant Proc 22 (2): 442–443

Transplant Int (1992) 5 [Suppl 1]: S274–S277

TRANSPLANT
International
© Springer-Verlag 1992

The use of FK506 and RS61443 for reversal of small-bowel rejection

M. J. Stangl[1], **C. Gräb**[2], **T. Fischer**[2], **H. Mebert**[2], **M. Weiß**[3], and **C. Hammer**[2]

[1] Chirurgische Klinik und Poliklinik der LMU München, Klinikum Großhadern,
[2] Institut für Chirurgische Forschung der LMU München,
[3] Institut für Pathologie der LMU München, München, Federal Republic of Germany

Successful clinical small-bowel transplantation is still difficult to achieve [3, 6]. Two features render the small intestine unique among vascularised solid organ grafts. First, the bowel contains a large amount of lymphoid tissue within the Peyer's patches, mesenteric lymph nodes, and intraepithelial lymphocytes, which are thought to mediate graft-versus-host disease and provide a major stimulus for the recipient's immune system [10]. Unfortunately, mere surgical reduction of these tissues, by using segmental allografts, does not furnish any immunological advantage [12]. Second, the small bowel lacks specific serum markers such as blood urea nitrogen (BUN) in the kidney or bilirubin in liver transplantation. Clinical signs such as fever, pain, or tenderness of the abdomen may indicate an already advanced destruction of the graft. Therefore, very potent immunosuppressive regimens are necessary to avoid small-bowel allograft rejection or even to reverse an ongoing rejection process. Cyclosporin was shown in small and large animal models to control rejection reactions sufficiently [4, 13]. However, there are two even more promising immunosuppressive agents currently under investigation. FK506, a macrolide lactone isolated from *Streptomyces tsukubaensis*, leads to long-term survival of small-bowel allografts in a rodent model and has already been used in a few clinical small-bowel transplantations [11, 14]. RS61443, a mycophenolic acid morpholinoethylester, selectively inhibits T- and B-cell proliferation [9]. We have investigated the use of FK506 and RS61443 for the reversal of small-bowel allograft rejection in a small animal model.

Key words: FK506 – RS61443 – Small-bowel rejection

Methods

The experimental *animals* were adult male rats of the inbred Lewis (LEW) (RT1[1]) and Brown Norway (BN) (RT1[n]) strains, weighing from 180 to 280 g. In each instance, BN rats served as donors and LEW rats as recipients of grafts.

The *operative procedure* involved the orthotopic transplantation of the entire small bowel, with end-to-side anastomoses of the superior mesenteric artery and the portal vein of the graft to the infrarenal aorta and vena cava, respectively, of the recipient. After revascularization of the graft, the small bowel of the recipient was resected to an extent equivalent to the length and type of the allograft. The allograft was interposed by means of two end-to-end intestinal anastomoses.

Five *experimental groups* were formed according to the different immunosuppressive regimens. All animals received a basic immunosuppression with cyclosporin A (CyA; 10 mg/kg) for the first 5 postoperative days. In groups 2–5 all animals were treated from day 13–15 postoperatively with CyA, FK506, or RS61443. Biopsies were taken from each animal on days 13, 16, and 25 postoperatively and at sacrifice.

Group 1 ($n = 13$) animals did not receive any further immunosuppressive therapy.
Group 2 ($n = 11$) recipients received CyA again on days 13–15 postoperatively as a dose of 10 mg/kg.
Group 3 ($n = 9$) rats were treated from day 13–15 postoperatively with a dose of FK506 2 mg/kg.
In group 4 ($n = 3$), a rescue therapy was started on day 13 with 20 mg/kg RS61443 and stopped on day 15.
In group 5 ($n = 9$) RS61443 was administered in a dose of 40 mg/kg on the same days as in group 4.

Determination of rejection. Complete rejection of the allograft was easily determined because it led to the death of the recipient in each instance.

Graft-versus-host reaction (GvHR). All animals were monitored daily for clinical signs of GvHR (redness of ears, snout, and paws, hair loss, diarrhea). Spleen, lymph nodes, liver, and host intestine were examined histologically at the time of autopsy or sacrifice.

Skin grafting. Full-thickness skin grafts, 2.5 cm², of the abdominal wall [2] from homozygous donor animals were prepared. These were then sutured into position on the recipient's neck using an interrupted 4/0 silk suture. The grafts were inspected daily, and rejection was declared when more than 50 % of the graft surface had become scabby or necrotic.

Offprint requests to: Dr. Manfred J. Stangl, Chirurgische Klinik und Poliklinik der LMU München, Klinikum Großhadern, Marchioninistr. 15, 8000 München 70, Federal Republic of Germany

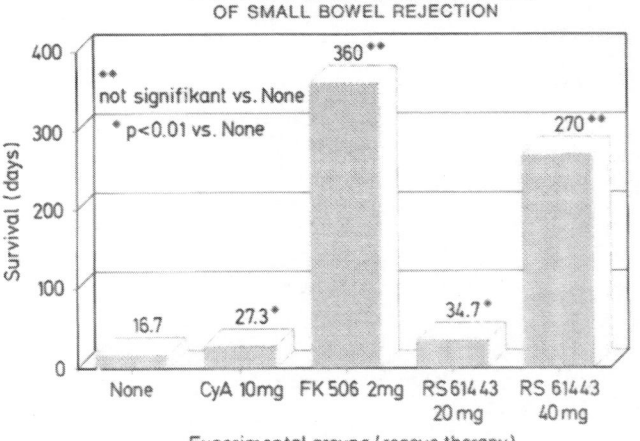

Fig. 1. Survival times of small-bowel allograft recipients after rescue therapy with cyclosporin A (CyA), FK506, or RS61443

Fig. 3. Mesenteric lymph node from a transplanted small intestine on postoperative day 13 (see text)

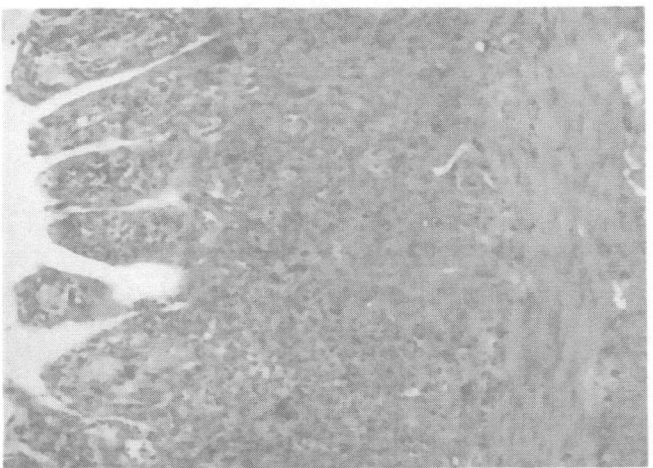

Fig. 2. Small-bowel allograft on the postoperative day 13 after short-term CyA therapy (see text)

Histology examination. The small-bowel graft with its mesentery and lymph nodes as well as the recipient's own mesenteric lymph nodes, spleen, and liver were obtained at the time of autopsy or at the time of sacrifice. The specimens were fixed in formalin and prepared for light microscopy study with H & E staining.

Statistical analysis. All results were expressed as mean and SEM. Student's t-test was performed for the calculation of P values.

Results

Animals that received only the basic immunosuppression regimen with CyA (10 mg/kg) for 5 days died from rejection reaction after an average of 16.7 ± 1.7 days. Recipients receiving an immunosuppressive therapy with either CyA (10 mg/kg) or RS61443 (20 mg/kg) from day 13–15 postoperatively in addition to the basic immunosuppression showed a prolonged survival. But finally all animals died from rejection on day 27.3 ± 4.8 in the CyA group or day 34.7 ± 1.5 in the RS61443 (20 mg) group (Fig. 1). The difference was not statistically significant in the CyA group ($P > 0.05$), but it was in the RS61443 group ($P < 0.05$). All rats in groups 3 and 5 which received a rescue therapy with either FK506 (2 mg) or RS61443 (40 mg) showed an indefinite survival ($P < 0.01$). Animals that were sacrified after more than 360 days (in group 3) or 270 days (in group 5) revealed no signs of a rejection reaction.

Pathohistology study

The biopsy studies taken on the 13th postoperative day showed a thickening of the small-bowel wall in all animals and a fibrotic encapsulation of the mesenteric lymph node. Histology sections of the transplanted small bowel revealed a severe lymphocyte infiltration into the lamina propria and a shortening and blunting of the villi. In addition, there was an almost complete loss of goblet cells in the villous epithelium (Fig. 2). In the mesenteric lymph nodes we found a follicular hyperplasia with an increased number of germinal centers and a sinus histiocytosis (Fig. 3). After a 3-day treatment with either FK506 or RS61443, the histology sections taken on the 25th and 36th day, respectively, showed an almost complete recovery of the small bowel and lymph node architecture (Figs. 4–7).

Graft-versus-host disease

None of the animals showed clinical signs of GvHR. This was the case before the animals received rescue therapy as well as thereafter. Examinations of host tissue (spleen, lymph nodes, liver) on days 13, 16, 25, and at sacrifice revealed no histological signs of GvHR such as loss of architecture, depletion of lymphoid cells, or periportal lymphocytic infiltration.

Skin grafts

Three animals from groups 3 and 5 received a skin graft more than 270 days after small intestine transplantation and cessation of immunosuppressive therapy. No clinical

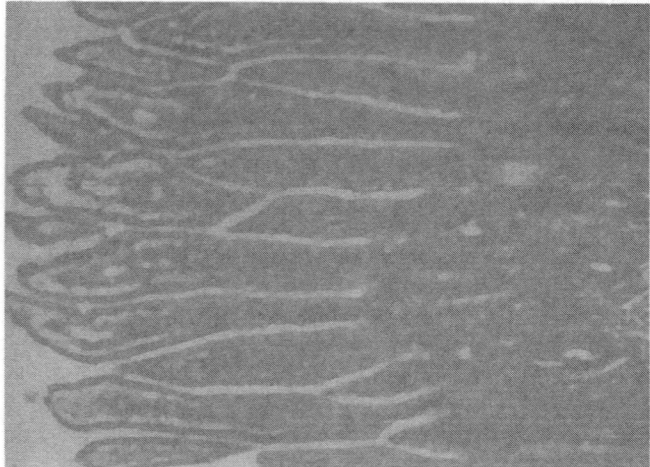

Fig. 4. Small intestine after rescue therapy with FK506 (25th day); regular height of the villi with only little edema and cellular infiltration

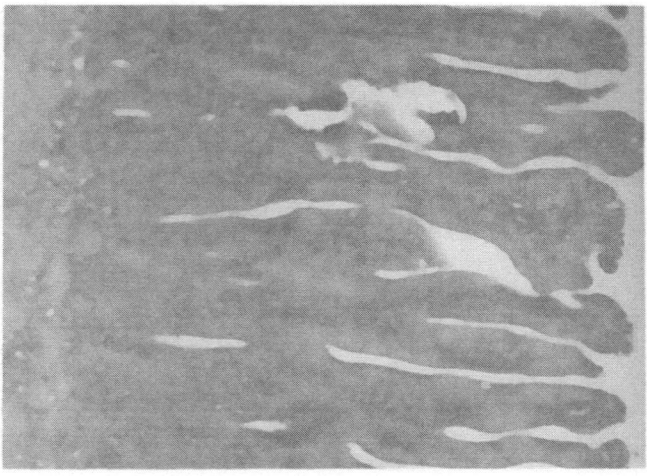

Fig. 6. Small-bowel allograft after rescue therapy with RS61443 (day 36); normal length of the villi with only minor cellular infiltration

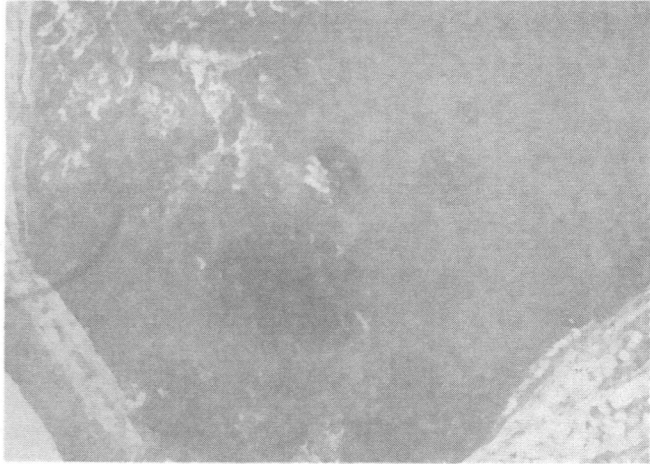

Fig. 5. Mesenteric lymph node on the day 25 after FK506 treatment; slight sinus histiocytosis and dispersed architecture

Fig. 7. Mesenteric lymph node after therapy with RS61443 (day 36); regular architecture with no signs of rejection reaction

or histological signs of rejection were seen at the time of skin grafting. All skin grafts were rejected between day 10 and 14 after transplantation. However, this rejection reaction had no influence on the function, integrity, or histological appearance of the small-bowel graft.

Discussion

The new immunosuppressive drugs FK506 and RS61443 have increased the hope that small-bowel transplantation will become a clinical reality in the near future. FK506 acts similarly to CyA and inhibits the production of interleukin (IL-2, IL-4, IL-5), interferon (IFNτ), and tumor necrosis factor (TNFα) from stimulated mononuclear cells [1]. Studies in rats have shown that FK506 inhibits lethal, acute GvHR [7] and leads to indefinite survival of small-bowel transplant recipients after a short course of treatment [11]. RS61443, a semisynthetic derivative from mycophenolic acid, inhibits inosine 5'-monophosphate dehydrogenase and guanosine monophosphate synthetase and thereby specifically depresses the "de novo" syn-

thesis of nucleic acid [5]. As stimulated T- and B-lymphocytes depend on this "de novo" pathway, RS61443 inhibits their activation. RS61443 prolongs graft survival in experimental heart transplantation [9].

In our study we have tested both drugs for their ability to reverse an ongoing rejection reaction. All animals receiving either FK506 or RS61443 on day 13 postoperatively showed a destruction of the mucosa, a thickening of the small-bowel wall, and a marked cellular infiltration. Just a 3-day treatment with FK506 and RS61443 completely abrogated the rejection process and led to an indefinite survival of all recipients. None of the animals showed any clinical side effects, such as retching, tremor, or decrease of spontaneous mobility [8]. However, the animals receiving RS61443 lost weight and suffered from infectious complications approximately 20 days after cessation of the treatment. None of the recipients died from these events, and clinical integrity could be restored by treatment with antibiotics. The rejection of all skin grafts without any influence on the transplanted small bowel indicates that FK506 and RS61443 produce a status of specific tolerance. The ability of the immune system to act against a new stimulus seems to be unaffected. Todo et al. [14] reported on 5 cases of successful clinical small-bowel transplantation using FK506. Four of these patients received a small-bowel allograft together with a liver; the protective potential of a liver transplant on a second graft, especially with a venous outflow into the portal vein, is still not clear. Nevertheless, these results are encouraging regarding the future of clinical small-intestine transplantation. In our model we have demonstrated the efficiency of FK506 and RS61443 to reverse an ongoing rejection reaction with an already destroyed graft architecture. These results are promising for the treatment of severe and otherwise uncontrollable rejection reactions and possibly even for the treatment of chronic rejection.

References

1. Andersson J, Nagy S, Groth C, Andersson U (1991) Effects of FK 506 or cyclosporin A on cytokine production studied in vitro at a single cell level. First International Congress on FK506, Pittsburgh, Penn., August 21–24
2. Billingham RE, Medawar PB (1951) The technique of free skin grafting in mammals. J Exp Biol 28: 3
3. Deltz E, Schroeder P, Schweizer E, Gebhardt H, Gundlach M, Hansmann ML, Leimenstoll G (1991) Experimental fundamentals and first clinical experiences in small bowel transplantation. Eur Surg Res 23: 130
4. Diliz-Perez HS, McClure J, Bedetti C, Hong HQ, de Santibanes E, Shaw BW, Thiel D van, Iwatsuki S, Starzl TE (1984) Successful small bowel allotransplantation in dogs with cyclosporine and prednisone. Transplantation 37 (2): 126–129
5. Franklin TJ, Cook JM (1969) The inhibition of nucleic acid synthesis by mycophenolic acid. Biochem J 113: 515
6. Goulet O, Revillon Y, Jan D, Brousse N, Ricour C (1991) Small bowel transplantation in children. Eur Surg Res 23: 130–131
7. Hoffman AL, Makowka L, Banner B, Cai X, Cramer DV, Pascualone A, Todo S, Starzl TE (1990) The use of FK 506 for small intestine allotransplantation. Transplantation 49: 483–490
8. Mong S (1991) Preclinical toxicolocy of FK 506. First International Congress on FK 506, Pittsburgh, Penn., August 21–24
9. Morris RE, Hoyt EG, Murphy MP, Eugui EM, Allison AC (1990) Mycophenolic acid morpholinoethylester (RS 61443) is a new immunosuppressant that prevents and halts heart allograft rejection by selective inhibition of T- and B-cell purine synthesis. Transplant Proc 22 (4): 1659–1662
10. Snell GD (1957) The homograft reaction. Ann Rev Microbiol 11: 439
11. Stangl MJ, Lee KKW, Starzl T, Land W, Schraut WH (1990) Specific tolerance induction with FK 506 after allogeneic small bowel transplantation. Langenbecks Arch Chir 323–326
12. Stangl MJ, Schraut WH, Moynihan HL, Lee T (1989) Rejection of ileal versus jejunal allografts. Transplantation 47: 424–427
13. Stangl MJ, Schraut WH, Moynihan HL, Lee TK, Lee KKW (1990) Effect of cyclosporine therapy in controlling the rejection of ileal versus jejunal allografts. Transplant Int 3: 149–155
14. Todo S, Tzakis A, Fung J, Abu-Elmagd K, Reyes J, Thiel D van, Starzl T (1991) Clinical small bowel transplantation under FK 506. First International Congress on FK 506, Pittsburgh, Penn., August 21–24

Graft Monitoring

TRANSPLANT
International
© Springer-Verlag 1992

Monitoring of cardiac graft recipients: comparison of in vivo activated, committed T lymphocytes in peripheral blood and in the graft

C. C. Baan[1], L. M. B. Vaessen[1], A. J. Ouwehand[2], P. Heyse[1], C. R. Daane[1], N. H. P. M. Jutte[1], F. H. J. Claas[3], and W. Weimar[1]

Department of [1] Internal Medicine I and [2] the Thorax Center, University Hospital Rotterdam-Dijkzigt, Rotterdam, and
[3] Department of Immunohaematology and Blood Bank, University Hospital Leiden, Leiden, The Netherlands

Abstract. The proliferative and cytotoxic capacity of peripheral blood lymphocytes (PBL) and the cytotoxic activity of lymphocytes propagated from endomyocardial biopsies (EMB) towards donor cells was used to identify in vivo activated, committed T cells. A series of 39 PBL samples and 38 EMB simultaneously taken from 20 patients after heart transplantation was cultured in interleukin 2 (IL-2) conditioned medium. The cytotoxic capacity of these cultures against donor cells was tested in a 4-h chromium-51 release assay. From a comparable patient group, 224 samples were evaluated for donor reactivity by a primed lymphocyte test (PLT). Analysis showed that PBL cultures hardly ever contained committed cytotoxic T lymphocytes (cCTL, 2/39) or committed proliferative T lymphocytes (cPTL, 1/224). In contrast, significantly more EMB cultures (17/38, $P < 0.001$, χ^2 test) demonstrated donor-directed cytotoxicity. This was especially found during rejection (11/17 vs 6/21 without rejection, $P = 0.05$). These results show that after heart transplantation, committed cells are mainly found in the graft.

Key words: Heart transplantation – Rejection monitoring – Committed T lymphocytes

Despite previous attempts to correlate morphologic and phenotypic changes of T lymphocytes in the peripheral blood lymphocytes (PBL) with allograft rejection, histologic evaluation of endomyocardial biopsies (EMB) remains the only reliable method for the diagnosis of cardiac rejection. Results of diagnostic studies in PBL were conflicting and did not provide information about the function and specificity of these T cells [2, 3, 7]. We have recently demonstrated that the lymphocyte growth obtained from EMB cultured in interleukin (IL-2) conditioned medium correlates with the histologic rejection grade [5] and that the majority of the in vivo activated, committed T lymphocytes showed cytotoxicity against donor antigen-committed T lymphocytes [1]. In this report, we analyzed whether the presence of committed T lymphocytes in PBL and their proliferative or cytotoxic ability to react against donor cells was associated with rejection episodes. The specific cytotoxicity of PBL cultures was compared with cytotoxic reactivity patterns from lymphocytes isolated from EMB obtained at the same time.

Patients and methods

Patients were diagnosed by histologic criteria according to Billingham for acute rejection in EMB. All cardiac transplant recipients received cyclosporin A (CsA) and low-dose steroids as immunosuppressive therapy.

We analyzed 39 (Ficoll-Hypaque isolated) PBL and 38 EMB samples simultaneously taken from 20 heart transplant patients. The PBL and EMB samples were expanded in IL-2 containing medium and tested in a 4-h chromium-51 release assay for cytotoxic reactivity as reported previously [5]. As targets we used donor B-LCL, third party B-LCL (Epstein-Barr virus transformed B-lymphocyte cell lines) and lymphokine-activated killer (LAK) and natural killer (NK) sensitive target cell line K562 to detect committed cytotoxic T lymphocytes (cCTL) in the cultures. Cold target inhibition studies with K562 were performed to confirm the allospecificity of the cCTL derived from the cultured PBL. A fixed number of cold K562 (2.5×10^4) was added to 2.5×10^3 hot K562 or donor B-LCL cells. Control values were established by adding unrelated cold PHA blasts to hot target cells.

From a comparable patient group we tested 20 pretransplant and 224 post-transplant PBL samples with a standard primed lymphocyte test (PLT) [9] against donor and third party spleen cells to detect cPTL in PBL.

Results

We grew sufficient cells from 19/38 EMB (10 patients) and from all PBL ($n = 39$, 20 patients) for the analysis of donor-directed cytotoxicity.

All cultured PBL samples showed LAK-like nonspecific cytotoxicity since the cultures killed K562 and vari-

Offprint requests to: C. C. Baan, Department of Internal Medicine I, Bd299, University Hospital Rotterdam-Dijkzigt, Dr. Molewaterplein 40, 3015 GD Rotterdam, The Netherlands

Table 1. Cultures containing committed cytotoxic T lymphocytes in peripheral blood lymphocytes (PBL) and endomyocardial biopsies (EMB) in relation to periods of acute rejection (AR)

	Number of cultures (%)		
	AR$^-$	AR$^+$	P value[a]
PBL	0/23 (0)	2/16 (12)	n.s.
EMB	6/21 (28)	11/17 (65)	0.05

[a] χ^2 test

ous B-LCL. In 2/16 (12%) PBL cultures taken at the time of or followed by acute rejection, we identified cCTL after cold target inhibition with K562 (Table 1). Significantly more (11/17, 65%) of the corresponding EMB cultures were cytotoxic against donor antigens ($P < 0.01$, χ^2 test). The EMB cultures did not lyse the NK-sensitive cell line K562. None of the 23 PBL cultures, taken during periods of immunologic quiescence, contained cCTL. In contrast, we observed donor-directed cytotoxicity in 6/21 (28%) of the EMB cultures ($P = 0.02$) taken in the absence of rejection. This proved to be significantly lower than was found during acute rejection (6/21 vs 11/17, $P = 0.05$).

In cases in which there was histologic evidence of rejection, 1/40 of the PBL samples showed a significant proliferative response when stimulated with donor cells compared with pretransplant samples. None of the other PBL samples ($n = 184$, no rejection) demonstrated primed lymphocyte responses against donor antigens. Third party stimulator cells did not induce proliferation of the PBL in the PLT.

Discussion

We demonstrated that the in vitro proliferative or cytotoxic capacity of PBL cultures towards donor antigens was negligible even at the time of or prior to an acute rejection. A significantly higher proportion of the corresponding EMB cultures showed cytotoxicity against donor antigens. The number of EMB cultures containing cCTL was correlated with histologic diagnosis of rejection. These data clearly demonstrate that committed lymphocytes are only seldom present and indicate that committed alloreactive cells have a preference for the allograft. Similar results obtained with limiting dilution analysis of alloreac-

tive precursor cytotoxic T lymphocytes (pCTL) were reported from human cardiac graft infiltrating cells [8] and cCTL in mouse sponge grafts [4]. Another recent report suggested that the increased frequencies of circulating donor-specific pCTL were associated in a predictive manner with rejection. However, the measurement of pCTL in PBL had no predictive value as no difference was found between clinically relevant (myocytolysis) and irrelevant (infiltrate only) rejection episodes [6]. We conclude that the immune status of the PBL is no reflection of the histologic and functional changes in the EMB. Therefore, monitoring of the PBL for the diagnosis of rejection in heart transplant recipients remains an illusion.

References

1. Baan CC, Ouwehand AJ, Vaessen LMB, Jutte NHPM, Balk AHMM, Mochtar B, Claas FHJ, Weimar W (1991) The clinical relevance of HLA matching in heart transplantation: impact on rejection and donor-directed cytotoxicity of graft infiltrating lymphocytes. Transplant Proc (in press)
2. Hammer C, Reichenspurner H, Ertel W, Lerch C, Plahl M, Brendel W, Reichart B, Uberfuhr R, Welz A, Kempkes BM (1984) Cytological and immunologic monitoring of cyclosporine-treated human heart recipients. Heart Transplant 3: 228–232
3. Jutte NHPM, Hop WCJ, Daane CR, Essed CE, Weimar W, Simoons ML, Bos E (1990) Cytoimmunologic monitoring of heart transplant recipients. Clin Transplant 4: 297–300
4. Orosz CG, Horstemeyer B, Zinn NE, Bishop DK (1989) Development and evaluation of limiting dilution analysis technique that can discriminate in vivo alloactivated cytotoxic T lymphocytes from their native CTL precursor. Transplantation 47: 189–194
5. Ouwehand AJ, Vaessen LMB, Baan CC, Jutte NHPM, Balk AHMM, Essed CE, Bos E, Claas FHJ, Weimar W (1991) Alloreactive lymphoid infiltrates in human heart transplants. Hum Immunol 30: 50–59
6. Reader JA, Burke MM, Counihan P, Kirby JA, Adams S, Davies MJ, Pepper JR (1990) Noninvasive monitoring of human cardiac allograft rejection. Transplantation 50: 29–33
7. Roodman ST, Miller LW, Tsai CC (1988) Role of interleukin 2 receptors in immunologic monitoring following cardiac transplantation. Transplantation 45: 1050–1056
8. Suitters AJ, Rose ML, Dominguez MJ, Yacoub MH (1990) Selection for donor-specific cytotoxic T lymphocytes within the allografted human heart. Transplantation 49: 1105–1109
9. Zeevi AJ, Fung TR, Zerbe C, Kaufman BS, Rabin BP, Griffith RL, Hardesty L, Duquesnoy RJ (1986) Allospecificity of activated T cells grown from endomyocardial biopsies from heart transplant patients. Transplantation 41: 620–626

Transplant Int (1992) 5 [Suppl 1]: S283–S285

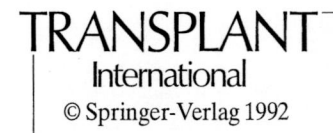

TRANSPLANT
International
© Springer-Verlag 1992

Intercellular adhesion molecule 1 (ICAM-1) induction on hepatocytes is an early marker of acute liver allograft rejection

I. Lautenschlager, K. Höckerstedt, and P. Häyry

Transplantation Laboratory, Fourth Department of Surgery, University of Helsinki, Helsinki, Finland

Abstract. Intercellular adhesion molecule 1 (ICAM-1) induction on hepatocytes was investigated in relation to immune activation of acute liver allograft rejection. Twelve liver recipients undergoing an episode of acute rejection were monitored by frequent fine needle aspiration biopsy (FNAB) study. All episodes were reversible, and the lymphocyte and lymphoid blast predominated with a high peak of inflammation (6.9 ± 4.0 corrected increment units). The rejections were treated with a high dose of steroids, and the inflammation subsided within 1 week. ICAM-1 was demonstrated from FNAB preparations by a monoclonal antibody and immunoperoxidase staining. ICAM-1 was not detected on the hepatocytes immediately after transplantation but was always seen during rejection. ICAM-1 appeared 1–5 days before the onset of inflammation in the FNAB. The intensity of ICAM-1 expression increased towards the peak of inflammation and subsided thereafter. ICAM-1 induction on hepatocytes appears to be linked with a very early phase of immune activation and can be considered an early marker for acute liver allograft rejection in the FNAB.

Key words: Liver allograft rejection – ICAM-1 induction – Hepatocytes

Intercellular adhesion molecule 1 (ICAM-1), a ligand for lymphocyte function antigen (LFA-1), is a cell surface glycoprotein with important functions in leucocyte adhesion and the cell-cell interactions of the inflammatory processes [1]. The expression of ICAM-1 is upregulated by several cytokines, such as IL-1, TNF-α and INF-γ, and it is produced at the early phase of lymphoid activation [2]. Expression of ICAM-1 on hepatocytes has also been demonstrated on biopsy histology during liver allograft rejection [3, 4]. Although the role of adhesion molecules in liver rejection is not yet clear, they are upregulated by the cytokines produced during the cascade of immune activation of acute rejection.

The hallmark of acute liver allograft rejection monitored by the fine needle aspiration biopsy (FNAB) method is the appearance of a lymphocyte and lymphoid blast-dominated inflammatory infiltrate in the graft [5]. The cellular findings in the FNAB correlate with clinical signs and biochemical markers of acute liver rejection, but the cellular hallmarks of rejection are usually seen 1–3 days before the clinical diagnosis of rejection is established [5].

In this study the ICAM-1 induction on hepatocytes was investigated in relation to the immune activation of acute liver allograft rejection monitored by frequent FNABs. The induction of ICAM-1 was correlated with the appearance of lymphoid activation in the graft, and the downregulation of ICAM-1 expression was correlated with the disappearance of inflammation during anti-rejection treatment.

Patients and methods

Patients. Twelve liver transplant recipients treated with combinations of azathioprine (1–2.5 mg/kg daily), cyclosporine (3–10 mg/kg daily) and methylprednisolone (0.5–2 mg/kg daily) for basic immunosuppression (triple therapy CyA, Aza, MP) underwent an inflammatory episode of acute rejection monitored by fine needle aspiration biopsy (FNAB). The recipients received high-dose MP (3 mg/kg daily) as the anti-rejection therapy for 5 days. All rejections were reversible with steroids. No infections occurred during the rejection episodes.

FNAB and blood specimens. The liver allografts were monitored with FNAB from the day of transplantation at 1 to 3-day intervals. The method for performing and processing FNABs of liver [6] and corresponding blood specimens is similar to that described for renal allografts [7]. The inflammation associated with rejection was quantified from May-Grunwald-Giemsa (MGG) stained cytocentrifuge preparations by the increment method and expressed in corrected increment units (CIU) [7].

Offprint requests to: I. Lautenschlager, Transplantation Laboratory, Fourth Department of Surgery, University of Helsinki, Haartmaninkatu 3, SF-00290 Helsinki, Finland

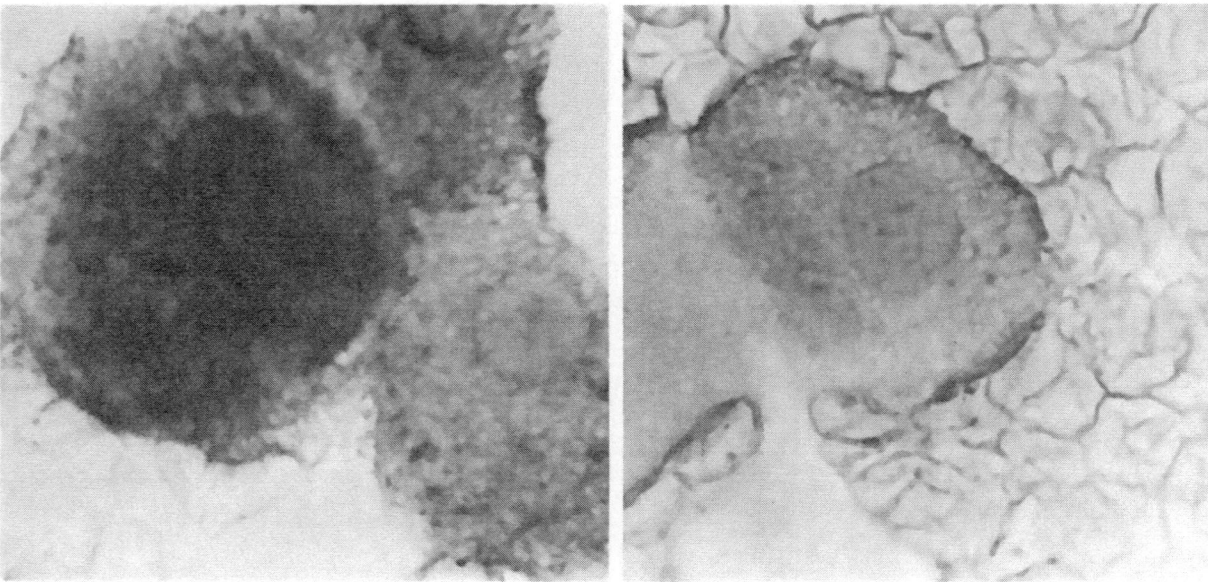

Fig. 1 a, b. An intense expression of intercellular adhesion molecule 1 (ICAM-1) on hepatocytes (score 3) at the peak of lymphoid activation (**a**), and a negative for staining ICAM-1 of hepatocytes after the inflammatory episode of rejection (**b**) demonstrated by monoclonal antibody and immunoperoxidase techniques

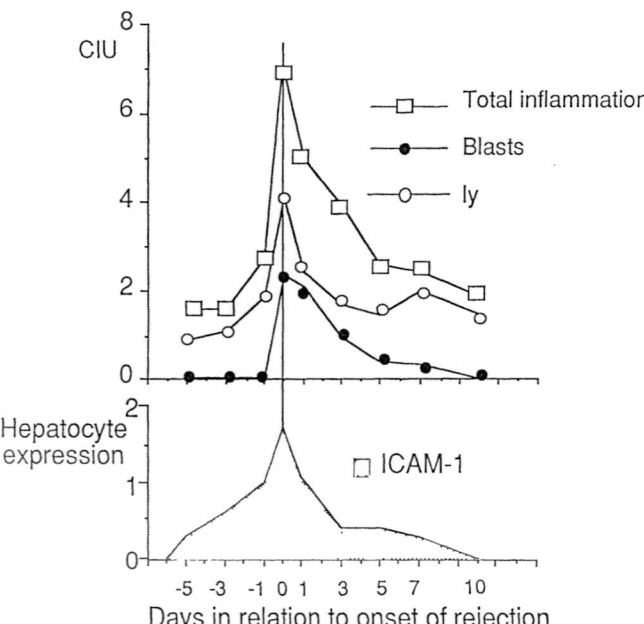

Fig. 2. Inflammatory profiles of 12 episodes of acute rejection expressed in corrected increment units (CIU). The major inflammatory cell components of total inflammation are lymphocytes *(ly)* and lymphoid blast cells. The induction and the intensity of ICAM-1 expression (scored from 1 to 3) is demonstrated in relation to onset of immune activation of rejection seen in the biopsy study

Demonstration of ICAM-1. For further analysis of ICAM-1 expression, a three-layer indirect immunoperoxidase technique and a monoclonal antibody to ICAM-1 were used. A monoclonal antibody against CD54 (ICAM-1) (Immunotech, Marseille, France) was employed. The cytocentrifuge preparations of liver FNABs were first incubated with the monoclonal mouse antibody, then with the peroxidase-conjugated rabbit antimouse antibody (Dako, Copenhagen, Denmark) and thereafter treated with a peroxidase-conjugated goat antirabbit antibody (Tago, Burlingame, Calif.). The reaction was revealed by AEC (3-amino-9-ethyl carbatzole) solution containing hydrogen peroxide. Mayer's hemalum was used for counterstaining. The intensity of positive staining was scored from 1 to 3.

Results

The rejection episodes appeared during the first postoperative month (6–27 days). All episodes demonstrated a high peak of inflammation (1.6 ± 0.8 CIU before, 6.9 ± 4.0 CIU at the peak and 1.9 ± 0.9 CIU after the episode), and subsided within 1 week. The inflammatory infiltrate consisted mainly of lymphocytes (0.9 ± 0.6 CIU before, 4.1 ± 1.8 CIU at the peak and 1.5 ± 0.9 CIU after the episode) and lymphoid blast cells (2.3 ± 2.5 CIU at the peak), with a minor involvement of mononuclear phagocytes. All rejection episodes were reversible, and the inflammation subsided with a high dose of MP in 5–7 days.

ICAM-1 was not detected in the FNABs obtained immediately after transplantation but was always seen during rejection. The expression of ICAM-1 on hepatocytes was induced 1–5 days before the onset of inflammation. The intensity of ICAM-1 expression (scored from 1 to 3) increased towards the peak of inflammation (0.3 ± 0.5 on day 5, 0.6 ± 0.7 on day 3, 1.0 ± 0.6 on day 1 before the onset and 1.7 ± 0.8 at the peak of inflammation) and subsided slowly thereafter. Some expression of ICAM-1 (0.3 ± 0.6) was still recorded on day 7, but absolutely negative staining for ICAM-1 was always seen 10 days after the onset of rejection and the administration of anti-rejection therapy (Fig. 1). The cytological findings of lymphoid activation in acute liver allograft rejection thus closely correlated with the intensity of ICAM-1 on hepatocytes. However, ICAM-1 induction on hepatocytes preceded the other markers of rejection in the FNAB (Fig. 2).

Discussion

The expression of ICAM-1 on hepatocytes has been demonstrated in biopsy histology during liver rejection [3, 4]. In our study, the frequent FNAB monitoring made it possible to investigate the induction of ICAM-1 expression in relation to immune activation of liver allograft rejection. ICAM-1 induction was recorded at a very early phase of immune activation in the graft. The up-regulation of ICAM-1 even preceded the lymphoid activation.

ICAM-1 and its complementary adhesion molecule LFA-1, expressed on lymphocytes and on other leukocytes, are important in the cell-cell interactions and in T-cell activation at the early phase of inflammatory processes. Also, the antigen presentation of the cells is dependent on ICAM-1, in addition to major histocompatibility complex (MHC), and co-expression of those molecules is needed for T-cell activation [8].

The role of adhesion molecules in the anti-allograft response is thus obvious, as well as the induction of those molecules during the immune activation of rejection. On the other hand, ICAM-1 expression has also been demonstrated in biopsy histology of liver from recipients with bacterial and viral infections [4] and may thus be considered as an unspecific marker of immune processes. Though unspecific, ICAM-1 induction on hepatocytes is an early marker for acute liver allograft rejection in the FNAB.

References

1. Marlin SD, Springer TA (1987) Purified intercellular adhesion molecule-1 (ICAM-1) is a ligand for lymphocyte function associated antigen-1 (LFA-1). Cell 51: 813–819
2. Dustin ML, Staunton DE, Springer TA (1988) Supergene families meet the immune system. Immunol Today 9: 213–215
3. Adams DH, Hubscher SG, Shaw J, Rothlein R, Neuberger JM (1989) Intercellular adhesion molecule 1 on liver allografts during rejection. Lancet II: 1122–1125
4. Steinhoff G, Behrend M, Pichlmayr R (1990) Induction of ICAM-1 on hepatocyte membranes during liver allograft rejection and infection. Transplant Proc 22: 2308–2309
5. Lautenschlager I, Höckerstedt K, Ahonen J, Eklund B, Isoniemi H, Korsbäck C, Pettersson E, Salmela K, Scheinin TM, Willebrand E von, Häyry P (1988) Fine needle aspiration biopsy in the monitoring of liver allografts. II. Applications to human liver allografts. Transplantation 46: 47–53
6. Lautenschlager I, Höckerstedt K, Häyry P (1991) Fine needle aspiration biopsy in the monitoring of liver allografts. Transplant Int 4: 54–61
7. Häyry P, Willebrand E von (1981) Practical guidelines for fine needle aspiration biopsy of human renal allografts. Ann Clin Res 13: 288–306
8. Altman DM, Hogg N, Trowsdale J, Wilkinson D (1989) Cotransfection of ICAM-1 and HLA-DR reconstitutes human antigen-presenting cell function in mouse L cells. Nature 338: 512–514

Transplant Int (1992) 5 [Suppl 1]: S 286–S 289

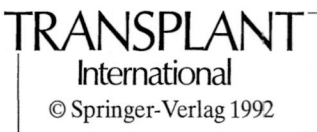

TRANSPLANT
International
© Springer-Verlag 1992

Lung transplantation:
pulmonary cell lysis mediated by alveolar mononuclear cells

A. C. Cunningham, J. A. Kirby, I. W. Colquhoun, and J. H. Dark

Department of Surgery, The Medical School, University of Newcastle upon Tyne NE2 4HH, United Kingdom

Abstract. Methods were developed to monitor graft rejection in a porcine model of unilateral lung transplantation. The ability of peripheral blood mononuclear cells and lavage-derived mononuclear cells to lyse donor pulmonary tissue was determined by standard chromium release assays at various times after transplantation. Effective antigraft activity was observed in the local environment of a rejecting graft, but not in the periphery. Since transplant rejection is a reversible process, with the administration of suitable immunosuppressive regimes frequently restoring graft function, it was reasoned that immunological assays based on the lysis of individual cells may not be relevant to the in vivo situation. We therefore describe an assay of the lung barrier function; perturbations of the tight intraepithelial junctions which compose the air-blood barrier can be determined in vitro by the measurement of transmonolayer resistance values.

Key words: Graft monitoring – Lung transplantation – Alveolar epithelium – Tissue resistance

Monitoring a transplanted organ is essential for the early diagnosis and effective treatment of rejection. Lung grafts can be physically observed by radiography or transbronchial biopsy [1, 2], their function can be monitored or immunological assays can be performed to determine the responsiveness of the recipient's immune system to the donor tissue.

A great deal of interest has been generated in the possibility of using bronchial lavage fluid for the diagnosis of lung allograft rejection. It has been shown that the mononuclear cells present in lavage fluid are recruited from the periphery, that the frequencies of donor-specific cytotoxic T lymphocytes in both the periphery and the local environment of a rejecting rat lung allograft increase after transplantation, and that mononuclear cells present within a lavage are effectively cytotoxic against donor but not

third-party splenic lymphocytes [3–5]. However, it is also clear that the response of the immune system to a foreign graft can often appear similar to that mounted to a pathogen, and consequently great care must be taken in the interpretation of the results.

There are clear advantages in the use of donor graft tissues rather than donor splenic cells for the measurement of recipient anti-donor immunoreactivity. This approach allows responses to both donor tissue-specific and major histocompatibility antigens to be quantified. In this study, we investigated the cytotoxic ability of lavage-derived mononuclear cells (LDMC) and peripheral blood mononuclear cells (PBMC) against donor pulmonary cells in a porcine model of unilateral lung transplantation.

Since acute rejection is frequently a reversible process, immunological assays which measure the irreversible cytolysis of donor cells may not be applicable to in vitro investigation of the clinical situation. We report an assay of pulmonary tissue function which makes use of the fact that the tight junctions between alveolar epithelial cells can be measured in vitro by the determination of transmonolayer electrical resistance values. The interepithelial cell tight junctions are largely responsible for maintaining the blood-air permeability barrier essential for normal lung function [6, 7].

Materials and methods

Single lung transplants were performed in Gottingen minipigs (30–40 kg; Froxfield Farms, Hants, UK). Heart-lung blocks were retrieved from donors following perfusion with modified Euro-Collins solution; the left lung was dissected from the block and transplanted into the recipient (mean ischaemic time of 220 min, $n = 4$). Animals were immunosuppressed with azathioprine, cyclosporin A and prednisolone. The right lung was immersed into RPMI 1640 medium (Northumbria Biologicals, Northumberland, UK) on ice. Within 4 h a 2-cm³ portion of the tissue was chopped and digested overnight by stirring with collagenase (Sigma, Dorset, UK) at 1 mg/ml (w/v) in RPMI 1640 (Northumbria Biologicals). After digestion, the material was washed twice by centrifugation and propagated in D-valine minimal essential medium (Gibco, Renfrewshire, UK) supplemented with 15% (v/v) heat-inactivated fetal calf serum (FCS),

Offprint requests to: Dr. A. C. Cunningham

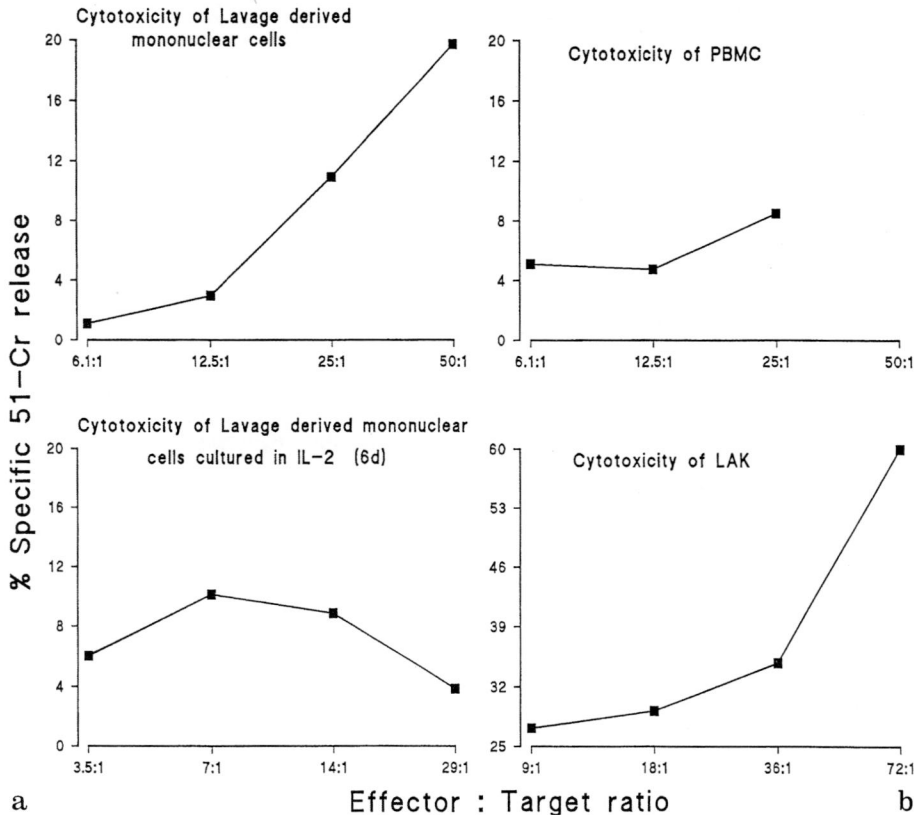

Fig. 1. Specific cytotoxicity of lavage-derived mononuclear cells (LDMC) and peripheral blood mononuclear cells (PBMC) towards pulmonary cells 1 week after transplantation. Each point represents the mean of triplicate determinations. *LAK*, lymphokine-activated killer cells; *IL-2*, interleukin 2

$1 \times 10^{-4} M$ HEPES (Northumbria Biologicals), $2 \times 10^{-3} M$ glutamine (Northumbria Biologicals), 10^5 U/l penicillin (Sigma), 100 mg/l streptomycin (Sigma), insulin-transferrin-sodium selenite (Sigma), $5 \times 10^{-8} M$ hydrocortisone (Sigma) and $3 \times 10^{-8} M$ triiodothyronine (Sigma) at 37 °C in an atmosphere of 5 % CO_2. Cells with a cobblestone morphology were purified by differential detachment using trypsin-ethylene diamine tetra-acetic acid (Northumbria Biologicals). Cell monolayers were cultured on 10-mm diameter tissue culture inserts (Nunc; Gibco, Renfrewshire, UK) by seeding each insert with 5×10^5 cells in 0.5 ml of the D-valine culture medium. Trans-monolayer resistance values were measured using an ohmmeter and 'chopstick' electrodes (Millicell-ERS, Millipore), as described previously [8].

Samples of peripheral blood (collected in sterile universals containing 100 U of heparin; Sigma) and bronchial lavage fluid (obtained by washing with approximately 20 ml RPMI 1640 medium through a fibreoptic bronchoscope wedged into a limiting bronchus of an anaesthetized recipient) were taken from recipient animals at regular intervals after transplantation. PBMC were prepared by centrifugation over a Ficoll-Metrizoate (400 g; Lymphoprep; Nycomed, W. Midlands, UK) density gradient [9]; the interfacial cells were recovered, washed and resuspended in RPMI 1640 culture medium supplemented with 10 % (v/v) heat-inactivated FCS, $1 \times 10^{-4} M$ HEPES and antibiotics. Lymphokine-activated killer (LAK) cells were generated from these by incubation in culture medium supplemented with recombinant interleukin 2 (IL-2) (50 U/ml; Boehringer Mannheim, East Sussex, UK) for 5 days. LDMC were obtained by centrifugation (400 g). Adherent cells (presumably alveolar macrophages) were removed by resuspending the cell pellet in culture medium and incubating in 25-cm³ flasks (Falcon) at 37 °C in a humid atmosphere of 95 % air and 5 % CO_2 for at least 60 min. Donor pulmonary cells were labelled with 200 μCi of $Na_2^{51}CrO_4$ for 90 min, washed twice with RPMI 1640 and once with culture medium, resuspended at 2×10^4/ml and used as the targets in cytotoxicity assays. Effector cells (PBMC, LAK, LDMC or LDMC cultured in 50 U/ml IL-2 for 5 days) were incubated with the chromium-labelled pulmonary target cells at various effector: target ratios for 4 h at 37 °C in round-bottomed microtitre plates (Nunc) in a total volume of 200 μl. The plates were then centrifuged for 5 min at 50 g and

the supernatants harvested for γ-counting (LKB, 1272 Clinnigamma). Maximal chromium release was estimated by lysing the target cells with 10 μl of Triton X-100 followed by freezing and thawing the samples. The cytolytic capacity of each culture was expressed in terms of percentage specific release of ^{51}Cr [10]:

% specific ^{51}Cr release =

$$\frac{(\text{experimental }^{51}Cr \text{ release} - \text{spontaneous }^{51}Cr \text{ release})}{\text{maximal }^{51}Cr \text{ release} - \text{spontaneous }^{51}Cr \text{ releaseright})} \times 100$$

The effects of incubating 2×10^6 LAK or unstimulated porcine splenic cells (in 0.5 ml of culture medium) on the trans-monolayer resistance values of pulmonary cell monolayers cultured on tissue inserts was also determined.

Results

It was demonstrated that LDMC from an animal undergoing rejection were effectively cytotoxic against donor pulmonary cells, whereas PBMC were not. After culture in IL-2 for 5 days, PBMC were capable of lysing the donor pulmonary cells, presumably due to non-specific LAK function. The LDMC were not cytotoxic following culture in IL-2; this may have been due to the inhibitory effects of any pulmonary surfactant or alveolar macrophages remaining in the culture. The results presented in Fig. 1 are from an animal 7 days after transplantation; partial consolidation of the transplanted lung was observed by radiography at that time. One week later, it was demonstrated that the LDMC caused an increase in the maximum specific chromium release liberated from donor pulmonary cells; it had increased from 20 % (Fig. 1) to 40 % (Fig. 2b). However, LDMC from the native lung were also effective-

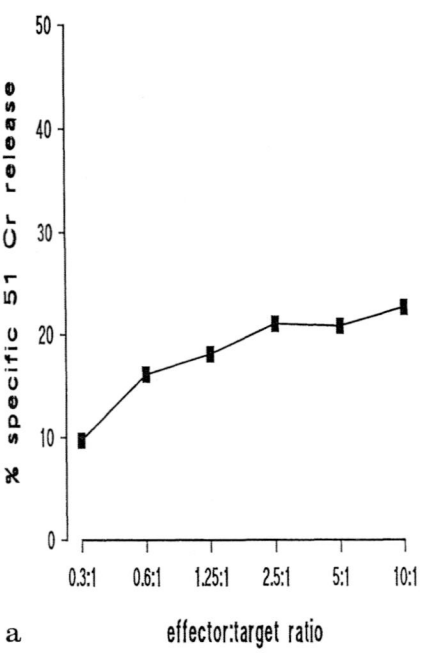

a

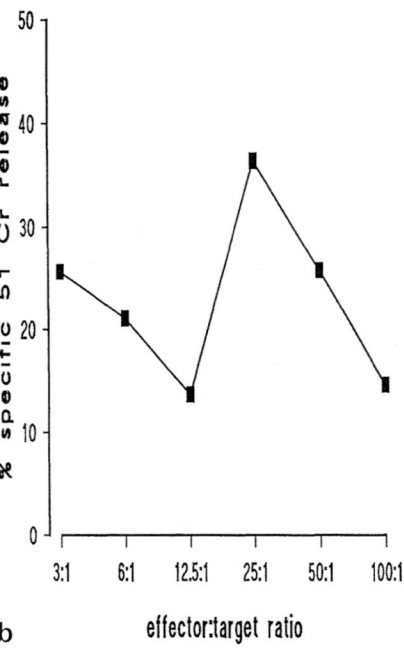

b

Fig. 2. a Specific cytotoxicity of LDMC from the native lung 2 weeks after transplantation. **b** Specific cytotoxicity of LDMC from the allograft 2 weeks post transplant. Each point represents the mean of triplicate determinations

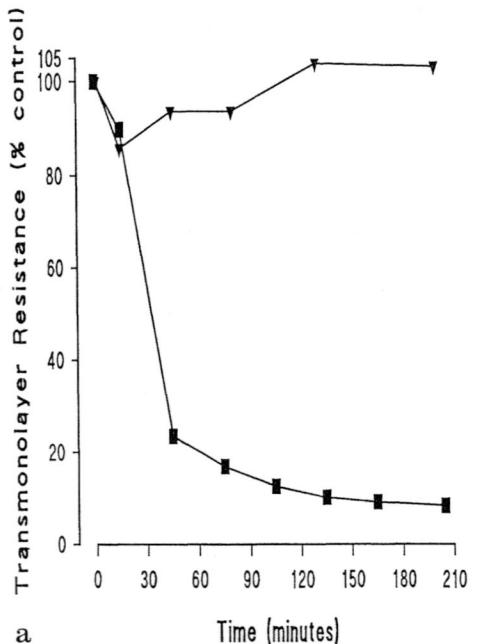

a

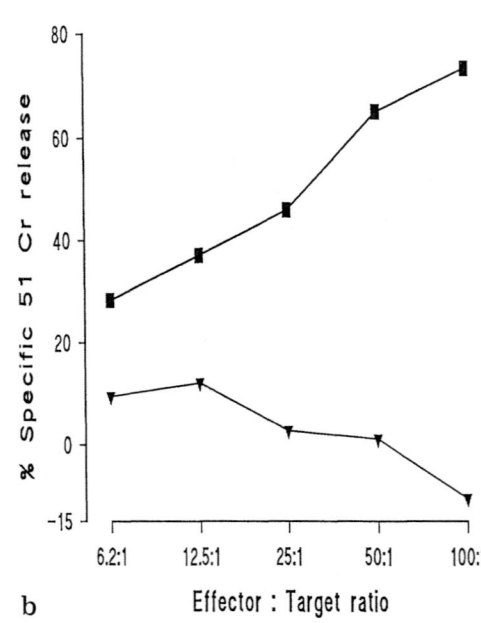

b

Fig. 3. a Representative results showing the effect on transmonolayer resistance values of adding 2×10^6 LAK (■) or porcine splenic cells (▼) to confluent porcine pulmonary cells. **b** Representative results showing the cytotoxicity of LAK cells (■) or splenic mononuclear cells (▼) towards porcine pulmonary cells. Each point represents the mean of triplicate determinations

ly cytotoxic against the donor pulmonary cells (Fig. 2a); subsequent investigation showed that the animal had developed bacterial pneumonia.

Porcine pulmonary cells cultured on inserts developed high trans-monolayer resistance values which generally reached a plateau on the 5th day of culture. At this time, the average value was 5500 Ω. The fact that primary porcine pulmonary cell monolayers produced high trans-monolayer resistance values provides good evidence that this cell population retains epithelioid characteristics.

The addition of LAK cells to the monolayers at an approximate effector: target cell radio of 4:1 caused an 80% reduction in the trans-monolayer resistance values within a 60-min period (Fig. 3a). Control experiments performed with unstimulated splenic mononuclear cells showed no change in resistance. In a standard 4-h chromium release

assay, similar LAK cells caused a 73% specific chromium release at an effector: target cell ratio of 100:1; cytotoxicity was less pronounced at ratio of 6.2:1, with only 28% of the cells being lysed within the assay period (Fig. 3b). Incubation with control splenic lymphocytes resulted in no significant cytolysis (less than 15% specific chromium release).

Discussion

Effective anti-graft cell cytotoxic activity was detected in immune cells derived by lavage of the local environment of a rejecting lung graft, but this activity was not observed in peripheral immune cells. This result indicates the great potential of bronchoalveolar lavage, which allows direct sampling of the active immune cells from within rejecting tissue. However, it was not possible to use these cytotoxicity assays to differentiate between infection and rejection, as LDMC from the infected, non-transplanted lung were also cytotoxic for donor pulmonary cells. It is possible that donor-specific lymphocytes activated during the process of rejection elsewhere in the body were recruited non-specifically to the inflamed site of the infection and were recovered by the lavage technique.

Activated porcine immune cells were capable of impairing the barrier function of cultured pulmonary cells (Fig. 3a); this process reflects dysfunction of the tight junctions between the cells. Unstimulated mononuclear immune cells had no effect on the barrier function of pulmonary cells. These results indicate that in vitro assays of epithelial tissue function may be more relevant to the analysis of the pulmonary rejection process, since the measurement of cytotoxic activity by the standard chromium release assays simply reflects the lysis of individual cells.

Acknowledgements. We are grateful to the Chest, Heart and Stroke Association and the Moorgate Trust Fund for providing financial support of this work.

References

1. Higenbottam T, Stewart S, Penketh A, Wallwork J (1988) Transbronchial lung biopsy for the diagnosis of rejection in heart-lung transplant patients. Transplantation 46: 532–539

2. Slieman C, Groussard O, Mal H, Duchatelle J-P, Dubois F, Darne C, Baldeyrou P, Jebrak G (1991) Clinical use of transbronchial biopsy in single lung transplantation. Transplantation 51: 927–928

3. Kirby JA, Wood A, Reader JA, Isted K, Hynd J, Hawkes D, Hudson L, Pepper JR (1985) Origin and immunological hyporeactivity of canine alveolar lymphocytes. Immunology 55: 531–537

4. Kirby JA, Pepper JR, Reader JA, Corbishley CM, Hudson L (1986) Precursor frequency of donor-specific lymphocytes recovered from canine lung transplants. Clin Exp Immunol 63: 334–342

5. Kirby JA, Parfett GJ, Reader JA, Pepper JR (1988) Lung transplantation in the rat: a model for study of the cellular mechanisms of allograft rejection. Immunology 63: 369–372

6. Rochat T, Casale J, Hunninghake GW, Peterson MW (1988) Neutrophil cathepsin G increases permeability of cultured type II pneumocytes. Am J Physiol 255: C603–C611

7. Cheek JM, Kim K-J, Crandall ED (1989) Tight monolayers of rat alveolar epithelial cells: bioelectric properties and active sodium transport. Am J Physiol 256: C688–C693

8. Kirby JA, Morgan JC, Shenton BK, Lennard TWJ, Proud G, Taylor RMR (1991) Renal allograft rejection: functional impairment of kidney epithelial cell monolayers mediated by lymphokine-activated killer cells and by complement. Transplantation 51: 891–895

9. Boyum A (1968) A one-stage procedure for the isolation of granulocytes and lymphocytes from human blood: general sedimentation properties of white blood cells in a 1 g gravity field. Scand J Clin Lab Invest 21 [Suppl 97]: 77

10. Brunner KT, Mauel J, Cerrotini J-C, Chapuis B (1968) Quantitative assay on immune lymphoid cells on 51-chromium labelled allogeneic targets in vitro: inhibition by isoantibody and by drugs. Immunology 14: 181–187

Transplant Int (1992) 5 [Suppl 1]: S 290–S 295

TRANSPLANT
International
© Springer-Verlag 1992

Nonspecific hemolytic effector of activated macrophages as activation marker of allograft rejection

M. Ishibashi, A. Moutabarrik, H. Kameoka, Y. Takano, H. Jiang, Y. Kokado, and S. Takahara

Department of Urology, Osaka University Medical School, Osaka, Japan

Abstract. The aim was to assess a nonspecific hemolytic effector of activated monocytes/macrophages, designated spontaneous plaque-forming cell (SPFC), as an activation marker in allograft rejection. An in vitro study on the immunologic characteristics of SPFC monocytes in man and an in vivo study in Lewis rats as to the monitoring of SPFC generation of allograft infiltrating cells with or without immunosuppression were conducted. Hemolysis of SPFC was mediated by CR3 adhesion molecules, detected by Mo-1 and OKM10 monoclonal antibodies. Hemolysis of SPFC was nonspecific, and nonrosette-forming T cells with autologous erythrocytes (non-ARFC-T) acted as suppressor T cells inhibiting SPFC-hemolysis against autologous erythrocytes. A 6-day course of immunosuppression with a daily dose of cyclosporin A (CyA) 10 mg/kg and of FK506 1 mg/kg suppressed the SPFC generation to the level of syngeneic control. In contrast, peak SPFC generation coincided with rejection, and the degree of SPFC generation reflected the grade of histoincompatibility. The present findings suggested that SPFC-activated monocytes/macrophages may be one of the activation markers in allograft rejection and lead to a new concept of graft rejection and self or nonself discrimination mediated by nonspecific, hemolytic SPFC effectors and suppressor T cells inhibiting autoreactivity.

Key words: Activated monocytes/macrophages – Hemolysis – Complement receptor 3 (CR3) of adhesion molecules – Allograft rejection – Self or non-self discrimination

As immunologic activation markers of allograft rejection, interleukin 2 (IL-2) receptor expression [4, 14, 21], major histocompatibility complex (MHC) expression [5], release of cytokines such as interferon-γ or TNF-α/β from activated T cells [15, 3], and activated macrophages were studied in rats and man [4, 6, 16, 17]. We found a new effector of activated monocytes or macrophages in man [7–11] and designated it spontaneous plaque-forming cell, SPFC, because SPFC undergoes hemolysis nonspecifically and without the addition of exogenous complement. The involvement of SPFC in human renal allograft rejection [10] and the suppression of SPFC generation by various immunosuppressive agents in normal human subjects [11] were reported.

The activated macrophage is one of the activation markers in allograft rejection in rats and man [4, 6, 16, 17]. However, since the definite immunologic understanding of cytolysis by activated macrophages is obscure, any strategy for the suppression of activated macrophages is not immediately forthcoming. We have detected SPFC in rats [12, 18]. Human SPFC is reproducible in allogeneic stimulation in vitro [9] and may be an objective tool in studying immunologic characteristics of activated monocytes or macrophages in vitro or in vivo.

To assess the role of the SPFC of activated monocytes/macrophages in allograft rejection, two kinds of experiments were performed. In one, the in vitro immunologic characteristics of the SPFC-monocyte effector of activated monocytes/macrophages in man was studied, and in the other, in vivo SPFC generation in rat allograft rejection with or without immunosuppression was attempted. These studies have demonstrated that a new concept of self or nonself discrimination can be proposed by understanding the immunologic characteristics of the SPFC effector and that SPFC might be one of the activation markers in allograft rejection.

Materials and methods

The spontaneous plaque-forming cell assay was described previously [9, 11]. Autologous or allogeneic target erythrocytes in a monolayer and effector cells, approximately $5–10 \times 10^3$, were mixed and incubated at 37°C for 3 h in a microplate using serum-free Hanks' solution for the SPFC assay, and then the number of hemolytic plaques

Offprint requests to: Dr. M. Ishibashi, Department of Urology, Osaka University Medical School, Fukushima 1-1-50, Fukushima-ku, Osaka 553, Japan

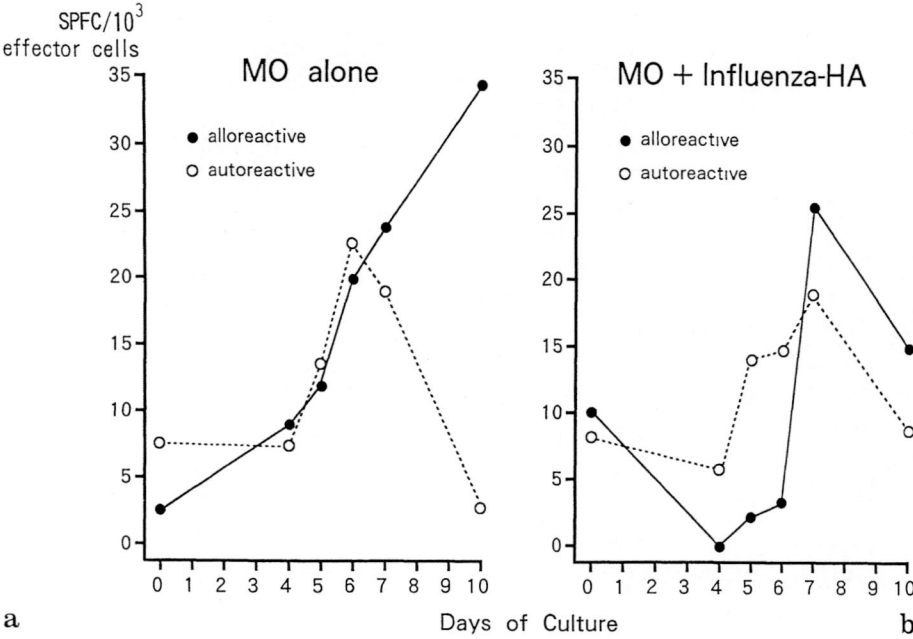

Fig. 1. Kinetics of spontaneous plaque-forming cells (SPFC) generation, in vitro, of monocytes *(MO)* enriched alone (with antigen) and monocytes enriched with influenza hemagglutinin *(HA)*, containing 14 chick cell hemagglutinins. Enriched monocytes of normal subjects, suspended in RPMI1640 supplemented with 20 % AB serum, were cultured, and the number of SPFC generated in cultured monocytes were determined against autologous and allogeneic erythrocytes

(SPFC) was determined under an inverted microscope. The number of SPFC per 10^6 effector cells was calculated.

Monoclonal antibody (mAb) Mo-1(904) (IgG1), directed against the α-chain (CD11b) of CR3 [13], was a gift of Dr. J. Griffin (Dana-Farber Cancer Center, Boston, Mass.); mAb OKM10 (IgG2b), directed against the α-chain (CD11b) [23], was a gift of Dr. P. Rao (Ortho Pharmaceutical, Raritan, N.J.); and mAb 3G8 (IgG1), directed against the low avidity Fc receptor of neutrophils (FcRIII, CD16) [1] was purchased from Medarex. The F(ab')$_2$ of mAB Mo-1 was prepared by Dr. T. Kinoshita (Osaka University Medical School, Suita, Osaka, Japan).

Rats and skin transplantation. The H-1 incompatible combination of ACI and Lewis and the H-1 compatible combination of F344 and Lewis were selected. A 9-week-old male Lewis rat was the recipient of the allograft skin transplantation, and a male ACI or F344 rat of the same age was the donor. The procedure of skin transplantation was described previously [18].

Immunosuppressive agents. Cyclosporin was a gift of Sandoz Pharmaceutical (Basel, Switzerland), FK506 was a gift of Fujisawa Pharmaceutical (Osaka, Japan), and prednisolone was a gift of Shionogi & Co. (Osaka, Japan). Immunosuppressive agents were administered subcutaneously for 6 days from day 0 to day 5 after skin transplantation. Each agent was mixed with arabic gum and saline to a final concentration of 5%.

Cell preparation. Peripheral blood mononuclear cells (PBMC) of normal human subjects or of rats were separated by Ficoll-Conray (d = 1.078) gradient centrifugation. Human enriched monocytes (MO) and T lymphocytes were fractionated by Percoll discontinuous gradient centrifugation. Rosette-forming T cells with autologous erythrocytes (ARFC-T) or MO cells were fractionated by the method of Tomonari et al. [20]. Allograft infiltrating cells were separated by the enzymatic methods described previously [18].

Results

I. Immunologic characteristics of the SPFC-monocyte effector of activated monocytes/macrophages in man

To evaluate the SPFC-monocyte effectors of activated monocytes or macrophages involved in allograft rejection, the mechanism of nonspecific hemolysis of SPFC-effectors was investigated. Secondly, since nonspecific hemolysis of SPFC is also autoreactive, the mechanism of self or nonself discrimination preventing hemolysis against autologous erythrocytes in SPFC-effector limbs was studied. Thirdly, T-cell-dependent and T-cell-independent SPFC generation in vitro was demonstrated.

Table 1. SPFC generation in vitro was regulated in a T-lymphocyte-dependent or T-lymphocyte-independent manner. Autorosette-forming cells of T cells (ARFC-T) as helper cells and non-ARFC-T as suppressor cells acted on SPFC generation. SPFC effectors of monocytes were generated without participation of T lymphocytes, and enrichment of ARFC in the monocyte culture resulted in loss of SPFC generation

	Coculture of monocytes and T cells for 7 days (ratio of MO to T = 1:5)	SPFC generation per 10^6 cultured cells	
T-cell-dependent SPFC generation		Autoreactive	Alloreactive
	MO + unfractionated T cells	2333	1417
	MO + ARFCT cells	11467	16513
	MO + non-ARFC-T cells	333	500
T-cell-independent SPFC generation	Culture of monocytes, fractionated or not, for 7 days		
	MO alone	10500	4333
	ARFC-MO alone	0	0
	non-ARFC-MO alone	11000	21500

Table 2. Suppressor activity (%) of nonautorosette-forming T cells (non-ARFC-T) against autoreactive hemolysis of SPFC. Autoreactive SPFC were selectively inhibited by non-ARFC-T

Nonspecific SPFC effector	Ratio of cultured MO as effector to non-ARFC-T as suppressor cells	
	1:1	5:1
Autoreactive SPFC	100.0%	92.0%
Alloreactive SPFC	100.0%	−8.3%

T-cell-dependent or -independent SPFC generation in vitro. The SPFC are generated in vitro in 6–7 days of culture with or without antigen stimulation, and only monocytes are differentiated into SPFC effectors of activated monocytes or macrophages (Fig. 1). On the 7th day of culture, the peak of SPFC generation, which showed nonspecific hemolysis, was found in monocytes cultured with influenza virus or without antigen. On day 10 of culture, the SPFC generated in monocytes cultured alone showed spontaneously diminished autoreactivity and augmented alloreactivity, while the SPFC generated in monocytes cultured with influenza virus showed a different reactivity profile except for the same peak of nonspecific reactivity. The reactivity found in the present study suggested the presence of regulating cells among the monocytes.

As shown in Table 1, SPFC were generated by different regulating cells, i.e., rosette-forming T cells with autologous erythrocytes (ARFC-T) as helper cells or non-ARFC-T as suppressor cells which regulate SPFC generation, and monocytes themselves, independently of T cells. A fraction of ARFC receptor-bearing monocytes resulted in the loss of SPFC generation, which suggests that ARFC receptor-bearing monocytes might be suppressor monocytes. The SPFC showed nonspecific hemolysis against autologous and allogeneic target erythrocytes.

Nonautorosette-forming T lymphocytes inhibiting autoreactive SPFC-hemolysis. Erythrocytes have the function of clearing pathogens, and a nonspecific SPFC effector against erythrocytes is useful for clearing erythrocytes with pathogens. Meanwhile, any persisting autoreactivity of SPFC might be harmful to autologous tissues such as vascular endothelium bearing erythrocyte antigens. In Table 2, the suppressor activity of nonauto-rosette-forming T cells (non-ARFC-T) against autoreactive SPFC is shown. Since one non-ARFC-T inhibited five SPFC effector cells, it was as effective as suppressor T cells. Figure 1 suggests that suppressor monocytes might participate in preventing the autoreactivity of SPFC.

Complement-receptor 3 of adhesion molecules involved in nonspecific hemolysis of SPFC-monocyte effector. CR3-adhesion molecules (CD11b/CD18) bind iC3b [23], zymosan, lipopolysaccharide (LPS) [22], and erythrocytes [19] as ligands. CR3 expresses two different epitopes [24], one that binds LPS or erythrocytes and is recognized by Mo-1 mAb and the other that recognizes iC3b and other proteinaceous ligands and is recognized by OKM10 mAb. We determined whether the mAb of Mo-1, Mo-1-F(ab')$_2$ or OKM10 was able to inhibit hemolysis of SPFC in the SPFC assay (Table 3). The numbers of SPFC

against autologous and allogeneic erythrocytes as target were suppressed by the Mo-1 and OKM10 mAb, respectively. The F(ab')$_2$-Mo-1 mAb also suppressed the hemolysis of SPFC. The inhibition of hemolysis of SPFC effectors generated in allogeneic stimulation was greater than that generated without antigen stimulation. The results confirmed that the epitope of CR3 recognized by the Mo-1 mAb binds directly to the erythrocyte, and the binding results in hemolysis by H_2O_2 released from activated SPFC-monocyte effectors.

II. Allograft rejection and SPFC response in rats

An SPFC was also demonstrated in PBMC and infiltrating cells of rejecting allograft, and not in the spleen, of rats. To assess the involvement of SPFC-monocyte effectors in allograft rejection, monitoring of the SPFC generation in the infiltrating cells of transplanted allograft skin with or without immunosuppression was performed.

Concomitant SPFC generation with skin allograft rejection and with histoincompatibility. The mean allograft survival times of the H-1 incompatible ACI-Lewis combination and the H-1 compatible F344-Lewis combination were 7.67 ± 0.82 and 10.50 ± 3.27 days, respectively. The kinetics of SPFC generation after skin transplantation is shown in Fig. 2. In the ACI-Lewis combination, the peak number of SPFC of infiltrating cells, separated from rejecting allograft skin, was $23\,850 \pm 1340 \times 10^6$ on day 6 after transplantation, and the day of peak SPFC generation coincided with the onset of acute irreversible rejection. In the F344-Lewis combination, the peak SPFC response was seen on days 6 and 10. Since two of the three allografts harvested on day 6 were rejected and all skin allografts studied on day 10 were rejected, it was likely that the pattern of SPFC generation was biphasic. The peak number of SPFC on day 10 was $11\,606 \pm 4235 \times 10^6$, and there was a significant difference in the peak number of SPFC between the ACI-Lewis and F344-Lewis combinations ($P < 0.05$, Student's t-test). As to the SPFC response of PBMC, the peak SPFC generation (3893 ± 1273 SPFC $\times 10^6$) of PBMC in the ACI-Lewis combination was seen on day 6 and that ($13\,440 \pm 3484 \times 10^6$) of

Table 3. CR3 (complement receptor 3, CD11b/CD18) involved in hemolysis of SPFC-monocyte effectors in man. Monoclonal antibodies Mo-1, Mo-1-F(ab')$_2$, or OKM10 at various dilutions were added and incubated for SPFC assay. The 50% suppression level of the number of SPFC per 10^6 effectors was expressed as IC 50 (ng/ml). As effector cells, an allogeneic PBMC mixture cultured for 7 days or antigen-unprimed cultured PBMC were used

Monoclonal antibody against CR3	Ligand	IC 50 (ng/ml) Suppression of SPFC by monoclonal antibody	
		Allo-MLC primed effector	Unprimed effector
Mo-1	LPS/RBC	43	167
MO-1-F(ab')$_2$		21	167
OKM 10	iC3b	84	167
3G8	FcRIII	>333	333

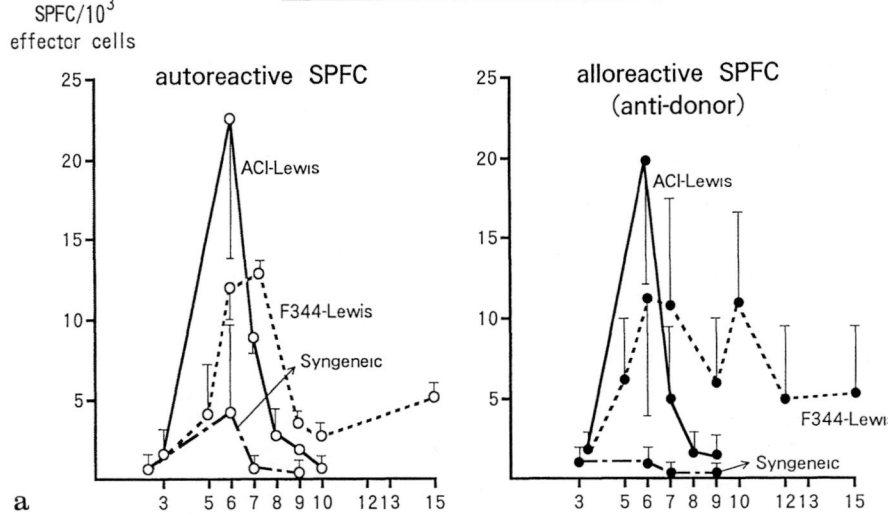

Graft Infiltrating Cells

SPFC/10³ effector cells

autoreactive SPFC

alloreactive SPFC (anti-donor)

ACI-Lewis

F344-Lewis

Syngeneic

a

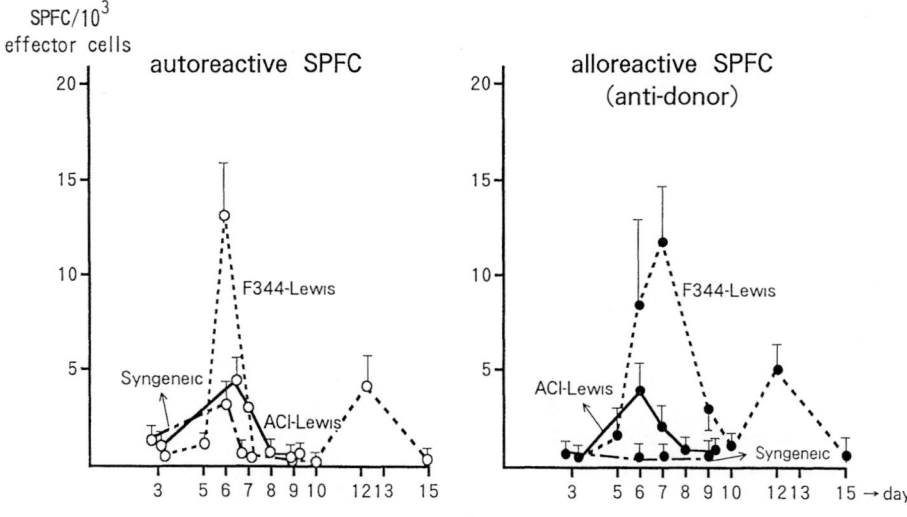

P B M C

SPFC/10³ effector cells

autoreactive SPFC

alloreactive SPFC (anti-donor)

F344-Lewis

Syngeneic

ACI-Lewis

b

Days after Transplantation

Fig. 2. Kinetics of SPFC generation, in vivo of graft infiltrating cells or PBMC of recipient Lewis rats receiving ACI H-1 incompatible (ACI-Lewis ———), F344 H-1 compatible (F344-Lewis -----), or syngeneic (Lewis-Lewis · · · · ·) skin transplantation. Autoreactive and alloreactive SPFC effectors of graft infiltrating cells and PBMC are shown

PBMC in the F344-Lewis combination was also found on day 6. In the syngeneic Lewis combination, the mean number of SPFC ($3190 \pm 4294 \times 10^6$) was observed on day 6, though the number of SPFC was smaller than that in both allogeneic combinations. Therefore, the extent of SPFC generation of allograft cellular infiltration following allograft transplantation reflected the grade of histoincompatibility.

Like the SPFC in man, the SPFC found in rats also showed nonspecific hemolysis against autologous and allogeneic RBC. In heart transplantation in the ACI-Lewis combination, the same tendency was observed between peak SPFC generation on day 5 and onset of acute rejection.

Suppression of SPFC generation by administration of immunosuppressive agents. A 6-day course of subcutaneous administration of immunosuppressive agents, cyclosporine 10 mg/kg daily, FK506 1 mg/kg daily, or predniso-

lone 10 mg/kg daily, was given, and the SPFC generation of allograft cellular infiltrating cells was monitored. Both cyclosporine and FK506 were able to prolong allograft skin survival by more than 21 days in the ACI-Lewis combination. Prednisolone prolonged allograft skin survival by fewer than 3 days, both compared with untreated cases. Figure 3 shows that the SPFC generation of infiltrating cells harvested on day 6 was completely suppressed by cyclosporine and FK506 to the level of a syngeneic, untreated transplantation. Meanwhile, prednisolone showed a weak inhibitory effect on SPFC generation in graft infiltrating cells and in PBMC. The suppression of SPFC generation in PBMC following allograft skin transplantation coincided with that of graft infiltrating cells. These results suggested that potent immunosuppressants which inhibit T-cell activation, such as cyclosporine and FK506, but not prednisolone, were able to suppress the SPFC generation ability of graft cellular infiltrating cells as well as of PBMC.

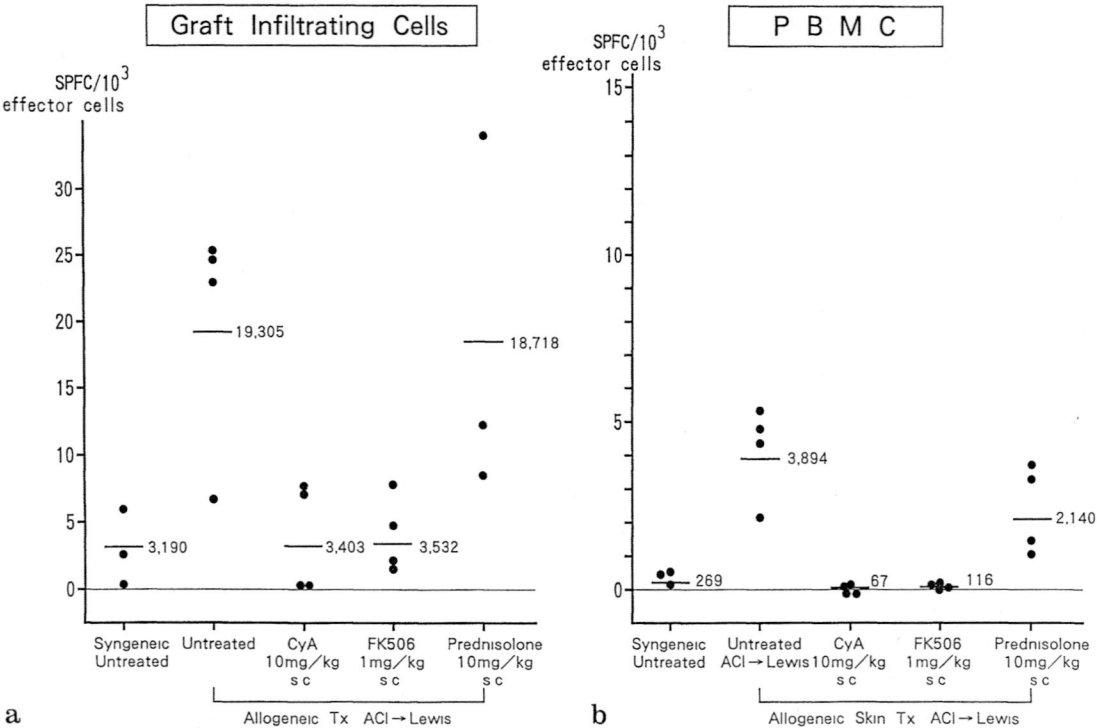

Fig.3. Effect of immunosuppressive drugs on SPFC generation in ACI-Lewis skin allograft transplantation. Cyclosporine *(CyA)*, FK506, or prednisolone, respectively, was administered for a 6-day course of subcutaneous treatment on days 0–5 after transplantation. On day 6, the number of SPFC generated per 10^6 of graft infiltrating cells or PBMC was determined

Discussion

Activated macrophages were reported as one of the activation markers of allograft rejection in man and in rats. SPFC represent a unique effector of activated monocytes or macrophages in that nonspecific hemolysis by SPFC is mediated by the direct recognition of erythrocyte antigens or iC3b on tissues via an epitope of the CR3-adhesion molecule. The immunologic mechanism of graft destruction by activated macrophages might be explained by the concept of a network for the regulation of SPFC generation. In the effector phase of activated macrophages, SPFC recognize antigenic determinants of erythrocytes on the vascular endothelium via an epitope of CR3 expressed on the SPFC with or without local complement activation on the target endothelial tissues. Though the SPFC undergo hemolysis, nonspecifically releasing H_2O_2, suppressor T lymphocytes (detected as non-ARFC-T) or suppressor monocytes might inhibit autoreactive SPFC effectors. If the determinants of erythrocytes expressed on the allograft which are recognized by CR3 molecules are close to those of self-erythrocytes, acceptance of allograft tissues might be easily induced by the participation of suppressor cells. According to the present concept of self or nonself discrimination on the effector level as described by nonspecific SPFC effector and suppressor cells inhibiting autoreactivity, the mechanism of allograft rejection or acceptance might be clarified.

Furthermore, the SPFC have the heterogenous function of effector cells, because they express different epitopes of CR3 for iC3b and erythrocytes. Local complement activation on target tissue, either in the absence or in the presence of antibody, forms iC3b, and SPFC binds to target tissues via CR3 molecules to iC3b and erythrocytes on targets and finally undergoes hemolysis or induces cytolysis. Since the SPFC express a Fc receptor, binding of the SPFC with antibody across the target tissue might induce phagocytosis or cytolysis.

The SPFC generation is regulated in a T-lymphocyte-dependent or T-lymphocyte-independent manner in man. As to the regulation of SPFC generation in rats, the present findings revealed that the degree of SPFC generation reflected the grade of histoincompatibility, which induces T-cell activation to various degrees, and that potent immunosuppressants which inhibit T-cell activation suppressed SPFC generation of allograft infiltration. It is suggested that SPFC generation is also regulated by T cells in rats. Our previous study [12] as to the effect of FK506 on SPFC generation in rats also demonstrated that a dose of FK506 of less than 0.3 mg/kg daily suppressed graft infiltration of the SPFC but failed to suppress SPFC generation of the PBMC. Also, tumor necrosis factor (TNF)-β [2], released from activated T cells and promoting the accumulation of inflammatory cells in inflammatory sites, might be involved in the regulation of SPFC generation of graft infiltrating cells. Therefore, nonspecific SPFC-monocytes might be one of the activation markers of allograft rejection.

References

1. Fleit HB, Wright SD, Unkeless JC (1982) Human neutrophile Fcr receptor distribution and structure. Proc Natl Acad Sci USA 79: 3275–3279

2. Gamble JR, Harlan JM, Klebanoff SJ, Vadas MA (1985) Stimulation of the adherence of neutrophils to umbilical vein endothelium by human recombinant tumor necrosis factor. 82: 8667–8671

3. Halloran PF, Cockfield SM, Madrenas J (1989) The mediators of inflammation (interleukin 1, interferon-r, and tumor necrosis factor) and their relevance to rejection. Transplant Proc 21: 26–30

4. Hancock WW, Lord RH, Colby AJ, Diamanstein T, Rickles FR, Diskstora C, Hogg NZ, Tilney NL (1987) Identification of IL-2R T cells and macrophages within rejecting rat cardiac allografts, and comparison of the effects of treatment with anti-IL2R monoclonal antibody or cyclosporine. J Immunol 138: 164–170

5. Harris HW, Gill TJ III (1986) Expression of class I transplantation antigens. Transplantation 42: 109–117

6. Häyry P, Willebrand E von, Parthenais E, Nemlander A, Soots A, Lautenschlager I, Alfordy P, Renkonen R (1984) Immunol Rev 77: 85–142

7. Ishibashi M, Ichikawa Y, Sagawa S, Takaha M, Sonoda T, Inou K (1984) Immunologic studies of red cell antigens in the renal transplant patient. Transplant Proc 16: 1509–1511

8. Ishibashi M, Ichikawa Y, Takaha M, Sonoda T (1985) Monocyte-mediated hemolytic response in renal transplant patients. Transplant Proc 17: 2644–2647

9. Ishibashi M, Kokado Y, Takahara S, Ichikawa Y, Sonoda T (1987) Cellular immune response agaist human red blood cell antigens and renal allograft rejection. Transplant Proc 19: 4511–4515

10. Ishibashi M, Kokado Y, Takahara S, Ichikawa Y, Sonoda T (1988) Novel effector monocyte against human RBC antigens invading rejected renal allograft. Transplant Proc 20: 285–288

11. Ishibashi M, Jiang H, Kokado Y, Takahara S, Sonoda T (1989) Immunopharmacologic effect of immunosuppressive agents explored by a new effector-monocyte generation assay. Transplant Proc 21: 1854–1858

12. Ishibashi M, Moutabarrik A, Kameoka H, Takano Y, Jiang H, Kokado Y, Takahara S, Sonoda T (1991) Effect of FK506 on generation of activated macrophages invading rejected skin allografts in rats: discrepancy of in vitro versus in vivo effect of FK506. Transplant Proc (in press)

13. Letvin NL, Todd RR III, Palley LS, Schlossman SF, Griffin JD (1983) Conservation of myeloid surface antigens on primate granulocytes. Blood 61: 408–410

14. Lord RHH, Padberg WM, Hancock WW, Kupiec-Weglinski JW, Tilney NL (1989) Correlation of macrophage and NK cell numbers with "activation markers" in rat cardiac allografts. Transplant Proc 21: 449–450

15. Lowley RP, Magghesco DM, Blackburn JH (1985) Immune mechanisms in organ allograft rejection. IV. Delayed-type hypersensitivity. Immunol Rev 77: 167–184

16. Macoherson GC, Christmas SE (1984) The role of the macrophage in cardiac allograft rejection in the rat. Immunol Rev 77: 143–166

17. Mason DW, Dallman MJ, Arthur RP, Morris PJ (1984) Mechanisms of allograft rejection: the roles of cytotoxic T-cells and delayed-type hypersensitivity. Immunol Rev 77: 167–184

18. Moutabarrik A, Ishibashi M, Kameoka H, Takahara S, Kokado Y, Jiang H, Takano Y, Sonoda T (1992) Monocyte hemolytic activity as an immunologic indicator of allograft rejection in rat skin transplantation. Transplant Proc (in press)

19. Ross GD, Cain JA, Lachman PJ (1985) Membrane complement receptor type three (CR3) has lectin-like properties analogous to bovine conglutinin and functions as a receptor for zymosan and rabbit erythrocytes as well as a receptor for iC3b. J Immunol 134: 3307–3315

20. Tomonari K, Wakisaka A, Aizawa M (1980) Self recognition by autologous mixed lymphocyte reaction-primed cells. J Immunol 125: 1596–1602

21. Uchiyama T, Broder S, Waldmann TA (1981) A monoclonal antibody (anti-Tac) reactivity with activated and functionally mature human T cells. I. Production of anti-Tac monoclonal antibody and distribution of Tac(+) cells. J Immunol 126: 1393–1397

22. Wright SD, Jong MTC (1986) Adhesion-promoting receptors on human macrophages recognize *Escherichia coli* by binding to lipopolysaccharide. J Exp Med 164: 1876–1888

23. Wright SD, Rao PE, Van Voorhis WC, Craigmyle LC, Iida MA, Talle MA, Westberg EF, Goldstein G, Silverstein SC (1983) Identification of the C3bi receptor on human monocytes and macrophages by using monoclonal antibodies. Proc Natl Acad Sci USA 80: 5699–5703

24. Wright SD, Levin SM, Jong MTC, Chad Z, Kabbash LG (1989) CR3 (CD11b/CD18) expresses one binding site for Arg-Gly-Asp-containing peptides and a second site for bacterial lipopolysaccharide. J Exp Med 169: 175–183

Transplant Int (1992) 5 [Suppl 1]: S 296–S 299

TRANSPLANT
International
© Springer-Verlag 1992

Relation of suppressor activity to lymphocyte subsets, in vitro IL-2R expression, and biopsy results in cardiac transplant patients

N. Schnitzler[1], H. Völker[2], B. Geörger[1], H.-G. Leusch[1], and S. Markos-Pusztai[1]

[1] Institute of Medical Immunology, [2] Medical Clinic I, Medical Faculty of the Technical University Aachen, Aachen, Federal Republic of Germany

Abstract. Nonspecific suppressor activity of peripheral blood mononuclear cells (PBMC) was determined from 8 patients preoperatively and 22 patients subsequent to heart transplantation. Whereas no correlation was found between any defined lymphocyte subsets, in vitro interleukin-2 (IL-2) production, and IL-2R expression, or biopsy-proven rejection and suppressor cell activity when data obtained on the same day as the suppressor assay were analysed, the phytohemagglutinin – but not the concanavalin A induced, in vitro IL-2 production – was significantly enhanced ($P < 0.02$) in patients with evidence of concomitant rejection. In contrast, a significant correlation between diminished, nonspecific suppression and rejection was found when the results of biopsies performed up to 2 ($P < 0.0075$) and 4 ($P < 0.0033$) weeks after the investigation of suppressor cell activity were compared. We conclude that periodic determination of the suppressor functional status may be useful to discriminate between patients at low or high risk for graft rejection after heart transplantation.

Key words: Nonspecific suppressor function – Interleukin 2 production – Rejection – Heart transplantation

Suppressor cells play important regulatory roles in the feedback control of immunological functions and, among other factors, a privotal role in transplantation tolerance. Nonspecific suppressor mechanisms have been demonstrated to act under a variety of experimental circumstances, including some that are of potential clinical relevance. Suppressor cells and specific and nonspecific suppressor functions were demonstrated using different cell systems in allograft recipients [3, 5, 14]. In addition, a reduced B-cell response after mitogenic stimulation, probably due to T suppressor cells, indicated a good graft acceptance in renal transplant patients [16]. Furthermore, after cadaveric kidney transplantation, cyclosporin-treated recipients showed a preserved suppressor function and a significantly lower incidence of acute rejection episodes when compared with patients on azathioprine and antilymphocyte serum [2].

In the course of monitoring the lymphocytes of cardiac transplant patients, we found that analysis of circulating cell subsets has only a restricted value in the diagnosis of rejection because of the high individual variability, although a high and constant level of CD57 and CD8 coexpressing cells showed a significant correlation ($P < 0.025$) with the number of rejection episodes (unpublished data). It was suggested that this natural killer (NK) cell subset represents an immature stage in the NK lineage, is much less efficient in the cytotoxic assay than $CD8^- CD57^+$ cells [1], and can also mediate suppression in different in vitro systems such as to act as suppressors of B-cell differentiation [13].

These results altogether prompted us to examine the inducibility of suppressor cell activity in the peripheral blood mononuclear cells (PBMC) of patients after heart transplantation. In addition, the correlation between cytoimmunological data, in vitro interleukin 2 (IL-2) production, and in vitro expression of IL-2 receptors (IL-2R) on T cells and the results of the suppressor assays in relation to graft rejection was analysed.

Materials and methods

A total of 144 consecutive biopsies were obtained from 22 heart allograft recipients. The patients received cyclosporin, azathioprine, and prednisone for baseline immunosuppression. At the time of the biopsy, venous blood samples were collected in heparinized tubes. Biopsy results were graded according to Kemnitz et al. [8].

Enumeration of lymphocyte subsets. Two colour fluorescence analysis was performed with the whole blood technique on a FACScan cytometer (Becton Dickinson) using monoclonal reagents directly conjugated either with fluorescein or phycoerythrin.

Offprint requests to: Prof. S. Markos-Pusztai, Institute of Medical Immunology, Medical Faculty, Pauwelsstrasse 30, W-5100 Aachen, Federal Republic of Germany

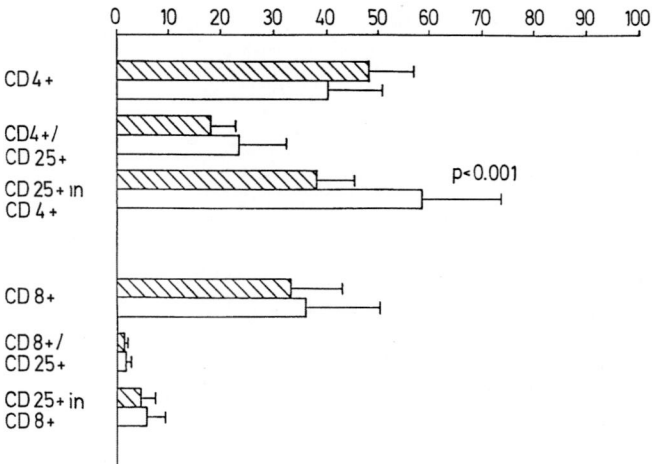

Fig. 1. Comparison of percentages (mean ± 1 SD) of CD4+, CD4+/CD25+, CD8+, and CD8+/CD25+ cells as well as the calculated proportion of the CD25+ cells within the CD4+ and CD8+ subsets in patients preoperatively ⊠ and after heart transplantation ▢. Number of specimens analysed was 8 and 32, respectively

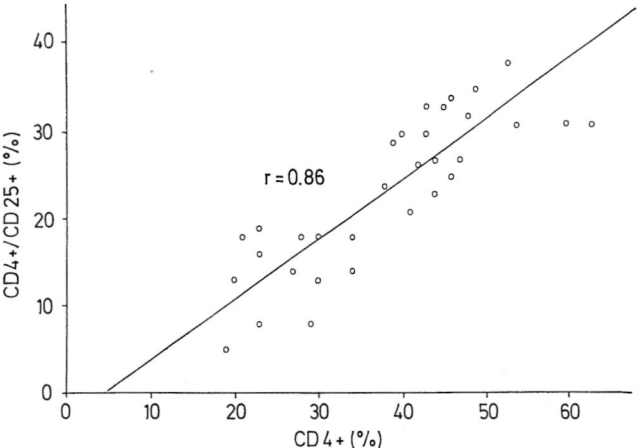

Fig. 2. Correlation between frequencies of the CD4+ cells and the IL-2R (CD25+)-expressing CD4+ cells

For cell culture methods PBMC were fractionated from the heparinized blood by Ficoll-Hypacue centrifugation. Cells were cultured in tissue culture medium consisting of RPMI 1640 supplemented with penicillin 100 U/ml, streptomycin 100 μg/ml, 2 mM glutamine, and 10% human AB serum.

IL-2 production and assay. For IL-2 production, PBMC (10^6/ml) were cultured in 12×75 mm culture tubes with and without 5 μg/ml phytohemagglutinin (PHA) or concanavalin A (ConA). After 24 h at 37°C in 5% CO_2 in air, the culture supernatant was harvested and frozen at −70°C until assayed. The indicator cells for measuring the IL-2 activity of the supernatants were of IL-2-dependent PHA blasts and prepared as previously described [11]. For the assay, indicator cells (100 μl; 4×10^5/ml) were placed in microtiter plates with a serial dilution of either the supernatants or recombinant IL-2 (Boehringer Mannheim, FRG). Cultures were incubated for 48 h at 37°C in 5% CO_2, and proliferation was measured by the incorporation of tritiated thymidine (Amersham) (0.5 μCi/well) over the last 16 h of the culture period. Results were expressed in U/ml by comparison with the standard curve.

Suppressor cell induction. Some 1×10^6/ml PBMC were treated with 20 μg/ml ConA and incubated in culture medium for 48 h and were compared with nontreated control cells. Autologous responder cells derived from the same sample were incubated during the induction phase of effector cells in culture medium. After the incubation period, ConA-activated and -nonactivated cells were washed three times with 30 mM α-methyl-D-mannoside (Sigma Chemical). Then, 50 μl of 1×10^6/ml responder and 50 μl of 1×10^6/ml effector cells were mixed and with and without 10 μg/ml PHA incubated at 37°C in 5% CO_2 in air for 3 days in microculture plates in quadruplicate. Controls, consisting of all cell populations alone with and without PHA were also prepared. Sixteen hours before harvesting, 0.5 μCi of tritiated thymidine was added to each well. The suppressor index (SI) was calculated according to the following formula:

$$SI = \frac{\text{cpm of responder cells with ConA} - \text{activated cells}}{\text{cpm of responder cells with ConA} - \text{nonactivated cells}} \times 100$$

Analysis of data and statistical methods. Mean values and standard deviations were calculated by Student's t-test and statistical analysis by χ^2 test.

Results

IL-2R expression on CD4+ and CD8+ cells

The analysis of the data obtained by cytoimmunological monitoring did not reveal any significant correlation between the different lymphocyte subsets and biopsy-proven rejection (data not shown). Correspondingly, in contrast to previous studies [4, 12], no correlation was found between the percentage of IL-2R-expressing T cells and rejection. As the preferential expression of IL-2R was demonstrated on CD4+ T cells in healthy adults [6], but only a few data are available on the distribution of the CD25 antigen-positive cells within the CD4+ or CD8+ T cells after heart transplantation [12], we studied the expression of this marker by means of two-colour fluorescence of the T-cell subsets in a group of patients before and after transplantation. Whereas an insignificant increase of CD4+ T cells was observed postoperatively, the proportion of IL-2R-expressing cells showed a significant increase from 38.0% ± 9.8% to 58.6% ± 15.7% ($P < 0.001$) within the CD4+ T cell subsets without a concomitant elevation of the CD25 antigen-expressing CD8+ cells (Fig. 1). Additionally, as shown in Fig. 2, there was a significant relationship of the percentage of CD4+/CD25+ cells to the percentage of CD4+ cells; thus, an enhancement of the IL-2R expression reflected only the relative rise of the inductor/helper cell subset.

In vitro induction of IL-2. Whereas the in vitro induction of IL-2R expression after PHA or allogeneic cell stimulation failed to correlate with a positive biopsy result (data not shown), the inducibility of IL-2 production after stimulation by PHA but not by ConA correlated significantly with biopsy specimens positive for acute rejection (Fig. 3).

Suppressor cell function. Some 84 suppressor cell inductions were carried out over 11 months, and the results were compared with data from the simultaneous examination of cell subsets, in vitro IL-2 production, in vitro IL-2R expression, and biopsies. No relationship could be established in any case between the grade of nonspecific suppression and the results of the above investigations. In contrast, analysing the frequency of rejection episodes at 2 and 4 weeks after the suppressor cell assay, a significant correlation was found between biopsy-proven rejection and suppressor activity, when taking a cut-off value for the suppressor index (SI) of $\leq 60\%$ (Fig. 4).

Figure 5 shows the SI of 8 patients before transplantation and of the transplant recipients classified according to the grading of the histological findings. As in the case of a negative histological result and inconspicuous clinical state no biopsy was performed within 2 weeks, only a small number of SI data classified as 0 were evaluable, although 34 out of the 84 suppressor assays showed a

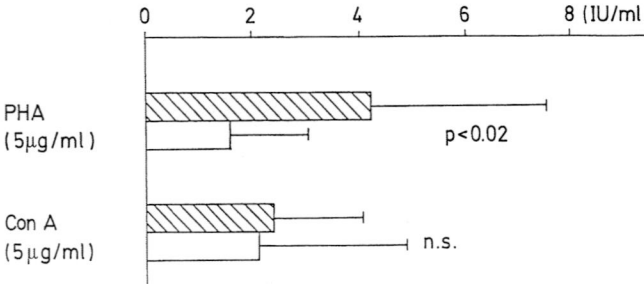

Fig. 3. Comparison of the mean values ± 1 SD of the in vitro IL-2 (U/ml) production induced by PHA and ConA in heart transplantation patients with ($\boxtimes$, $n = 11$) and without ($\square$, $n = 12$) biopsy-proven rejection. Blood samples were taken on the day of biopsy

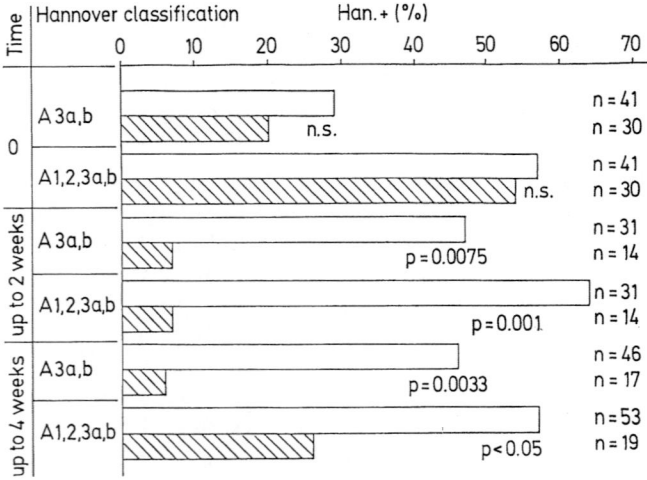

Fig. 4. Frequencies of biopsy-proven rejection and suppressor cell function. Patients were grouped according to the level of suppressor index (SI) $> 60\%$ $\boxtimes$ and $\leq 60\%$ $\square$. Frequencies of biopsy results graded as A3a, b or A1, 2, 3a, b are shown in relation to the time intervals between the suppressor cell assay and examination of the biopsy

SI $> 60\%$. Patients who did not experience rejection by up to 2 weeks exhibited a pronounced suppressor activity, and all patients with evidence of mild (A1, 2), moderate or severe rejection (A3a, 3b), except for one, showed a diminished suppressor cell activity. Furthermore, whereas a comparably lower suppressor activity was demonstrated when the patient's biopsy results were graded as in the early phase of resolving (5a) or in the late phase of resolving (5b), the distribution of SI found was similar to that in the group of patients tested preoperatively. Although the positive predictive value of a SI $\leq 60\%$ revealing a rejection of 3a or 3b was only 0.65 for up to 2 and 0.57 for up to 4 weeks, because the inducibility of suppressor cell activity was also diminished in the resolving phase of rejection, the negative predictive value was 0.93 and 0.94, respectively.

Discussion

Our observations demonstrate a better correlation between the histological findings and the investigation of cellular immunological functions, such as suppressor cell activity or IL-2 production, than the analysis of lymphocyte subsets in heart transplant patients. Previous studies have also failed to show a consistent correlation between different noninvasive techniques, such as cytoimmunological monitoring, expression of activation markers, or serum levels of sIL-2R, and rejection severity after solid-organ transplantation [7, 9, 17, 18]. The partially contradictory results can be explained by the intrinsic normal individual variability, in addition to the alterations due to processes other than rejection, e.g., infection. These disappointing findings suggest a poor and perhaps transient correlation between the features of circulating cells and immunological events in allograft.

Whereas neither the direct estimation nor the in vitro inducibility of IL-2R-expressing T cells correlated with the biopsy results, we found a significantly enhanced IL-2 production concomitant with a positive histological assessment in a restricted number of patients. Additionally, the analysis of IL-2R expression on T-cell subsets by means of the CD25-specific monoclonal antibody which detects the α-chain of the receptor revealed a close relationship of the proportion of IL-2R-expressing helper cells to the proportion of CD4 + cells. However, no correlation between the IL-2R-expressing cells and the rejection or suppressor function was established. Since IL-2

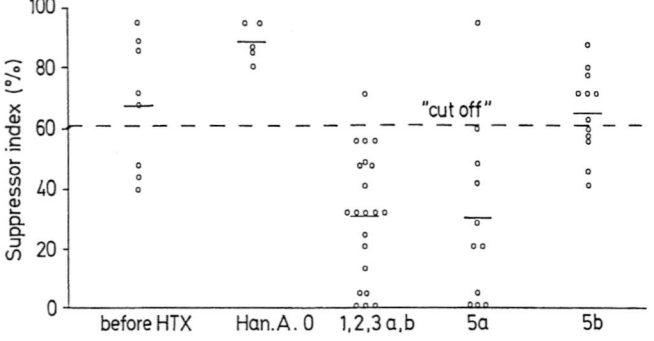

Fig. 5. Suppressor cell function from heart allograft patients. The SI results are shown for preoperative patients and are then grouped in accordance with rejection status as defined by biopsies examined between days 5 and 14 after investigation of suppressor function. *Dotted line* represents cut-off value for high ($< 60\%$) and low ($\leq 60\%$) SI

signal transduction is supposed to be transmitted via the β-chain but not the α-chain of IL-2R, evaluation of both high- and intermediate-affinity receptor-expressing cells might be more useful in monitoring transplant patients' lymphocytes, as discussed recently by Niguma et al. [10].

Although the relationship of mitogen-induced suppressor T cells to physiologically relevant suppressor function is unclear, heart allograft recipients displaying an efficient nonspecific suppressor acivity seemed to be protected from rejection in the subsequent 2–4 weeks. In addition, the failure of a correlation between biopsy-proven rejection and low SI (at time 0) suggests that the determination of different parameters such as circulating cells or humoral factors outside the allograft might not be helpful markers in the diagnosis of rejection.

To identify patients at risk of rejection, it seems to be more important to define the relative state of homeostasis between the recipient and allograft under conditions which favour tolerance induction, such as immunosuppressive therapy. The ability to display an effective hyporesponsiveness in the sense of a feedback downregulation of effector mechanisms demands to a certain degree the maintenance of immunoregulatory competence. This 'suppressor sparing effect' was postulated as one of the advantages of cyclosporine therapy [15]. In conclusion, we suggest that the periodic determination of the suppressor functional status may be useful to discriminate between patients at low or high risk for graft rejection after heart transplantation.

Acknowledgment: We express our thanks to Drs. J. Kemnitz, Institute for Pathology, Medical University of Hannover, and C. J. Kirkpatrick, Institute for Pathology, Medical Faculty of RWTG Aachen, for obtaining results of biopsy investigations.

References

1. Abo T, Cooper MD, Balch CM (1982) Characterization of HNK-1 (Leu-7) human lymphocytes. I. Two distinct phenotypes of human NK cells with different cytolytic capability. J Immunol 129: 1752

2. Brando B, Civati G, Busnach G, Grillo C, Minetti L (1984) T suppressor cell function in cyclosporine-treated renal transplant recipients. Transplant Proc 16: 1639–1641

3. Charpentier BM, Bach M-A, Lang P, Fries D (1983) Expression of OKT 8 antigen and Fcγ receptors by suppressor cells mediating specific unresponsiveness between recipient and donor in renal-allograft-tolerant patients. Transplantation 36: 495–501

4. Fieguth HG, Haverich A, Hadam M, Kemnitz J, Dammenhayn L (1989) Correlation of interleukin-2 receptor positive circulating lymphocytes and acute cardiac rejection. Transplant Proc 21: 2517–2518

5. Harada M, Ueda M, Nakao S, Kondo K, Odaka K, Shiobara S, Matsue K, Mori T, Matsuda T (1986) Nonspecific suppressor T cells cause decreased mixed lymphocyte culture reactivity in bone marrow transplant patients. J Immunol 137: 428–432

6. Jackson AL, Matsumoto H, Janszen M, Maino V, Blidy A, Shye S (1990) Restricted expression of p55 interleukin 2 receptor (CD25) on normal T cells. Clin Immunol Immunopathol 54: 126–133

7. Jutte NHPM, Daane R, Bemd JMG van den, Hop WCJ, Essed CE, Simoons ML, Bos E, Weimar W (1989) Cytoimmunological monitoring to detect rejection after heart transplantation. Transplant Proc 21: 2519–2520

8. Kemnitz J, Cohnert T, Schäfers HJ, Helmke M, Wahlers T, Herrmann G, Schmidt RM, Haverich A (1987) A classification of cardiac allograft rejection. A modification of the classification by Billingham. Am J Surg Pathol 11: 503–515

9. Mooney ML, Carlson P, Szentpetery S, Duma RJ, Markowitz SM (1990) A prospective study of the clinical utility of lymphocyte monitoring in the cardiac transplant recipient. Transplantation 50: 951–954

10. Niguma T, Sakagami K, Kawamura T, Haisa M, Fujiwara T, Kusaka S, Uda M, Orita K (1991) Expression of the interleukin 2 receptor β chain (p75) in renal transplantation – applicability of anti-interleukin 2 receptor β chain monoclonal antibody. Transplantation 52: 296–302

11. Pusztai-Markos S, Hauss K (1989) In vitro effect of different antimicrobial agents on IL-2 production and IL-2 receptor expression of human lymphocytes. In: Gillissen G, Opferkuch W, Peters G, Pulverer G (eds) The influence of antibiotics on the host-parasite relationship III. Springer-Verlag, Berlin Heidelberg New York, pp 245–254

12. Roodman ST, Miller LW, Tsai CC (1988) Role of interleukin 2 receptors in immunologic monitoring following cardiac transplantation. Transplantation 45: 1050–1056

13. Tilden AB, Abo T, Balch CM (1983) Suppressor cell function of human granular lymphocytes identified by the HNK-1 (Leu 7) monoclonal antibody. J Immunol 130: 1171–1175

14. Waer M, Vanrenterghem Y, Schueren E van der, Michielsen P, Vandeputte M (1985) Phenotypic and functional analysis of suppressor cells in renal transplant recipients receiving cyclosporine A or preoperative total lymphoid irradiation. Transplant Proc 17: 2539–2542

15. Wang BS, Heacock EH, Chang-Xue Z, Tilney NL, Strom TB, Manick JA (1982) Evidence for the presence of suppressor T lymphocytes in animals treated with cyclosporin A. J Immunol 128: 1382–1385

16. Weimer R, Daniel V, Pomer S, Opelz G (1989) B lymphocyte response as an indicator of acute renal transplant rejection. Transplantation 48: 572–575

17. Wijngaard PLJ, Meulen A van der, Schuurman H-J, Gmelig Meyling FHJ, Heyn A, Borleffs JCC, Jambroes G (1989) Cytoimmunological monitoring for the diagnosis of acute rejection after heart transplantation. Transplant Proc 21: 2521–2522

18. Young JB, Windsor NT, Smart FW, Kleiman NS, Weilbaecher DG, Noon GP, Nelson DL, Lawrence EC (1991) Inability of isolated soluble interleukin-2 receptor levels to predict biopsy rejection scores after heart transplantation. Transplantation 51: 636–641

TRANSPLANT
International
© Springer-Verlag 1992

β_2-Microglobulinuria as an early sign of cytomegalovirus infection following renal transplantation

J. Steinhoff[1], A. Feddersen[1], W. G. Wood[1], J. Hoyer[1], G. Bein[2], G. Wiedemann[1], L. Fricke[1], and K. Sack[1]

Departments of [1] Internal Medicine and [2] Immunology and Transfusion Medicine, Medical University of Lübeck, Lübeck, Federal Republic of Germany

Abstract. The frequency of cytomegalovirus infection was studied in a prospective study of 106 kidney recipients. The detection of cytomegalovirus-immediate-early-antigen and cytomegalovirus-immunoglobulin (IgM) antibodies in serum was used as the reference method and showed that 23.6 % (25/106) of all patients were infected. In addition, four urinary proteins (IgG and transferrin as glomerular markers and α_1-microglobulin and β_2-microglobulin as tubular markers) were quantitatively measured in 24-h urine samples from all of the patients using an immunoluminometric assay (ILMA). In all cytomegalovirus infection cases a pronounced but isolated increase of urinary β_2-microglobulin excretion was observed. In 20 of 25 infected patients, the β_2-microglobulinuria occurred 1–21 days (median 5.0) earlier than the appearance of the cytomegalovirus-immediate-early-antigen in blood. Thus, it can be seen that the quantitative measurement of β_2-microglobulin in urine is useful for the early detection of cytomegalovirus infection following renal transplantation.

Key words: Renal transplantation – Cytomegalovirus – Proteinuria – β_2-Microglobulin – Cytomegalovirus-immediate-early-antigen

Florid disease in cytomegalovirus (CMV)-infected patients usually presents a much smaller diagnostic challenge than CMV infection in an early form, and the real value of a diagnostic test lies in its predictive value before the severe complications of CMV infection arise. The detection of CMV infection in patients who have successfully undergone a renal transplantation has been improved during the past few years because florid CMV infection is associated with the concomitant occurrence of CMV-immediate-early-antigen (CMV-IEA) in blood.

This is important as in patients under immunosuppression with cyclosporin following renal transplantation, a significant increase of IgM antibodies is unlikely to occur. In such patients, the otherwise typical neutropenia is not a useful diagnostic criterion when cyclosporine, azathioprine, and prednisolone are used in combination to achieve immunosuppression.

Clinical criteria such as fever, myalgia, or arthralgia are not pathognomonic. The rapid and early diagnosis of CMV is of decisive importance because of the lethal complications (e. g., pneumonia) or irreparable damage (e. g., retinitis). In a few studies, tubular proteinuria accompanying CMV infection has been observed [4, 7]. However, this observation has not led to further prospective investigations.

Grundy et al. found that CMV is coated with β_2-microglobulin before renal excretion [5]. However, the diagnostic possibilities arising from this statement were not examined. It has been shown that a pathological β_2-microglobulinuria can both appear in patients with cyclosporin intoxication and accompany renal transplant rejection [1]. In previous studies, we have not been able to confirm these observations [9]. Here we report a prospective study performed to evaluate the diagnostic value of β_2-microglobulinuria in CMV-infected patients following renal transplantation.

Methods

In a prospective study started in July 1989 on 106 kidney recipients to date, the "glomerular" proteins immunoglobulin G (IgG) and transferrin as well as the selected "tubular" proteins α_1-microglobulin and β_2-microglobulin were measured in the urine. During hospitalization, these analytes were measured daily. Prior to analysis, the urine was centrifuged for 10 min at 3000 min^{-1}, and the proteins were measured immediately after centrifugation. Additionally, creatinine in urine and serum was evaluated colorimetrically using the Jaffe method without prior deproteinisation. Quantitative analysis of urinary proteins were made with immunoluminometric assays (ILMA) which have been developed in this laboratory. The assays function using the "sandwich technique" in which the liquid antibody is la-

Offprint requests to: Dr. J. Steinhoff, Department of Internal Medicine, Medical University of Lübeck, Ratzeburger Allee 160, W-2400 Lübeck, Federal Republic of Germany

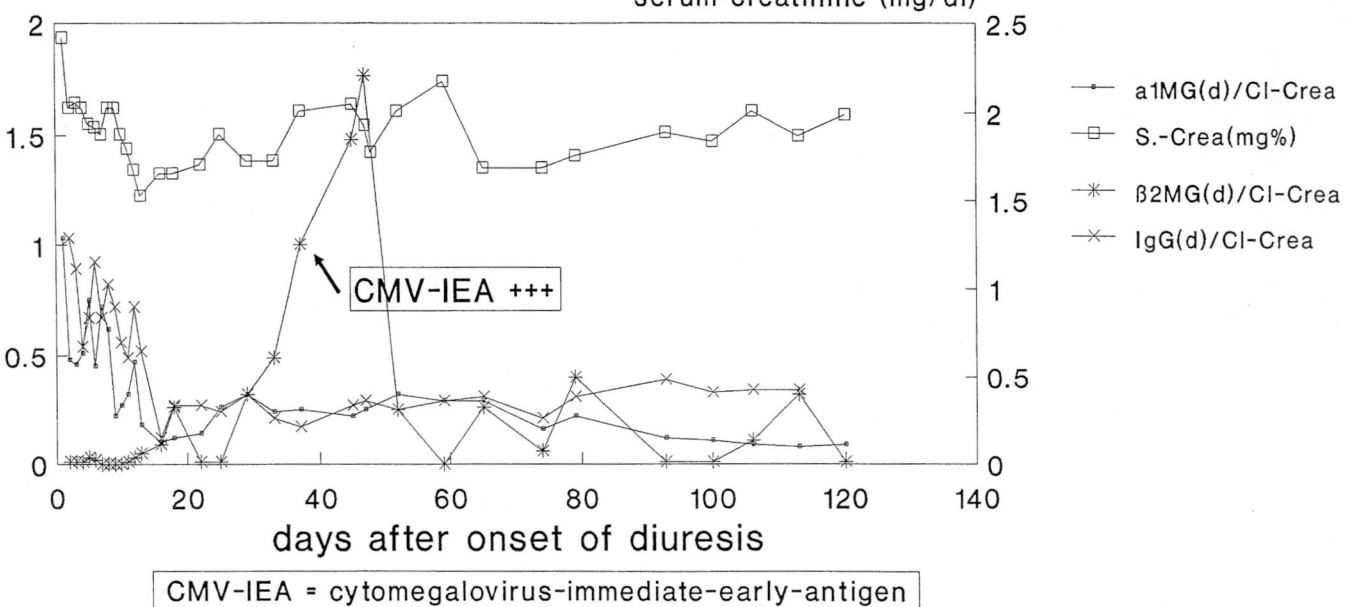

serum creatinine (mg/dl)

CMV-IEA +++

days after onset of diuresis

CMV-IEA = cytomegalovirus-immediate-early-antigen

- a1MG(d)/Cl-Crea
- S.-Crea(mg%)
- β2MG(d)/Cl-Crea
- IgG(d)/Cl-Crea

Fig. 1. Course of proteinuria in a 52-year-old patient with a cytomegalovirus (CMV) infection. After transplantation, at first typical mixed proteinuria without β_2-microglobulin excretion. On day 37 the detection of CMV-IEA was first positive. An isolated increase in β_2-microglobulin was seen, however, several days before. Other marker proteins (immunoglobulin IgG and α_1-microglobulin) showed little change

belled with a luminogen. All measurements were made in duplicate on a semiautomatic 250-sample luminometer (LB 952T/16; Berthold, Wildbad, FRG). Detailed descriptions of these assays have already been published [10, 11]. The adjustment of the urinary pH to above 7.0, which is often recommended for measurements of β_2-microglobulin [8], was not done for two reasons: Firstly, interference with other protein assays could not be excluded, and secondly, the β_2-microglobulin seems to be more stable in the urine of CMV-infected patients in general [5].

Patient-derived data were expressed as a quotient of the daily protein excretion (mg/day) to the actual individual creatinine clearance (ml/min) and was measured daily. Then the ratios between the actual quotient were compared with the previous quotient in the same patient and any significant increases or decreases logged for diagnostic purposes.

All patients received the same immunosuppressive therapy (prednisolone 25-7.5 mg/day, azathioprine 2 mg/kg daily, cyclosporin 3–5 mg/kg daily). Therapeutic cyclosporin levels in whole blood were normally between 80 and 120 ng/ml when measured with a specific radioimmunoassay (RIA; Sandoz). The CMV-IEA in the peripheral blood leukocytes was determined histochemically using the alkaline phosphatase/antialkaline phosphatase technique (APAAP) [2]. In our experience the APAAP method provides a higher diagnostic specificity and sensitivity for labeling CMV-IEA-positive leukocytes than the method described by van der Bij [3]. If at least 2 out of 400000 leukocytes were labeled, the CMV-IEA test was considered to be positive.

CMV-IgM antibodies were evaluated by a routine enzyme immunoassay. In hospitalized patients, the CMV-IEA and CMV-IgM antibody levels were determined weekly. In patients followed up in the outpatient clinic, the tests were made each time they attended.

Results

To judge cytomegaloviremia, the diagnostic criterion was a positive CMV-IEA test in blood. Out of 106 renal transplant recipients 25 were considered CMV infected

(23.6%). One of these 25 patients showed a positive CMV-IEA test following treatment with methylprednisolone, which had been given to counteract acute renal transplant rejection. The other 24 patients had been treated with antithymocyte-globulin (ATG), either against renal transplant rejection (7 patients) or because of a high immunological risk accompanying repeated renal transplantation (17 patients).

Figure 1 shows the typical development of the β_2-microglobulinuria and its temporal course following the first positive CMV-IEA test in the blood. Note here that neither the "tubular" marker protein α_1-microglobulin nor the "glomerular" marker protein IgG showed significant alterations.

In all of the CMV-IEA-positive cases, an isolated (at least three fold) increase of β_2-microglobulin excretion was observed. Only in 4 cases were slight increases in IgG and in 6 cases, slight increases in α_1-microglobulin seen.

Table 1 shows the time course of the first appearance of β_2-microglobulinuria, CMV antibodies in serum, and CMV-IEA in blood (day 0). With the exception of 5 cases, increases of β_2-microglobulin in urine were found considerably earlier than or at the same time as CMV-IEA in the blood. The CMV-IgM antibody in the serum appeared much later.

Only in CMV infections is an *isolated* increase of β_2-microglobulinuria to be found. β_2-microglobulinuria was also observed in patients with renal transplant rejections and during urosepsis; however, in these patients the β_2-microglobulinuria was associated with general "tubular" proteinuria (α_1-microglobulinuria). In patients with renal transplant rejection, initial "glomerular" proteinuria was followed by extensive "tubular" proteinuria. In renal transplant recipients suffering from urosepsis, extensive

Table 1. The time relation between the appearance of CMV-imme-diate-early-antigen in blood (day 0 = CMV-IEA detection) and the detection of CMV-IgM antibody in serum and β_2-microglobulinuria expressed in days before (−) or after (+) appearance of CMV-IEA

Patient	β_2-MG	CMV-IgM	CMV-IgG Donor/recipient
1	− 3	+ 3	+ / −
2	− 5	+ 9	+ / −
3	− 4	+ 4	+ / −
4	− 9	> 10	+ / −
5	− 1	+ 2	+ / +
6	− 5	> 10	+ / −
7	− 1	> 10	+ / −
8	− 8	> 10	+ / −
9	− 15	> 10	+ / +
10	− 6	> 10	+ / −
11	0	> 10	+ / −
12	− 8	> 10	+ / −
13	+ 4	+ 9	+ / +
14	− 7	+ 8	+ / −
15	− 6	> 10	+ / −
16	− 9	> 10	+ / +
17	0	> 10	+ / −
18	− 4	> 10	− / −
19	− 21	> 10	+ / −
20	− 3	> 10	+ / −
21	− 8	+ 6	+ / +
22	0	> 10	+ / −
23	− 5	> 10	+ / −
24	+ 2	> 10	+ / −
25	− 9	> 10	+ / −

The CMV-antibody constellation of donor and recipient at the time of transplantation is shown in the last column

"tubular" proteinuria was observed. In patients with acute cyclosporin nephrotoxicity, no changes in proteinuria were seen [9].

The specificity of an isolated β_2-microglobulinuria during CMV infection is 100 %. The sensitivity is 80 %, when related to the occurrence of CMV-IEA in blood.

Discussion

Our study results found no general tubular proteinuria during CMV infection. More interestingly, an *isolated* (at least three fold) increase of β_2-microglobulin excretion only occurred in CMV-infected patients. Moreover, in 20 out of 25 CMV-infected patients, the β_2-microglobulinuria occurred up to 21 days (median 5.0) earlier than the appearance of CMV-IEA in the blood. Thus, the detection of isolated β_2-microglobulinuria is specific for CMV infection and is useful in the early diagnosis of CMV infection in renal transplant recipients.

The underlying pathomechanisms causing β_2-micro-globulinuria in CMV infection are not clear. Grundy and coworkers [5] reported that the β_2-microglobulin coats the CMV, resulting in a stable complex. It could be shown that β_2-microglobulin was at higher concentrations in the sediment than in the supernatant, which supports the results of Grundy et al.

Thus, it can be concluded that the CMV-β_2-microglo-bulin complex is to be found in the sediment because of the higher weight of the viral complex and that it can be measured in a β_2-microglobulin assay [5].

It seems to be an advantage not to alkalinize the urine because most of the "unspecific" and instable "tubular" β_2-microglobulin is not supposed to be detectable in acid urine, whereas the more stable "CMV-specific" β_2-micro-globulin can be measured.

Measuring β_2-microglobulin alone is not sufficient to diagnose a CMV infection, as β_2-microglobulinuria can also be found after successful antirejection therapy as well as following bacterial infections of the urinary tract [9, 11]. Nevertheless, in such cases, a general tubular proteinuria, but not an isolated increase of β_2-microglobulin, is to be observed [9].

References

1. Bäckmann L, Ringden O, Björkhen I, Lindbäck B (1986) Increased serum β_2-microglobulin during rejection, cyclosporine-induced nephrotoxicity, and cytomegalovirus infection in renal transplant recipients. Transplantation 42: 368
2. Bein G, Bitsch A, Hoyer J, Kirchner H (1991) The detection of human cytomegalovirus immediate early antigen in peripheral blood leucocytes. J Immunol Methods (in press)
3. Bij W van der, Torensma R, Son WJ van, Anema J, Schirm J, Tegzess AM, The TH (1988) Rapid immunodiagnosis of active cytomegalovirus infection by monoclonal antibody staining blood leucocytes. J Med Virol 25: 179
4. Boesken W, Schmidt M, Jontofrohn R (1975) Proteinuria as diagnostic marker after human kidney transplantation. EDTA 11: 333
5. Grundy JE, McKeating JA, Sanderson AR, Griffith PD (1988) Cytomegalovirus and β_2-microglobulin in urine specimens. Transplantation 45: 1075
6. Immich H Medizinische Statistik. Schattauer, Stuttgart, p 259
7. Jensen H (1972) Proteinuria. A survey. Dan Med Bull 19: 89
8. Odlind B, Backman U, Forbes MA, Cooper EH (1988) Proteinuria after renal transplantation. Contrib Nephrol 68: 149
9. Steinhoff J, Feddersen A, Wood WG, Hoyer J, Sack K (1991) Glomerular proteinuria as an early sign of renal-transplant rejection. Clin Nephrol 35: 255
10. Wood WG (1989) Radioimmunoassay versus nicht-radioisotopischer Immunoassay 1989 – Pro und Contra. Lab Med 13: 345
11. Wood WG, Herhahn D, Steinhoff J, Feddersen A, Schulz E, Sack K (1990) The diagnostic relevance of specific urinary proteins after renal transplantation. Ärztl Lab 36: 260

Xenografting

Transplant Int (1992) 5 [Suppl 1]: S 305–S 306

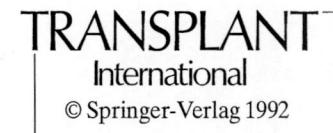

TRANSPLANT
International
© Springer-Verlag 1992

Perfusion of rabbit hearts with human blood results in immediate graft thrombosis, a temporally distinct component of hyperacute rejection

J. Forty, R. Hasan, N. Cary, D. J. G. White, and J. Wallwork

Papworth Hospital, Cambridge, UK

Hyperacute discordant xenograft rejection can be simulated by a blood-perfused working isolated heart [2]. The survival of the heart is dependent on its functional integrity, and the preparation is thus sensitive to early myocardial damage.

Perfusion of rabbit hearts with human blood produces immediate graft destruction by a thrombotic process which is a distinct component of hyperacute rejection.

Key words: Heart graft thrombosis – Hyperacute rejection

Methods

Hearts of 1.7 kg New Zealand White rabbits were perfused with rabbit or human group AB blood. Blood of either species was collected into heparin (6500 units/l) and was reduced to a haematocrit of 25%. Human blood was unmodified, or had previously perfused another heart, or had been treated as detailed below. A log-rank analysis of survival of the six hearts in each group was performed.

Complement was depleted by the additon of 10 μg purified cobra venom factor (CoF) [3] to 240 ml plasma. Platelets were removed (99.5%) with a Pall RC50 filter. Platelet activating factor was inactivated by addition of WEB 2170, a specific antagonist. Anti-rabbit antibody (ARA) was absorbed from plasma by incubation with rabbit blood cells for 80 min at 4 °C.

Hearts were perfused as working preparations [2] until functional failure. Lytic human ARA titres were measured before and after perfusion [2]. Complement classical pathway activity was measured using the CH50 technique [3]. Hearts were examined after perfusion by conventional and immunohistological methods (IgG, IgM, C3, C4, C9).

Results

Homologous perfusion resulted in organ survival for 300 min with no functional change. Hearts perfused with human blood failed at 1 min ($P < 0.001$). This failure was characterized by cessation of coronary flow and an ischaemic appearance and ECG. Examination of hearts revealed platelet occlusion of small vessels and immediate deposition of interstitial IgG, endothelial IgM and C3, 4 and 9. This event has been termed immediate graft thrombosis (IGT). Heart perfused with modified human blood did not thrombose.

Blood which had previously perfused another heart produced rejection at a median time of 20 min ($P < 0.001$). Perfusion with platelet-free blood resulted in rejection at a median time of 22 min ($P < 0.001$). Platelet activating factor block with WEB 2170 produced rejection at a median time of 20 min ($P < 0.001$). Perfusion with blood from which the ARA had been absorbed resulted in rejection at a median time of 33 min ($P < 0.001$).

Examination of rejected hearts revealed neutrophil and lymphoid infiltrates. Interstitial IgG and endothelial IgM were again seen. C9 was deposited in excess or absence of C4. Treatment with CoF delayed organ failure to a median time of 207 min ($P < 0.001$). No C3, 4 or 9 was seen. Organ survival is summarized in Fig. 1.

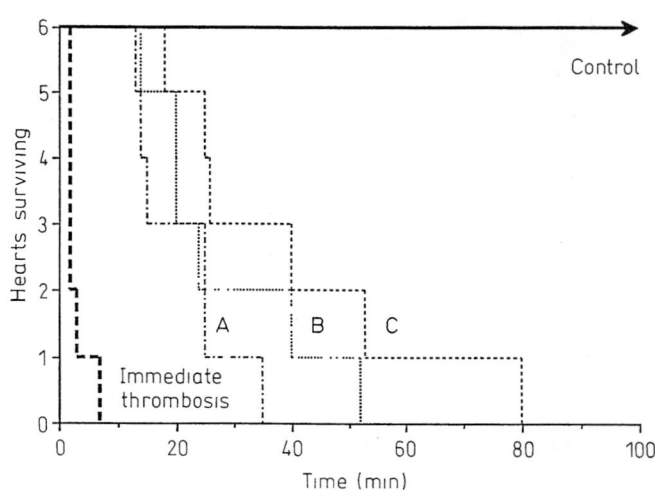

Fig. 1. Organ survival. *A,* WEB 2170; *B,* platelet free; *C,* antibody absorbed

Offprint requests to: J. Forty, Department of Cardiothoracic Surgery, Freeman Hospital, Newcastle-upon-Tyne, UK

Discussion

Rejection in this species combination has two components. The first is immediate and thrombotic, and can be prevented by removal of platelets or inhibition of platelet activating factor. Removal of IgM anti-rabbit antibody also presents the thrombosis but has no effect on subsequent rejection. The central part played by complement, by whichever pathway, is confirmed by the prevention of both IGT and subsequent events by treatment with CoF. Immediate graft thrombosis, then, is a process initiated by IgM anti-rabbit antibody and mediated by complement by its classical pathway. It is then effected by platelet activating factor presumably of endothelial origin and the formation of platelet plugs. Heart which are rejected in the absence of IGT have C9 deposition in excess C4 suggesting that the alternative pathway of complement is responsible for this second process. This hypothesis has been confirmed in other studies [1].

The assumption that hyperacute discordant xenograft rejection is the consequence of heterophile antibody [6, 7] is in part confirmed. However, a distinction has been made between immediate thrombosis and another rapid event mediated by the alternative pathway of complement. The potential importance of this pathway has been commented upon by other investigators [4, 5].

The distinction that has been made between immediate graft thrombosis and alternative pathway mediated rejection in discordant organ perfusion has been made only with the use of a new, sensitive technique.

References

1. Forty J, Hasan R, Carey N, White DGJ, Wallwork J (1992) Transplant Proc (in press)
2. Forty J, White DJG, Wallwork J (1992) (in press)
3. Harrison RA, Lachman PJ (1986) In: Weir DM, Herzenberg LA, Blackwell C (eds) Handbook of experimental immunology, 4th edn, vol 1. Blackwell, Oxford, p 39
4. Johnston PS, Lim SML, Wang MW, Wright L, White DJG (1991) Transplant Proc 23: 877–879
5. Miyagawa S, Hirose H, Shirakura R, et al (1988) Transplantation 46: 825–830
6. Perper RJ, Najarian JS (1966) Transplantation 4: 377–388
7. Platt JL, Vercellotti GM, Dalmasso AP, et al (1990) Immunol Today 11: 450–457

Transplant Int (1992) 5 [Suppl 1]: S 307–S 310

TRANSPLANT
International
© Springer-Verlag 1992

Allogeneic heart transplantation following xenogeneic bridging

A. Schütz[1], **J. Pratschke**[2], **M. Breuer**[1], **C. Hammer**[2], **M. Engelhardt**[1], **U. Brandl**[1], **R. Babic**[3], **B. Reichart**[1], and **B. M. Kemkes**[1]

[1] Department of Cardiac Surgery, [2] Institute for Surgical Research, and
[3] Institute for Pathology, Ludwig-Maximilians-University, Klinikum Großhadern, Munich, FRG

Abstract. Xenografting seems to be a solution to bridge the time intervals when an essential allograft cannot be obtained. A subsequent allograft was never tried. Eight dogs (20–24 kg) of 2 years of age underwent right cervical heart transplantation. Donors were silver foxes (3–4 kg). The animals were treated by triple drug therapy consisting of cyclosporin A, methylprednisolone and azathioprine in clinical dosages. For control, six recipients received allogeneic heart transplantation (AHTP) and the identical immunosuppression. After rejection of the xenograft, a second allogeneic heart was anastomosed to the same right cervical vessels. Routine histology and immunohistology were performed. Thromboxane B2 and 6-keto-prostaglandin F1a were determined daily in peripheral blood. After final rejection sensitization of the recipient was controlled by haemagglutination tests. Survival times of the xenografts were 9.6 ± 1.2. The subsequent hearts under the same therapy beat for 4.5 ± 5.0 days. The average survival time of control hearts was 18 ± 1.9 days. The five hyperacute second allografts showed signs of humoral rejection by absence of inflammation. The release of thromboxane B2 was different in hyperacute, accelerated or cellular rejection. In contrast to the long-functioning grafts, thromboxane B2 persisted during hyperacute rejection at a high level. However 6-keto-prostaglandin F1a showed no significant differences between long-time survivors and hyperacute rejecting hearts. After xenogeneic transplantation all recipients showed haemagglutinating titres between 1:4 and 1:16. Allogeneic grafts have different kinetics of rejection following xenogeneic heart transplantation (XHTP) compared with control hearts. Thromboxane B2 seems to be an important mediator in hyperacute rejection. This type of rejection is not associated with a change in 6-keto-prostaglandin F1a levels. These results indicate, that xenogeneic bridging under a common immunosuppressive regimen could lead to accelerated rejection of the following allograft. Under this condition clinical bridging is not advisable.

Key words: Allogeneic heart transplantation – Xenogeneic bridging

The continuing shortage of human donor hearts has led to the suggestion that hearts from appropriate animal species could be used for bridging a time interval in which a desperately needed heart allograft is not available. The question raised was whether such an intermediate XHTP would jeopardize the success and survival time (SVT) of the following AHTP, due to the sensitization with xenogeneic heart antigen. The aim of this study was to determine the SVT of allografts after XHTP and the rejection type occurring after xenogeneic bridging uder standardized immunosuppression (IS) using a fox/dog model. In addition a potential correlation between thromboxane B2 (TxB2), 6-keto-PGF$_{1a}$ liberation and the type of rejection was investigated.

Materials and methods

XHTP was performed on nine mongrel dogs of 20 to 25 kg aged under 2 years. Xenogeneic donors were silver foxes of 3–4 kg. After rejection of the sensitizing xenografts, the second allogeneic heart was anastomosed onto the same cervical vessels. Adult beagles of 10–12 kg served as donors for the AHTP. As control group, six AHTP were performed under the same conditions. The operation technique has previously been described, as has the anaesthesia [16]. The sensitization to the xenograft was monitored by haemagglutination of fox red blood cells. All transplanted grafts were under continuous observation for the first 3 h. Blood samples were drawn every 15 min during the first postoperative hours, and subsequently daily. The samples for TxB2 and 6-keto-PGF$_{1a}$ were centrifuged at 4°C and stored at −70° until use.

Histopathology

The rejected hearts were explanted with the recipients still alive. Sections of standardized areas were stained with HE, methylgreen pyronin and PAS. Ischaemic necroses within the first 6 h were demonstrated by succinate dehydrogenase (SDH) staining, modified according to previously described methods [3, 14]. AR was graded ac-

Offprint requests to: A. Schütz, M. D., Department of Cardiac Surgery, University of Munich, Klinikum Großhadern, Marchioninistr. 15, 8000 Munich 70, FRG

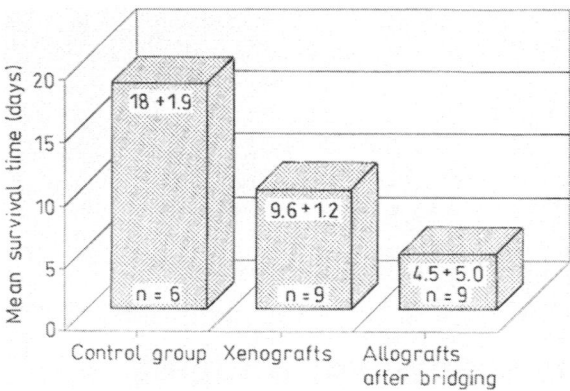

Fig.1. Average graft survival time of xenogeneic, control and subsequent allogeneic hearts

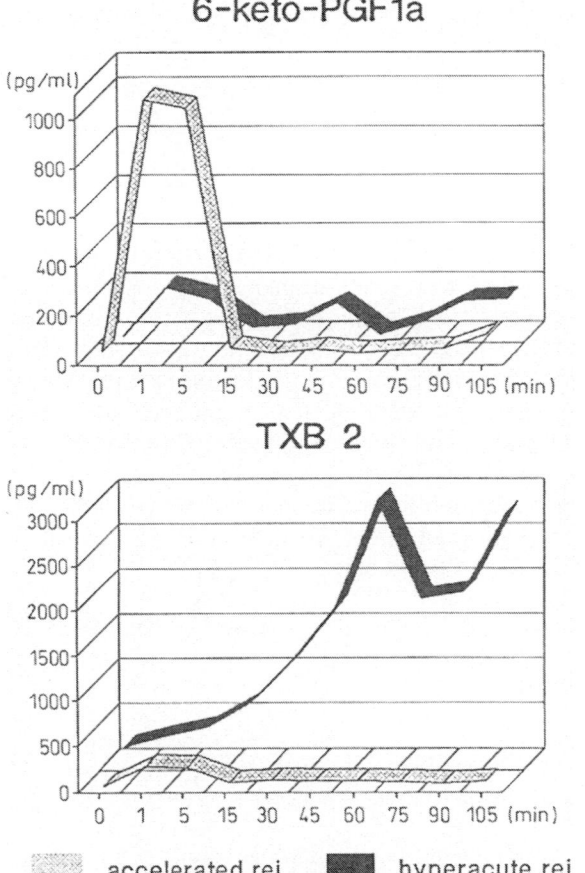

Fig.2. Liberation of TxB2 and 6-keto-PGF$_{1a}$ plotted against time after opening the anastomoses. During hyperacute rejection a sharp increase in TxB2 could be observed, while 6-keto-PGF$_{1a}$ remained at the orginal level. In contrast the accelerated rejection shows an increase in 6-keto-PGF$_{1a}$ and unchanged levels of TxB2

cording to Billingham et al. [4]. Monoclonal antibodies directed against canine B cells, CD3 positive cells, monocytes and IgM were visualized with peroxidase conjugated antibodies [11].

Immunosuppression

Allogeneic and xenogeneic recipients were immunosuppressed in the same fashion using a triple drug therapy. Prior to perfusion of the graft the recipients received MP i. v. 250 mg and AZA i. v. 50 mg. The

trough blood levels of CyA ranged between 500 and 700 ng/ml. AZA 1.25 mg/kg and MP 0.25 mg/kg were given daily. Imipenem/cilastatin (Zienam) was injected i.v. for the first 5 days followed by benzylpenicillin i. m. for another 7 days in order to prevent infections.

Results

All 9 XHTP and the following AHTP were performed without surgical problems and became perfused uniformly after connection with the blood circulation. Four xenogeneic and three allogeneic hearts showed spontaneous contractions, and two xenogeneic and six allogeneic grafts needed defibrillation. The controls functioned as described previously [15]. SVT of the control group (Fig.1) was 18 ± 1.9 days. Xenogeneic fox hearts for 9.6 ± 1.2 days (Fig.1). In contrast the subsequent allografts survived only 4.5 ± 5.0 days (Fig.1), with a range between 105 min and 14 days. The observed immunoreactions were classified as hyperacute ($n = 5$), accelerated ($n = 3$) and acute rejection ($n = 1$). The haemagglutination titre after sensitization by XHTP varied between 1:4 and 1:16. There was no correlation between the level of the haemagglutinating titre and the type of rejection which occurred after the second transplantation.

Hyperacute rejected grafts

Hyperacute rejection (HXR) was defined as rejection within less than 48 h. According to this definition, five hearts (55.5%) were rejected hyperacutely. Visible evidence of AR was present after about 30 min of haemoperfusion in three cases. During the course of AR the hearts became progressively enlarged, livid and finally cyanotic. Routine histological examination of the rejected hearts revealed no signs of cellular rejection in terms of infiltration. In this type of rejection focal ischaemic necroses were observed in two cases. In three cases even with SDH no significant morphological changes could be detected. Congestion of arterioles with platelets and RBC was a rare and inconstant feature. Discrete extravascular haemorrhage and perivascular oedema could be detected in all cases. Immunohistology showed IgM-producing plasma cells, but no infiltration by monocytes or CD3-positive cells. Traces of IgM were found around muscle cells and predominantly on the endothelium of vessels. Levels of TxB2 increased continuously during the first hour in all cases (Figs. 2 and 3). After a moderate reduction it reached a second peak, lasting to the final stage of rejection in three cases. In the other recipients with HXR, TxB2 concentration increased immediately after reperfusion and remained at a high level until final rejection. In contrast the levels of 6-keto-PGF$_{1a}$ did not change in this group.

Accelerated rejection

The three accelerated rejected hearts (33.3%) showed a cellular infiltrate corresponding to grade 2–4. Only distinct focal ischaemic necroses could be found, in contrast extravascular haemorrhage with large infiltrates of B cells and monocytes was characteristic. Thrombi consisting of

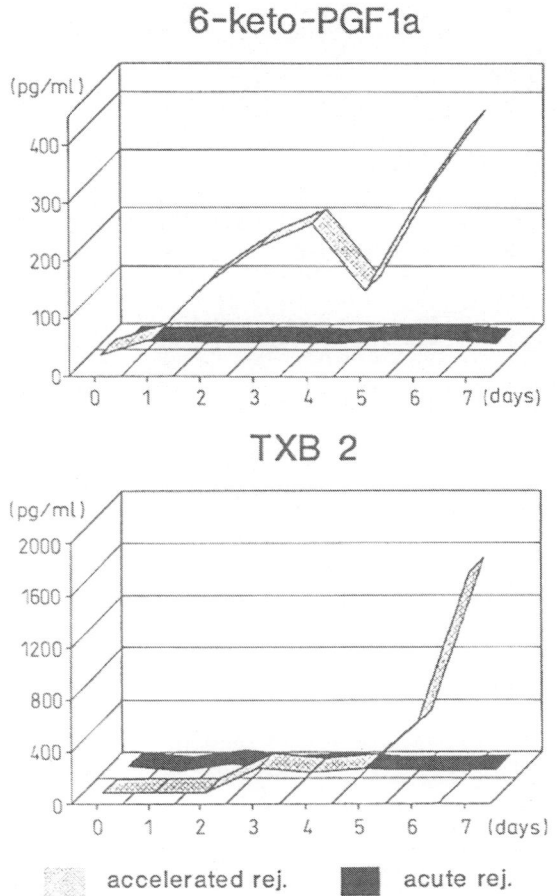

Fig. 3. Time course of daily TxB2 and 6-keto-PGF$_{1a}$ levels during accelerated and acute rejection. During the final stage of accelerated rejection TxB2 increased and 6-keto-PGF$_{1a}$ showed only slight alteration. In the case of acute rejection neither 6-keto-PGF$_{1a}$ nor TxB2 changed

immunosuppressive drugs have pushed xenotransplantation into a new era [8, 9]. Preformed natural antibodies [7] and cross-species antibodies, generated in response to transplantation, blood transfusion or pregnancy, interfere with this type of organ transplantation. It was, however, not clear whether these antibodies also cross-react with allografts. Investigations into bridging time in the clinical situation have been published using artificial organs [5]. Allogeneic transplantation following xenografting could not be attempted up to now due to previously described unsolved problems [2]. Experiments in rodents have been described. However, the size of the recipients made transplantation of two consecutive organs of the same type impossible [10]. The fox-to-dog model represents an adequate model to examine a bridging procedure. The animals are large enough to receive two consecutive transplants at the same site. Fox and dog are closely related species and according to their evolutionary and genetic background comparable with the baboon – man system [8]. Antigenic similarity induces the formation of anti-fox antibodies which have partial identity with antigens of the canine relative, the dog [17]. This is postulated to be the explanation for the histological findings revealing a purely humoral rejection mechanism in five cases, comparable with the mechanism found after sensitization with an allograft [6, 13]. In the case of HXR immunohistology showed that antibodies are reacting predominantly with the endothelium of the donor graft's vessels. Some of the allografts were rejected by cellular and humoral mechanisms in an accelerated fashion. As described in previous experiments, single allogeneic transplanted hearts follow a mainly cellular rejection of the acute type. One juvenile allograft in our study resulted in a SVT close to that of unsensitized recipients. The rejection mechanism was of the cellular type with confluent myocytolyses and haemorrhage.

These findings were confirmed by the liberation of TxB2, which was only found during HXR. High levels of TxB2 were reached after reperfusion of the allograft, when HXR occurred, but not during cellular events. The failure to detect an increase in 6-keto-PGF$_{1a}$ levels in HXR may be attributed to damage to the endothelium caused by antibodies and complement activation. On the other hand, the damage of the endothelium activates thrombocytes and leads to liberation of TxB2. The mediation of cardiac ischaemia by TxB2 released from platelets is well described [12]. We suggest that cardiac ischaemia, caused by such potent vasoconstrictors as TXB2 and possibly endothelin [1], is an important factor in HXR cases. These findings would lead to the suggestion that organs from closely related species are of clinical value because of the relatively long survival time. This procedure, however, might be dangerous due to the close antigenicity. The antibodies directed against the xenogeneic species recognize similar targets on the subsequent allogeneic graft and are thus able to jeopardize the prospective permanent allograft. Without more information about possible immunosuppression or modulation of both allogeneic and xenogeneic graft rejection, this bridging should not be ventured in a clinical situation at the present time under conventional triple drug therapy.

fibrinogen or platelets and RBC were found occasionally. Immunohistology showed a massive deposit of IgM predominantly around muscle cells, endothelium of vessels and perivascular tissue, suggesting that a mixed rejection type with strong humoral participation occurred. TxB2 and 6-keto-PGF$_{1a}$ showed no significant alterations during the first postoperative hours and days (Figs. 2 and 3). While TxB2 increased rapidly 1 day prior to final rejection, 6-keto-PGF$_{1a}$ levels altered little.

Acute rejection

The AHTP of the control group showed typical severe cellular rejection. One juvenile AHTP after bridging reacted in the same way as described for the control group. Interstitial haemorrhage and widespread myocytolysis were found. Only slight B-cell infiltrates and accumulations of IgM could be detected.

Discussion

Organ availability is a worsening problem in clinical transplantation. The shortage of human organs has prompted trials for the use of organs from other species. New, potent

References

1. Addonizio P, Wetstein L, Fisher C (1982) Mediation of cardiac ischaemia by thromboxanes released from human platelets. Surgery 2: 292–297
2. Baily L, Nehlsen-Cannorella S, Conception W, et al (1985) Baboon to human cardiac xenotransplantation in a neonate. JAMA 23: 3321–3329
3. Bajusz E, Jasmin G (1964) Histochemical studies on the myocardium following experimental interference with coronary circulation in the rat. Acta Histochem 18: 222–237
4. Billingham ME, Cary N, Hammond E, et al (1990) A working formulation for the standardization of nomenclature in the diagnosis of heart and lung rejection: Heart rejection study group. Heart Transplant 6: 587–593
5. Devries WC, Anderson JL, Joyce LD, et al (1984) Clinical use of the total artificial heart. N Engl J Med 310: 273–278
6. Forbes RDC, Kuramochi T, Guttmann J, et al (1982) A controlled sequential morphologic study of hyperacute cardiac allograft rejection in the rat. Surgery 3: 292–297
7. Hammer C (1987) Isohaemaglutinins and preformed natural antibodies in xenogeneic organ transplantation. Transplant Proc 6: 4443–4447
8. Hammer C (1989) Evolutionary considerations in xenotransplantation. In: Hardy M (ed) Xenograft 25. Elsevier Science, Amsterdam, pp 115–125
9. Hammer C, Saumweber D, Krombach F (1989) Xenotransplantation in canines. In: Hardy M (ed) Xenograft 25. Elsevier Science, Amsterdam, pp 67–85
10. Knechtle S, Kolbeck P, Tsuchimoto S, et al (1987) Hepatic transplantation into sensitized recipients: Demonstration of hyperacute rejection. Transplantation 43: 8
11. Krombacher K, Happel M, Grosse-Wilde H (1991) Recognition of monocyte associated antigens in the dog. Tissue Antigens 37: 21–25
12. Masashi Y, Akihiro I, Tomohisha I, et al (1988) Primary structure, synthesis and biological activity of rat endothelin, an endothelium-derived vasoconstrictor peptide. Proc Natl Acad Sci USA 85: 6964–6967
13. Mullerworth MH, Lixfeld W, Rose A, et al (1972) Hyperacute rejection of heterotopic heart allografts in dogs. Transplantation 3: 570–575
14. Pearse AGE (1960) Histochemistry. Theoretical and applied. Churchill
15. Schütz A, Kemkes BM, Kugler C, et al (1990) Kinetics and dynamics of acute rejection after heterotopic heart transplantation (abstract). J Heart Transplant 9: 63
16. Schütz A, Breuer M, Engelhardt M, et al (1991) Heterotopic cervical heart transplantation with unsensitized vs. presensitized donors ('Domino'): Comparison of kinetics in acute rejection. Texas Heart Inst J (in press)
17. Vriesendorp HM, Westbroek DL, D'Amaro J et al (1973) Joint report of 1st international workshop on canine immunogenetics. Tissue Antigens 3: 145–172

Transplant Int (1992) 5 [Suppl 1]: S 311–S 312

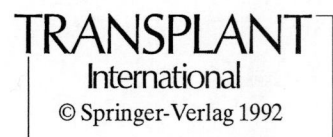

TRANSPLANT
International
© Springer-Verlag 1992

Activation of the alternative pathway of complement is an important component of hyperacute rejection of rabbit hearts by human blood

J. Forty, R. Hasan, N. Cary, D. J. G. White, and J. Wallwork

Papworth Hospital, Cambridge, UK

Hyperacute discordant xenograft rejection can be simulated by blood perfused working isolated heart [1]. The survival of the heart is dependent on its functional integrity, and the preparation is thus sensitive to early myocardial damage.

Perfusion of rabbit hearts with human blood results in immediate graft destruction by a thrombotic process. Prevention of this process results in rapid rejection at about 20 min by the alternative pathway of complement.

Key words: Heart graft thrombosis – Hyperacute rejection – Alternative pathway of complement

Methods

Hearts of 1.7 kg New Zealand White Rabbits were perfused with rabbit or human group AB blood. Blood of either species was collected into heparin (6500 units/l) and was reduced to a haematocrit of 25 %. Human blood was unmodified, or had previously perfused another heart, or had been treated as detailed below. A log-rank analysis of survival of the six hearts in each group was performed.

Complement was inactivated by the addition of 10 μg purified cobra venom factor (CoF) [3] to 240 ml plasma. Alternative pathway inactivation alone was produced by heating plasma at 50 °C for 20 min to destroy factor B. Anti-rabbit antibody (ARA) was absorbed from human plasma by incubation with rabbit blood cells for 80 min at 4 °C.

Hearts were perfused as working preparations [1] until their functional failure. Lytic human ARA titres were measured before and after perfusion [1]. Complement classical pathway activity was measured by the CH50 technique [3]. Hearts were examined after perfusion by conventional and immunohistological methods (IgG, IgM, C3, C4, C9).

Results

Homologous perfusion resulted in organ survival of 300 min with little functional change. Hearts perfused with human blood underwent immediate graft thrombosis

(IGT) ($P < 0.001$). This is initiated by IgM anti-rabbit antibody and the classical pathway of complement, is mediated by platelet activating factor and is effected by platelets [2]. Hearts perfused with human blood modified as above did not undergo this immediate process.

In systems where IGT was prevented, rejection occurred at a median time of 20 min ($P < 0.001$) [2]. Examination of rejected hearts showed neutrophil and lymphoid infiltrates with interstitial IgG and endothelial IgM deposits. C9 deposition was in excess of C4.

Perfusion with blood, complement-inactivated with CoF, delayed organ failure to a median time of 207 min ($P < 0.001$). No C3, 4 or 9 was seen. Perfusion with heat-inactivated blood resulted in survival to 300 min with little functional change ($P < 0.001$). IgM, IgG and C3 were deposited. Classical pathway CH50 remained normal. Rejection at a median time of 33 min still occurred with blood from which the ARA had been absorbed. No IgM was seen in these hearts though the interstitial IgG remained. C3 was present as was C9 in excess of C4. Organ survival is summarized in Figure 1.

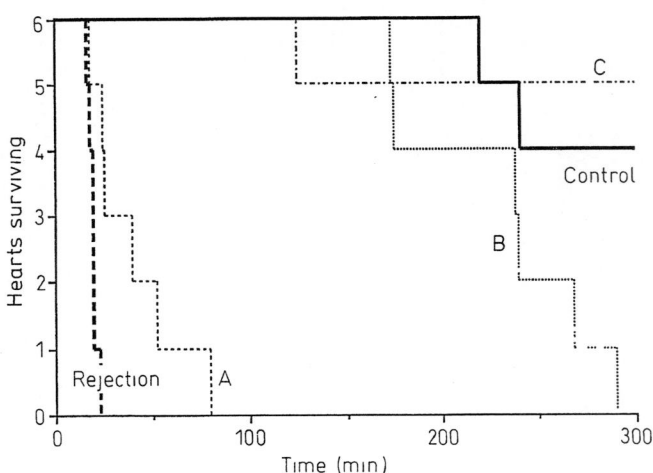

Fig. 1. Organ survival. *A*, antibody absorbed; *B*, complement inactivated; *C*, alternative pathway inactivated

Offprint requests to: J. Forty, Department of Cardiothoracic Surgery, Freeman Hospital, Newcastle-upon-Tyne, UK

Discussion

Hearts which had been rejected at about 20 min in the absence of IGT had C9 deposition in excess of C4 suggesting that activation of the alternative pathway of complement had occurred. The part played by complement, by whichever pathway, is confirmed by the prevention of rejection by complement inactivation with CoF. The important role of the alternative pathway of complement is demonstrated by the prevention of rejection by heart inactivation, to destroy factor B and inactivate this pathway, despite the presence of normal plasma titres and deposition of anti-rabbit antibody and a normal classical pathway CH50. Failure of absorption of heterophile antibody to prevent rejection confirms the unimportance of this antibody in this second component of rejection.

The distinction that has been made between immediate graft thrombosis, a classical pathway process, and rejection by the alternative pathway in discordant organ perfusion has been made possible only by the use of a new, sensitive technique.

The assumption that hyperacute discordant xenograft rejection is the consequence of a heterophile antibody [6] has been challenged [4, 5]. These results suggest that rejection is multifactorial and that an important component is mediated by the alternative pathway of complement.

References

1. Forty J, White DJG, Wallwork J (1991)
2. Forty J, Hasan R, Cary N, White DGJ, Wallwork J (1991) Transplant Proc
3. Harrison RA, Lachman PJ (1986) In: Weir DM, Herzenberg LA, Blackwell C (eds) Handbook of experimental immunology, 4th edn. Blackwell, Oxford
4. Johnston PS, Lim SML, Wang MW, Wright L, White DJG (1991) Transplant Proc 23: 877–879
5. Miyagawa S, Hirose H, Shirakura R, et al (1988) Transplantation 46: 825–830
6. Perper RJ, Najarian JS (1966) Transplantation 4: 377–388

Transplant Int (1992) 5 [Suppl 1]: S 313–S 317

TRANSPLANT
International
© Springer-Verlag 1992

Inhibition of rejection of hamster-to-rat heart xenografts

R. Hasan, J. van den Bogaerde, J. Forty, L. Wright, J. Wallwork, and D. J. G. White

Papworth Hospital, Cambridge, UK

Abstract. Prolonged survival of concordant organ xenografts as typified by hamster-to-rat heart transplants is difficult to produce. Studies have revealed that T cells are not primarily involved in rejecting such xenografts and that the rat recipients produce high titres of lytic anti-hamster antibodies. In this study, 200 hamster-to-rat cardiac xenografts performed in 30 different experiments revealed that cyclophosphamide (CyP) and cyclosporin A (CyA) could inhibit this antibody production. CyP alone was relatively ineffective in prolonging graft survival (the median survival time was 14 days versus 3 days in untreated controls). Combining CyP and CyA virtually abolished rejection in this model. Four critically timed doses of CyP combined with continuous CyA resulted in recipients not producing anti-hamster antibodies, despite cessation of CyP therapy, and prolonged graft survival time (median survival time was more than 100 days). Cessation of CyA at 60 and 100 days resulted in the rejection of the xenografts and the appearance of the rat anti-hamster antibodies. Xenografts in recipients given only one or two doses of CyP (and continuous CyA) had a median survival time of 7 and 12 days respectively. However xenograft rejection in rats given only 1 or 2 doses of CyP could be averted by complement depletion using a 3-week course of cobra venom factor (CoF) starting on day 4 or day 7 post-transplantation respectively. Discontinuation of CoF after 3 weeks did not result in graft rejection. These results showed that immunosuppressive therapies directed at inhibiting antibody production may be of value in preventing rejection of concordant xenografts. Short-term complement depletion could rescue xenografts from rejection such that rescued grafts appear to be accommodated.

Key words: Hamster-to-rat xenograft – Cyclophosphamide – Cyclosporin A – Cobra venom factor – Complement – Concordant xenograft

Xenografts have been categorized as discordant or concordant [5]. The discordant category is that species combination in which rejection of organ xenografts is hyperacute, with vascular lesions similar to those seen in second-set allografts. In the concordant category, rejection occurs at a tempo and with morphological characteristics similar to first-set allografts. In this study the immunologic processes involved in the rejection of concordant hamster-to-rat xenografts were investigated.

Current immunosuppressive regimes used in transplantation are designed to inhibit the predominantly cellular processes which are responsible for first-set rejection of allografts. The application of these protocols in both experimental and clinical xenografting has been disappointing [24, 30]. While graft prolongation has been achieved in combinations where donor and recipient were phylogenetically very closely related such as wolf to dog [9, 12], goat to sheep [25], hare to rabbit [8] and chimpanzee to man [29], results in more distantly related species though still concordant such as hamster to rat [33], monkey to baboon [6] or baboon to man [32] have been disappointing. Those regimes which do produce prolongation of such xenografts rely on immune ablative procedures, the mechanisms of which cannot be fully analyzed because of their multifunctional nature [15, 16]. The transplantation of organs from hamster to rat has been extensively studied as a model of concordant xenograft rejection [7, 14, 16, 21, 37]. Previous workers have not been able to achieve long term xenograft survival consistently in this species combination, in spite of the ablation of T cell mediated immune responses [11, 36]. However, the depletion of complement in rat recipients of hamster heart in combination with continuous cyclosporin A (CyA) therapy has resulted in some long term survival [37]. Additionally, the kinetics of the anti-hamster antibody response in untreated or T cell deficient recipients [17] in conjunction with the demonstration of binding of these antibodies to the rejected grafts, has suggested an important role for antibody as well as complement in the rejection of these concordant xenografts. These data indicate that inhibition of anti-graft antibody production might extend xenograft survival in this model.

Offprint requests to: R. Hasan, Department of Surgery, Addenbrookes Hospital, Hills Road, Cambridge CB2 2QQ, UK

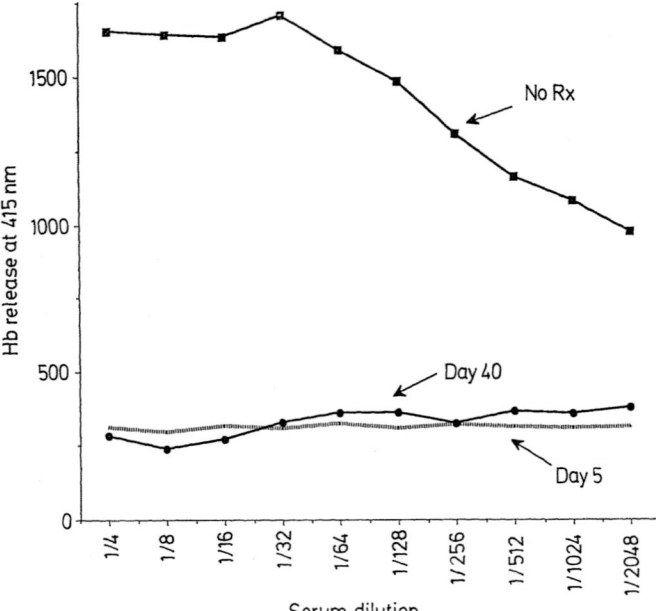

Fig. 1. Lytic anti-hamster antibody in cyclophosphamide and cyclosporin A treated rat recipients of a hamster heart xenograft on days 5 and 40 compared with antibody levels on day 5 in an untreated recipient

This study was designed to investigate the possibility of suppressing pharmacologically anti-hamster antibody production in rat recipients of hamster heart xenografts using cyclophosphamide (CyP) because of its known ability to inhibit antibody production via selective action on rapidly proliferating B cell blasts [34]. We also explored the feasibility of rescuing concordant xenografts from rejection.

Materials and methods

Animals. Syrian hamsters (80–110 g) were used as heart donors (Wright Brothers, Essex, UK) and PVG rats (220–250 g) as recipients (Bantin and Kingman, Hull, UK).

Cardiac transplants. Heterotopic cardiac transplants were placed into the neck of recipients vascularizing the xenograft on a pedicle of the external jugular and carotid vessels using the cuff technique as previously described [13].

Immunosuppressive agents. Cyclophosphamide (CyP) was freshly prepared in distilled water at 10 mg/ml from 100 mg vials (Degussa Pharmaceuticals, Cambridge), injected intraperitonealy and the excess discarded. CyA (a gift from Dr. J. F. Borel, Sandoz Ltd, Basel, Switzerland) was dissolved in olive oil and administered intramuscularly at 20 mg/kg on alternate days (i.e. 10 mg/kg daily). Cobra venom factor (CoF) was prepared as previously described in aliquots of 0.5 mg/ml and administered intramuscularly at a dose of 0.5 mg/kg on alternate days (i.e. 0.25 mg/kg daily). Cobra venom was prepared as previously described in 0.5 mg/ml aliquots and injected intramuscularly at 0.5 mg/kg on alternate days (i.e. 0.25 mg/kg daily) [37].

Antibody titres. Lytic antibody titers were measured in the serum of recipient rats, using hamster red blood cells as targets and baby rabbit serum as a source of complement. Cell lysis was assayed by haemoglobin release into complement fixation diluent as measured on a spectrophotometer [37].

Statistical analysis. Groups of survivors were compared using the Mann Whitney test [18], with significance achieved with P value less than 0.01.

Results

Untreated rats rejected hamster hearts in a median of 3 days (group 1, Table 1). Very high titres of anti-hamster antibodies in excess of 1/2048 were detected in these animals (Fig. 1). Animals receiving CyP only at a dose of 40 mg/kg on day 1 followed by 20 mg/kg twice weekly for 4 weeks ($n = 10$), (group 2, Table 1) survived significantly longer (median survival time of 14 days) than the untreated group ($P < 0.01$). In this group, five animals rejected their xenografts while three died with beating hearts during therapy. The remaining two recipients completed the course of treatment (28 days), but died 1 week later with beating xenografts.

A series of experiments were performed to verify the optimum dosage of CyP (Hasan et al., manuscript submitted) necessary to suppress antibody production. It was found that four critically timed doses of CyP (days 1, 2, 5 and 8) was sufficient to prevent rejection by the effect of suppressing anti-hamster antibodies; 60% of recipients survived long term (> 100 days) while the remaining 40% of recipients died of infection with beating xenografts (group 3, Table 1). There were no detectable anti-hamster antibodies in any rat recipient receiving CyP and CyA therapy up to 30 days after the last dose of CyP (Fig. 1).

Table 1. Survival of hamster heart xenografts in rats treated with cyclophosphamide (CyP) and cyclosporin A (CyA)

Group	Therapy	Survival in days	N	MST
1	Untreated	3, 3, 3, 3, 3, 3, 3, 3, 4, 4	10	3
2	CyP (4 wks)	3[a], 4[a], 11[a], 12, 14, 14, 18, 20, 35[a], 35[a]	10	14
3	CyP (one dose) + CyA	7, 7, 7, 7, 7, 7, 8, 8, 9, 9	10	7
4	CyP (two doses) + CyA	11, 11, 11, 12, 12, 12, 12, 12, 13, 13	10	12
5	CyP (four doses) + CyA	10[a], 18[a], 27[a], 61[a], (> 100 × 6)	10	> 100

[a] Recipient died with beating xenograft
MST, Median survival time

Table 2. Survival of hamster hearts in rat recipients treated with one and two doses of cyclophosphamide (CyP) and continuous cyclosporin A (CyA) when they are rescued by a 3-week course of cobra venom factor (CoF) starting on day 4 and day 7 respectively

Group	Therapy	Survival in days	N	MST
6	CyP (one dose) + CyA + CoF (on day 4 for 3 weeks)	4[a], 17, 18, 21, 38, (60 × 5)	10	49
7	CyP (two doses) + CyA + CoF (on day 7 for 3 weeks)	38, 40, (60 × 8)	10	60

[a] Recipient died with beating xenograft
MST, Median survival time

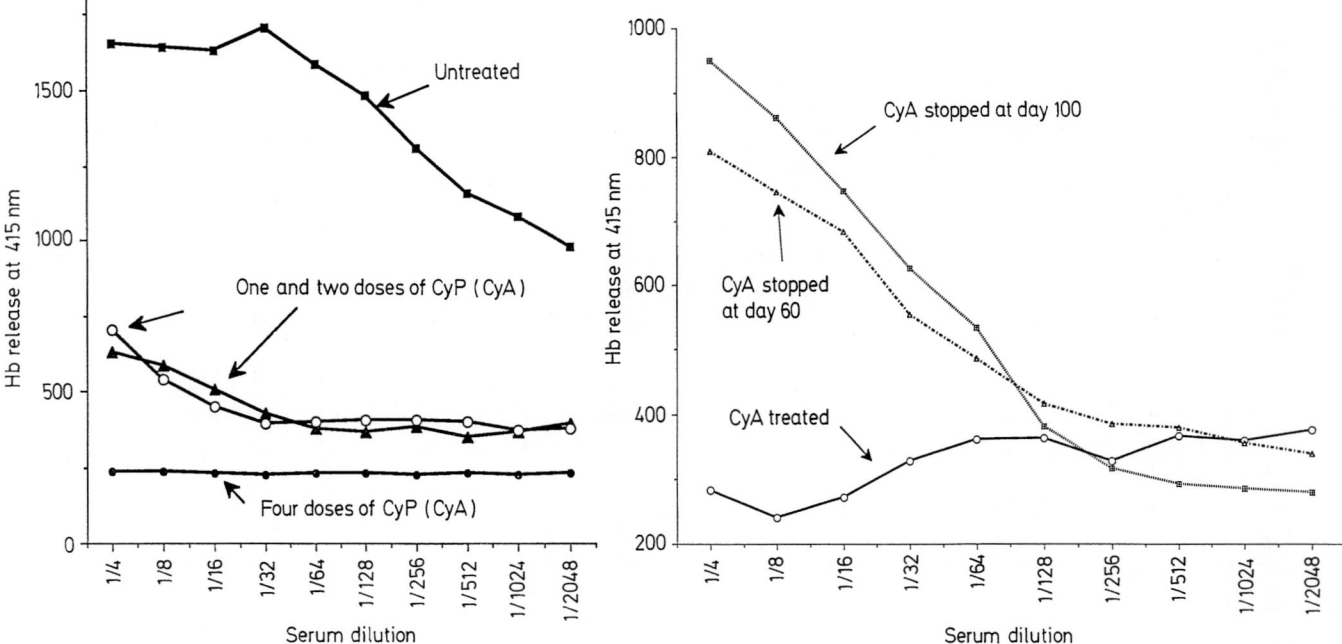

Fig. 2. Lytic anti-hamster antibody in cyclophosphamide (one and two doses) and cyclosporin A treated rat recipients of a hamster heart xenograft at the time of rejection compared with antibody levels on day 12 in recipients who had four doses of cyclophosphamide and continuous cyclosporin A. Peak lytic anti-hamster antibody in untreated rat recipients on day 5 is shown for comparison

Fig. 3. Lytic antibody in rat recipients of hamster heart xenograft who had cyclosporin therapy discontinued on day 60 and day 100 post-transplantation. Antibodies were measured at the time of rejection. As a control, antibody levels were measured in a recipient rat on day 40 while it was still receiving cyclosporin

In an attempt to eliminate the infective complications, the CyP dosage was reduced to one (the day before transplantation) or two (the day before the operation and on the second post-operative day) doses only, but this was not sufficient to suppress antibody production and the xenografts survived for a median of 7 or 12 days respectively (groups 4 and 5, Table 1). Antibody in these animals was detectable at a titre of 1/16 compared to a total absence in recipients who had four doses (Fig. 2). A rescue therapy was attempted in which recipients given 1 or 2 doses of CyP as described above were treated with CoF either on day 4 (1 dose group) or day 7 (2 doses group) post-transplantation. This therapy was successful in averting the rejection. Furthermore, when CoF was discontinued after 3 weeks the grafts continued to survive (Table 2).

The role of continued CyA therapy was examined in two experiments. A group of 10 recipients (out of 13) treated with four doses of CyP, and CyA at 10 mg/kg daily survived for 60 days. These recipients then had the CyA therapy discontinued. All the transplanted hearts were rejected with a median survival time of 11 days following

the discontinuation of CyA (group 1, Table 3). A second group of 10 recipients, who received the same CyP and CyA therapy, with xenografts surviving more than 100 days had the CyA therapy discontinued at day 100. All the recipients rejected the transplanted hearts with a median survival time of 19.5 days following the withdrawal of CyA therapy (group 2, Table 3). In these two groups anti-hamster antibodies could be demonstrated in the recipients at the time of rejection (Fig. 3).

Discussion

The data described here demonstrated that judicious treatment of rat recipients of hamster heart xenografts with a combination of CyP and CyA inhibited the production of anti-species antibodies and produced long-term xenograft survival. Furthermore it seems likely that these two events were causally linked. Insufficient doses of cyclophosphamide produced some prolongation of graft survival but all the grafts were rejected due probably to the development of antibodies although the titres were less than those in untreated recipients. Prevention of graft rejection in the face of the imminent appearance of anti-species antibodies was achieved by a short-term depletion of complement with CoF (3-week course).

Others have demonstrated the importance of antibodies in the rejection of concordant xenografts [3, 4, 10, 19, 23]. In addition, measures designed to decrease antibody production in rats are able to produce an increase in the survival of hamster heart xenografts. These measures involve the use of splenectomy with or without cyclo-

Table 3. Survival of hamster heart xenografts in rats after discontinuation of cyclosporin A (CyA)

Group	Therapy	Survival in days	N	MST
1	CyP (4 doses) + CyA 10 mg/kg CyA stopped at day 60	8, 9, 9, 10, 11, 11, 15, 18, 20, 20	10	11
2	CyA stopped at day 100	17, 17, 17, 18, 18, 21, 21, 23, 23, 23	10	19.5

CyP, Cyclophosphamide; MST, median survival time

sporin A [22] or 15-deoxyspergualin alone or combined with splenectomy or total lymphoid irradiation [19, 28, 35] but they were unsuccessful in producing long-term survival in this concordant combination (survival ranged from 7–40 days). The demonstration of some long-term survival of hamster xenografts in CyA-treated complement-depleted recipients, implicates complement in the rejection of concordant xenografts [37]. In addition, very high anti-graft antibody titers and antibody binding to transplanted hamster hearts were shown in these animals. The use of one or two doses of CyP depressed this antibody production but was not sufficient to prevent it and rejection occured. Complement depletion with CoF in such animals prevented this rejection.

This offers an exciting possibility for the future, since concordant xenograft recipients could be monitored by measuring anti-species antibodies and if they appear, then complement depletion for a short period should prevent rejection. The depletion of C3 disarms both the alternative and classical complement pathway. Both pathways have been shown to be involved in the rejection of discordant xenografts [20, 27, 31]. One question addressed by this study was whether alternative complement activation was able to cause destruction of these concordant xenografts. The data reported here showed that combination therapy with CyP and CyA completely inhibited anti-hamster antibody production, did not affect complement activity and yet produced significant prolongation of hamster heart xenograft survival. This confirmed that unlike the discordant models previously studied, [31, 20] destruction in this concordant model was not caused by the alternative pathway of complement.

These data also showed that the anti-xenograft antibody response could be inhibited by a short pulse of CyP and continuous CyA therapy. Monotherapy with CyP resulted in significant prolongation of the xenografts but was insufficient to produce long-term survival. Combined CyP and CyA was capable of producing long-term survival in this model with total absence of rat anti-hamster antibodies for the duration of CyA therapy. However, discontinuation of CyA at 60 or 100 days post-transplantation resulted in rejection of the xenografts and the emergence of anti-hamster antibodies. These results strongly suggested a major role for anti-species antibodies in the rejection of concordant xenografts and that the combined therapy of CyP and CyA produced long-term survival by suppressing this antibody production.

Data from this and other publications showing the importance of antibody-mediated rejection in "concordant" xenografts, has clouded the original distinction between concordant and discordant xenografts [5]. Although hyperacute, "antibody-driven" complement-mediated xenograft rejection is apparently unique to "discordant" combinations [26], similarities in the histological appearance and rejection mechanisms between discordant and certain concordant xenograft combinations places the value of the original "first-set allograft" (concordant) and "second-set allograft" (discordant) definition in some doubt [1]. To resolve this difficulty we would propose a subdivision of concordant xenografts into "difficult" and "easy" depending on whether antibody-mediated rejec-

tion ("difficult concordant"), or T cell mediated rejection ("easy concordant") is of primary importance. This is of practical significance, since baboon to human transplants, which represent the most likely combination for clinical xenografting in the immediate future, would appear to be "difficult concordant" xenografts according to histological and immunological data currently available [2]. By the same criteria, chimpanzee to man [29] would fall in the "easy concordant" category. The extrapolation of results obtained from rodents to clinical practice is ill advised, yet the data reported here suggest that similar studies in primates need to be undertaken to establish the possibility of using this clinically applicable therapy to prevent xenograft rejection in man and the preliminary results using the above therapeutic regimens are encourging.

References

1. Bailey LL, Nehlsen-Cannarella SL (1986) Observations on cardiac xenotransplantation. Transplant Proc 18 3 [Suppl 2]: 88–92
2. Bailey Ll, Nehlsen-Cannarella SL, Concepcion W, Jolley WB (1985) Baboon-to-human cardiac xenotransplantation in a neonate. JAMA 245: 3321–3329
3. Bogman MJ, Berden JM, Hagemann JM, Maass CN, Koene RP (1980) Patterns of vascular damage in the antibody-mediated rejection of skin xenografts in the mouse. Am J Pathol 100: 727–737
4. Bouwman E, Bruin RF, Marquet RL, Jeekel J (1989) Prolongation of graft survival in hamster to rat xenografting. Transplant Proc 21: 540–541
5. Calne R (1970) Organ transplantation between widely disparate species. Transplant Proc 2: 550–553
6. Cooper DKC, Rose AG (1989) Experience with experimental xenografting in primates. In: Hardy MA (ed) Xenograft 25. Elsevier Science Publication (Biomedical Division), Amsterdam, The Netherlands
7. DeMasi R, Alqaisi M, Araneda D, Nifong W, Thomas J, Gross U, Sawson M, Thomas JM (1990) Revaluation of total lymphoid irradiation and cyclosporine therapy in the syrian hamster-to-lewis rat cardiac xenograft model. Transplantation 49: 639–662
8. Dieperink H, Steinbruchel D, Starklint H, Larsen S, Kemp E (1987) Improvement in hare-to-rabbit kidney transplant survival. Transplant Proc 19: 1140–1142
9. Duswald KH, Scheel JV, Hammer C, Brendel W (1976) Long-term graft survival in the xenogenic system wolf-dog. Res Exp Med (Berl) 167: 255–266
10. Ertel W, Reichenspurner H, Hammer C, Welz A, Uberfuhr P, Hemmer W, Reichart B, Gokel M, Brendel W (1984) Heterotransplantation in closely related species: a model for humoral rejection. Transplant Proc 16: 1258–1261
11. Gudas VM, Carmichael PG, Morris RE (1989) Comparison of the immunosuppressive and toxic effects of FK 506 and cyclosporin in xenograft recipients. Transplant Proc 21: 1072–1073
12. Hammer C, Chaussey C, Welter H, Weinbacher J, Hobel G, Brendel W (1981) Exceptionally long survival time in xenogeneic organ transplantation. Transplant Proc 13: 881–884
13. Heron I (1971) A technique for accessory cervical heart transplantation in rabbits and rats. Acta Pathol Microbiol Immunol Scand [A] 79: 366–372
14. Homan WP, Williams KA, Fabre JW, Millard PJ, Morris P (1981) Prolongation of cardiac xenograft survival in rats receiving cyclosporin A. Transplantation 31: 164–166
15. Kemp E, Dieperink H, Jensenius J, Koch C, Larsen S, Madsen H, Nielsen B, Starklint H, Steinbruchel DA (1990) Hope for successful xenografting by immunosuppression with monoclonal antibody against CD4, total lymphoid irradiation and cyclosporine. Scand J Urol Nephrol 24: 79–80

16. Knetchle SJ, Halperin EC, Bollinger RR (1987) Xenograft survival in two species combination using total lymphoid irradiation and cyclosporin. Transplantation 43: 173–175

17. Lim SML, Li SQ, Wee A, Chong SM, Hu A, Rauff A, White DJG (1991) Both concordant and discordant heart xenografts are rejected by athymic(nude) rats with the same tempo as in T cell competent animals. Transplant Proc 23: 581–582

18. Mann HB, Whitney DR (1947) On a test of whether one of two random variables is statistically larger than the other. Ann Math Statist 18: 50–60

19. Marchman WAD, DeMasi R, Taylor D, Carrobi A, Larkin E, Alqaisi M, Thomas F (1991) Therapy with 15-deoxyspergualin and total lymphoid irradiation blocks xenograft rejection and antibody formation after xenografting. Transplant Proc 23: 210–211

20. Miyagawa S, Hirose H, Shirakura R, Yoshihumi N, Nakata S, Kawashima Y, Seya T, Matsumoto M, Uenaka A, Kimtamura H (1988) The mechanism of discordant xenograft rejection. Transplantation 46: 825–830

21. Moden M, Valdivia LA, Gotoh M, Hasuike Y, Kubota N, Kanai T, Okamura J, Mori T (1987) Hamster-to-rat orthotopic liver transplant. Transplantation 43: 745–746

22. Monden M, Valdivia LA, Goton M (1989) A crucial effect of splenectomy on prolonging cardic xenograft survival in combination with cyclosporine. Surgery 105: 535–542

23. Nakajima K, Sakamoto K, Ochiai T, Asano T, Isono K (1989) Effects of 15-deoxyspergualin and FK506 on the histology and survival of hamster-to-rat cardiac xenotransplantation. Transplant Proc 21: 546–548

24. Nakajima K, Sakamoto K, Ochiai T, Nagata M, Asano T, Isono K (1988) Prolongation of cardiac xenograft survival in rats treated with 15-deoxyspergualin alone and in combination with FK506. Transplantation 45: 1146–1148

25. Perper RJ, May J, Way L, Najarian JS (1965) Experimental renal heterotransplantation in closely related species. Fed Proc 24: 573

26. Perper RJ, Najarian JS (1966) Experimental renal heterotransplantation I. in widely divergent species. Transplantation 4: 377–388

27. Platt JL, Vercellotti GM, Dalmasso AP, Matas AJ, Bolman RM, Najarian JS, Bach FH (1990) Transplantation of discordant xenografts: a review of progress. Immunol Today 11: 450–456

28. Pruitt SK, Halperin EC, Bollinger RR (1991) The effect of 15-deoxyspergualin on hamster-to-rat cardiac xenograft survival. Transplant Proc 23: 585–586

29. Reemtsma K, McCracken DH, Schilegel JU, Pearl MA, Pearce CW, DeWitt CW, Smith PE, Hewitt RL, Flinner RL, Oscar-Creech Jr (1964) Renal heterotransplantation in man. Ann Surg 160: 384–410

30. Sakakibara N, Click RE, Condie RM, Jamieson SW (1989) Rejection/acceptance of xenografts. Transplant Proc 21: 524–526

31. Schilling A, Land W, Pratschke E, Pielsticker K, Brendel W (1976) Dominant role of complement in the hyperacute xenograft rejection reaction. Surg Gynecol Obstet 142: 29–32

32. Starzl TE, Marchioro TL, Peters GN, Kirckpatrick CH, Wilson WEC, Porter KA, Rifkind D, Ogden DA, Hitchcock CR, Waddell WR (1964) Renal heterotransplantation from baboon to man: experience with 6 cases. Transplantation 2: 752–776

33. Thomas FT, DeMasi RJ, Araneda D, Marchman W, Alqaisi M, Larkin EW, Condie RM, Carobbi A, Thomas JM (1990) Comparative efficacy of immunosuppressive drugs in xenografting. Transplant Proc 22: 1083–1085

34. Turk JL, Poulter LW (1972) Effects of cyclophosphamide on lymphoid tissue labelled with 5-iodo-2-deoxyuridine ^{125}I and Cr-51. Int Arch Allergy 43: 620–629

35. Valdivia LA, Monden M, Gotoh M, Nakano Y, Tono T, Mori T (1990) Evidence that deoxyspergualin prevents sensitization and first-set cardiac xenograft rejection in rats by suppression of antibody formation. Transplantation 50: 132–136

36. van den Bogaerde JB, White DJG, Roser B, Kampinga JR, Aspinall R (1990) In vitro and in vivo effects of monoclonal antibodies against T-cells subsets in allogenic and xenogeneic responses in the rat. Transplantation 50: 915–920

37. van den Bogaerde JB, Aspinall R, Wright L, Wang MW, Carey N, White DGJ (1991) The induction of long term survival of hamster heart xenografts in rats. Transplantation 53: 15–20

Transplant Int (1992) 5 [Suppl 1]: S 318–S 319

TRANSPLANT
International
© Springer-Verlag 1992

Perfusion of rabbit hearts with pig blood results in complement mediated hyperacute xenograft rejection

J. Forty, D. J. G. White, and J. Wallwork

Papworth Hospital, Cambridge, UK

Investigation of hyperacute rejection of discordant xenografts has been hampered by the lack of a model for the study of rapid time course events. In vivo models are unsuitable for observation of early rejection processes and, along with most ex-vivo perfusion preparations, are insensitive since no functional demand is placed on the organ which may have undergone extensive damage whilst still appearing viable. For this reason a blood perfused isolated working heart preparation has been developed [1]. With left atrial and left ventricular loading the heart performs measurable work as it ejects into a mock circulation with both afterload and compliance components. When cardiac function is compromised the heart is no longer able to eject against the fixed afterload and both cardiac output and coronary circulation cease with resultant organ failure. The model is thus highly sensitive to minimal organ damage and has an easily identifiable endpoint. In the present study, we used this preparation to study the discordant species combination of rabbit hearts perfused with pig blood.

Key words: Blood perfused isolated working heart preparation – Rabbit hearts – Rabbit blood – Pig blood

Methods

Hearts of 1.7 kg New Zealand White rabbits were perfused with either rabbit blood collected into heparin (6500 units/l) and with the haematocrit reduced to 25 %, or similarly collected and treated pig blood either unmodified or complement depleted with cobra venom factor (CoF). There were four hearts in each perfusion group. Hearts were perfused until functional damage caused their failure. A log-rank analysis of survival was performed.

Complement depletion was achieved by the addition of 10 µg purified CoF [2] to 240 mls plasma. Lytic pig anti-rabbit antibody

(ARA) titres were measured before and after perfusion by a haemolytic method [1]. Complement classical pathway activity was measured with a CH50 technique [2]. Hearts were examined after failure by conventional and immunohistological methods (IgG, IgM, C3).

Results

Rabbit hearts perfused with rabbit blood survived for a median time of 271 min. Perfusion with unmodified pig blood resulted in organ rejection at a median time of 13 min ($P < 0.001$). Total complement haemolytic activity (CH50) and ARA titre was unchanged during perfusion. Conventional histology revealed lymphoid and neutrophil cell infiltrates and immunofluorescence showed interstitial IgG and endothelial deposits of IgM and C3. Perfusion with pig blood treated with CoF (complement activity completely removed) produced survival of a median time of 175 min ($P < 0.001$). The myocardium remained normal and IgG and IgM were deposited but no C3 was seen. Organ survival is summarised in Fig. 1.

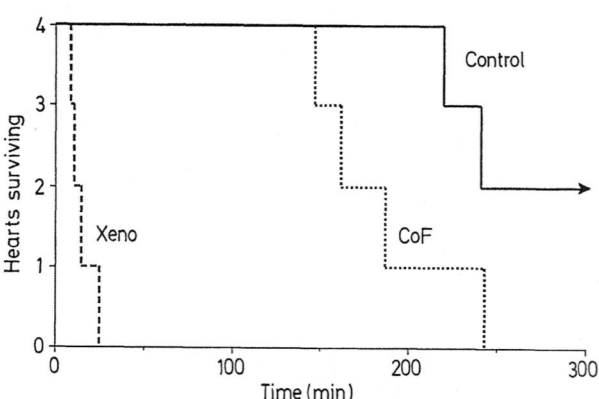

Fig. 1. Survival of rabbit hearts perfused with rabbit blood (auto), pig blood (xeno) and complement depleted pig blood (CoF)

Offprint requests to: J. Forty

Discussion

A sensitive perfusion model for the investigation of rapid time course events has been developed and has been used to simulate hyperacute discordant rejection of rabbit hearts by pig blood. Prevention of rejection by complement inactivation and the detection of C3 on the perfused myocardium demonstrated the central role of complement in the process. No conclusion could be made, however, concerning the relative importance of the classical and alternative pathways of complement. Further analysis of rejection in this species combination is prevented by the lack of immunological reagents for the investigation of pig blood. The sensitivity of this technique will permit detailed analysis of the components of rejection of rabbit hearts by human blood where a wider range of immunological tools is available.

References

1. Forty J, White DJG, Wallwork J (1991) A technique for perfusion of an isolated working heart to investigate hyperacute discordant xenograft rejection. In press
2. Harrison RA, Lachman PJ (1986) Complement Technology. In: Weir DM, Herzenberg LA, Blackwell C (ed) Handbook of Experimental Immunology, vol 1, 4th edn. Blackwell, Oxford, p 39

Transplant Int (1992) 5 [Suppl 1]: S 320–S 322

TRANSPLANT
International
© Springer-Verlag 1992

Antibody binding to endothelial and epithelial antigens triggers pig-to-rabbit xenograft rejection and its absence results in atypical complement deposition

I. R. Marino[1], S. Celli[1], G. Ferla[2], H. R. Doyle[1], N. Maggiano[3], G. Zetti[1], and P. Musiani[4]

[1] Department of Surgery, University Health Center of Pittsburgh, University of Pittsburgh, and the Veteran's Administration Medical Center, Pittsburgh, Pennsylvania, USA [2] Department of Surgery of the University of Milan, Milan, Italy [3] Department of Pathology of the Catholic University, Rome, Italy [4] Department of Pathology of the University of Chieti, Chieti, Italy

Abstract. In pig-to-rabbit kidney xenograft (PRKX), endothelial antigen determinants (EAD) are immediately recognized by IgG and IgA, while IgM does not react with them. The purpose of this study was to investigate the different roles of IgG, IgA, IgM, and complement in the hyperacute rejection of a PRKX model. Nine isolated Landrace pig kidneys were each perfused with 10 ml normal New Zealand rabbit serum. Perfusates (serum A) were collected after discarding the first 0.5 ml. Serum A and rabbit complement were then incubated for 30 min with frozen sections of normal pig kidney. After washing with buffer solution all the specimens were treated for immunohistochemistry. Three frozen sections of normal Landrace pig kidney and three samples of normal New Zealand rabbit serum were used as controls. Immunohistochemical analysis of the nine perfused kidneys demonstrated IgG, IgA and C3 deposition on the peritubular and glomerular vascular endothelium. No IgM reactivity was shown. In the frozen sections exposed to serum A, immunofluorescence showed minimal IgG, IgA and C3 reactivity while IgM deposition was clearly evident on the tubular epithelium. Immunofluorescence of frozen sections exposed to rabbit complement, done by fluorescein-labeled goat anti-rabbit C3 antibodies were positive only in the glomerular endothelium. The same rabbit complement was active in antibody dependent cytotoxicity on human T cells. Our results indicated that in the PRKX model, IgG and IgA acted as preformed antibodies recognizing endothelial EAD. IgM did not bind to any endothelial molecules, but recognized antigens located on the brush border of the tubular epithelium. Furthermore, in this model, absence of antigen-antibody complexes resulted in atypical complement deposition.

Key words: Xenotransplantation – Natural antibodies – Hyperacute rejection

Transplantation is currently the treatment of choice for several end-stage organ diseases [10–13]. Considering that the increasing demand for human organs for transplantation far exceeds their availability, xenogeneic transplantation is probably the most realistic solution to the problem [1, 3]. Hyperacute rejection of discordant xenografts is triggered by natural antibodies binding to endothelial antigen determinants (EAD) of the graft, and by complement activation [1]. We have already reported [7–9] that IgG and IgA are responsible for triggering the hyperacute rejection of the pig kidney in a pig-to-rabbit kidney xenograft model (PRKX). In PRKX, EADs are immediately recognized by IgA and IgG, while IgM does not react with them [7–9]. The purpose of this study was to investigate the different roles played by IgG, IgA, IgM and complement in the hyperacute kidney rejection of PRKX. We were interested in identifying the antigen determinants recognized by the different Ig classes, and in ascertaining whether complement can be activated in the absence of antibody binding.

Materials and methods

Five female Landrace pigs weighing 2.0–2.5 kg were used as donors from which nine kidneys were harvested. The donor operation technique has already been reported in detail elsewhere [7]. The kidneys underwent an initial vascular isolation in situ. The infrarenal aorta and the left renal vein were cannulated in order to perfuse the left kidney, while the suprarenal aorta and the cava were cannulated in order to perfuse the right kidney. Fifteen New Zealand female rabbits weighing 4.1–5.0 kg were used as donors of a total of 180 ml normal rabbit serum. Of this normal rabbit serum 90 ml was used to perfuse the nine isolated Landrace pig kidneys (10 ml each). The perfusion of the kidneys was performed through the aorta; 10 ml rabbit serum was infused in each kidney (serum A), and then collected through the renal vein (left kidney) or through the cava (right kidney). The first 0.5 ml of each perfusate was discarded. Following the perfusion with serum A, kidney tissue samples were taken and embedded in the optimum cutting temperature medium (Miles Scientific, Naperville, Ill.), Snap frozen in liquid nitrogen, sectioned and prepared for immunohistochemical analysis. The sections were incubated with fluorescein isothiocyanate conjugated (FICT) goat

Offprint requests to: Ignazio R. Marino, M. D. Transplantation Institute, Department of Surgery, University of Pittsburgh, 3601 Fifth Avenue, Suite 5C, Pittsburgh, Pennsylvania 15213, USA

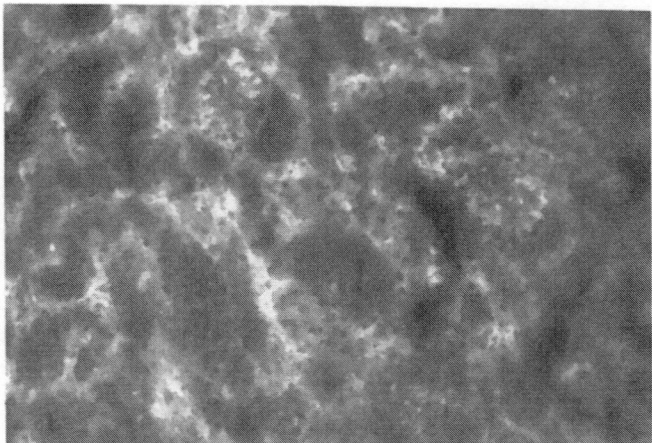

Fig. 1. Immunohistochemical analysis of a Landrace pig kidney perfused with normal New Zealand rabbit serum. The fluorescence staining was performed with goat anti-rabbit IgG. IgG deposits were present in the peritubular capillary walls and in the glomerular capillary loops ($\times 20$). Deposits of IgA were present with similar distribution. Ig deposits were absent from the tubular epithelium

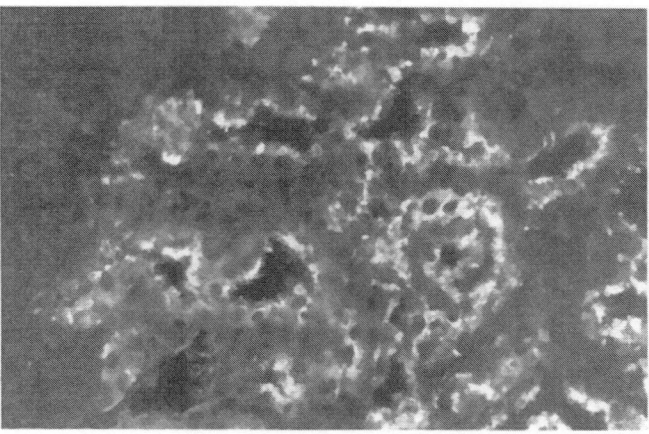

Fig. 2. Immunohistochemical analysis of a frozen section of tissue samples of Landrace pig kidney exposed to serum A (New Zealand rabbit serum infused through the renal artery of an isolated Landrace pig kidney and then collected from the renal vein). The fluorescence staining was performed with goat anti-rabbit IgM. IgM deposits are evident on the tubular epithelium ($\times 40$)

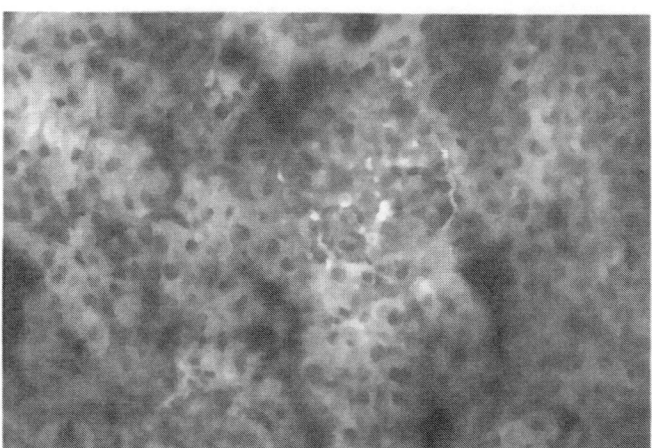

Fig. 3. Immunohistochemical analysis of a frozen section of Landrace pig kidney exposed to rabbit complement. The fluorescence staining was performed with fluorescein-labeled anti-rabbit C3 antibodies. Complement deposition is evident on the glomerular endothelium, while the other tissues did not take the stain ($\times 40$)

anti-rabbit IgM, IgA, IgG, and C3 (Cappel, Organon Teknika, Veedijk, Belgium) for 60 min at room temperature, in a moist chamber.

Three female Landrace pigs weighing 2.0–2.5 kg were then used as donors from which three kidneys were procured. These three kidneys were used to prepare tissue samples of normal pig kidney. They were embedded in the optimum cutting temperature medium (Miles Scientific, Naperville, Ill.), frozen in liquid nitrogen and maintained at $-80\,^{\circ}\mathrm{C}$. Fifteen sections, 5 µm thick each, were then prepared from the frozen tissue. They were thaw-mounted on slides coated with poly-L-Lysine hydrobromide (Polysciences, Warrington, Pa.), and allowed to air dry for 3 h. Finally, they were fixed for 10 min in 100% acetone. Of these 15 sections, 10 were incubated for 30 min with serum A. The remaining five sections were incubated at $37\,^{\circ}\mathrm{C}$ with rabbit complement (Low-toxic-M, Cederlane, Ontario). The sections were then washed with buffer solution and incubated with FICT goat anti-rabbit IgM, IgA, IgG, and C3 (Cappel, Organon Teknika, Veedijk, Belgium) for 60 min at room temperature, in a moist chamber. Three frozen sections of normal pig kidneys that were incubated with three different samples of normal New Zealand rabbit serum were used as controls.

Results

Immunohistochemical analysis of nine Landrace pig kidneys perfused with serum A confirmed the results obtained in our previous in vivo and in vitro study [7–9]. Specifically, IgG, IgA and C3 deposition were evident with uniform distribution on the endothelium of the peritubular capillaries, and on the glomerular endothelium (Fig. 1). No IgM deposition was shown on the vascular endothelium. Immunohistochemical analysis of the ten frozen sections of tissue samples of normal pig kidneys exposed to serum A showed minimal IgG, IgA, and C3 reactivity was compared with the deposition obtained when perfusing normal pig kidneys with normal rabbit serum. Instead, IgM deposition was clearly evident on the tubular epithelium (Fig. 2). Immunofluorescence of the frozen sections exposed to rabbit complement, done by fluorescein-labeled anti-rabbit C3 antibodies demonstrated complement granular deposition only on the glomerular endothelium, while the other tissues did not take the stain (Fig. 3). The same rabbit complement was active in antibody-dependent cytotoxicity reactions on human T cells.

Discussion

Hyperacute rejection mechanisms in discordant xenogeneic transplantation are still unclear [3]. It is recognized that preformed antibodies mediate the hyperacute rejection of solid organs in discordant species combinations [2, 6, 10, 11]. However, it seems that the classes of Ig involved in the process are different in all the discordant xenogeneic transplantation models. IgM plays a primary role in mediating the rejection in many species combinations [4,5]. In our previous reports [7–9] we have demonstrated that in a PRKX, IgA and IgG act as preformed antibodies and trigger the hyperacute rejection process by recognizing antigen determinants on the vascular endothelium. In this model, rabbit IgM does not react with the pig kidney vascular endothelium, but it recognizes antigen determinants located on the brush border of the tubular epithelium. This

S322

happens at least 120 min following xenograft reperfusion [9]. The present study established that, at least in our model, preformed antibodies binding to endothelial targets (IgA and IgG) were different from those binding to epithelial targets (IgM). In fact, the fluorescence studies on the Landrace pig kidney, perfused with normal New Zealand rabbit serum, reproduced the fluorescence pictures obtained previously by our in vivo study [7]. The incubation of sections of normal Landrace pig kidneys with serum A demonstrated clearly two facts. First, that the passage of the New Zealand rabbit serum through the vascular bed of the Landrace pig kidney was characterized by IgG and IgA deposition on the capillary endothelium. Consequently, the effluent collected was IgG and IgA deprived. IgM was normally present in serum A because it did not bind to any endothelial antigen determinants. On the other hand IgM deposition was evident on the tubular epithelium when the sections of normal Landrace pig kidneys were incubated with serum A. Furthermore, in this model, in the absence of antigen-antibody complexes, complement deposits were detectable only on the glomerular endothelium. The endothelium of the peritubular capillaries did not show any complement deposition in the absence of antibody. In vivo [7–9], in PRKX the hyperacute rejection cascade starts as early as 15 min after kidney reperfusion in the wall of the peritubular capillaries. The glomeruli withstand antibody and complement activity longer than do the peritubular capillaries and this results in damage only 60–120 min after the organ reperfusion. The significance of the early complement deposition that we obtained in vitro on the glomerular endothelium remains uncertain and further studies should be conducted to clarify this point.

Acknowledgements. This study was supported by research grants from the Veterans Administration and Project Grant No. DK 29961 from the National Institutes of Health, Bethesda, Maryland, and by C.N.R. Target Project, Biotechnology and Bioinstrumentation, Rome, Italy.

References

1. Auchincloss H Jr (1988) Xenogeneic transplantation. Transplantation 46: 1–20
2. Calne RY (1970) Organ transplantation between widely disparate species. Transplant Proc 2: 550–553
3. Cooper DKC, Kemp E, Reemtsma K, White DJG (1991) Xenotransplantation. Springer-Verlag, New York, NY
4. Fischel RJ, Bolman RM III, Platt JL, Najarian JS, Bach FH, Matas AJ (1990) Removal of IgM anti-endothelial antibodies results in prolonged cardiac xenograft survival. Transplant Proc 22: 1077–1078
5. Gambiez L, Weill BJ, Chereau CH, Calmus Y, Houssin D (1990) The hyperacute rejection of guinea pig to rat heart xenografts is mediated by preformed IgM. Transplant Proc 22: 1058
6. Kissmeyer-Nielson F, Olsen S, Peterson VP, Fjeldborg O (1966) Hyperacute rejection of kidney allografts associated with pre-existing humoral antibodies against donor cells. Lancet II: 662–665
7. Marino IR, Ferla G, Celli S, Stieber A, Muttillo I, Maggiano N, Mazzaferro V, Perrelli L, Musiani P (1990) Hyperacute rejection in renal discordant xenograft (pig-to-rabbit): model assessment and rejection mechanisms. Transplant Proc 22: 1071–1076
8. Marino IR, Ferla G, Celli S, Stieber A, Muttillo I, Maggiano N, Perrelli L, Musiani P (1991) In vivo and in vitro study of hyperacute rejection mechanism of renal discordant xenograft. Transplant Proc 23: 620–622
9. Marino IR, Celli S, Ferla G, Stieber A, Maggiano N, Musiani P (1991) Histopathological, immunofluorescent and electromicroscopical features of hyperacute rejection in discordant xenotransplantation. In: Cooper DKC, Kemp E, Reemtsma K, White DJG (eds) Xenotransplantation. Springer-Verlag, New York
10. Starzl TE (1964) Experience in Renal Transplantation. Saunders, Philadelphia
11. Starzl TE (1969) Experience in Hepatic Transplantation. Saunders, Philadelphia
12. Starzl TE, Iwatsuki S, Thiel DH van, Gartner JC, Zitelli BJ, Malatack JJ, Schade RR, Shaw BJ Jr, Hakala TR, Rosenthal JJ, Porter KA (1982) Evolution of liver transplantation. Hepatology 2: 614–636
13. Terasaki PI (1990) Clinical Transplants. UCLA Tissue Typing Laboratory, Los Angeles

Preservation

Transplant Int (1992) 5 [Suppl 1]: S 325–S 326

TRANSPLANT
International
© Springer-Verlag 1992

The influence of an improved preservation solution on prognostic factors for graft survival in pediatric liver transplantation

P. M. J. G. Peeters, E. M. ten Vergert, S. Pisarski, C. M. A. Bijleveld, R. P. Bleichrodt, and M. J. H. Slooff

Liver Transplant Group, University Hospital Groningen, Department of Surgery, Groningen, The Netherlands

Abstract. We investigated the influence of Eurocollins (EC) and University of Wisconson solution (UW) on prognostic factors for graft survival after pediatric liver transplantation. The 1-year graft survival was studied for 30 patients in which 38 transplantations were performed between 1982 and 1988. We preserved 19 grafts in EC and the other 19 grafts in UW solution. For grafts preserved in EC, the median preservation time was 5 h compared to 10.8 h for grafts preserved in UW solution ($P < 0.01$). Graft survival at 1 year was equivalent in both groups (63 %). No significant differences were observed between the two groups for the following variables: patient diagnosis, child-pugh score, age, operative time, anhepatic phase, blood loss, morbidity, ICU stay, donor age and graft survival. Multivariate analysis indicated that in the EC group anhepatic phase, blood loss and preservation time were significant predictors of graft survival whereas in the UW group, none of these factors appeared to be significant. We concluded that UW was superior to EC solution in pediatric liver transplantations because it allowed longer preservation times, the length of the anhepatic phase was less important and the tolerance for blood loss seemed to be extended.

Key words: Liver preservation – UW/EC preservation solution – Prognostic factors – Graft survival

Until 1987, Eurocollins solution (EC) was the most frequently used solution for clinical liver transplantation. EC allowed preservation times up to a maximum of about 10 h [1, 2] making liver transplantation a non-elective procedure performed mostly during the night hours. Extending the preservation time of the liver beyond 9 h often caused delayed and poor graft function affecting the prognosis of the patient. The introduction of the University of Wisconson solution (UW) by Belzer and his associates allowed for significantly longer preservation times with-

out negatively affecting the function of the graft [3]. Nowadays, preservation times of between 12 and 24 h are not exceptional making liver transplantation an elective procedure. Additionally, the results of liver transplantation have shown improvement with UW [4, 5]. The purpose of the present study was to examine whether the use of either the EC or UW solution had any effect on factors predicting graft survival after pediatric liver transplantation.

Patients and methods

Between March 1982 and March 1990, 38 transplantations were performed in 30 patients: 23 whole, 7 reduced and 8 segmental grafts were implanted. Of these, 19 grafts were preserved in the Eurocollins solution (EC group) whereas the other 19 grafts were preserved in the University of Wisconson (UW) solution.

During this time period the same protocols for immunosuppressive therapy and infection prevention were employed except for 3 transplants. Immunosuppressive therapy was instituted by means of a quadruple regimen. Azathioprine was given in a dose of 3 mg/kg daily. Prednisolone was started in a dose of 4 mg/kg daily and quickly tapered down to a dose of 0.5 mg/kg. Cyclosporine A was started as soon as the creatinine clearance was above 50 ml/min (corrected for body surface). Dosages were adjusted according to the serum levels. During the first 4 weeks, we aimed at levels of 200–250 ng/l and thereafter at levels of 100–150 ng/l. Additionally, cyclophosphamide was given during the 1st postoperative week.

Infection prevention was performed by means of selective decontamination of the bowl (SDB). SDB was carried out by administering three oral non-absorbable antibiotics; polymixin E (100 mg qid), tobramycin (80 mg qid) and amfotericin B (500 mg qid). Since eliminating the gram negative bacteria and fungi takes some time, prophylactic parenteral antibiotics (tobramicin and cefotaxim) were given during the first 48 h after the transplantation.

For the EC and UW groups preservation times ranged from 3.5 to 7 h and from 3.3 to 18.5 h, respectively. The median preservation time for the EC group was 5 h and for the UW group, 10.8 h ($P < 0.01$).

In order to study the influence of the EC and UW solution on prognostic factors of graft survival, a logistic regression model was used. All patients were followed for at least 1 year after transplantation. The proportion of grafts surviving for 1 year was 0.63 for both groups. The following prognostic factors were considered: child-pugh score, recipient and donor age, operative time, preservation time, blood loss and anhepatic phase.

The Mann-Whitney test and chi-square test were used to test the differences between the EC and UW group for the following variables: recipient and donor age, anhepatic phase, child-pugh score,

Offprint requests to: P. M. J. G. Peeters, Liver Transplant Group, University Hospital Groningen, Department of Surgery, Oostersingel 59, 9713 EZ Groningen, The Netherlands

Table 1. Characteristics of the liver recipient, liver donor and transplant procedure. Continuous variables are expressed as median values (ranges); discrete variables as frequencies (%)

	EC solution $(n = 19)$[a]	UW solution $(n = 19)$
1. Recipient age (years)	3.3 (0.17–16.0)	1.7 (0.3–16.0)
2. Donor age (years)	6.0 (0.58–20.0)	5.5 (0.3–44.0)
3. Anhepatic phase (min)	75.0 (40.0–310.0)	85.0 (55.0–175.0)
4. Child-Pugh score	9 (6–14)	11 (6–14)
5. Operative time (min)	370.0 (260.0–480.0)	328.0 (245.0–480.0)
6. Blood loss (cl)	960.0 (180.0–4410.0)	570.0 (140.0–3190.0)
7. ICU (days)	5.5 (1.0–88.0)	9.0 (1.0–62.0)
8. Complications (Yes)	15 (78.9 %)	11 (57.9 %)
9. Diagnosis[b]	10 (71.4 %)	6 (37.5 %)

[a] No. of transplanted patients in EC and UW group was 14 and 16, respectively

[b] Diagnosis: 1 = biliary atresia, 2 = others

Table 2. Significant predictors of graft survival after pediatric liver transplantation in the EC group

Predictors**	Estimated regression coefficients* EC Solution
Constant	4.50
Anhepatic fase	0.24
Blood loss	− 0.66
Preservation time	− 0.37

* $P < 0.05$

** Chi-square for testing the hypothesis that all regression coefficients are zero = 17.39, 7 degrees of freedom, $P < 0.05$

operative time, blood loss, ICU stay, complications and patient diagnosis. Values at $P < 0.05$ were considered to be significant.

Results

In order to make a comparative statement about prognostic factors we looked for possible differences between the EC and UW group in the distributions of characteristics relevant for graft survival. Details of the donor, recipient and operation characteristics are given in Table 1. Statistical analyses revealed that there were no significant differences between the EC and UW group with respect to these factors. Thus, both the type of patients, recipients, and the operation characteristics were similar and the groups were comparable. A logistic model was then used to examine the influence of prognostic factors on at least 1-year graft survival for the EC and UW group, separately. Variables entered into the model included blood loss, recipient and donor age, operative time, anhepatic phase, child-pugh score and cold ischemia time. By means of a backward stepwise selection procedure, those factors were selected which significantly effected graft survival. In the EC group, anhepatic phase, blood loss and preservation time were significant predictors of at least 1-year graft survival (Table 2) whereas none of the seven variables appeared to be significant predictors in the UW group.

Before using the three significant factors for predictive purposes, it was important to test the adequacy of the model. In the present study the number of transplantations was small enough to question the appropriateness of

using the chi-square statistic for interpreting the fitness of the model. Therefore, a different, though related, indication of the strength of the estimated regression coefficients in Table 2 was obtained by testing the null hypothesis that all regression coefficients were zero [6]. This hypothesis was rejected (chi square = 17.39, degrees of freedom 7, $P < 0.05$) which indicated that the relationship between anhepatic phase, blood loss and preservation time and the 1-year graft survival was statistically significant for grafts which were preserved in the EC solution.

Discussion

Although previous studies have shown the superiority of the UW over the EC solution for clinical liver transplantation [4], the significance of this new preservation solution on the prognosis of the graft was unknown. In this study the effect of the UW preservation solution on prognostic factors for graft survival after pediatric liver transplantation was investigated.

The EC and UW group were comparable on a variety of variables; recipient and donor age, anhepatic phase, child-pugh score, operative time, blood loss, ICU stay, complications and patient diagnosis. There was a significant difference between the preservation times for the EC and UW group. Logistic regression analysis revealed that in the EC group, anhepatic phase, blood loss and preservation time were significant predictors for (at least) 1-year graft survival. In the UW group, none of the variables entered into the regression model were significantly associated with graft survival.

These results clearly showed that the introduction of the UW solution allows a longer preservation time without negatively affecting graft prognosis. This results in more efficient transplant programs. There is more time for preoperative patient preparation. The length of the anhepatic phase is of less importance in the UW era compared to the EC era, providing more time for reconstructions or adaptations of the graft and hemostatis of the liver bed. Finally, the tolerance for blood loss appears to be extended in patients with livers preserved in the UW solution which may leave the patient in a stronger position for coping with preoperative disasters.

References

1. Benichou J, Halgrimson CG, Weil R III, Koep LJ, Starzl TE (1977) Canine and human liver preservation for 6 to 18 hr by cold infusion. Transplantation 24: 407–411
2. Belzer FO, Southhard JH (1988) Principles of solid-organ preservation by cold storage. Transplantation 45: 673–676
3. Olthoff KM, Millis JM, Imagawa DK, Nuess BJ, Derus LJ, Rosenthal JT, Milewicz AL, Busuttil RW (1992) Comparisons of UW solution and Euro-collins for cold preservation of human liver grafts. Transplantation 49: 284–290
4. Kalayoglu M, Sollinger HW, Stratta RJ, d'Allesandro AM, Hoffman RM, Pirsch JD, Belzer FO (1988) Extended preservation of the liver for clinical transplantation. Lancet I: 617–619
5. Yanaga K, Tzakis AG, Starzl TE (1989) Personal experience with the procurement of 132 liver allografts. Transplant Int 2: 137–142
6. Aldrich JH, Nelson FD (1984) Lineair Probability, Logit and Probit models. Sage Publications Inc, Beverly Hills, Los Angeles

Transplant Int (1992) 5 [Suppl 1]: S 327–S 328

TRANSPLANT
International
© Springer-Verlag 1992

Multivisceral cluster transplantation in the rat

M. Knoop[2], R. Steffen[1], and P. Neuhaus[1]

[1] Department of Surgery, Free University of Berlin, [2] University Hospital Rudolf Virchow, Berlin, FRG

Transplantation of multivisceral grafts has evolved recently as a new therapeutic modality for hepatopancreatobiliary malignancies [1, 2]. The mutual interactions between the liver, pancreas, small bowel and the recipient organism after cluster grafting are not clearly understood and deserve further experimental evaluation. We present a technique for combined hepatopancreaticoduodenal cluster transplantation in the rat. The cluster grafts consisted of a pancreaticoduodenal graft and an orthotopic arterialized liver graft. A separate arterial anastomosis of the liver and a bile duct anastomosis were not necessary. Bile and exocrine pancreas secretions drained over the duodenal conduit of the graft into the recipients jejunum via an end-to-side anastomosis.

Key words: Multivisceral grafts – Hepatopancreaticoduodenal cluster transplantation – Rat

Materials and methods

Outbred male Wistar rats of 250–300 g body weight were used as donors and recipients. All operations were performed under ether anesthesia using a clean, non-sterile technique. Surviving animals were sacrified 72 h post-transplant and underwent autopsy. In the donor, the pancreaticoduodenal part of the cluster was prepared following mainly the original pancreaticoduodenal grafting described by Lee [3]. The pancreas was freed from its attachments to the omentum and the colon. The splenic vessels and the left gastric artery were ligated and the liver was mobilized. Before starting an in situ hypothermic perfusion, an aortic segment giving off the celiac axis and the superior mesenteric artery were prepared and the infrahepatic vena cava and the aorta were crossclamped. The whole cluster was perfused with 40 ml saline at 4 °C using a 16-gauge i. v. catheter. The graft was removed and stored in saline at 4 °C.

Offprint requests to: M. Knoop, MD, Chirurgische Klinik, Universitätsklinikum Rudolf Virchow, Augustenburgerplatz 1, 1000 Berlin 65, FRG

In the recipient, hepatectomy was performed as for liver transplantation. The cluster graft was placed orthotopically with regard to the liver into the recipient. After completion of the suprahepatic vena cava anastomosis, the anhepatic phase was finished by restoration of the venous blood flow through the hepatic part of the graft. The infrahepatic vena cava was anastomosed end-to-end and the arterial pedicle was sutured end-to-side to the infrarenal recipient aorta. Then the arterial perfusion of the pancreaticoduodenal part and the liver was reestablished. Finally, the exocrine drainage was reestablished by suturing the open end of the distal duodenum to the first jejunal log of the recipient in end-to-side technique with 6-0 running nylon sutures.

Results

A total of 25 transplants were performed establishing the technique. The portal clamping time averaged 16 min; the mean cold storage time was 25 min. While no problems were encountered in the donor, 6 recipients died during the procedure, the reasons being failure of the end-to-side portoportal anastomosis due to hemorrhage or stenosis with resulting splanchnic congestion and irreversible shock. Eight animals died 4–24 h post-transplantation without signs of hemorrhage and with patent anastomoses. One animal died after 2 days of peritonitis caused by intestinal perforation. Ten recipients were well at 72 h and all anastomoses were patent at autopsy.

Discussion

Four demanding vascular, anastomoses can be performed with an acceptable operation time, and the anhepatic time of less than 20 min allows the recipient to recover from splanchnic congestion after clamping of the portal vein. Functional impairment of the rat pancreas does not occur by warm ischemia at 37 °C prolonged up to 90 min [4]. In our experiments revascularization of the pancreaticoduodenal part of the cluster occurred after 40 min and was therefore within safe limits. This model represents a new technique for multivisceral grafting in the rat with a simultaneous retrieval of liver, pancreas and duodenum en bloc.

The immunology and preservation of composite grafts can be studied with this experimental procedure.

References

1. Starzl TE, Rowe MI, Todo S, Jaffe R, Tzakis A, Hoffman AL, Esquivel C, Porter KA, Venkataramanan N, Makowka L, Duquesnoy R (1989) Transplantation of multiple abdominal viscera. Jama 261: 1449–1457
2. Starzl TE, Todo S, Tzakis A, Podesta L, Mieles L, Demetris A, Teperman L, Selby R, Stevenson W, Stieber A, Gordon R, Iwatsuki S (1989) Abdominal organ cluster transplantation for the treatment of upper abdominal malignancies. Ann Surg 210: 374–386
3. Lee S, Tung KSK, Koopman SH, Chandler JG, Orloff MJ (1972) Pancreaticoduodenal transplantation in the rat. Transplantation 13: 421–425
4. Schulak JA, Franklin WA, Stuart FP, Reckard CR (1983) Effect of warm ischemia on segmental pancreas transplantation in the rat. Transplantation 35: 7–11

Transplant Int (1992) 5 [Suppl 1]: S329–S335

TRANSPLANT
International
© Springer-Verlag 1992

Reperfusion rather than storage injury predominates following long-term (48 h) cold storage of grafts in UW solution: studies with Carolina Rinse in transplanted rat liver

W. Gao[1], R. J. Currin[2], J. J. Lemasters[2], H. D. Connor[1], R. P. Mason[3], and R. G. Thurman[1]

[1] Laboratory of Hepatobiology and Toxicology, Department of Pharmacology
[2] Laboratories of Cell Biology, Department of Cell Biology and Anatomy, The University of North Carolina at Chapel Hill, NC 27599, USA
[3] Laboratory of Molecular Biophysics, NIEHS, NIH Research Triangle Park, NC 27709, USA

Abstract. Both storage injury and reperfusion injury have been reported in association with liver transplantation; however, which predominates is not clear. Therefore, these studies were designed to evaluate whether Carolina Rinse, which minimizes reperfusion injury following orthotopic liver transplantation in the rat, would be effective after long-term (48 h) storage of grafts in University of Wisconsin (UW) cold storage solution where sufficient time for development of storage injury exists. Livers were rinsed with either Ringer's solution or Carolina Rinse solution immediately prior to completion of implantation surgery. In the Ringer's group, 30-day survival was high following 24 h of cold storage (4/5) but was very low after 48 h (1/16). Importantly, survival was increased significantly (5/14) when grafts were rinsed with carolina Rinse following 48 h of cold storage. In both groups, parenchymal cells appeared normal by scanning electron microscopy, excluded trypan blue, and released SGOT at values only slightly above the normal range immediately (i.e., less than 5 min) after 48 h of cold storage. However, SGOT values rose steadily during the 1st hour postoperatively following reperfusion in the Ringer's rinse group and reached levels around 1,000 U/l. In addition, nonparenchymal cells were not labelled with trypan blue following storage, but significant labelling occurred within 1 h. Both SGOT release and nonparenchymal cell injury were reduced significantly when grafts were rinsed with Carolina Rinse prior to completion of surgery. Liver injury assessed histologically 24 h postoperatively was also reduced about 50 % by Carolina Rinse. Oxidative stress appeared to be involved, since radical adducts, most likely of lipid origin, were trapped during the first 5 min after reperfusion with the spin trapping technique and detected by electron paramagnetic resonance spectroscopy. Lipid radical formation was reduced nearly completely on reperfusion by Carolina Rinse. Since Carolina Rinse improved survival of liver grafts following long periods of cold storage and reduced lipid radical formation and hepatocellular injury, we concluded that a reperfusion injury rather than a storage injury predominates following orthotopic transplantation of livers stored for long periods of time in cold UW solution.

Key words: Carolina Rinse – Reperfusion injury – Orthotopic rodent liver transplantation – Lipid radical adducts

With the development of University of Wisconsin (UW) cold storage solution in the late 1980's [2], the storage time of liver for transplantation was extended from 8–10 h to up to 20–24 h [23]. However, despite this improvement, primary graft non-function still occurs [14].

Several years ago we demonstrated that a selective injury to hepatic nonparenchymal cells occurred following cold storage and reperfusion in vitro and in vivo [7, 8, 21]. Reperfusion injuries have also been demonstrated in many organs, including heart, lung, kidney and pancreas, and have been reported to exacerbate the rejection reaction in liver [15]. Studies on the pathophysiological mechanisms involved in reperfusion injury in liver have focused on damage to endothelial cells [7, 8], activation of Kupffer cells [6, 21], adherence of leukocytes [20], as well as disturbances in the microcirculation [22] and activation of the coagulation system [13]. It is possible that activated Kupffer cells produce toxic mediators such as proteases, toxic radicals, leukotrienes and tumor necrosis factor [18]. Oxygen radicals could be involved, since xanthine and hypoxanthine, substrates for superoxide radical formation, accumulate during cold storage [17] and free radicals could be formed postoperatively when oxygen is reintroduced [9].

Since UW solution increases the time of cold storage, it has been reasoned that injury to the graft occurs during cold storage. In support of this idea, the hepatic ultrastructure of the liver is altered during cold storage. However, recent studies with Carolina Rine indicate that reperfu-

Offprint requests to: Ronald G. Thurman, Lab. of Hepatobiology and Toxicology, Department of Pharmacology, CB # 7365, FLOB. The University of North Carolina, Chapel Hill, NC 27599-7365, USA

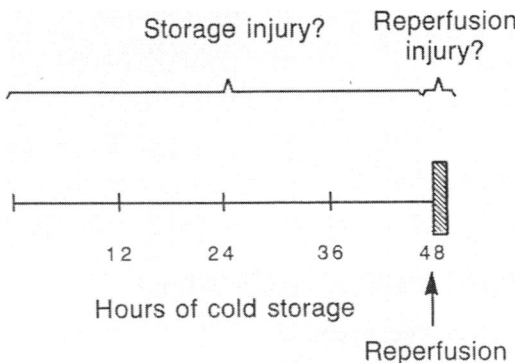

Fig. 1. Scheme contrasting storage and reperfusion injury following orthotopic liver transplantation

sion injury also occurs [10, 13, 22]. While it is generally accepted that changes which occur during cold storage probably trigger reperfusion injury, whether reperfusion or storage injury predominates following transplantation has not been clarified (Fig. 1). This is an important distinction, since whether the focus in the future is on storage or rinse solutions depends on the type of injury that predominates. Therefore, these studies were designed to determine whether Carolina Rinse, which minimizes reperfusion injury, would be effective after long-term (48 h) immersion of liver grafts in cold UW solution where storage injury would have sufficient time to develop.

Methods

Transplantation. Liver transplantation was performed under ether anesthesia using a technique essentially as described by Kamada [19]. Syngenic female Lewis rats (175–200 g) were used to eliminate rejection. For electron paramagnetic resonance (EPR) spectroscopy, inbred female Sprague-Dawley rats (175–200 g) were used. Briefly, 0.5 ml Ringer's solution with 100 units of heparin was injected into the donor vena cava and the liver was flushed with 3–5 ml of cold UW solution. Subsequently, cuffs were placed on the portal vein and subhepatic vena cava of the donor liver. Grafts were stored at 0–4 °C for 24 or 48 h in UW solution and were rinsed either with 3–5 ml Ringer's solution or Carolina Rinse. The composition of Carolina Rinse is as follows: NaCl (115 ml), KCl (5 mM), CaCl$_2$ (1.3 mM), KH$_2$PO$_4$ (1 mM) MgSO$_4$ (1.2 mM), allopurinol (1 mM), desferrioxamine mesylate (1 mM), glutathione (3 mM), nicardipine (2 μM), adenosine (1 mM), fructose (10 mM), glucose (10 mM), hydroxyethyl starch (50 g/l), insulin (100 U/l), MOPS (20 mM), pH 6.5, mOsm/l 290–305 [10, 13]. Subsequently, livers were implanted by connecting the suprahepatic vena cava with a running suture, inserting cuffs into appropriate vessels without rearterialization, and anastomosing the bile duct with an intraluminal splint. The explantation required less than 6 min, and the ischemic interval due to clamping of the portal vein during implantation did not exceed 15 min. Surviving animals were sacrificed after 30 days for histology.

Serum enzymes. Blood samples were drawn from the vena cava at 0, 5, 15, 30, 60, and 180 min after the clamp on the portal vein was removed. Sera were separated by centrifugation and kept at −20 °C for enzyme measurements. Serum glutamic oxaloacetic transaminase (SGOT) was assayed by standard enzymatic procedures [3].

Tissue ultrastructure. Rats were sacrificed 24 h postoperatively and livers were fixed with 1% paraformaldehyde in Krebs-Henseleit buffer, embedded in paraffin, and processed for light microscopy. Sections were stained with hematoxalin and eosin. Liver damage was scored using a scale of 0–5 based on the degree of necrosis and 0–2 based on six structural parameters: cellular swelling, acidophilic inclusions, nuclear pyknosis, cellular deposition, cytoplasmic vacuolization, and sinusoidal dilatation (maximal score = 17). Where indicated, the vital dye trypan blue was infused into livers for 5 min at the end of experiments, followed by fixation of the liver with 1% paraformaldehyde in Krebs-Henseleit buffer. Livers were processed for light microscopy and sections were stained with eosin only so that nuclei of dead cells could be identified [1].

For scanning electron microscopy, livers fixed with 2% paraformaldehyde: 2% glutaraldehyde were cut into 1 cm cubes and placed overnight in cold secondary fixative containing 2% glutaraldehyde in 0.1 M sodium phosphate buffer, pH 7.4. The tissue was then washed in water, dehydrated in graded ethanol, and critical-point dried in carbon dioxide. The dried tissue was cut manually with a razor blade, mounted on an aluminum stub, coated with gold-palladium using a sputter evaporator, and viewed in a JEOL 820 scanning electron microscope [16].

Spin trapping of free radicals. Following cold storage in UW solution, the liver was implanted and an O$_2$-saturated solution of α-phenyl N-tert-butyl nitrone (PBN; 15 mM) in saline, or Carolina Rinse was infused into the portal vein at a rate of 0.3 ml/min immediately after the clamp on the portal vein was opened. Four to five 1 ml samples of blood were collected immediately from the suprahepatic vena cava, and serum was separated by centrifugation and frozen in liquid nitrogen.

Serum was extracted based on methods used in studies of reperfusion injury to heart [4, 5]. Samples in chloroform were placed in a 3.0 mm i.d. quartz EPR tube, bubbled with nitrogen for 5 min, and placed in the EPR cavity. A varian E-109 spectrometer equipped with a TM$_{110}$ cavity was used. Instrument conditions were 20-mW microwave power, 0.68-G modulation amplitude and 80-G scan width for all analyses. Scan time was 1.0 h with an 8-s time constant.

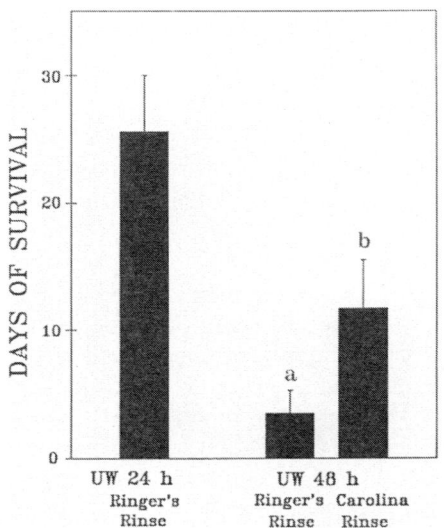

Fig. 2. Effect of Carolina Rinse on postoperative survival of livers stored in University of Wisconsin (UW) cold storage solution for 48 h. Livers were rinsed and stored in UW cold storage solution at 0–4 °C for 24 h (survival conditions) or 48 h (non-survival conditions). Following storage, livers were rinsed with 3 to 5 ml of either cold Ringer's or Carolina Rinse solution and implanted immediately. Survival was assumed to be permanent when rats were alive 30 days postoperatively. **a** $P < 0.05$ for comparison with livers stored under survival conditons; **b** $P < 0.05$ for comparison with Ringer's group of livers stored under non-survival conditons. Mean ± SEM for 5 to 16 livers in each group

Results

Calronina Rinse increases survival following long-term storage in UW solution. The purpose of these studies was to determine whether liver graft injury occurs predominantly during cold storage (i.e., while in cold UW solution) or following reperfusion after implantation (Fig. 1). Carolina Rinse was designed to minimize reperfusion injury and was used to address this question. Average survival time of livers stored in UW solution 24 h prior to implantation and rinsed with Ringer's solution was approximately 25 days (i.e., survival conditions; Fig. 2). In this model, survival for 30 days is considered permanent. In contrast, when the time of storage in UW solution was extended to 48 h, the length of survival declined dramatically to less than 3 days when grafts were rinsed with Ringer's solution (i.e., nonsurvival conditions). However, when Carolina Rinse was substituted for Ringer's as the rinse solution, average survival time increased significantly by approximately 3-fold (Fig. 2).

Comparison of hepatocellular injury following cold storage with cold storage plus reperfusion. Liver injury was also assessed in these studies by release of transaminases into the blood. At the initiation of reperfusion, SGOT levels were low in livers stored for 48 h in UW solution and rinsed with either Ringer's solution or Carolina Rinse (Fig. 3). However, enzyme release increased sharply to values around 1000 U/l during the 1st hour of reperfusion in the Ringer's group and reached peak values of over 1200 U/l. When Carolina Rinse was substituted for

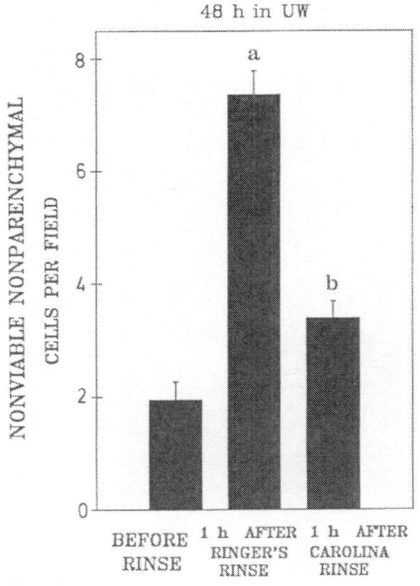

Fig. 4. Effect of Carolina Rinse on nonparenchymal cell injury following long-term cold storage and reperfusion. Livers were reperfused with oxygenated Krebs-Henseleit bicarbonate buffer (pH 7.4, 37 °C) either before implantation or 1 h postoperatively. The flow rate was initially 15 ml/min and was increased to 30 ml/min over 2 min. After 5 min of reperfusion, trypan blue (0.5 mM) was added and perfusion was continued for 7 min. Livers were flushed with buffer for 5 min, and tissue was fixed and stained as described in Methods. Trypan blue-positive nonparenchymal cell nuclei in eosin-stained sections were counted in 8 random microscopic fields. Total cells were determined in H & E sections. **a** $P < 0.05$ for comparison with nontransplant group. **b** $P < 0.05$ for comparison with either nontransplant or Ringer's groups. Mean ± SEM for 4 to 6 livers per group

Ringer's solution, maximal transaminase release was diminished approximately 2-fold.

Infusion of the vital dye trypan blue allows easy identification of irreversibly damaged cells. Liver stored for 48 h in UW solution and fixed immediately sustained minimal cell injury (i.e., only about 3% of parenchymal cells were stained with trypan blue; data not shown). Nonparenchymal cell injury was also minimal immediately following surgery (Fig. 4). However, nonparenchymal cell injury increased 3 to 4-fold 1 h following surgery if the graft had been rinsed with Ringer's solution. This nonparenchymal cell injury was reduced dramatically by Carolina Rinse (Fig. 4).

Liver damage was also assessed 24 h postoperatively on a histological score as described in Methods. In livers stored for 48 h in UW solution and rinsed with Ringer's solution, the liver damage index 24 h postoperatively was around 7.5 (Fig. 5). In livers stored under similar conditions but rinsed with Carolina Rinse, however, the index was reduced significantly by almost 50%.

To evaluate the effect of reperfusion on hepatic ultrastructure, scanning electron microscopy was performed. Livers were stored for 48 h in UW solution, rinsed either with Ringer's solution or Carolina Rinse, fixed 15 min postoperatively and processed for electron microscopy. As expected, at this early time point following reperfusion, parenchymal cells exhibited near normal morphology (i.e., cell death was minimal; data not shown).

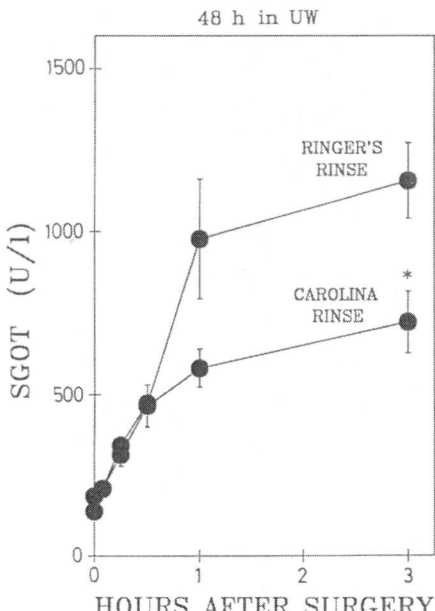

Fig. 3. Effect of Carolina Rinse on serum enzyme release from livers stored under non-survival conditions. Blood samples were collected via the inferior vena cava at 0, 5, 15, 30, 60 and 180 min postoperatively. SGOT activity was measured as described in Methods. Blood pressure was maintained by infusion of up to 3 ml of 5% albumin in Ringer's solution via the tail vein. Mean ± SEM for 4 livers in each group

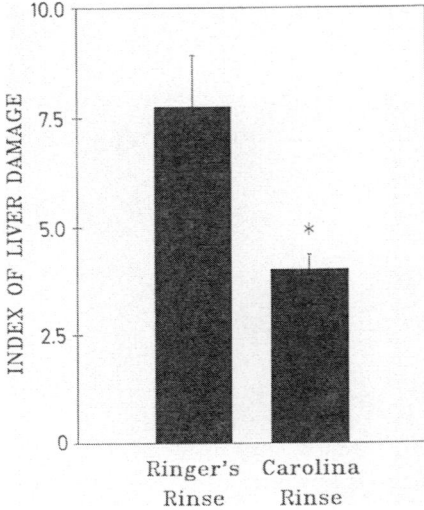

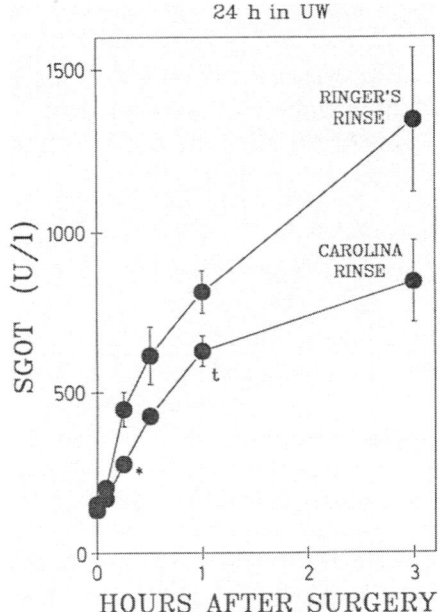

Fig. 5. Effect of Carolina Rinse on postoperative liver damage. Index of liver damage was determined 24 h postoperatively as described in Methods. Mean ± S.E.M. for 4 livers in each group. * $P < 0.05$ compared to the Ringer's rinse group

Fig. 7. Effect of Carolina Rinse on serum enzyme rlease by livers stored under survival conditions. Conditions as in Fig. 3 except that livers were stored in cold UW solution for 24 h (survival conditions). Mean ± SEM for 6 to 10 livers in each group

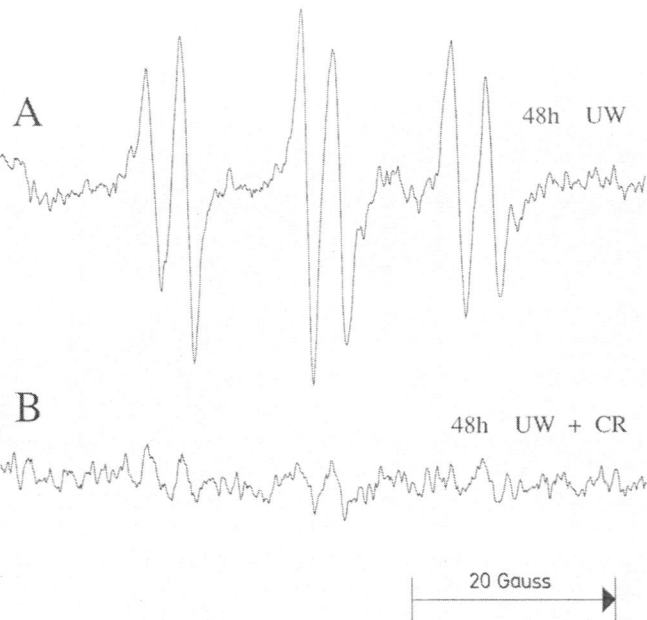

Fig. 6 A, B. Representative EPR spectra of radical adducts in chloroform extracts of serum from transplanted livers stored in cold UW solution for 48 h. Livers were transplanted, spin trap was infused, blood was collected for 5 min, and EPR analysis was performed as described in Methods. **A** livers stored for 48 h in UW solution and rinsed with Ringer's solution before implantation surgery. **B** liver stored for 48 h in UW solution and rinsed with Carolina Rinse solution

Inhibition of radical adduct formation by Carolina Rinse. Since oxygen and oxygen radicals have been implicated in the mechanism of reperfusion injury [13], experiments utilizing electron paramagnetic resonance (EPR) spectroscopy were designed to determine if free radicals were formed as a result of reperfusion following orthotopic liver transplantation. When livers were stored for 48 h in UW solution and reperfused with oxygenated blood con-

taining the spin trap PBN, the immediate effluent leaving the liver contained high levels of PBN radical adducts, as indicated by the appearance of a robust six-line EPR signal (Fig. 6). Computer simulation of the data indicated that two carbon-centered radical adducts were present, and the hydrophobic behavior of these species in extraction and sample preparation suggested strongly that they were lipid-derived radicals. Carolina Rinse, which contains reagents which inhibit radical formation, suppressed the radical adduct signal nearly completely (Fig. 6).

Effect of Carolina Rinse on SGOT release following 24 h of storage in UW solution. In the clinic, most human livers are stored for less than 24 h before transplantation; therefore, we compared the effect of Ringer's Rinse, which is used currently to remove cardiotoxic potassium contained in UW solution, with the effect of Carolina Rinse on transaminase release during reperfusion following 24 h of storage in UW solution. SGOT release increased following reperfusion with Ringer's rinse, increasing gradually from approximately 150 to 1200 U/l over 3 h. Carolina Rinse tended to reduce values at all time points examined (Fig. 7).

Discussion

Definition of storage and reperfusion injury. Storage injury is defined as any alteration in the liver that occurs *during* the period of cold storage (see Fig. 1). This is sometimes referred to erroneously as a preservation injury since preservation means "to keep safe, alive, or free from injury". To avoid this contradiction in terms, storage injury is used as a more appropriate term to describe damage which occurs during cold storage. On the other hand, reperfusion

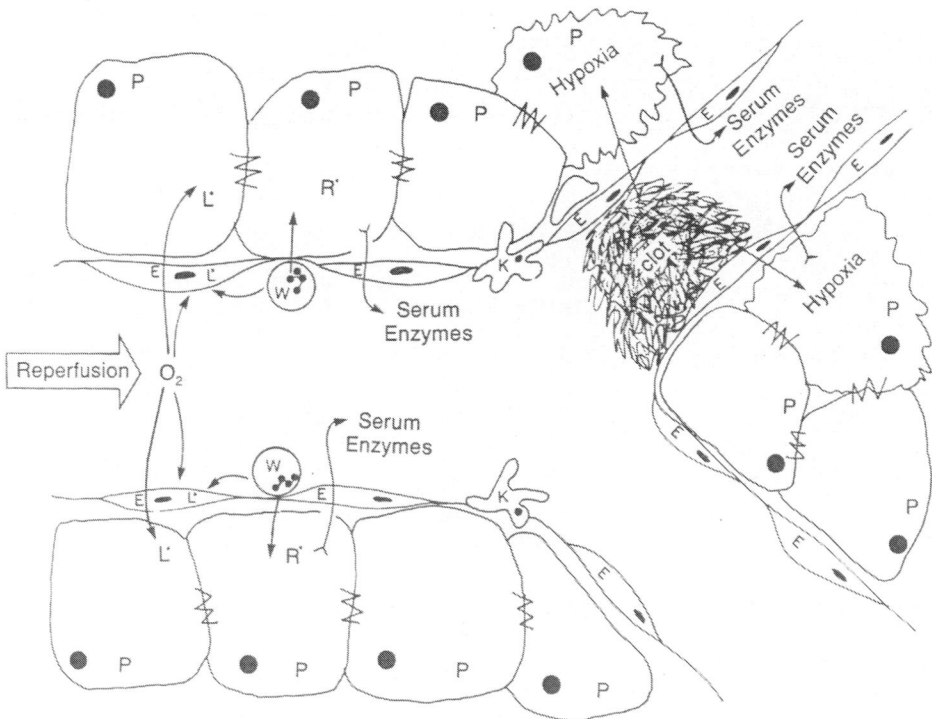

Fig. 8. Scheme depicting possible mechanisms of reperfusion injury to the graft following orthotopic liver transplantation. *P*, parenchymal cell; *E*, endothelial cell; *K*, Kupffer cell; *W*, white blood cell; $L\cdot$ and $R\cdot$, lipid and other free radicals

injury is broadly defined as any pathophysiological alteration in the liver which occurs *after* surgery but narrowly refers to radical-mediated events which occur upon reflow which may be due to oxygen [22]. Obviously, changes that occur in the cold most likely trigger the subsequent reperfusion injury.

There is considerable variation in times of cold storage which allow maximal survival. In the rat, times range from 4 to 24 h [12, 20] for reasons that may relate to the time of ischemia during surgery. In this study, 24 h in UW solution resulted in complete survival (Fig. 2). Thus, the rat can be as suitable a model as the dog and human where maximal cold storage times which result in 100 % survival are also around 24 h.

Reperfusion injury rather than storage injury predominated after 48 h in UW solution. As mentioned in the introduction, an oxygen-dependent reperfusion injury has been described in the orthotopic rat liver transplantation model [22]. Further, since cold storage time has been extended significantly over times for Euro-Collins by the introduction of UW solution and because alterations in hepatic ultrastructure have been observed immediately

following cold storage [23], it has been assumed that injury occurs during cold storage. As mentioned above, 48 h of cold storage was used in this study to allow sufficient time for injury to develop. However, based on several criteria of hepatic viability assessed in this study, it was clear that significant damage did not occur during the 48 h of cold storage in UW solution but rather developed during the 1st hours after reperfusion (i.e., it was a reperfusion injury). Specifically, cells excluded trypan blue and had near normal SGOT values immediately after 48 h of cold storage in UW solution, indicating that they were not injured irreversibly during cold storage (Figs. 3, 4). However, massive injury was detected 1 h following reperfusion (e.g., serum enzymes increased gradually over about 1 h postoperatively). This observation was very important since it defined the time course of the reperfusion injury and led to the inescapable conclusion that a reperfusion injury occured following long-term cold storage in UW solution only after oxygenated blood reentered the organ following transplantation.

A second argument that a reperfusion injury predominated comes from studies with Carolina Rinse. Carolina Rinse was developed specifically to prevent reperfusion

Table 1. Time course of pathophysiologic changes on reperfusion

System	Detection after reperfusion (min)	Reference
Free radical formation	5	Fig. 6; Connor et al. (1991) Transplantation, submitted
Clotting time decreased and platelet count down	5	Gao et al. (1991) Transplantation, in press
Endothelial cell death	7–15	Caldwell-Kenkel et al. (1988) Hepatology 10: 292–299
Leukocyte adhesion	15	Takei et al. (1991) Transplantation 51: 959–65
Kupffer cell activation	30	Caldwell-Kenkel et al. (1991) Cells of the hepatic sinusoid, in press
Hepatocyte injury	15–60	Fig. 3

injury and contains adenosine [11] as well as antioxidants and radical scavengers [13]. In this study the postoperative increases in trypan blue labelling of nonparenchymal cells and serum enzyme release were diminished significantly by Carolina Rinse (Figs. 3, 4). Thus, it was concluded that survival was affected by what occured during reperfusion, making the evaluation of cold storage solutions based on survival outcome questionable.

Radical-mediated endothelial cell killing rather than parenchymal cell death correlated with graft survival. Interestingly, in livers stored under survival conditions (24 h; Fig. 7), the time course of SGOT release postoperatively (i. e., parenchymal cell injury) was identical in livers stored under non-survival (48 h) conditions. Thus, reperfusion injury to *parenchymal cells* did not correlate directly with survival. This is important clinically, since serum enzymes are a common measure of postoperative outcome. On the other hand, survival did correlate with nonparenchymal cell injury (Fig. 4). More appropriate indices related specifically to survival will need to be identified in the future.

It is accepted that hypothermia is the basic principle on which existing liver preservation methods depend. By reducing the metabolic demand of the tissue for nutrients and oxygen, the period during which anoxic tissue retains viability is lengthened. However, cold ischemia causes alterations in the organ which most likely are responsible for reperfusion injury. For example, ATP degradation leads to high cellular concentrations of xanthine which could enhance superoxide production and thus injure the cell when oxygen is reintroduced. Indeed, on reoxygenation, free radicals are formed in minutes (Fig. 8) followed by endothelial cell injury ([9]; Table 1), Kupffer cell activation [6] and leukocyte adhesion. Only much later does loss of parenchymal cell function occur. In support of this hypothetical sequence of events, Connor et al. [9] have demonstrated that free radical formation in the early postoperative minutes correlates with survival.

Alternatively, the clotting system may be involved (Fig. 8). In a previous study, we have demonstrated that clotting time decreased as soon as 5 min postoperatively under nonsurvival conditions [13]. Further, in this study massive microthrombi were observed by electron microscopy 15 min after revascularization. On the other hand, SGOT values did not increase maximally until about 1 h postoperatively. Thus, one alternative explanation for early graft injury is that damaged endothelial cells stimulate platelet aggregation. This could stimulate clotting, block the microcirculation and lead to hypoxia which could ultimately kill parenchymal cells.

Can reperfusion injury be treated with Carolina Rinse? Carolina Rinse contains antioxidants and was shown in this study to diminish free radical formation and endothelial cell death and to decrease parenchymal cell injury dramatically following long-term cold storage in UW solution (Figs. 3, 6). The efficacy of Carolina Rinse is apparently due to its ability to prevent free radical formation in the liver during the 1st minutes following surgery [9] as well as an apparent extrahepatic effect of adenosine on survival [11]. Thus, Carolina Rinse might be a valuable adjunct to

UW solution in reducing postoperative graft injury clinically. Currently, a limited clinical trial to evaluate Carolina Rinse is underway at the Mayo clinic.

Acknowledgement. This work was supported, in part, by NIH grants DK-37034 and AA-03624.

References

1. Belinsky SA, Popp JA, Kauffman FC, Thurman RG (1984) Trypan blue uptake as a new method to investigate hepatotoxicity in periportal and pericentral regions of the liver lobule. Studies with allyl alcohol in the perfused liver. J Pharmacol Exp Ther 230: 755–760
2. Belzer FO, Southard JH (1988) Principles of solid-organ preservation by cold storage. Transplantation 45: 673–676
3. Bergmeyer HU (1988) Methods of Enzymatic Analysis. Academic Press, New York
4. Bolli R, Jeroudi MO, Patel BS, DuBose CM, Lai EK, Roberts R, McCay PB (1989) Direct evidence that oxygen-derived free radicals contribute to postischemic myocardial dysfunction in the intact dog. Proc Natl Acad Sci USA 86: 4695–4699
5. Bolli R, Patel BS, Jeroudi MO, Lai EK, McCay PB (1988) Demonstration of free radical generation in "stunned" myocardium of intact dogs with the use of the spin trap α-phenyl N-tert-butyl nitrone. J Clin Invest 82: 476–485
6. Caldwell-Kenkel JC, Currin RT, Gao W, Tanaka Y, Thurman RG, Lemasters JJ (1991) Reperfusion injury to livers stored for transplantation: Endothelial cell killing and Kupffer cell activation. In: Wisse E, Knook DL, McCuskey RS, (eds) Cells of the Hepatic Sinusoid III. The Kupffer Cell Fndn., Rijswijk, The Netherlands, (In Press)
7. Caldwell-Kenkel JC, Currin RT, Tanaka Y, Thurman RG, Lemasters JJ (1989) Reperfusion injury to endothelial cells following cold ischemic storage of rat liver. Hepatology 10: 292–299
8. Caldwell-Kenkel JC, Thurman RG, Lemasters JJ (1988) Selective loss of nonparenchymal cell viability after cold ischemic storage of rat livers. Transplantation 45: 834–837
9. Connor HD, Gao W, Nukina S, Lemasters JJ, Mason RP, Thurman RG (1991) Free radicals are involved in graft failure following orthotopic liver transplantation: An EPR spin trapping study. Transplantation (submitted)
10. Currin RT, Toole JG, Thurman RG, Lemasters JJ (1990) Evidence that Carolina rinse solution protects sinusoidal endothelial cells against reperfusion injury after cold ischemic storage of rat liver. Transplantation 50: 1076–1078
11. Gao W, Hijioka T, Lindert KA, Caldwell-Kenkel JC, Lemasters JJ, Thurman RG (1991) Adenosine is a key component in Carolina rinse responsible for reducing graft failure after orthotopic liver transplantation in the rat. Transplantation, (In Press)
12. Gao W, Lemasters JJ, Thurman RG (1991) The second generation of Carolina rinse, Solution II, improves graft survival following orthotopic liver transplantation in the rat by preventing reperfusion injury. Transplant Int (submitted)
13. Gao W, Takei Y, Marzi I, Lindert KA, Caldwell-Kenkel JC, Currin RT, Tanaka Y, Lemasters JJ, Thurman RG (1991) Carolina Rinse solution: A new strategy to increase survival time after orthotopic liver transplantation in the rat. Transplantation, (In Press)
14. Greig PD, Woolf GM, Sinclair SB, Abecassis M, Strasberg SM, Taylor BR, Blendis LM, Superina RA, Glynn MFX, Langer B, Levy GA (1989) Treatment of primary liver graft nonfunction with prostaglandin E₁. Transplantation 48: 447–453
15. Howard TK, Klintmalm GBG, Cofer JB, Husberg BS, Goldstein RM, Gonwa TA (1990) The influence of preservation injury on rejection in the hepatic transplant recipient. Transplantation 49: 103–107
16. Lemasters JJ, Stemkowski CJ, Ji S, Thurman RG (1983) Cell surface changes and enzyme release during hypoxia and reoxygenation in isolated, perfused rat liver. J Cell Biol 97: 778–786

17. Marzi I, Zhong Z, Zimmermann FA, Lemasters JJ, Thurman RG (1989) Xanthine and hypoxanthine accumulation during storage may contribute to reperfusion injury following liver transplantation in the rat. Transplant Proc 21: 1319–1320

18. Nolan JP (1981) Endotoxin, reticuloendothelial function, and liver injury. Hepatology 1: 458–465

19. Sumimoto R, Jamieson NV, Kamada N (1990) Examination of the role of the impermeants lactobionate and raffinose in a modified UW solution. Transplantation 50: 573–576

20. Takei Y, Marzi I, Gao W, Gores GJ, Lemasters JJ, Thurman RG (1991) Leukocyte adhesion and cell death following orthotopic liver transplantation in the rat. Transplantation 51: 959–965

21. Thurman RG, Lindert KA, Cowper KB, te Koppele JM, Currin RT, Caldwell-Kenkel JC, Tanaka Y, Gao W, Takei Y, Marzi I, Lemasters JJ (1991) Activation of Kupffer cells following liver transplantation. In: Wisse E, Knook DL, McCuskey RS, (eds) Cells of the hepatic sinusoid III. Kupffer Cell Fndn., Rijswijk, The Netherlands, (In Press)

22. Thurman RG, Marzi I, Seitz G, Thies J, Lemasters JJ, Zimmermann FA (1988) Hepatic reperfusion injury following orthotopic liver transplantation in the rat. Transplantation 46: 502–506

23. Todo S, Nery J, Yanaga K, Podesta L, Gordon RD, Starzl TE (1989) Extended preservation of human liver grafts with UW solution. JAMA 261: 711–714

Transplant Int (1992) 5 [Suppl 1]: S 336–S 339

TRANSPLANT
International
© Springer-Verlag 1992

Prolonged rat pancreas preservation using a solution with the combination of histidine and lactobionate

T. Urushihara[1,2], R. Sumimoto[1], K. Sumimoto[1], N. V. Jamieson[3], M. Ikeda[1], H. Ito[4], H.-Q. Hong[1], Y. Fukuda[1], and K. Dohi[1]

[1] Second Department of Surgery, Hiroshima University School of Medicine, 1-2-3 Kasumi Minami-ku, Hiroshima 734, Japan
[2] Department of Surgery, Addenbrooke's Hospital, Cambridge, England
[4] First Department of Pathology, Hiroshima University, School of Medicine, 1-2-3 Kasumi Minami-ku, Hiroshima 734, Japan

Abstract. A newly formulated solution consisting of lactobionate with or without histidine was tested in the preservation of the rat pancreas. Adult male Lewis rats weighing 120–250 g were used as donors and recipients. Fifty-four rat pancreas transplants were performed to investigate the effectiveness of this test solution and to compare it with the standard University of Wisconsin (UW) solution. The final osmolarity of the new test solution was 290–320 mosmol/l. This solution had a higher sodium content and lower potassium content (Na: 110 mEq/l, K: 50 mEq/l). Adenosine, insulin, hydroxyethyl starch and dexamethasone, which are components of the UW solution, were not present in this test solution. Histidine was used as a buffer. Rat pancreases were stored at 4°C in either standard UW solution, or high-Na$^+$-histidine solution, or high-Na$^+$-lactobionate solution for 48 h and 72 h prior to heterotopic transplantation into rats with streptozotocin-induced diabetes mellitus. Functional success rates for rats receiving pancreases that had been preserved in high-Na$^+$-histidine and in high-Na$^+$-lactobionate solutions at 4°C were 100% (5/5) and 100% (7/7) after 48 h preservation, and 50% (4/8) and 14% (1/7) after 72 h preservation, respectively. By contrast, standard UW solution gave only a 44% (4/9) success rate after 48 h preservation and a 0% (0/8) success rate after 72 h preservation. These results demonstrated that the high-Na$^+$-histidine solution was superior to standard UW solution for rat pancreas preservation. This was probably due to the buffer, histidine, which prevented the acidosis of ischemic tissue during the period of preservation.

Key words: Pancreas preservation – Rat – Modified UW solution – Histidine – HL solution

It has been well established both by experimental models and clinically that University of Wisconsin (UW) solution is a highly effective preservation solution suitable not only for the liver [1, 2], kidney [3] and pancreas [4, 5], but also for the heart [6, 7]. Nevertheless, the mechanism for this remains unclear. Earlier studies by the present authors [8–13] and others [14–16] have demonstrated that not all components of the original UW solution are necessary. The effectiveness of UW solution is still maintained in the study of rat [10, 11, 15, 16], rabbit [8] and human [9] liver preservation, and rat pancreas [13] and kidney preservation [14], if hydroxyethyl starch (HES) and some pharmacological additives are omitted from the solution. We have shown previously that the effectiveness of UW is dependent mainly on the presence of the lactobionate anion and this effectiveness can be maintained or even improved by the use of different sugar moieties or altered cation composition in the preservation of rat liver and pancreas [10, 13].

Our recent experiments have demonstrated the relatively high viscosity of the UW solution due to the presence of HES [8, 11]. It is probable that this feature makes the processing of initial perfusion slow and harmful to the organs because of the outflow block after reflow in rat and dog liver experiments [11, 17, 18]. The relatively limited buffering capacity of the UW solution may also be a disadvantage when preservation time is prolonged. Therefore, a new preservation solution was developed containing lactobionate, but removing those components which are unnecessary or injurious (HES, adenosine, insulin, raffinose) and adding histidine to enhance the buffering capacity. This solution, consisting of histidine and lactobionate, is called HL solution. By using this HL solution we have obtained satisfactory survival in rats receiving liver transplants after 24 h cold (4°C) storage. In the present study we described our experience in the use of this type of solution for long-term rat pancreas preservation. The effectiveness of this solution in rat pancreas preservation was compared with that of standard UW solution, high-Na$^+$-UW solution [13] and Eurocollins [EC] solution.

Offprint requests to: Takashi Urushihara M. D., Second Department of Surgery, Hiroshima University School of Medicine, 1-2-3 Kasumi Minami-ku, Hiroshima 734, Japan.

Table 1. Composition of test solutions. (mmol/l). Penicillin and streptomycin were added to both solutions. They were filter-sterilized by a 0.22 μm filter, stored in sealed glass containers, kept in a refrigerator at 4°C and used within 1 week

Solution	high-Na$^+$-lactobionate solution	high-Na$^+$-Histidine solution
Na-Lactobionate	110	110
MaSO$_4$	5	5
K-KH$_2$PO$_4$	25	25
Raffinose	30	0
Histidine	0	30
Glutathione	3	3
Allopurinol	1	1
Adenosine	5	0
Na$^+$ (mEq/l)	110 ± 5	110 ± 5
K$^+$ (mEq/l)	45 ± 5	45 ± 5
Osmolarity (mOsm/l)	315 ± 5	295 ± 5
pH	7.4	7.4

Table 2. The results of 48- and 72-h rat pancreas preservation using Belzer UW solution, Eurocollins solution, high-Na$^+$-lactobionate solution and high-Na$^+$-histidine solution. Belzer UW solution (ViaSpan) was from Du Pont Japan and Eurocollins solution, from Green Cross Corporation Japan

Experimental groups	Preservation time	Functional success rate	K value
Belzer UW solution	48 h (n = 9)	44 % (4/9)	2.41 ± 0.73
	72 h (n = 8)	0 % (0/8)	–
Eurocollins solution	48 h (n = 5)	20 % (1/5)	1.16
	72 h (n = 5)	0 % (0/5)	
High-Na$^+$-lactobionate solution	48 h (n = 7)	100 % (7/7)	2.23 ± 0.56
	72 h (n = 7)	14 % (1/7)	1.65
High-Na$^+$-histidine solution	48 h (n = 5)	100 % (5/5)	2.35 ± 0.74
	72 h (n = 8)	50 % (4/8)	2.37 ± 0.53

Materials and methods

Inbred LEW rats (Charles River, Japan) weighing 120–250 g were used as donors and recipients. The methods of total pancreatectomy and heterotopic pancreas transplantation were as we have described previously [13]. Donor segmental pancreas grafts were perfused in situ via the aorta with 2 ml of the test solution containing 20 units of heparin and stored in the test solution at 4°C in a refrigerator. After either 48 h or 72 h of cold preservation, donor pancreases were transplanted heterotopically into the right side of the neck of recipient rats which had been previously rendered diabetic by the administration of streptozotocin (65 mg/kg, i.v.). Graft endocrine function was evaluated by measuring non-fasting blood glucose values on days 1, 3, 5, 7 and 14 post-transplant and performing an intravenous glucose tolerance test (IVGTT) on the 14th post-operative day, following administration of 0.5 g glucose/kg body weight. Normal graft function was defined as random blood glucose values consistently below 200 mg/dl and K values exceeding 1.0 on IVGTT.

The composition of our high-Na$^+$-lactobionate solution with or without histidine is shown in Table 1. Magnesium sulphate, glutathione and allopurinol were present at concentrations of 20, 3 and 1 mmol/l, respectively, as in the original UW solution. The final osmolarity of both solutions was 290–320 mosmol/l. The pH was adjusted to 7.4 at room temperature.

The buffering capacity was defined as the number of milliequivalents per liter of H$^+$ required to cause a decrease of 1 pH unit from the initial pH of the solution. This pH change was determined by plotting pH (measured at 15°C) when 1 l of test solution was titrated with 0.1 M HCl. The viscosity of the test solution was measured at 4°C with an Ostwald viscosity meter and expressed as a ratio against distilled ion exchanged water. Statistical analysis was performed using Fisher's test to compare the results of different experimental groups.

Results

A total of 54 rat pancreas transplants were performed and no recipient animals were excluded from the experimental groups. The outcome of these experimental groups is summarized in Table 2. In the 48 h preservation groups, all grafts preserved in high-Na$^+$-lactobionate solution and high-Na$^+$-histidine solution showed normal endocrine function (7/7 vs. 5/5) whereas four out of nine grafts preserved in Belzer UW solution recovered normal function and one out of five grafts showed normal function using EC solution. In the 72-h preservation group using the high-Na$^+$-histidine solution, four out of eight recipients showed satisfactory graft function, while only one out of seven pancreases preserved in high-Na$^+$-lactobionate solution demonstrated normal graft function. Following 72-h preservation, none of the grafts preserved in Belzer UW solution (0/8) or EC solution (0/5) resulted in normal endocrine function. The differences were statistically significant for the 72-h preservation group, on comparing UW solution with the high-Na$^+$-histidine solution ($P < 0.05$) but not quite so on comparing the high-Na$^+$-lactobionate solution with the high-Na$^+$-histidine solution.

According to our laboratory parameters, the buffering capacities of UW solution, EC solution and high-Na$^+$-histidine solution were 11.0, 20.0 and 20.4 mEq/l per pH unit, respectively (Fig. 1). The viscosity of each solution, expressed as a ratio compared with deionized water, was 3.32 for the UW solution, 1.21 for the EC solution and 1.20 for the high-Na$^+$-histidine solution (Fig. 2).

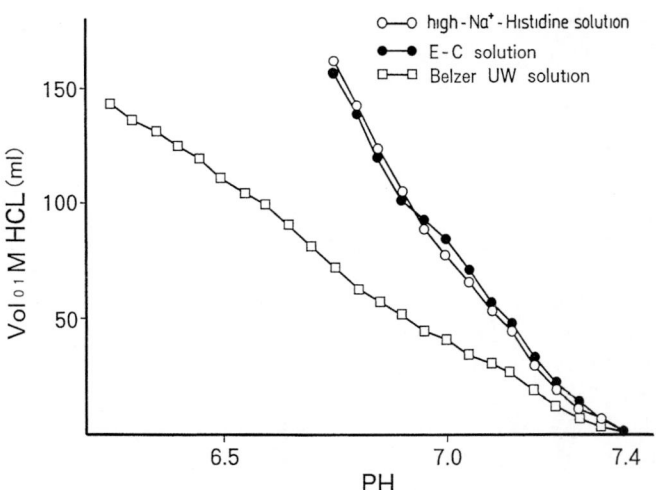

Fig. 1. The buffering capacity of the solutions. One liter of each solution was titrated with 0.1 M HCl, and pH measured at 15°C sequentially and plotted out. High-Na$^+$-histidine solution represents a substantially greater buffering capacity than does Belzer UW solution. E-C = Eurocollins

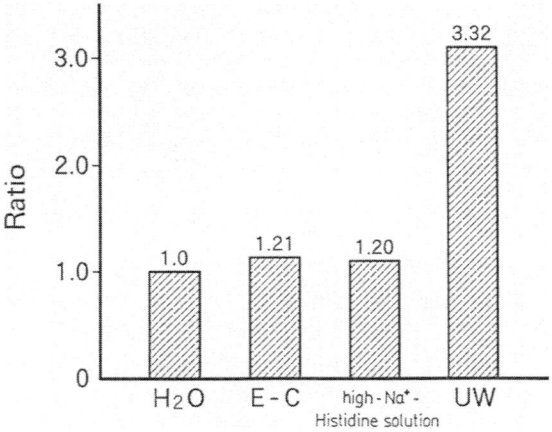

The viscosity of test solutions

Fig. 2. The viscosity was expressed as a ratio compared with deionized water. EC solution and high-Na$^+$-histidine solution have similar ratios at 1.21 and 1.20, respectively, while Belzer UW solution has a substantially higher viscosity at 3.32. *E-C* = Eurocollins

Discussion

In our previous report the effectiveness of UW solution was significantly improved by altering the cation composition from high-K$^+$ to high-Na$^+$ content in the rat liver preservation study [10]. This was also the case in the rat pancreas preservation study [13]. Using the high-Na$^+$ solution, similar improved results over standard UW solution have also been reported in dog liver, kidney and pancreas [19] as well as in human liver preservation studies [9]. This improvement with the high-Na$^+$ solution may be due to the reduction in potassium content leading to decreased vasoconstriction, minimized endothelial cell injury, and ameliorated microcirculation during the initial phase of reperfusion.

It should be pointed out that substitution of the amino acid histidine for raffinose improved survival rates although not to a statistically significant degree. Histidine has pK values of 1.78, 5.97 and 8.97 and appears to be a highly effective buffer in the physiological pH range. A higher concentration of histidine (90 mmol/l) with 20 mmol KH$_2$PO$_4$ has previously been shown to result in a potent buffering capacity (buffering capacity: 28 mEq/l per pH unit). But even at the lower concentration of histidine used in the present study, buffering capacity (20.4 mEq/l per pH unit) was adequately maintained and exceeded that of the original UW solution. This was also noted in EC solution. This improved buffering capacity may be the reason for the improved survival when using the high-Na$^+$-histidine solution.

Raffinose is a trisaccharide and was present in the original UW solution to suppress cell edema during cold storage [20]. However, the relatively low concentration of raffinose (30 mmol/l) in the standard UW solution can be replaced by an equimolar concentration of glucose, without reducing the effectiveness of lactobionate based solutions, in the preservation of rat liver and pancreas [11, 13]. Even a higher concentration of raffinose (190 mmol/l) can be replaced by either equimolar sucrose or glucose in a

phosphate buffer based solution in rat liver preservation without loss of effect [21]. The sugar component, irrespective of its molecular weight does not, therefore, appear essential to the preservative capacity of solutions in rat organs. Indeed the present results indicated that a simple sugar moiety may not really be necessary, as far as our new preservation solution is concerned. Replacement of raffinose with histidine cause little difference to the viscosity of the solution (1.22 vs 1.2) and was unlikely to be responsible for the improvement in survival rates noted in this study.

In conclusion, the present results indicated that our new solution used in combination with histidine and lactobionate was more effective than standard UW solution or high-Na$^+$ UW solution in rat pancreas preservation. The mechanism for this action should be further clarified.

References

1. Kalayoglu M, Sollinger HW, Stratta RJ, et al (1988) Extended preservation of the liver for clinical transplantation. Lancet I:617
2. Todo S, Nery J, Yanaga K, Podesta L, Gordon RD, Starzl TW (1989) Extended preservation of human liver grafts with UW solution. JAMA 261:711
3. Ploeg RJ, Coosens D, Vreugdenhil P, McAnulty JF, Southard JH, Belzer FO (1988) Successful 72-hour cold storage kidney preservation with UW solution. Transplant Proc 20:935
4. Wahlberg JA, Southard JH, Belzer FO (1986) Development of a cold storage solution for pancreas transplantation. Cryobiology 23:477
5. Wahlberg JA, Love R, Landegaard L, et al (1987) Successful 72-hour preservation of the canine pancreas. Transplantation 43:5
6. Makowka L, Zerbe TR, Chapman F, et al (1989) Prolonged rat cardiac preservation with UW lactobionate solution. Transplant Proc 21:1350
7. Wicomb WN, Collins GM (1989) Twenty-four-hour rabbit heart storage with UW solution; effects of low flow perfusion, colloid and shelf storage. Transplantation 48:6
8. Jamieson NV, Lindel S, Sundberg R, Southard JH, Belzer FO (1988) An analysis of the components in UW solution using the isolated perfused rabbit liver. Transplantation 46:512
9. Jamieson NV, Johnston PS, O'Gray JG, et al (1990) Clinical use of UW solution or simplified liver preservation solution prior to transplantation in 179 human livers. Transplant Proc 22:2088
10. Sumimoto R, Jamieson NV, Wake K, Kamada N (1989) 24-hour rat liver preservation using UW solution and some simplified variants. Transplantation 48:1
11. Sumimoto R, Jamieson NV, Kamada N (1990) Examination of the role of the impermeants Lactobionate and Raffinose in a modified UW solution. Transplantation 50:573
12. Sumimoto R, Kamada N, Jamieson NV, et al (1991) A comparison of a new solution combining histidine and lactobionate with UW solution and Eurocollins for rat liver preservation. Transplantation 51:589
13. Urushihara T, Sumimoto R, Jamieson NV, et al (1991) A comparison of some simplified lactobionate preservation solution with standard UW solution and Eurocollins solution for pancreas preservation. Transplantation. In press
14. Biguzas M, Jabloski P, Howden BO, et al (1990) Evaluation of UW solution in rat kidney preservation. II The effect of pharmacological additives. Transplantation 49:1051
15. Marshall VC, Howden B, Jablonski P, Scott DF, Thomas AC, Cham C, Biguzas M, Walls K (1990) Analysis of UW solution in a rat liver transplant model. Transplant Proc 22:503

16. Yu W, Coddington D, Bitter-Suermann H (1990) Rat liver preservation I. The components of UW solution that are essential to its success. Transplantation 49:1060

17. Jamieson NV, Sundberg R, Lindell S, et al (1988) Preservation of the canine liver for 24–48 hours using simple cold storage with UW solution. Transplantation 46:517

18. Jamieson NV (1991) Improved preservation of the liver for transplantation. Alimentary Pharmacol Ther. In press

19. Moen J, Claesson K, Pienaar H, et al (1989) Preservation of dog liver, kidney and pancreas using the Belzer-UW solution with a high sodium and low potassium content. Transplantation 47:940

20. Belzer FO, Southard JH (1988) Principles of solid-organ preservation by cold storage. Transplantation 45:673

21. Kobayashi T, Sumimoto R, Shimada et al (1991) Effective of sugars in the preservation solution on liver storage in rats. Cryobiology 21:1350

Transplant Int (1992) 5 [Suppl 1]: S 340–S 342

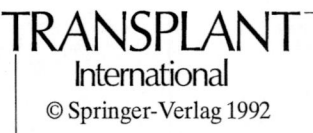
TRANSPLANT
International
© Springer-Verlag 1992

The impact of liver preservation in HTK and UW solution on microcirculation after liver transplantation

F. Walcher, I. Marzi, and V. Bühren

Department of Surgery, University of Saarland, Homburg/Saar, Germany

Abstract. Severe microcirculatory disturbances due to endothelial cell damage and leukocyte adherence during reperfusion of transplanted livers are considered to contribute to early graft failure. Since the degree of reperfusion injury after liver transplantation depends on the length of preservation time and the solution used for preservation, the aim of our study was to assess three solutions with respect to microvascular perfusion and leukocyte adhesion. Therefore, rat livers were stored up to 24 h in Euro-Collins (EC), University of Wisconsin (UW), or histidin-tryphtophan-ketoglutarate (HTK) solutions prior to orthotopic transplantation. The livers were studied in situ 60 min postoperatively using intravital fluorescence video microscopy. Using simple syringe flushing (10 ml), sinusoidal perfusion decreased below 50 % in EC preserved livers after 8 h preservation, in HTK preserved livers after 16 h preservation, and remained higher than 70 % in livers preserved in UW up to 24 h. Permanent adhesion of leukocytes was increased more rapidly in organs after 1, 8, 16, and 24 h preservation in HTK (16 %, 15 %, 34 %, and 49.7 % ± 4.7 %) compared to those preserved in UW (15 %, 18 %, 17 %; and 32.7 % ± 3.3 %; $P < 0.05$). Using a 10-fold volumn of the organ weight of HTK solution during the harvesting procedure, with an 8 min equilibration period, sinusoidal perfusion (39.6 ± 4.7 %) and leukocyte adhesion (42.7 ± 3.1 %) were not improved after 24 h. In contrast, equilibration with a volumn of approximately 40-times the liver weight improved sinusoidal perfusion (70.8 % ± 2.7 %; $P < 0.01$) and leukocyte adhesion (24.9 % ± 3.1 %; $P < 0.01$) significantly. Thus, using HTK solution, simple flushing prior to long-term cold storage resulted in microcirculatory disturbances when compared to UW solution. Larger volumns of HTK solution with an additional equilibration period of 8 min, however, reduced leukocyte adhesion and improved sinusoidal perfusion to a similar degree as UW solution.

Key words: Liver transplantation – Preservation solutions – UW solution – HTK solution – Leukocyte adherence – Microcirculation

Reperfusion injury to sinusoidal endothelial cells and microcirculatory disturbances have been observed after liver transplantation in recent years [3, 9, 11]. Subsequent adhesion of leukocytes leading to organ injury as well as microcirculatory perfusion failure were considered to contribute to primary nonfunction or poor function of liver grafts [19]. The degree of reperfusion injury and microcirculatory disturbances, however, depend on the period of cold storage prior to transplantation and the preservation solution used. In the late 1980s, the University of Wisconsin cold storage solution (UW) [1] was introduced and has replaced Euro-Collins solution in many centers allowing significantly longer preservation times [13]. In 1990, histidine-tryphtophane-ketoglutarate solution (HTK), developed by Bretschneider [2], was used successfully for clinical liver transplantation [4].

A comparative study using intravital fluorescence microscopy after rat liver transplantation by our group has shown recently that UW and HTK solutions comparably reduce microcirculatory disturbances, and both are superior to Euro-Collins (EC) solution [10]. This study, however, was performed after cold storage of livers for 1 h in a standard liver transplantation model. The aim of the present study was, therefore, to assess microcirculation and leukocyte adhesion in transplanted rat liver after cold storage periods of up to 24 h.

Materials and methods

Fed female Lewis rats (HAN, Hanover, FRG) weighing 220–250 g were used as donors and recipients to exclude immunological interference ($n = 3$–7/group). In the first part of the study, the livers were harvested after flushing the organs with 10 ml of ice-cold Euro-Collins (Fresenius, Bad Homburg, Germany), UW (DuPont, Waukegan, Illinois, USA), and HTK (Custodiol, Dr. F. Köhler Chemie, Alsbach, Germany), respectively (syringe flushing). The

---

Offprint requests to: I. Marzi, Dept. of Surgery, University of Saarland, D-6650 Homburg/Saar, FRG

organs were stored in the cold for 1 to 24 h, except those in EC solution which were stored only for 1 and 8 h. Since equilibration with HTK solution for at least 6 min has been suggested by Bretschneider [2], we modified the havesting procedure in the second part of the study. In two additional groups, livers were perfused for 8 min with a volumn of 10–12 times the liver weight or 40–45 times the liver weight. To keep all other experimental conditions constant (e.g., equilibration time of 8 min), the larger volumn was applied by elevating the bottle of the cold storage solution (40 cm and 100 cm, respectively). To prevent rewarming of the solution during perfusion, a cooling system was used.

All livers were transplanted orthotopically according to the technique described earlier [6]. The rats were anaesthetized with pentobarbital sodium (30 mg/kg i.p.) 60 min after surgery, and the liver was exposed under an intravital microscope (Nikon MM1; Düsseldorf, Germany; 545 nm filter, $20 \times$ water immersion objective) achieving a final magnification of $330 \times$, as described recently [9]. After injection of the leukocyte marker, acridine orange (1 μmol/kg; Sigma Chemicals, Deisenhofen, Germany), 5–8 pericentral fields of the liver lobule were recorded continuously for 30 s using a CCD camera (Cohu, FK 6990, Fa. Pieper, Schwerte, Germany) and an S-VHS video recording system (Panasonic, NV-FS1, Japan). Using off-line frame-by-frame analysis, sinusoidal perfusion and adhesion of leukocytes were analysed. Data of permanently adherent leukocytes, defined as white blood cells adhering at least 20 s to the sinusoidal wall, were given as percentage of all labelled and observed leukocytes [10].

Results

The hepatic microcirculation was disturbed in all groups as reflected by the decrease in sinusoidal perfusion (Table 1). The sinusoidal perfusion rate declined to below 50 % in the EC solution group after 8 h preservation and in the HTK solution group after 16 h preservation, while UW preserved livers still had a perfusion rate above 70 % after 24 h of cold storage. Adhesion of leukocytes, which

Table 1. Microcirculation and permanent leukocyte adhesion after cold storage in EC, HTK and UW as investigated 1 h after liver transplantation

Solution	EC		HTK				UW			
Storage time (hours)	1	8	1	8	16	24	1	8	16	24
Microcirculation (%)	84	47	89	83	59	37	93	81	74	73
Leukocyte adhesion (%)	34	45	16	15	34	50	15	18	17	33

was significantly increased after 8 h of cold storage in EC solution, rose substantially in livers stored for 16 h in HTK and in livers stored for 24 h in UW. Thus, cold storage with HTK solution after simple flushing with 10 ml resulted in a significant reduction in sinusoidal perfusion and an increase in adhesion of leukocytes compared with UW solution under identical conditions (Figs. 1 and 2). A larger volumn of HTK solution (approx. $10 \times$ liver weight) did not improve sinusoidal perfusion (Fig. 1) and leukocyte adhesion (Fig. 2). However, high volumn equilibration (approx. $40 \times$ liver weight), allowed a significant improvement of the microvascular perfusion (Fig. 1) and attenuation of leukocyte adhesion (Fig. 2). Using this procedure, the data were comparable with those of the UW group with no statistical difference.

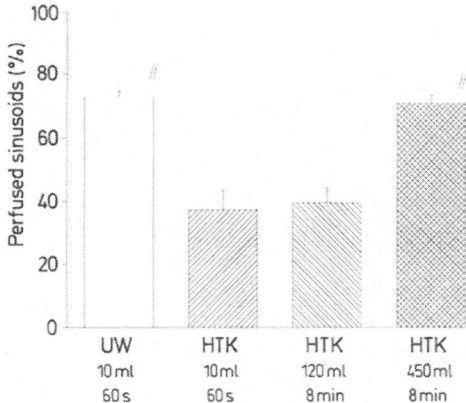

Fig. 1. Sinusoidal perfusion after 24 h of cold storage in UW and HTK solution. Application procedure as indicated and described in Methods. Data are expressed as mean ± SEM. #, $P < 0.05$

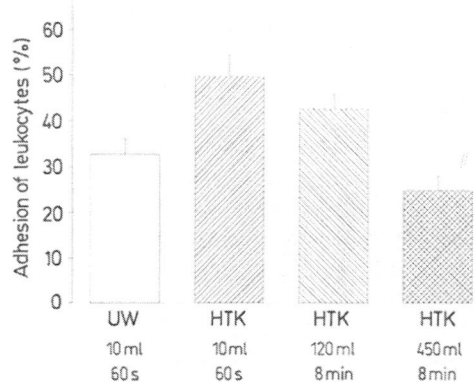

Fig. 2. Leukocyte adhesion after 24 h of cold storage in UW and HTK solution. Application procedure as indicated and described in Methods. Data are expressed as mean ± SEM. #, $P < 0.05$

Discussion

During reperfusion of liver grafts, endothelial cell injury has been demonstrated [3, 11] and has been suggested to cause microcirculatory failure of the transplanted organ [19]. On the other hand, activation of liver macrophages has been demonstrated after cold storage and transplantation of rat livers [18]. The macrophages most likely release inflammatory mediators (e.g., PAF, leukotrienes) deteriorating further microvascular perfusion [20]. Microvascular perfusion failure is due partly to an increased expression of adhesion sites (e.g., GMP140, ELAM-1, ICAM-1) on endothelial cells [14] and can be induced by inflammatory mediators generated during the reperfusion period [7]. Subsequently, activated leukocytes emigrate into the tissues, and organ destruction can be expected [8]. Indeed, increased adhesion of leukocytes and microcirculatory disturbances have been shown after rat liver transplantation using in vivo fluorescence microscopy techniques, even after 1 h of cold storage in EC, UW, and HTK solutions [10]. Since long-term preservation is becoming more important clinically, the aim of this study was to evaluate its effect on hepatic microcirculation after transplantation.

The results of this study demonstrated clearly the superiority of UW and HTK solution over EC solution after liver preservation up to 8 h with respect to sinusoidal perfusion and number of adherent leukocytes. This is consistent with other experimental and clinical studies comparing UW solution in liver [12, 13, 17] and HTK solution in kidney transplantation with Euro-Collins solution [5]. The benificial effects have been attributed in part, to prevention of cell swelling and free-radical-mediate reperfusion injury by impermeant and antioxidant ingredients [1, 15] and the histidine/histidine chloride buffering system in HTK solution [2, 16].

The second part of the study demonstrated the importance of different application procedures using UW and HTK solution. Whereas organ protection with UW was achieved with simple flushing (10 ml) only, HTK solution required equilibration with a high volumn for 8 min to achieve comparable results (Figs. 1, 2). This method of application of HTK solution was based on the extensive studies of Bretschneider [2]. He noted that the extracellular fluid in the HTK solution has low potassium levels, which facilitates flushing by the prevention of potassium induced vasoconstriction. Moreover, the viscosity of the HTK solution is lower than that of the UW solution, containing hydroxyl-ethyl starch as impermeant [1]. To achieve an equilibration of the extracellular space, a volumn of 20 times the organ weight with a pressure of 120 cm was used successfully for kidney protection [2]. In clinical liver transplantation with cold ischemia times up to 12.5 h, 9–10 l HTK solution were given via the portal vein and the aorta for 6–8 minutes with good results [4]. In this experimental study, HTK solution was only comparable with UW solution when a substantially higher volumn was used. The reasons why such a large volumn was needed to reduce microcirculatory failure significantly in this animal model remain unclear. This needs to be evaluated in further studies.

Acknowledgements. This study was supported in part by a grant from the Deutsche Forschungsgemeinschaft (Ma 1119/2-1).

References

1. Belzer FO, Southard JH (1988) Principles of solid-organ preservation by cold storage. Transplantation 45:673–676
2. Bretschneider HJ, Helmchen U, Kehrer G (1988) Nierenprotektion. Klin Wochenschr 66:817–827
3. Caldwell-Kenkel JC, Thurman RG, Lemasters JJ (1988) Selective loss of nonparenchymal cell viability after cold ischemic storage of rat livers. Transplantation 45:834–837
4. Gubernatis G, Pichlmayr R, Lamesch P, Grosse H, Bornscheuer A, Meyer H-J, Ringe B, Farle M, Bretschneider HJ (1990) HTK-solution (Bretschneider) for human liver transplantation. Langenbecks Arch Chir 375:66–70
5. Kallerhoff M (1989) Nierenprotektion in Anlehnung an das Verfahren zur Myokardprotektion nach Bretschneider im Vergleich zum Euro-Collins Verfahren. Z Transplantationsmedizin 1:15–33
6. Kamada N, Calne RY (1979) Orthotopic liver transplantation in the rat. Technique using cuff for portal vein anastomosis and biliary drainage. Transplantation 28:47–50
7. Kubes P, Suzuki M, Granger DN (1990) Platelet-activating factor-induced microvascular dysfunction: Role of adherent leukocytes. Am J Physiol 258:G158–G163
8. Lawrence MB, Springer TA (1991) Leukocytes roll on a selectin at physiologic flow rates: Distinction from and prerequisite for adhesion through integrins. Cell 65:859–873
9. Marzi I, Takei Y, Knee J, Menger MD, Gores GJ, Bhren V, Trentz O, Lemasters JJ, Thurman RG (1990) Assessment of reperfusion injury by intravital fluorescence microscopy following liver transplantation in the rat. Transplant Proc 22:2004–2005
10. Marzi I, Walcher F, Bhren V, Menger MD, Knee J, Trentz O (1991) Microcirculatory disturbances and leucocyte adherence in transplanted livers after cold storage in Euro-Collins, UW and HTK solutions. Transplant Int 4:45–50
11. Marzi I, Zhong Z, Lemasters JJ, Thurman RG (1989) Evidence that graft survival is not related to parenchymal cell viability in rat liver transplantation: The importance of nonparenchymal cells. Transplantation 48:463–468
12. Momii S, Koga A, Eguchi M, Fukuyama T (1989) Ultrastructural changes in rat liver sinusoids during storage in cold Euro-Collins solution. Virchows Arch [B] 57:393–398
13. Olthoff KM, Millis JM, Imagawa DK, Nuesse BJ, Derus LJ, Rosenthal JT, Milewicz AL, Busuttil RW (1990) Comparison of UW solution and Euro-Collins solutions for cold preservation of human liver grafts. Transplantation 49:284–290
14. Pober JS, Cotran RS (1990) The role of endothelial cells in inflammation. Transplantation 50:537–544
15. Southard JH, Gulik TM van, Ametani MS, Vreugdenhil PK, Lindell SL, Pienaar BL, Belzer FO (1990) Important components of the UW solution. Transplantation 49: 251–257
16. Sumimoto R, Kamada N, Jamieson NV, Fukuda Y, Dohi K (1991) A comparison of a new solution combining histidine and lactobionate with UW solution and Eurocollins for rat liver preservation. Transplantation 51:589–593
17. Takaoka F, Brown MR, Ramsay MAE, Paulsen AW, Brajtbord D, Klintmalm GB (1990) Intraoperative evaluation of EuroCollins and University of Wisconsin preservation solutions in patients undergoing hepatic transplantation. Transplantation 49:544–547
18. Takei Y, Marzi I, Kauffman FC, Lemasters JJ, Thurman RG (1990) Increase in survival time of liver transplants from injury by protease inhibitors and a calcium channel blocker, nisoldipine. Transplantation 50:14–20
19. Thurman RG, Marzi I, Seitz G, Thies J, Lemasters JJ, Zimmermann FA (1988) Hepatic reperfusion injury following orthotopic liver transplantation in the rat. Transplantation 46:502–506
20. Wake K, Decker K, Kirn A, Knook DL, McCuskey RS, Bouwens L, Wisse E (1989) Cell biology and kinetics of Kupffer cells in the liver. Int Rev Cytol 118:173–230

Transplant Int (1992) 5 [Suppl 1]: S 343–S 344

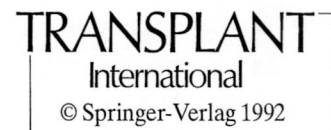

TRANSPLANT
International
© Springer-Verlag 1992

Myocardial preservation with the UW solution.
First European results in clinical heart transplantation

S. Demertzis, T. Wahlers, H.-J. Schäfers, J. Wippermann, M. Jurmann, J. Cremer, and A. Haverich

Division of Thoracic and Cardiovascular Surgery, Hannover Medical School, Hannover, Federal Republic of Germany

Abstract. In recent years, there is a growing body of evidence that the University of Wisconsin (UW) solution offers many advantages in organ preservation with regard to preservation quality and time. We, therefore, conducted the first European prospective, randomized, clinical trial comparing myocardial performance after preservation with UW and St. Thomas Hospital (ST) solution. Preliminary results indicated superior heart function after preservation with UW solution.

Key words: Cardiac transplantation – Myocardial preservation – UW solution

Throughout the last 3 years the overall number of heart transplantations has reached a plateau, reflecting mainly the limited number of the potential donors available [2]. In kidney and liver transplantation the use of the University of Wisconsin solution (UW) has led to a significant prolongation of ischemic times [3, 5]. Since improved results were also obtained after experimental cardiac preservation with UW solution [1, 4], we initiated a prospective, randomized clinical trial to compare myocardial performance after preservation with St. Thomas Hospital solution (ST) and UW solution.

Patients and methods

From December 1990 to April 1991, 18 patients undergoing orthotopic heart transplantation were included in this prospective randomized study. Patients were randomized according to the preservation solution used. In both groups, there were 8 males and 1 female. Mean age for the ST group was 45.5 ± 16.1 years and for the UW group, 42.3 ± 14.8 years (n.s.). A total of 11 patients had a dilative cardiomyopathy (DCM), 6 in the ST and 5 in the UW group, and 2 patients had an ischemic cardiomyopathy (ICM), 1 in each group.

Offprint requests to: Stefanos Demertzis, M.D., Division of Thoracic and Cardiovascular Surgery, Hannover Medical School, Konstanty-Gutschow-Str. 8, D-3000 Hannover 61, FRG

One patient underwent re-transplantation for accelerated graft coronary disease, while two patients in the UW group had an hypertrophic, non-obstructive cardiomyopathy.

Immunosuppression in all patients was based on 3-drug therapy, including cyclosporine A, azathioprine and prednisone. Both groups were compared with regard to donors' and recipients' pre- and postoperative data (age, interval from brain death to organ procurement, catecholamine support), and operation data (ischemic time, aortic clamp time, reperfusion time, spontaneous heart activity). Preoperative parameters were as follows: age, diagnosis, catecholamine support, cardiac output (CO) and pulmonary vascular resistance (PVR). Postoperative data included: right heart catheterization and CO determination via Swan-Ganz-catheter 2, 8 and 12 h postsurgery, as well as cumulative drug support. Statistical analysis was performed with ANOVA or Fisher's exact test.

Results

None of the patients died perioperatively. There were no significant differences regarding donor and preoprative recipient data: mean donor age was 26.1 ± 8 years vs 29.9 ± 5 years, brain death to harvesting interval was 15.4 ± 4 vs 10.9 ± 6 h for the ST and UW groups respectively. Mean preoperative CO was 4.4 ± 1.4 l/min for the ST and 4.2 ± 0.8 l/min for the UW group. Mean PVR was 208 ± 70 dyn/s $\cdot$ cm^{-5} for the ST and 268 ± 110 dyn/s $\cdot$ cm^{-5} for the UW group. No significant differences could be demonstrated with regard to the operation data: mean ischemic time was 168.3 ± 26 min for the ST and 139.5 ± 75 min for the UW group. The mean aortic cross-clamp time was 37.3 ± 6 min for the ST and 35.6 ± 19 min for the UW group. The mean reperfusion time was 37.8 ± 15 min for the ST and 29.8 ± 7 min for the UW group. Spontaneous activity during reperfusion resumed in 2 hearts in the ST and in 5 in the UW group ($P \le 0.05$). Defibrillation attempts averaged 2 in the ST vs 0.7 in the UW group ($P \le 0.05$). Significant differences were revealed with regard to the central venous pressure (CVP) 12 h postsurgery and pulmonary capillary wedge presure (PCWP) 8 and 12 h postsurgery: CVP 12 h was 13.7 ± 3.4 mm Hg vs 6.9 ± 4.3 mm Hg for the ST and UW groups respectively. At 8 h the PCW was

13 ± 4.7 mm Hg vs 7.6 ± 4.3 mm Hg and at 12 h 14.8 ± 3.5 mm Hg vs 7.6 ± 4.3 mm Hg in the ST and UW groups respectively ($P \leq 0.05$). Compared to patients in the UW group, patients in the ST group needed significantly more adrenaline to achieve hemodynamic stability (0.42 ± 0.23 vs 0.2 ± 0.11 µg/kg per min) and more nitroglycerine (7 ± 1 vs 2 ± 1.2 mg/kg per min) for effective preload reduction.

Discussion

In recent years, there has been growing evidence that UW solution offers many advantages in organ preservation with regard to preservation quality and time. After an encouraging initial experimental experience we proceeded to a prospective, randomized clinical trial, comparing early postoperative cardiac performance after preservation with ST and UW solution. The lower filling pressures at 8 and 12 h postoperatively at similar cardiac output values and the significantly lower drug support as well as the higher incidence of spontaneous defibrillation reflected superior graft function in the UW group. In conclusion, preliminary results of this first European prospective, randomized clinical study indicated improved myocardial preservation by use of UW solution.

References

1. Demertzis S, Siclari F, Erhorn U, Haverich A (1991) Improved myocardial recovery after 8 hours of cold global ischemia with UW-solution compared to St. Thomas Hospital solution with and without "hot shot" reperfusion. J Heart Lung Transplant 10:156
2. Kriett JM, Kaye MP (1991) The registry of the International Society for Heart and Lung Transplantation: Eighth official report – 1991. J Heart Lung Transplant 10:491–498
3. Ploeg RJ, van Bockel JH, Langendijk PTH, Groenewegen M, van der Woude FJ, Persijn G, Thorogood J, Hermans J (1991) A randomized clinical trial comparing preservation with UW solution and EuroCollins solution in cadaveric kidney transplantation. In: Ploeg RJ (ed) Preservation of kidney and pancreas with the UW solution. The Hague, Pasmans Offsetdrukkerij B. V., pp 156–184
4. Swanson DK, Psaoglu I, Berkoff HA, Southard JA, Hegge JO (1988) Improved heart preservation with UW preservation solution. J Heart Transplant 7:456–467
5. Todo S, Nery J, Yanga K, Podesta L, Gordon RD, Starzl TE (1989) Extended preservation of human liver grafts with UW solution. JAMA 261:711–714

Transplant Int (1992) 5 [Suppl 1]: S 345–S 350

TRANSPLANT
International
© Springer-Verlag 1992

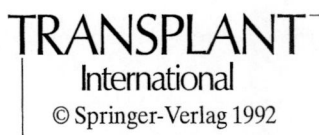

Protection by pentoxifylline against graft failure from storage injury after orthotopic rat liver transplantation with arterialization

S. Bachmann[1], **J. C. Caldwell-Kenkel**, **R. T. Currin**, **S. N. Lichtman**[1], **R. Steffen**[3], **R. G. Thurman**[2] and **J. J. Lemasters**[1]

Departments of Cell Biology & Anatomy, [1] Pediatrics, and [2] Pharmacology, University of North Carolina at Chapel Hill, North Carolina, USA, and [3] Department of Surgery, Free University of Berlin, Berlin, FRG

Abstract. Destruction of the endothelial cell lining and activation of Kupffer cells after reperfusion limits the safe storage of livers for transplantation surgery. Tumor necrosis factor-alpha (TNF) release by activated Kupffer cells may contribute to graft failure from storage injury. Accordingly, we evaluated whether pentoxifylline, which suppresses macrophage TNF release, would improve graft survival after orthotopic rat liver transplantation with arterialization. Livers from syngeneic Lewis rats were stored for 12–24 h in cold UW solution. Prior to implantation, the livers were flushed with cold Ringer's solution or warm Carolina rinse solution B. With either rinse, pentoxifylline treatment of graft recipients significantly improved graft survival. Combined use of pentoxifylline (50 mg/kg for 5 days) and Carolina rinse solution doubled the safe storage time to 24 h. Acidotic pH and antioxidants were essential components of Carolina rinse solution that acted synergistically with pentoxifylline. Pentoxifylline was also shown to suppress TNF release by lipopolysaccharide (LPS)-stimulated cultured rat Kupffer cells. Thus, pentoxifylline may protect against primary non-function and failure of grafts from storage injury by suppressing excessive TNF release by activated Kupffer cells. However, neutralization of TNF with excess anti-TNF antibody did not improve survival. This may mean that depletion of TNF is as deleterious as excess TNF production. Alternatively, other Kupffer cell secretions [e.g., interleukin-1 (IL-1), interleukin-6 (IL-6) and other cytokines] may be involved in the pathogenesis of graft failure. In conclusion, pentoxifylline could protect against graft failure from storage injury.

Key words: Carolina rinse solution – Endothelium – Kupffer cells – Liver transplantation – Organ preservation – Pentoxifylline – Reperfusion injury – Tumor necrosis factor

Liver transplantation is an accepted therapy for children and adults with end-stage liver disease and is increasing worldwide. With the development of University of Wisconsin (UW) cold storage solution, human livers can now be preserved under cold ischemic conditions for more than twice the length of time as with Euro-Collins solution which had been used previously [2, 20, 30]. Despite the improvement in UW solution, disturbances in liver function and histology attributable to storage injury commonly occur postoperatively. Moreover, primary graft non-function still occurs in 5–15 % of patients [17, 19].

Liver graft failure after prolonged storage involves a reperfusion injury to non-parenchymal cells: sinusoidal endothelial cells lose viability and Kupffer cells become activated by several structural and functional criteria [5, 6, 8, 9, 21, 28]. By contrast, parenchymal structure, function and viability are well maintained. Moreover, reperfusion injury occurs to liver grafts in vivo even under conditions where long-term graft survival is assured [29]. Nonparenchymal cell injury seems to lead to marked microcirculatory disturbances, including inhomogeneous reflow, hypoperfusion, and leukocyte margination, which may lead to ischemia and inflammation [8, 27]. In addition, Kupffer cells that have been activated by ischemia/reperfusion are likely to release tumor necrosis factor and other cytokines into the general circulation [13]. Release of cytokines may account for severe systemic problems associated with primary non-function, including coagulopathy, pulmonary infiltration, and multiple organ failure [22].

Recently, a new solution, Carolina rinse solution, has been developed to prevent reperfusion injury to livers stored for transplantation surgery [14]. In vitro, Carolina rinse solution prevents reperfusion-induced killing of endothelial cells, and in vivo, it improves graft survival markedly after orthotopic rat liver transplantation [1, 14, 16]. Improved survival has been associated with preservation of endothelial cell ultrastructure, suggesting that protec-

Offprint requests to: John J. Lemasters, Laboratories for Cell Biology, Department of Cell Biology & Anatomy, School of Medicine, University of North Carolina at Chapel Hill, Campus Box 7090, 236 Taylor Hall, Chapel Hill, North Carolina 27599-7090, USA

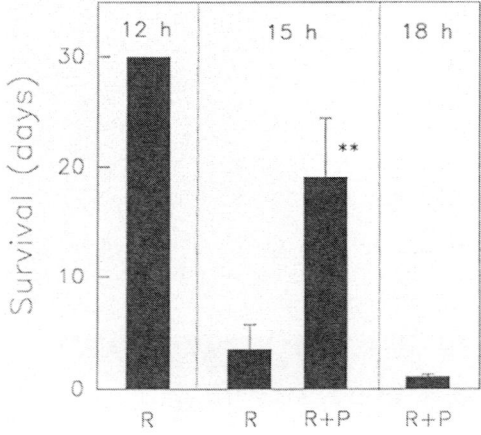

Fig. 1. Improvement by pentoxifylline in graft survival after orthotopic rat liver transplantation. Rat livers were stored for 12–18 h in UW solution and transplanted as described in Materials and methods. Liver grafts were rinsed with Ringer's solution and implanted into untreated recipient rats *(R)* or rats pretreated with a single dose of pentoxifylline *(R + P)*. ** *P* < 0.01 by Students *t*-test compared to *R*. Mean survival times ± SE from 6–13 experiments per group

tion is mediated, at least in part, by prevention of lethal reperfusion injury to endothelial cells.

Pentoxifylline is a drug which has long been used to treat peripheral vascular disease [31]. More recently, pentoxifylline has been shown to suppress tumor necrosis factor-alpha (TNF) release by macrophages [25], to inhibit TNF-mediated inflammatory action [26], and to be effective clinically in graft-versus-host disease after bone marrow transplantation [3]. Accordingly, we evaluated the effect of pentoxifylline on graft survival after rat liver transplantation in order to test the hypothesis that the release of TNF by Kupffer cells contributes to graft failure from storage injury. Our results indicated that pentoxifylline is indeed protective. Significantly, protection was achieved through treatment of the recipient animal, without any change in organ harvesting and storage conditions.

Materials and methods

Orthotopic rat liver transplantation with arterialization – surgery. Rat livers were transplanted under ether anesthesia essentially as described by Steffen et al. [24]. To avoid immunologic interference, syngeneic male Lewis rats (250–300 g) were used. In the donor operations, donor livers were flushed via the portal vein with chilled UW solution, cuffs were attached, and the explants were placed in an ice water bath immersed in storage solution. At the end of storage, donor livers were rinsed with 30 ml of cold Ringer's solution or Carolina rinse solution B at 28–30 °C. Carolina rinse solution B contained 115 mM NaCl, 5 mM KCl, 1.3 CaCl₂, 1 mM KH_2PO_4, 50 g/l modified hydroxyethyl starch, 1 mM allopurinol, 1 mM desferrioxamine mesylate, 3 mM glutathione, 2 µM nicardipine, 200 µM adenosine, 10 mM fructose, 10 mM glucose, 100 U/l insulin, and 20 mM MOPS [3-(N-morpholino)propanesulphonic acid] buffer, pH 6.5 [1]. In some experiments, Carolina rinse solution was modified by adjusting its pH to 7.4 or by omitting the antioxidants (allopurinol, desferrioxamine, and glutathione). Implantation surgery required 60 min. During this time the portal vein was clamped for

15 min and the inferior vena cava for not more than 20 min. Rats were given food and water ad libitum postoperatively. Average days of survival (with 30 days as a maximum) was used as an index of experimental outcome.

Treatment of recipient rats with pentoxifylline and anti-TNF antisera. Pentoxifylline was injected intraperitoneally (i. p.) into recipient animals in doses of 50 mg/kg, 1 h preoperatively. In some experiments, the dosage was repeated daily for 4 more days. In preliminary experiments, we compared recipient treatment with donor plus recipient treatment and donor treatment alone. Donor treatment produced no improvement in survival, whereas donor plus recipient treatment was no different than recipient treatment alone.

In other experiments, recipient animals were administered antisera via the penile vein under anesthesia at the beginning of the implantation operation. Two antisera were used: rabbit anti-mouse TNF polyclonal antibody and hamster anti-mouse TNF monoclonal IgG. Both antisera were obtained from Genzyme Corp. (Boston, Mass.) and cross reacted with rat TNF. Polyclonal antibody (1 ml) was diluted into 1 ml RPMI before injection. Monoclonal antibody (0.1 ml of a 2 mg/ml solution) was diluted into 0.5 ml RPMI before use.

Kupffer cell culture and measurement of TNF. Kupffer cells were isolated from Sprague-Dawley rats (300–350 g) by collagenase digestion and purified by counter-flow elutriation by modification of the technique described by Irving et al. [18]. Purified Kupffer cells were cultured overnight in 96-well microtiter plates (500 000 cells/well) with RPMI-1640 media supplemented with 20 % fetal calf serum and 10 mM HEPES [4-(2-hydroxyethyl)-piperazine ethanesulfonic acid] at 37 °C in humidified air/5 % CO_2. The next day, cultures were incubated for 1 h with various concentrations of pentoxifyline before the addition of 400 ng/ml lipopolysaccharide (LPS). After 8 h, supernatants were removed and stored at – 70 °C. TNF of thawed samples was measured using an ELISA kit (Genzyme, Boston, Mass.) and was expressed as pg equivalents of mouse recombinant TNF-alpha.

Materials. Nicardipine and modified hydroxyethyl starch (Pentafraction) were gifts of DuPont/Merck Pharmaceuticals (Wilmington, Del.) Pentoxifylline was the gift of Hoechst-Roussel Pharmaceuticals, (Somerville, N.J.). Lipopolysaccharide from *E. coli* was purchased from Sigma Chemical (St. Louis, Mo.). Other reagents were obtained from standard commercial sources.

Results

Protection by pentoxifylline against graft failure. For liver grafts stored 12 h in UW solution and rinsed with cold Ringer's solution, long-term graft survival after transplantation approached 100 % (Fig. 1). In contrast, after 15 h storage, no recipient rat survived longer than a day. This poor survival improved dramatically when recipient rats were pretreated with a single dose of pentoxifylline (50 mg/kg, i. p., 2 h preoperatively). However, pentoxifylline could not prevent graft failure after 18 h storage.

Survival was also much improved when grafts were rinsed with Carolina rinse solution instead of Ringer's solution (Fig. 2). After 18 h storage in UW solution, average survival time was more than 10 times that of the Ringer's-rinsed group (compare with Fig. 1). After 24 h storage, however, survival once again was lost. In contrast to our findings with Ringer's rinse, single dose pentoxifylline did not significantly improve survival of Carolina rinse-treated livers after 24 h storage. However, when the preoperative dose of pentoxifylline was followed by daily in-

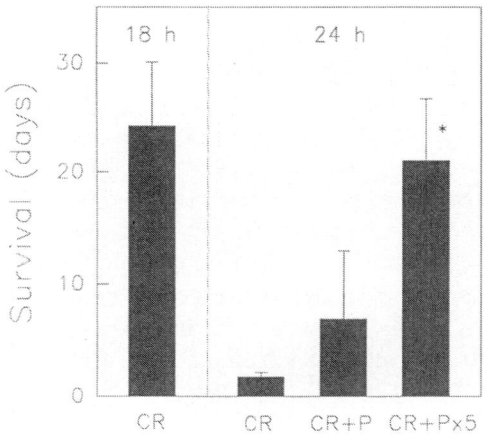

Fig. 2. Survival of liver grafts stored in UW solution and rinsed with Ringer's solution. Liver grafts were rinsed with Carolina rinse solution B after 18 or 24 h cold storage in UW solution and implanted into untreated recipient rats *(CR)*, rats pretreated with a single dose of pentoxifylline *(CR + P)*, or rats treated with five daily doses of pentoxifylline *(CR + Px5)*. * *P* < 0.05 by Student's *t*-test compared to *CR*. There were five to six experiments per group

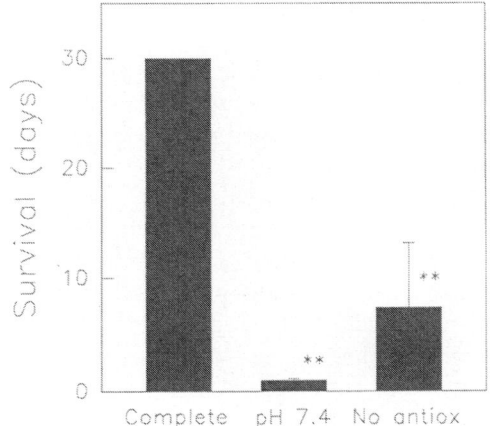

Fig. 3. Loss of survival at pH 7.4 or after omission of antioxidants from Carolina rinse solution. Liver grafts were stored for 18 h in UW solution and transplanted into recipient rats pretreated with a single dose of pentoxifylline. Prior to implantation, grafts were rinsed with complete Carolina rinse solution B *(Complete)*, Carolina rinse solution adjusted to pH 7.4 *(pH 7.4)*, or Carolina rinse solution containing no allopurinol, desferrioxamine or glutathione *(No antiox)*. ** *P* < 0.01 by Student's *t*-test compared to Complete. There were five to six experiments per group

jections for an additional 4 days, survival of Carolina rinse-treated livers increased significantly after 24 h storage.

Importance of acidotic pH and antioxidants in Carolina rinse solution for graft survival. Single dose pentoxifylline did not improve survival of liver grafts rinsed with Carolina rinse solution. To explore the hypothesis that pentoxifylline might be acting in the same way as components of Carolina rinse solution, we investigated the consequence of deleting specific components of Carolina rinse

on survival of pentoxifylline-treated graft recipients. Previously, we have found that the acidotic pH of Carolina rinse solution was critically important in preventing lethal reperfusion injury to endothelial cells after storage and reperfusion of isolated rat livers [5, 13]. To determine whether acidotic treatment remained important when pentoxifylline was used, we rinsed 18 h-stored livers with Carolina rinse solution adjusted to pH 7.4 prior to implanting livers into pentoxifylline-treated recipient rats (Fig. 3). Under these conditions, long-term survival went from 100 % to 0 % (Fig. 3). Similarly, we investigated the importance of antioxidants in Carolina rinse solution, since in vitro and in vivo studies have shown oxygen free radical generation by Kupffer cells after long-term storage and reperfusion [5, 12]. When antioxidants (allopurinol, desferrioxamine, glutathione) were deleted from Carolina rinse solution, survival of pentoxifylline-treated recipient rats again fell drastically (Fig. 3). Thus, we conclude that the beneficial effects of pentoxifylline seemed unrelated to prevention of pH-dependent endothelial cell killing or to suppression of oxygen free radical formation.

Suppression by pentoxifylline of TNF release by Kupffer cells. To explore the possibility that pentoxifylline suppresses TNF release by Kupffer cells, we exposed cultured rat Kupffer cells to LPS. This treatment caused TNF release into the medium to increase more than 25-fold over untreated cells (Fig. 4). Pentoxifylline suppressed LPS-stimulated TNF release by more than 70 % in a dose-dependent fashion. Half-maximal suppression of TNF release was achieved with about 10 μM pentoxifylline.

Lack of protection by TNF antisera against graft failure after liver transplantation. To test further the hypothesis that pentoxifylline-sensitive TNF release contributes to graft failure from storage injury, transplant recipients

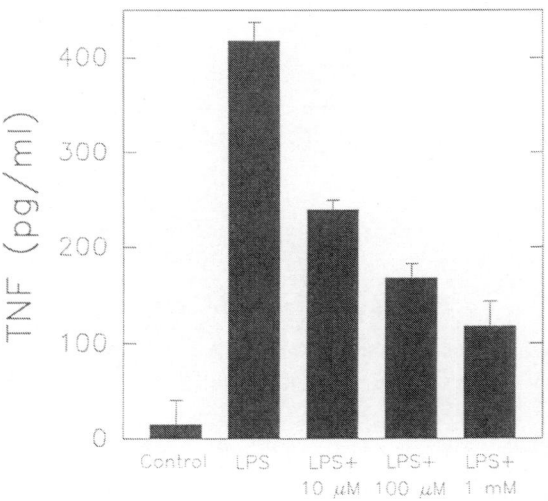

Fig. 4. Suppression by pentoxifylline of TNF release by LPS-stimulated cultured rat Kupffer cells. Kupffer cells cultured overnight were incubated for 8 h as described in Materials and methods. Cells were exposed to LPS (400 ng/ml) and 10–1000 μM pentoxifylline as indicated

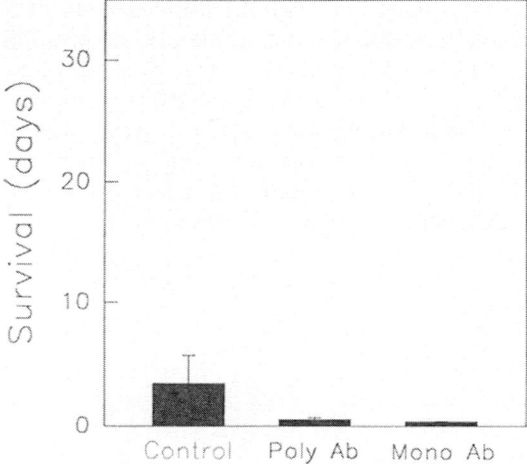

Fig. 5. Lack of protection against graft failure by anti-TNF antisera. Liver grafts were stored for 15 h in UW solution, rinsed with Ringer's rinse, and implanted into untreated rats *(Control)*, rats injected with anti-TNF polyclonal antibody *(Poly Ab)*, or rats injected with anti-TNF monoclonal antibody *(Mono Ab)*. There were two to three experiments per Ab group

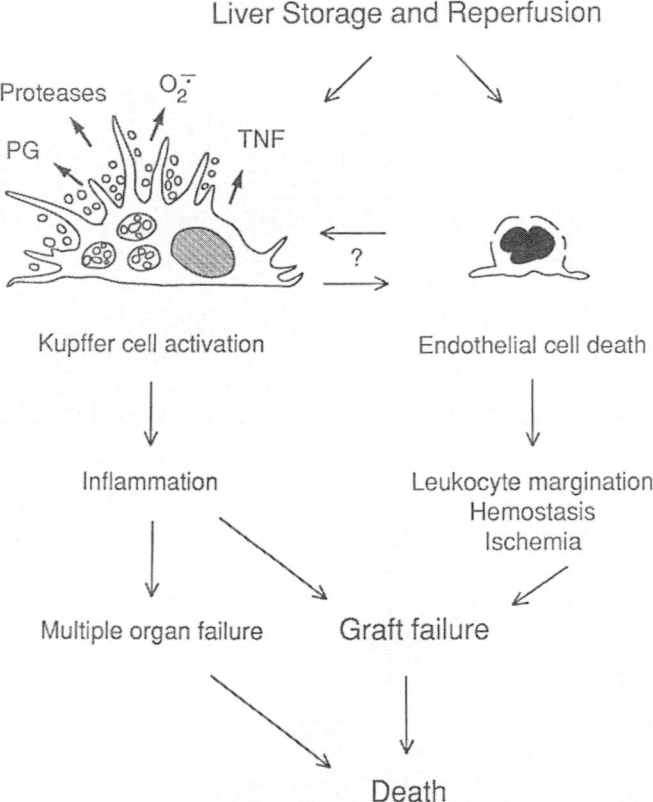

Fig. 6. Schematic picture of storage and reperfusion injury to liver. See text for details. *PG,* prostaglandin; O_2^-, superoxide radical; *TNF,* tumor necrosis factor

were pretreated with anti-TNF antisera. Under the conditions employed (storage for 15 h, rinse with Ringer's solution), neither polyclonal nor amonoclonal antisera improved graft survival (Fig. 5). If anything, average time of survival trended lower.

Discussion

Primary graft failure (primary non-function) remains a serious complication of liver transplantation surgery, occurring in about 5–15 % of cases. Graft failure is generally attributed to suboptimal conditions during harvesting and storage and to pathology in the donor liver, such as fatty infiltration, but the exact mechanisms are unknown. As shown by the present work, storage time is a very important determinant of graft success. Under controlled laboratory conditions employing syngeneic animals, only 3 h difference in storage time determined the success or failure of orthotopic rat livers transplantations (Figs. 1 and 2). In out-bred human populations under far less controlled conditions, it is unlikely that the response to storage time would be so consistent. Thus, mechanisms causing failure of rat livers after prolonged cold ischemic storage may be similar to those underlying idiopathic primary graft failure in human transplantation.

The present study demonstrated, for the first time, that pentoxifylline treatment of recipient rats could protect against graft failure from storage injury (Figs. 1 and 2). The only other drug showing possible efficacy against primary graft failure is prostaglandin E1 [17]. Since it is well documented that pentoxifylline is safe to humans, there is a possible use for the drug as a routine pre- and postoperative medication to minimize the incidence of primary non-function. Such a prophylactic use might have other benefits, as pentoxifylline also reduces the nephrotoxicity of cyclosporin and amphotericin, agents typically given to transplant patients [4, 32].

The beneficial effects of pentoxifylline were synergistic with Carolina rinse solution. Together, recipient treatment with pentoxifylline and rinsing of implants with Carolina rinse solution doubled safe preservation times (Figs. 1 and 3). Pentoxifylline is unlikely to act as an antioxidant, since pentoxifylline-treated recipient rats died when antioxidants were removed from Carolina rinse (Fig. 3). Similarly, pentoxifylline may not protect against pH-related injury to endothelial cells, since no animal survived when the pH of Carolina rinse solution was increased from pH 6.5 to pH 7.4.

A likely scenario is that pentoxifylline suppresses cytokine formation by Kupffer cells activated by storage and reperfusion. In cultured Kupffer cells, pentoxifylline strongly suppressed TNF release after stimulation with LPS (Fig. 4). Moreover, serum TNF increases in transplant recipients with failing liver grafts ([23], and data not shown). Against this hypothesis is the observation that neutralization of TNF with excess antibody did not improve graft survival (Fig. 5). This may mean that depletion of TNF was as deleterious as excess TNF production. Alternatively, other Kupffer cell secretions (e.g., IL-1, IL-6 and other cytokines) may be involved in the pathogenesis of graft failure.

Pentoxifylline is also a hemorrheologic agent which improves microcirculation in vasoocclusive disease [31]. It improves hepatic function and reduces enzyme release after hypothermic preservation of isolated rat livers in vitro, an effect associated with increased blood flow and reduced vascular resistance [10]. Since microcirculatory disturbances are prominent in failing liver grafts [15, 27], pentoxifylline may enhance graft survival by improving hepatic blood flow. By whatever mechanism, the benefit of pentoxifylline extends beyond the initial period of reperfusion, since pentoxifylline was more effective given daily over 5 days than when given as a single preoperative does (Fig. 2).

The present work also extended our in vivo analysis of the ingredients of Carolina rinse solution that contribute to its success. Previously, we have shown that Carolina rinse solution loses efficacy if adenosine is omitted [1, 15, 16]. The present work showed that efficacy was also lost if either antioxidants or acidotic pH were removed (Fig. 3). These findings suggested strongly that multiple mechanisms underlie liver graft failure from storage injury. As illustrated in Fig. 6, liver storage and reperfusion led to endothelial cell killing and Kupffer cell activation. Endothelial cell death promotes leukocyte margination, hemostasis, microcirculatory disturbances, and ischemia. Kupffer cell activation leads to inflammation, release of toxic soluble mediators, and possibly multiple organ failure. These parallel mechanisms both contribute to graft failure and death of recipient animals. It seems probable, therefore, that prevention of endothelial cell killing (acidotic pH), neutralization of oxygen free radicals (antioxidants), suppression of Kupffer cell release of TNF (pentoxifylline), and vasodilation (adenosine) together account for the efficacy and synergism of pentoxifylline and Carolina rinse solution.

In conclusion, pentoxifylline and Carolina rinse solution used together doubled storage times of rat livers in UW solution. Such treatments may become useful clinically in extending storage times of human livers, in reducing the incidence of primary graft failure, and improving graft function postoperatively.

Acknowledgements. We thank Mr. John Williams of Genzyme Corporation for helpful discussions and access to anti-TNF antisera. This work was supported, in part, by grant DK 37034 from the National Institutes of Health. J.C.C.-K. was the recipient of Individual National Research Service Fellowship DK 08094 from the National Institutes of Health.

References

1. Bachmann S, Caldwell-Kenkel JC, Oleksy I, Thurman RG, Lemasters JJ (1991) Prevention by warm Carolina rinse solution of graft failure from storage injury after orthotopic rat liver transplantation with arterialization. Transplant Int submitted
2. Belzer FO, Southard JH (1988) Principles of solid-organ preservation by cold storage. Transplantation 45:673–676
3. Bianco J, Nemunaitis J, Brown B, Aimgren J, Ballard B, Andrews F, Appelbaum FR, Buckner CD, Shields T, Singer J (1990) Pentoxifylline (PTX) and GM-CSF decrease TNF-alpha levels in patients undergoing allogeneic bone marrow transplantation (BMT). Blood 76 [Suppl 1]
4. Brunner LJ, Vakiei K, Iyer LV, Luke DR (1989) Prevention of cyclosporine-induced nephrotoxicity with pentoxifylline. Ren Fail 11:97–104
5. Caldwell-Kenkel JC, Coote A, Currin RT, Thurman RG, Lemasters JJ (1991) Activation of oxygen radical formation by Kupffer cells in rat livers stored for transplantation surgery. Gastroenterology 100:726
6. Caldwell-Kenkel JC, Currin RT, Tanaka Y, Thurman RG, Lemasters JJ (1989) Reperfusion injury to endothelial cells following cold ischemic storage of rat livers. Hepatology 10:292–299
7. Caldwell-Kenkel JC, Currin RT, Tanaka Y, Thurman RG, Lemasters JJ (1991) Kupffer cell activation and endothelial cell damage after storage of rat livers: effects of reperfusion. Hepatology 13:83–95
8. Caldwell-Kenkel JC, Thurman RG, Lemasters JJ (1988) Selective loss of non-parenchymal cell viability after cold ischemic storage of rat livers. Transplantation 45:834–837
9. Chazouilleres O, Ballet F, Chretien Y, Marteau P, Rey C, Maillard D, Poupon R (1989) Protective effect of vasocilators on liver function after long hypothermic preservation: a study in the isolated perfused rat liver. Hepatology 9:824–829
10. Colletti LM, Remick DG, Burtch GD, Kunkel SL, Strieter RM, Campbell DA (1990) The role of tumor necrosis factor alpha in the pathophysiologic alterations following hepatic ischemia/reperfusion injury. J Clin Invest 85: 1936–1943
11. Connor HD, Gao W, Nukina S, Lemasters JJ, Mason RP, Thurman RG (1991) Free radicals are involved in graft failure following orthotopic liver transplantation in the rat: an EPR spin trapping study. In preparation
12. Currin RT, Thurman RG, and Lemasters JJ (1990) Importance of individual components of Carolina Rinse for protection against lethal reperfusion injury to non-parenchymal cells after storage of rat livers for transplantation surgery. Symposium and Poster Abstracts: XIII International Congress of the Transplantation Society, p 592
13. Currin RT, Toole JG, Thurman RG, Lemasters JJ (1990) Evidence that Carolina rinse solution protects sinusoidal endothelial cells against reperfusion injury after cold ischemic storage of rat liver. Transplantation 50:1076–1078
14. Gao W, Hijioka T, Lindert KA, Caldwell-Kenkel JC, Lemasters JJ, Thurman RG (1991) Evidence that adenosine is a key component in Carolina rinse responsible for reducing graft failure after orthotopic liver transplantation in the rat. Transplantation, in press
15. Gao W, Takei Y, Marzi I, Lindert KA, Caldwell-Kenkel JC, Currin RT, Tanaka Y, Lemasters JJ (1991) Carolina rinse solution: a new strategy to increase survival time after orthotopic liver transplantation in the rat. Transplantation, in press
16. Greig PD, Woolf GM, Sinclair SB, Abecassis M, Strasberg SM, Taylor BR, Blendis LM, Superina RA, Glynn MR, Langer B, Levy GA (1989) Treatment of primary liver graft nonfunction with prostaglandin E1. Transplantation 48:447–453
17. Irving MG, Roll FJ, Huang S, Bissell DM (1984) Characterization and culture of sinusoidal endothelium from normal rat liver: lipoprotein uptake and collagen phenotype. Gastroenterology 87:1233–1247
18. Kahn D, Esquivel CO, Makowka L, Machigal-Torres M, Yunis E, Iwatsuki S, Starzl TE (1989) Causes of death after liver transplantation in children treated with cyclosporine and steroids. Clin Transplant 3:150–155
19. Kalayoglu M, Hoffman RM, D'Alessandro AM, Pirsch JD, and Belzer FO (1989) Clinical results in liver transplantation using UW solution for extended preservation. Transplant Proc 21: 3487–3488
20. Lemasters JJ, Caldwell-Kenkel JC, Currin RT, Tanaka Y, Marzi I, Thurman RG (1989) Endothelial cell killing and activation of Kupffer cells following reperfusion of rat livers stored in Euro-Collins solution. In: Wisse E, Knook DL, Decker K (eds) Cells of the Hepatic Sinusoid, vol 2. Kupffer Cell Foundation, Rijswijk, The Netherlands, pp 277–280
21. Ringe B, Pichlmayr R, Lubbe N, Bornscheuer A, Kuse E (1988) Total hepatectomy as temporary approach to acute hepatic or primary graft failure. Transplant Proc 20 [Suppl 1]:552–557
22. Savier E, Shedlofsky SI, Lemasters JJ, Thurman RG (1991) Release of tumor necrosis factor following rat liver transplantation is increased by nisoldipine. 5th Congress of the European Society for Organ Transplantation, Book of Abstracts, in press

S350

23. Steffen R, Ferguson DM, Krom RAF (1989) A new method for orthotopic rat liver transplantation with arterial cuff anastomosis to the recipient common hepatic artery. Transplantation 48:166–168

24. Strieter RM, Remick DG, Ward PA, Spengler RN, Lynch JP, Larrick J, Kunkel SL (1988) Cellular and molecular regulation of tumor necrosis factor-alpha production by pentoxifylline. Biochem Biophys Res Commun 155: 1230–1236

25. Sullivan GW, Carper HT, Novick WJ, Mandell GL (1988) Inhibition of the inflammatory action of interleukin-1 and tumor necrosis factor (alpha) on neutrophil function by pentoxifylline. Infect Immun 56:1722–1729

26. Takei Y, Marzi I, Gao W, Gores GJ, Lemasters JJ, Thurman RG (1991) Leukocyte adhesion and cell death following orthotopic liver transplantation in the rat. Transplantation 51:959–965

27. Takei Y, Marzi I, Kauffman FC, Currin RT, Lemasters JJ, Thurman RG (1990) Increase in survival time of liver transplants by protease inhibitors and a calcium channel blocker, nisoldipine. Transplantation 50:14–20

28. Thurman RG, Marzi I, Seitz G, Thies J, Lemasters JJ, Zimmerman F (1988) Hepatic reperfusion injury following orthotopic liver transplantation in the rat. Transplantation 46:502–506

29. Todo S, Nery J, Yanaga D, Podesta L, Gordon RD, Starzl TE (1989) Extended preservation of human liver grafts with UW solution. JAMA 261:711–714

30. Ward A, Clissold SP (1987) Pentoxifylline. A review of its pharmacodynamic and pharmacokinetic properties, and its therapeutic efficacy. Drugs 34:50–97

31. Wasan KM, Vadiel K, Lopez-Berestein G, Verani RR, Luke DR (1990) Pentoxifylline in amphotericin B toxicity rat model. Antimicrob Agents Chemother 34:241–244

Transplant Int (1992) 5 [Suppl 1]: S 351–S 356

TRANSPLANT
International
© Springer-Verlag 1992

Pulmonary mechanics after cardio-pulmonary transplantation, an experimental study

J. P. Carteaux[1], P. M. Mertes[1], C. Dopff[1], J. Borrely[1], T. Hubert[2], R. Peslin[3], and J. P. Villemot[2]

[1] Laboratoire de Chirurgie expérimentale, Faculté de Médecine,
[2] Service de Chirurgie Cardiaque et Transplantation, C. H. U. de Brabois,
[3] INSERM U. 14, Plateau de Brabois, Vandœuvre les Nancy, France

Abstract. An experimental model was developed in pigs (weight: 25 ± 2 kg), to evaluate pulmonary mechanics during the first 2 h of reperfusion following heart-lung transplantation. We studied two groups with three transplantations each: group A (45 min of preservation) and group B (6 h of preservation). After rinsing out the heart-lung mass by the injection of a cold intracellular solution ($K^+ = 115$ mEq/l) into the aorta and the pulmonary artery, the organs were removed and conserved in a cold environment ($0.5\,°C$). The orthotopic heart-lung transplantation was carried out using extra-corporeal circulation. Pulmonary mechanics were evaluated before and after transplantation by measuring the pulmonary compliance (C), and the aero-dynamic resistance (R) with an interrupted air flow technique.

Cardiorespiratory assistance	Group A	Group B
C: 1 h of reperfusion	$- 17.2\% \pm 7.04$	$- 20.8\% \pm 12.4$
C: 2 h of reperfusion	$- 30.3\% \pm 4.6$	$- 32.2\% \pm 2.6$
R: 1 h of reperfusion	$+ 130.8\% \pm 116.9$	$+ 301.5\% \pm 60.7$
R: 2 h of reperfusion	$+ 193.7\% \pm 80$	$+ 372.5\% \pm 190.7$

The duration of ischaemia appeared to be a pernicious factor in cardiopulmonary function. In all cases, the protection protocol of the heart-lung block had allowed a cutting-off of the cardiorespiratory assistance. However, there were major pulmonary mechanical perturbations, associated with a reduction in the pulmonary compliance and a very important increase in the aerodynamic resistance.

Key words: Cardiopulmonary transplantation – Pulmonary mechanics

The advances in cardiac transplantation following the introduction of Cyclosporine A, and the encouraging results of cardiopulmonary transplantation in primates resulted in the initiation of the cardiopulmonary transplantation programme in humans at Stanford in 1981 [6]. Despite the evolution of this procedure [1], a number of problems remain; these include patient selection, short conservation period of the heart-lung block, post-operative immunosuppression, and identification and treatment of bouts of rejection and infection. An increase in the conservation period of the heart-lung block by several hours would allow one to use th donors more effectively, to optimize the compatibility of the donor and recipient, to reduce transport costs, and finally, to defuse the sense of urgency characteristic of such operations.

The difficulty with this particular domain of organ preservation is the need for total and immediately functioning transplanted organs. The removal of the heart-lung block and its subsequent preservation cause modifications in pulmonary physiology which are important during the reperfusion phase and possibly account for the success of the surgical procedure [2–4]. The aim of this work was to study the modifications in pulmonary mechanics (compliance and resistance), appearing after the conservation of the heart-lung graft in a cold plegic solution of the intracellular type at a stable low temperature during the initial hours of reperfusion.

Materials and methods

We studied 3-month-old piglets weighing 25 ± 2 kg. Six orthotopic cardio-pulmonary transplants were carried out under extracorporeal circulation (ECC). The animals were divided into two groups (A and B), depending on the pre-implantation conservation period of the heart-lung graft. Group A represented those grafts ($n = 3$) conserved for 45 min, whilst group B consisted of those conserved for over 6 h ($n = 3$).

The donor animal was premedicated with ketamin (Ketalar), 12 mg/kg intramuscularly, 1 h before surgery. General anaesthesia was induced by the intravenous (IV) administration of disodium pentobarbital (Nesdonal), 3 mg/kg, and of alcuronium chloride (Alloferine), 0.5 mg/kg. The animal was then intubated and artificially ventilated ($FiO_2 = 75\%$). After a median sternotomy had been performed, the heart-lung block was dissected and the animal heparinised (3 mg/kg IV). A cannula (Bardik) was introduced into the

Offprint requests to: J. P. Carteaux, Service de Chirurgie cardiaque et Transplantation, C. H. U. Brabois, 54500 Vandœuvre les Nancy, France

Table 1. Cardiopneumoplegic solution

K^+	115	mEq
Na^+	10	mEq
CA^{++}	0.025	mEq
CI^-	15	mEq
HCO^{3-}	10	mEq
HPO^{4-}	85	mEq
H^2PO^4	15	mEq
Gluconate	0.025	mEq
Glucose	35	g

pulmonary artery. The cardioplegic cannula was positioned in the aortic root, and blood was drawn and stored for possible use during the reperfusion phase. Following aortic clamping, simultaneous cardioplegia and pneumoplegia was achieved. The right and left auricles were opened to allow the evacuation of the plegic solutions and to bring about a dilation of the cardiac cavities. Gentle manual ventilation was maintained to ensure a proper distribution of the pneumoplegia. The pneumoplegia was halted when the lungs became discoloured. The cardioplegia and pneumoplegia were performed with an intracellular type, cold crystalloid solution (at 2°C) (Table 1). After sectioning the trachea beneath the tracheal plane and the aorta above the aortic plane, the heart-lung block was removed from the thorax and placed in a sterile hermetic bag, and immersed in a saline solution at 0.5°C for conservation.

Cardio-pulmonary transplantation

The recipient animal was anaesthetised and ventilated in a similar fashion to the donor. Following a median sternotomy and dissection of the vessels at the base of the heart, systemic heparin was administered at a dose of 3 mg/kg IV and an ECC was installed between the ascending thoracic aorta and the vena cava. The extracorporal circulation circuit, which consisted of a bubble oxygenator (shiley 100 A) was primed with a solution containing crystalloid (Ringer) and macromolecular (Plasmion) solutes and sodium bicarbonate (14 part per thousand).

The heart and lungs of the recipient piglet were excised and the heart-lung block of the donor was implanted into the thorax of the recipient, according to the technique of Reitz et al. The aorta was unclamped and the aorta, cardiac cavities and the pulmonary artery were purged of air. The heart was defibrillated and manual ventilation with the aid of a souple balloon was effected for a few minutes. Artificial ventilation with a positive end-expiratory pressure of 4 cmH2O was then established. A perfusion of isoprenatine (Isuprel) was started; its flow rate being a function of the cardiac frequency.

Monitoring

During the experiment, the ECG was monitored and the arotic pressure was measured with a catheter placed in the aorta, via the right carotid artery. The pulmonary artery pressure was measured with a catheter placed in the trunk of the pulmonary artery and the left auricular pressure was measured by a catheter placed in the left auricle (pressure gauge: physiological transducer AE840). These parameters were measured in the anaesthetised donor animal and in the recipient animal after 1, 2 and 3 h of reperfusion. The coagulation times (Hemochron 400 R) were recorded while the ECC functioned.

Blood gases were measured (Radiometer ABL 4) from samples drawn from a catheter in the left carotid artery and electrolyte (Na^+, K^+, Cl^-) and plasma protein levels were measured by standard techniques (Prisma). These parameters were measured in the donor animals before excision and in the recipient animals during the first 3 h of reperfusion. The blood gases and biochemical analyses (Na^+, K^+, Cl^-, plasma proteins) were presented for experiments 3, 4, 5 and 6 only). For technical reasons, these measurements could not be performed under the conditions described above for experiments 1 and 2.

Evaluation of pulmonary mechanics

Pulmonary compliance and resistance were measured in the donor animal before excision of the graft and in the recipient animal after transplantation with the thorax and pleura open, and under the ventilation conditions described previously. Before each measurement, a bronchial aspiration was performed.

Technical details (Fig. 1). The transpulmonary pressure was measured with a differential manometer [Statham PM5 (± 70 cmH2O)] connected to the intratracheal tube and to atmospheric pressure, as the thorax and pleura were open. A pneumotachogram was added to obtain the spirogram. All the data were recorded on a chart recorder. The calibration of the pressure line was achieved with the aid of an inclined-water manometer. The calibration of the flow rate line was achieved with a calibrated syringe (3 l) and by an integration method [15].

Calculation of compliance and resistance. The compliance and resistance were calculated from a respiratory cycle containing two zero-flow points (A and B). The first zero-flow point (A) was that at the end of expiration. The second zero-flow point (B) was obtained by suddenly clamping the intratracheal tube at the end of inspiration. Compliance (C) was calculated as the ratio of pulmonary volume

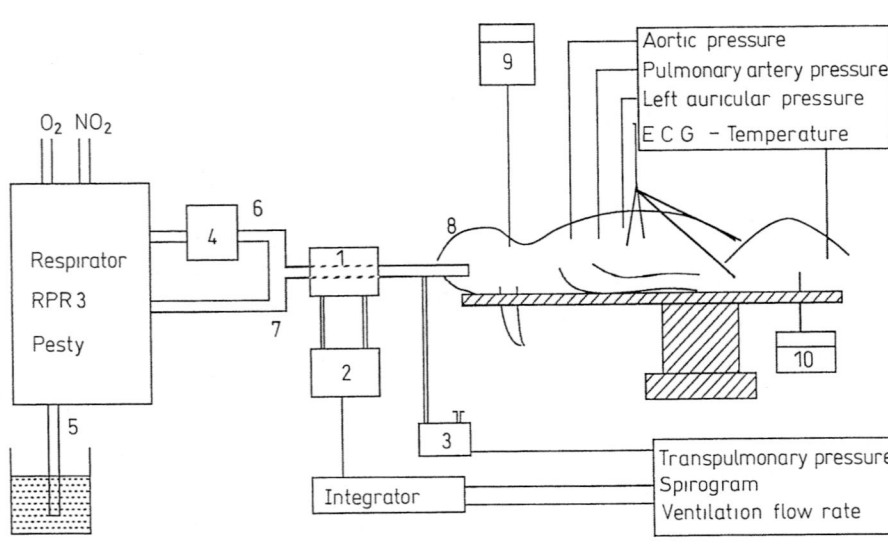

Fig. 1. Measurement techniques for compliance and resistance. *1* Pneumotachograph FLEISCH nº *1, 2* differential manometer STAHAM PM283, *3* differential manometer STATHAM PM5, *4* humidifierheater, *5* expiratory circuit outlet, *6* inspiratory circuit, *7* expiratury circuit, *8* intratracheal tube, *9* perfusion, *10* urine probe

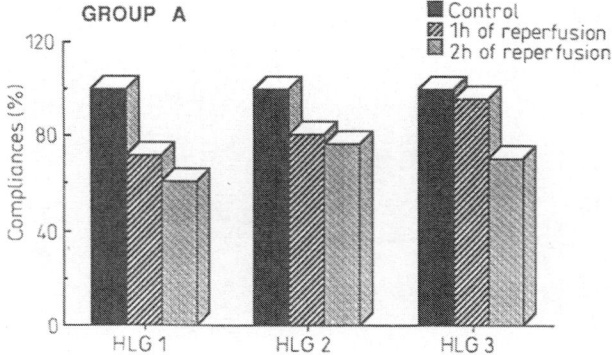

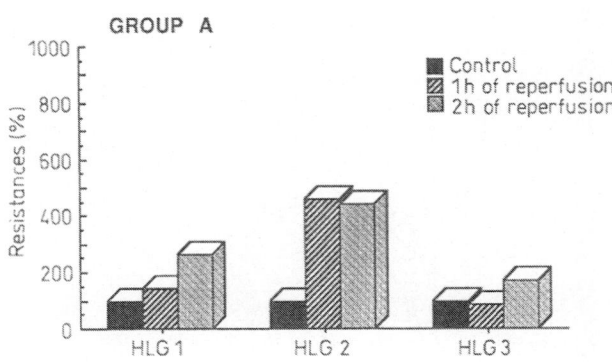

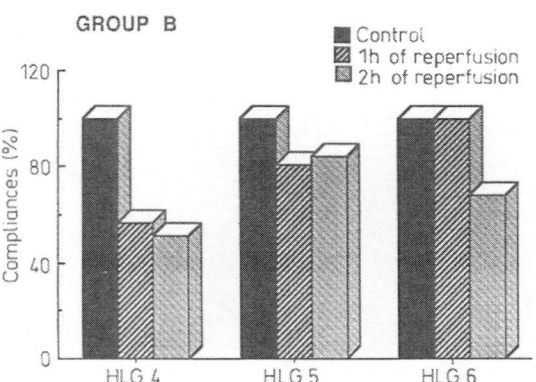

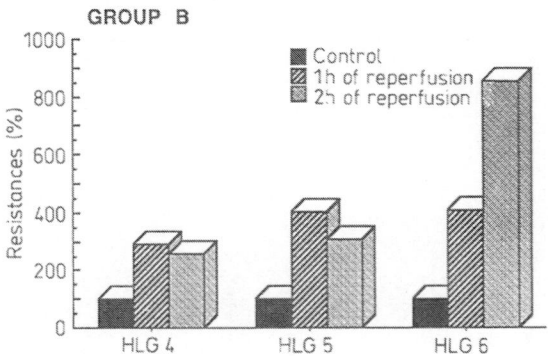

Fig. 2. Evolution of pulmonary compliance, after 1 and 2 hours of reperfusion for each of the heart-lung grafts (HLG) in group 1 (GA: 45 min of conservation) and in group B (GB: 6 hours of conservation)

Fig. 3. Evolution of pulmonary resistance after 1 and 2 hours of reperfusion for each of the heart-lung grafts (HLG) in group A (GA: 45 min of conservation) and in group B (GB: 6 hours of conservation)

variation (Δ V), (read from the spirogram) and the difference in transpulmonary pressures (of elastic origin) between points (A) and (B). (C = ΔV/ΔP1).

Resistance (R) was calculated as the ratio of (1) the difference in transpulmonary pressure (of dynamic origin) (Δ P2) between the transpulmonary pressure measured at (B) and the transpulmonary pressure measured at the moment of clamping the intratracheal tube, and (2) the inspiratory flow rate (Δ di) observed immediately after clamping the intratracheal tube. The result was corrected for the resistance of the intratracheal tube (Rp) [(R = (ΔP2/ΔDi) − Rp)].

Pulmonary compliance and resistance were calculated for the donor animal before excision and for the recipient animal after 1 and 2 h of reperfusion. The results of the pulmonary mechanics were calculated as the mean of the measurements carried out over two respiratory cycles.

Presentation of results

Results are presented as a percentage of control values and expressed as mean ± standard error of mean (SEM).

Results

The conservation time of the heart-lung grafts for the animals in group B was 351.6 ± 18.9 min and 46 ± 5.1 min for the animals in group A. The conservation temperature varied between 0.5 and 2 °C. The cardio-pulmonary assistance period for the animals in group A was 56.6 ± 2 min, whereas that for group B animals was 88.3 ± 35.4 min.

Pulmonary mechanics results (Figs. 2 and 3). In group A, compliance decreased by 17.2 ± 7.4 % after the 1st h of reperfusion and by 30.3 ± 4.6 % after 2 h of reperfusion. In a similar manner, compliance in group B decreased by 20.8 ± 12.4 % and 32.2 ± 2.6 % after 1 and 2 h of reperfusion, respectively. In group A, the resistances increased by 130.8 ± 116.9 % after the 1st h of reperfusion and by 193.7 ± 80 % after the 2nd h. In group B, the resistances increased by 301.5 ± 60 % and 372.5 ± 190.7 % in the same time scale.

Our study population was too small to allow confidence in statistical results. However, the results were sufficiently homogeneous to allow us to make several comments. In all experiments, pulmonary compliance decreased, although the period of conservation did not appear to influence the extent of the decrease. Similarly, in all experiments, pulmonary resistance was seen to increase during reperfusion. This increase was greater in group B (6 h of conservation).

Haemodynamic results (Fig. 4). The haemodynamic behaviour of groups A and B appeared to be identical during reperfusion. However, in the two groups, there were differences between the per-perfusion measurements and those of the control animals. There was an increase in the cardiac frequency, in the left auricular pressure and in the mean pulmonary arterial pressure. The mean aortic pressure diminished during reperfusion, whilst the systolic

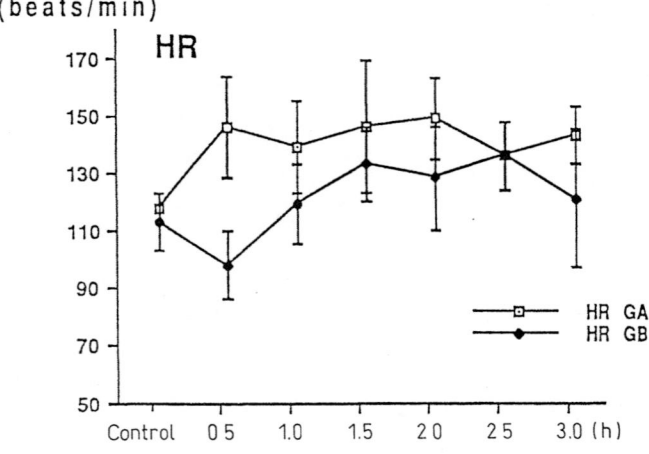

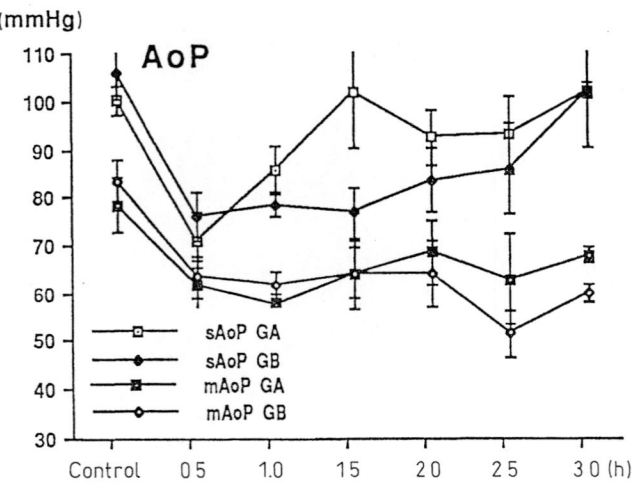

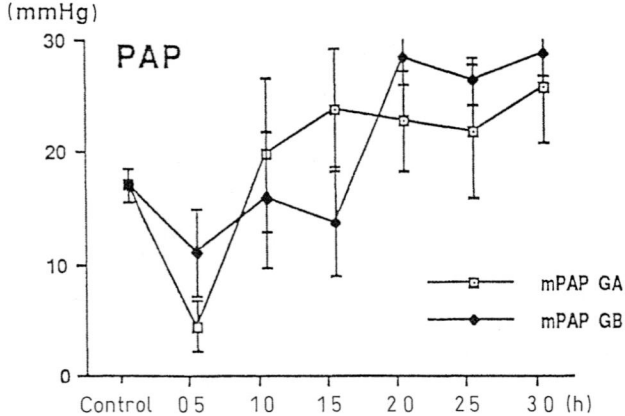

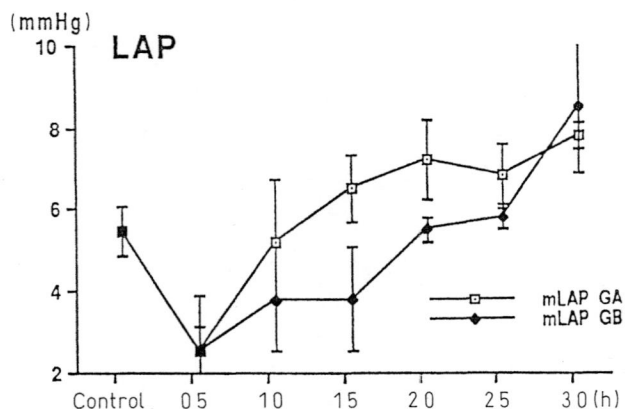

Fig. 4. Average heart rate (HR), aortic pressure (AOP), pulmonary artery pressure (PAP) and left atrial pressure (LAP) for the two groups during control conditions, and 1, 2, and 3 hours of reperfusion. Mean, m; Systolic, s. Group A (GA): 45 min of conservation; Group B (GB): 6 h of conservation

---

aortic pressure exhibited a value close to that of the control animals.

Arterial blood gas results (Fig. 5). The PaO_2 remained greater than 200 mmHg during the experiment. The $PaCO_2$ was maintained at approximately 40 mmHg. A metabolic acidosis set in progressively at the end of reperfusion.

Biochemical results. Figure 6 illustrates the average evolution of the electrolytes and plasma proteins during the experiments. The plasma proteins decreased once the extracorporeal circulation was established, probably due to haemodilution. During the reperfusion phase, the protein concentration remained constant.

Discussion

We retained the use of a single plegic solution, rich in potassium, because of its capacity to assure pulmonary protection [6, 13]. Moreover, experimental studies have shown that this solution also ensures long-term cardiac protection [17, 22]. The logic for using such a solution is that active ionic transfers at low temperature are interrupted, and hence, ionic concentration gradients on either side of the cellular membrane are avoided [12]. In addition, the hyperosmolarity of the solution allows for stabilisation of the membrane and thus, a decreased ionic exchange [19]. Our haemodynamic results confirmed the capacity of such a solution to preserve the myocardial function over a 6 h period. The pulmonary mechanical perturbations (increased resistances, reduced compliances as well as an increased pulmonary artery pressure) reflected the degree of pulmonary insult sustained. Experimental studies on dogs have shown similar results [2, 3].

The drop in pulmonary compliance may be interpreted in several ways. All the pulmonary tissue constituents contribute to the elastic properties of the lung. The most important of these are the connective tissues (elastine, reticuline, collagen) as well as the pleura, the arteries and pulmonary veins. Previous studies have shown that the plasto-elastic properties of the tissue deformations are only moderately disturbed after the excision and cooling of the lungs [3]. Moreover, the state of vascular congestion only affects slightly the pressure-volume relationship of lungs excised from cats [5]. However, interstitial or intraalveolar pulmonary oedema, through the perturbations developed along the dimensions of the elastic elements and through the perturbations developed along the dimension of the elastic elements and through the geome-

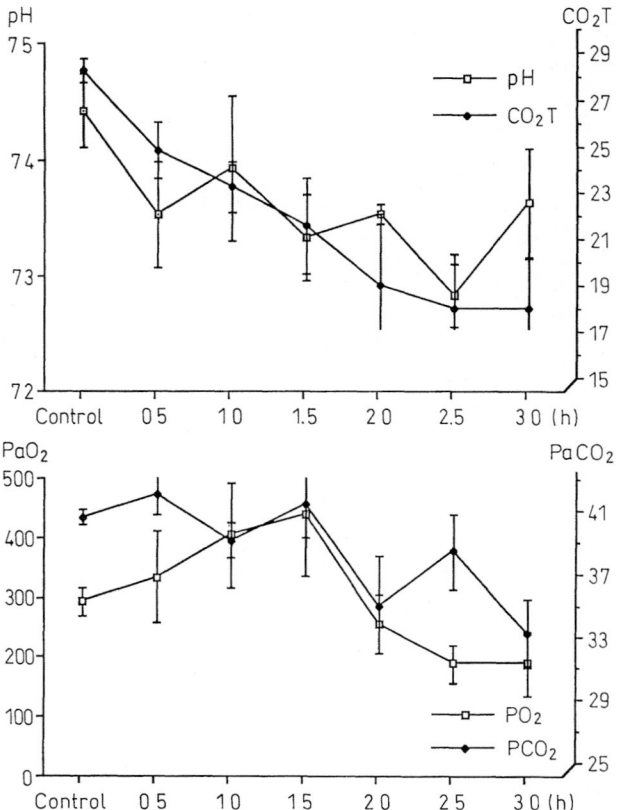

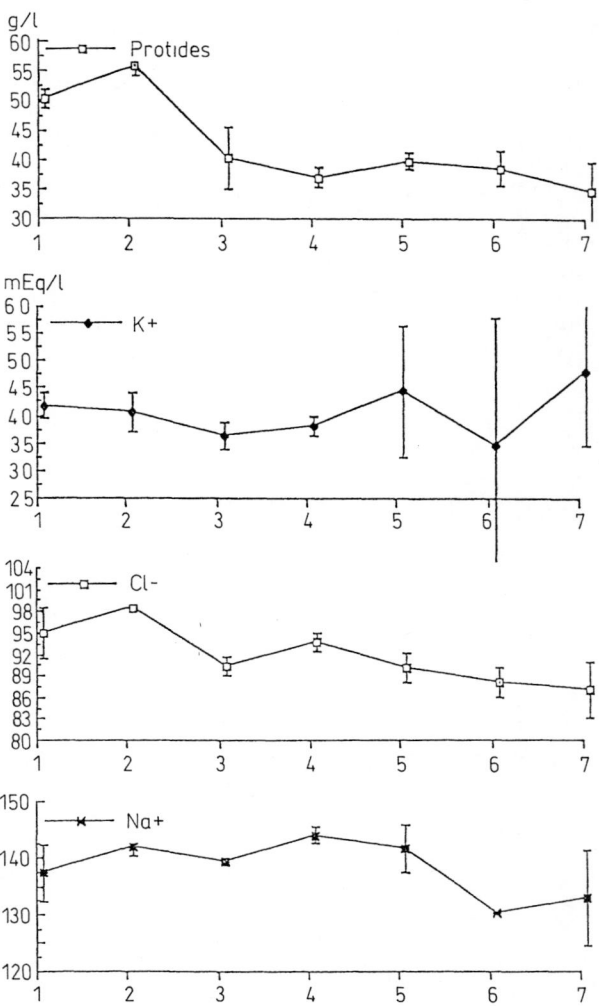

Fig. 5. Arterial blood gas, results. Average pH, CO2T, PaO2, PaCO2 during control conditions and reperfusion. (Experiment 3, 4, 5, and 6)

Fig. 6. Protides, K⁺, Cl⁻, Na⁺ plasmatic concentrations. *1,* Donor anesthesia; *2,* Receiver anesthesia; *3,* Beginning of ECC; *4,* Beginning of the reperfusion; *5,* 1 h of reperfusion; *6,* 2 h of reperfusion; *7,* 3 h of reperfusion

trical disposition of the surfaces separating the air from the liquid, bring about important modifications of the pulmonary mechanical properties in the form of reduced distensibility [10].

Pulmonary resistance increased in a regular manner during reperfusion. The period of ischaemia evidently had a deleterious effect on pulmonary resistance. Pulmonary resistance results from two forces: tissue friction and the resistance developed as air flows done the airways. As with compliance, the tissue component may be disturbed by the alteration of the interstitial geometry related to the oedema. The loss of bronchial vascularisation [2] and above all, the presence of interstitial oedema, predispose to increased airway resistance; in fact, the dynamic resistances of the respiratory pathways depend upon the calibre of these serial pathways. The calibre expresses not only the resting diameter of the structures concerned, their rigidity and their muscular tension, but also the transmural pressure which manifests itself on the wall lining [11].

Improvements in pulmonary characteristics following cardio-pulmonary transplantation appear after 10 h of reperfusion. This phenomenon is, therefore, most likely to be related to the reabsorption of the reperfusion oedema. The measurement of these constants in man, 7 weeks after cardio-pulmonary transplantation, shows a return to normal levels [14].

Acknowledgements. We are grateful to Dc C. Saunier, J. P. Gille and C. Duvivier for their suggestions. Technical assistance was provided

by J. Baumgarten, B. Wiedenkeller, C. Pierron, J. M. Horras and C. Jenot.

References

1. Coperland JG (1987) Heart Lung Transplantation: Current status. Ann Thorac Surg 43:2–3
2. Dawkins KD, Jamieson SW (1986) Pulmonary function of the transplanted human lung. Ann Rev Med 37:263–269
3. Edward P, Radford JR (1964) Static mechanical properties of mammalian lungs. Handbook of Physiology. American Physiological Society, Washington, D. C.
4. Feeley TW, Mihm FG, Dowing TP, Sadeghi AM, Baumgartner WA, Reitz BA, Shumway NE (1986) Hypothermic preservation of the heart and lungs with Collins solution: effect on respiratory function following heart-lung allotransplantation in dogs. Ann Thorac Surg 41:301–306
5. Frank NR, Radford EP, Wittenberger JL (1959) Static volume pressure interrelations of the lung and pulmonary blood vessels in excised cat's lung. J Appl Physiol 14:167–173
6. Jameison SW, Reitz BA, Oyer PE, Billingham E, Modry D, Baldwin JC, Stinsor EB, Hunt S, Theodore J, Bieber CP, Shumway NE (1983) Combined heart and lung transplantation. Lancet I:1130–1132
7. Konertz W, Saka B, Bernard A Orthotopic heart transplantation in pig after 24 hours hypothermic storage in eurocollins-solution. Dept Cardiovascular surgery university Kiel, West Germany. Tirés à part

8. Lazar HL, Painvin GA, Robert AJ (1986) Myocardial preservation. Surg Clin North Am 66:467–475
9. Morishita Y, Saigenji H, Higashi T, Umebayashi Y, Taira A, Goto M (1985) Function of the transplanted canine heart after prolonged preservation by simple immersion. Heart Vessels 1: 220–224
10. Petit JM Applications de la mécanique pulmonaire à l'exploration fonctionelle. L'exploration fonctionelle pulmonaire: technique d'étude et application clinique. Editions Médicales, Flamarion
11. Petit JM Aspects physiologiques de la mécanique thoracopulmonaire. L'exploration fonctionnelle pulmonaire: technique d'étude et application clinique. Editions Médiales, Flamarion
12. Reitz BA, Brody WR, Hickey PR, Michaleis LL Protection of the heart for 24 hours with intracellular (High K^+) solution and hypothermia. Surg Forum 149–51
13. Sharp JT, Griffith GT, Bunnel IL, Greene DG (1958) Ventilatory mechanics in pulmonary oedemas in man. J Chir Invest 37:111
14. Theodore J, Jamieson SW, Burke CM, Reitz BA, Stinson EB, Kessel A van, Dawkins KD, Herran JH, Oyer PE, Hunt SA, Shumway NE, Robin ED (1984) Physiologic aspects of human heart-lung transplantation. Pulmonary function status of the post-transplanted lung. Chest 86:349–357
15. Varene P, Vieilleford H, Saumon G, Lafosse JE (1974) Etalonnage de pneumotachographe par méthode intégrale. Bull Physiopathol Respir 10:349–360

Transplant Int (1992) 5 [Suppl 1]: S 357–S 361

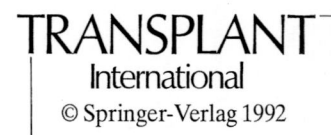

© Springer-Verlag 1992

Simplified microvascular suture techniques for rat liver transplantation as a microsurgical model with arterial blood supply

B. Dippe[1], **D. Kreisel**[1], **H. Petrowsky**[1], **O. Richter**[1], **S. Krueger**[2], **D. von Heimburg**[1], **M. Schneider**[2], **E. Hanisch**[1], **H. J. C. Wenisch**[1], **A. Encke**[1]

Departments of [1] General Surgery and [2] Pathology, University of Frankfurt Medical Center, Frankfurt/Main, Germany

Abstract. The methods for liver transplantation in the rat mainly used do not include reconstruction of the arterial blood supply to the liver. Furthermore, to ensure a short anhepatic phase these methods almost all entail specially developed cuff anastomoses in the recipient operation instead of the conventional microvascular suture technique. Thus an acceptable survival rate can be attained in the experimental animals. This detailed description of simplified microvascular suture techniques is intended to present an alternative to the cuff anastomoses used almost exclusively. In the donor operation with this method, the liver is dissected with an arterial pedicle including the abdominal segment of the aorta, and the liver is flushed in situ not only via the portal vein, but also via the hepatic artery. The organ is implanted in the recipient animal using simplified microvascular suture reconstruction of the arterial blood supply to the liver. Use of telescopic spectacles with 2-fold magnification has proven to be adequate for the entire procedure. With mastery of this method of rat liver transplantation, the average duration of the anhepatic phase is about 20 min, substantially below the 30-min limit which is critical for the survival of the experimental animals. The donor operation requires about 60 min, and the recipient operation 70 to 80 min. With this method, the spectrum of investigations on liver transplantation which are possible in the rat is substantially extended in that clinical conditions can be reproduced very much more exactly by combination of portal and arterial in-situ flushing in the donor operation and rearterialization of the transplant in the recipient operation, as compared to the transplanted rat liver being supplied only with portal venous blood.

Key words: Rat liver transplantation – Arterial reconstruction – Microvascular suture techniques

---

Offprint requests to: Dr. B. Dippe, Department of General Surgery, University of Frankfurt Medical Center, Theodor-Stern-Kai 7, D-6000 Frankfurt/Main 70, Germany

The necessity of keeping the anhepatic phase of the recipient operation in rat liver transplantation under 30 min led to the development of cuff techniques for anastomosis of vessels. Since rearterialization of the transplant is not crucial for survival of the rat, most experimental models for rat liver transplantation do not provide for a reconstruction of the arterial blood supply to the liver [1, 5, 6, 8–12].

The present paper describes in detail our method for orthotopic rat liver transplantation, which adheres to the principles of microvascular suture techniques for vascular anastomoses. For reconstructing the arterial blood supply of the transplant, it is necessary, during the donor operation, to prepare the liver with an arterial pedicle which includes the abdominal segment of the aorta. Furthermore, in situ perfusion is performed not only via the portal vein, but also via the hepatic artery. The organ is implanted in the recipient using simplified and thus rapidly executed microvascular suture techniques for all vascular anastomoses.

This method including portal and arterial in-situ flushing in the donor and rearterialization of the transplant in the recipient can be employed for a broad spectrum of investigations on liver transplantation, since clinical conditions are reproduced with greater accuracy in comparison to other methods.

Materials and methods

The halogenated methyl-ethyl ether enflurane is used as the anesthetic agent, which is especially indicated for liver surgery. A pediatric Satinsky clamp, which is suitable for the suprahepatic vena cava, is an integral part of the microsurgical instruments. Small mosquito clamps are applied for the portal vein and infrahepatic vena cava, while microvascular clips are apt for the aorta. Ligatures are performed with 5–0 silk and vessels are sutured with 7–0 or 8–0 monofilament material.

Donor operation

The preparatory steps of hepatectomy in the donor have been extensively described [1, 2, 5–8, 12]; therefore, only essential modifications

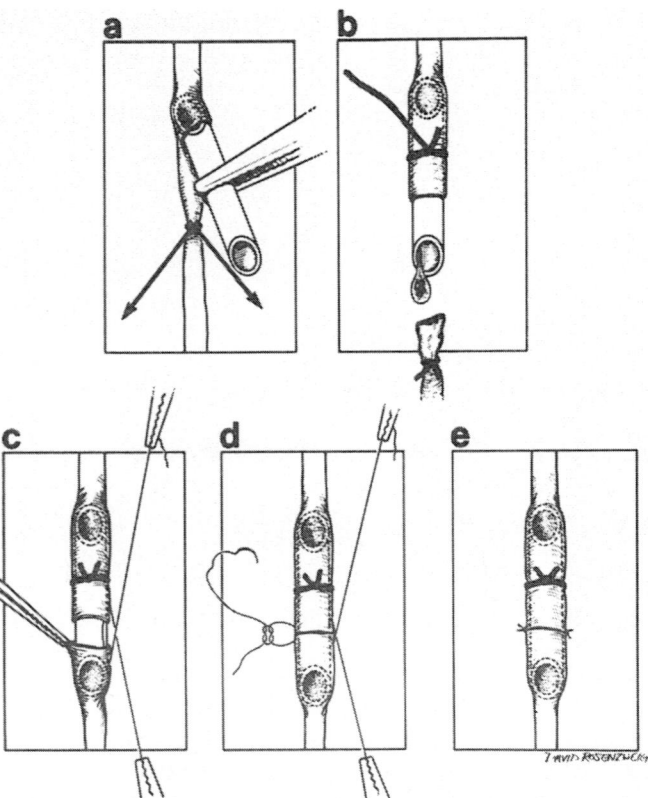

Fig. 1a–e. Reconstruction of the bile duct. **a,b** Introduction and fixation of a splint in the donor operation. **c–e** Choledocho-choledo-chostomy with splint technique and additional suturing in the recipient operation, with use of traction sutures

are reported. The liver is prepared with an arterial pedicle which includes the abdominal aorta. All branches of the aorta between the diaphragm and the bifurcation into the common iliac arteries are ligated and cut, while the celiac trunk is preserved. Additionally, the hepatic artery is isolated in its course to the hilus after the splenic artery and the left gastric artery have been ligated and dissected.

An angiocatheter, (about 8 mm long, beveled at both ends) is introduced with over two thirds of its length in the lumen at a distance from the liver and fixed with one ligature, followed by the complete separation of the duct (Figure 1a, b).

Antecedent to the beginning of in-situ perfusion of the liver two mosquito clamps are applied to the infrahepatic vena cava above the right renal vein. Division of the infrahepatic vena cava is followed by clamping of the portal vein at the junction of the splenic vein. Flushing begins with the introduction of the perfusion catheter (14-gauge angiocatheter) into the transversely incised portal vein. The perfusion pressure equals the physiologic pressure in the portal vein of the rat [1]. For simultaneous arterial perfusion, 2 to 3 ml of the perfusate are injected into the caudal end of the aorta.

Application of two traction sutures (7–0) for the later anastomosis of the suprahepatic vena cava during the recipient operation represents the last step of the donor operation; these sutures are fixed to the vessel wall with a surgical knot (Figure 2a). The liver is removed at the clamp on the intrahepatic vena cava and is placed in the preservation bath without removing this clamp.

Recipient operation

After the steps preparing for the removal of the recipient's liver, which are basically analogous to the procedure for donor hepatectomy [1, 2, 5, 8–12] the anhepatic phase begins when the infrahepatic vena cava is clamped at the junction of the right renal vein and the portal vein at the

junction of the splenic vein (with mosquito clamps from the right side of the rat); and finally, the pediatric Satinsky clamp is applied to the suprahepatic vena cava. A diaphragm cuff is included in the clamp. Removal of the liver begins with the circular excision of the suprahepatic vena cava at its entry to the liver. Next, the portal vein is cut at the bifurcation into its two main branches, followed by the dissection of the infrahepatic vena cava at its juncture with the liver. After the liver has been removed and before the transplant is introduced, the dissection board is rotated through 180°. The donor organ is placed in the anatomically correct position by means of the clamp on the infrahepatic vena cava.

Anastomosis of the suprahepatic vena cava (running suture with 7–0, Figure 2b–f). With traction sutures already having been applied to the transplant at the end of the donor operation, it is considerably easier to approximate the suprahepatic stumps of the vena cava by placing two corner sutures. We begin to perform the running suture with the thread of one of the corner sutures, from the inside of the posterior wall. As in the venous anastomoses that follow, there is no need for also sewing the suture from the outside to the inside. At the opposite corner this suture is brought to the outside of the recipient vena cava. Without tying a knot with the opposite corner suture, we continue the running suture on the anterior wall, applying a single interlocking stitch which maintains tension on the posterior wall until the anterior line is completed. For the elimination of air bubbles, the vessel lumen is flushed before completing the anastomosis.

Anastomosis of the portal vein (running suture with 8–0, Figure 3) and reperfusion of the transplant. The dissection board is rotated back into its original position. The corner sutures for the anastomosis of the

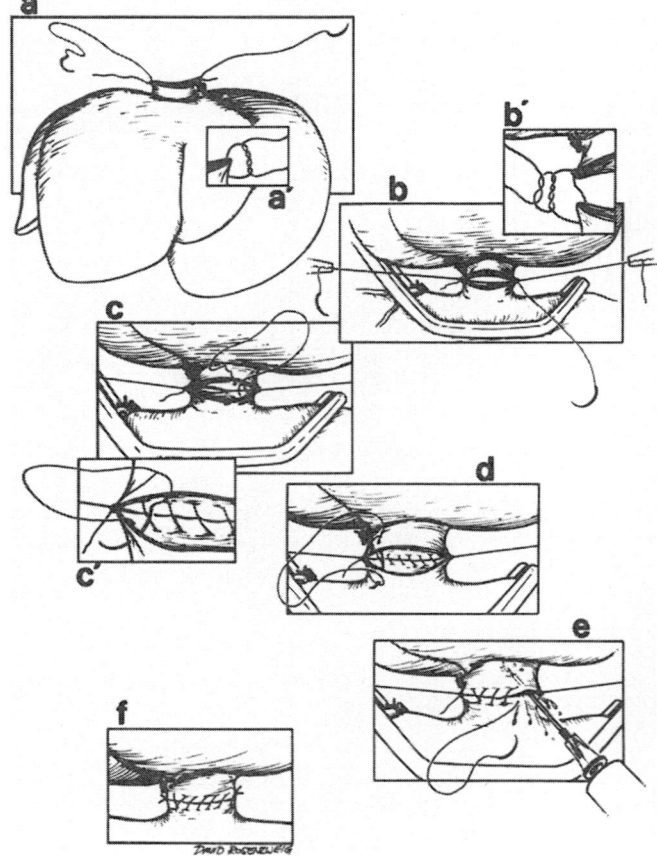

Fig. 2a–f. Anastomosis of the suprahepatic vena cava. **a** Application and tying of traction sutures at the end of the donor operation. **b** Application of corner sutures. **c** Suture of posterior wall from inside. **d** Interlocking stitch at start of suturing of anterior wall. **e** Flushing of lumen of the anastomosis. **f** Completed anastomosis

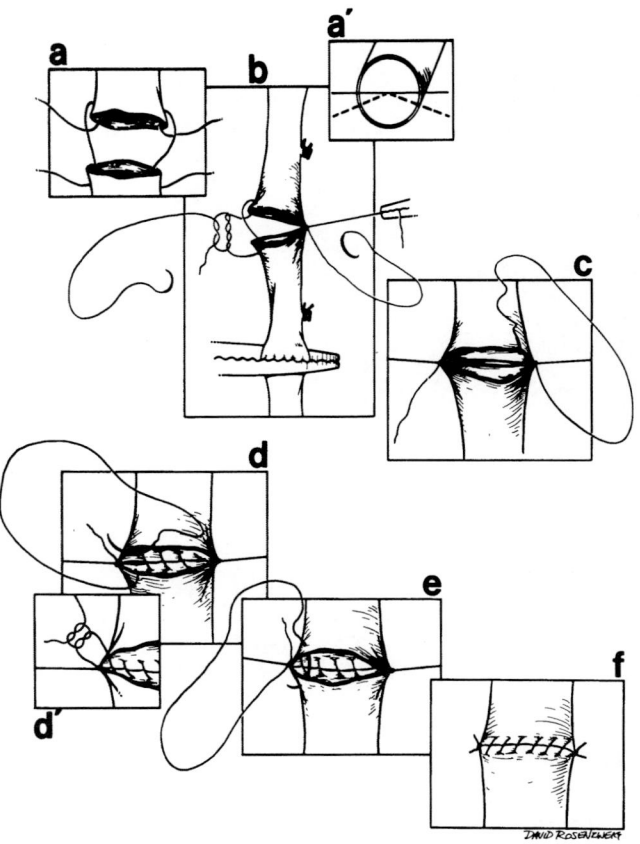

Fig. 3 a–f. Anastomosis of the portal vein. **a, b** Application of corner sutures. **c, d** Suture of posterior wall from inside. **e** Suture of anterior wall. **f** Completed anastomosis

portal vein are placed at about 120° and thus the anterior wall is flaccid, while the posterior one is stretched. It is advisable to place the corner stitches on both stumps from the inside toward the outside. Due to an indistinct view of the collapsed venous tissue, this procedure not only proves to be time-saving, but also makes it possible to locate the opposite corners with greater accurary, without affecting adversely the quality of the anastomosis. The ligated junction of the gastroduodenal vein which is located on the left side of both recipient and donor vessels serves as an orientation and helps to avoid any

twisting. Three to four stitches are performed on the posterior wall from the inside with the thread of one of the corner sutures (Fig. 4); this suture is then brought to the outside and tied to the short end of the second corner suture, and then continues to be used for suturing the anterior wall (Fig. 4). Immediately after the completion of the anastomosis of the portal vein, the anhepatic phase ends with removal of the clamps from the portal vein and suprahepatic vena cava.

Anastomosis of the infrahepatic vena cava (running suture with 8–0). The infrahepatic vena cava is sutured, after the two clamps have been placed in parallel, with a technique analogous to the anastomosis described for the portal vein (Fig. 5). However, in contrast to the portal anastomosis the corner stitches should be applied in the conventional way; i.e., the end of the vein on the transplant should be sutured from the outside to the inside, and the recipient end, from the inside to the outside.

Anastomosis of the infrarenal aorta of the recipient and of the arterial pedicle of the transplant (side-to-end, running suture with 8–0). Following isolation, clamping and longitudinal incision of the aortal segment lying directly caudal to the ventrally crossing left renal vein, a side-to-end anastomosis with the arterial pedicle of the transplant is performed. For the aortotomy, application of corner sutures, and suturing of the left lateral wall, it is required to place the dissection board sideways, with the head of the rat near the right hand of the operator; for suturing of the right lateral wall, it is turned in the opposite direction (with the head of the rat on the left).

Choledocho-choledochostomy (with use of a splint, two single button sutures with 8–0, Fig. 1 c–e). After the ligature on the bile duct of the recipient has been cut, a traction suture on the left side of both stumps is applied to approximate them. While introducing the free end of the splint into the recipient's duct, simultaneously applied tension to the left corner suture prevents the separation of the stumps, so that the right corner suture can be placed and tied. By tying the left corner suture the choledocho-choledochostomy is completed. The recipient operation is concluded with flushing the abdominal cavity and closing the abdominal wall.

Results

With increasing practice, our most recent perioperative mortality was 12,9% (this figure applied to the most recent 186 transplantations). With mastery of this method of rat liver transplantation, the average duration of the an-

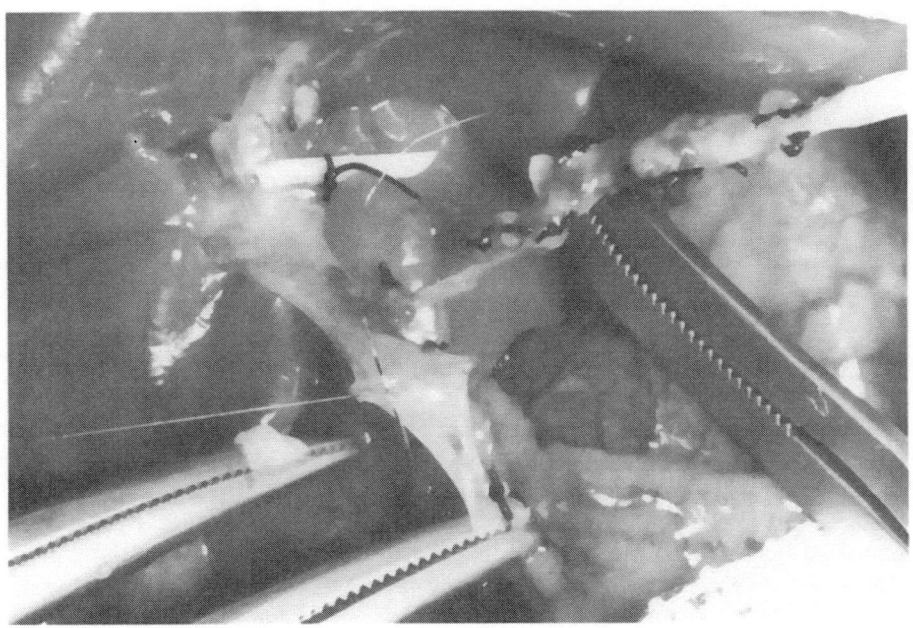

Fig. 4. Anastomosis of the portal vein. Completed suture of posterior wall, first stitch on the anterior wall. On the *right* in the figure, arterial pedicle, which includes the abdominal segment of the donor aorta, for arterial reattachment of the transplant

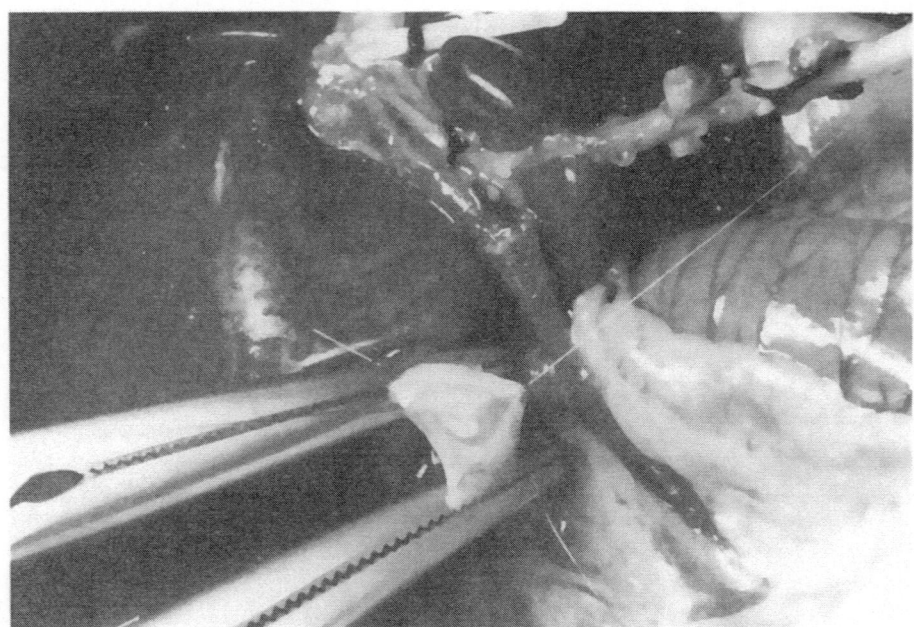

Fig. 5. Anastomosis of the infrahepatic vena cava. On the *right* in the figure, reperfused transplant with completed anastomosis of portal vein

hepatic phase is about 20 min, and thus substantially below the 30-min limit which is critical for the survival of the experimental animals [2, 5]. The donor operation requires about 60 min, and the recipient operation, between 70 and 80 min. Since rearterialization of the liver is not essential for survival of the animals, the technique described here can be applied alternatively without restoring the arterial blood supply; in this case particularly the donor operation is shortened considerably.

Discussion

This technique of orthotopic rat liver transplantation represents a further development of the technique described by Lee et al. [7, 8] and is based on the principle of microsurgical suturing for vascular anastomoses. The following technical details, which simplify the procedure, are the basis for a short anhepatic phase during the recipient operation:

1. The donor operation is finished with the application of traction sutures for anastomosis of the suprahepatic vena cava. By keeping the clamp on the infrahepatic vena cava in place ex-situ, the manipulation of the transplant during the anatomically correct insertion into the recipient site, is simplified.
2. In all vessel anastomoses, the circular suture is applied with only one of the corner sutures. For all venous anastomoses, the posterior wall is sewn from the inside; the corner suture used does not need to be brought from the outside to the inside in addition when the running suture is begun. An apparently more cumbersome and time-consuming alternative is the reconstruction of the portal vein with suturing of the anterior wall, subsequent rotation of the anastomosis, and suturing of the posterior wall from the outside [1, 12].

3. The corner sutures in the anastomosis of the portal vein are sewn from the inside to the outside on both ends, contrary to the conventional procedure. Taking the collapse of the venous tissue into consideration, which interferes with visibility, this procedure not only saves time, but also makes it possible to locate the corners more precisely without affecting adversely the quality of the anastomosis.

Choledocho-choledochostomy with the aid of a splint was originated by Zimmermann et al. [12]. The traction-suture technique is a useful addition, because it prevents the recipient bile duct from sliding back from the splint.

Postoperative morbidity and mortality after liver transplantation in the rat, to the extent that they are caused by the operative procedure, are due mainly to complications in the bile duct; since the hepatic artery represents the only arterial blood supply for the bile duct, rearterialization of the transplant lowers considerably the rate of bile duct complications [2–4].

Furthermore, the conditions of clinical transplantation are reproduced more accurately with the combination of portal and arterial perfusion in situ during the donor operation, and with the arterial reconstruction during the recipient operation, than is the case when the transplant is supplied only via the portal vein. Elimination of rejection phenomena by means of a syngeneic donor-recipient combination renders rat transplantation models especially valuable for experimental investigations on organ ischemia, reperfusion and preservation. However, restoration of a physiological blood supply appears to be an essential prerequisite for such investigations on a rat model for orthotopic liver transplantation. A cuff anastomosis proposed by Hasuike et al. [3] for rearterialization of the transplanted rat liver involving a right nephrectomy of the recipient introduces further stress and anatomic variation in the experimental animals.

By providing a detailed description of simplified microvascular suture techniques, an alternative to the almost exclusively used cuff anastomoses is presented. Although the cuff methods can be learned somewhat more quickly, the disadvantages outweigh the advantages from our point of view. Cuff anastomoses differ from the clinical procedure, require relatively long vessel stumps, can be used only for end-to-end attachments, and necessitate additional ex-situ preparation of the vessel ends of the donor organ. It would appear that the cuff technique [10, 11] is more demanding and more subject to complications than is the suture technique especially for anastomosis of the suprahepatic vena cava.

In conclusion, physiologic conditions for the graft are restored extensively with the technique described. Furthermore, high survival rates can be attained. We consider this model to be appropriate for most studies involving liver grafting in the rat.

References

1. Castaing D, Houssin D, Bismuth H (1980) Hepatic and Portal Surgery in the Rat. Masson, Paris–New York
2. Engemann R (1985) Technique for orthotopic rat liver transplantation. In: Thiede A, Deltz E, Engemann R, Hamelmann H (eds) Microsurgical models in rats for transplantation research. Springer, Berlin Heidelberg, pp 69–75
3. Hasuike Y, Monden M, Valdivia LA, Kubota N, Gotoh M, Nakano Y, Okamura J, Mori T (1988) A simple method for orthotopic liver transplantation with arterial reconstruction in rats. Transplantation 45: 830–832
4. Howden B, Jablinski P, Grossman H, Marshall VC (1989) The importance of the hepatic artery in rat liver transplantation. Transplantation 47: 428–431
5. Kamada N, Calne RY (1979) Orthotopic liver transplantation in the rat; technique using cuff for portal vein anastomosis and biliary drainage. Transplantation 28: 47–50
6. Kamada N (1987) Technique in the rat. In: Calne RY (ed) Liver Transplantation. Grune and Stratton, London, pp 25–34
7. Lee S, Charters AC, Chandler JG, Orloff MJ (1973) A technique for orthotopic liver transplantation in the rat. Transplantation 16: 664–669
8. Lee S, Charters AC, Orloff MJ (1975) Simplified technic for orthotopic liver transplantation in the rat. Am J Surg 130: 38–40
9. Marni A, Ferrero ME (1988) A four-technique comparative study of orthotopic liver transplantation in the rat. Am J Surg 156: 209–213
10. Miyata M, Fischer JH, Fuhs M, Isselhard W, Kasai Y (1980) A simple method for orthotopic liver transplantation in the rat; cuff technique for three vascular anastomoses. Transplantation 30: 335–338
11. Tsuchimoto S, Kusumoto K, Nakajima Y, Kakita A, Uchino J, Natori T, Aizawa M (1988) Orthotopic liver transplantation in the rat; a simplified technique using the cuff method for suprahepatic vena cava anastomosis. Transplantation 45: 1153–1155
12. Zimmermann FA, Butcher GW, Davies HS, Brons G, Kamada N, Tuerel O (1979) Techniques for orthotopic liver transplantation in the rat and some studies of the immunologic responses to fully allogeneic liver grafts. Transplant Proc 11: 571–577

Transplant Int (1992) 5 [Suppl 1]: S 362–S 365

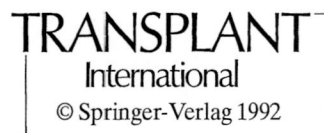

TRANSPLANT
International
© Springer-Verlag 1992

The second generation of Carolina Rinse, solution II, improves graft survival following orthotopic liver transplantation in the rat by preventing reperfusion injury

W. Gao[1], J. J. Lemasters[2], and R. G. Thurman[1]

[1] Laboratory of Hepatobiology and Toxicology, Department of Pharmacology, [2] Laboratories of Cell Biology, Department of Cell Biology & Anatomy, The University of North Carolina at Chapel Hill, Chapel Hill, USA

Abstract. Carolina Rinse solution was designed to minimize reperfusion injury following orthotopic liver transplantation. Carolina Rinse blocks reperfusion-induced endothelial cell killing, diminishes postoperative enzyme release and improves survival dramatically. Adenosine and mildly acidotic pH were identified as key components. Here we report results with a simplified formulation, Carolina Rinse II, which contains extracellular inorganic ions similar to Ringer's solution, adenosine, as well as antioxidants and radical scavengers (allopurinol, glutathione and desferrioxamine). In this study, 44 rat livers were explanted and stored for 12 h in University of Wisconsin (UW) cold storage solution (non-survival conditions). Control livers were rinsed with 15 ml cold Ringer's solution just prior to completion of implantation surgery. In this control group, average 30-day survival was poor (8%). However, survival was increased to around 60% when grafts were rinsed with Carolina Rinse II. Survival was not improved significantly by rinsing the graft with Ringer's solution containing antioxidants and radical scavengers with adenosine omitted (about 30%). Peak SGOT values of nearly 3000 U/l, measured 1–3 days postoperatively in the Ringer's rinse control group, were decreased 4- to 5-fold both by Carolina Rinse II and by Ringer's solution containing antioxidants. On the other hand, the addition of adenosine to Ringer's solution improved survival (around 60%) but did not decrease the postoperative elevation of serum enzymes significantly. Thus, it appears that adenosine was necessary for optimal survival whereas antioxidants and radical scavengers were needed to prevent injury to the transplanted graft. These data were consistent with the hypothesis that at least two mechanisms, one involving the liver and a second one non-hepatic, are responsible for post-transplant pathophysiology. Carolina Rinse II also reduced the postoperative elevation in serum enzymes 2- to 3-fold in livers stored under survival conditions (e. g., for 8 h in UW solution). This study demonstrated convincingly that a very simple rinse solution, Carolina Rinse II, improved survival significantly and minimized graft injury following orthotopic liver transplantation.

Key words: Carolina Rinse II – Orthotopic liver transplantation – Graft survival – Reperfusion injury

It has been demonstrated previously that an oxygen-dependent reperfusion injury occurs in the rat model of orthotopic liver transplantation [21]. Nonparenchymal cell injury characterized by loss of viability of sinusoidal endothelial cells and activation of Kupffer cells occurrs following cold storage and reperfusion which precede graft failure [5–7, 9, 18, 19]. Accordingly, a new rinse solution, Carolina Rinse, was developed to minimize reperfusion injury following cold storage [9, 12, 13]. Carolina Rinse, which is mildly acidic [8, 14], contains extracellular inorganic ions at concentrations similar to blood; a calcium channel blocker to inhibit Kupffer cell activation [20]; and antioxidants and radical scavengers (allopurinol, glutathione and desferrioxamine) to minimize O_2 radical formation. Carolina Rinse also contains adenosine to improve the microcirculation [10] and fructose to supply energy under hypoxic conditions [1]. Indeed, by rinsing liver grafts with Carolina Rinse, postoperative enzyme release is minimized and survival is improved dramatically following orthotopic liver transplantation in models with and without rearterialization [2, 12, 13]. However, in the non-rearterialized model the efficacy of Carolina Rinse is lost when adenosine is omitted [11]. The importance of adenosine is further emphasized when donor livers are rinsed simply with Ringer's solution containing adenosine. Under these conditions, average survival time is improved as effectively as with Carolina Rinse [4]. Importantly, while adenosine is as effective as Carolina Rinse at improving survival, it does not prevent liver injury. Thus, we reasoned that a simple combination of adenosine with

Offprint requests to: Ronald G. Thurman, Lab. of Hepatobiology and Toxicology, Department of Pharmacology, CB # 7365, FLOB, The University of North Carolina, Chapel Hill, NC 27599-7365, USA

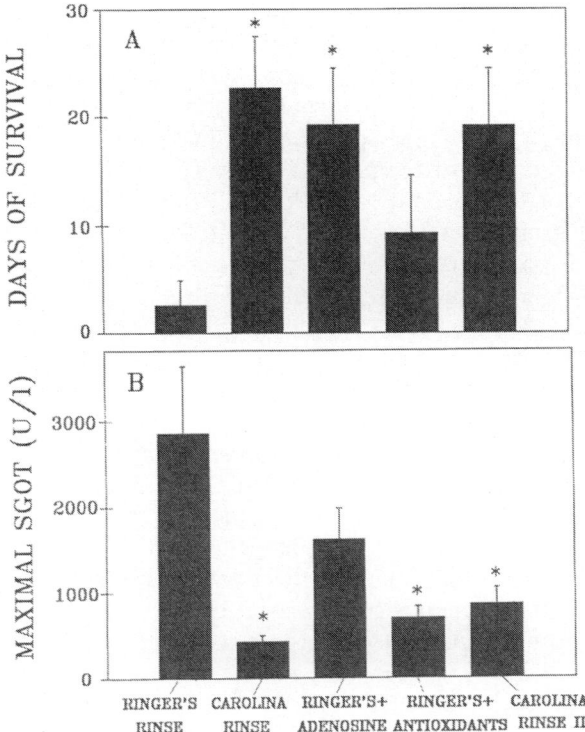

Fig. 1 A, B. Effect of Carolina Rinse II on postoperative survival. **A** Livers were rinsed and stored in UW cold storage solution at 0–4 °C for 12 h (non-survival conditions). After storage, livers were rinsed with 15 ml of either cold Ringer's solution, Carolina Rinse, Ringer's with antioxidants and radical scavengers (1.0 mM allopurinol, 1.0 mM desferrioxamine, 3.0 mM glutathione), Ringer's with 0.1 mM adenosine, or Carolina Rinse II (see Table 1). Graft survival was assumed to be permanent when rats were alive 30 days postoperatively. *P < 0.05 for comparison with Ringer's rinse group. n = 7–13 per group. **B** Blood samples were collected postoperatively via the tail vein of recipient rats at 2 day intervals during the first week and at weekly intervals thereafter. SGOT activity was measured as described in Methods. Data represent maximal values observed 1–3 days postoperatively. *P < 0.05 compared to Ringer's rinse group. n = 4–6 per group

antioxidants and radical scavengers might both improve survival and minimize postoperative hepatic injury. Therefore, this study was designed to determine the effect of Carolina Rinse II, a simple solution developed to meet these criteria, on graft injury and survival following orthotopic liver transplantation in the rat.

Methods

Transplantation. Liver transplantations were performed under ether anesthesia using a technique described by Zimmermann [22] and Kamada [17]. Syngenic female Lewis rats (175–200 g) were used to eliminate immunologic interference. Briefly, livers were removed and cuffs were placed on the portal vein and subhepatic vena cava of donor livers. Grafts were stored at 0–4 °C for 12 h in University of Wisconsin (UW) solution and were rinsed either with 15 ml of Ringer's solution, Ringer's solution containing adenosine (0.1 mM) or antioxidants, Carolina Rinse, or Carolina Rinse II. Subsequently, livers were implanted by connecting the suprahepatic vena cava with a running suture, inserting cuffs into appropriate vessels, and anastomosing the bile duct with an intraluminal splint. The explantation required less than 6 min, and the ischemic interval due to clamping the

portal vein during the implantation procedure did not exceed 15 min. Surviving animals were sacrificed after 30 days for histology.

Serum enzymes. Following transplantation, blood samples were drawn from the tail vein at 2-day intervals during the first 7 days and at weekly intervals thereafter. Sera were separated by centrifugation and kept at −20 °C for subsequent enzyme measurements. Serum glutamic oxaloacetic transaminase (SGOT) was assayed by standard enzymatic procedures [3].

Histology. Livers were fixed 24 h postoperatively with 1 % paraformaldehyde in Krebs-Henseleit buffer and processed for histology. Sections were stained with hematoxalin and eosin. Liver damage was scored using a scale of 0–5 based on the degree of necrosis and 0–2 based on six structural parameters: cellular swelling, acidophilic nuclear inclusions, nuclear pyknosis, cellular deposition, cytoplasmic vacuolization, and sinusoidal dilatation (maximal score = 17). The degree of damage to the lung was expressed as a percentage of the microscopic area exhibiting infiltration of inflammatory cells.

Results

Composition of Carolina Rinse and Carolina Rinse II. Carolina Rinse II contains adenosine to improve survival and antioxidants to prevent liver injury (Table 1). The original Carolina Rinse formulation contains modified hydroxyethyl starch (pentastarch) for oncotic support against interstitial edema, antioxidants and radical scavengers, as well as extracellular inorganic ions at concentrations similar to those found in blood and Ringer's solution. Carolina Rinse also contains fructose and glucose plus insulin to diminish hypoxic injury and a dihydropyridine-type calcium channel blocker. Further, Carolina Rinse is mildly acidotic because small decreases in pH have been shown to reduce hypoxic injury to hepatocytes [8]. In contrast, Carolina Rinse II is a simple solution which only contains extracellular inorganic ions similar to Ringer's solution, adenosine, antioxidants and radical scavengers (Table 1). Like the original formulation, Carolina Rinse II is acidotic.

Effects of Carolina Rinse II on graft function and survival. After 12 h cold storage in UW solution (non-survival conditions), livers were rinsed with Ringer's solution, Carolina Rinse, Ringer's containing adenosine, Ringer's with antioxidants, or Carolina Rinse II. In the Ringer's rinse group, average survival was only 8 % (Fig. 1). Similar results were obtained when grafts were rinsed with Ringer's containing antioxidants or with Carolina Rinse with adenosine deleted (data not shown). In contrast, Carolina Rinse, Ringer's containing adenosine, and Carolina Rinse II increased survival dramatically to 60–75 %. Peak SGOT levels reached values around 3000 U/l in the Ringer's rinse group 24 h following implantation surgery. Surprisingly, values were also very high in the Ringer's containing adenosine group. In the Carolina Rinse group, however, the peak SGOT was only around 800 U/l. Similar results were obtained with Ringer's solution containing antioxidants and with Carolina Rinse II. Histological evaluation showed that damage to the liver and lung was also decreased 2- to 3-fold by Carolina Rinse II (Table 2). Furthermore, in livers stored under more relevant clinical conditions of survival (8 h in UW), Carolina Rinse II re-

Table 1. Composition of Carolina Rinse and Carolina Rinse II

Component	Carolina Rinse	Carolina Rinse II
NaCl	115.0 mM	102.7 mM
KCl	5.0 mM	4.0 mM
CaCl$_2$	1.3 mM	1.8 mM
KH$_2$PO$_4$	1.0 mM	–
MgSO$_4$	1.2 mM	–
Sodium Lactate	–	27.4 mM
Allopurinol	1.0 mM	1.0 mM
Desferrioxamine	1.0 mM	1.0 mM
Glutathione	3.0 mM	3.0 mM
Nicardipine	2.0 µM	–
Adenosine	1.0 µM	0.1 mM
Fructose	10.0 mM	–
Glucose	10.0 mM	–
Hydroxyethyl Starch	50.0 g/l	–
Insulin	100.0 U/l	–
MOPS	20.0 mM	–
pH	6.5	< 6.5
mosmd/l	290–305	273

Table 2. Effect of Carolina Rinse II on index of liver and lung damage. Livers were transplanted as described in Methods following 12 h (non-survival conditions) cold storage in UW solution. Rats were sacrificed 24 h postoperatively for histology. The index of liver and lung damage was scored as described in Methods. Mean ± S.E.M. for 4 livers and lungs in each group

Group	Liver damage score	Lung damage %
Ringer's Rinse	9.5 ± 0.7	72.5 ± 4.8*
Carolina Rinse II	6.9 ± 0.5*	52.0 ± 6.2*

* $P < 0.05$ for comparison with Ringer's rinse group

Table 3. Rationale for Carolina Rinse II

Addition	Hepatic mechanism (SGOT)	Extra-hepatic mechanism (Survival)
Adenosine	–	+
Antioxidants, radical scavengers	+	–
Carolina Rinse II (adenosine + antioxidants and radical scavengers)	+	+

Effective as rinse at improving (+) or not improving (–) the parameter being evaluated. All additions except Carolina Rinse II were in Ringer's solution

duced postoperative SGOT release 2- to 3-fold compared with Ringer's rinse (1255 vs 464 U/l).

Discussion

The development of UW cold storage solution extended the time of liver graft preservation for up to 30 h [16]. Primary nonfunction of livers stored in UW solution still occurs in about 15 % of liver transplant patients [15]. The effects of the rinse solution on graft injury were not studied until recently and may be very important. Following cold storage, Ringer's solution is used by most transplant treams to remove potassium contained in the UW solu-

tion; however, rinsing with Ringer's solution, even for short periods of time, can cause graft edema [13]. Since an oxygen-dependent reperfusion injury occurs in the rat model of orthotopic liver transplantation [21], rinsing with well-designed solutions could reduce reperfusion injury. Accordingly, a new rinse soution, Carolina Rinse, was designed to minimize reperfusion injury following orthotopic liver transplantation. Indeed, Carolina Rinse improved graft survival from 4 % to 56 % and reduced maximal postoperative SGOT release 3-fold compared with Ringer's solution. Carolina Rinse also diminished postoperative sinusoidal endothelial cell damage assessed by electron microscopy [13]. Thus, Carolina Rinse is a superior alternative to Ringer's solution in vivo, protecting liver grafts from reperfusion injury.

Interestingly, removal of the calcium channel blocker or elevating the pH did not diminish the efficacy of Carolina Rinse in the non-arterialized model; however, when adenosine was omitted, Carolina Rinse no longer improved survival [10]. Further, rinsing with Ringer's containing 0.1 mM adenosine was as effective as Carolina Rinse at improving postoperative survival although postoperative SGOT values were not reduced significantly and the endothelium was ragged (Table 3). On the other hand, survival was not improved significantly by Ringer's containing antioxidants alone, yet postoperative SGOT values were decreased 4- to 5-fold. These results indicated that adenosine is an essential component of Carolina Rinse and is needed to improve survival (i. e., the extrahepatic mechanism), and that oxygen radicals may be involved in a second mechanism (i. e., the hepatic mechanism) responsible for graft injury. On reperfusion, antioxidants and radical scavengers are necessary to minimize reperfusion injury to the liver. Indeed, Carolina Rinse II, designed with these criteria in mind, improved graft survival from 8 % to around 60 % and reduced postoperative SGOT values nearly 3-fold compared with the control Ringer's rinse group. Since Carolina Rinse II is a simple solution composed of inexpensive ingredients, it represents a practical way to reduce postoperative reperfusion injury following live transplantation.

Acknowledgement. This work was supported, in part, by NIH grant DK-37034.

References

1. Anundi I, King J, Owen DA, Schneider H, Lemasters JJ, Thurman RG (1987) Fructose prevents hypoxic cell death in liver. Am J Physiol 253: G390–G396
2. Bachmann S, Oleksy I, Thurman RG, Lemasters JJ (1991) Improved graft survival using warm Carolina Rinse solution after orthotopic rat liver transplantation with rearterlization. Gastroenterology (In Press)
3. Bergmeyer HU (1988) Methods of Enzymatic Analysis. Academic Press, New York
4. Bird RP, Droper HH (1984) Comparative studies on different methods of malonaldehyde determination. Methods Enzymol 105: 299–305
5. Caldwell-Kenkel JC, Currin RT, Tanaka Y, Thurman RG, Lemasters JJ (1989) Reperfusion injury to endothelial cells following cold ischemic storage of rat liver. Hepatology 10: 292–299
6. Caldwell-Kenkel JC, Currin RT, Tanaka Y, Thurman RG, Lemasters JJ (1991) Kupffer cell activation and endothelial cell

damage after storage of rat livers: Effects of reperfusion. Hepatology 13: 83–95

7. Caldwell-Kenkel JC, Thurman RG, Lemasters JJ (1988) Selective loss of nonparenchymal cell viability after cold ischemic storage of rat livers. Transplantation 45: 834–837

8. Currin RC, Gores GJ, Thurman RG, Lemasters JJ (1989) Protection by acidotic pH against anoxic injury in perfused rat liver. FASEB J 3: A626

9. Currin RT, Toole JG, Thurman RG, Lemasters JJ (1990) Evidence that Carolina Rinse solution protects sinusoidal endothelial cells against reperfusion injury after cold ischemic storage of rat liver. Transplantation 50: 1076–1078

10. Gao W, Caldwell-Kenkel JC, Lemasters JJ, Thurman RG (1990) Adenosine rinse reduces graft failure after orthotopic liver transplantation in the rat. Hepatology 12: 839

11. Gao W, Hijioka T, Lindert KA, Caldwell-Kenkel JC, Lemasters JJ, Thurman RG (1991) Adenosine is a key component in Carolina Rinse responsible for reducing graft failure after orthotopic liver transplantation in the rat. Transplantation (In Press)

12. Gao W, Takei Y, Marzi I, Currin RT, Lemasters JJ, Thurman RG (1991) Carolina Rinse solution increases survival time dramatically after orthotopic liver transplantation in the rat. Transplant Proc 23: 648–650

13. Gao W, Takei Y, Marzi I, Lindert KA, Caldwell-Kenkel JC, Currin RT, Tanaka Y, Lemasters JJ, Thurman RG (1991) Carolina Rinse solution: A new strategy to increase survival time after orthotopic liver transplantation in the rat. Transplantation (In Press)

14. Gores GJ, Nieminen A-L, Fleishmann KE, Dawson TL, Hermann B, Lemasters JJ (1988) Extracellular acidosis delays onset of cell death in ATP-depleted hepatocytes. Am J Physiol 255: C315–C322

15. Greig PD, Woolf GM, Sinclair SB, Abecassis M, Strasberg SM, Taylor BR, Blendis LM, Superina RA, Glynn MFX, Langer B, Levy GA (1989) Treatment of primary liver graft nonfunction with prostaglandin E_1. Transplantation 48: 447–453

16. Jamieson NV, Sundberg R, Lindell S, Laravuso R, Kalayogu M, Southard JH, Belzer FO (1988) Successful 24- to 30-hour preservation of the canine liver: a preliminary report. Transplant Proc 20: 945–947

17. Kamada N, Calne RY (1979) Orthotopic liver transplantation in the rat. Technique using cuff for portal vein anastomosis and biliary drainage. Transplantation 28: 47–50

18. Lemasters JJ, Caldwell-Kenkel JC, Currin RT, Tanaka Y, Marzi I, Thurman RG (1989) Endothelial cell killing and activation of Kupffer cells following reperfusion of rat liver stored in Euro-Collins solution. In: Wisse E, Knook DL, Decker K (eds) Cells of the Hepatic Sinusoid II. The Kupffer Cell Fndn., Rijswijk, The Netherlands, pp 277–280

19. Takei Y, Marzi I, Kauffman FC, Cowper KB, Lemasters JJ, Thurman RG (1990) Prevention of early graft failure by the calcium channel blocker nisoldipine: Involvement of Kupffer cells. Transplant Proc 22: 2202–2203

20. Takei Y, Marzi I, Kauffman FC, Currin RT, Lemasters JJ, Thurman RG (1990) Increase in survival time of liver transplants by protease inhibitors and a calcium channel blocker, nisoldipine. Transplantation 50: 14–20

21. Thurman RG, Marzi I, Seitz G, Thies J, Lemasters JJ, Zimmermann FA (1988) Hepatic reperfusion injury following orthotopic liver transplantation in the rat. Transplantation 46: 502–506

22. Zimmermann FA, Butcher GW, Davies HS, Brons G, Kamada N, Turel O (1979) Techniques of orthotopic liver transplantation in the rat and some studies of the immunologic response to fully allogeneic liver grafts. Transplant Proc 1: 571–577

Transplant Int (1992) 5 [Suppl 1]: S 366–S 369

TRANSPLANT
International
© Springer-Verlag 1992

Efficacy of PGI$_2$ analog in preventing ischemia reperfusion damage of liver grafts from living donors

S. Goto[1], Y. I. Kim, K. Kawano, T. Kai and M. Kobayashi

[1] Department of Surgery I, Oita Medical College, Oita, Japan

Abstract. In living-related transplantation, warm ische-mia/reperfusion damage (IRD) of liver grafts is inevitable during harvesting. In this study, we investigated the effects of prostacyclin (PGI$_2$) on IRD of liver grafts in the rat liver transplant model. Donor rats underwent 30-min warm ischemia of part of the liver (right lateral and medial lobes). After 10 min of reflow, the ischemic partial livers were flushed with Ringer's lactate and immediately transplanted into untreated recipients. Donor animals were divided into two groups: group I received vehicle, and group II received PGI$_2$ analog OP-41483 (OP, 500 ng/kg per min, i. v.) during the donor operation. One-week survival was studied and cellular adenine nucleotide levels of donor livers were assayed by high-performance liquid chromatography (HPLC). Donor treatment with PGI$_2$ analog group II significantly improved 1-week survival (86 %), in comparison with the controls group I (25 %). The levels of total adenine nucleotides (TAN, μmol/g dry wt) of the grafts just before implantation were well maintained by PGI$_2$ treatment (12.22), as compared with the controls (10.36). In summary, PGI$_2$ treatment of the donor maintained high energy metabolism of the liver graft after IRD and improved the survival of recipients after transplantation. Our study suggested that PGI$_2$ treatment of donors improves viability in liver grafts from living donors thus and increases graft availability for transplantation.

Key words: Living related transplantation – Warm ischemia/reperfusion damage – Prostacyclin

Recently, the shortage of hepatic grafts for children has prompted the use of reduced-sized grafts from adults and the use of living-related liver donors. These complicated donor-harvesting procedures result in an increased incidence of warm ischemia/reperfusion damage (IRD) to liver grafts and a decrease in graft viability. It is of utmost importance that living-donor hepatectomy is performed safely. Besides, one of the major reasons for retransplantation is the primary nonfunction of a graft resulting from warm IRD. Therefore, the alleviation of warm IRD during donor harvesting would be of benefit in liver transplantation.

Prostacyclin (PGI$_2$) and its analogs have several physiological actions such as antiplatelet aggregation [1], vasodilation [2] and cytoprotection [3], and our group as well as others have shown that they are protective in warm ischemia [4] or cold preservation of the liver [5–7]. The aim of this study was to investigate the effects of a stable PGI$_2$ analog (OP-41483) on graft viability after IRD, in particular in a setting of living-related transplantation.

Materials and methods

Transplantation procedure. Male Wistar rats, weighing 200–300 g were used as donors and recipients. In a setting of IRD during harvesting of liver grafts from living donors, a temporary normothermic IRD was induced by methods described previously by our group [8]. Briefly, the left portal vein and hepatic artery of the donor rats were occluded with a microvessel clip 15 min after the abdomen was opened. After 30 min of liver ischemia, the vascular clip was released and the right and caudate lobes were excised, leaving behind only the ischemic left lateral and median lobes. After 10 min of reflow, the donor left lateral and median lobes were flushed with Ringer's lactate and immediately transplanted into untreated recipients without arterialization (Fig. 1). Details of the technique of liver removal and orthotopic liver transplantation have been described previously [9]. To estimate technical standards, results from eight fresh reduced-sized-liver transplants were added.

Experimental protocol. Donor rats were divided into two groups: group I received vehicle, and group II received PGI$_2$ analog (OP-41483, 500 ng/kg per min, i. v.) continuously from soon after the abdomen was opened to the removal of the donor graft. OP-41483 (OP) [15-cyclopentyl-w-pentanor-5(E)-carbacyclin; Ono Pharmaceutical, Osaka, Japan] was dissolved in Ringer's lactate at 2.5 μg/ml. Fifteen rat liver transplants were performed in both groups for the preliminary 1-week survival study. Donor liver tissue specimens (50 mg–100 mg) were taken after opening the abdomen, after 30 min ischemia and after harvesting (just before implantation) for the determination of adenine nucleotide tissue concentrations.

Offprint requests to: Shigeru Goto, M. D., Department of Surgery 1, Oita Medical College, Oita, 879-56, Japan

Schematic diagram of the experiment (Donor)

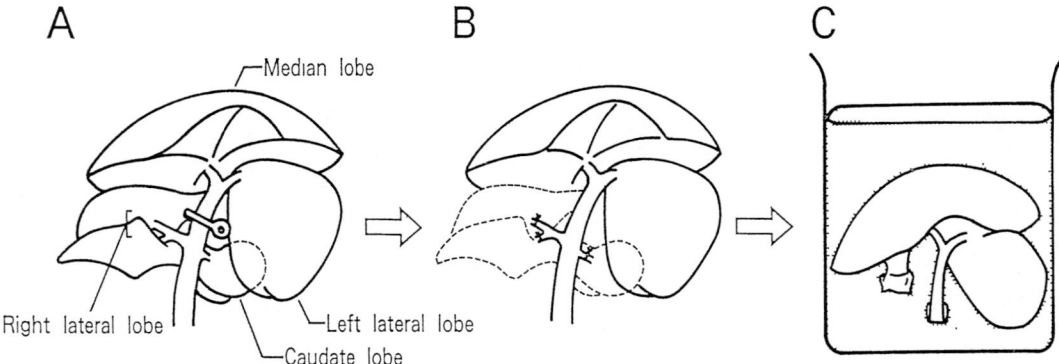

Fig.1. A Schematic diagram for the induction of warm IRD liver during donor operation. Afferent vessels were occluded by a small clip. **B** After 30 min, the clip was released and right lateral and caudate lobes were removed. **C** After 10 min reflow, the reduced liver was flushed with 10 ml of cold Ringer's lactate and stored in 50 ml Ringer's lactate at 4 °C prior to implantation

Measurement of adenine nucleotides. The concentrations of adenine nucleotides in donor livers were measured by a modification of the technique described by Kamiike et al. [10]. Adenosine triphosphate (ATP), adenosine diphosphate (ADP) and adenosine monophosphate (AMP) were measured by high-performance liquid chromatography (HPLC) on an anion exchanger column, DEAE-2SW (4.6 × 250 mm, Toyo Soda Manufacturing), equilibrated with 0.38 M phosphate buffer, pH 6.56. The energy charge was calculated according to the formula proposed by Atkinson [11]; energy charge (EC) = (ATP + 0.5 ADP)/(ATP + ADP + AMP). Total adenine nucleotides (TAN) levels were calculated by the following formula: TAN = ATP + ADP + AMP.

Statistical analysis. Fisher's exact test and Student's *t*-test were utilized for determining significant differences in the survival rate and in the ATP and cyclic nucleotide levels respectively.

Results

One-week survival rates for the two groups of animals are shown in Table 1. In group I, 25 % of rats (2/8) survived; four animals died of liver failure within 24 h of transplantation and two rats died between the 1st and 3rd days. In contrast, PGI₂ treatment of the donor (group II) markedly improved 1-week survival (86 %, 6/7), which was statistically significantly higher than that of the control group I (Fisher's exact test, $P < 0.01$). The 1-week survival of eight animals grafted with 70 % of fresh liver was 100 % (8/8), which indicated that the technical problems were completely overcome.

Figures 2–5 show the changes in adenine nucleotide concentrations in the livers biopsied at the end of the 30 min ischemia or just before implantation. The cellular ATP levels in the livers of both groups showed a marked decrease at the end of the 30 min ischemia, and returned to 60–70% of the pre-ischemia levels after donor harvesting (after 30 min ischemia and 10 min reflow) (Fig. 2). At the end of the 30 min ischemia, ATP [1.76 (SD = 0.58)

μmol/g dry wt] in PGI₂-treated livers in group I was significantly higher than that of the control group [0.98 (0.20) μmol/g dry wt]. However, there was no significant difference in the ATP levels of liver grafts in the two groups just before implantation. On the other hand, the ADP levels in the livers decreased gradually after ischemia and returned gradually to normal after reperfusion without a significant difference between the two groups (Fig. 3). A significant increase in AMP [6.82 (0.86) μmol/g dry wt] was observed in PGI₂-treated livers at the end of the 30 min ischemia, as compared with that [5.44 (0.44) μmol/g dry wt] of the control group (Fig. 4). But, there was no significant difference in AMP levels of liver grafts in the two groups before implantation.

In contrast, the TAN levels in PGI₂-treated liver were 11.55 (1.44) μmol/g dry wt at the end of 30 min ischemia, and 12.22 (1.29) μmol/g dry wt before implantation, which were significantly higher than those of the control group 8.85 (0.36) μmol/g dry wt and 10.36 (0.90) μmol/g dry wt respectively (Fig. 5). No significant differences were observed in the energy charge (EC) of the two groups at the end of ischemia or after donor harvesting.

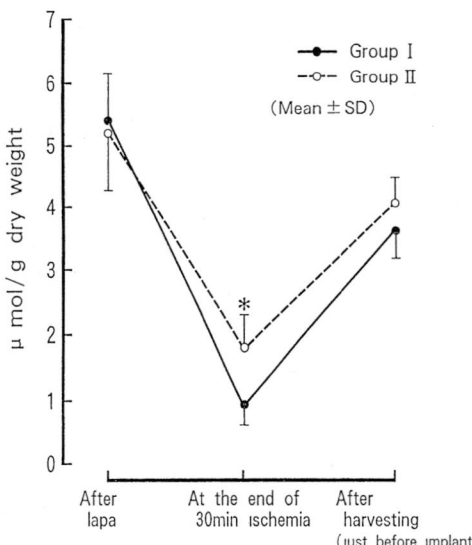

Fig. 2. Changes in hepatic cellular contents of adenosine triphosphate (ATP) in donor livers. Small specimens were taken at the times indicated during donor operation. Values are means for five experiments. (●) Group I; (○) Group II. *$P < 0.05$ vs Group I

S368

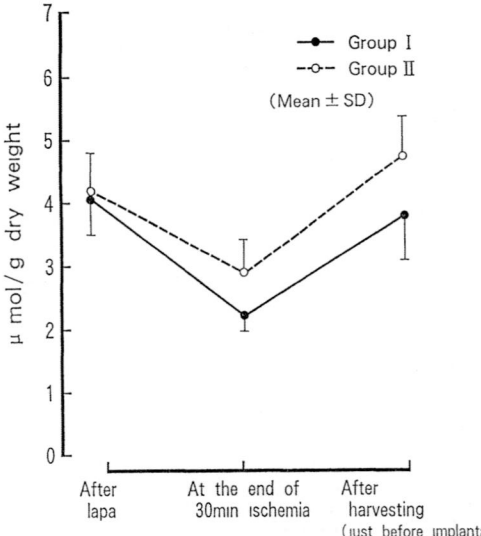

Fig. 3. Changes in cellular contents of adenosine diphosphate (ADP) in donor livers. The data were obtained from the same extracts as for Fig. 1. Values are means for five experiments. (●) Group I; (○) Group II

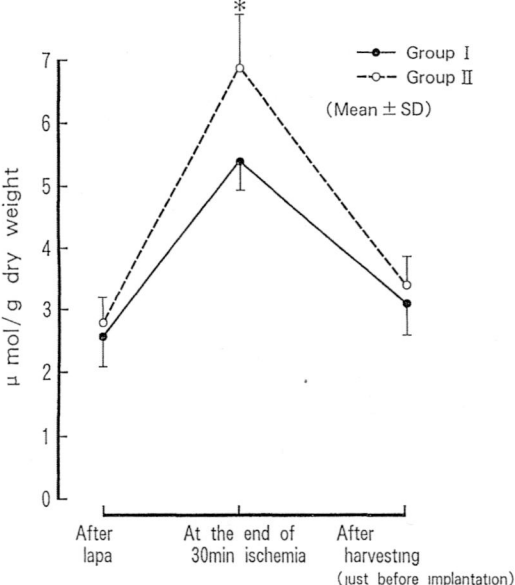

Fig. 4. Changes in cellular contents of adenosine monophosphate (AMP) in donor livers. The data were obtained from the same extracts as for Fig. 1. Values are means for five experiments. (●) Group I; (○) group II; *P < 0.05 vs group I

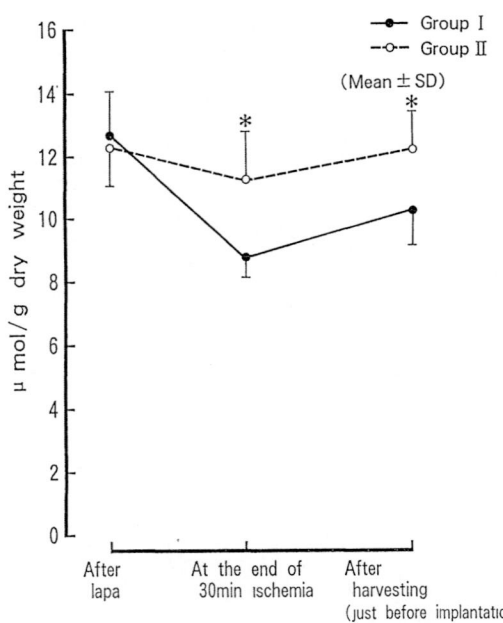

Fig. 5. Cellular total adenine nucleotides (TAN; ATP + ADP + AMP) levels soon after laparotomy, at the end of 30 min ischemia and after harvesting (just before implantation). Values are means for five experiments. (●) Group I; (○) group II; *P < 0.05 v.s. group I

livers in the rat after cold preservation for 24 h with the combined use of OP-41483 and lactobionate solution [7]. In the present study, we tested the effects of OP-41483 on graft viability after warm IRD in a rat liver transplant model.

Sumimoto et al. [14] have indicated that 30 min is the critical time for warm ischemia during the donor operation in the rat liver transplant model. In our present study, the effects of OP-41483 on a 30-min ischemic insult and 10-min reperfusion injury during the donor operation were assessed by the survival of the transplanted rats, and by measuring cellular adenine nucleotides in the donor liver. Donor treatment with PGI₂ improved the 1-week survival (86% vs 25% in the control group), and this correlated with well maintained levels of TAN.

A relationship between energy metabolism and the extent of ischemic tissue damage has been demonstrated in experimental models [15, 16]. However, our results demonstrated that there were no significant differences in levels of ATP, ADP and AMP between PGI₂-treated liver

Discussion

In living-related transplantation, both the liver graft and the liver remaining in the living donor have to remain viable. Therefore, the grafts from living donors are easily exposed to warm IRD, in addition to cold ischemic injury. PGI₂ and its analogs protect the liver against warm ischemic insult [4] and are efficacious in cold preservation [5–7]. However, its major drawback is that it is highly unstable [12], with ureliable results. The synthetic compound, OP-41483 is stable for more than 20 days even at 60°C and is independent of the pH of the solution and has similar pharmacological effects to those of native PGI₂ [13]. In a previous study, we succeeded in transplanting

Table 1. One-week survival rates of rats grafted with fresh liver grafts, or liver grafts exposed to warm IRD

	One-week survival (%)	Causes of death (xn)
Fresh liver grafts	8/8 (100)	
Liver grafts exposed to IRD		
Group I (vehicle treatment of donor)	2/8 (25)	bleeding (1) liver failure (3) obstructive jaundice (2)
Group II (PGI₂ treatment of donor)	6/7 (86)*	bleeding (1)

*P < 0.01 vs group I
IRD, Ischemia reperfusion damage

grafts and untreated grafts after harvesting (just before implantation). Kamiike et al. [10] have demonstrated that TAN levels of human donor grafts correlated and predicted the graft viability after transplantation, in comparison with ATP levels. This was confirmed by our result that TAN levels of IRD-induced grafts were well maintained by PGI$_2$ treatment, and this reflected the graft survival after transplantation.

The exact cytoprotective mechanism of PGI$_2$ at the cellular level has been investigated by others [3, 17]. Sikujara et al. [4] have indicated that PGI$_2$ is capable of protecting the liver from 75-min ischemic insult. Although the livers were not subsequently transplanted, they concluded that elevated ATP and cyclic nucleotide levels of PGI$_2$-treated livers played an important role in successful cytoprotection during ischemia. In our present study, elevated levels not only of ATP but also AMP at the end of 30-min ischemia were observed in PGI$_2$-treated livers. During warm ischemia of the liver, AMP is degraded rapidly to xanthine via adenosine, inosine, hypoxanthine [18]. Although the levels of degradation products such as purine catabolites were not measured in our study, our results suggested that degradation of ATP to urate was more retarded by PGI$_2$ treatment at the AMP to adenosine step at the end of 30 min ischemia, which may contribute to well maintained TAN levels of the graft after harvesting (just before implantation).

In summary, our data suggested that PGI$_2$-treatment of donors maintained graft viability before and after transplantation. Future clinical application of PGI$_2$ during donor harvesting from not only cadavers but also living donors may contribute to maximal utilization of available donor grafts.

Acknowledgements. This work was supported by a grant for paediatric research (63-A-05) from the Ministry of Health and Welfare and Grant-in-Aid (A-01440054) for general scientific research from the Ministry of Education of Japan.

References

1. Dusting GJ, Moncada S, Vane JR (1977) Prostacyclin (PGX) is the endogeneous metabolite responsible for relaxation of coronary arteries induced by arachidonic acid. Prostaglandins 13: 3–15
2. Higgs EA, Higgs GA, Moncada S, Vane JR (1978) Prostacyclin (PGI$_2$) inhibits the formation of platelet thrombi in arteroles and venules of the hamster cheek pouch. Br J Pharmacol 63: 535–539
3. Araki H, Lefer AM (1980) Cytoprotective actions of prostacyclin during hypoxia in the isolated perfused cat liver. Am J Physiol 238: H176–H181
4. Sikujara O, Monden M, Toyoshima, Okamura J, Kosaki G (1983) Cytoprotective effects of prostaglandin I$_2$ on ischemia-induced hepatic cell injury. Transplantation 36: 238–243
5. Monden M, Fortner JG (1982) Twenty-four-and 48-hour canine liver preservation by simple hypothermia with prostacyclin. Ann Surg 196: 38–42
6. Toledo-Pereyra JH (1984) Role of prostaglandins (PGI$_2$) in improving the survival of ischemically damaged liver allografts. Trans Am Soc Artif Intern Organs 30: 390–394
7. Goto S, Kim YI, Kodama Y et al. (1991) The beneficial effect of a stable prostacyclin analog (OP-41483) on rat liver preserved for 24 hours with lactobionate solution. Transplantation in press
8. Kawano K, Kim YI, Kaketani K, Kobayashi M (1989) The beneficial effect of cyclosporine on liver ischemia in rats. Transplantation 48: 759–764
9. Goto S, Kim YI, Shimada T, Kawano K, Kobayashi M (1991) The effects of pretransplant cyclosporine therapy on rats grafted with twelve-hour cold-stored liver. With special reference to reperfusion injury. Transplantation (in press)
10. Kamiike W, Budelski M, Steinhoff G, Ringe B, Lauchart W, Pichlmayer R (1988) Adenine nucleotide metabolism and its relation to organ viability in human liver transplantation. Transplantation 48: 138–143
11. Atkinson DE, Walton GM (1967) Adenine triphosphate conservation in metabolic regulation. J Biol Chem 242: 3239–3243
12. Dusting GJ, Moncada S, Vane JR (1977) Disappearance of prostacyclin in the circulation of the dog. Br J Pharmacol 62: 414–417
13. Yui Y, Takatsu Y, Hattori R, Kawai C, Osaki Y, Yoshida T (1985) A new stable prostacyclin analogue OP41483 (15-cyclopentyl-w-pentanor-5(e)-carbacyclin). Jpn Circ J 49: 571–575
14. Sumimoto K, Inagaki K, Yamada K, Kawasaki T, Dohi K (1988) Reliable indices for the determination of viability of grafted liver immediately after orthotopic transplantation. Transplantation 46: 506–509
15. Kamiike W, Watanabe F, Hashimoto T et al. (1982) Changes in cellular levels of ATP and its catabolites in ischemic rat liver. J Biochem 91: 1349–1356
16. Marubayashi S, Takenaka M, Dohi K, Ezaki H, Kawasaki T (1980) Adenine nucleotide metabolism during hepatic ischemia and subsequent blood reflow periods and its relation to organ viability. Transplantation 30: 294–298
17. Ozaki N, Tokunaga Y, Wakashiro S, et al. (1988) Evaluation of cytprotective drugs for liver preservation by pyridine nucleotide fluorometry. Surgery 104: 98–103
18. Harvey PRC, Iu S, McKeown CMB, Petrunka CN, Ilson RG, Strabrg SM (1988) Adenine nucleotide tissue concentrations and liver allograft viability after cold preservation and warm ischemia. Transplantation 45: 1016–1020

Transplant Int (1992) 5 [Suppl 1]: S370–S373

TRANSPLANT
International
© Springer-Verlag 1992

Heart and lung preservation using a new solution; UCLA Formula

M. Hachida, H. Koyanagi, and M. Endo

Department of Cardiovascular Surgery, Heart Institute of Japan, Tokyo Womens' Medical College, Tokyo, Japan

Abstract. Heart and lung preservation is a significant barrier in clinical heart and lung transplantation. In a previous study, we have shown that UCLA Formula, modified from cardioplegic solution, has a favorable effect on lung preservation. In this study, we evaluated the effect of the simultaneous flushing method using UCLA Formula alone on both heart and lung preservation. We conducted six experiments using 18 mongrel dogs, weighing 20–28 kg. In the donor animals, the heart and lungs were each flushed with 500 ml of cold UCLA Formula, using two catheters, one inserted into the ascending aorta and the other into the main pulmonary artery. After the heart and lung block was trimmed, orthotopic cardiac transplantation and single left lung transplantation were independently performed on different recipients following preservation for 4.3 h in the case of the heart and 7.5 h in the case of the lung. Thus, the function of the preserved organs was independently assessed using cardiac output and left ventricular end-diastolic pressure (LVEDP) with constant central venous pressure (CVP) in heart transplantation, and arterial gas analysis and the relationship between inspiratory pressure and expiratory tidal volume in lung transplantation. These measurements were performed before harvesting and 1 h and 4 h after transplantation. After heart transplantation cardiac output showed no significant deterioration. No significant differences in gas analysis and the pressure-volume curve were seen after lung transplantation. In conclusion, the simultaneous flushing method using the UCLA Formula may offer reliable preservation for both heart and lung in preparation for transplantation.

Key words: Heart transplant – Lung transplant – Organ preservation

The greatest single problem facing combined heart and lung transplantation is the shortage of suitable donor or-

gans. In particular, the difficulty of prolonged preservation of the heart and lung is a major barrier for distant donor procurement [1, 2]. Our previous studies have shown that a new solution, UCLA Formula, is effective in prolonging lung preservation up to 12 h [3, 4]. Furthermore, since this solution was originally modified from a cardioplegic solution, it is possible to preserve both the heart and lung by perfusion with the same solution. In this study, we assessed the efficacy of UCLA Formula in prolonging the ischemic time in both heart and lung preservation.

Materials and methods

Eighteen mongrel dogs, weighing from 20–28 kg, were used in this study. Heart and lung grafts were obtained from six dogs. To assess the organ viability following preservation, orthotopic heart transplantation was performed in six dogs and single lung transplantation was performed in the remaining six dogs. The animals were assigned randomly to each experiment.

The donor animals were anesthetized by intravenous administration of sodium pentobarbital, 30 mg/kg. After endotracheal intubation and ventilatory support, a median sternotomy was performed. The heart and both lungs were freed of mediastinal attachments and the animal was given heparin (3 mg/kg). Two catheters were placed into the ascending aorta from the right common carotid artery and the main pulmonary artery. These catheters were connected to bottles containing UCLA Formula. After inflow occlusion was produced and the respirator discontinued, the aorta and trachea were clamped. The heart was perfused with 500 ml of cold UCLA Formula (4 °C) at a pressure of 100 mm Hg, and both lungs were perfused with 500 ml of cold UCLA Formula (4 °C) at 50 cm of H_2O pressure (Fig. 1). A small incision was made in the inferior vena cava and the left atrium to drain the perfused solution. Topical cooling was also applied with ice slush inserted into the chest cavity.

After 5–10 min of perfusion, the carotid arteries were divided and an incision was made in the aortic arch. The incision was carefully extended to the posterior mediastinum and the heart and lung block was excised at both venae cavae, the ascending aorta, and the trachea just above the carina. Subsequently, the heart and lung block was immersed in cold saline (4 °C) and stored in the refrigerator at 4 °C after being double wrapped in a sterile plastic bag. After 4 h of preservation, the heart and lung block was taken out and trimmed for orthotopic heart transplantation. The remaining lungs were fur-

Offprint requests to: Mitsuhiro Hachida, 8-1 Kawada-cho, Shinjuku, Tokyo, Japan 162

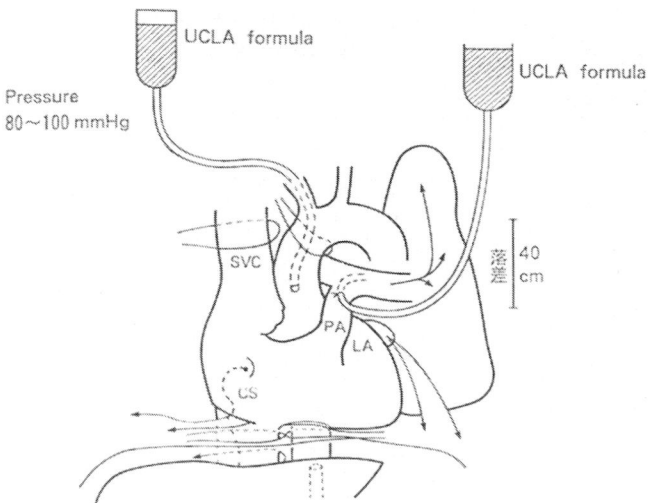

Fig. 1. Experimental model

ther preserved at 4°C in the refrigerator. Orthotopic heart transplantation was performed in six dogs in the usual manner after the 4 h of preservation. During the surgical procedure, the donor heart was continuously perfused with approximately 200 ml of cold UCLA Formula (4°C) at 50 cm H_2O pressure.

Single left lung transplantation was performed in six dogs, using the remaining preserved left lung as a donor graft. The surgical technique has been described previously [3]. Throughout the surgical procedure, the lung was wrapped in a cold towel and slowly perfused with approximately 100 ml of UCLA Formula to maintain it at a low temperature and to avoid mechanical damage to the graft. Mean ischemic time was 4.3 h in the heart and 7.6 h in the lung.

Measurements. The viablity of the preserved heart was evaluated by measuring cardiac output (CO) and left ventricular end-diastolic pressure (LVEDP) with a constant central venous pressure (CVP). The pretransplant values were obtained immediately after the median sternotomy was performed on the donor animal. Hemodynamic data including blood pressure, cardiac output, LVEDP, and CVP were measured with the catheter directly introduced into the ascending aorta and left ventricle. A 7F Swan-Ganz catheter was inserted into the main pulmonary artery to measure the cardiac output by the thermo-dilution method and to monitor pulmonary artery pressure. These measurements were performed while the CVP was adjusted to 7 cm H_2O by the use of transfusion and diuretics. Arterial blood gases including pH, oxygen tension (PO_2) and carbon dioxide tension (PCO_2) were examined periodically throughout and after the transplantation.

To assess the preserved left lung viability after the transplantation, blood gas analysis, including PO_2 and PCO_2, and the pulmonary pressure-volume curve with a contra-lateral occlusion test were used as indicators. Each animal was placed on a pressure-controlled respirator (Mark 7, Bird Products, Palm Springs, Calif.) with an inspiratory oxygen fraction (FiO_2) of 0.5. The inspiratory pressure was adjusted to 7, 10, 15, and 20 cm H_2O and the expiratory tidal volume was simultaneously recorded while the right pulmonary artery and bronchus were tightly clamped with a non-clashing vascular calmp. Throughout the operation, approximately 1000 ml of lactated Ringer's solution were infused.

All measurements were repeated at each interval of the preharvesting operation, and at 1 h and 4 h after the transplantation.

Solution. The UCLA Formula used in this study was made in our laboratory prior to each experiment. It contained glucose 50 gm/l regular insulin 80 U/l, NaH_2PO_4 0.6 gm/l, Na_2HPO_4 6.4 gm/l, KCL 1.5 gm/l, Mannitol 2.5 gm/l, autologous serum 30 ml/l, and verapamil 10 mg/l (Table 1). The concentrations of electrolytes in the solution

were: Na, 60 mEq/l and K, 30 mEq/l. The pH and osmolarity were 7.4 and 350 mosmol, respectively. The serum used in the solution was derived from blood from the same animal used as a donor.

All results are expressed as mean ± standard deviation of the mean. Paired and unpaired *t*-tests were used to assess statistical significance. Analysis of variance was used to determine the significance of differences between the experimental groups. Differences were considered to be statistically significant at a probability value less than 0.05.

Results

The mean ischemic time was 4.3 ± 0.5 h in the heart and 7.5 ± 0.7 h in the lung. Figure 2 demonstrates the cardiac output, LVEDP and CVP at the pretransplant and postoperative periods. CVP was maintained at 7 cm H_2O during the measurements. Cardiac output was 4.01 ± 1.36 l/min in the pretransplant period, 3.26 ± 0.68 l/min at 1 h, and 3.24 ± 0.26 l/min at 4 h after the heart transplantation these changes were not significant. LVEDP was 7.1 ± 0.8 mm Hg in the pretransplant period, 6.5 ± 0.86 mm Hg at 1 h, and 7.4 ± 1.2 mm Hg at 4 h after the transplantation. These changes were not significant. Thus, there was no significant difference between the pretransplant, and posttransplantation values of cardiac output and LVEDP under constant CVP following 4.3 h of heart preservation in UCLA Formula.

The preserved lung was examined while the left pulmonary artery and bronchus were totally occluded. The PO_2 tension (FiO_2 0.5) was 293.7 ± 38.3 mm Hg in the pretransplant period, 310 ± 62.7 mm Hg at 1 h, and 235.0 ± 87.8 mm Hg at 4 h postoperatively. These changes were not significant (Fig. 3). PCO_2 tension was 24.6 ± 7.2 mm Hg in the pretransplant period, 26.2 ± 9.4 mm Hg at 1 h, and 33.2 ± 9.3 mm Hg at 4 h postoperatively. These changes were not significant. Thus, no significant difference was observed between each period in PO_2 and PCO_2 after lung transplantation following 7.5 h lung preservation in UCLA Formula.

The relationship between inspiratory pressure and expiratory tidal volume was evaluated in each period (Fig. 4). The expiratory tidal volume at a pressure of 20 cm H_2O was 475 ± 55.9 ml in the pretransplant period, 437.0 ± 165.9 ml at 1 h, and 536.7 ± 101.5 ml at 4 h postoperatively; at a pressure of 15 cm H_2O the expiratory tidal volume was 330.0 ± 71.6 ml in the pretransplant period, 352.5 ± 71.6 ml at 1 h, 366.7 ± 54.0 ml at 4 h postopera-

Table 1. Constitution of UCLA Formula

Glucose	(gm/l)	50
Insulin	(U/l)	80.0
Na_2HPO_4	(gm/l)	6.4
NaH_2PO_4	(gm/l)	0.6
KCl	(gm/l)	1.5
Mannitol	(gm/l)	2.5
Verapamil	(mg/l)	10.0
Serum	(ml/l)	30.0
pH		7.4
Na	(mEq/l)	60
K	(mEq/l)	30
Osmolarity	(mosmol)	350

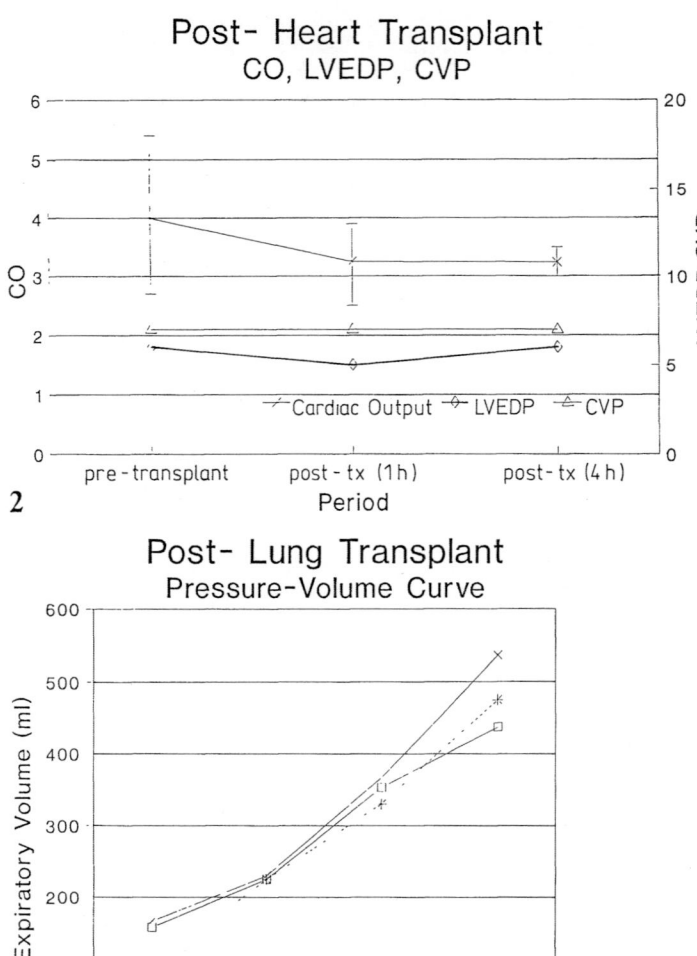

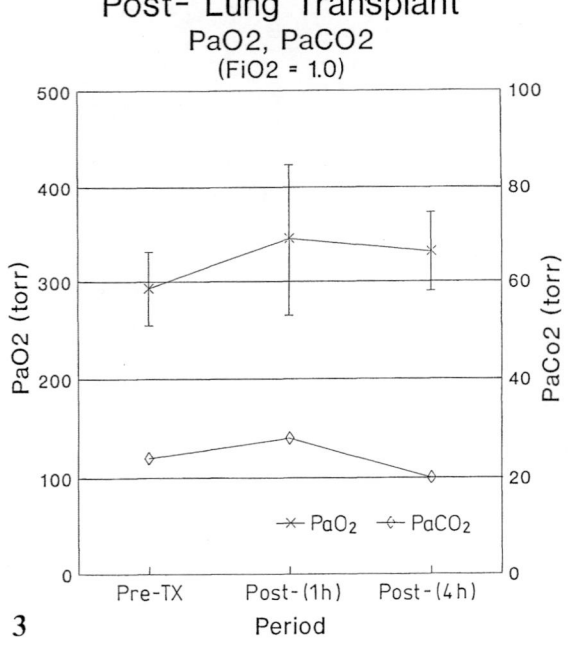

Post- Heart Transplant
CO, LVEDP, CVP

2

Post- Lung Transplant
Pressure-Volume Curve

4

Post- Lung Transplant
PaO2, PaCO2
(FiO2 = 1.0)

3

Fig. 2. Assessment of the donor heart preserved with UCLA Formula. Cardiac output and LVEDP were measured with a constant CVP (7 cm H₂O). There was no significant difference between pre- and post-transplantation *(tx)* value (paired and unpaired *t*-test)

Fig. 3. Assessment of the donor lung preservation with UCLA Formula. PO₂, PCO₂ showed no significant deterioration after transplantation *(Tx)* (paired and unpaired *t*-test)

Fig. 4. The relationship between inspiratory pressure and expiratory tidal volume. There was no significant difference between pre- and post-transplantation *(Tx)* values (paired and unpaired *t*-test)

tively; at a pressure of 10 cm H_2O, this was 225 ± 71.2 ml pretransplant, 225.0 ± 94.1 ml at 1 h, and 230.0 ± 46.3 ml at 4 h postoperatively; at a pressure of 7 cm H_2O, this was 102.5 ± 17.8 ml pretransplant, 157.5 ± 99.6 ml at 1 h, and 166.7 ± 51.2 ml at 4 h postoperatively. The tidal volume at each inspiratory pressure was not significantly different among the three groups. Therefore, no significant deterioration was detected in heart and lung following preservation in UCLA Formula.

Discussion

An effective method of organ preservation is crucial for both lung and combined heart-lung transplantation [5–8]. Of the many solutions that have been tested, no solution has been effective in both heart and lung [9]. Up until now, the heart and lung have been independently perfused with different solutions. The lungs could be preserved for 4 h with Euro-Collins' solution, which consists of intra-cellu-

lar components. In contrast, approximately 4 h of heart preservation was obtained with various cardioplegic solutions of extra-cellular composition [9]. We can assume that approximately 60 ml of the remaining solution in each lung graft is flushed into the heart after reperfusion, and since extra-cellular solutions contain high amounts of potassium, there may be an unfavorable effect on the donor heart graft. In cases where single lung transplantation and orthotopic transplantation are performed by sharing a heart and lung from the same donor animal, which are preserved using conventional solutions, a similar deteriorating effect may occur in the native heart upon flushing of the remaining solution in the donor lung. As UCLA Formula contains 30 mEq/l of potassium (vs 115 mEq/l in Euro-Collins' solution which is made of intracellular composition) and is beneficial for both heart and lung preservation, the drastic interaction of the different solutions during preservation and the deleterious effect on the heart after the reperfusion might be prevented by using the same extra-cellular solution. Therefore, we believe that flushing the heart and lungs with the same extracellular solution may be the optimal method for preservation.

The major role of a pulmoplegic solution is to provide prompt hypothermia to the whole lung without toxicity to the various types of specialized cells in the lung tissue. In particular, the effect of solutions on alveolar type II cells are the most critical because these cells play an important role in synthesis, storage, and secretion of the alveolar surfactant [10]. Using the viability of these cells as an indicator, we have investigated the effect of various solutions in vitro [11]. We found that GIK solution, which has been used as a cardioplegic solution, was the most effective solution for the pulmonary alveolar cells. Furthermore, in 1986, we demonstrated the beneficial effect of the Ca channel blocker, verapamil, on lung preservation. In that study, tissue damage caused by ischemia was significantly reduced by adding verapamil [12]. Based upon these experimental experiences, we composed the new solution, UCLA Formula, for lung preservation. Using this solution, 12 h of lung preservation was achieved.

UCLA Formula is based on the GIK (Glucose-Insulin-Potassium) solution, which was originally developed as a cardioplegic solution [13]. The effect of glucose, insulin, and potassium in heart preservation has received much attention over the years. In fact, it has been reported that glucose and insulin enhance the rate of anaerobic glycolysis, reverse ion loss, alter membrane electrophysiologic impairment, decrease plasma free fatty acid concentration, and alter plasma osmolarity. Furthermore, insulin reduces sodium permeability and stimulates active Na ion efflux. Hess and colleagues have suggested that glucose in GIK may also act as a scavenger of oxygen free radicals [14]. Because the energy source of the ischemic lung is exclusively dependent on anaerobic glycolysis, the presence of sufficient glucose in the solution plays an important role in supplying this energy. Because of these beneficial effects, we considered that the GIK solution might be an optimal solution for protecting the ischemic lung from injury. On the basis of these experimental experiences, we used this solution for simultaneous heart and lung preservation in the present study.

To assess the heart and lung function independently following each preservation, we evaluated the heart with orthotopic heart transplantation, and the lung with single lung transplantation using a contra-lateral occlusion test. As a result, the parameters we used in this study showed no significant deterioration in the heart and lung after the preservation. Although we have achieved 12 h of lung preservation using this Formula, the results of the present study suggest that UCLA Formula was effective not only in the lung preservation, but also in heart preservation. In conclusion, the simultaneous flushing method using the UCLA Formula may offer reliable preservation for both heart and lung transplantation. We studied 4 h of heart preservation and 7 h of lung preservation using the UCLA Formula in this study. We will continue to investigate the limitation of preservation time in the heart and lung using UCLA Formula.

Acknowledgements. We express our appreciation to Miss Barbara Levine and Miss Keiko Satake for excellent secretarial assistance in preparing this manuscript.

References

1. Fragomeni LS, Kaye MP (1988) The Registry of the International Society for Heart Transplantation: Fifth Official Report – 1988. J Heart Transplant 7: 249–253
2. Harjula A, Baldwin JC, Stanes VA, Shumway NE (1987) Proper donor selection for heart and lung transplantation: the Stanford experience. J Thorac Cardiovasc Surg 94: 874–880
3. Hachida M, Morton DL (1989) A new solution (UCLA Formula) for lung preservation. J Thorac Cardiovasc Surg 97: 513–521
4. Hachida M, Morton DL (1989) Lung function after prolonged lung preservation. J Thorac Cardiovasc Surg 97: 911–919
5. Hardestry RL, Griffith BP (1987) Autoperfusion of the heart and lung for preservation during distant procurement. J Thorac Cardiovasc Surg 93: 11–18
6. Kontos GJ, Adachi H, Borkon AM, Reitz BA (1987) A non-flush core-cooling technique for successful cardiopulmonary preservation in heart and lung transplantation. J Thorac Cardiovasc Surg 94: 836–842
7. Griffth BP, Hardesty RL, Trento A (1987) Heart and lung transplantation: lessons learned and future hopes. Ann Thorac Surg 43: 6
8. Emery RW, Cork RC, Levinson MM (1986) The cardiac donor: six year experience. Ann Thorac Surg 41: 356–362
9. Haverich A, Scott WC, Jamieson SW (1985) Twenty years of lung preservation – A review. J Heart Transplant 4: 230–240
10. Said SI (1985) The pulmonary circulation and acute injury. Furuta, New York, pp 18–27
11. Hachida M, Hoon DSB, Morton DL (1988) A comparison of solutions for lung preservation using pulmonary alveolar type II cell viability. Ann Thorac Surg 45: 643–646
12. Hachida M, Morton DL (1988) The protection of ischemic lung with verapamil and hydralazine. J Thorac Cardiovasc Surg 95: 178–183
13. Opie LH, Bruyneel K, Owens (1970) Effect of glucose, insulin and potassium infusion on tissue metabolic changes within first hour of myocardial infarction in baboon. Circulation 52: 49–57
14. Hess ML, Okabe E, Poland J, Warner M, Stewart JR, Greenfield LJ (1983) Glucose, insulin potassium protection during the course of hypothermic global ischemia and reperfusion: a new proposed mechanism by the scavenging of free radicals. J Cardiovasc Pharmacol 5: 35–43

Transplant Int (1992) 5 [Suppl 1]: S 374–S 378

TRANSPLANT
International
© Springer-Verlag 1992

Antagonisation of platelet activating factor – a new therapeutic concept for improvement of organ quality in lung preservation

S. W. Hirt, Th. Wahlers, M. Jurmann, L. Dammenhayn, R. Rohde, and A. Haverich

Division of Thoracic and Cardiovascular Surgery, Hannover Medical School, Hannover, Federal Republic of Germany

Abstract. The release of platelet activating factor (PAF) is thought to be one of the most important pathophysiological pathways in the development of ischemic lung injury. We investigated the use of a PAF antagonist (PAF-a) in a canine model in reducing PAF-mediated pulmonary dysfunction following lung preservation and transplantation. Twelve combined heterotopic heart and orthotopic left lung allotransplantations were performed after 6 h of cold ischemia. Following administration of prostacyclin (PGI$_2$), Euro-Collins solution (EC) was used for pulmonary artery flush in all donors, while in six animals the PAF-a, WEB 2170 BS, was administered to the donor (0.15 mg/kg for 30 min), to the storage solution (0.3 mg/kg) and to the recipient during reperfusion for a total of 6 h (0.3 mg/kg per h) EC/PAF-a). In all donors myocardial preservation was achieved using St. Thomas Hospital solution. Postoperatively, cardiorespiratory function was evaluated seperately for donor and recipient organs at an FiO$_2$ of 0.4 for a maximum of 12 h. The quality of lung preservation was assessed by means of postoperative oxygenation (pO$_2$), pulmonary artery pressure (PAP) and pulmonary vascular resistance index (PVRI). In the EC/PAF-a group, pO$_2$ of the donor lung was significantly elevated ($P < 0.01$) and PVRI was significantly lower ($P < 0.05$) when compared to the EC group, while PAP showed no significant differences between both groups and throughout the entire postoperative course. We concluded that a significant improvement in the current clinical standard for lung preservation could be obtained by the application of WEB 2170 BS in combination with EC flush as demonstrated by improved oxygenation and lower PVRI of the transplantated organs.

Key words: PAF-antagonist – Prostacyclin – Euro-Collins solution – Heart and lung transplantation

---

Offprint requests to: Stephan W. Hirt, M. D., Division of Thoracic and Cardiovascular Surgery, Hannover Medical School, Konstanty-Gutschow-Strasse 8, D-3000 Hannover, FRG

Initially, attempts at lung transplantation failed in the early postoperative period due to the poor preservation quality of the transplanted organs [1]. Several methods for distant organ procurement have been succesfully established [2–5]. Currently, pulmonary artery flush perfusion with Euro-Collins solution (EC) in combination with prostacyclin (PGI$_2$) pretreatment is most frequently used for lung preservation [6–9] and acceptable results are achieved clinically within ischemia times of up to 4 h [10].

Elevated concentrations of platelet activating factor (PAF), released by circulating polymorphonuclear leucocytes and pulmonary macrophages, account for pulmonary tissue injury resulting in bronchoconstriction, oxygen free radical generation, elevated pulmonary vascular resistance and microvascular leakage [11, 12]. Synthetic PAF-antagonists (PAF-a) were initially developed for the treatment of small airways disease [13], but due to the major involvement in the pathophysiology of pulmonary dysfunction various other indications – septic shock, graft rejection, pulmonary preservation and transplantation – were investigated throughout further evaluation [11, 13–15]. Since most of these problems are encountered in reperfusion injury we investigated the prevention of PAF-induced pulmonary dysfunction after lung transplantation in a canine model by the addition of a PAF-a (WEB 2170 BS). This was combined with our current clinical setup for lung preservation as represented by pulmonary artery flush with EC after previous systemic administration of PGI$_2$.

Materials and methods

Twenty-four mongrel dogs were divided in 2 groups of six donors and six weight-matched recipients each. All animals were cared for in compliance with the "Principles of Laboratory Animal Care" formulated by the National Society for Medical Research and the "Guide for the Care and Use of Laboratory Animals" published by the National Institutes of Health (NIH Publication No. 85-23, revised 1985).

The dogs were anaesthetized and ventilated with 40% oxygen and 60% nitrous oxide using a positive endexspiratory pressure

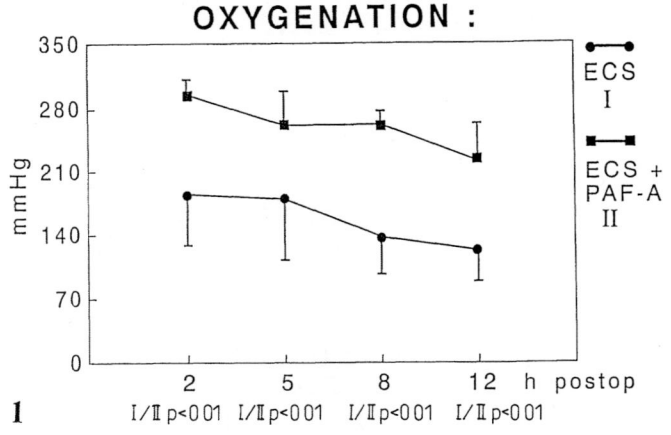

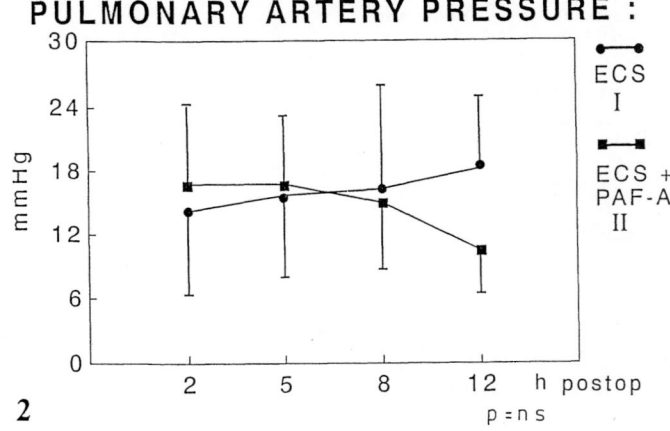

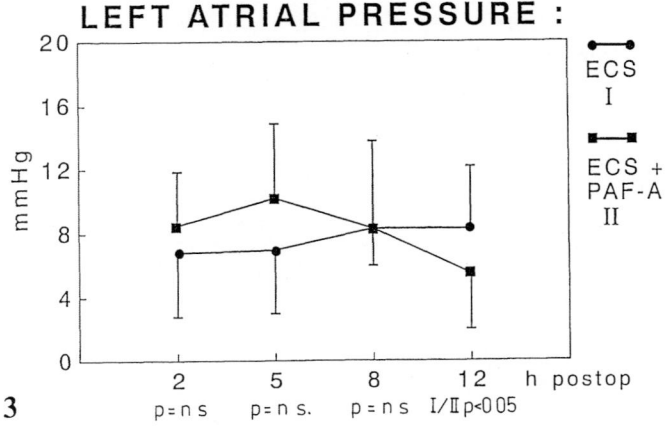

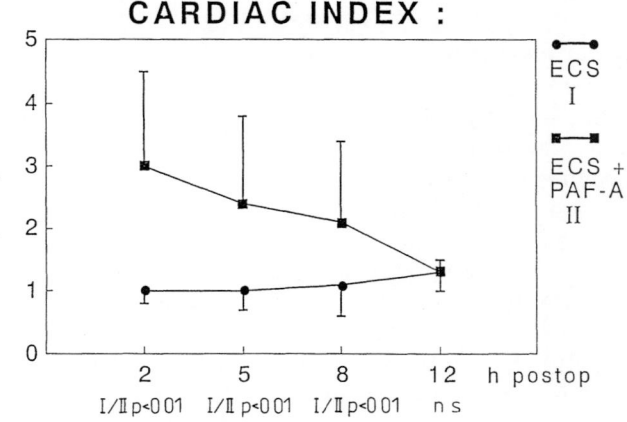

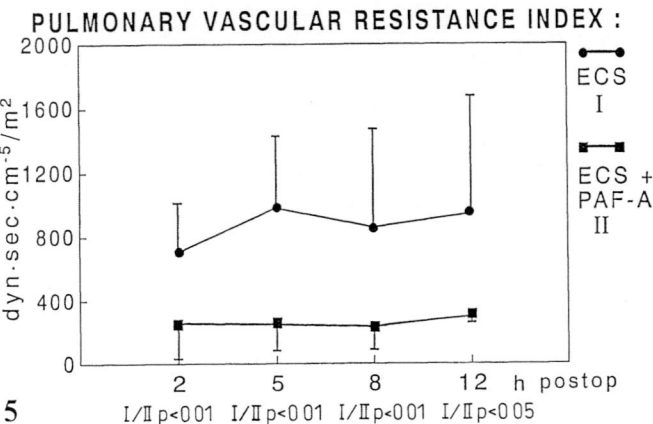

Fig. 1. Postoperative donor left atrial pO₂-values (mean ± SD)

Fig. 2. Postoperative donor mean pulmonary artery pressure (PAP) (mean ± SD)

Fig. 3. Postoperative donor left atrial pressure (LAP) (mean ± SD)

Fig. 4. Postoperative donor cardiac index (CI) (mean ± SD)

Fig. 5. Postoperative donor pulmonary vascular resistance index (PVRI) (mean ± SD)

(PEEP) of 5 cm H₂O. The operative technique for donor and recipient operation has been described previously by Wahlers et al. [6]. Donor animals were divided into 2 groups according to the method of pulmonary preservation. In both groups pulmonary artery flush perfusion was performed with EC (60 ml/kg at 4 °C) after previous intravenous administration of PGI₂ over a 10 min period (20 ng/kg per min), while additionally, in group II, WEB 2170 BS was administered to the donor, added to the storage solution and administered to the recipient during reperfusion (Table 1). For cardioplegia, St. Thomas Hospital solution (20 ml/kg at 4 °C) was used in all donors. The organ block was immersed in cold EC without further dissection and stored at 4 °C for about 5 h.

The recipient animals were prepared during the organ storage period. Briefly, a left pneumonectomy was performed and the donor heart with the adjacent left lung were transplanted as has been described in earlier studies [6, 16]. Anastomoses were performed end-

to-side between the donor's and recipient's superior vena cava (SVC) and the donor's descending aorta was sutured end-to-side to the proximal part of the recipient's descending aorta. Ligation of the recipient's SVC proximal to the anastomosis after 30 min of reperfusion provided a separation of the donor and recipient pulmonary circulation. The donor's trachea was intubated with an endotracheal tube inserted through the 2nd intercostal space and ventilated separately (oxygen 40 %/nitrous oxide 60 %, tidal volume: 10 cc/kg, respiratory rate: 12/min, PEEP: 5 cm H₂O). The chest was closed temporarily.

Arterial pressure (AP) was measured in the carotid artery, and heart rate (HR), central-venous pressure (CVP), pulmonary artery pressure (PAP), left atrial pressure (LAP), cardiac output (CO) and left atrial blood gas analysis (BGA) were obtained separately every hour in the donor's and the recipient's circulation until the postoperative course was terminated after 12 h or the animal died. Calculation of cardiac index (CI) and pulmonary vascular resistance index (PVRI) were performed according to standard formula. Data are expressed as mean values ± standard deviation (SD). To exclude influences of baseline data on postoperative results, analysis of covariance (ANCOVA) was performed. P values less than 0.05 were considered significant.

Results

No significant differences were found between the donor data – except for the oxygenation – and the ischemia time (Table 2). The CVP was adjusted in both groups to approximately 6–8 mmHg for the entire postoperative course. No recipient animal died during the first 8 h postoperatively, however one animal in the EC group (group I) and two dogs in the EC/PAF-a group (group II) died between 8 and 12 h postoperatively. Causes for premature deaths were progressive cardiac failure or dysrhythmias in all cases.

Significantly improved oxygenation of the donor lung after transplantation was observed in the EC/PAF-a (group II) group compared to the EC group (group I) throughout the entire postoperative period (Fig. 1). In both groups mean values of left atrial pO_2 were stable during the first 6 h after transplantation and decreased significantly in the later postoperative course from 190 ± 56 mmHg at 2 h to 123 ± 34 mmHg at 12 h in group I ($P < 0.05$), and 296 ± 17 mmHg at 2 h and 223 ± 47 mmHg at 12 h in group II ($P < 0.05$). Comparing mean pO_2 values of the donor lung before harvesting and early postoperatively, a reduction in oxygenation of 61 % was noted in group I versus only 23 % in group II.

Mean postoperative PAPs ranged from 14.2 ± 7.3 mmHg at 2 h to 18.3 ± 6.7 mmHg at 12 h in group I, and from 16.8 ± 7.3 mmHg at 2 h to 10.5 ± 4.9 mmHg at 12 h in group II (Fig. 2). While in group I a slight, but not significant increase was found in PAP throughout the postoperative period, PAP decreased in group II, but this was not significant. Comparing the corresponding postoperative PAP values of both groups, no significant differences were found at any time. Analysis of postoperative LAP values of both groups revealed a statistically significant difference only at 12 h postoperatively (group I: 8.3 ± 3.9 mmHg versus 5.5 ± 3.5 mmHg in group II, $P < 0.05$) (Fig. 3).

Cardiac index (CI) was elevated in group II compared to group I and this difference was significant during the first 8 h postoperatively (CI at 2 h: group I, 1.06 ± 0.29 l/min/m^2, group II, 2.98 ± 1.45 l/min/m^2, $P < 0.01$; at 5 h: group I, 1.04 ± 0.43 l/min/m^2, group II, 2.41 ± 1.38 l/min/m^2, $P < 0.05$; and at 8 h: group I, 1.15 ± 0.62 l/min/m^2, group II, 2.12 ± 1.32 l/min/m^2, $P < 0.05$). While CI was stable in both groups during this time, in the later postoperative course CI decreased in group II ($P < 0.05$). Despite this decrease in CI, values in group II were still elevated compared with group I, but the differences were no longer significant (CI at 12 h: group I, 1.05 ± 0.23 l/min/m^2; group II, 1.32 ± 0.20 l/min/m^2, n.s.) (Fig. 4).

The pulmonary vascular resistance index (PVRI) was elevated postoperatively in both groups and ranged be-

Table 1. Groups investigated

I ($n = 6$)	Pulmonary artery flush with cold Euro-Collins-solution (60 ml/kg) after prostacyclin pretreatment (20 ng/kg/min) (storage: ECS)
II ($n = 6$)	Pulmonary artery flush ($\cong$ I) + PAF-antagonist WEB 2017 BS (Donor: 0.15 mg/kg/30 min, recipient: 0.3 mg/kg/h for 6 h, Storage solution: ECS + 0.3 mg/kg WEB 2170 BS)

Table 2. Donor and procurement data (mean ± SD)

	Group I (EC)	Group II (EC/PAF-a)	
Body weight (kg)	23.2 ± 2.8	23.8 ± 3.8	n.s.
PAP (mmHg)	15.7 ± 4.8	16.8 ± 5.0	n.s.
LAP (mmHg)	9.0 ± 3.4	7.3 ± 4.6	n.s.
CI (l/min/m^2)	3.89 ± 1.07	3.45 ± 1.50	n.s.
PVRI (dyn s cm^{-5} m^2)	197 ± 29	196 ± 85	n.s.
pO$_2$ (mmHg)	190 ± 10	270 ± 25	$P < 0.01$
Perfusion pressure (mmHg)	13.5 ± 5.5	11.7 ± 3.4	n.s.
Ischemia time (min)	$368 + 30$	$338 + 18$	n.s.

PAP, pulmonary artery pressure; LAP, left atrial pressure; CI, cardiac index; PVRI, pulmonary vascular resistance index; pO$_2$, arterial oxygen tension; EC, Euro-Collins solution; PAF-a, PAF antagonist; n.s., not significant

tween 705 ± 313 dyn s cm^{-5} m^2 at 2 h and 947 ± 732 dyn s cm^{-5} m^2 at 12 h in group I and between 296 ± 268 dyn s cm^{-5} m^2 at 2 h and 300 ± 40 dyn s cm^{-5} m^2 at 12 h in group II (Fig. 5). PVRI values in group I were elevated at all times postoperatively compared with the corresponding values for group II. These differences reached statistical significance at 2, 5, and 8 h postoperatively.

Between the two groups no significant differences were found in the recipient data during the postoperative course comparing corresponding values of CI, PAP, LAP and PVRI, except for a significant decrease in the pO$_2$ values in both groups ($P < 0.05$).

Discussion

In the past, different methods and techniques for lung procurement and preservation have been developed and used in clinical transplantation. However, donor core cooling by means of extracorporeal circulation [5, 17] and single flush perfusion of the pulmonary artery using either Euro-Collins solution [2, 6–10] or cold blood [4], are currently used by most lung transplant centers. The EC flush is combined with the systemic administration of prostaglandins to the donor immediately before harvesting, since Jurmann et al. have demonstrated that the addition of PGI$_2$ provides pulmonary vasodilatation resulting in better distribution of the crystalloid flush and improved postoperative graft function [18]. Despite satisfactory clinical results in lung transplantation, with mean ischemia times of up to 4 h [10] multiple efforts have been made to prolong the ischemic tolerance of the lung. In particular, the use of oxygen free radical scavengers [19, 20] and the use of University of Wisconsin solution for lung preservation [21] have been studied recently.

We investigated, in canine model, the effects of the PAF-antagonist WEB 2170 BS in combination with EC flush perfusion after PGI_2 pretreatment on the postoperative graft function compared to EC + PGI_2 alone. In both experimental groups, EC was administrated with a perfusion volume of 60 ml/kg at 4°C and perfusion pressures according to the native PAP were used, since Haverich et al. have demonstrated the advantages of the high volume low pressure pulmonary artery flush with respect to homogeneous fluid distribution and uniform organ cooling [7]. Heterotopic heart- and orthotopic single lung-transplantation was performed, since extracorporeal circulation can be omitted throughout the implantation [6, 16]. Another advantage of the model is based on the separation of donor and recipient circulation, because organ deterioration does not directly lead to the recipient's death and reperfusion injury can be studied more extensively.

For quantification of lung preservation quality, left atrial pO_2, PAP and PVRI were considered, since various experimental studies have demonstrated that these parameters are most suitable for assessment of posttransplant lung function [6, 7, 22]. Analysis of lung water content was not performed, because a minor sensitivity can be expected when compared to functional parameters [23]. Our results demonstrated that the use of WEB 2170 BS in combination with EC flush resulted in a significantly improved postoperative oxygenation of the transplanted lung. In addition, comparing donor pO_2 values before harvesting and early postoperatively only the slightest impairment of oxygenation was noted in the EC/PAF-a group. Comparing corresponding PAP and LAP values between both groups and throughout the postoperative course no significant differences or changes were observed except for the PAP at 12 h postoperatively ($P < 0.05$). However, using identical myocardial protection in both groups, the higher CI in the EC/PAF-a group without corresponding increase in PAP probably reflects a better preservation of the pulmonary vascular bed resulting in a significantly lower PVRI during the first 8 h postoperatively. Similar results have been described by Conte and Foegh using the PAF-a BN 52021 in long term lung preservation in a canine model [14].

The excellent post-transplant lung function using the PAF-a WEB 2170 BS might be due to improved donor organ preservation as well as reduced reperfusion injury. It can be speculated that the PAF release by circulating leucocytes and alveolar macrophages is probably one of the most important pathophysiologic pathways activated during perfusion, ischemic storage and reperfusion of the lungs. PAF-induced oxygen free radical generation and liberation of vasoactive substances may be attenuated by the addition of PAF-antagonists resulting in better oxygenation and lower pulmonary vascular resistance.

In conclusion, the use of the PAF-a, WEB 2170 BS, in combination with EC flush in lung transplantation provided significantly improved postoperative oxygenation and lower pulmonary vascular resistance when administered to the donor before harvesting, to the storage solution and to the recipient during reperfusion as demonstrated in a canine heterotopic heart- and orthotopic left lung-transplant model after 6 h of cold ischemia.

Acknowledgements. The statistical analysis was performed by R. Rohde, and WEB 2170 BS was kindly supplied by Dr. Blank, Boehringer Ingelheim, Germany.

References

1. Haverich A, Scott WC, Jamieson SW (1985) Twenty years of lung preservation – a review. J Heart Transplant 4: 234
2. Jamieson SW, Stinson EB, Oyer PE, Reitz BA, Baldwin J, Modry D, Dawkins K, Theodore J, Hunt S, Shumway NE (1984) Heart-lung transplantation for irreversible pulmonary hypertension. Ann Thorac Surg 38: 554
3. Ladowski JS, Kapelanski DP, Theodori MF, Stevenson WC, Hardesty RL, Griffith BP (1985) Use of autoperfusion for distant procurement of heart-lung allografts. Heart Transplant 3: 330
4. Hakim M, Higgenbottam T, Bethune D, Cory-Pearce R, English TAH, Kneeshaw J, Wells FC, Wallwork J (1988) Selection and procurement of combined heart and lung grafts for transplantation. J Thorac Cardiovasc Surg 95: 474
5. Yacoub MH, Khaghani A, Banner N, Tajkarimi S, Fitzgerald M (1989) Distant organ procurement for heart and lung transplantation. Transplant Proc 21: 2548
6. Wahlers Th, Haverich A, Fieguth HG, Schäfers HJ, Takayama T, Borst HG (1986) Flush perfusion using Euro-Collins solution vs cooling by means of extracorporeal circulation in heart-lung preservation. J Heart Transplant 5: 89
7. Haverich A, Aziz S, Scott WC, Jamieson SW, Shumway NE (1986) Improved lung preservation using Euro-Collins solution for flush perfusion. Thorac Cardiovasc Surg 34: 368
8. Stuart RS, Monte S, Baumgartner WA, Hutchins GM, Borkon AM, Reitz BA, Galloway EJ (1984) Successfull 4 hour hypothermic lung storage with Euro-Collins solution, a simplified model assessing preservation. Heart Transplant 3: 346
9. Feeley TW, Mihm FG, Downing TP, Sadeghi AM, Baumgartner WA, Reitz BA, Shumway NE (1986) Hypothermic preservation of the heart and lungs with Collins solution: effect on cardiorespiratory function following heart-lung allotransplantation in dogs. Ann Thorac Surg 41: 301
10. Haverich A, Wahlers Th, Schäfers HJ, Ziemer G, Cremer J, Fieguth HG, Borst HG (1990) Distant organ procurement in clinical lung- and heart-lung transplantation. Eur J Cardiothorac Surg 4: 245
11. Camussi G, Salvidio G (1988) Platelet-activating factor in graft rejection. Prog Biochem Pharmacol 22: 106
12. Handley DA, Velen RG van, Melden MK, Saunders RN (1984) Evaluation of dose and route effects of platelet activating factor-induced extravasation in the guinea pig. Thromb Haemost 52: 34
13. Pretolani M, Lefort J, Malànchere E, et al. (1987) Interference by the novel PAF-acether antagonist WEB 2086 with the bronchopulmonary responses to PAF-acether and to active and passive anaphylactic shock in guinea pigs: Eur J Pharmacol 140: 311
14. Conte JV, Ramwell PW, Foegh ML (1990) Lung Preservation: A new indication for a PAF antagonist, BN 52021. In: O' Flaherty JT, Ramwell PW (eds) PAF antagonists: new developments for clinical application. Gulf Publishing Company, Houston, pp 129–137
15. Heuer H, Casals-Stenzel J, Stransky W, Weber KH (1988) Alterations in the lung of the guinea pig induced by platelet activating

S 378

factor and its inhibition by specific antagonists of the hetrazepine type (WEB 2170 and STY 2108). Allergy 43. [Suppl 7]: 72

16. Schäfers HJ, Dammenhayn L, Wahlers Th, Fieguth HG, Haverich A (1987) Heterotopic heart-unilateral left lung transplantation in dogs. Ann Thorac Surg 44: 145

17. Kontos GJ, Adachi H, Borkon AM, Cameron DE, Baumgartner WA, Hutchins GM, Brawn J, Reitz BA (1987) A no flush, core-cooling technique for successful cardiopulmonary preservation in heart lung transplantation. J Thorac Cardiovasc Surg 94: 836

18. Jurmann MJ, Dammenhayn L, Schäfers HJ, Wahlers Th, Fieguth HG, Haverich A (1987) Prostacyclin as an additive to single crystalloid flush. Improved pulmonary preservation in heart-lung transplantation. Transplant Proc 19: 4103

19. Cremer J, Jurmann M, Dammenhayn L, Wahlers TH, Haverich A, Borst HG (1989) Oxygen free radical scavengers to prevent pulmonary reperfusion injury after heart-lung transplantation. J Heart Transplant 8: 330

20. Detterbeck FC, Keagy BA, Paull DE, Wilcox BR (1990) Oxygen free radical scavengers decrease reperfusion injury in lung transplantation. Ann Thorac Surg 5: 204

21. Hirt SW, Wahlers Th, Jurmann M, Dammenhayn L, Kemnitz J, Haverich A University of Wisconsin-versus Euro-Collins solution for lung preservation. Ann Thorac Surg (in press)

22. Veith FJ, Crane R, Torres M, Colon I, Hagstrom JWC, Pinsker K, Koerner SK (1976) Effective preservation and transportation of lung transplants. J Thorac Cardiovasc Surg 72: 97

23. Naka Y, Shirakura R, Matsuda H, Nakata S, Kawaguchi N, Fukushima S, Nakano S, Kawashima Y (1990) Canine heart-lung transplantation after 24 hours of hypothermic preservation. Eur J Cardiovasc Surg 4: 499

Transplant Int (1992) 5 [Suppl 1]: S379–S381

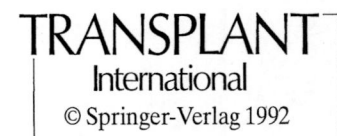

TRANSPLANT
International
© Springer-Verlag 1992

Usefulness of ^{31}P-MRS as a method of evaluating the viability of preserved and transplanted rat liver

Y. Kanetsuna, S. Fujita, T. Tojimbara, S. Fuchinoue, S. Teraoka, and K. Ota

3rd Department of Surgery, Tokyo Women's Medical College, 8-1 Kawada-cho, Shinjuku-ku, Tokyo, Japan

Abstract. We used phosphorus-31 magnetic resonance spectroscopy (^{31}P-MRS) to evaluate the viability of transplanted rat liver. Wistar rats were used as donors and recipients. The donor livers were preserved in saline (group 1), Euro-Collins solution (group 2), or in University of Wisconsin (UW) solution (group 3) for 3 and 6 h in groups 1, 2 and 3 and for 9 h in groups 2 and 3. Thereafter the livers were orthotopically transplanted. ^{31}P-MRS spectra were measured after portal reperfusion. Finally, all the recipients were divided into survivors and non-survivors. Survival rates were better in group 3 than in groups 1 and 2. In the 9-h-preserved livers, the livers in group 3 showed a significantly higher β-ATP/Pi ratio than those in group 2. Comparing survivors and non-survivors in the 6-h-preserved livers in group 2, survivors' livers showed significantly higher β-ATP/Pi ratio than those of non-survivors. We concluded that ^{31}P-MRS is a useful method for assessing viability of rat liver grafts.

Key words: ^{31}P-MRS – β-ATP/Pi ratio – Liver transplantation – Graft viability

Phosphorus-31 nuclear magnetic resonance spectroscopy (^{31}P-MRS) is a noninvasive technique for monitoring the energy metabolism of tissues and organs at the cellular level. With this method, we evaluated the viability of preserved and transplanted rat liver and studied the relationship between ^{31}P-MRS and prognosis.

Materials and methods

A total of 72 male Wistar rats, weighing 250–400 g were used as donors and recipients. All animals were treated according to the ethical rule for experimental animals of Tokyo Women's Medical College, and all operations were performed under ether anaesthesia.

Offprint requests to: Yukiko Kanetsuna, M.D., 3rd Department of Surgery, Tokyo Women's Medical College, 8-1 Kawada-cho, Shinjuku-ku, Tokyo 162, Japan

Prior to excision, the donor livers were perfused with saline via the portal vein. Then the livers were excised and perfused with each preservation solution. The livers were preserved at 4°C in saline (group 1), in Euro-Collins solution (EC) (group 2), or in University of Wisconsin (UW) solution (group 3) for 3 and 6 h in groups 1, 2 and 3 and for 9 h in groups 2 and 3. In group 1, the 6-hour-preserved livers showed such a low survival rate that 9-hour-preservation was not performed. After cold storage, the livers were orthotopically transplanted using the Kamada method. ^{31}P-MRS spectra were measured before the donor hepatectomy (control), and every 10 min from 15 to 105 min after portal reperfusion. Finally, all the recipients were divided into survivors (recipients surviving more than 48 h after transplantation) and non-survivors.

^{31}P-MRS spectra were recorded using a 2.1 Tesla bore superconducting magnet interfaced with a spectrometer (BEM 250/80, Otsuka Electronics, Osaka, Japan) operating at 34.45 MHz for phosphorus and 85.12 MHz for protones. A surface coil was placed on the surface of the liver graft. ^{31}P-MRS spectra were attained using a radiofrequency of 34 μsec wave length applied every 2 s. For each study, data from 300 scans were accumulated and summed to produce each spectrum. β-ATP/Pi ratios were calculated from the peak areas. The data were statistically analyzed with two sample *t*-test.

Results

The mean β-ATP/Pi ratio in the controls was 1.18 ± 0.16 (mean ± SD). Table 1 shows the number of survivors and

Table 1. The number of survivors and non-survivors in each group

	Preservation time	Survivors	Non-survivors	Total	Survival rate
Group 1					
Saline	3 h	7	1	8	0.88
Saline	6 h	4	5	9	0.44
Group 2					
EC	3 h	8	1	9	0.89
EC	6 h	7	3	10	0.70
EC	9 h	6	3	9	0.67
Group 3					
UW	3 h	8	2	10	0.80
UW	6 h	6	2	8	0.75
UW	9 h	8	1	9	0.89

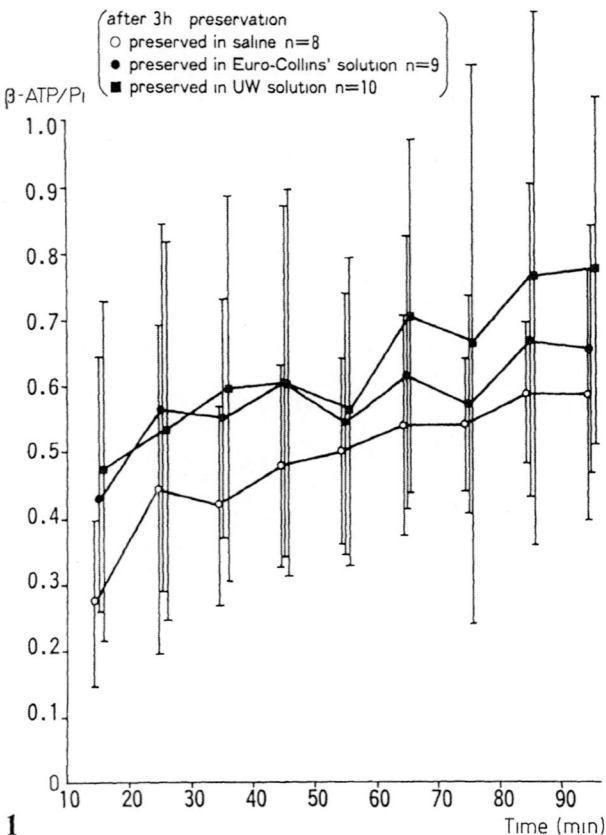

Change in β-ATP/Pi ratio after portal reperfusion
(mean±SD)

after 3h preservation
○ preserved in saline n=8
● preserved in Euro-Collins' solution n=9
■ preserved in UW solution n=10

β-ATP/Pi

Time (min)

1

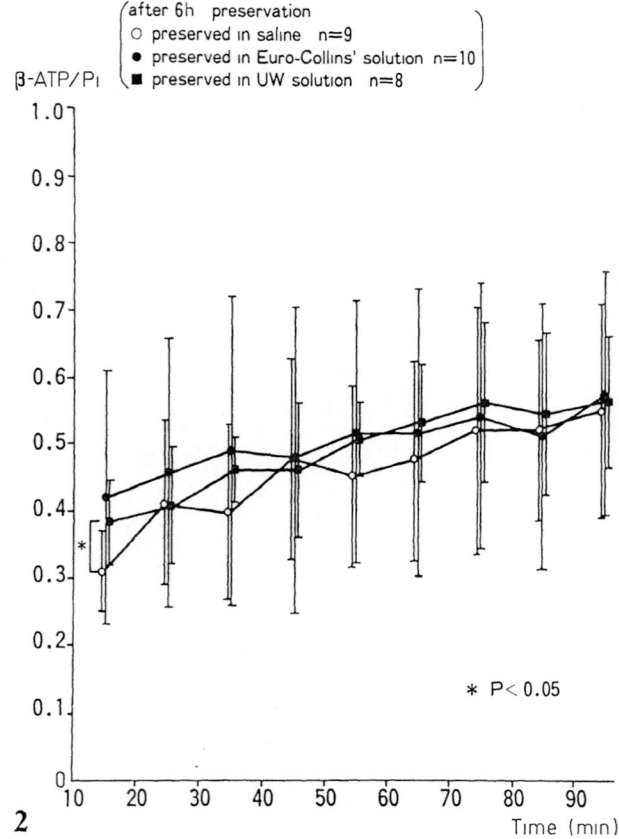

Change in β-ATP/Pi ratio after portal reperfusion
(mean±SD)

after 6h preservation
○ preserved in saline n=9
● preserved in Euro-Collins' solution n=10
■ preserved in UW solution n=8

β-ATP/Pi

* P< 0.05

Time (min)

2

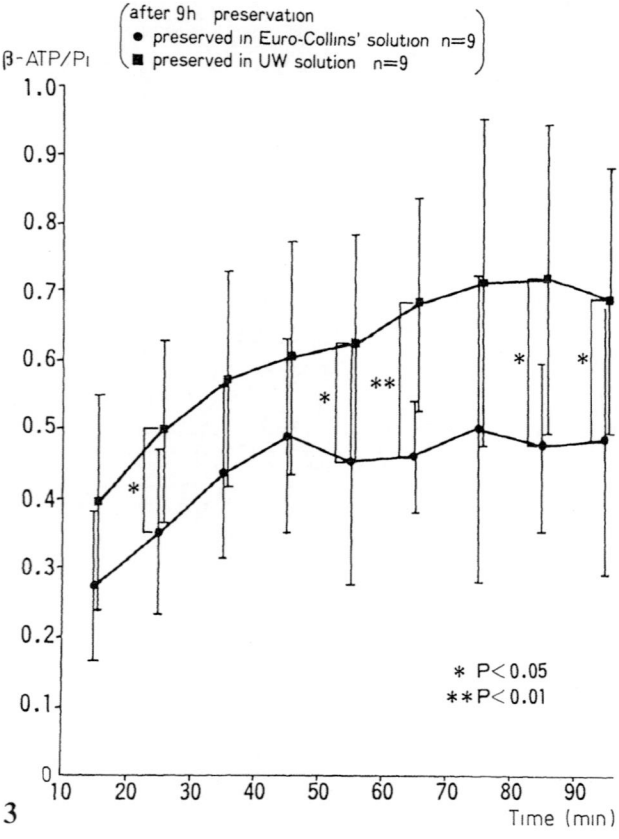

Change in β-ATP/Pi ratio after portal reperfusion
(mean±SD)

after 9h preservation
● preserved in Euro-Collins' solution n=9
■ preserved in UW solution n=9

β-ATP/Pi

* P< 0.05
**P< 0.01

Time (min)

3

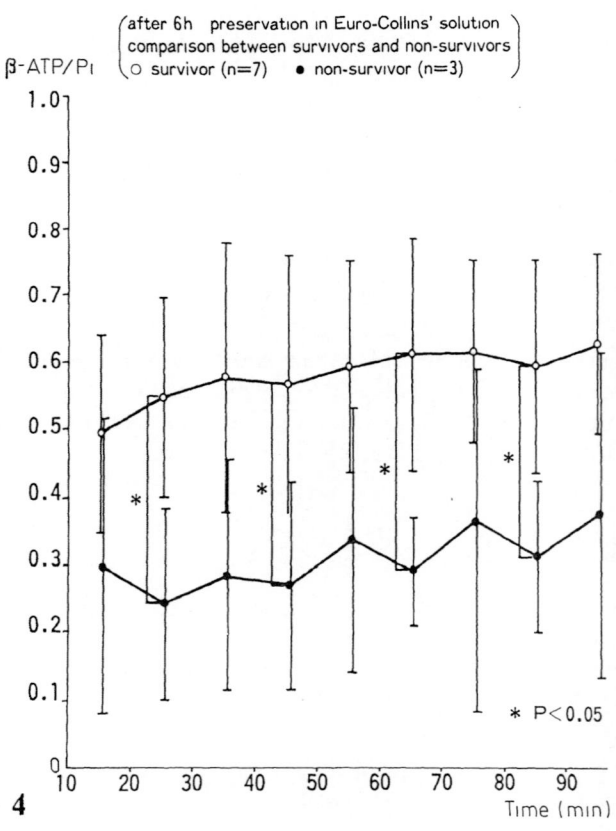

Change in β-ATP/Pi ratio after portal reperfusion
(mean±SD)

after 6h preservation in Euro-Collins' solution
comparison between survivors and non-survivors
○ survivor (n=7)   ● non-survivor (n=3)

β-ATP/Pi

* P< 0.05

Time (min)

4

non-survivors in each group. In the saline-preserved group (group 1), the survival rate decreased to 44 % in the 6-h-preserved group. In the EC-preserved group (group 2), the survival rate decreased to 67 % in the 9-h-preserved group. However, in the UW-preserved group (group 3), recipients showed high survival rates until 9 h of preservation.

After 3 h preservation, no significant difference in β-ATP/Pi ratio was observed between the three groups (Fig.1), while after 6 h preservation, a significant difference was observed only at 15 to 25 min after portal reperfusion (Fig.2). After 9 h preservation, liver grafts in group 3 showed significantly ($P < 0.05$) higher β-ATP/Pi ratios than those in group 2 at 25, 55, 65, 85, and 95 min after portal reperfusion (Fig.3).

Comparing survivors and non-survivors, after 6 h preservation in EC (group 2), a significant difference was observed in the β-ATP/Pi ratio (Fig.4). In this case, survivors' liver grafts showed significantly higher β-ATP/Pi ratios at 25, 45, 65, and 85 min after the portal reperfusion.

Discussion

Liver transplantations are increasing in number and have been established as the treatment for end-stage liver disease. Although many studies evaluating graft viability have been reported, the results remain controversial. Even now, primary nonfunction occurs in about 5–10 % of liver transplants, reflecting a poor prognosis and the need for retransplantation. It has been suggested that graft viability is dependent upon its capacity to regenerate ATP, the energy source indispensable for protein synthesis, res-

toration of ion gradients, bile production, other factors in metabolism [1, 2].

The measurement of hepatic phosphorus metabolites and inorganic phosphate by ^{31}P-MRS has been performed widely using perfusion models, and it has been proven to be an excellent, objective, noninvasive method for assessing the energy status of liver grafts. In this study, we used ^{31}P-MRS to evaluate the viability of preserved and transplanted rat liver using the β-ATP/Pi ratio which is regarded as reflecting energy availability. The survival rate in group 2 was higher than that in group 1, and it was highest in group 3. Although no significant difference existed in the grafts transplanted after 3 h preservation, the β-ATP/Pi ratios after transplantation in group 2 and 3 were higher than those in group 1 but not significantly so. After 9 h preservation, β-ATP/Pi ratios after transplantation in group 3 were higher than those in group 2 after portal reperfusion. Thus, after 9 h preservation, UW-preserved livers had more satisfactory results compared with those of EC-preserved livers. In the 6-hour-EC-preserved group, survivors' livers showed significantly higher β-ATP/Pi ratios after portal reperfusion compared with those of non-survivors. Therefore, we concluded that the capacity of ATP regeneration at an early stage, namely, 15–105 minutes after portal reperfusion is important in predicting the subsequent recovery of graft function.

We concluded that ^{31}P-MRS could be used in evaluating graft viability and in predicting graft nonfunction at an early stage.

Fig.1. Change in β-ATP/Pi ratio after portal reperfusion after 3 h preservation

Fig.2. Change in β-ATP/Pi ratio after portal reperfusion after 6 h preservation

Fig.3. Change in β-ATP/Pi ratio after portal reperfusion after 9 h preservation

Fig.4. Change in β-ATP/Pi ratio after portal reperfusion after 6 h preservation in EC-solution

References

1. Lanir A, Clouse ME, Lee RGL (1987) Liver preservation for transplant. Evaluation of hepatic energy metabolism by ^{31}P-NMR. Transplantation 43: 786–790
2. Palombo JD, Pomposelli JJ, Fechner KD, Blackburn GL, Bistrian BR (1991) Enhanced restoration in UW solution by provision of adenosine during reperfusion. Transplantation 51: 867–873
3. Momii S, Koga A (1990) Time related morphological changes in cold-stored rat livers. Transplantation 50: 745–750
4. McKeown CM, Edwards V, Phillips MJ, Petrunka CN, Stersberg SM (1988) Sinusoidal lining cell damage: the critical injury in cold preservation of liver allografts in the rat. Transplantation 46: 178–191

Transplant Int (1992) 5 [Suppl 1]: S 382–S 387

TRANSPLANT
International
© Springer-Verlag 1992

Predictive value of liver tissue flow in assessment of the viability of liver grafts after extended preservation in pigs

Y. I. Kim[1], T. Kai[1], K. Kawano[1], S. Goto[1], Y. Kodama[2], F. Yasunaga[2], M. Takeyama[2], S. Akizuki[3], N. Kamada[4], and M. Kobayashi[1]

[1] Departments of Surgery I, [2] Hospital Pharmacy, and [3] Pathology, Oita Medical College, Oita, Japan
[4] Department of Experimental Surgery, The National Children's Medical Research Centre, Tokyo, Japan

Abstract. The crucial damage in cold storage of liver allografts is to the hepatic sinusoidal lining (microcirculation). Using different solutions, we studied whether determinations of graft tissue flow were valuable in estimating the viability of liver grafts. Twenty-three pairs of female pigs underwent orthotopic liver transplantation and were assigned to five groups according to the cold preservation time or solutions used: in group I the liver grafts were stored in Euro-Collins solution (EC) for 4 h ($n = 3$), in group II the grafts were stored in EC for 12 h ($n = 5$), in group III the donor was pretreated with azathioprine (AZA), 1 mg/kg per day, orally (PO) for 3 days before harvesting and the graft was implanted after 12 h cold storage with EC ($n = 6$), in group IV the graft was stored in modified University of Wisconsin solution (mUW) for 4 h ($n = 3$), and in group V the graft was stored in mUW for 24 h ($n = 6$). Liver tissue blood flow (LTBF) was measured, using a laser doppler device, at 60 min after recirculation of the graft. In the case of EC preservation, LTBF (ml/100 g of liver tissue per min) correlated well with 4-day survival: 21.2 ± 3.0 ml/100 g of tissue per min mean $\pm$ SD, in group I (3/3, 100 %); 10.0 ± 2.8 ml/100 g of tissue per min in group II (0/5, 0 %); and 19.1 ± 3.4 ml/100 g of tissue per min in group III (5/6, 83.3 %) ($P < 0.05$, group II vs I and III). All grafts with LTBF of more than 15 ml/100 g tissue per min functioned well. However, changes in microcirculation of the mUW-stored livers did not correlate with early function of the graft: 23.0 ± 2.3 ml/100 g of tissue per min in group IV (4-day survival; 3 of 3, 100 %) and 23.5 ± 9.1 ml/100 g of tissue per min in group V (0 of 6, 0 %). This was accompanied by graft dehydration during storage and an increased number of erythrocytes in the hepatic sinusoids post-recirculation. We concluded that assessment of liver tissue flow by LDF was very helpful and easy to apply in predicting liver graft failure in the case of preservation with Euro-Collins solution. However, LTBF should be carefully evaluated as a marker of liver graft viability when the liver graft is preserved with mUW.

Key words: Liver transplantation – Liver tissue flow – Laser doppler flowmetry – Euro-Collins solution – Modified University of Wisconsin solution – Liver graft function

In recent years, there has been growing evidence that the integrity of non-parenchymal cells plays a crucial role in liver graft function after extended cold preservation [1–4]. Cold ischemia damages hapatic sinusoidal endothelium preferentially, which becomes particularly vulnerable when exposed to reflow of the recipient's circulation. Subsequently, the loss of viability of sinusoidal endothelial cells can cause severe microcirculatory disturbances with tissue hypoperfusion, finally compromising parenchymal hepatocyte function, resulting in liver graft failure. In this context, we postulated a correlation between the state of hepatic microcirculation and liver graft viability following hepatic transplantation. Therefore, in this study we investigated whether assessment of hepatic microcirculation is efficacious in predicting early function and survival of liver allografts post-transplantation. To test our hypothesis, we used different periods and solutions for liver preservation. Liver tissue blood flow (LTBF) was assessed by laser doppler flowmetry (LDF).

Materials and methods

Transplantation procedure. We used 23 pairs of female mongrel pigs (18–36 kg) in this study. After intratracheal intubation, liver transplantation was performed under general anesthesia with a mixture of oxygen (2 l/min), nitrous oxide (2 l/min), and fluothane (0.2 %). The technique of pig liver allografting has been described in detail elsewhere [5]. Briefly, the donor liver was removed after systemic heparinization (2000 units) by cooling via the portal vein and celiac axis with 1.5 l of preservation solution (4°C). A total of 1.4 l of solution was perfused through the portal vein and 100 ml through the celiac artery. The biliary tree was flushed with 50 ml of solution. The graft was stored in a refrigerator at 4°C. The recipient hepatectomy

Offprint requests to: Y. I. Kim, Department of Surgery I, Oita Medical College, Oita, 879-55, Japan

Table 1. Outcomes following orthotopic transplantation of liver treated with different solutions and periods of preservation (mean ± SD)

Group	Total ischemia time (h) (n)	Survival (days)	LTBF (ml/100 g tissue per min) (n)	4-day survival (%)
I (EC/4 h)	4.1 ± 0.2 (3)	5, 29, 8	21.2 ± 3.0 (n = 3)	3/3 (100)
II (EC/12 h)	12.6 ± 0.5 (5)	0, 0, 0, 0, 2	10.0 ± 2.8[*] (n = 4)	0/5[**] (0)
III (EC-AZA/12 h)	12.6 ± 0.3 (6)	6, 4, 4, 8, 9, 0	19.1 ± 3.4 (n = 6)	5/6 (83)
IV (mUW/4 h)	4.0 ± 0.6 (3)	6, 6, 11	23.0 ± 2.3 (n = 3)	3/3[***] (100)
V (mUW/24 h)	24.9 ± 0.6 (6)	0, 0, 0, 0, 0, 0	23.5 ± 9.1 (n = 6)	0/6 (0)

$P < 0.05$, [*] vs all other groups, [**] vs groups I and III and [***] vs group V

was carried out with a pump-driven venous bypass connecting the portal and external iliac veins and the external jugular vessel following heparinization (2000 units). The bypass blood flow was maintained above 30 ml/min per kg with a Bio-pump (Bio Medicus, Minn). Arterial and central venous cannulation in the recipient was carried out via a cervial and groin cutdown for monitoring, blood sampling and administration of fluids and medication. Calcium gluconate (850 mg), sodium bicarbonate (40 mEq), and protamine sulfate (10 mg) were administered intravenously (IV) when the blood flow was restored. The donor liver was orthotopically implanted with a suprahepatic vena caval anastomosis (Prolene 4-0), followed by the portal vein anastomosis (cuff technique). Immediately before the completion of the portal vein anastomosis, the graft was flushed via the portal vein with 500 ml of lactated Ringer's solution. Following revascularization, the vena caval anastomosis below the liver (cuff technique) and hepatic artery (Prolene 6-0) was performed. The bile duct was anastomosed by telescoping using a stent. The animals received a constant IV infusion of lactated Ringer's solution (30 ml/kg per h) during surgery and approximately 1000 ml of the same solution postoperatively. They were first fed 24 h after revascularization. One unit of blood was transfused from donor to recipient as the sole coagulation support. Cefamandole (1 g) was given IV daily until day 3.

Experimental protocols. Euro-Collins (EC) and modified University of Wisconsin solutions (mUW) (the additives of original UW solution, adenosine, glutathione, allopurinol, insulin and dexamethasone, and a colloid-5% hydroyethyl starch were omitted) [6] were chosen. The animals were divided into five groups. In group I (EC/4 h, n = 3), the liver graft was stored in EC and implanted 4 h following harvesting. In group II (EC/12 h, n = 5), the liver was stored in EC for 12 h. In group III (EC-AZA/12 h, n = 6), the donor was pretreated with azathioprine (AZA), 1 mg/kg per day, orally (PO) for 3 days, and the graft was preserved as in group II. In group IV (mUW/4 h, n = 3), the liver was preserved in mUW and implanted after harvesting as in group I. In group V (mUW/24 h, n = 6), the liver was transplanted after 24 h of cold storage in mUW.
Parameters and statistics. The 4-day survival rate and liver tissue blood flow (LTBF) were studied as well as graft weight change, histology, coagulation and serum biochemistry. LTBF was measured during donor harvesting and at 1 h after portal venous reflow of the graft with a laser doppler device (model BPM 403A, TSI, St. Paul, Minn.). A representative estimate was the mean of 3 to 6 determinations which were provided by randomly placing the probe in different areas in the same liver. For histology, graft biopsy specimens were stained with hematoxylin and eosin and examined by an independent pathologist (SA). All values were given as mean ± SD. Statistical analysis was made by using the chi-square test or Student's *t*-test. A P value of less than 0.05 was considered to be statistically significant.

Results

The outcomes of the liver transplants are described in Table 1. All animals receiving transplants approximately 4 h after liver harvesting were alive for more than 5 days (groups I and IV). In contrast, no pig survived beyond 2 days in the EC/12 h (group II) and the mUW/24 h groups (group V). Five of six pigs survived more than 4 days in group III (EC-AZA/12 h) in which the donor was pretreated with AZA. The hepatoprotective effect of AZA pretreatment has been discussed elsewhere [4].

Figure 1 shows the changes in liver tissue flow (LTBF) of the allografts during the transplantation procedure. In the case of storage in EC, the LTBF post-recirculation was significantly higher in the EC-AZA/12 h group (group III), which showed improved animal survival, than that in group II (EC/12 h) which had poor graft survival; all eight grafts (five in group III and all three livers in group I) with LTBF of more than 15 ml/100 g of liver tissue per min functioned well post-implantation. However, all pigs died on the day of surgery in the mUW/24 h group (group V) in spite of a well-maintained flow of the graft tissue.

As shown in Fig. 2, there was no correlation between the transaminase levels and animal survival in the EC groups (groups I, II and III). In the groups treated with mUW, AST was significantly higher in the non-surviving pigs (group V) than that in the pigs with improved survival (group IV). There were no differences in prothrombin values among the groups.

Liver weight changes during cold preservation are shown in Fig. 3. It is of note that the liver grafts in mUW groups (IV and V) lost weight significantly during storage, when compared with the changes in EC groups (I, II and III).

Representative livers at the end of preservation and 1 h after implantation are shown in Fig. 4. As shown in Fig. 4B and C, EC preservation for 12 h caused substantial swelling of hepatocytes. There was substantial damage to the graft after re-flow of blood for 1 h (eosinophilic and fatty degeneration of hepatocytes, parenchymal haemorrhage, and diffuse neutrophil infiltration in the sinusoids) (Fig. 4B'). This was significantly ameliorated by AZA

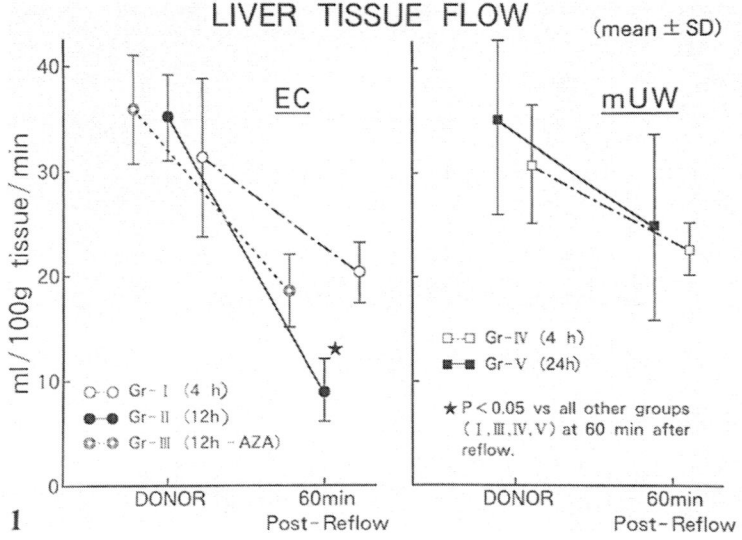

LIVER TISSUE FLOW (mean ± SD)

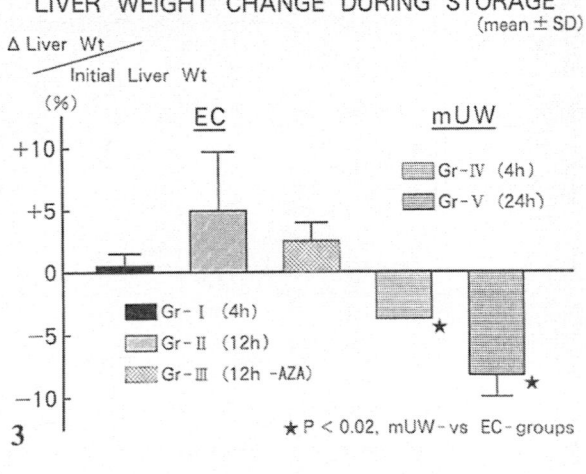

LIVER WEIGHT CHANGE DURING STORAGE (mean ± SD)

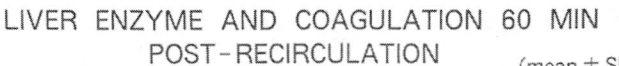

LIVER ENZYME AND COAGULATION 60 MIN POST-RECIRCULATION (mean ± SD)

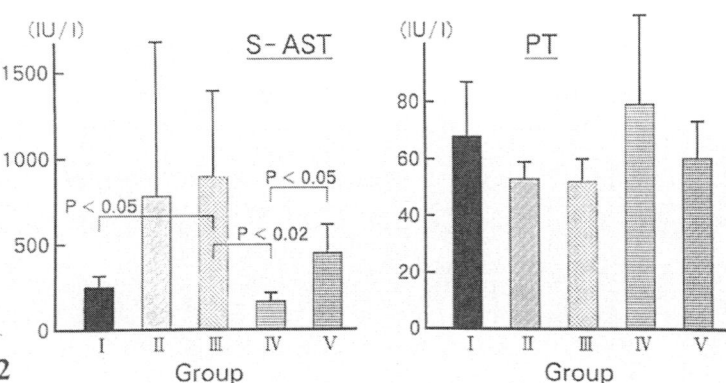

Fig. 1. Tissue flow of the liver graft (LTBF) during harvesting and 60 min after implantation

Fig. 2. Values for serum aspartate aminotransferase (S-AST) and prothrombin time (PT) 60 min after transplantation of the liver graft. The numbers examined in groups I–V were 3, 4, 6, 3, and 6, respectively

Fig. 3. Changes in weight of the liver graft during cold preservation. The numbers examined in groups I–V were 3, 5, 6, 3, and 6, respectively

pretreatment in donors (Fig. 4 C'). In comparison with EC-stored liver, mUW storage caused marked shrinkage of parenchymal hepatocytes with subsequent dilatation of sinusoidal spaces (Fig. 4 D). An increased number of erythrocytes were found in the sinusoidal lumen at 60 min after transplantation (Fig. 4 D').

Discussion

To date, no parameters are available for early, accurate forecasting of liver graft failure; therefore, the patient's condition becomes critical when emergency retransplantation is needed. Biochemical assessment, such as hepatic enzyme release, energy status, and biopsy findings, are unpredictable or time-consuming procedures, and thus not practical on clinical grounds [7–10]. There was no correlation in the present study between animal survival and serum levels of transaminase (AST) when the graft was preserved with Euro-Collins solution.

Hepatic sinusoidal endothelium is the first target tissue facing reflow of the recipient's circulation, therefore, injury to the microvasculature is the primary effect of ischemia/reperfusion insult of the liver graft [1–4]. The parenchymal hepatocytes are subsequently damaged because of disturbances in metabolic exchanges through the sinusoidal endothelium. Indeed, evidence has accumulated that the integrity of the hepatic endothelial cells plays a key role in graft viability, particularly in the case of early ischemia/reperfusion. Therefore, it would be reasonable to speculate that assessment of hepatic microcirculation could be a marker of graft function. In line with this hypothesis, Manner et al. [11] have reported recently that the state of graft tissue perfusion correlates well with preservation damage in pig liver transplantation. They suggest, using H2-clearance technique and HTK solution, that assessment of hepatic microcirculation (30 min post-transplantation) is efficacious in predicting early function and survival of liver grafts.

Our results showed that LTBF was very effective in predicting the viability of liver grafts when preserved with

Fig. 4. Representative livers **A–D** at the end of cold preservation and **A'–D'** 60 min after implantation. **A** and **A'** group I (EC/4 h), **B** and **B'** group II (EC/12 h), **C** and **C'** group III (EC-AZA/12 h), **D** and **D'** group V (mUW/24 h) (Hematoxylin and eosin, ×90)

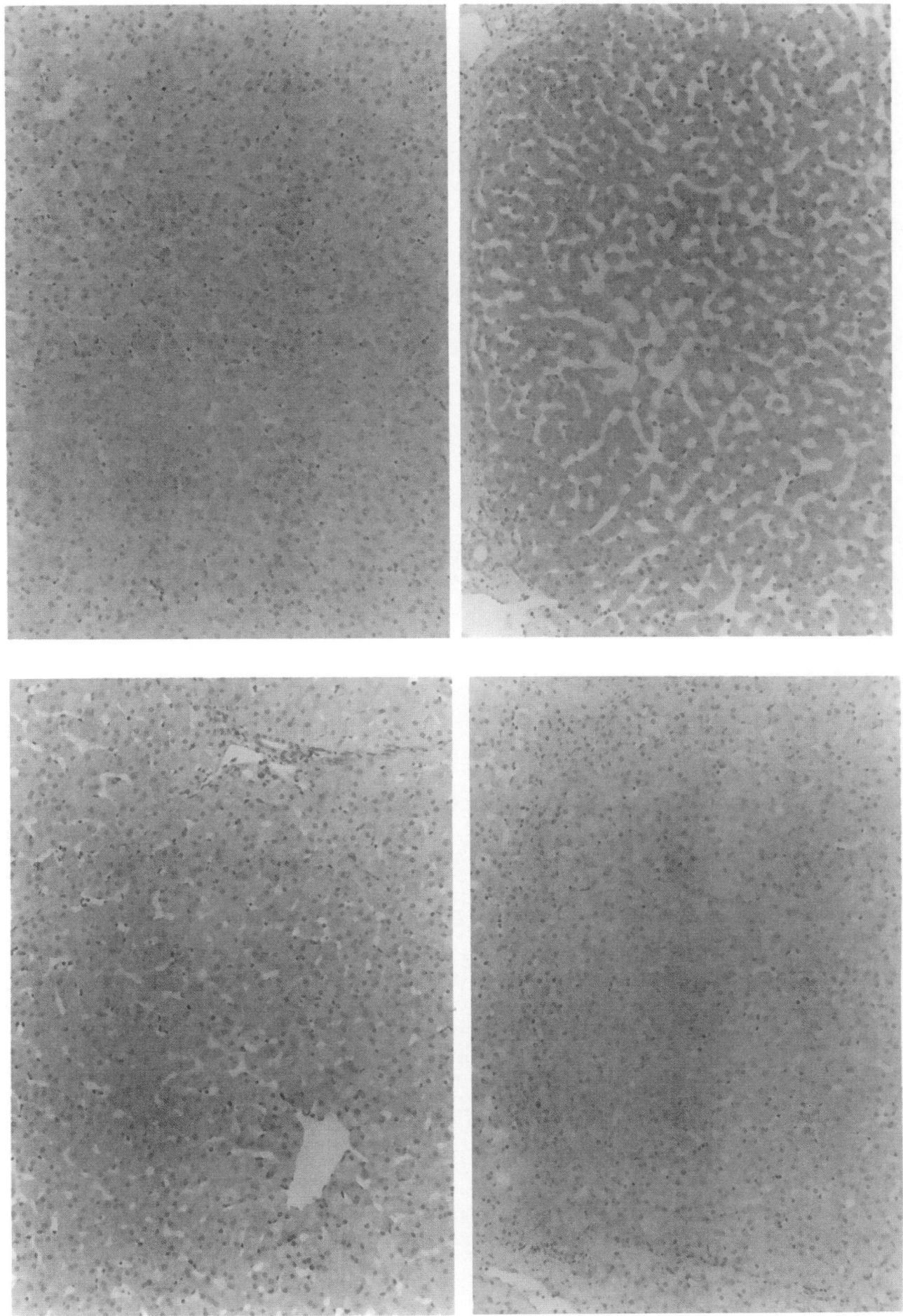

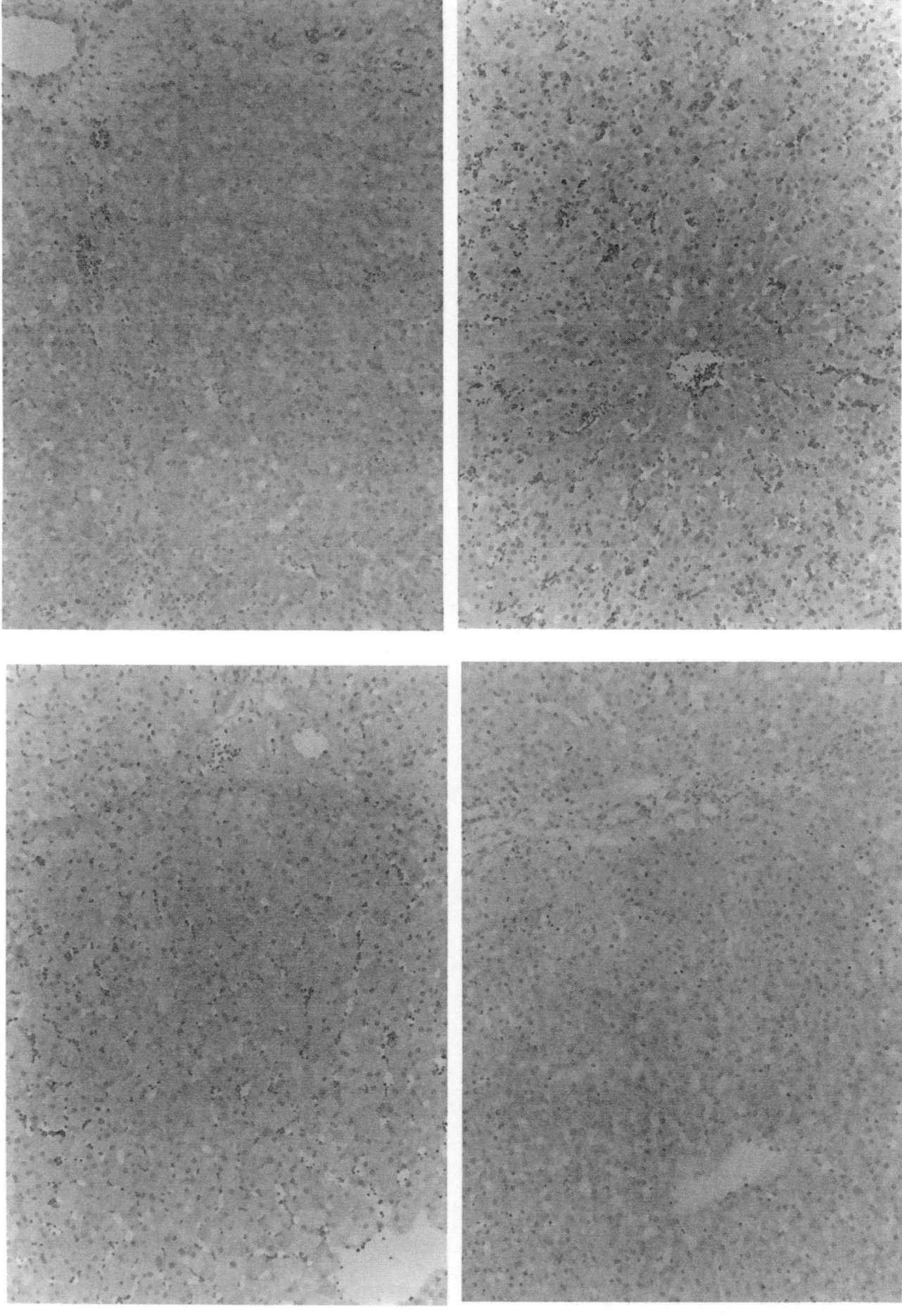

the Euro-Collins solution; all grafts with LTBF of more than 15 ml/100 g of liver tissue per min functioned well. However, changes in microcirculation of the mUW-stored liver did not correlate with the function of the graft. One explanatation may be the significant graft dehydration induced by mUW. We hypothesize that shrinkage of parenchymal hepatocytes temporarily ameliorated hepatic microcirculation by widening the sinusoidal lumen early during graft recirculation. Another possibility may have to do with our measurement technique (LDF). Since LDF is able to monitor blood flow in a small surface range of liver tissue ($1–2\ mm^3$), it is possible that the small volume of tissue in which LDF measures perfusion is not always representative of total hepatic blood flow [12]. This is of importance in the case of early estimation of the graft recirculation when the state of hepatic microcirculation can be different from site to site or particularly between the deep and surface portion of the allografts. We should be able to estimate more accurately the state of microcirculation if LTBF is evaluated later, in other words, a few hours post-transplantation or at the time of closure of the abdomen. Based on our data, we concluded that assessment of liver tissue flow by LDF is very helpful and easy to apply for predicting liver graft failure in the case of Euro-Collins preservation. However, LTBF should be carefully evaluated as a marker of liver graft viability when the liver graft is preserved in mUW.

Acknowledgements. The authors wish thank Professor M. Ito and Mr. Y. Magari, Department of Laboratory Medicine, Oita Medical College, Oita, Japan, for assistance and Miss M. Arakane for preparing the manuscript. This work was supported by a Grant-in-Aid (A-01440054) for general scientific research from the Ministry of Education of Japan.

References

1. McKeown CMB, Edwards V, Phillips MJ, Harvey PRC, Petrunka CN, Strasberg SM (1988) Sinusoidal lining cell damage: The critical injury in cold preservation of liver allografts in the rats. Transplantation 46: 178–191
2. Caldwell-Kenkel JC, Currin RT, Tanaka Y, Thurman RG, Lemasters JJ (1989) Reperfusion injury to endothelial cells following cold ischemic storage of rat livers. Hepatology 10: 292–299
3. Thurman RG, Marzi I, Seitz G, et al. (1988) Hepatic reperfusion injury following orthotopic liver transplantation in the rat. Transplantation 46: 502–506
4. Kim YI, Kawano K, Goto S, et al. (1991) Beneficial effect of pretreatment with azathioprine on warm and cold ischemia of the swine liver. Transplant Proc 23: 2201–2203
5. Calne RY (1987) Technique in the pig. In: Calne RY (ed) Liver Transplantation. Grune & Stratton, Orlando, Fla., pp 9–16
6. Goto S, Kim YI, Kodama Y, et al. The beneficial effect of a stable prostacyclin analog (op-41483) on rat liver preserved for 24 hours with lactobionate solution. Transplantation, in press
7. Fath JJ, Ascher NL, Konstantinides FN, et al. (1984) Metabolism during hepatic transplantation: indicators of allograft function. Surgery 96: 664–673
8. Kamiike W, Burdelski M, Steinhoff G, Ringe B, Lauchart W, Pichlmayr R (1988) Adenine nucleotide metabolism and its relation to organ viability in human liver transplantation. Transplantation 45: 138–143
9. Ray RA, Lewin KJ, Colonna J et al. (1988) The role of liver biopsy in evaluating acute allograft dysfunction following liver transplantation. Hum Pathol 19: 835–848
10. Forster J, Greig PB, Glynn MFX, et al. (1989) Prediction of graft function following liver transplantation. Transplant Proc 21: 3356–3357
11. Manner M, Shult W, Senninger N, Machens G, Otto G (1990) Evaluation of preservation damage after porcine liver transplantation by assessment of hepatic microcirculation. Transplantation 50: 940–943
12. Shepherd AP, Riedel GL, Kiel JW, Haumschild DJ, Maxwell LC (1987) Evaluation of an infrared laser-Doppler blood flowmeter. Am J Physiol 252: G832–G839

Transplant Int (1992) 5 [Suppl 1]: S 388–S 390

TRANSPLANT
International
© Springer-Verlag 1992

Successful 96-hour preservation of the canine pancreas

Y. Kuroda, Y. Fujino, A. Morita, Y. Tanioka, Y. Suzuki, T. Kawamura, Y. Ku, and Y. Saitoh

First Department of Surgery, Kobe University School of Medicine, Kobe, Japan

Abstract. We tested the preservation of the pancreas for 96 h by a modified two-layer (UW solution/perfluorochemical) cold storage method (group 1) in the canine model of pancreas autotransplantation and compared this with an original two-layer (Euro-Collins' solution/perfluorochemical) cold storage method (group 2) and simple cold storage method with UW solution (group 3). A graft was considered functioning if the dog had a normal blood glucose for at least 5 days after transplantation. The functional success rates after preservation for 72 h were 100%, 100% and 80% for groups 1, 2 and 3 respectively. On the other hand, the functional success rates for groups 1, 2 and 3 after preservation for 96 h were 75%, 0% and 0% respectively. The mean K value of 96-hour preserved grafts for group 1 at 2 weeks after transplantation was 1.52 ± 0.30 compared with 1.98 ± 0.48 before preservation. Biopsies of grafts from group 1 showed almost normal pancreatic architecture even after preservation for 96 h. In addition, biopsies of grafts preserved for 96 h in group 1 at 4 weeks after transplantation showed almost normal endocrine tissue with mild fibrosis of the exocrine tissue. This study demonstrated the possibility of preserving the pancreas for 96 h prior to transplantation.

Key words: Pancreatic transplantation – University of Wisconsin solution – Perfluorochemical – Preservation for 96 h

To reduce ischemic cell injury and tissue edema during simple cold storage of the pancreas, we have developed a two-layer [Euro-Collins' solution (EC)/perfluorochemical (PFC)] cold storage method [1], that continuously supplies sufficient oxygen to the pancreas during preservation [2], and extends preservation time of the canine pancreas with EC for up to 72 h [3]. On the other hand, a new flush-out and preservation solution, University of Wisconsin solution (UW solution), has been developed to reduce cell swelling during preservation [4, 5] and also extends the preservation time of the canine pancreas for up to 72 h [6].

Although the exact mechanism of action of UW solution and the two-layer method in pancreatic preservation is not yet clear, we used UW solution as a flush-out and preservation solution in place of EC in the two-layer cold storage method and examined the possibility of extending the preservation time of canine pancreas for more than 72 h. In this paper, we report the success of 96-hour preservation of the canine pancreas by a modified two-layer (UW solution/PFC) cold storage method.

Materials and methods

Mongrel dogs of both sexes, weighing 12–18 kg were used for the experiments. Perfluorodecaline, which is one of the PFCs, was a kind gift of Dr. K. Yokoyama (The Green Cross Corporation, Osaka, Japan). UW solution was purchased from E. I. Du Pont de Nemours, Waukegan, Ill., USA.

Operation procedures. Anesthesia was induced and maintained with sodium pentobarbiturate (25 mg/kg). After the abdomen was opened, a left lobectomy of the pancreas with the splenic artery and vein attached was meticulously performed, followed by splenectomy. The segmental pancreatic graft was washed with 50 ml of cold heparinized EC (1000 units/50 ml EC or UW solution) through the splenic artery and autotransplanted in the neck after preservation, as has been described previously [7], excising the remainder of the pancreas at the time of autotransplantation. After the operation, the dogs received saline with 10% glucose (30 ml/kg) and parenteral penicillin (25 mg/kg) for 3 days. After 3 days, standard kennel diets were given.

Preservation method. The two-layer cold storage method was performed as has been described previously by our group [1, 3]. The pancreatic graft was floated on the PFC, covered with EC or UW solution in a styrofoam box packed with ice and oxygenated throughout the storage period (Fig. 1).

Offprint requests to: Yoshikazu Kuroda, M. D., First Department of Surgery, Kobe University School of Medicine, 7-5-2, Kusunoki-cho, Chuo-ku, Kobe 650, Japan

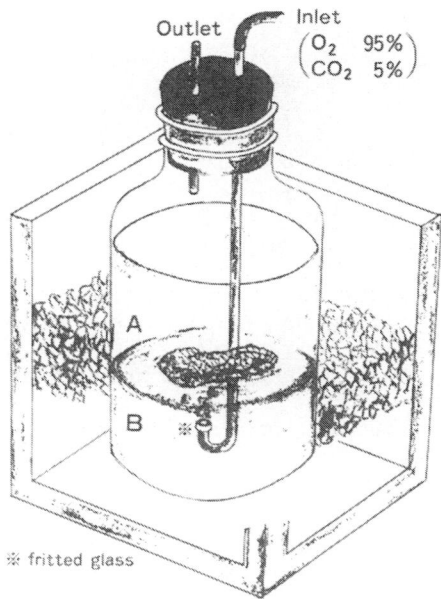

Fig. 1. The two-layer cold storage method. Oxygenation was continued through the fritted glass to PFC throughout the storage period, the pancreatic graft being surrounded by cold UW solution or EC and PFC in a styrofoam box packed with ice. *A*, UW solution or EC; *B*, perfluorochemical

Functional studies. Blood glucose concentration was determined daily during the 1st postoperative week after autotransplantation and biweekly thereafter. Intravenous glucose tolerance tests (IVGTT) were performed at 2 weeks after transplantation. Maintenance of normoglycemia for at least 5 days after transplantation was considered successful preservation [8].

Histological studies. Biopsies of the pancreatic grafts were taken at the time of the original operation, after 72 or 96 h preservation, at 4 weeks after transplantation and at autopsy. The tissue was fixed in Zamboni's solution, paraffin-embedded and stained with hematoxylin and eosin.

Experimental protocol. Four groups of dogs were studied. There were three experimental groups in which all dogs received segmental autografts that were stored at 4°C by the modified two layer (UW/PFC) method (group 1), the original two-layer (EC/PFC) method (group 2) and the simple cold storage method with UW solution (group 3) for 72 or 96 h. The groups were subdivided depending on the storage time: 1A, modified two-layer method for 72 h ($n = 5$); 1B, modified two layer method for 96 h ($n = 8$); 2A, original two layer method for 72 h ($n = 5$); 2B, original two layer method for 96 h ($n = 8$); 3A, simple cold storage method with UW solution for 72 h ($n = 5$); 3B, simple cold storage method with UW solution for 96 h ($n = 8$).

Table 1. Functional success rate in canine segmental pancreatic autografts after preservation at 4°C

Group	Preservation time (h)	Preservation method	Functional grafts No. transplants	Success[a] rate (%)
1A	72	UW/PEC	5/5	100
2A	72	EC/PFC	5/5	100
3A	72	UW	4/5	80
1B	96	UW/PFC	6/8	75
2B	96	EC/PFC	0/8	0
3B	96	UW	0/8	0

[a] Maintenance of normoglycemia for at least 5 days after transplantation was considered successful preservation [8]

Results

After preservation for 72 h, the functional success rate of groups 1A, 2A and 3A were 100% (5/5), 100% (5/5) and 80% (4/5), respectively. But after 96 h preservation, only group 1B was successful, with a success rate of 75% (6/8), and groups 2B and 3B were unsuccessful, 0% (0/8) and 0% (0/8) respectively (Table 1). One of eight dogs in group 1B died of thrombosis 5 days after transplantation and one died of a cause unrelated to the graft. The mean K values of group 1B at 2 weeks after transplantation was 1.52 ± 0.30 compared with 1.98 ± 0.42 before preservation. Biopsies of grafts from group 1B showed almost normal pancreatic architecture. In addition, biopsies of grafts from group 1B at 4 weeks after transplantation showed almost normal pancreatic architecture with minimal fibrotic changes in the exocrine tissue.

Discussion

In order suppress cell swelling or tissue edema, a new flush and preservation solution, UW solution, has been developed using a high molecular weight anion (lactobionate) and a high molecular weight saccharide (raffinose) as impermeants [4, 5] and this extends the preservation time of the canine pancreas for up to 72 h [6]. On the other hand, we have developed a two-layer (EC/PFC) cold storage method to reduce ischemic cell injury and maintain cellular integrity [1] and this also extends preservation time for up to 72 h in the canine pancreas [3]. Since preservation of the canine pancreas for 96 h by either the simple cold storage method with UW solution or the original two-layer (EC/PFC) cold storage method was unsuccessful but a combination of UW solution and the two-layer method made 96-hour preservation possible, it seemed reasonable to suppose that the mechanism of action of UW solution and the two-layer method in preservation of the canine pancreas are different and additive although the precise mechanisms of action of UW solution and the two-layer method are not clear. Recently, we have established that the two-layer method maintains high ATP tissue concentrations in the canine pancreas during and at the end of the cold storage period [2] and we have also established that there is a correlation between high ATP tissue concentrations and good post-transplant results after preservation by the two-layer method [9]. In addition, Pegg et al. [10] have clearly demonstrated that the provision of sufficient oxygen by retrograde oxygen persufflation to rabbit kidney allows the continued production of ATP in sufficient quantity to permit improved maintenance of cellular function. It is not clear whether maintenance of a high ATP tissue concentration during preservation by the two-layer method is a primary determinant of successful preservation or merely reflects the preservation of mitochondrial function during cold storage. The mechanism of action of the two-layer method in canine pancreatic preservation is currently being investigated by our group.

Acknowledgement. This work was supported by a grant from the scientific research fund from the Ministry of Education, Japan.

Reference

1. Kuroda Y, Kawamura T, Suzuki Y, Fujiwara H, Yamamoto K, Saitoh Y (1988) A new simple method for cold storage of the pancreas using perfluorochemical. Transplantation 46: 457

2. Kuroda Y, Fujino Y, Kawamura T, Suzuki Y, Fujiwara H, Saitoh Y (1990) Mechanism of oxygenation of pancreas during preservation by two layer (Euro-Collins' solution/perfluorochemical) cold storage method. Transplantation 49: 694

3. Kawamura T, Kuroda Y, Suzuki Y, et al. (1989) Seventy-two-hour preservation of the canine pancreas by the two-layer (Euro-Collins' solution/perfluorochemical) cold storage method. Transplantation 47: 776

4. Wahlberg JA, Southard JH, Belzer FO (1986) Development of a cold storage solution for pancreas preservation. Cryobiology 23: 477

5. Jamieson NV, Lindell S, Sundberg R, et al. (1988) An analysis of the component in UW solution using the isolated perfused rabbit liver. Transplantation 46: 512

6. Wahlberg JA, Love R, Landegaard J, Southard JH, Belzer FO (1987) 72-hour preservation of the canine pancreas. Transplantation 43: 5

7. Kuroda Y, Orita K, Iwagaki S, et al. (1987) A new technique of pancreatic exocrine diversion to the esophagus in canine segmental pancreatic autotransplantation. Transplantation 44: 583

8. Abouna GM, Heil JE, Sutherland DER, Najarian JS (1988) Factors necessary for successful 48-hour preservation of pancreas grafts. Transplantation 45: 270

9. Kuroda Y, Fujino Y, Morita A, Ku Y, Saitoh Y Correlation between high adenosine triphosphate tissue concentration and a good posttransplant outcome of the canine pancreas graft after preservation by a two-layer cold storage method. Transplantation (in press)

10. Pegg DE, Foreman J, Hunt CJ, Diaper MP (1989) The mechanism of action of retrograde oxygen persufflation in renal preservation. Transplantation 48: 210

Transplant Int (1992) 5 [Suppl 1]: S 391–S 394

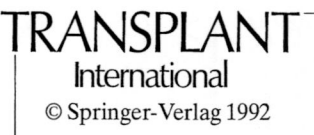
TRANSPLANT
International
© Springer-Verlag 1992

The mechanism of action of the two-layer (Euro-Collins' solution/perfluorochemical) cold storage method in canine pancreas preservation

Y. Kuroda, Y. Fujino, A. Morita, Y. Tanioka, Y. Suzuki, T. Kawamura, Y. Ku, and Y. Saitoh

First Department of Surgery, Kobe University School of Medicine, Kobe, Japan

Abstract. To clarify the mechanism of action of a two-layer [Euro-Collins' solution (EC)/perfluorochemical (PFC)] cold storage method in the preservation of the pancreas, pancreatic viability and tissue concentrations of adenosine triphosphate (ATP) were examined in the canine model of pancreatic autotransplantation after preservation for 24 and 48 h by simple cold storage in EC (group 1), the two-layer, EC/PFC, method (group 2) and the two-layer, EC + 2, 4 dinitrophenol (DNP)/PFC, method (group 3). DNP is an uncoupler of oxidative phosphorylation. Maintenance of normoglycemia for at least 5 days after transplantation was considered a successful preservation. After preservation for 24 h, the functional success rates of groups 1, 2 and 3 were 100% (4/4), 100% (5/5) and 80% (4/5) respectively. One of five dogs in group 3 died of a cause unrelated to the pancreas. ATP tissue concentrations in group 2 were significantly higher than in group 1 (7.47 ± 0.47 μmol/g dry weight vs 1.41 ± 0.53 μmol/g dry weight, $P < 0.01$) and ATP tissue concentrations in group 3 were significantly lower than in group 2 (1.25 ± 0.37 μmol/g dry weight vs 7.47 ± 0.47 μmol/g dry weight, $P < 0.01$). It was apparent that ATP was not an essential factor for successful 24-hour preservation of the canine pancreas in EC because all the pancreatic grafts except one of five grafts in group 3 remained viable after preservation for 24 h, regardless of ATP tissue concentrations. On the other hand, after preservation for 48 h, the functional success rates for groups 1, 2 and 3 were 0% (0/4), 100% (4/4) and 0% (0/3) respectively. ATP tissue concentrations in group 2 were significantly higher than in group 1 (7.91 ± 1.21 μmol/g dry weight vs 1.21 ± 0.31 μmol/g dry weight, $P < 0.01$) and ATP tissue concentrations in group 3 were significantly lower than in group 2 (0.61 ± 0.07 μmol/g dry weight vs 7.91 ± 1.21 μmol/g dry weight, $P < 0.01$). It was clear that preservation of the pancreas for 48 h was unsuccessful by simple cold storage in EC (group 1) and the two-layer method (group 2) made preservation for 48 h possible by increasing ATP tissue concentrations. However, DNP (group 3) inhibited the synthesis of ATP and the effectiveness of the two-layer method for 48-hour preservation of the pancreas. It was clear that maintenance of high ATP tissue concentrations during preservation was essential for the successful preservation of the canine pancreas in EC by the two-layer method for more than 48 h. We concluded that an adequate supply of oxygen to the pancreas during preservation by the two-layer method led to sufficient production of ATP to maintain cellular integrity and permitted the improvement of pancreatic preservation.

Key words: Preservation of the pancreas – 48 h – Adenosine triphosphate – Perfluorochemical

To reduce ischemic cell injury and maintain cellular integrity during cold preservation of the pancreas, we have developed a two-layer [Euro-Collins' solution (EC)/perfluorochemical (PFC)] cold storage method [1] that provides sufficient oxygen to the pancreas during preservation [2] and succeeds in preserving the canine pancreas in EC for 48–72 h [1, 3], although EC is effective only for preserving the canine pancreas for 24 h [1–4]. Since oxygen is one of essential metabolites depleted in the ischemic organ, it seems reasonable to suppose that the oxygenation of the pancreas during preservation by the two-layer method is essential in reducing ischemic cell injury and extending the preservation time. In addition, since the oxygenation of the pancreas by the two-layer method leads to the maintenance of high adenosine triphosphate (ATP) tissue concentrations [2] and there is direct correlation between high ATP tissue concentrations after preservation by the two-layer method and good post-transplant outcome [5] it is also reasonable to think that provision of sufficient oxygen to the pancreas by the two-layer method allows the continued production of ATP, maintains cellular integrity and prolongs the preservation time. But it is not clear whether maintenance of high ATP tissue concentrations

Offprint requests to: Yoshikazu Kuroda, M. D., First Department of Surgery, Krobe University School of Medicine, 7-5-2, Kusunoki-cho, Chuo-ku, Kobe 650, Japan

Table 1. Effect of DNP on viability of pancreatic graft after simple cold storage for 48 h

Group	Preservation solution	Preservation time (h)	Functional grafts No. transplants	Success rate[a] (%)
A_1	EC	24	5/5	100
A_2	EC + DNP	24	3/3	100
B_1	UW	48	4/4	100
B_2	UW + DNP	48	3/3	100

[a] Maintenance of normoglycemia for at least 5 days after transplantation was considered viable pancreas graft [7]

by the two-layer method is a primary determinant to success in extension of the preservation time or merely reflects well-preserved mitochondrial function during cold storage. To clarify this problem, we set up our study so that the pancreatic graft was sufficiently oxygenated but production of ATP was blocked by 2,4 dinitrophenol (DNP), an uncoupler of oxidative phosphorylation, during preservation by the two-layer method and examined the viability of the pancreas following transplantation. The purpose of this study was to clarify the mechanism of action of the two-layer cold storage method in preservation of the canine pancreas.

Materials and methods

Mongrel dogs of both sexes, weighing 12–18 kg were used for the experiments. Perfluorodecaline, one of the PFCs, was a kind gift of Dr. K. Yokoyama (The Green Cross Corporation, Osaka, Japan). A Shim-pack was purchased from Shimazu Manufacturing. Chemicals were from Sigma.

Operation procedures. Anesthesia was induced and maintained with sodium pentobarbiturate (25 mg/kg). After the abdomen was opened, a left lobectomy of the pancreas with the splenic artery and vein attached was meticulously performed, followed by splenectomy. The segmental pancreatic graft was washed with 50 ml of cold heparinized EC (1000 units/50 ml EC) or cold heparinized EC containing 0.2 mM 2,4 dinitrophenol (DNP) through the splenic artery and preserved. After preservation, the pancreatic graft was washed with saline and autotransplanted in the neck as described previously [6], excising the remainder of the pancreas at the time of autotransplantation. After surgery, the dogs received saline with 10 % glucose (30 ml/kg) and parenteral penicillin (25 mg/kg weight) for 3 days. After 3 days, standard kennel diets were given.

Functional studies. Blood glucose concentration was determined daily during the 1st postoperative week after autotransplantation and biweekly thereafter. Maintenance of normoglycemia for at least 5 days after transplantation was considered successful preservation [7].

Measurement of adenine nucleotides. High performance liquid chromatography on a reverse-phase column of Shim-pack CLC-ODS (6 × 150 mm), equilibrated with 0.1 M phosphate buffer, pH 6.0, containing 1 % methanol was employed to separate and quantitate adenine nucleotides.

Tissue extraction method for adenine nucleotides. At the end of preservation, a piece of pancreas was rapidly frozen with bronze tongs in liquid nitrogen and kept at − 70 °C until analysis. Lyophilized tissues were ground to a powder using a mortar and pestle. Dry tissue powder (200 mg) was then homogenized in 3 ml ice cold 0.5 N perchloric

acid. The precipitated protein was removed by centrifugation, and 500 μl of supernatant was neutralized by the additions of 50 μl 1.0 N $KHCO_3$ and 50 N Tris. Following centrifugation, 10 μl of supernatant was injected into the high performance liquid chromatography for analysis.

Preservation method and experimental protocol. In experiment 1 we examined the cytotoxic effect of DNP on the viability of the pancreatic graft during simple cold storage for 48 h. The pancreatic grafts were preserved by simple cold storage in EC (group A_1, $n = 5$) or EC + 0.2 mM DNP (group A_2, $n = 3$) for 24 h or University of Wisconsin solution (UW) (group B_1, $n = 4$) or UW + 0.2 mM DNP (group B_2, $n = 3$) for 48 h and then autotransplanted. It has been well established that EC is effective in preserving the canine pancreas for 24 h [1–4], and UW is effective in preserving the canine pancreas for 72 h [5, 8]. In experiment 2 we examined the effect of DNP on the viability and ATP tissue concentration of the pancreatic graft after preservation by the two-layer method. The two-layer cold storage method was performed as has been described previously [1–3]. There were six experimental groups in which all dogs received segmental autografts that were stored at 4 °C by simple cold storage in EC (group 1) or the two-layer (EC/PFC) cold storage method (group 2) or the two-layer cold storage method plus DNP (EC + DNP/PFC) (group 3) for 24 h or 48 h.

Data analysis. All values were expressed as the mean ± SD. Differences between groups were tested by the Student's t-test.

Results

Cytotoxic effect of DNP on the pancreatic graft after simple cold storage for 48 h. After preservation by simple cold storage in EC (group A_1) or EC + DNP (group A_2) for 24 h or in UW (group B_1) or UW + DNP (group B_2) for 48 h, the pancreatic grafts were autotransplanted. The functional success rates of groups A_1, A_2, B_1, and B_2 were 100 % (5/5), 100 % (3/3), 100 % (4/4) and 100 % (3/3) respectively. It was clear that the concentration of DNP used here (0.2 mM) was not lethal for pancreatic grafts during simple cold storage for at least up to 48 h (Table 1).

Effect of DNP on the viability and ATP tissue concentrations of pancreas grafts after preservation by the two-layer method (Table 2). After preservation for 24 h, the functional success rates of groups 1, 2 and 3 were 100 % (4/4), 100 % (5/5) and 80 % (4/5) respectively. One of five dogs in group 3 died of a cause unrelated to the pancreas. ATP tissue concentrations in groups 1, 2 and 3 after cold preservation were 1.41 ± 0.53 ($n = 4$) μmol/g dry weight, 7.47 ± 0.47 ($n = 5$) μmol/g dry weight and 1.25 ± 0.37 ($n = 4$) μmol/g dry weight respectively.

Although ATP tissue concentrations in group 2 were significantly higher than in group 1 ($P < 0.01$) and ATP tissue concentrations in group 3 was significantly lower than in group 2 ($P < 0.01$), all the pancreatic grafts except one of five grafts in group 3 remained viable for 24 h regardless of the preservation method. It was apparent that ATP was not an essential factor for successful 24-h preservation of the canine pancreas in EC. On the contrary, after preservation for 48 h, the functional success rates of groups 1, 2 and 3 were 0 % (0/4), 100 % (4/4) and 0 % (0/3) respectively. It was clear that 48-h preservation of the canine pancreas was unsuccessful using simple cold storage with EC [1–4] and the two-layer method made preservation for 48 h possible [1–3]. However, DNP inhibited the effectiveness of the two-layer method in 48-hour pres-

Table 2. Effect of DNP on viability and ATP tissue concentrations of pancreatic grafts after preservation by the two-layer method

Group	Preservation method	Preservation time (h)	Functional grafts no. transplants	Success rate[a] (%)	ATP tissue concentration (μmol/g dry weight)
1	EC	24	4/4	100	1.41 ± 0.53
	EC	48	0/4	0	1.21 ± 0.31
2	EC/PFC	24	5/5	100	7.47 ± 0.47*
	EC/PFC	48	4/4	100	7.91 ± 1.21*
3	EC + DNP/PFC	24	4/5	80	1.25 ± 0.37
	EC + DNP/PFC	48	0/3	0	0.61 ± 0.07

[a] Maintenance of normoglycemia for at least five days after transplantation was considered viable pancreas graft [7]
* $P < 0.01$, compared with groups 1 and 3

ervation of the pancreas. ATP tissue concentrations in groups 1, 2 and 3 after cold preservation were 1.21 ± 0.31 ($n = 4$) μmol/g dry weight, 7.91 ± 1.21 ($n = 4$) μmol/g dry weight and 0.61 ± 0.07 ($n = 3$) μmol/g dry weight respectively. ATP tissue concentrations in group 2 were significantly higher than in group 1 ($P < 0.01$) and ATP tissue concentrations in group 3 were significantly lower than in group 2 ($P < 0.01$). Thus the two-layer method facilitated ATP synthesis in the pancreas during preservation [2, 4] and ATP production in the pancreas was inhibited by DNP. It was clear that maintenance of high ATP tissue concentrations during preservation was essential for successful preservation of the canine pancreas in EC by the two-layer method for more than 48 h.

Discussion

The simple cold storage of the canine pancreas with so-called "intracellular solutions", EC [4], Collins' solution [9–12] and Sack's solution [13] is effective for preservation for 24 h but not for preservation for more than 48 h. However provision of sufficient oxygen to the pancreas during preservation by the two-layer method [1, 2] has made it possible to preserve the canine pancreas with EC for up to 72 h [3]. Since the oxygenation of the pancreas by the two-layer method leads to the maintenance of high ATP tissue concentrations [2], this maintenance of high ATP tissue concentrations could have an essential role in maintaining cellular integrity and contributing to successful preservation of the canine pancreas in EC for more than 48 h by the two-layer method. On the other hand, high ATP tissue concentrations could be a secondary phenomenon and not essential for successful preservation of the pancreas for more than 48 h because the pancreas can be preserved for more than 48 h without any significant ATP present in simple cold storage with a UW [8] and a silica-gel filtered plasma [13, 14]. To clarify this problem, we set up our study so that the pancreas was sufficiently oxygenated but production of ATP was blocked by DNP during the two-layer storage period and we examined the viability of the pancreas following autotransplantation. The results showed clearly that maintenance of ATP tissue concentrations during preservation were essential for successful preservation of the pancreas in EC for more than 48 h by the two-layer cold storage method. But it remains unclear

how ATP is utilized in maintaining cellular integrity during cold preservation by the two-layer method. This problem is currently being investigated. We concluded that the oxygenation of the pancreas during preservation by the two-layer method led to a production of ATP sufficient for maintaining cellular integrity and permitting the improvement of pancreatic preservation. In kidney preservation, the provision of sufficient oxygen by retrograde oxygen persufflation improves the preservation of canine kidneys that have suffered warm ischemia prior to preservation [15–17]. Whether the two-layer cold storage method might have a role in the preservation of the pancreas subjected to warm ischemia is inknown and is also under investigation.

Acknowledgement. This work was supported by a grant from the scientific research fund of the Ministry of Education, Japan.

References

1. Kuroda Y, Kawamura T, Suzuki Y, Fujiwara H, Yamamoto K, Saitoh Y (1988) A new simple method for cold storage of the pancreas using perfluorochemical. Transplantation 46: 457
2. Kuroda Y, Fujino Y, Kawamura T, Suzuki Y, Fujiwara H, Saitoh Y (1990) Mechanism of oxygenation of pancreas during preservation by a two-layer (Euro-Collins' sulution/perfluorochemical) cold storage method. Transplantation 49: 694
3. Kawamura T, Kuroda Y, Suzuki Y, et al. (1989) Seventy-two-hour preservation of the canine pancreas by the two-layer (Euro-Collins' solution/perfluorochemical) cold storage method. Transplantation 47: 776
4. Amiel J, Peraldi D, Bernard JL, LΦubiere R, Raymond G, Mouiel J (1984) Successful pancreatic allograft in dog after 24-hour cold ischemia. Transplant Proc 16: 126
5. Kuroda Y, Fujino Y, Morita A, Ku Y, Saitoh Y Correlation between high ATP tissue concentration and good posttransplant outcome of the pancreas graft after a two-layer cold storage method. Transplantation (in press)
6. Kuroda Y, Orita K, Iwagaki S, et al. (1987) A new technique or pancreatic exocrine diversion to the esophagus in canine segmental pancreatic autotransplantation. Transplantation 44: 583
7. Abouna GM, Heil JE, Sutherland DER, Najarian JS (1988) Factors necessary for successful 48-hour preservation of pancreas grafts. Transplantation 45: 270
8. Wahlberg JA, Love R, Landegaard L, Southard JH, Belzer FO (1987) 72-hour preservation of the canine pancreas. Transplantation 43: 5
9. Westbroek DL, de Gruyl J, Dijkhuis CM, et al. (1974) Twenty-four-hour hypothermic preservation: perfusion and storage of

S394

the duct-ligated canine pancreas with transplantation. Transplant Proc 6: 319

10. de Gruyl J, Westbroek DL, Macdicken I, Ridderhof E, Verschoor L, van Strik R (1977) Cryoprecipitated plasma perfusion preservation and cold storage preservation of duct-ligated pancreatic allografts. Br J Surg 64: 490

11. Baumgartner D, Sutherland DER, Heil JE, Zweber B, Awad EA, Najarian JS (1980) Cold storage of segmental canine pancreatic grafts for 24 hours. J Surg Res 29: 248

12. Florack G, Sutherland DER, Dunning M, Zweber B, Najarian JS (1984) Function of segmental pancreas grafts subjected to warm ischemia prior to hypothermic preservation. Transplant Proc 16: 111

13. Toledo-Pereyra LH, Chee M, Condie RM, Najarian JS, Lillehei RC (1979) Forty-eight hour hypothermic storage of whole canine pancreas allografts: improved preservation with a colloid hyperosmolar solution. Cryobiology 16: 221

14. Florack G, Sutherland DER, Heil J, Zweber B, Najarian JS (1982) Long-term preservation of segmental pancreas autografts. Surgery 92: 260

15. Fischer JH, Czerniak A, Hauer U, Isselhard W (1978) A new simple method for optimal storage of ischemically damaged kidneys. Transplantation 25: 43

16. Ross H, Escott ML (1979) Gaseous oxygen perfusion of the renal vessels as an adjunct in kidney preservation. Transplantation 28: 362

17. Rolles K. Foreman J, Pegg DE (1984) Preservation of ischemically injured canine kidneys by retrograde oxygen persufflation. Transplantation 38: 102

Transplant Int (1992) 5 [Suppl 1]: S 395–S 397

TRANSPLANT
International
© Springer-Verlag 1992

Improvement of liver preservation by the calcium channel blocker nisoldipine. An experimental study applying intravital microscopy to transplanted rat livers

I. Marzi, F. Walcher, and V. Bühren

Chirurgische Universitätsklinik, Homburg/Saar, Germany

Abstract. It has been shown recently that inclusion of the calcium channel blocker nisoldipine to University of Wisconsin (UW) solution significantly improves survival after rat liver transplantation. To further elucidate the mechanisms involved, rat livers were stored for 1 h in UW solution with or without the addition of 1.4 μM nisoldipine (Miles, West Haven, Conn., USA). The liver grafts were investigated in vivo 90 min after transplantation by intravital fluorescence microscopy. Sinusoidal perfusion was reduced in all sublobular regions of the liver in the UW group (e.g. portal area: $76.7 \pm 2.1\%$) and in the nisoldipine group ($85.8 \pm 1.5\%$). Diameters of liver sinusoids were comparably reduced in the UW and nisoldipine groups indicating that nisoldipine did not cause vasodilatation. Adhesion of leukocytes, however, rose significantly after liver transplantation particularly in periportal regions ($25.8 \pm 2.5\%$) compared to controls ($17.1 \pm 2.8\%$; $P < 0.05$). Adhesion of leukocytes was reduced when nisoldipine was included in UW solution ($13.3 \pm 1.7\%$; $P < 0.05$). Administration of latex particles, which were given in additional experimental groups, demonstrated an impressive increase in phagocytic activity of Kupffer cells after liver transplantation in periportal and pericentral areas ($161 \pm 14\%$ and $184 \pm 19\%$ of controls). Phagocytosis was significantly reduced by nisoldipine in the periportal region ($101 \pm 10\%$; $P < 0.01$). Thus, the beneficial effect of nisoldipine was most pronounced in periportal regions, where the majority of Kupffer cells are located and leukocyte adhesion was at a maximum.

Key words: Liver preservation – Microcirculation – Leukocyte adhesion – Liver transplantation – Macrophage activation – Calcium channel blocker

Liver preservation and outcome of liver transplantation has been improved dramatically in the past years. With the introduction of new preservation media, such as the University of Wisconsin cold storage solution (UW) [1],

preservation time could be extended thus allowing better organization and distribution of donor organs. However, primary nonfunction of liver grafts, which is the most serious complication of the transplantation procedure, still remains a critical problem [5]. Reperfusion injury to the transplanted organ has been suggested as a reason for primary nonfunction as well as for the poor quality of liver grafts [21].

Experimental studies in perfused and transplanted livers have shown a particular pattern of reperfusion injury after cold ischemia to the individual cell populations of the liver. Sinusoidal endothelial cells loose viability immediately after reperfusion, depending on the time of cold storage [4, 13, 15] while resident liver macrophages become activated under identical conditions [3, 20]. On the other hand, hepatic parenchymal cells tolerate cold ischemia significantly longer without morphological or functional losses [13]. Destruction of parenchymal cells most likely takes place subsequently, when their nutrition is disrupted, e. g. by microcirculatory failure [21]. There is evidence that oxygen free radicals contribute to reperfusion injury after liver transplantation [10, 16]. Furthermore, a rise in intracellular calcium during reperfusion has been proposed to contribute to cell injury [8] and to be involved in the activation of macrophages and the release of inflammatory mediators [17, 18]. Indeed, inclusion of the calcium channel blocker, nisoldipine, in a preservation solution improved survival rates significantly after rat liver transplantation. Part of this effect has been attributed to the prevention of Kupffer cell activation by nisoldipine [19].

The aim of our study was to evaluate the effect of nisoldipine on hepatic microcirculation, leukocyte adhesion and activity of Kupffer cells. Therefore, transplanted rat livers were investigated in vivo by fluorescence microscopy after cold storage in UW solution containing nisoldipine.

Materials and Methods

Liver transplantations were performed in Lewis rats (HAN, Hannover, Germany) weighing 200–230 g according to the technique described by Kamada [6]. The livers were stored for 60 min in UW sol-

---

Offprint requests to: I. Marzi, Department of Surgery, University of Saarland, D-6650 Homburg/Saar, Germany

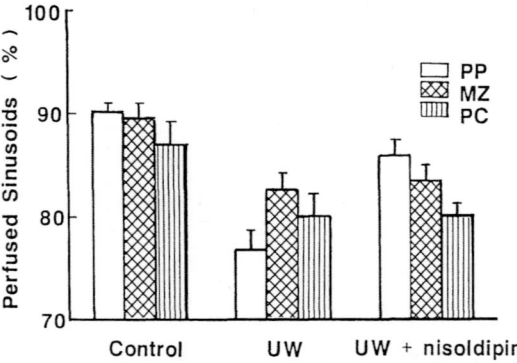

Fig. 1. Percentage of perfused sinusoids in sublobular regions of the liver. Discrimination of portal *(PP)*, midzonal *(MZ)*, and pericentral *(PC)* area was at a third of the distance between the centers of the portal and central field. Mean ± SEM

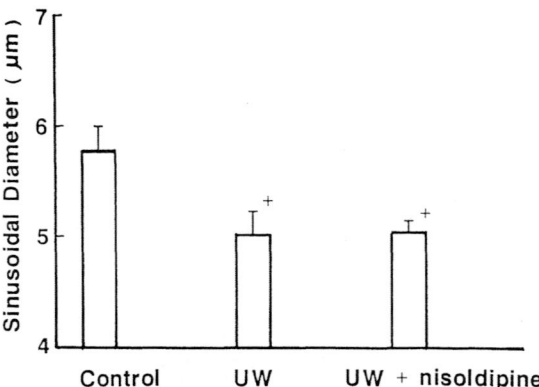

Fig. 2. Diameters of liver sinusoids. A circle with a radius of 150 μm was drawn around the central veins and diameters of all crossing sinusoids were measured. Mean ± SEM. + $P < 0.05$ versus control group

ution at 4°C with or without the addition of nisoldipine (1.4 μM; Miles, New Haven, Conn.) prior to transplantation.

Leukocyte adhesion and sinusoidal perfusion were studied by intravital fluorescence microscopy 90 min after reperfusion of the liver grafts and in sham-operated controls ($n = 6$ per group). Using pentobarbital anesthesia (30 mg/kg), the abdomen was opened and the left liver lobe exposed on a plexiglas stage for intravital microscopy (Leitz Orthoplan, Wetzlar, Germany; 545 nm filter; 12× eye piece, 10×/20× water immersion objectives, final magnification ×310 or ×815), as has been described recently [11,12]. After injection of acridine orange (0.9 mg/ml; Sigma, Deisenhofen, Germany), a leukocyte marker, 5–6 liver lobules were studied for 30 s each at the sublobular level, e.g. periportal, midzonal, and pericentral areas. Off-line analysis of video-recorded experiments allowed the determination of perfused sinusoids and permanently adherent leukocytes, defined as leukocytes with an adhesion time longer than 20 s [12].

Macrophage activity was assessed by the injection of latex particles ($260*10^6$; 0.8 μm; Polysciences, St. Goar, Germany) in a separate experimental series containing similar groups ($n = 6$ per group). Latex particles taken up by macrophages were measured in 5–6 periportal and pericentral areas of the liver 15 min after injection.

Data were given as mean ± SEM. Statistical significance was evaluated using ANOVA and Students *t*-test as appropriate.

Results

Sinusoidal perfusion was reduced by about 10% after liver transplantation, particularly in the periportal area. The addition of nisoldipine to the UW solution attenuated

sinusoidal perfusion slightly, as shown in Fig. 1. The diameters of sinusoids of 150 μm around the central veins were significantly reduced in both transplantation groups compared to controls (Fig. 2). There were no changes in sinusoidal diameters the UW + nisoldipine group. Adhesion of leukocytes rose after liver transplantation in all sublobular regions. This effect was significantly reduced in the periportal region when nisoldipine was added to UW solution (Table 1).

In an additional experimental series, phagocytosis of latex particles was higher in periportal ($316 ± 22/mm^2$) than in pericentral regions ($166 ± 13/mm^2$) in the control group. Compared to these values ($= 100\%$), transplantation after cold storage in UW solution resulted in a substantial rise in phagocytozed latex beads in periportal ($161 ± 14\%$) and pericentral ($184 ± 19\%$) regions. After inclusion of nisoldipine in the UW solution, phagocytosis of latex beads was significantly reduced in periportal ($102 ± 10\%$; $P < 0.01$) and in pericentral areas ($137 ± 27\%$).

Discussion

As indicated by the number of perfused sinusoids and diameters of hepatic sinusoids, transplantation of livers 1 h after cold storage in UW solution led to a moderate reduction in sinusoidal perfusion, which was slightly improved by nisoldipine. However, it seems obvious that this effect cannot account for the improved survival under identical conditions as has been shown previously [19]. Therefore, the action of the calcium channel blocker must be different from a direct effect on the microvascular perfusion.

It is well known that tissue macrophages, such as the Kupffer cells, release a variety of inflammatory mediators with the potential of influencing leukocyte adhesion and the microcirculation [22]. Since it has been shown that Kupffer cells are activated after cold storage [20] and transplantation [9], one aim of this study was to evaluate the activity of Kupffer cells in vivo after transplantation. Therefore, we used fluorescence labelled latex particles, as described by McCuskey et al. [14]. Uptake of latex particles has been observed in a ratio of 2:1 in periportal and pericentral areas, reflecting the physiological distribution of tissue macrophages [2]. In our study, the significant increase in both regions after transplantation was completely blocked by nisoldipine in the portal area and reduced in the central area. This suggests, that the benefical effect of the calcium channel blocker was due to prevention of

Table 1. Adhesion of leukocytes in sublobular regions of the liver. Percentage of leukocytes adherent longer than 20 s to the sinusoidal wall are expressed as percentage of all observed leukocytes. Data are given as mean ± SEM

Group	Periportal	Midzonal	Pericentral
Control	17.1 ± 2.8	11.3 ± 1.3	5.5 ± 0.8
UW	25.8 ± 2.5	16.7 ± 2.5	13.8 ± 2.4
UW/nisoldipine	13.3 ± 1.7	16.7 ± 2.5	6.4 ± 0.8

* $P < 0.05$ UW versus UW plus nisoldipine group

macrophage activation thereby reducing locally or systemically acting mediators, e. g. leukotrienes or cytokines [17, 18].

The pattern of leukocyte adhesion after liver transplantation with maximal adhesion in the portal regions supports the idea that the release of adhesion promoting mediators by Kupffer cells induces leukocyte adhesion. Indeed, the decrease in adherent leukocytes was maximal periportally (Table 1), where most of the Kupffer cells are located [2]. Because firm adhesion of leukocytes is necessary for leukocyte emigration and tissue injury [7], this sequence of events may explain the protective action of nisoldipine.

The results of this study indicated that the benefical effect of the calcium channel blocker nisoldipine on survival as shown by Takei et al. [19] was not due to its action on the microvasculature, e. g. on vasodilatation. It seems, however, that prevention of macrophage activation results in a reduced adhesion of leukocytes with attenuation of the postischemic liver injury. Thus, inclusion of a calcium channel blocker in preservation solutions may be useful in the clinical situation.

Acknowledgements. This work was supported by a grant from the Deutsche Forschungsgemeinschaft (DFG Ma 1119/2-1).

References

1. Belzer FO, Southard JH (1988) Principles of solid-organ preservation by cold storage. Transplantation 45: 673–676
2. Bouwens L, Baekerland M, de Zanger R, Wisse E (1986) Quantitation, tissue distribution and proliferation kinetics of Kupffer cells in normal rat liver. Hepatology 6: 718–722
3. Caldwell-Kenkel JC, Currin RT, Tanaka Y, Thurman RG, Lemasters JJ (1989) Reperfusion injury to endothelial cells following cold ischemic storage of rat livers. Hepatology 10: 292–299
4. Caldwell-Kenkel JC, Thurman RG, Lemasters JJ (1988) Selective loss of nonparenchymal cell viability after cold ischemic storage of rat livers. Transplantation 45: 834–837
5. Greig PD, Woolf GM, Sinclair SB, Abecassis M, Strasberg SM, Taylor BR, Blendis LM, Superina LA, Glynn MFX, Langer B, Levy GA (1989) Treatment of primary liver graft nonfunction with prostaglandin E₁. Transplantation 48: 447–453
6. Kamada N, Calne RY (1979) Orthotopic liver transplantation in the rat. Technique using cuff for portal vein anastomosis and biliary drainage. Transplantation 28: 47–50
7. Lawrence MB, Springer TA (1991) Leukocytes roll on a selectin at physiologic flow rates: Distinction from and prerequisite for adhesion through integrins. Cell 65: 859–873
8. Lemasters JJ, Diguiseppi J, Nieminen A-L, Herman B (1987) Blebbing, free Ca + + and mitochondrial membrane potential preceding cell death in hepatocytes. Nature 325: 78–81
9. Marzi I, Cowper KC, Lindert K, Lemasters JJ, Thurman RG (1991) Methyl palmitate prevents Kupffer cell activation and improves survival after orthotopic liver transplantation in the rat. Transplant Int 4 (in press)
10. Marzi I, Knee J, Bühren V, Menger MD, Trentz O (1991) Reduction by superoxide dismutase of leukocyte adherence after liver transplantation. Surgery 110 (in press)
11. Marzi I, Takei Y, Knee J, Kenger MD, Gores GJ, Bühren V, Trentz O, Lemasters JJ, Thurman RG (1990) Assessment of reperfusion injury by intravital fluorescence microscopy following liver transplantation in the rat. Transplant Proc 22: 2004–2005
12. Marzi I, Walcher F, Bühren V, Menger MD, Harbauer G, Trentz O (1991) Microcirculatory disturbances of transplanted livers due to cold storage in Euro-Collins, UW, and HTK solution. Transplant Int 4: 45–50
13. Marzi I, Zhong Z, Lemasters JJ, Thurman RG (1989) Evidence that graft survival is not related to parenchymal cell viability in rat liver transplantation: The importance of nonparenchymal cells. Transplantation 48: 463–468
14. McCuskey RS, Urbaschek R, McCuskey PA, Urbaschek B (1982) In vivo microscopic studies of the responses of the liver to endotoxin. Klin Wochenschr 60: 749–751
15. Momii S, Koga A, Eguchi M, Fukuyama T (1989) Ultrastructural changes in rat liver sinusoids during storage in cold Euro-Collins solution. Virchows Arch [B] 57: 393–398
16. Olson LM, Klintmalm GB, Husberg BS, Nery JR, Whitten CW, Paulsen AW, McClure R (1988) Superoxide dismutase improves organ preservation in liver transplantation. Transplant Proc 20: 961–964
17. Reynolds CH (1988) 5-Lipoxygenase and leukotriene synthesis: effects of calcium ions and of inhibitors. Prostaglandins 36: 59–68
18. Suttles J, Giri JG, Mizel SB (1990) Il-1 secretion by macrophages. Enhancement of Il-1 secretion and processing by calcium ionophores. J Immunol 144: 175–182
19. Takei Y, Marzi I, Kauffman FC, Lemasters JJ, Thurman RG (1990) Increase in survival time of liver transplants from injury by protease inhibitors and a calcium channel blocker, nisoldipine. Transplantation 50: 14–20
20. Thurman RG, Lindert KA, Cowper KC, Te Koppele JM, Dawson TL, Currin RT, Caldwell-Kenkel JC, Tanaka Y, Gao W, Takei Y, Marzi I, Lemasters JJ (1991) Activation of Kupffer cells following liver transplantation. In: Wisse E, Knook DL, McCuskey RS (eds) Cells of the hepatic sinusoids. vol. 3. The Kupffer Cell Foundation, Rijswijk, The Netherlands, p.
21. Thurman RG, Marzi I, Seitz G, Thies J, Lemasters JJ, Zimmermann FA (1988) Hepatic reperfusion injury following orthotopic liver transplantation in the rat. Transplantation 46: 5020–506
22. Wake K, Decker K, Kirn A, Knook DL, McCuskey RS, Bouwens L, Wisse E (1989) Cell biology and kinetics of Kupffer cells in the liver. Int Rev Cytol 118: 173–230

Transplant Int (1992) 5 [Suppl 1]: S 398–S 402

TRANSPLANT
International
© Springer-Verlag 1992

The calcium channel blocker nisoldipine minimizes the release of tumor necrosis factor and interleukin-6 following rat liver transplantation

E. Savier[1], S. I. Shedlofsky[3], A. T. Swim[3], J. J. Lemasters[2], and R. G. Thurman[1]

[1] Laboratory of Hepatobiology and Toxicology Department of Pharmacology
[2] Laboratory for Cell Biology, Department of Cell Biology and Anatomy, The University of North Carolina at Chapel Hill, Chapel Hill, USA
[3] Veterans Affairs Hospital, University of Kentucky, Lexington, USA

Abstract. Kupffer cells, when activated, release toxic cytokines such as tumor necrosis factor (TNF), which can cause tissue injury. Takei et al. have reported that nisoldipine, a calcium channel blocker which decreases phagocytotic activity by Kupffer cells, also diminishes liver and lung injury and dramatically improves survival following liver transplantation [27]. Therefore, we studied the effect of nisoldipine on the time course of TNF and interleukin-6 (IL-6) release following cold storage and liver transplantation in the rat. Livers were stored under survival and non-survival conditions in cold Euro-Collins solution in the presence or absence of nisoldipine (1.4 µM). After storage, the effluent was collected for determination of cytokines. The liver was then transplanted orthotopically and serum was collected at various time intervals for up to 5 h. In the effluent, TNF levels were very low in both the control and nisoldipine-treated groups and IL-6 was not measurable. Furthermore, when livers were stored under survival conditions and transplanted (liver stored in the cold for 4 h), serum TNF (2 U/ml) and IL-6 (350 U/ml) values were minimal in both the control and nisoldipine-treated groups. In contrast, when livers were stored under non-survival conditions and transplanted (liver stored in the cold for 10 h), TNF levels increased to 15 ± 2 U/ml, 150 min after graft reperfusion, an increase which was prevented by nisoldipine (6.5 U/ml). Serum IL-6 levels were also elevated 300 min after transplantation in livers stored for 10 h. Nisoldipine also reduced the release of this cytokine. Serum transaminases (SGOT) were elevated to values around 2000 U/l 5 h following transplantation. In the nisoldipine-treated group, values were lower between 60 and 300 min. In the lung, interstitial and alveolar edema and cellular infiltration were detectable 5 h postoperatively and were diminished by nisoldipine. These data confirmed that TNF and IL-6 release were minimal following cold storage and transplantation of livers stored

under survival conditions, but were elevated transiently after transplantation under non-survival conditions. Nisoldipine prevented cytokine release, most likely by blocking the activation of Kupffer cells, which may explain how it decreases liver and lung injury very early following liver transplantation.

Key words: Nisoldipine – Tumor necrosis factor – Interleukin-6 – Liver transplantation

Although liver transplantation is now performed routinely in children and adults, the risk of primary non-function still occurs with an unacceptably high frequency [12]. Primary non-function can compromise postoperative recovery and necessitate retransplantation. The mechanism is not well understood, but it is likely that Kupffer cells, the hepatic macrophages, are involved since they are activated following cold storage and reperfusion [28]. When activated, macrophages release toxic mediators including cytokines such as tumor necrosis factor (TNF) as well as eicosanoids [10]. TNF has been implicated in lung injury [7, 16] and in shock states involving multiple organ failure [4], and it is released following warm ischemia [7] and rejection [31]. Nisoldipine, a calcium channel blocker, decreases phagocytosis of Kupffer cells, diminishes liver and lung injury 24 h following liver transplantation and improves survival [27]. We asked, then, whether injury to liver and lung following transplantation involves the release of TNF and if TNF release is affected by nisoldipine. Furthermore, almost no information is available on the release of other cytokines immediately following liver transplantation. Interleukin-6 (IL-6) may also influence postoperative outcome since it is involved in the acute phase response [13] as well as in the regulation of the immune system [2]. Therefore, we investigated the time course of release of TNF and IL-6 following liver transplantation.

Methods

Orthotopic liver transplantation. Inbred Lewis rats (180–220 g, female) were used to exclude immunological rejection and were transplanted according to the procedure described by Zimmermann [33]

Offprint requests to: Ronald G. Thurman, Laboratory of Hepatobiology and Toxicology, Department of Pharmacology, Faculty Laboratory Office Building, CB # 7365, University of North Carolina at Chapel Hill, Chapel Hill, NC 27599-7365, USA

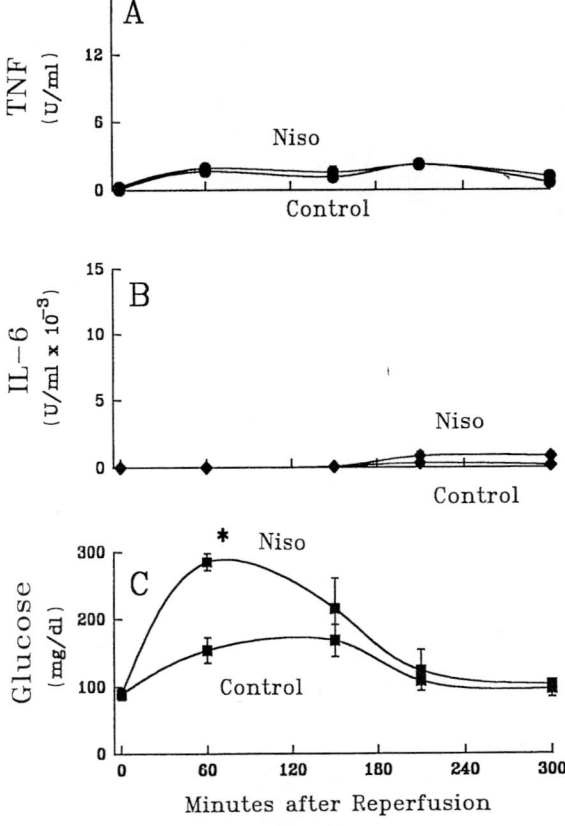

SURVIVAL CONDITIONS

A
TNF (U/ml)

Niso

Control

B
IL-6 (U/ml x 10^{-3})

Niso

Control

C
Glucose (mg/dl)

* Niso

Control

Minutes after Reperfusion

Fig.1A–C. Effect of nisoldipine on TNF, IL-6 and glucose release following transplantation under survival conditions. Livers stored for 4 h in cold Euro-Collins solution (i.e., survival conditions) were transplanted as described in Methods. TNF, IL-6 and glucose were measured in the effluent collected after storage (minute 0) and in recipient rat serum collected at various times. Rats were randomized between an untreated control group and a nisoldipine-treated group. Nisoldipine (*Niso;* 1.4 μM) in DMSO was added to Ringer's and Euro-Collins solutions during explantation and storage only. Nisoldipine was a kind gift of Miles, Inc. (West Haven, Conn.). Reperfusion was initiated by opening the portal vascular clamp. Mean ± SEM, * $P < 0.05$ ($n = 3$–6 per group)

and Kamada [17]. Rats were anesthetized lightly with ether, and surgery was performed under clean conditions. The explantation procedure included incision of the skin, sectioning of the hepatic ligaments, insertion of a splint (polyethylene tubing, PE 10) into the bile duct and dissection of the portal vein and inferior vena cava. The portal vein was then clamped and the liver was rinsed with 10 ml of Ringer's solution at 4°C followed by 15 ml of Euro-Collins solution at 4°C. Livers were then removed and immersed in Euro-Collins solution at 1°C and cuffs were placed on the portal vein and inferior hepatic vena cava before storage for 4 h (survival conditions) or 10 h (non-survival conditions). Implantation was performed by connecting the suprahepatic vena cava with a running suture, inserting cuffs into the appropriate vessels, and anastomosing the bile duct with an intraluminal splint. Grafts were rinsed with 5 ml of Ringer's solution at 21°C before reperfusion, and the effluent was collected. Ischemia of the gut due to clamping the portal vein did not exceed 20 min. Ringer's solution (5 ml) was infused via the tail vein during implantation.

Blood glucose levels were measured in whole blood collected from the superior vena cava with reagent strips (Chemstrip, Boehringer Mannheim) and quantified with an Accu-Check II

monitor. Serum glutamate oxaloacetate transaminase (SGOT) activity was measured enzymatically [3].

Blood sample collection and cytokine assays. The rat was anesthetized lightly with ether, the right external jugular vein was exposed and a glass micropipet (Corning) was inserted into the superior vena cava via the jugular vein to collect blood (400 μl) at 60, 150, 210 and 300 min after graft reperfusion. The protease inhibitor aprotinin (3 U/ml) was added to the effluent and blood samples and sera were stored at − 70°C until assayed. The cytotoxicity of TNF was assayed in L-M fibroblasts incubated with serum or effluent in the presence of 1 μg/ml actinomycin D as described elsewhere [19]. IL-6 was measured using the growth stimulation of B-9 cells as described by Aarden [1]. Results from unknown samples were compared with curves prepared from authentic standards.

Lung histology. Rats were sacrificed 5 h postoperatively, and lungs were fixed by immersion in 2 % paraformaldehyde in Krebs-Henseleit buffer, emmbedded in paraffin, and processed for light microscopy. Sections were stained with hematoxylin and eosin. Lung injury was indexed on a scale from 0 to 2 for interstitial edema, alveolar hemorrhage and infiltration of inflammatory cells (maximal score = 6).

Statistics. Data are presented as mean ± SEM Statistical analyses were performed using Students' *t*-test [26]. The criterion for significance was $P < 0.05$.

Results

Release of cytokines and glucose following transplantation under survival conditions

Following 4 h of storage in Euro-Collins, all rat recipients survived (4 of 4), – survival conditons. Blood levels of TNF, IL-6 and glucose were measured at various time points during the first five h postoperatively and are depicted in Fig. 1. In the rinse effluent and in sera from livers stored under survival conditions and transplanted, TNF levels were detectable but low (less than 4 U/ml) in samples from both control and nisoldipine-treated groups (Fig. 1A). IL-6 was not detectable in the effluent, but reached levels between 150 and 1500 U/ml 300 min after graft reperfusion (Fig. 1B). However, there were no statistical differences between the groups under these conditions.

Following sham-operation (i.e., surgery as described in Methods without graft implantation), levels of TNF and IL-6 were similar to values observed following control transplantation of livers stored for 4 h in Euro-Collins. Highest values of TNF (2.68 ± 0.1 U/ml, $n = 4$) were found 60 min after the operation. IL-6 reached 366 ± 72 U/ml at 150 min, and blood glucose was increased to 164 ± 26 mg/dl.

A transient hyperglycemia occurred 60 min following graft reperfusion which was significantly greater in the nisoldipine group (Figs. 1C and 2C). Treatment of the donor rat with gadolinium chloride, a procedure which selectively destroys Kupffer cells [5], prevented the postoperative increase in blood glucose (data not shown). This observation indicated that the transient hyperglycemia observed following transplantation involved rapid release of prostanoids from Kupffer cells [24] which are known to stimulate phosphorylase A, causing glucose release from

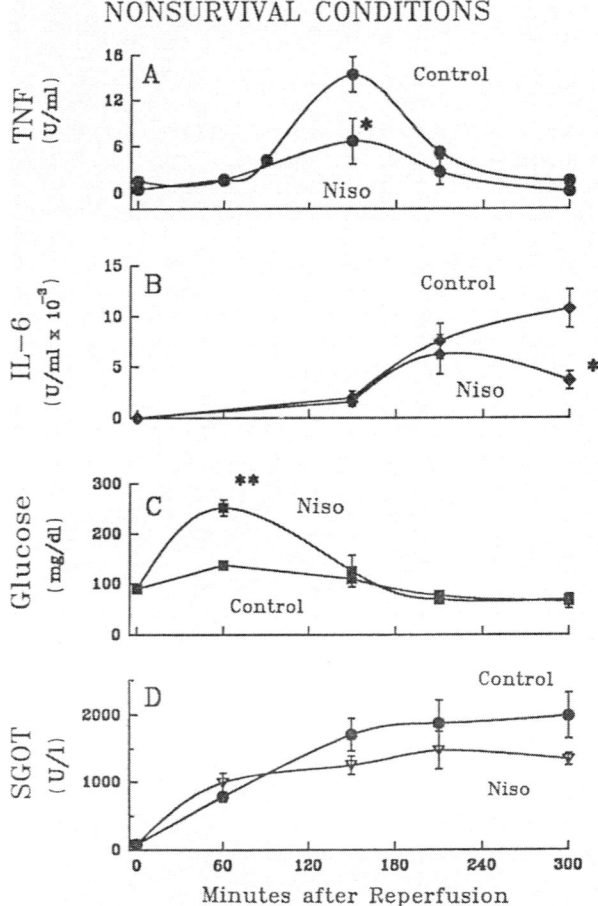

NONSURVIVAL CONDITIONS

Fig. 2 A–D. Effect of nisoldipine on TNF, IL-6, glucose and SGOT release following transplantation under non-survival conditions. Livers stored for 10 h in cold Euro-Collins solution (i.e., non-survival conditions) were transplanted, and TNF, IL-6, glucose and SGOT were measured postoperatively as described in Methods and in the legend of Fig. 1. Mean ± SEM, * $P < 0.05$; ** $P < 0.01$ ($n = 4$–5 per group)

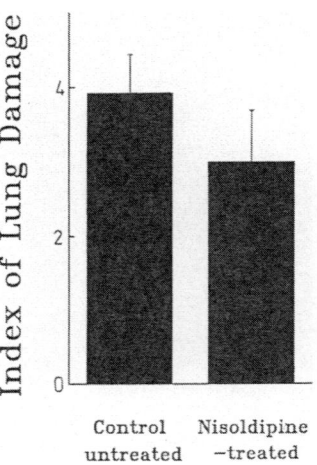

Fig. 3. Effect of nisoldipine on early postoperative lung injury. Five hours following liver transplantation under non-survival conditions (10 h storage in Euro-Collins), rats were sacrificed and their lungs were fixed and evaluated histologically as described in Methods. Nisoldipine was added to the storage solution as described in the legend of Fig. 1. Mean ± SEM, ($n = 5$–6 per group)

parenchymal cell glycogen stores [21]. Surprisingly, nisoldipine stimulated glucose release (Fig. 1 C and 2 C) for reasons that remain unclear. A partial agonist effect of the drug may be involved [14].

Nisoldipine prevented postoperative cytokine release in livers stored under non-survival conditions

Following 10 h of storage, survival was poor (3 of 8) – non-survival conditions. In the graft effluent, TNF was minimal in both the control (0.5 U/ml) and the nisoldipine-treated groups (1.5 U/ml). Following transplantation under these conditions, TNF levels in the blood increased slowly, beginning 90 min following graft reperfusion and reaching values of around 15 U/ml at 150 min before declining to basal levels at 210 min (Fig. 2 A). Importantly, this increase was prevented by nisoldipine. IL-6 reached values around 10000 U/ml 5 h following transplantation, a phenomenon which was also minimized by nisoldipine (Fig. 2 B).

Nisoldipine decreased transaminase release and lung injury

Following 10 h of storage and reperfusion, serum glutamate oxaloacetate transaminase (SGOT) increased gradually in both the control and nisoldipine groups. Between 60 and 300 min postoperatively, SGOT values were higher (ca. 2000 U/l) in the control than in the nisoldipine-treated group (1300 U/l; Fig. 2 D). Under non-survival conditions, lung edema and cellular infiltration were prominent 5 h postoperatively. Nisoldipine reduced this injury by about 25 % (Fig. 3).

Influence of explantation time on TNF release

Between two series of transplantations under survival conditions performed after 12 and 18 months of surgical training, explantation time decreased from 26 to 15 min. When the data were compared, a significant positive correlation was found between the explantation time and TNF levels measured 60 min after graft reperfusion (Fig. 4). Thus, surgical conditions during explantation of the liver in the donor rat influenced TNF release in the recipient.

Discussion

Tumor necrosis factor release following graft reperfusion

TNF is a toxic mediator present in the blood during pathological states [4]. We observed that TNF was released a few hours (Fig. 2 A) following liver transplantation under non-survival conditions raising the question: what factors influence TNF release after reperfusion of the graft? Two factors, explantation time in the donor (Fig. 4) and duration of cold storage (compare Figs. 1 A and 2 A), appeared important in this study.

One hypothesis is that during explantation of the liver, manipulation of the gut may increase the release of bacteria and endotoxin (LPS) into the portal blood, which is known to activate TNF production [4]. Therefore, a

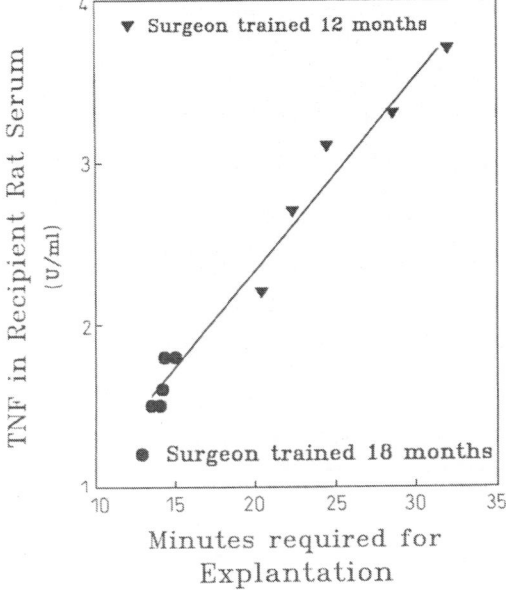

Fig. 4. Effect of explantation time on TNF release. Livers stored for 4 h in cold Euro-Collins solution (i.e., survival conditions) were transplanted orthotopically as described in Methods. TNF was measured in sera of recipient rats 60 min after graft reperfusion as described in Methods. The explantation time was the time from incision of the skin to immersion of liver in cold Euro-Collins. *Triangles:* surgeon trained 12 months (250 transplantations). *Circles:* surgeon trained 18 months (400 transplantations). Coefficient of the linear regression, $r = 0.99$, $P < 0.01$

longer explantation time would be expected to increase hepatic exposure to LPS in the transplant model, leading to greater TNF release after storage and reperfusion (Fig. 2 A). In support of this hypothesis, a dose-dependent release of TNF has been observed in vivo following the injection of LPS [22]. Therefore, it is likely that LPS release into the circulation during explantation contributes to TNF release following transplantation. Thus, by measuring LPS in the donor, it may be possible to predict the clinical outcome in the recipient.

When explantation time was kept constant and duration of cold storage was changed from 4 to 10 h, TNF release increased from minimal to high values (Figs. 1 A and 2 A). Endotoxemia produced by clamping the portal vein [23] cannot explain the high levels of TNF under non-survival conditions since surgical time was identical in the survival and non-survival groups. One possibility is that cold storage influences cells responsible for TNF release. Many studies have reported that cold storage and reperfusion activate Kupffer cells [20, 27, 28], and it is known that macrophages (e. g. Kupffer cells) release TNF when activated [4, 10]. Therefore, it seems reasonable to propose that TNF release following transplantation involves activation of Kupffer cells. Activation may sensitize Kupffer cells to LPS. Another possibility for explaining the release of TNF only under non-survival conditions may be an alteration in regulation of TNF synthesis. Endothelial cells release PGE$_2$ [20], which suppresses TNF synthesis [18]. Cold storage followed by reperfusion injures endothelial cells substantially [6]; therefore, loss of endothelial cell

viability would be expected to decrease PGE$_2$ and allow uncontrolled synthesis of TNF.

Nisoldipine prevented cytokine release and minimized postoperative injury

Following transplantation under survival conditions, TNF release and liver and lung injury were minimal (data not shown). In contrast, under non-survival conditions, TNF was elevated and liver (Fig. 2 D) and lung injury occurred (Fig. 3), raising the question of whether TNF produces liver and lung injury directly. SGOT was released before the peak of TNF levels occurred (Fig. 2 A and D); therefore, at least part of the hepatic injury observed was TNF-independent and most likely involved other mechanisms such as the production of lipid radicals on reperfusion [8, 29]. However, nisoldipine treatment decreased TNF (Fig. 2 A) and also lowered SGOT release with a similar time course (after 60 min). Moreover, nisoldipine tended to reduce lung injury after 300 min; however, values were only decreased significantly after 24 h (Figs. 2 D and 3; [27]). Thus, it is possible to hypothesize that protection by nisoldipine involves TNF. The beneficial effect of nisoldipine following transplantation is not totally understood, but several arguments support the hypothesis that it prevents Kupffer cell activation (see Fig. 5). Kupffer cells have calcium channels [15] and nisoldipine blocks TNF release in isolated Kupffer cells [9]. Moreover, nisoldipine prevents stimulation of phagocytosis by Kupffer cells in the perfused liver following cold storage [27]. White cells also release TNF [4]; however, because nisoldipine is very lipophilic and since the liver was rinsed before reperfusion, the concentration of the drug in the recipient blood

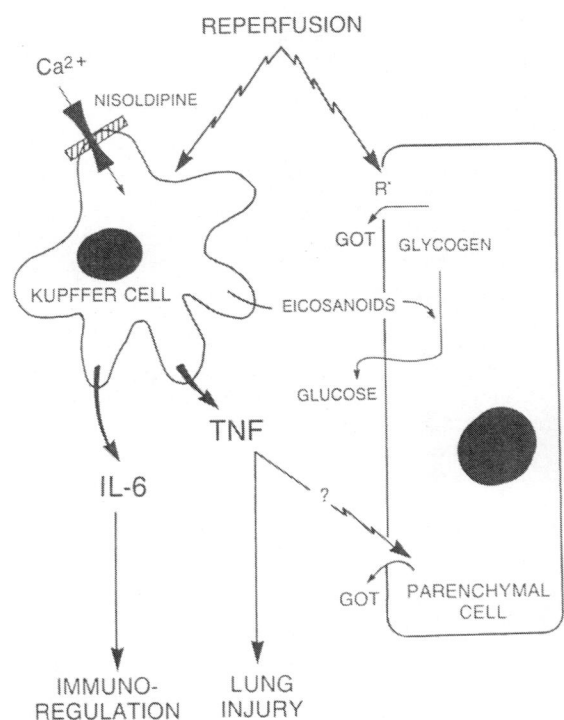

Fig. 5. Scheme depicting cytokine release on reperfusion. *R*, lipid free radicals; *GOT*, serum enzymes

should be too low to affect TNF release by leukocytes directly. Therefore, it is likely that the major site of action of nisoldipine is the Kupffer cell. Prevention of TNF release by Kupffer cells may decrease postoperative injury, as shown in this study (Figs. 2 D and 3). In support of this hypothesis, TNF has been implicated in other models of liver [30, 32] and lung injury [7, 16]; however, TNF does not appear to cause hepatic injury directly [30, 32]. Thus, the effect of nisoldipine may be complex and involve factors in addition to TNF. To illustrate this point, nisoldipine also decreased IL-6 (Fig. 2 B). It is not known whether the IL-6 detected in this study was derived from donor liver nonparenchymal cells or from recipient blood cells. High levels of IL-6 observed under non-survival conditions may be increased either my TNF or other cytokines [25] or result from decreased clearance. IL-6 may affect transplant outcome directly since it regulates synthesis of most of the hepatic acute phase proteins (i.e., fibrinogen) and can stimulate lymphocyte differentiation [2, 11]. More studies are necessary to determine the consequences of cytokine release on liver function and rejection following transplantation.

Acknowledgements. This work was supported in part by a grant (DK-37034) from NIH. ES held a fellowship from the French Fondation de Rothschild.

References

1. Aarden LA, de Groot ER, Schaap OL, Landsdorp PM (1987) Production of hybridoma growth factor by human monocytes. Eur J Immunol 17: 1411–1416
2. Akira S, Hirano T, Taga T, Kishimoto T (1990) Biology of multifunctional cytokines: IL 6 and related molecules (IL 1 and TNF). FASEB J 4: 2860–2867
3. Bergmeyer HU (1988) Methods of Enyzmatic Analysis. Academic Press, New York
4. Beutler B, Cerami A (1988) The history, properties, and biological effects of cachectin. Biochemistry 27: 7575–7582
5. Bouma JMW, Smit MJ (1989) Gadolinium chloride selectively blocks endocytosis by Kupffer cells. In: Wisse E, Knook DL, Decker K (eds) Cells of the hepatic sinusoid II. The Kupffer Cell Foundation, Rijswijk, The Netherlands, pp 132–133
6. Caldwell-Kenkel JC, Currin RT, Tanaka Y, Thurman RG, Lemasters JJ (1989) Reperfusion injury to endothelial cells following cold ischemic storage of rat liver. Hepatology 10: 292–299
7. Colletti LM, Burtch GD, Remick DG, Kunkel SL, Strieter RM, Guice KS, Oldham KT, Campbell DA (1990) The production of tumor necrosis factor alpha and the development of a pulmonary capillary injury following hepatic ischemia/reperfusion. Transplantation 49: 268–272
8. Connor HD, Gao W, Nukina S, Lemasters JJ, Mason RP, Thurman RG (1991) Free radicals are involved in graft failure following orthotopic liver transplantation: An EPR spin trapping study. Transplantation (submitted)
9. Currin RT, Lichtman SN, Thurman RG, Lemasters JJ (1991) Pentoxifylline, adenosine, prostaglandin E₁ and nisoldipine inhibit tumor necrosis factor release from LPS-stimulated rat Kupffer cells. Hepatology (in press)
10. Decker K (1990) Biologically active products of stimulated liver macrophages (Kupffer cells). Eur J Biochem 192: 245–261
11. Ford HR, Hoffman RA, Tweardy DJ, Kispert P, Wang S, Simmons RL (1991) Evidence that production of interleukin-6 within the rejecting allograft coincides with cytotoxic lymphocyte-T development. Transplantation 51: 656–661
12. Greig PD, Woolf GM, Sinclair SB, Abecassis M, Strasberg SM, Taylor BR, Blendis LM, Superina RA, Glynn MFX, Langer B,

13. Heinrich PC, Castell JV, Andus T (1990) Interleukin-6 and the acute phase response. Biochem J 265: 621–636
14. Hess P, Lansman JB, Tsien RW (1984) Different modes of Ca channel gating behavior favoured by dihydropyridine Ca agonists and antagonists. Nature 311: 538–544
15. Hijioka T, Rosenberg RL, Lemasters JJ, Thurman RG (1991) Rat Kupffer cells contain voltage-dependent calcium channels: Studies with Bay K-8644. FASEB J 5: A1390
16. Hocking DC, Phillips PG, Ferro TJ, Johnson A (1990) Mechanisms of pulmonary edema induced by tumor necrosis factor-α. Circ Res 67: 68–77
17. Kamada N, Calne RY (1979) Orthotopic liver transplantation in the rat. Technique using cuff for portal vein anastomosis and biliary drainage. Transplantation 28: 47–50
18. Karck U, Peters T, Decker K (1988) The release of tumor necrosis factor from endotoxin-stimulated rat Kupffer cells is regulated by prostaglandin E₂ and dexamethasone. J Hepatology 7: 352–361
19. Kramer SM, Carver ME (1986) Serum-free in vitro bioassay for the detection of tumor necrosis factor. J Immunol Methods 93: 201–206
20. Kuiper J, Zijlstra FJ, Kamps JAAM, Berkel TJC van (1988) Identification of prostaglandin D₂ as the major eicosanoid from liver endothelial and Kupffer cells. Biochim Biophys Acta 959: 143–152
21. Kuiper J, Zijlstra FJ, Kamps JAAM, Berkel TJC van (1989) Cellular communication inside the liver. Biochem J 262: 195–201
22. Mathison JC, Wolfson E, Ulevitch RJ (1988) Participation of tumor necrosis factor in the mediation of gram negative bacterial lipopolysaccharide-induced injury in rabbits. J Clin Invest 81: 1925–1937
23. Miyata T, Todo S, Imventarza O, Furukawa H, Starzl TE (1989) Endogenous endotoxemia during orthotopic liver transplantation in dogs. Transplant Proc 21: 3861–3862
24. Post S, Goerig M, Otto G, Manner M, Senninger N, Kommerell B, Herfarth C (1990) Prostanoid release in experimental liver transplantation. Transplantation 49: 490–494
25. Schindler R, Mancilla J, Endres S, Ghorbani R, Clark S, Dinarello CA (1990) Correlations and interactions in the production of interleukin-6 (IL-6), IL-1, and tumor necrosis factor (TNF) in human blood mononuclear cells: IL-6 suppresses IL-1 and TNF. Blood 75: 40–47
26. Steel RGD, Torrie JH (1980) Principles and procedures in statistics: A biometric approach. McGraw-Hill, New York
27. Takei Y, Marzi I, Kauffman FC, Currin RT, Lemasters JJ, Thurman RG (1990) Increase in survival time of liver transplants by protease inhibitors and a calcium channel blocker, nisoldipine. Transplantation 50: 14–20
28. Thurman RG, Cowper KB, Marzi I, Currin RT, Lemasters JJ (1988) Activation of Kupffer cells by storage of the liver in Euro-Collins solution. Hepatology 8: 261
29. Thurman RG, Marzi I, Seitz G, Thies J, Lemasters JJ, Zimmermann FA (1988) Hepatic reperfusion injury following orthotopic liver transplantation in the rat. Transplantation 46: 502–506
30. Tiegs G, Wolter M, Wendel A (1989) Tumor necrosis factor is a terminal mediator in galactosamine/endotoxin-induced hepatitis in mice. Biochem Pharmacol 38: 627–631
31. Tilg H, Vogel W, Aulitzky WE, Herold M, Königsrainer A, Margreiter R, Huber C (1990) Evaluation of cytokines and cytokine-induced secondary messages in sera of patients after liver transplantation. Transplantation 49: 1074–1080
32. Wang JF, Wendel A (1990) Studies on the hepatotoxicity of galactosamine/endotoxin or galactosamine/TNF in the perfused mouse liver. Biochem Pharmacol 39: 267–270
33. Zimmermann FA, Butcher GW, Davies HS, Brons G, Kamada N, Turel O (1979) Techniques of orthotopic liver transplantation in the rat and some studies of the immunologic response to fully allogeneic liver grafts. Transplant Proc 1: 571–577

Levy GA (1989) Treatment of primary liver graft nonfunction with prostaglandin E₁. Transplantation 48: 447–453

Transplant Int (1992) 5 [Suppl 1]: S 403–S 407

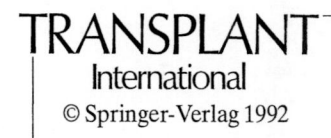

TRANSPLANT
International
© Springer-Verlag 1992

Comparison of HTK- and UW-solution for liver preservation tested in an orthotopic liver transplantation model in the pig

R. Steininger, E. Roth, P. Holzmüller[1], H. Reckendorfer[2], T. Grünberger, M. Sperlich[3], H. Burgmann[3], E. Moser[1], W. Feigl[2], F. Mühlbacher

I. Chirurgische Universitätsklinik, [3] Institut für Medizinische Physiologie, [1] Institut für Medizinische Physik,
Vienna University Medical School Wien, Austria
[2] Pathologisch-Bakteriologisches Institut der Allgemeinen Poliklinik, Mariannengasse 10, A-1090 Wien, Austria

Abstract. The aim of this experimental study was to compare the preservation potency of University of Wisconsin (UW) and HTK (Bretschneider) solutions in an orthotopic liver transplantation (OLT) model in pigs. Livers were harvested using an in situ perfusion technique, where organs were flushed with the solution being tested, stored on ice – cold storage (CS) – for 2 or 24 h and then transplanted. Parameters monitored were liver enzymes in serum, hepatic water content, high energy phosphates, nuclear magnetic resonance (NMR) relaxation time T2, light microscopy and bile production. CS for 24 h is an extreme in pig liver preservation and is not compatible with animal survival. Biopsies showed drastic morphological changes and grafts did not produce bile in either group. (Bile production 2 h CS: HTK, 5.6 ± 1.8 ml/h; UW, 4.7 ± 2.3 ml/h) Enzyme release after reperfusion (ΔSGOT, ΔLDH) was higher in long-term preservation. Hepatic tissue water content significantly decreased during CS in UW preserved livers. Edema alter reperfusion (ΔH_2O: HTK 24 h = + 5.6%, UW 24 h = + 4.8%) and regeneration capacity after reperfusion (UW 2 h = 63%, HTK 2 h = 55%, UW 24 h = 30%, HTK 24 h = 30%) were not significantly different. However, we did not observe major differences in preservation potency between the solutions tested. Differences were correlated, rather, with length 9 time of CS, than with the solution used. Therefore, HTK solution seemed to be a low potassium containing alternative to UW solution.

Key words: Comparison of HTK and UW solution – Liver preservation – Liver transplantation – Pig

The introduction of University of Wisconsin (UW) solution in solid organ preservation has had a major impact, particularly on the logistics of liver transplantation. Since this solution permits the storage of canine livers for 48 h [8] and human livers for 24 h [16], orthotopic liver transplantation has changed from an emergency procedure to a semielective procedure and, therefore, UW solution is currently standard in clinical liver transplantation. However, the histidine-buffered tryptophan ketoglutarate solution of Bretschneider (HTK), originally designed for cardioprotection and in clinical use for many years in heart surgery, has recently entered the field of solid organ preservation. Clinical trials are presently being carried out on its use in preservation of the kidney [3] and recent reports claim this solution is also very effective in preservation of the liver [13]. The results of organ preservation in the cold for these two solutions are quite different. One key component in UW solution seems to be the appropriate concentration of impermeants, counteracting hypothermic-induced cell swelling, whereas HTK solution contains very effective buffer systems, using the principal of equilibration of the extracellular space without any impermeants. The aim of this experimental study was to compare some aspects of the preservation potency of UW and HTK solutions in short- (2 h) and long-term (24 h) cold storage (CS) in an orthotopic liver transplantation (OLT) model in the pig. Efficacy of preservation was evaluated by monitoring the following parameters during the procedure: histological examination of liver specimens, hepatic tissue water content, high energy phosphate levels, graft nuclear magnetic resonance NMR relaxation time T2, enzyme release and bile production after reperfusion.

Materials and methods

Young, white large pigs of the German land race weighing 20–25 kg (mean 22.5 ± 2.6 kg) of either sex were used as donors and recipients. After a fasting period of 24 h, livers were harvested from the donors using an in situ perfusion technique. Organs were flushed by gravity with the test solution (4°C) by giving 1 l via the aorta (pressure = 120 cmH$_2$O) and 1 l via the portal vein (pressure = 25 cmH$_2$O). HTK preserved organs were flushed with an additional 2 l via the portal vein at the backtable, according to the recommendation of the manufacturer, to achieve equilibration of the extracellular space.

Offprint requests to: R. Steininger, I. Chirurg. Universitätsklinik Wien, Alserstrasse 4, A-1090 Wien, Austria

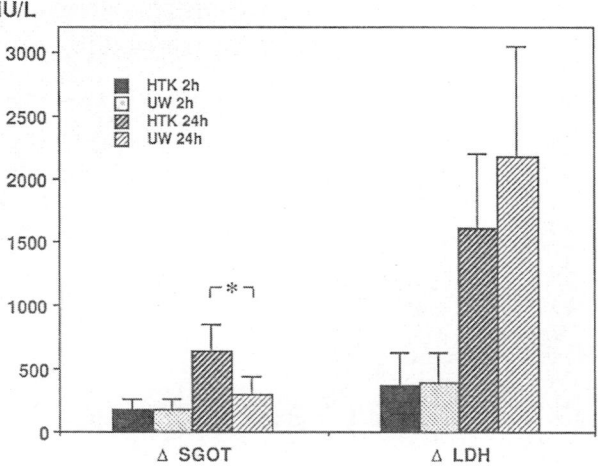

IU/L

Fig. 1. Changes in SGOT and LDH after reperfusion (IU/l). Significant changes in ΔSGOT and ΔLDH in short- and long term HTK, and in ΔLDH in short- and long-term UW preserved grafts. There was a smaller ΔSGOT in 24 h UW preserved liver (* $P < 0.05$) as compared to 24 h HTK preserved livers

The livers were stored in an additional 500 ml of the same solution in two sterile plastic bags, packed on ice (0–4 °C) and subjected to a short or a long time of cold storage (CS). Groups were as follows: short-time preservation (CS = 2 h): HTK $n = 3$, UW $n = 4$; long-time preservation (CS = 24 h): HTK $n = 6$, UW $n = 6$.

At the end of the preservation period, the livers were transplanted orthotopically using a standard technique. A passive venovenous bypass from the end of the portal vein to the internal jugular vein was used during the anhepatic period. Before completing the infrahepatic caval anastomosis, all grafts were washed out via the portal vein with 500 ml Haemaccel to remove the preservation fluid. This step was necessary only in UW preserved livers containing high levels of potassium, but was done also in HTK preserved organs to keep experimental conditions comparable. Reperfusion of the liver was carried out simultaneously via the hepatic artery and the portal vein. Hemodynamic conditions were monitored by continuous registration of CVP and arterial blood pressure. Animals with hemodynamic instability, especially during reperfusion, were excluded. Blood samples (collected from a catheter in the jugular vein) and liver excision biopsies were obtained at the beginning of the donor operation (normal), at the end of cold storage (CS) before and after the Haemaccel flush, immediately before reperfusion (WIT), and 30 min and 2 h after reperfusion. For clarity, only the data of three points of greatest interest during the procedure were compared: normal, end of CS and 30 min after reperfusion. Liver enzymes in serum were estimated by using comercially available kits. For histological examinations, liver biopies were fixed in 4.5 % formol, prepared for light microscopy and stained with HE and CAB. Bile was collected quantitatively by insertion of a catheter into the common bile duct of the graft. For estimation of overall hepatic tissue water content, liver specimens were blotted and weighed immediately after excision (mean wet weight of sample 27.8 ± 9 mg) and then reweighed again after drying at 90 °C for 36 h. Hepatic tissue water content is given as the difference between wet and dry weight of liver specimens. High energy phosphate levels of liver tissue were assessed by high performance liquid chromatography (HPLC). In preparation for HPLC analysis using an LKB HPLC system (LKB-Produktor AB, Bromma, Sweden), tissue samples were weighed and immediately homogenized in 3 ml of 8 % perchloric acid [4]. The homogenate was centrifuged for 10 min at 3000 rpm, the supernatant was collected and adjusted to pH 6.0 using 4 M KOH. After passing through a 0.45 μm acro-disk filter (Sartorius Göttingen, FRG), 20 μl of the sample was applied to a reverse phase column (LKB 2134 UltroPac Li- Chromosorb RP-18.5 μm 4.0 × 250 mm) and eluted at a flow speed of

0.5 ml/min with 0.2 M NaH$_2$PO$_4$, 0.025 M tetrabutylammoniumhydroxyde, 18 % methanol (v/v), pH 6.0. Peaks were detected at 254 nm by an ultraviolet detector (LKB 2151 variable wavelength monitor) and recorded on a LKG 2210 recorder. Each peak was assigned by comparison with retention times of authentic compounds. The concentration of nucleotides was estimated by measuring the peak area. Energy charge (EC) was calculated according to the formula by Atkinson [1]. Proton nuclear magnetic resonance (NMR) spin-spin relaxation time T2 was determined 30 min after biopsy excision using a low resolution1H-NMR spectrometer (Minispec pc 120, 0.47 T Bruker, Karlsruhe, FRG) and applying a CPMG pulse sequence (TE = 2 ms, N = 100, Tr = 3.0 s, 9 averages) [11]. Measurement temperature was 37 °C. A monoexponential model was fitted for quantitative data analysis.

Statistical analysis. Mean values and standard deviations are given in the results section. Differences were analysed by means of *t*-test or by Mann-Whitney U test (nonparametric data). Probability values of $P < 0.05$ were considered to be statistically significant.

Results

Histological examinations. In all cases, we could differentiate clearly between long- and short-term preservation, because of major differences in the morphological findings after reperfusion. However, it was impossible to find major differences between organs preserved in HTK or UW. When the length of CS was 2 h, all specimens (UW and HTK) showed a normal hepatic architecture with normal sinusoidal structure at the end of CS. Also on reperfusion, there was no evidence for the occurrence of severe hemorrhage or detachement of endothelial cells. After 24 h of CS in both groups (UW and HTK), a regular organisation of the hepatic lobules and considerable sinusoidal dilatation with pyknosis of some sinusoidal endothelial cells was observed. Hepatocytes were quite intact, except for the occurrence of moderate microvesicular steatosis. After flushing the grafts with Haemaccel to remove the preservation fluid, a marked detachment of sinusoidal lining cells with accompanying enlargement of the spaces of Disse was seen. At 30 min after reperfusion, drastic morphological changes were obvious in liver specimens from both groups. The hepatocytes were spread by sinus' full of blood, with pyknosis of the nucleus in several cells, there was necrosis of numerous single cells and areas with hepatocyte apoptosis. In addition, we found considerable areas of hemorrhage in the portal tracts and even in the walls of hepatic veins. Numerous sinusoidal lining cells were detached from the underlying hepatocytes with condensed nuclei and pyknosis.

Bile production. Long-term preserved grafts did not produce any bile in the first h after reperfusion after preservation in either UW or HTK. Short-term preserved organs immediately produced comparable amounts of well-colored bile in both groups. (HTK, 5.6 ± 1.8 ml; UW, 4.7 ± 2.3 ml).

Liver enzymes. Changes in GOT and LDH are depicted in Fig. 1 as the differences between concentrations 30 min after reperfusion and normal values. There were significant differences in ΔSGOT and ΔLDH between short-

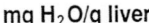

mg H$_2$O/g liver

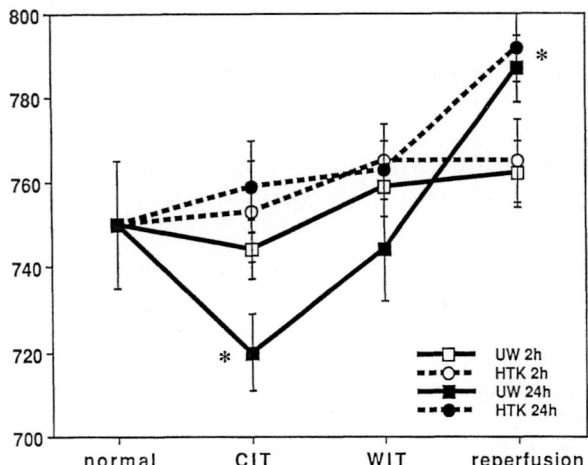

Fig. 2. Hepatic tissue water content at the end of cold storage *(CIT)*, immediately before *(WIT)* and 30 min after reperfusion (mgH$_2$O/g liver). There was significantly (* $P < 0.05$) less water content in 24 h UW preserved grafts at the end of CIT. There was marked edema after reperfusion in all livers stored for 24 h (* $P < 0.05$)

Δ EC

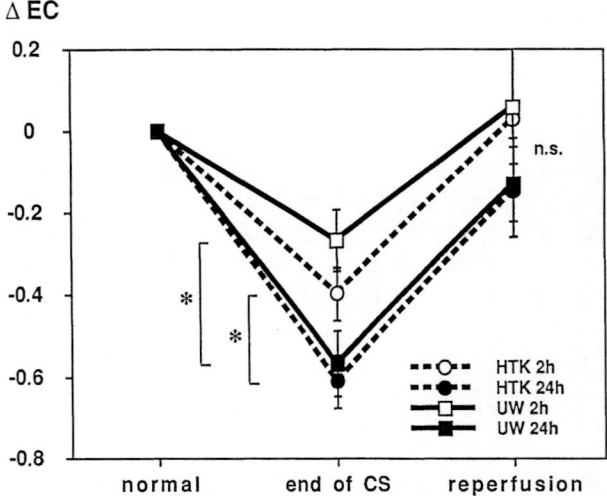

Fig. 4. Changes in energy charge *(EC)* of liver tissue at the end of CS and after reperfusion. EC = ATP + 0.5 ADP/ATP + ADP + AMP. There were significantly different EC levels at the end of CS between long- and short-term preserved grafts (* $P < 0.05$). There was good restoration of EC after reperfusion in grafts stored for 24 h. No major effect of the solution used was observed

% ATP

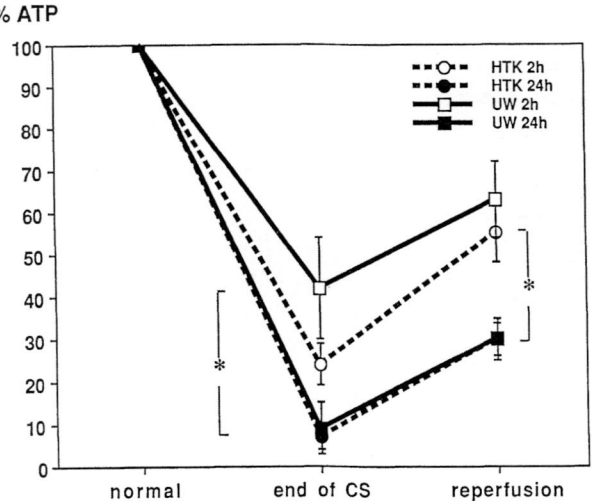

Fig. 3. ATP (% of normal) in liver tissue at the end of CS and after reperfusion. There was significantly less ATP in long-term preserved grafts after CS and after reperfusion (* $P < 0.05$). No major effect of the preservation solutions was observed

and long-term preservation in HTK (ΔSGOT, 174 ± 86 IU/l vs 639 ± 207 IU/l; ΔLDH, 363 ± 264 IU/l vs 1611 ± 590 IU/l; $P < 0.01$) and in ΔLDH between short- and long-term preservation in UW (383 ± 239 IU/l vs 2179 ± 869 IU/l, $P < 0.01$), but no significant difference was observed in ΔSGOT levels between UW (179 ± 82 IU/l vs 297 ± 133 IU/l). Comparison of UW and HTK solutions for the same preservation time showed no differences in enzyme release despite lower ΔSGOT levels in the 24 h UW group as compared to the 24 h HTK group ($P < 0.05$).

Tissue water content. In organs preserved for 2 h, hepatic tissue water content was found to be in the normal range in the HTK as well as in the UW group at the end of CS and also after reperfusion (Fig. 2). Normal hepatic tissue water content was found to be 750.8 ± 16 mg H$_2$O/g liver.

Long-term UW preserved livers showed a significant decrease in tissue water content at the end of CIT (720.5 ± 9.5 mg H$_2$O/g liver; $P < 0.01$ compared to normal), whereas in long-term HTK preserved organs no major changes were detectable after 24 h of CS (763.2 ± 7.8 mg H$_2$O/g liver). There was a significant difference between the water content of HTK preserved organs and UW preserved organs at the end of CS. Marked tissue edema, both in UW and in HTK preserved grafts (789.2 ± 8.7 mg H$_2$O/g liver vs 792.2 ± 8.3 mg H$_2$O/g liver, $P < 0.01$ compared to normal) was observed after reperfusion with no significant difference between the groups.

High energy phosphates. Due to the large scatter of data obtained from normal pig liver (ATP, 7.26 ± 0.94 µmol/g dry liver tissue; EC, 0.719 ± 0.063), the percentage of normal values (for ATP) and differences from normal values (for EC) were used for comparison between the groups and results are shown in Figs. 3 and 4. After 2 h of CS, ATP levels dropped to 24.1 ± 5 % in HTK and to 42.2 ± 12 % in UW preserved livers ($P < 0.05$) and were significantly lower ($P < 0.05$) after 24 h of CS in HTK (6.9 ± 3.2 %) and UW preserved grafts (9.2 ± 5.5 %). On reperfusion of the organ, ATP levels increased in short-term preserved organs to 54.8 ± 7.3 % (HTK) and 62.7 ± 9.4 % (UW) and in long-term preserved organs to 30.1 ± 4.1 % (HTK) and 30.0 ± 5.5 % (UW), indicating significant differences ($P < 0.05$) only for the length of preservation and not for the solution used. Energy charge dropped by 0.39 ± 0.06 (HTK) and 0.27 ± 0.07 (UW) after 2 h and by 0.61 ± 0.06 (HTK) and 0.57 ± 0.08 (UW) after 24 hours CS. After reperfusion EC returned to normal in short-term and to near normal values in long-term preserved organs. These changes were not significant.

Spin-spin relaxation time T2. Due to the large scatter of data obtained from normal pig liver (T2 = 46.5 ± 4.1 ms) only the use of Δ values was appropriate. At the end of CS, long-term UW preserved livers showed a marked decrease in T2. There was no change in the HTK group. (HTK 2 h, -1.9 ± 3.3 ms; HTK 24 h, -0.34 ± 4.9 ms; UW 2 h, -1.1 ± 3.4 ms; UW 24 h, -8.2 ± 2.9 ms). There was a highly significant correlation between ΔT2 and Δ water content (HTK, $r = 0.80$; UW, $r = 0.85$; $P < 0.001$) for both storage solutions. Also highly significant correlations were detected between ΔT2, ΔATP and Δ EC for UW. (ΔT2/ΔATP, $r = 0.75$, $P < 0.005$; ΔT2/ΔEC, $r = 0.73$, $P < 0.005$).

Discussion

In a review of the principles of solid organ preservation [2] Belzer and Southard have suggested, that an effective and appropriate flushout solution should have a composition that (1) minimizes hypothermic induced cell swelling, (2) prevents intracellular acidosis (3) prevents the expansion of the interstitial space during the flushout period, (4) prevents injury from oxygen free radicals and (5) provides substrates for regenerating high-energy phosphate compounds during reperfusion. The aim of our study was to evaluate points (1), (3), and (5) of these principals, determining tissue water content and high energy phosphate levels in an experimental model in the pig. Using a large animal model, the conditions of human liver transplantation were well imitated, with similar operative trauma, a second warm ischemic period during grafting and similar sized vessels for anastomosis. Furthermore, we examined time-periods during the procedure, where the quality of the preservation solution had a major impact on liver viability and the influence of factors unrelated to preservation were minimal. Therefore, this model should be suitable for the comparison of preservation solutions. Looking at morphology and bile production after reperfusion, there was marked damage to the grafts stored for 24 h as early as 30 min after reperfusion, whereas the appearance and function of livers stored for 2 h was quite normal. Furthermore, tissue edema, as monitored by hepatic water content, indicated considerable disturbance of cell membrane integrity. In this study CS for 24 h seemed to result in liver damage independent of the protective effect of the solution used. However, a certain regeneration capacity of high energy phosphates was also obvious in long-term preserved grafts, as shown by an increase in ATP and EC levels after reperfusion. Hepatocytes are thought to be relatively resistant and to be involved only secondarily in ischemia-reperfusion injury [17]. Good energy restoration early after reperfusion and minimal changes in cell-morphology of the hepatocytes confirmed these findings. Preventing micro-circulatory disturbances by maintaining the integrity of endothelial and sinusoidal lining cells during CS appears to be very important for liver preservation [7, 12]. Several reports have been published concerning damage to endothelial cells by using flushout solutions for organ preservation [9, 10]. In our study, in both groups (HTK and UW), after 24 h of CS, the first signs of injury were already evident in sinusoidal endothelial cells at the end of CS. Looking for a quick viability parameter to distinguish, before reperfusion, between good and poor donor livers we investigated T2 relaxation times, and found correlations with tissue water content and high energy phosphate levels. However, these promising results were obtained from a small series and the value of this method has to be confirmed in further studies. Most of the parameters monitored in our study could clearly differentiate between short- and long-term preservation. Comparing HTK and UW solution by means of hepatic water content, it was evident that in grafts preserved in HTK, tissue water content remained in the normal range even after long-term preservation; UW solution was able to draw water from the tissues during CS, but edema after reperfusion was also found to be in the normal range. Although UW solution contains adenosine, which has been found to be an effective substrate for the resynthesis of ATP, we did not observe any major differences in the regeneration capacity of high energy phosphates in our model. The effectiveness of adenosine was demonstrated by using isolated cell models of organ preservation and the importance of adenosine in UW solution is still debated [14]. Comparing HTK and UW solutions in the preservation of the pig liver, we did not observe a major advantage in using one or other of the solutions. A solution that offers greater buffering capacity and uses the principle of equilibration would have greater preservation potency. This would be achieved by a solution stressing the osmotic force during CS. First attempts to combine histidine and lactobionate in a new solution are reported to be very effective [15]. Therefore, the HTK solution seems to be a low potassium containing alternative to the UW solution. The first promising results in clinical liver preservation with HTK solution confirm our results [5, 6].

References

1. Atkinson DE (1968) The energy charge of the adenylate pool as a regulatory parameter; interaction with feed back modifiers. Biochemistry 7:4030–4036
2. Belzer FO, Southard JH (1988) Principles of solid organ preservation by cold storage. Transplantation 45:673–676
3. Groenewoud AF, Isemer FE, Stadler J (1989) A comparison of early function between kidney grafts protected with HTK solution versus Euro-Collins solution. Transplant Proc 21:1243–1244
4. Gruber W, Moellering H, Bergmeyer HU (1974) Bestimmung von ADP, ATP sowie Summe GTP + ITP in biologischem Material. In: Bergmeyer HU (ed) Methoden der enzymatischen Analyse. Verlag Chemie, Weinheim 7:351–355
5. Gubernatis G, Kemnitz J, Oldhafer KJ, Hauss J, Pichlmayr R (1991) Extended cold preservation time of a human liver graft by using the cardioplegic HTK solution (Bretschneider). Transplant Proc 5:560–561
6. Gubernatis G, Pichlmayr R, Lamesch P, Grosse H, Bornscheuer A, Meyer HJ, Ringe B, Farle M, Bretschneider HJ (1990) HTK-solution (Bretschneider) for human liver transplantation. Langenbecks Arch Chir 375:66–70
7. Holloway CMB, Harvey PRC, Strasberg SM (1990) Viability of sinusoidal lining cells in cold preserved rat liver allografts. Transplantation 49:225–229
8. Jamieson NV, Sundberg R, Lindell S, Claesson K, Moen J, Vreugdenhil PK, Wight DGD, Southard JH, Belzer FO (1988)

Preservation of the canine liver for 24–48 hours using simple cold storage with UW solution. Transplantation 46:517–522

9. Lahnborg G, Bracher M, Hickman R, Terblanche J (1989) Disturbances of reticulo-endothelial function following experimental liver transplantation. Eur Surg Res 21:129–136

10. Mc Keown CMB, Edwards V, Phillips MJ, Harvey PRC, Petrunka CN, Strasberg SM (1988) Sinusoidal lining cell damage, the critical injury in cold preservation of liver allografts in the rat. Transplantation 46:178–191

11. Moser E, Gomiscek G, Schuster J, Echsel H (1989) Systematic investigation of degradation effects on spin-spin relaxation times in mouse liver by low resolution NMR. Physiol Med NMR 21:133–144

12. Pienaar BH, Stapleton GN, Bracher M, Lotz Z, Innes CR, Fourie J, Hickman R (1991) Six-hour porcine liver storage without flushing or perfusion. Transplantation 52:38–43

13. Pichlmayr R, Bretschneider HJ, Kirchner E (1988) Ex situ Operation an der Leber – Eine neue Möglichkeit in der Leberchirurgie. Langenbecks Arch Chir 373:122–126

14. Southard JH, Gulik TM van, Ametani MS, Lindell SL, Pienaar BL, Belzer FO (1990) Important components of the UW solution. Transplantation 49:251–257

15. Sumimoto R, Kamada N, Jamieson NV, Fukuda Y, Dohi K (1991) A comparison of a new solution combining histidine and lactobionate with UW solution and Eurocollins for rat liver preservation. Transplantation 51:589–593

16. Todo S, Nery J, Yanaga K, Podesta L, Gordon RD, Starzl TE (1989) Extended preservation of human liver grafts with UW solution. JAMA 261:711–714

17. Wu D, Piche D, Huet PM, Viallet A (1989) The surprising resistance of hepatocytes to cold ischemia. Hepatology 10:623–628

Transplant Int (1992) 5 [Suppl 1]: S 408–S 410

TRANSPLANT
International
© Springer-Verlag 1992

A comparison of histadine lactobionate solution with University of Wisconsin solution for rat liver and heart preservation

R. Sumimoto[1], K. Dohi[1], Y. Fukuda[1], T. Urushihara[1], K. Sumimoto[1], and N. Kamada[2]

[1] Second Department of Surgery, Hiroshima University, School of Medicine, Hiroshima, Japan
[2] Department of Experimental Surgery, National Children's Medical Research Center, Tokyo, Japan

Abstract. We developed a new solution mainly composed of Na-lactobionate and histidine (HL) and compared the effectiveness of this solution with that of University of Wisconsin (UW) solution using orthotopic liver and heterotopic heart transplantation in rats. The new solution has a higher sodium content and a lower potassium content (Na, 90 mEq/l; K, 45 mEq/l) than UW. Hydroxyethyl starch, adenosine, dexamethasone and insulin are not included. Buffering capacity is increased by adding histidine (90 mM/l) together with KH_2PO_4 (20 mM/l). Rat liver was perserved in either UW or HL solution hypothermically for 24 h and then transplanted orthotopically into the recipient rat. The heart was preserved in either solution for 18 h and transplanted heterotopically into the recipient rat. The 1-week survival rate for rats receiving livers preserved in UW for 24 h at 4°C was 29% (5/17). In contrast, the new solution (HL) gave a 78% (11/14) survival rate ($P < 0.01$). The 1-week heart graft survival rate, using UW solution was 50% (3/6), following 18-h cold preservation, whereas all hearts (7/7) continued to beat for over a week using new HL solution ($P < 0.05$). These results demonstrated that the new HL solution, with a substantial buffering capacity, was superior to UW solution in rat liver and heart preservation.

Key words: Rat liver preservation – Rat heart preservation – UW solution – Histidine – Buffering capacity

University of Wisconsin (UW) solution has had a great impact in the field of organ transplantation and preservation [5, 6]. However, clinical heart preservation has not benefited from it, and there still appears to be some room left for its further improvement. We have shown that the UW solution has a high viscosity, a high potassium content, and a low buffering capacity as compared with con-

ventional preservation solutions such as EuroCollins solution, citrate solution and phosphate-buffered sucrose solution. These limiting factors undermine ideal long-term preservation. By ameliorating these points it is, therefore, possible to develop a better preservation solution than standard UW solution. In this experiment we described the use of a new solution composed mainly of Na-lactobionate and histidine (HL) and compared the effect of this solution with standard UW solution employing the orthotopic rat liver and heterotopic heart transplant models.

Materials and methods

Male Wistar rats for liver transplantation and Lewis rats for heart transplantation were used as donors and recipients respectively.

Rat liver preservation and transplantation. Following the intravenous injection of 200 units of heparin, the donor liver was perfused in situ with 3–5 ml of chilled test solution via the portal vein. The liver was preserved hypothermically (4°C) in a beaker containing the test solution for 24 h and then transplanted orthotopically into the recipient rat according to the modified techniques originally described by Kamada [7]. Arterial reconstruction was not performed. One-week survival rates were compared.

Rat heart preservation and transplantation. Following the injection of 200 units of heparin, the donor heart was initially perfused in situ with 5 ml of chilled test solution via the suprahepatic vena cava and excised. The heart was perfused with 2 ml of chilled test solution by manual injection via the aortic root and immersed in the test solution at 4°C. After 18 h of storage, the heart was transplanted in the right side of the neck of the recipient animal according to the modified techniques described by Heron [3]. Graft survival was judged by inspecting and palpating the heart. One-week graft survival rates were compared.

Test solution. The composition of HL solution and standard UW solution is shown in Table 1. The solutions contain penicillin and streptomycin and were filter sterilized and stored at 4°C and used within 1 week of preparation.

Offprint requests to: Ryo Sumimoto, M.D., 2nd Department of Surgery, School of Medicine, Hiroshima University, 1-2-3, Kasumi Minami-ku, Hiroshima 730, Japan

Table 1. Composition of UW and HL solutions (mM/l)

K-lactobionate	100	
Na-lactobionate		90
Histidine		90
Na-KH$_2$PO$_4$	25	
K-KH$_2$PO$_4$		20
Raffinose	30	25
MgSO$_4$	5	5
Glutathione	3	3
Adenosine	5	
Allopurinol	1	1
Insulin	100 U/l	
Hydroxyethyl starch	5 g%	
Na (mEq/l)	30	90
K (mEq/l)	120	45
Osmolarity	320–330	320–330
pH	7.4	7.4

Table 2. The viscosity of UW, EC and HL solutions. Values are means ($n = 6$ per group)

H$_2$O	UW solution	EC solution	HL solution
1.0	3.32	1.21	1.33

Table 3. The buffering capacity (mEq/l/per pH unit) of UW, EC, PBS and HL solutions. Values are shown as means ($n = 3$ per group)

UW solution	EC solution	PBS solution	HL solution
11	20	30	28

Viscosity. The viscosity of the test solution was measured at 4°C using an Ostwald viscosity meter and expressed as a ratio in comparison with the value for deionized water (Table 2).

Buffering capacity. The buffering capacity of the solutions was defined as the number of milliequivalents per liter of H + required to produce a decline of one pH unit from the initial pH of the test solution. This was determined by plotting the pH (measured at 15°C) when 1 l of test solution was titrated with 0.1 M HCl (Table 3).

Tissue water content. Samples of liver tissue were taken immediately before initial flushing and folowing 24 h and 48 h of cold preservation. The tissue was weighed immediately to give wet weight and then reweighed after being dried overnight in an oven at 105°C to give the dry weight. The tissue water content could then be calculated from the following formula:

$$\text{tissue water content} = \frac{(wet\ weight - dry\ weight)}{wet\ weight} \times 100\,(\%)\ \text{(Table 4)}$$

pH change. The pH change in each test solution was measured at 15°C before and after 24 and 48 h of liver preservation using a pH meter (Table 5).

Results

The results are shown in Tables 2–6. This new solution has a lower viscosity (1.33 vs. 3.32) and a substantial buffering capacity (30 vs. 10 mEq/l per pH unit) as compared with that of standard UW solution. The results of pH change in the preservation solution surrounding the graft suggested

Table 4. Tissue water content (liver) (%). Values are shown as means with SD ($n = 6$ per group)

	Before flush	After 24 h	After 48 h
UW solution	72.0 ± 0.4	67.8 ± 0.3	67.6 ± 0.7
HL solution	71.6 ± 0.8	67.9 ± 0.5	68.4 ± 0.6

Table 5. The pH values of the preservation solution surrounding the graft. Values are shown as means with SD ($n = 6$ per group)

	Before immersion	After 24 h	After 48 h
UW solution	7.40	7.20 ± 0.03	7.16 ± 0.02
HL solution	7.40	7.38 ± 0.05	7.35 ± 0.04

Table 6. % Graft survival. Rat livers or hearts were preserved for the indicated time and transplanted. Survival was considered 100% if graft was functioning on the 7th day post-transplant. Values given are surviving grafts/total

	UW	HL
Liver 24 h	29% (5/17)	78% (11/14)*
Heart 18 h	50% (3/6)	100% (7/7)**

* $P < 0.05$ vs UW
** $P < 0.05$ vs UW

that the combined histidine-KH$_2$PO$_4$ buffer was more effective than the phosphate buffer alone in UW solution.

Hearts preserved in UW solution for 18 h developed a dark red appearance shortly after reperfusion. Three out of six heart grafts failed within 1 week. In contrast, all heart grafts preserved in HL solution retained a normal light pink color after revascularization and effective beating commenced. All seven grafts continued to beat for over a week.

The livers preserved in UW for 24 h developed a mottled appearance on reperfusion, suggesting an area of no reflow and subcapsular hemorrhage. The 1-week survival rate for UW was 29%. Using HL solution, 78% of the rats receiving livers preserved for 24 h survived for over 1 week. In this group, livers rapidly resumed normal color and showed an even perfusion.

Discussion

Since the introduction of UW solution in 1986, preservation times of solid organs have ben markedly extended in animal experiments [5, 14] and in the clinical situation [6, 13]. Nevertheless, it is still unclear whether and to what extent all components contribute to the effect of the UW solution. From our earlier experiments using the rat liver transplant model, we can safely conclude that the dramatic effect of the UW solution results from the use of lactobionate as an anion and the inclusion of fresh glutathione as a radical scavenger [1, 11, 12]. The effect of the other pharmacological components, if any, is masked under the effect of these two components. Moreover, the apparent limitations of the UW solution are as follows: (1) UW has a high viscosity due to the inclusion of hydroxyethyl starch which does not permit rapid organ perfusion,

(2) the high potassium cation content in the UW solution produces vasoconstriction and endothelial cell injury when used in the initial perfusion [8, 10], and (3) the substantially small buffering capacity of the UW solution augments intracellular acidosis during cold storage that can be deleterious to cell viability if the preservation times are extended.

Histidine has pK values of 1.78, 5.97 and 8.97 and appears to be a highly effective buffer in the physiological pH range. This amino acid can be safely added to the preservation solution without raising the electrolyte content or the osmolarity. Bretschneider's solution [2], which consists primarily of histidine with low concentrations of sodium and potassium, has been widely used experimentally and clinically in the heart, liver [9], and kidney [4]. The HL solution was thus formulated by combining constituents from our previous experiments with lactobionate-based solutions, with histidine as a buffer, to produce a solution containing, what we believed to be, the most important components included in the UW solution and Bretschneider's solution. Although UW solution has been shown to preserve effectively abdominal organs, clinical heart preservation has not benefitted from these advances in preservation, the best results being obtained with a modified UW solution experimentally.

These experiments clearly demonstrated that when using a solution in which Na-lactobionate and histidine were combined it was possible to produce results which were superior to the standard UW solution in rat liver and heart preservation. Although the mechanism of action of histidine has not been fully defined, the results with HL merit investigation and trials in larger animals and in man.

References

1. Boudjema K, Gulik TM, Lindell SL, Vreugdenhil PS, Southard JH, Belzer FO (1990) Effect of oxidized and reduced glutathione in liver preservation. Transplantation 50:948–951

2. Heinemeyer D, Belles G, Stapenhorst K (1987) Intracellular pH measurements during cardiac arrest in ventricular myocardium by Bretschneider's cardioplegic solution HTK and St. Thomas Hospital solution with and without procaine. Thorac Cardiovasc Surg 35:48

3. Heron I (1971) A technique for accessory cervical heart transplantation in rabbits and rats. Acta Pathol Microbiol Scand 79:366

4. Ismer FE, Ludwig A, Schunck O, Bretschneider HJ, Peiper HJ (1988) Kidney procurement with the HTK solution of Bretschneider. Transplant Proc 20:885

5. Jamieson NV, Sunderberg R, Lindell S, Claesson K, Moen J, Vreugdenhil PK, Wight DGD, Southard JH, Belzer FO (1988) Preservation of the canine liver for 24–48 hour using simple cold storage with UW solution. Transplantation 46:517–522

6. Kalayoglu M, Sollinger HW, Stratta RJ, D'alessandro AM, Hoffmann RM, Pirsch JD, Belzer FO (1988) Extended preservation of the liver for clinical transplantation. Lancet 19:617

7. Kamada N, Calne RY (1979) Orthotopic liver transplantation in the rat. Technique using cuff for portal vein anastomosis and biliary drainage. Transplantation 28:47

8. Moen J, Claesson K, Pienaar H, Lindell S, Ploeg RJ, McAnulty JF, Vreugdenhil P, Southard JH, Belzer FO (1989) Preservation of dog liver, kidney and pancreas using the Belzer-UW solution with a high sodium and low-potassium content. Transplantation 47:940–945

9. Pichlmayr R, Bretschneider HJ, Kirchner E (1988) Ex situ Operation an der Leber – eine neue Möglichkeit in der Leberchirurgie. Langenbecks Arch Chir 20:122

10. Sumimoto R, Jamieson NV, Wake K, Kamada N (1989) 24-hour rat liver preservation using UW solution and some simplified variants. Transplantation 48:1–5

11. Sumimoto R, Jamieson NV, Kamada N (1990) Examination of the role of the impermeants lactobionate and raffinose in a modified UW solution. Transplantation 50:573–577

12. Sumimoto R, Jamieson NV, Kobayashi T, Fukuda Y, Dohi K, Kamada N (1991) The need for glutathione and allopurinol in the HL solution for rat liver preservation. Transplantation 52:565–567

13. Todo S, Nery, Yanaga K, Podesta L, Gordon RD, Starzl TW (1989) Extended preservation of human liver grafts with UW solution. JAMA 261:711–714

14. Wahlberg JA, Love R, Landegaard L, Southard JH, Belzer FO (1987) Successful 72 hour preservation of the canine pancreas. Transplantation 43:5–8

Transplant Int (1992) 5 [Suppl 1]: S411–S416

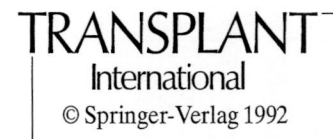

© Springer-Verlag 1992

The significant role of membrane stabilization in hypothermic cardioplegic cardiac preservation in a canine experimental model

Makoto Sunamori, Imad Sultan, Toshizumi Shirai, and Akio Suzuki

From the Department of Thoracic-Cardiovascular Surgery, Tokyo Medical and Dental University, School of Medicine, Tokyo, Japan

Abstract. Isolated mongrel hearts were preserved for 6 h at 5 °C followed by normothermic reperfusion for 2 h. The dogs were divided into three groups; K^+-cardioplegic solution alone, group C, $n = 7$; K^+-cardioplegic solution with lidocaine 200 mg/l, group L, $n = 7$; and K^+-cardioplegic solution with betamethasone 250 mg/l and lidocaine 200 mg/l, group B + L, $n = 7$. Ventricular fibrillation occurred early during reperfusion in all dogs in group C, in one of seven in group L, and in two of seven dogs in group B + L. The serum MB fraction of creatinine kinase (MB-CK), mitochondrial aspartate aminotransferase (m-AAT) and calcium overload were suppressed to a greater extent in both groups L and B + L during reperfusion compared to group C. Myocardial ATP, total adenine nucleotide, and creatine phosphate did not differ between the three groups at the end of reperfusion. Myocardial ADP and AMP declined significantly during reperfusion in group C, however, they remained unchanged in group B + L and increased in group L which showed significantly higher levels compared to group C. Left ventricular functional recovery during reperfusion was consistently better in both group L and B + L compared to group C. These results suggested that membrane stabilization prevents myocardial damage from hypothermia and cardioplegia and provides better myocardial viability and functional recovery in donor heart preservation.

Key words: Heart transplantation – Cardioplegic solution – Lidocaine – Betamethasone

The preservation of the donor heart is a major issue in cardiac transplantation. This falls within two objectives: to improve the early operative results and to increase the supply of donor hearts. Hypothermia has been widely accepted as a means of myocardial preservation since it reduces myocardial consumption of oxygen and metabolic demand. However, hypothermia below 15 °C inhibits the activity of membrane-bound ATPase resulting in ionic shifts across the sarcolemma [14] and inducing a change in the fluidity of the phospholipid layers of the membrane [7, 15].

The current method of cardioplegia is based largely on depolarization of the membrane of the myocyte. Under depolarized conditions, myocardial cells are exposed to unfavorable phenomena such as increased permeability and the accumulation of sodium and calcium, with subsequent cellular swelling. Calcium overload is thought to be one of the major causes of reperfusion injury [18]. The function of the myocardial membranes is severely modified under conditions of prolonged ischemia followed by reperfusion. The major problems during reperfusion include dysrrhythmias, depletion of high energy phosphate (HEP), ventricular dysfunction, and myocardial necrosis.

Lidocaine hydrochloride [2, 6, 10, 13, 17, 19, 22–24, 33] and betamethasone [9, 25, 29], one of the glucocorticoids, have been reported to have a significant effect on membrane stabilization in the myocardium via different mechanisms. Thus, our objective was to elucidate the effects of membrane stabilization with lidocaine alone or lidocaine plus betamethasone in preservation of the donor heart. We evaluated myocardial viability by assessing biochemical findings, cell ultrastructure, and left ventricular function in experimental hypothermic cardioplegic cardiac preservation.

Offprint requests to: Makoto Sunamori, M.D., Department of Thoracic-Cardiovascular Surgery, Tokyo Medical and Dental University, School of Medicine, 1-5-45, Yushima, Bunkyo-ku, Tokyo, 113, Japan

Materials and methods

Twenty-one mogrel dogs weighing between 8 and 21 kg were used in this experiment. All dogs were anesthetized with pentobarbital (approximately 30 mg/kg intravenously) to the suppression of corneal reflexes. Respiration was controlled with a positive-pressure ventilator. Ringer's lactate solution was infused intravenously to maintain a physiologic hemodynamic status. These animals received humane care as described in "Principles of Laboratory Animal Care" formulated by the National Society for Medical Research and the "Guide for the Care and Use of Laboratory Animals" prepared by the Na-

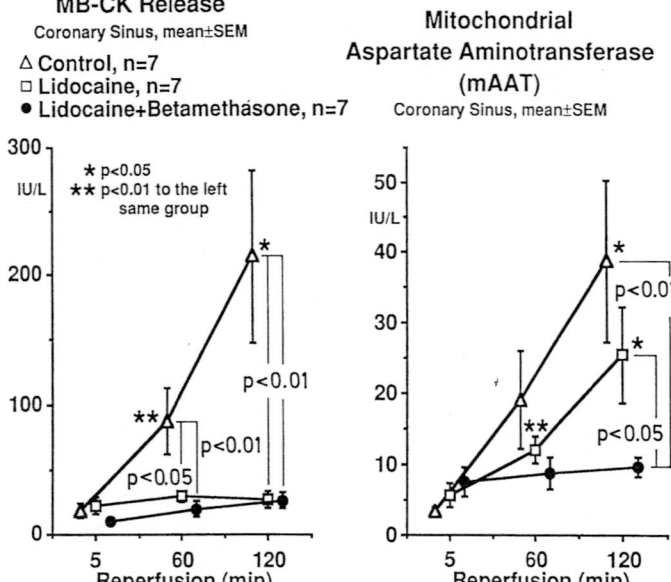

MB-CK Release
Coronary Sinus, mean±SEM
△ Control, n=7
□ Lidocaine, n=7
● Lidocaine+Betamethasone, n=7

Mitochondrial Aspartate Aminotransferase (mAAT)
Coronary Sinus, mean±SEM

Fig. 1. Myocardial enzyme release into coronary sinus. MB-CK during reperfusion was significantly suppressed in both groups L and B + L as compared to group C. mAAT remained unchanged in group B + L however, it increased significantly during the course of reperfusion in groups C and L

tional Academy of Sciences and published by the National Institutes of Health.

Procurement of the heart. After median sternotomy, the superior and inferior vena cava were encircled with 2–0 silk sutures at both proximal and distal ends for future ligation and division. The azygous vein was ligated and divided. Both common carotid arteries, the left subclavian artery, and the descending aorta were encircled with 2–0 silk both proximally and distally. The hili of the lungs were encircled with 00 silk bilaterally in each animal. An arterial canula (Fr # 10) was inserted through the proximal right subclavian artery. A venous canula

(Fr # 24) was placed in the right ventricle through the right atrial appendage. Approximately 500 ml of blood was withdrawn from the venous canula. This blood was saved with adequate heparinization for transfusion during reperfusion. The encircled arteries were ligated. The pulmonary hili were also ligated after ventilation was terminated. Immediately after aortic occlusion, cardioplegia was induced by infusion of cold (4 °C) cardioplegic solution via the arterial canula. The initial amount infused was 10 ml/kg. The superior and inferior vena cava were subsequently ligated and divided, and the heart was harvested.

Preservation of the heart. The heart was immersed in cold (4 °C) saline solution for 6 h. The cardioplegic solution (3 ml/kg) was infused every 60 min. The cardioplegic solution consisted of K^+ 20 mEq, Mg^{2+} 16 mM, Ca^{2+} 1 mM, mannitol 100 mM, and glucose 245 mM, per liter, osmolarity 450 mOsm, pH 7.50, adjusted by bicarbonate. One hour prior to reperfusion, a latex-balloon was placed in the left ventricle with a holding apparatus sutured in the mitral position. This balloon was connected to a transducer (Statham P23DB, Statham Instruments, Los Angeles, Calif.) to measure left ventricular pressure during reperfusion with a polygraph (Nihon Kohden, Tokyo). Special care was taken not to induce mechanical aortic regurgitation. For 30 min prior to reperfusion, the heart was exposed to room temperature without cold saline immersion.

Reperfusion. An additional mongrel dog was anesthetized and ventilated in the manner described earlier. The dog was maintained in physiologic cardio-pulmonary status with an infusion of Ringer's lactate solution. Both carotid arteries were canulated (Fr # 10), and these arterial lines were connected to the arterial canula placed in the preserved heart. A pressure transducer (Statham P23DB, Statham Instruments, Los Angeles, Calif.) and a magnetic flow meter (Nihon Kohden, Tokyo) for measurement of perfusion pressure and perfusion flow, respectively, were connected to the circulation. Coronary sinus blood flow was measured by a magnetic flow meter (Nihon Kohden, Tokyo) to obtain a close approximation of coronary blood flow. Blood from the canula placed in the right ventricle, and from the left ventricle vented at the apex was collected in a reservoir. This blood was infused back into a supporting dog by a pump and normothermia was maintained by a heat exchanger. Reperfusion was continued for 2 h. Defibrillation was applied when the heart developed ventricular fibrillation during early reperfusion. After 5 min

Table 1. Myocardial high energy phosphate

		Control $n = 7$	Lidocaine $n = 7$	Lidocaine + Betamethasone $n = 7$
Adenosine Triphosphate (ATP) µg/mg protein	Preservation 6 h	14.34 ± 1.50	$8.67 \pm 1.09^{*1}$	10.06 ± 5.20
	Reperfusion 2 h	13.28 ± 4.10	$13.34 \pm 1.58^{*3}$	14.29 ± 0.99
Adenosine Diphosphate (ADP) µg/mg protein	Preservation 6 h	4.51 ± 0.31	$2.34 \pm 0.36^{*2}$	$2.86 \pm 0.28^{*1}$
	Reperfusion 2 h	$2.58 \pm 0.31^{*3}$	$3.56 \pm 0.17^{*3}$	3.06 ± 0.34
Adenosine Monophosphate (AMP) µg/mg protein	Preservation 6 h	0.82 ± 0.11	0.55 ± 0.13	0.74 ± 0.12
	Reperfusion 2 h	$0.36 \pm 0.08^{*3}$	$0.71 \pm 0.09^{*1}$	0.56 ± 0.09
Total Adenine Nucleotide (TAN) µg/mg protein	Preservation 6 h	20.11 ± 1.61	$11.23 \pm 1.22^{*2}$	$13.49 \pm 2.24^{*1}$
	Reperfusion 2 h	16.32 ± 4.24	$17.52 \pm 1.22^{*3}$	17.99 ± 1.18
Creatine Phosphate (CP) µg/mg protein	Preservation 6 h	3.58 ± 0.64	2.85 ± 0.93	3.98 ± 0.77
	Reperfusion 2 h	$16.67 \pm 5.31^{*4}$	$16.14 \pm 3.40^{*3}$	$17.14 \pm 2.60^{*3}$

Mean ± SEM *1 $P < 0.05$, *2 $P < 0.01$ indicate significance vs control group, *3 $P < 0.01$, *4 $P < 0.05$ indicate significance vs preservation 6 h group

of reperfusion, all dogs were paced at 130 beats/minute. No cardiotonic drug was administered to any dog.

The 21 dogs were grouped as follows: group C (control, 7 dogs) received cardioplegic solution alone, group L (7 dogs) received cardioplegic solution together with lidocaine hydrochloride 200 mg/l, and group B + L (7 dogs) received cardioplegic solution together with both betamethasone 250 mg/l and lidocaine 200 mg/l.

At the end of both preservation and during reperfusion while the heart was beating and oxygenated, tissue was biopsied from the subendocardium of the left ventricle. These tissues were analyzed for myocardial content of adenosine triphosphate (ATP), adenosine diphosphate (ADP), adenosine monophosphate (AMP), creatine phosphate (CP), cyclic adenosine monophosphate (cAMP), cyclic guanosine monophosphate (cGMP) and calcium (Ca) by methods described elsewhere [30]. These tissues were also examined by electron microscopy to evaluate ultrastructural changes.

At 5, 60 and 120 min of reperfusion, coronary sinus venous blood was withdrawn through a venous canula. The serum MB fraction of creatine kinase (MB-CK) and mitochondrial aspartate aminotransferase (m-AAT) were measured. Left ventricular (LV) end-systolic pressure was measured with a balloon inflated with saline, using volumes of 10, 15, and 20 ml. The left ventricular end-systolic pressure-volume relation (ESPVR) was studied to evaluate the functional recovery of the left ventricle.

Data within each group was analyzed by the Student's paired t-test, and between groups by the Mann-Whitney test. A level of $P < 0.05$ was accepted as statistically significant.

Results

Basic data such as perfusion pressure and flow during reperfusion, coronary flow, hematocrit, temperature and weight of the LV were well matched between the groups.

Defibrillation was performed in all seven dogs in group C (2.43 times/dog), while one of the seven dogs in group L (0.29 times/dog), and two of the seven dogs in group B + L (0.29 times/dog) were defibrillated. All the dogs in each of the three groups survived 2 h of reperfusion.

Myocardial high-energy phosphate (HEP)

As shown in Table 1, myocardial ATP content in group L was significantly lower at the end of preservation than that of group C. Myocardial ATP in group L increased significantly during reperfusion, and its level was not significantly different from the other two groups. No significant difference in myocardial ATP was observed at the end of both preservation and reperfusion between group L and group B + L. Myocardial ADP in group L was significantly lower at the end of preservation and significantly higher at the end of reperfusion as compared to those in group C. Depletion of myocardial AMP in group C was significant, while myocardial AMP did not decline during reperfusion in both group L and group B + L. Myocardial AMP at the end of reperfusion in group L was significantly higher than that of group C. Myocardial total adenine nucleotide (TAN) in group C was significantly better maintained during preservation than that of group L. However, myocardial TAN did not differ at the end of reperfusion between the three groups. Myocardial CP increased significantly during reperfusion in all groups. However, no significant difference in CP was observed between the three groups at the end of either preservation or reperfusion.

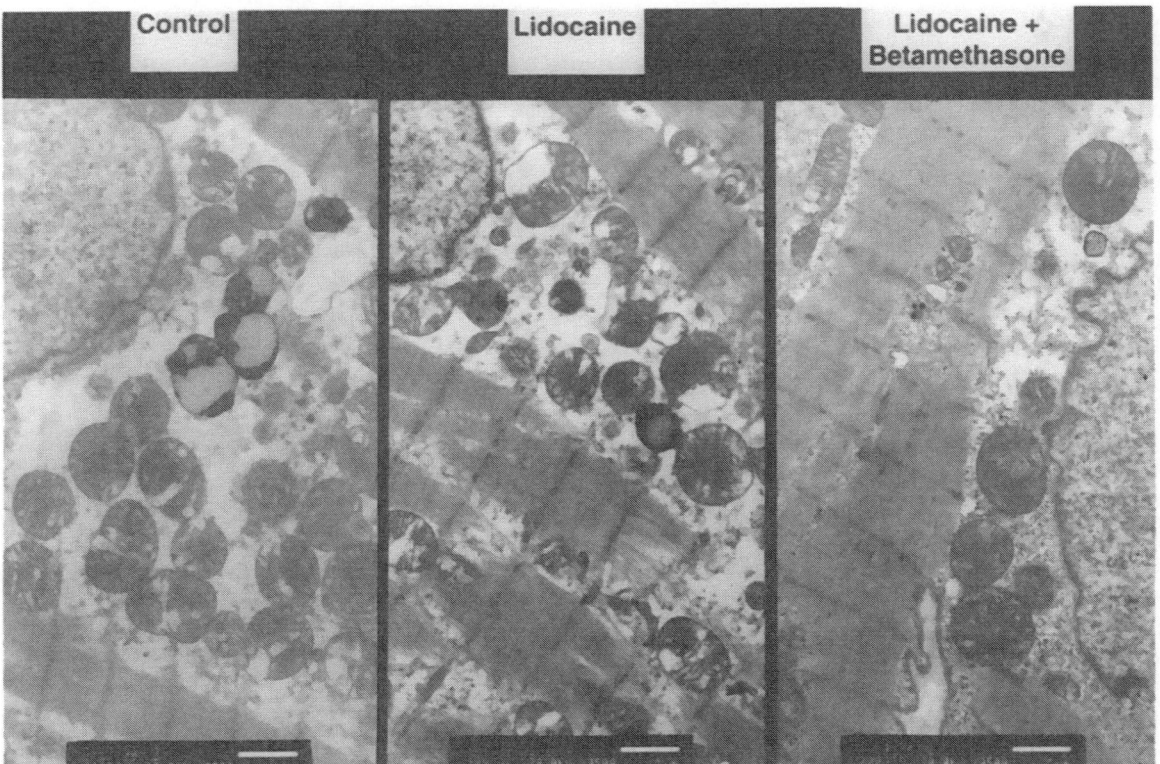

Fig. 2. Ultrastructure of the subendocardial layer of the left ventricle: *left,* group C; *middle,* group L; and *right,* group B + L. Mitochondrial disruption and swelling are observed in addition to interstitial edema in group C. Ultrastructure is well preserved in group B + L

Table 2. Myocardial cyclic monophosphate

		Control $n = 7$	Lidocaine $n = 7$	Lidocaine + Betamethasone $n = 7$
Cyclic Adenosine Monophosphate (cAMP) pmol/g	Preservation 6 h	2604 ± 137	2770 ± 154	2523 ± 389
	Reperfusion 2 h	1161 ± 338*	1033 ± 84*	1099 ± 435**
Cyclic Guanosine Monophosphate (cGMP) pmol/g	Preservation 6 h	15.0 ± 2.7	13.5 ± 2.8	15.8 ± 2.2
	Reperfusion 2 h	10.0 ± 2.0	5.8 ± 0.4**	5.0 ± 1.3* **

Mean ± SEM * $P < 0.01$, ** $P < 0.05$ indicates significance vs preservation 6 h group, *** $P < 0.05$ indicates significance vs control group

Table 3. Myocardial tissue calcium content, µg/g tissue, mean ± – SEM

	Control $n = 7$	Lidocaine $n = 7$	Lidocaine + Betamethasone $n = 7$
Preservation 6 h	50.7 ± 4.7	46.7 ± 5.4	39.6 ± 2.6*
Reperfusion 2 h	83.7 ± 13.2**	58.6 ± 4.2 **	50.5 ± 2.9 **

* $P < 0.05$ indicates significance vs control group, ** $P < 0.05$ indicates significance vs preservation 6 h group

Cyclic monophosphate. Tissue content of cyclic monophosphates is shown in Table 2. Tissue cAMP declined significantly during reperfusion in all three groups, and no significant difference in tissue cAMP was observed between the three groups at the end of either preservation or reperfusion. Tissue cGMP in both groups L and B + L declined significantly during reperfusion. Their levels at the end of reperfusion tended to be lower than those of group C.

Myocardial isoenzymes. As shown in Fig. 1, MB-CK and m-AAT in group C increased remarkably during the course of reperfusion, while MB-CK and m-AAT in both groups L and B + L remained unchanged or increased only slightly.

Tissue Ca. As shown in Table 3, tissue Ca increased significantly during reperfusion in all groups. Tissue Ca at the end of preservation tended to be lower in group L and was significantly lower in group B + L as compared to that in group C.

Ultrastructural change. Mitochondrial changes were minimal in both groups L and B + L at the end of reperfusion. On the other hand, moderate damage was observed in the cristae and membranes of mitochondria in group C. Myofibrils were well preserved in all groups. Representative pictures are shown in Fig. 2.

Left ventricular functional recovery. As shown in Fig. 3, the ESPVR at 2 h of reperfusion demonstrated satisfactory functional recovery in all groups. Better functional recovery of the left ventricle was observed in both groups L and B + L in the range of 5 to 20 ml of LV volume as compared to group C.

Discussion

The major myocardial problems encountered during reperfusion following ischemia are arrhythmia, depletion of HEP and substrates for myocardial metabolism, myocardial necrosis, and ventricular dysfunction. Hypothermic cardioplegia has become the standard procedure for myocardial protection of the donor heart. Cardiac arrest under hypothermia serves to reduce dramatically the rate of oxygen consumption and metabolic demand, and consequently slows various degradative processes within the myocardium [20]. However, hypothermia has deleterious effects on the myocardium: firstly, there is an alteration of membrane lipid bilayer structures, and secondly, there is an increase in ion permeability across the cell membranes. The cell membrane undergoes phase transition as the temperature is lowered [7, 15]: at 18°C, membrane lipids undergo a stabilizing phase change, but below 10°C, lipid crystallization can occur resulting in rupture of the membranes and an increase in ion permeability, particularly for sodium and calcium [1, 16]. This process is significantly modified in ischemia-reperfusion. As for the mechanism of the increase in membrane permeability during hypothermia, it is well documented that hypothermia

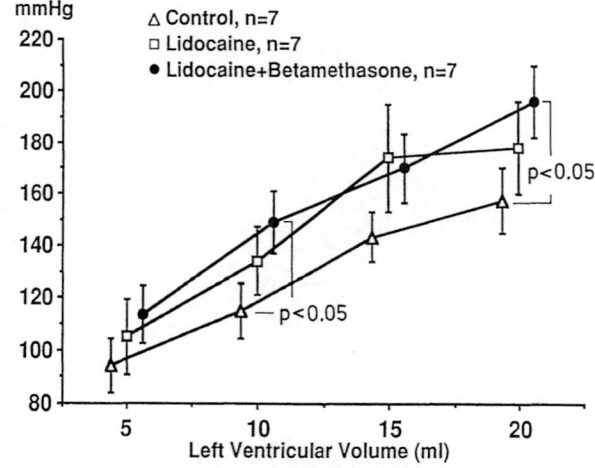

Fig. 3. Left ventricular functional recovery. This Fig. represents values at 2 h of reperfusion. ESPVR in group B + L is consistently better compared to group C

inactivates both enzyme systems of the Na-K ATPase and Ca ATPase located in the sarcolemma and sarcoplasmic reticulum, leading to possible loss of cell volume regulation and swelling [12]. Other ion pumps are probably also temperature-sensitive. The cardiac sarcolemma has, in addition to the Na-Ca exchange system, an ATP-dependent Ca transport system [4]. This system seems to have a higher affinity for Ca than does the Na-Ca exchange system, but a lower transport rate. Hypothermia depresses ATPase activity in tissues, and membrane-bound ATPase is inhibited at temperatures below 15 °C [14], thereby inactivating the Na-K pump so that sodium and water enter the cell and potassium moves out [12]. Through the Na-Ca exchange system, calcium influx is accelerated.

The current method of cardioplegia is based largely on depolarization of the membranes. When depolarized, myocardial cells are exposed to unfavorable phenomena such as increased permeability, the accumulation of sodium and calcium with subsequent cellular swelling, Ca overload, damage to subcellular organelles and ventricular fibrillation during reperfusion after ischemia. Calcium overload is thought to be one of the major causes of reperfusion injury [18]. The fundamental composition of our solution for cardiac preservation in this study is classified as a depolarizing type of solution. The resting membrane potential was estimated to be around -50 mV at 15 °C given the concentration of potassium in the solution of the control group. However, the hearts in the other two groups were preserved with the solution which contained lidocaine, 200 mg/l (approximately 1 mM/l) in addition to the solution administered to the hearts in the control group. Therefore, the hearts in both groups L and B + L may have had a slightly lower resting membrane potential, i.e. be more repolarized than the hearts in the control group. This electrophysiological difference in membrane potential between the groups suggests that the hearts in the former two groups are more resistant to ischemia than those of the latter. It is interesting to note that the hearts in the control group experienced a significantly higher incidence of ventricular fibrillation during early reperfusion than did the other two groups. Ventricular fibrillation is the most typical arrhythmia in early reperfusion following ischemia. It is proposed that the arrhythmia of early reperfusion results from an alteration of the Na^+-H^+-Ca^{2+}-exchange system [32]. Our results demonstrating inhibition of Ca overload and suppression of ventricular fibrillation during early reperfusion may be explained by these mechanisms.

Betamethasone protects ischemic myocardium by increasing coronary blood flow [29], and suppressing myocardial edema in an open heart model [28]. Furthermore, steroids stabilize lysosomal membranes [9, 25]. Lidocaine preserves mitochondrial oxidative phosphorylation [2], and inhibits cellular and subcellular damage from ischemia followed by reperfusion by stabilizing the membranes [17, 21]. Our previous investigations have suggested that combined pharmacological protection similar to that utilized in this investigation provides significant protection from prolonged cardioplegia followed by reperfusion [31].

The method of myocardial protection utilized in this investigation differed from the common method in clinical practice with respect to both the formula and frequency of injection of the cardioplegic solution. This study was conducted as a prospective animal experiment, and did include the use of a placebo; however, the data were analyzed in a blind fashion, particularly with regard to biochemical and ultrastructural changes.

Regarding the adenine nucleotide pool, HEP is catabolized during ischemia. The depletion of HEP and its intermediates leads to irreversible myocyte damage during reperfusion. Sukehiro et al. [27] have reported that ATP decreases to a level that is 50–60 % of normal during the first 6 h of preservation. Our results with myocardial ATP in this study were slightly lower than predicted by that observation. Those authors have also reported that ATP catabolism is less pronounced when the Bretschneider solution is used instead of the extracellular fluid-type hyperkalemic cardioplegic solution. Our results suggested that myocardial ATP and TAN did not differ within the three groups. During reperfusion, however, myocardial ADP and AMP did not decline, but either remained unchanged or rose significantly higher in hearts treated with membrane stabilization. This finding suggested that unfavorable leakage of AMP from cytosol could be prevented during reperfusion of the preserved heart with membrane stabilization. Coronary sinus plasma concentration of MB-CK in this study was significantly suppressed during reperfusion in the hearts treated with lidocaine or lidocaine + betamethasone. This finding clearly suggested that the hearts preserved with the aid of membrane stabilization experienced less injury during reperfusion following hypothermic cardioplegia than did hearts preserved with hypothermic cardioplegia alone. These data were further corroborated by the finding that the ultrastructure of the hearts treated with membrane stabilization was better preserved compared to hearts undergoing cardioplegia alone.

Ignarro et al. [8] and others [5] report that cGMP destabilizes lysosomal membranes while cAMP stabilizes them. In our study, tissue cAMP in all groups decreased slightly during the 6 h of preservation, and decreased significantly during reperfusion; however, no significant difference was observed between the three groups at the end of 2 h reperfusion. Tissue cGMP declined significantly during reperfusion in hearts treated with either lidocaine or lidocaine + betamethasone as compared to hearts of the control group. In addition, tissue levels of cGMP at the end of reperfusion in the former two groups tended to be lower than that of the control group. It has been reported that glucocorticoids inhibit the activity of guanylate cyclase [26] that catalyzes cGMP synthesis. Kuehl [11] has reviewed the meticulous interrelation between cyclic nucleotides and endogenous prostaglandins involving adenylate cyclase, phosphodiesterase, adenylate kinase and ATPase, which all influence intracellular cAMP levels. In this study, the addition of glucocorticoid to lidocaine did not demonstrate additional protection with regards to myocardial adenine nucleotide metabolism, but added significant protection in terms of mAAT and myocardial ultrastructure. Furthermore, the present study demonstrated better functional recovery of the left ventricle with the addition of lidocaine and betamethasone for membrane stabilization together with a lower content of myocardial cGMP, suggesting that further study of these phenomena is required.

Acknowledgements. The authors wish to express our gratitude to Mr. Tatsuyuki Nakamura for his excellent technical assistance.

References

1. Alto LE and Dhalla NS (1979) Myocardial cation contents during induction of calcium paradox. Am J Physiol 237: H13–H19
2. Baron DW, Sunamori M, Harrison CE Jr (1983) Preservation of oxidative phosphorylation by lidocaine in ischemic and reperfused myocardium. Adv Myocardiol 4: 567–573
3. Busuttil RW, George WJ (1978) Myocardial ischemia, cyclic nucleotides and lysosomal enzymes. Adv Cyclic Nucleotide Res 9: 629–645
4. Caroni P, Carafoli E (1980) An ATP-dependent Ca^{2+}-pumping system in dog heart sarcolemma. Nature 283: 765–767
5. Carr FK, Goldfarb RD (1980) Ischemia-induced canine myocardial lysosome labilization: the role of endogenous prostaglandins and cyclic nucleotides. Exp Mol Pathol 33: 36–42
6. Chance B, Mela L, Harris EJ (1968) Interaction of ion movements and local anesthetics in mitochondrial membranes. Fed Proc 27: 902–906
7. Flaherty FT, Schaff HV, Goldman RA, Gott VL (1979) Metabolic and functional effects of progresive degrees of hypothermia during global ischemia. Am J Physiol 236: H839–H845
8. Ignarro LJ, Krassikoff N, Slywka J (1973) Release of enzymes from a rat liver lysosome fraction: Inhibition by catecholamines and cyclic 3', 5'-adenosine monophosphate, stimulation by cholinergic agents and cyclic 3', 5'-guanosine monophosphate. J Pharmacol Exp Ther 186: 86–99
9. Jefferson TA, Glenn TM, Martin JB, Lefer AM (1971) Cardiovascular and lysosomal actions of corticosteroids in the intact dog. Proc Soc Exp Biol Med 136: 276–280
10. Johnson CL, Schwartz A (1969) Some effects of local anesthetics on isolated mitochondria. J Pharmacol Exp Ther 167: 365–373
11. Kuehl FA Jr (1974) Prostaglandins, cyclic nucleotides and cell function. Prostaglandins 5: 325–340
12. Leaf A (1973) Cell swelling. A factor in ischemic tissue injury. Circulation 48: 455–458
13. Lesnefsky EJ, van Benthuysen KM, McMurtry IF, Shikes RH, Johnston RB Jr, Horwitz LD (1989) Lidocaine reduces canine infarct size and decreases release of a lipid peroxidation product. J Cardiovasc Pharmacol 13: 895–901
14. Martin DR, Scott DF, Downer GL, Belzer FO (1972) Primary causes of unsuccessful liver and heart preservation: Cold sensitivity of the ATPase system. Ann Surg 175: 111–117
15. McMurchie EJ, Raison JK, Cairncross KD (1973) Temperature-induced phase changes in membranes of hearts: A contrast between the thermal responses of poikilotherms and homeotherms. Comp Biochem Physiol 44: 1017–1026
16. Mattiazi A, Nilson E (1976) The influence of temperature on the tissue course of the mechanical activity in rabbit papillary muscle. Acta Physiol 97: 310–318
17. Okamura T, Sunamori M, Suzuki A (1982) Protective effect of lidocaine in reperfused ischemic myocardium. Evaluation by hemodynamic and biochemical study. Jpn Circ J 46: 657–662
18. Opie LH (1991) Role of calcium and other ions in reperfusion injury. Cardiovasc Drug Ther 5: 237–248
19. Peck SL, Johnston RB, Horwitz LD (1985) Reduced neutrophil superoxide anion release after prolonged injusions of lidocaine. J Pharmacol Exp Ther 235: 418–422
20. Rosenfeldt FL, Hearse DJ, Cankovic-Darracott S, Braimbridge MV (1980) The additive protective effects of hypothermia and chemical cardioplegia during ischemic cardiac arrest in the dog. J Thorac Cardiovasc Surg 79: 29–38
21. Schaub RG, Lemole GM, Pinder GC, Black P, Stewart GJ (1977) Effects of lidocaine and epinephrine on myocardial preservation following cardiopulmonary bypass in the dog. J Thorac Cardiovasc Surg 74: 571–576
22. Schaub RG, Stewart G, Strong M, Ruotolo R, Lemole G (1977) Reduction of ischemic myocardial damage in the dog by lidocaine infusion. Am J Pathol 87: 399–414
23. Seeman P (1972) The membrane actions of anesthetics and tranquilizers. Pharmacol Rev 24: 583–655
24. Seppala AJ, Saris NEL, Gauffin ML (1971) Inhibition of phospholipase A-induced swelling of mitochondria by local anesthetics and related agents. Biochem Pharmacol 20: 305–313
25. Spath JA Jr, Lane DL, Lefer AM (1974) Protective action of methyprednisolone on the myocardium during experimental myocardial ischemia in the cat. Cir Res 35: 44–51
26. Steiner AL, Pagliara EA, Chase LR, Kipnis DM (1972) Radioimmunoassay for cyclic nucleotides. II. cAMP and cGMP in mammalian tissues and body fluids. J Biol Chem 247: 1114–1120
27. Sukehiro S, Dyszliewics W, Minten J, Wynants J, van Belle H, Flameng W (1991) Catabolism of high energy phosphates during long-term cold storage of donor hearts: effects of extra- and intracellular fluid-type cardioplegic solutions and calcium channel blockers. J Heart Lung Transplant 10: 387–393
28. Sunamori M (1978) Protective effect of betamethasone on the subendocardial ischemia after the cardiopulmonary bypass. J Cardiovasc Surg (Torino) 19: 291–310
29. Sunamori M, Harrison CE Jr (1980) Effect of betamethasone on mitochondrial oxidative phosphorylation in ischemic canine myocardium. Mayo Clin Proc 55: 377–382
30. Sunamori M, Amano J, Okamura T, Suzuki A (1982) Superior action of magnesium-lidocaine-l-aspartate cardioplegia to glucose-insulin-potassium cardioplegia in experimental myocardial protection. Jpn J Surg 12: 372–380
31. Sunamori M, Innami R, Amano J, Suzuki A, Harrison CE Jr (1988) Role of protease inhibition in myocardial preservation in prolonged hypothermic cardioplegia followed by reperfusion. J Thorac Cardiovasc Surg 96: 314–320
32. Tani M, Neeley JR (1989) Role of intracellular Na^+ in Ca^{2+} overload and depressed recovery of ventricular function of reperfused ischemic rat hearts. Possible involvement of H^+-Na^+ and Na^+-Ca^{2+} exchange. Circ Res 65: 1045–1056
33. Tosaki A, Balint S, Szekeres L (1988) Protective effect of lidocaine against ischemia and reperfusion-induced arrhythmia and shifts of myocardial Na, K, and Ca content. J Cardiovasc Pharmacol 12: 621–628

Transplant Int (1992) 5 [Suppl 1]: S417–S419

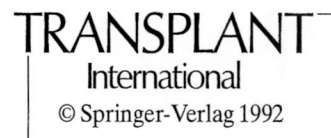

© Springer-Verlag 1992

Kupffer cell and hepatocyte function in rat transplanted liver

G. Svensson[3], M. Fjälling[1], J. Gretarsdottir[2], L. Jacobsson[2], and S. B. Holmberg[3]

Departments of Nuclear Medicine[1], Radiation Physics[2], and Transplantation Surgery[3] Sahlgrenska Hospital, Göteborg, Sweden

Abstract. The liver consists essentially of two compartments, parenchymal cells (PC) and non parenchymal cells (NPC) i. e. Kupffer cells, endothelial cells, fat storing cells and pit cells. PC remain after transplantation but NPC are eventually exchanged with host cells. Dynamic liver scintigraphy with albumin colloid, extracted by NPC, and IODIDA, extracted by PC, were tested to evaluate function as determined by clearance rates in these two cellular compartments. Experimental liver transplantation was performed in 15 syngeneic rats. Following transplantation, we performed dynamic liver scintigraphy with 0.5 ml 5 MBq ^{99m}Tc-Nanocoll and 0.5 ml 20 MBq ^{99m}Tc-IODIDA, 10 s per frame, 30 min for each examination. Percentage clearance rate, per minute was calculated from uptake curves over the liver. Uptake curves were nearly exponential and clearance rates could be estimated from a logarithmic plot of uptake versus time. The clearance rate was 25 ± 4 % per min (mean $\pm$ SD) for NPC and 32 ± 15 % per min for PC in controls. After liver transplantation it was 31 ± 7 % per min for NPC and 30 ± 15 % per min for PC. Dynamic liver scintigraphy with ^{99m}Tc-Nanocoll and ^{99m}Tc-IODIDA alloweds a separate assessment of the function of PC and NPC after experimental liver transplantation in rats.

Key words: Liver transplantation – Liver scintigraphy – Kupffer cells

The liver can be divided into two functional compartments. The parenchymal cells (PC) including hepatocytes and bile ducts are responsible for many metabolic functions and the production of bile. The non parenchymal cells (NPC) or sinusoidal cells include Kupffer cells (liver macrophages), endothelial cells, fat storing cells and pit cells (NK cells). The NPC have not only a metabolic role but also an important immunologic and surveillance function, since the liver sinusoids with fenestrated endothelial cells and Kupffer cells act as a "sieve", establishing contact with particulate matter including cells in the blood stream [5, 16]. According to analyses of liver biopsies posttransplantation NPC are replaced by host cells from the recipient bone marrow after liver tranplantation [13, 14]. This procedure of host cell replacement of NPC seems to influence graft rejection or tolerance [11, 13].

[99m]Tc-Nanocoll, an albumin colloid with a diameter of 50 nm, is used mainly for bone marrow imaging. Nanocoll is phagocytosed by macrophages and 70 % is accumulated in the liver by Kupffer cells. Dynamic liver scintigraphy and calculation of the clearance rate of ^{99m}Tc-Nanocoll has been used to measure RES macrophage phagocytic function [3, 5]. [99m]Tc IODIDA (N 2,6 diethyl 3-iodophenyl carbamoyl iminodiacetic acid) is an iminodiacetic acid derivative used to assess hepatocyte function and visualize the hepato-biliary system (HBS). It is excreted by the HBS and allows examination even with high bilirubinemia [2]. IODIDA is protein bound in the blood and transported to the space of Disse in the liver sinusoids by albumin. IODIDA enters the hepatocyte by a carrier-mediated non-sodium-dependant membrane transport mechanism similar to bilirubin [8]. Dynamic registration and calculation of the clearance rate from the blood of ^{99m}Tc IODIDA is used to measure liver PC uptake function in humans [1].

The aim of this study was to develop a method, in vivo, using dynamic liver scintigraphy for examining the function in these two liver compartments after experimental liver tranplantation.

Materials and methods

Animals. We used 8 control and 15 procedure syngeneic Wistar-FU rats weighing about 250 g in this study. They were fed water and pellets ad libitum and maintained on a normal day and night cycle.

Surgical procedure. Liver transplantation was performed according to Kamada and Sun-li on 15 normal Wistar/FU rats weighing about 250 grams. Atropine (0.1 mg/100 g body weight) was given for premedication and Buprenorphin (Reckitt & Colman, Hull, UK) was given as a postoperative analgesic. Ether was used for induction and

Offprint requests to: Stig B Holmberg, Dept of Surgery, Sahlgrenska Hospital, 413 45 Göteborg, Sweden

Table 1. Clearance rate, % per minute, (mean ± SD) by liver parenchymal cells (IODIDA) and liver non parenchymal cells (Nanocoll)

	Parenchymal cell	Non Parenchymal cell	n
Normal rats	32 ± 15	25 ± 4	8
Liver transplantation	30 ± 15	31 ± 7*	15

* $P = 0.02$ compared with normal rats

maintenance of anaesthesia in donor and recipient animals. No other durgs were used. Postoperatively, the rats maintained normal weight and feeding habits. Serum bilirubin and liver transaminases were within normal limits.

The technique of orthotopic liver transplantation in the rat without rearterialization (reanastomosis of the hepatic artery) was first described by Lee [9] and was performed in this study using a modified technique [10, 15]. In this rat model the vascular anastomosis is performed with a running suture technique and without using any cuffs. This model has proved reliable and acceptable for all types of biochemical and immunological studies of orthotopic liver transplantation [6, 7, 17].

Dynamic liver scintigraphy. The animals were anaesthetized with nembutal 60 mg/kg 2–60 days after liver transplantation. The rats were placed on a gamma camera after canulation of the jugular vein. Dynamic liver scintigraphy was performed after the injection of 0.5 ml 5 MBq ^{99m}Tc-Nanocoll i. v. and followed 30 min later by 0.5 ml 20 MBq ^{99m}Tc-IODIDA. Aquisition time was 10 s per frame for 30 min for each examination. Uptake curves were constructed by the Region Of Interest (ROI) over the liver on the gamma camera images. Calculation of clearance rate (k) was done using the formula:

$$\ln [1\text{-}U(t)/U_{final}] \text{ versus } t$$

where k is the slope in a least square fit of the plot. Q_0 = injected activity; t = time, U = uptake counts; U_{final} = final liver uptake

The clearance rate was calculated as the percentage uptake per minute. Uptake counts were measured in the ROI over the liver for the ^{99m}Tc-Nanocoll but the ROI was expanded to the include the intestines for the ^{99m}Tc IODIDA uptake count, since there was excretion into the intestines during this examination.

Results

The clearance rate in control rats was 25 ± 4 % per min (mean ± SD) for Nanocoll albumin colloid and 32 ± 15 % for IODIDA. After liver tranplantion the Nanocoll clearance rate was 31 ± 7 % and IODIDA clearance rate was 30 ± 15 % per min (Table 1). The clearance rate for Nanocoll was significantly elevated after liver transplantation ($P = 0.02$)

Discussion

There are more than 500 metabolic functions performed by the liver and liver function can be tested in many ways. Physiologic and anatomic studies suggest two main liver compartments, one essentially metabolic consisting of hepatocytes and bile ducts around the bile canaliculi and the other endothelial with sieving and immunologic functions around the liver sinusoids [16]. These two compartments fare differently after liver transplantation since liver biopsies after liver tranplantation have revealed that sinusoidal donor cells have been replaced by host bone marrow cells while parenchymal donor cells remain intact. These studies have used monoclonal antibodies directed at specific donor and recipient HLA-antigens. This exchange of donor cells with recipient cells might influence outcome after liver tranplantation or even initiate a host-versus-graft disease. Steinhoff et al. have shown that a complicated course post liver transplantion in humans is associated with an early exchange of donor sinusoidal cells [11–14].

Clearance studies of injected substanses with established affinity for different liver cells offer a physiologic in vivo model to study different liver functions. In vivo models allow for repeated examination during postoperative follow-up and are therefore suitable for examining processes in the liver that evolve over a period of weeks or months [1, 2, 8]. IODIDA is completely eliminated from the bloodstream by the liver and is one of several iminodiacetic acid substances used to examine the hepatic biliary system. IODIDA is highly protein bound and lipophilic and thus has almost no renal excretion. Hepatocyte uptake is competitive with bilirubin but there are additional uptake mechanisms. IODIDA can be used with a high bilirubinemia [1, 2, 8], in competion with spleen and bone marrow macrophages.

Due to Nanocoll's relative small colloid size, 50 nm, and large particle amount given, liver extraction is not complete on a first passage. Clearance rate is not wholly dependant on liver blood flow [3, 5]. This study used the total clearance rate for IODIDA and Nanocoll. A liver clearance rate (k_{liver}) can be calculated according to the formula

$$k_{liver} = k \times U_{final}/Q_0$$

Q_0 = injected activity; U_{final} = final liver uptake k_{liver} for IODIDA would be identical since U_{final} is completely (100 %) in the liver but k_{liver} for Nanocoll would only be about 70 % of the total clearance rate or about 18 % per min. The results in normal rats showed essentially the same total clearance rates but the liver clearance rate would be 40 % lower for Nanocoll. This supported different elimination mechanisms from the blood for the two test substances.

After liver tranplantation between syngeneic rats, with a short period of cold ischemia, no change was noted in the parenchymal function of the transplanted liver. There was a small but significant elevation of the non parenchymal cell clearance rate of Nanocoll. This might signify an activation of sinusoidal cells after transplantation [11]. In studies of clearance rates in normal and liver macrophage stimulated rats, a similar rise in the clearance rate of Nanocoll is noted [4]. Such macrophage activation is then correlated with cytotoxic ability against liver tumour growth.

Future studies will be aimed at studying more complicated experimental transplantation procedures such as longer periods of cold ischemia and possible reperfusion injuries or transplant rejection.

Acknowledgements. The authors wish to thank Lilian Karlsson for expert technical assistance with liver transplantation and liver scintigraphy.

References

1. Ekman M, Fjälling M, Holmberg SB, Persson H (1991) IODIDA clearance rate – a method for measuring hepatocyte uptake function. Transplant Proc (in press)
2. Hawkins RA, Hall T, Gambhir SS, Busuttil RW, Huang Sungcheng, Glickman S, Marciano D, Brown RKJ, Phelps ME (1988) Radionuclide evaluation of liver transplants. Semin Nucl Med 27: 199–212
3. Holmberg SB, Hafström Lo, Jacobsson L (1987) Phagocytosis and dynamic RES scintigraphy: an evaluation of commercial colloids in rats. Nucl Med Commun 8: 335–346
4. Holmberg SB, Hafström Lo, Jacobsson L (1988) RES macrophage stimulation and liver tumour growth in rats – evaluation with dynamic liver RES scintigraphy. Anticancer Res 6: 1291–1296
5. Holmberg SB, Hafström Lo, Forssell Aronsson E, Gretarsdottir J, Jacobsson L (1990) Vascular clearance by the reticuloendothelial system – measurement with two different-sized albumin colloids. Scand J Clin Lab Invest 50: 865–871
6. Kamada N, Davies HFFS, Wight D, Culank L, Rosen B (1983) Liver transplantation in the rat. Transplantation 35: 304–311
7. Kamada N, Calne RY (1983) A surgical experience with five hundred and thirty liver transplants in the rat. Surgery 93: 64–69
8. Krishnamurthy S, Krishnamurthy GT (1989) Technetium-99m-Iminodiacetic acid organic anions: review of biokinetics and clinical application in hepatalogy. Hepatology 9: 139–153
9. Lee S, Charters AC, Chandler JG, Orloff MJ (1973) A technique for orthotopic liver transplantation in the rat. Transplantation 16: 664–669
10. Lee S, Charters AC, Orloff MJ (1975) Simplified technique for orthotopic liver transplantation in the rat. Am J Surg 130: 38–40
11. Lemasters Jl, Caldwell-Kenkel JC, Currin RT, Tanaka Y, Marzi I, Thurman RG (1989) Endothelial cell killing and activation of Kupffer cells following reperfusion of rat liver stored in Euro-Collins solution In: Kirn A, Knook DL, Wisse E (eds) Cells of the hepatic sinusoid, vol 2. Kupffer Cell Foundation, Rijswijk, The Netherlands, pp 277–280
12. Paradis K, Blazar B, Sharp HL (1989) Rapid repopulation and maturation of Kupffer cells from the bone marrow in a murine bone marrow transplant model. In: Kirn A, Knook DL, Wisse E (eds) Cells of the hepatic sinusoid, vol 2. Rijswijk, The Netherlands
13. Steinhoff G, Behrend M, Sorg C, Wonigeit K, Pichlmayr R (1989) Sequential analysis of macrophage tissue differentiation and Kupffer cell exchange after human liver transplantation In: Kirn A, Knook DL, Wisse E (eds) Cells of the hepatic sinusoid, vol 2. Kupffer Cell Foundation, Rijswijk, The Netherlands, pp 406–409
14. Steinhoff G (1990) Major histocompatibility complex antigens in human liver transplants. Hepatology 11: 9–15
15. Svensson G, Aldenborg F, Karlberg I (1991) Effect of rearterialization on short-term graft function in orthotopic rat liver transplantation. J Eur Surg Res (in press)
16. Wisse E, de Zanger RB, Charles K, van der Smissen P, McCuskey RS (1985) The liver sieve: considerations concerning the structure and function of endothelial fenestrae, the sinusoidal wall and the space of Disse. Hepatology 5: 683–689
17. Zimmerman FA, Buther GW, Davies HS, Brons G, Kamada N, Turel O (1979) Techniques for orthotopic liver transplantation in the rat and some studies of the immunologic responses to fully allogenetic liver grafts. Transplant Proc 11: 571–577

Transplant Int (1992) 5 [Suppl 1]: S 420–S 423

TRANSPLANT
International
© Springer-Verlag 1992

A newly developed hydroxyl radical scavenger, EPC-K1 can improve the survival of swine warm ischemia-damaged transplanted liver grafts

T. Yagi, K. Sakagami, H. Nakagawa, Y. Takaishi, and K. Orita

First Department of Surgery, Okayama University Medical School, Okayama, Japan

Abstract. Using a swine orthotopic liver transplantation (SOLTx) model, we assessed the effect of a new hydroxyl radical scavenger EPC-K1 on warm ischemic damage of the liver graft and recipient survival. Animals were divided into 5 groups. The first group (control group 1) consisted of 5 pigs which were not operated on but served as controls for the indocianine green disappearance rate (K-ICG) determinations. In the second group (control group 2), 10 livers were transplanted without warm ischemia (WI) and the K-ICG values were measured. The third group (control group 3) was the main control group for the study groups and consisted of 5 liver transplants with 30 min of WI without any special treatment. The fourth and fifth groups served as study groups 1 and 2. Five transplants were carried out in each group, as in control group 3. In study group 1 recipients were treated with an additional 5 mg/kg i.v. EPC-K1 and in study group 2 with 20 mg/kg i.v. EPC-K1. Significant improvement in glutamic oxaloacetic transaminase (GOT) and lactate dehydrogenase (LDH) levels, K-ICG values and histological findings were observed in the EPC-K1 treated groups. The intravenous administration of this agent had a strong protective effect on warm ischemic damage after 30 min of WI and could significantly prolong the graft and recipient survival.

Key words: EPC-K1 – Hydroxyl radical – Liver transplantation – Warm ischemia – Reperfusion injury – K-ICG

Warm ischemic damage is one of the most troublesome and important aspects of organ transplantation which can contribute to the occurrence of pirmary nonfunction (PNF) [10]. Recently, many authors have reported that oxygen-free radicals, derived from warm ischemia damaged tissue, play a major role in reperfusion injury [3, 5]. Therefore, many kinds of radical scavengers, for example,

allopurinol and superoxide dismutase (SOD) have been investigated carefully in an effort to reduce warm ischemic damage.

A new compound, EPC-K1 L-ascorbic acid 2- [3, 4-di-hydro-2, 5, 7, 8-tetramethyl-2-(4, 8, 12-trimethyltridecyl)-2 H-1-benzopyran-6yl hydrogen phosphate] potassium salt, was developed by Senju Pharmaceutical Co., Ltd., Hyogo, Japan in 1989. EPC-K1 has a unique phosphodiester bond between Vitamin E and Vitamin C (Fig. 1). This compound has several properties that are of benefit in liver transplantation such as hydroxyl radical scavenging, human phospholipase A_2 blocking [4] and high affinity to liver tissue. In this study, we assessed whether this agent could prevent warm ischemic damage after liver transplantation and improve survival, using a swine orthotopic liver transplantation (SOLTx) model.

Materials and methods

We used 55 large white pigs weighing 20–25 kg (mean, 22.3 ± 1.26 kg) in this study and divided them into five groups. In control group 1, 5 pigs were used for measurement of the normal indocianine green disappearance rate (K-ICG). These animals were not operated on and only the K-ICG values were evaluated as described below. In control group 2, 20 pigs were paired and hepatic transplantation was carried out without warm ischemia (WI); warm ischemic time (WIT) was zero. The K-ICG values were evaluated. In control group 3, 10 other pigs were paired and hepatic transplantation was carried out with 30 min of WI. In study group 1, 10 pigs were paired and hepatic transplantation was carried out after 30 min of WI. Thy were given 5 mg/kg EPC-K1 as described below. In study group 2, 10 pigs underwent the same procedure as the pigs in study group 1 but the dose of EPC-K1 was increased to 25 mg/kg.

Liver transplantation protocol. After the donor liver was prepared for retrieval, in all groups except control group 2, warm ischemia was commenced by cross clamping and the intraperitoneal temperature was maintained at 37 °C by the continuous pouring of hot saline for 30 min. Then the graft was preserved in Euro-Collins solution until the recipient hepatectomy was performed and the graft was transplanted orthotopically into the recipient pig. The details of the whole transplantation procedure have been reported previously [9]. There were no statistically significant differences in body weights, total ischemic time and anhepatic time between the groups.

Offprint requests to: T. Yagi, M.D., First Department of Surgery, Okayama University Medical School, 2-5-1 Shikata-cho, Okayama 700, Japan

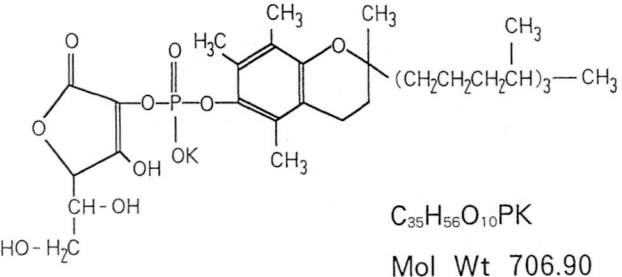

Fig. 1. Chemical structure of EPC-K1

$C_{35}H_{56}O_{10}PK$

Mol Wt 706.90

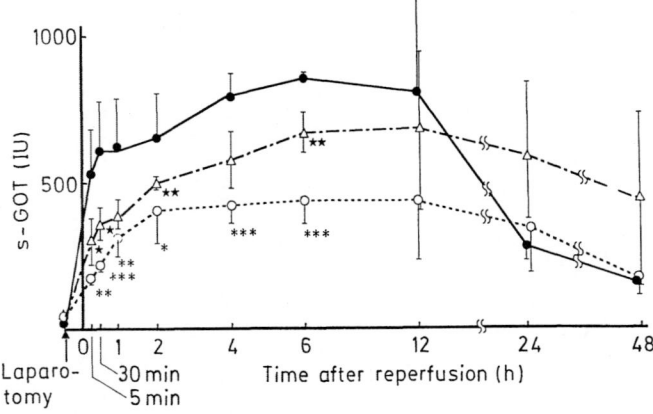

Fig. 2. Changes in serum GOT levels up to 48 h after reperfusion in three groups (mean ± SD). The serial serum GOT levels in treated groups were significantly lower than that in untreated group up to 6 h after reperfusion. * $P < 0.05$, ** $P < 0.02$, *** $P < 0.01$, study group 1 vs. control group 3; ★ $P < 0.05$, ★★ $P < 0.02$, study group 2 vs. control group 3). (Key ●—●, control group 3; ○---○, study group 1; △---△, study group 2)

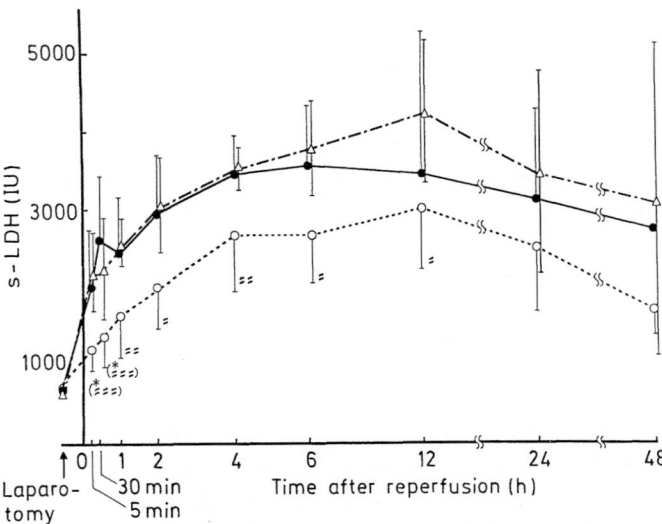

Fig. 3. Changes in serum LDH levels up to 48 h after reperfusion in three groups (mean ± SD). In serum LDH levels, significant suppression of s-LDH level was found only in study group 1. * $P < 0.05$ study group 1 vs. control group 3; # $P < 0.05$, # # $P < 0.02$ study group 1 vs. 2). Key ●—●, control group 3; ○---○, study group 1; △---△, study group 2)

EPC-K1 protocol. The animals were divided into three groups (control group 3, study groups 1 and 2). Recipient pigs in control group 3 ($n = 5$) served as controls and were not pre-treated prior to reperfusion. Pigs in study group 1 ($n = 5$) and study group 2 ($n = 5$) were pre-treated with a low dose of EPC-K1 (5 mg/kg) and a high dose

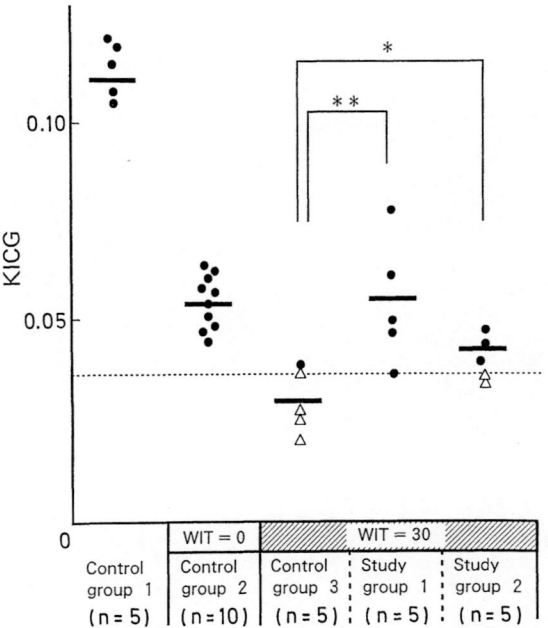

Fig. 4. The K-ICG values in normal pigs and in recipient pigs of SOLTx (mean ± SD). The first and second columns indicate K-ICG values in normal pigs (control 1 group, mean K-ICG value, 0.113 ± 0.006) and in the SOLTxed pigs without warm ischemic stress respectively (control group 2, 0.055 ± 0.006). The third to fifth columns show K-ICG values in recipients after 30 min of warm ischemia (0.030 ± 0.007, 0.055 ± 0.014, 0.040 ± 0.005). The *broken line* demonstrates the K-ICG value above which recipients survived for more than 1 week ($P < 0.01$). * $P < 0.05$, ** $P < 0.01$ (Key ●, cases surviving more than 1 week; △, cases dead within a week)

(20 mg/kg) respectively. EPC-K1 was administered 10 min prior to hepatectomy and 10 min prior to reperfusion in two equal doses.

Biochemical analysis and K-ICG. Analysis of graft function included serial serum glutamic oxaloacetic transaminase (GOT) and serum lactate dehydrogenase (LDH) measurements, and the determination of K-ICG values. K-ICG was calculated from three samples obtained at 5 min intervals after the bolus injection of indocianine green (0.5 mg/kg i.v.) which was administered just 30 min after reperfusion.

Histology. Biopsy specimens in control group 3, and study groups 1 and 2 were obtained 30 min after reperfusion from each transplanted liver. Blocks of tissue were fixed in 10% neutral-buffered formalin and were stained with hematoxylin and eosin for light microscopic examination.

Statistical analysis. Data are expressed as mean ± SD. Significance was tested using Student's t-test and the Chi-square test, taking $P = 0.05$ as the limit of significance.

Results

Biochemical analysis and K-ICG

Up to 6 h after reperfusion, significant suppression of elevation of serum GOT levels was observed in study groups 1 and 2 ($P < 0.05$) compared to control group 3 (Fig. 2). As shown in Fig. 3, the serum LDH level was suppressed in study group 1 up to 12 h after reperfusion but

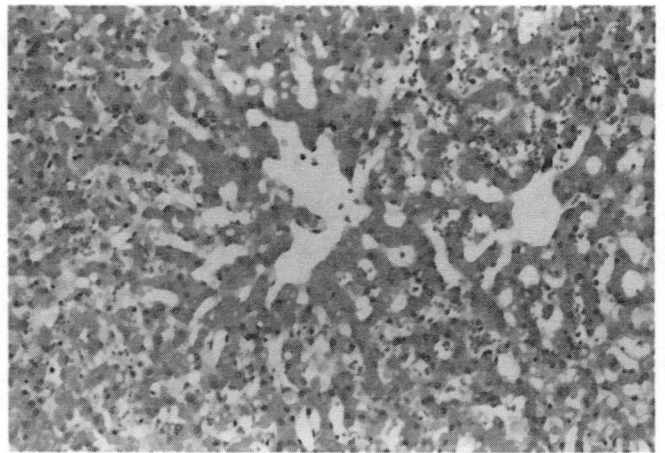

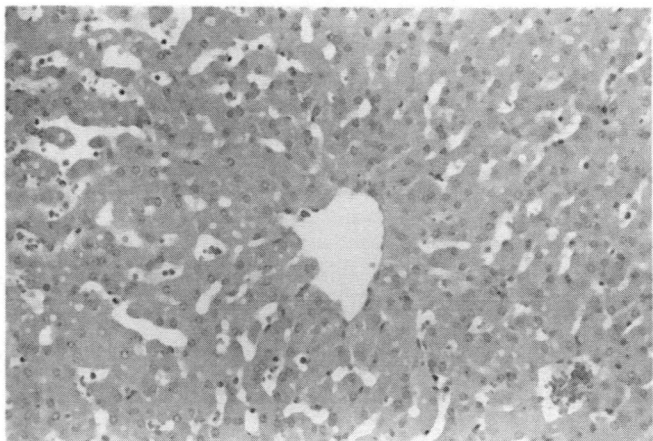

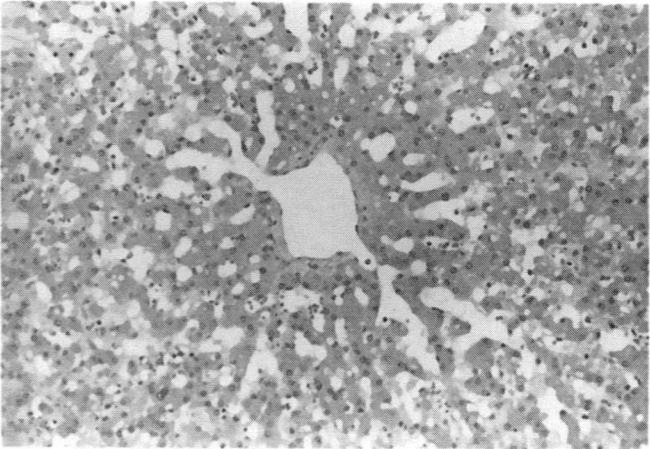

Fig. 5. Light micrographs of biopsy specimens 30 min after reperfusion (×168, H. E. staining). **A** Untreated group: marked disruption of hepatic architecture was observed in the centrilobular zone. Vacuolar degeneration of hepatocytes (HCs) and detachment of sinusoidal lining cells (SLCs) were seen. **B** EPC-K1 5 mg/kg i.v. group: almost normal structure was maintained. **C** EPC-K1 20 mg/kg i.v. group: the hepatic architecture was not disrupted, but vacuolar change of HCs and dissection of SLCs were observed in moderation

statistical significance was observed only between the two study groups ($P < 0.05$).

In control group 2 (WIT = 0), the mean K-ICG value following SOLTx surgery was decreased to almost half the value calculated in non-operated controls (Fig. 4). Furthermore, this decrease in mean K-ICG value was greater after 30 min of WIT as can be seen in Fig. 4. The mean K-ICG values in the study groups were significantly higher than in control group 3 (0.055 ± 0.014, and 0.040 ± 0.005 vs. 0.030 ± 0.007, $P < 0.01$, $P < 0.05$, Fig. 4).

Histology. As shown in Fig. 5, warm ischemic damage was marked in the centrilobular zone. Severe vacuolar degeneration of hepatocytes, congestion, dissection of the sinusoidal lining cells and disruption of hepatic architecture was observed in control group 3. In study group 1, the hepatic architecture remained almost normal. In study group 2, there were moderate vacuolar changes in the hepatocytes.

Survival. The survival rates for each group are presented in Table 1.

Discussion

It is well known that molecular oxygen generated in reperfused tissue can cause severe damage in previously ischemic tissue during organ transplantation, and the hydroxyl radical ($\cdot OH$) appears to be the most harmful oxygen-free radical because of its affinity for organic molecules and its low specificity. This effect may lead to primary non-function of the transplanted organ. It is suggested that the reperfused tissue itself and the neutrophils which flow into the graft after reperfusion are the sources of these oxygen-free radicals during transplant surgery [1]. Therefore, potent radical scavengers may facilitate the improvement of graft viability. EPC-K1 was synthesized as a specific hydroxyl radical scavenger, and it catalyzes reactions in vitro in a dose-dependent manner [7]. Furthermore, the latest study revealed that this agent could also scavenge the superoxide radical (O_2^-) derived from endotoxin-induced migrating neutrophils in the intraperitoneal space of the rat (unpublished data). The advantages of EPC-K1 in clinical use are, (1) it is a soluble and stable material suitable for injection, (2) it has high affinity for liver tissue, and (3) it has strong binding properties to cell membranes owing to its molecular similarity to lipid membrane molecules.

The released enzymes, represented by GOT and LDH, reflected the degree of oxidative cell injury. Elevation of GOT in the early phase was suppressed significantly by EPC-K1 regardless of dose. However, significant differences in LDH values were found only in recipients treated with 5 mg/kg EPC-K1 after 30 min of WI damage. This discrepancy between dose and effect was also noted in the K-ICG values, histological findings and survival rates.

The K-ICG value reflects liver function and hepatic blood flow and was regarded as a sensitive indicator of graft function in this study because recipients were jaundice-free. Most of the subjects who lived longer than 1 week showed a value of over 0.035, and the K-ICG value above which recipients survived for more than 1 week was 0.035 ($P < 0.01$). Both mean K-ICG values in the study groups were significantly better than that in control

Table 1. One-week survival rate in three experimental groups with 30 min of WI. Significant improvement of mean survival time (MST) and 1-week survival rate in EPC 5 mg/kg treated group (100%) was demonstrated

Groups	Treatment		WIT (min)	Survival (day)	MST (day)	1 week-survival rate (%)
Control group 3 (n = 5)	–		30	1, 1, 1, 2, 18	4.7 ± 6.7	20
Study group 1 (n = 5)	EPC-K1	5 mg/kg (i.v.)	30	7, 14, 16, 20, 48	24.3 ± 13.8*	100
Study group 2 (n = 5)	EPC-K1	20 mg/kg (i.v.)	30	3, 3, 7, 7, 9	6.4 ± 2.0	60

*; $P < 0.05$ (vs control group 3)

group 3, but the effect of low dose administration was somewhat superior to high dose administration.

Caldwell-Kenkel suggests that oxygen-free radical injury could explain the extensive cell death observed in the oxygen-rich periportal area compared to the oxygen-poor pericentral regions in the reperfused rat liver model after cold storage [2]. However in our histological study, the centrilobular zone was damaged more severely than the periportal zone after 30 min of WI. Some investigators have suggested that nonparenchymal cells may play an important role in the pathogenesis of oxygen-free radical injury [2, 6]. Marked detachment of sinusoidal lining cells and congestion increase the intrasinusoidal pressure, causing poor local circulation and creating anaerobic conditions. If vacuolation of hepatocytes, which is prominent in the centrilobular zone of the warm ischemia damaged graft, contributes to secondary changes in an effort to overcome the increased sinusoidal pressure, as Trowell has suggested [11], vacuolation may not be due to the anaerobic condition of hepatocytes during WIT, but may be the result of reperfusion injury that is mainly expressed in sinusoidal lining cells.

EPC-K1 effectively protected the grafts from warm ischemic damage and significantly improved clinical outcome. Increasing the dose of EPC-K1 from 5 mg/kg to 25 mg/kg surprisingly did not improve this effect (Table 1). This discrepancy may be explained by the detergent-like characteristics of EPC-K1, which may contribute to cytotoxity in higher doses. The only recognized side effect of EPC-K1 was a decrease in blood pressure at a dose above 25 mg/kg (i.v.) in a rat model (unpublished data). We did not observe any significant decrease in blood pressure following EPC-K1 injections in our model.

Three striking findings emerged from our present study: (1) EPC-K1 prevented warm ischemic damage after 30 min of WI in SOLTx and could significantly prolong the survival of the graft and recipient, (2) the intravenous administration of EPC-K1 suppressed significantly the increase in released enzymes, in line with the improvement of K-ICG values and histological findings and, (3) the protective effects of the agent were maximized at the dose of 5 mg/kg given intravenously. Further studies are required to confirm our findings and to establish a side effect profile of EPC-K1. The agent may prove to be a powerful oxygen-free radical scavenger in successful human liver transplantation.

Acknowledgements. The authors wish to express their sincere appreciation to Y. Kuribayashi from Senju Pharmaceutical Corp., Hyogo, Japan, for technical assistance and for providing EPC-K1.

References

1. Adkison D, Hollwarth ME, Benoit JN, Parks DA, McCord JM, Granger DN (1986) Role of free radicals in ischemia-reperfused injury to the liver. Acta Physiol Scand 548: 101–107
2. Caldwell-Kenkel JC, Currin RT, Tanaka Y, Thurman RG, Jemasters JJ (1989) Reprefusion injury to endotherial cells following cold ischemic storage of rat livers. Hepatology 10: 292–299
3. Granger DN, Rutili G, McCord JM (1981) Superoxide radicals in intestinal anemia. Gastroenterology 81: 22–29
4. Herbort CP, Okumura A, Mochizuki M (1989) Immunopharachological analysis of endotoxin-induced uveitis in the rat. Exp Eye Res 48: 693–705
5. Manson PN, Anthenelli RM, Im MJ, Bulkley GB, Hoopes JE (1983) The role of oxygen free radicals in ischemic tissue injury in island skin flaps. Ann Surg 198: 87–90
6. Marzi I, Zong Z, Zimmermann FA, Zemasters JJ, Thurman RG (1989) Xanthine and hypoxanthine accumulation during storage may contribute to reperfusion injury following liver transplantation in the rat. Transplant Proc 21: 1319–1320
7. Mori A, Edamatsu R, Kohno M, Ohmori S (1980) A new hydroxyl radical scavenger: EPC-K1. Neuroscience 15: 371–376
8. Ratch RE, Chuknyiska RS, Bulkley GB (1987) The primary localization of free radical generation after anoxia/reoxygenation in isolated endotherial cells. Surgery: 102–131
9. Sakagami K, Toda K, Nakai H, Higaki K, Morisaki F, Takasu S, Miichi N, Morisue M, Saito S, Miyazaki M, Fuchimoto S, Orita K (1987) Improved techniques for orthotopic liver transplantation: a preliminary study. Hiroshima J Med Sci 36: 211–217
10. Thurman RG, Rutili G, McCord JM (1981) Superoxide radicals in intestinal anemia. Gastroenterology 81: 22–29
11. Trowell OA (1946) The experimental production of watery vacuolation of the liver. J Physiol 105: 268–297

Transplant Int (1992) 5 [Suppl 1]: S 424–S 428

TRANSPLANT
International
© Springer-Verlag 1992

Kidney procurement from non-heartbeating donors: transplantation results

R. Schlumpf[1], **D. Candinas**[1], **A. Zollinger**[2], **G. Keusch**[3], **M. Retsch**[1], **M. Decurtins**[1], and **F. Largiadèr**[1]

[1] Department of Surgery, [2] Department of Anaesthesiology, [3] Department of Internal Medicine, University of Zurich Hospital, Rämistraße 100, CH-8091 Zurich, Switzerland

Abstract. To overcome the shortage of kidneyes (kdn's) available for transplantation we reactivated kdn procurement from non-heartbeating donors (NON-HBD). In this study, we reviewed our results with 34 kdn's from NON-HBD, transplanted between 1985 and 1991, and compared these with 34 control kdn's procured from heartbeating donors (HBD) matched for age, sex, primary graft or retransplant and transplant year. There was no difference in cold ischemia time, preservation solutions used, duration and type of preoperative dialysis, number of HLA mismatches and serum antibody levels between the two groups. The only significant findings were a lower diuresis in the last hour in the donors in the NON-HBD group, and a significantly higher serum creatinine level compared to the HBD group. The 1-year patient and graft survival rates were 89.4% and 84.9% for the HBD group, and 78% and 76.1% for the NON-HBD group respectively. There was need for dialysis support in the first posttransplant week in 10 out of 34 (29%) recipients in the HBD and 17 out of 34 (50%) recipients in the NON-HBD group. Primary non-function was observed in 1 of 34 (3%) recipients in the HBD group versus 3 of 34 (9%) in the NON-HBD group. None of the differences were statistically significant. There was also no difference in average serum creatinine levels at days 1, 3, and 7, at 1 month and at 1 year between the HBD and NON-HBD groups. In the NON-HBD group 6 of 34 kdn's (18%), 5 of which were retransplants, showed vascular rejection, 5 of them associated with haemolytic uremic syndrome (thrombotic microangiopathy); 2 of these 6 kdn's recovered, and 4 failed (2 with primary non-function). This important observation needs to be investigated further. The results is this study showed, however, that good short- and long-term results can be achieved with kdn's from NON-HBD. We concluded that organ procurement from NON-HBD is an adequate approach to an important cadaver donor source that in general is not effeciently used, but could significantly increase the number of kdn grafts in most transplant programs.

Offprint requests to: R. Schlumpf

Key words: Non-heartbeating donor – Vascular rejection – Hemolytic uremic syndrome

The shortage of donor kidneys [kdn] is the main cause for increasing waiting lists among patients awaiting a transplant and obliges to an efficient use of all donor sources. We have performed kdn retrieval from non-heartbeating donors [NON-HBD] in the recent past. In this study we reviewed our results with kdn's from NON-HBD and compared them with those from heartbeating donors [HBD].

Patients and methods

Study design

Between January 1985 and September 1991, 482 kdn were transplanted at our institution. During this period we procured 38 kidneys from 19 NON-HBD (14 kdn between 1985 and 1989, 10 kdn in 1990, and 14 kdn between January and September 1991); 34 were grafted at our clinic (4 elsewhere) and taken for retrospective analysis (NON-HBD group). For comparison we selected an equal number of kdn transplants who satisfied the following criteria: procurement only from HBD, recipients of the same sex, same age (same decade), same number of transplant (primary or retransplant) and same period (±6 months) of transplantation (HBD group).

Donor demographics

NON-HBD group. Donors suitable for postmortem kdn procurement are emergency patients dying from circulatory arrest as a consequence of either intractable hemorrhagic, – and rarely cardiogenic, shock, or of cardiovascular dysregulation caused by cerebral fatalities (or a combination in both). Most often these are trauma patients with fatal head injuries alone or combined with multitrauma, less frequently, they are patients suffering from nontraumatic intracerebral bleeding or ischemia and very seldom patients with heart disease. Some of these patients die in the ambulance or emergency room, others develop sudden circulatory instability in the intensive care unit and die in circulatory arrest. Since many hospitals require two electroencephalograms 24 h apart in order to use the patient as a HBD, most of these potential donors would be lost for organ procurement. However, nephrectomy can be performed after cardiac arrest. Whenever possible we brought these patients to the operating room before circulatory arrest had been established and procurement of the kdns was started immediately.

Of the 19 NON-HBD included in our study, 16 died from fatal head injury, 2 from ruptured cerebrovascular aneurysms and 1 from asphyxia. Of the 38 kdn's procured, 4 were shipped to other transplant centers, and 34 were transplanted in our institution and included in this study.

HBD group. Of the 34 donors in this group, 21 died from head injury, 6 from spontaneous cerebrovascular bleeding, 3 from cerebrovascular insult, 3 from anoxia and 1 from meningitis. All fullfilled the criteria for brain death and single or multiple organ procurement was performed under heartbeating conditions.

Table 1 gives a summary and comparison of other relevant donor data for both groups, i.e. donor age, need for catecholamines, diuresis during the last hour, serum creatinine level, presevation medium and cold ischemia time. Statistically relevant differences between the two donor groups were found for the last hour's diuresis which was significantly lower in the NON-HBD and for the serum creatinine levels which were significantly higher in the NON-HBD group. No significant differences were found for all other paramenters. Precise duration of warm ischemia time was not determined in most NON-HBD, because the exact moment when blood circulation ceased was not definable. Therefore, these data are not given for either group.

Donor operation

NON-HBD group. Heparin (20000 units) was given intravenously before cardiac arrest was established. A midline incision from the xiphoid to the pubis was performed followed by an incision of the posterior parietal peritoneum along the right colon. The right colon and the small bowel were mobilized and retracted superiorly and to the left. The distal vena cava and aorta were freed and the latter cannulated just above the bifurcation. The celiac axis, superior and inferior mesenteric arteries and inferior mesenteric vein were only ligated if their exposure was not time consuming. The proximal aorta was then isolated below the diaphragm, cross clamped and an in situ aortic flush was immediately initiated using either EuroCollins (EC) or University of Wisconsin (UW) solution. An incision in the distal vena cava allowed egress of cooling fluid. Care was taken that operating time to the beginning of the hypothermic flush was no more than 10 min. The kdn's and ureters were then mobilized. We did not usually carry out the en bloc removal of the kdn's but preferred to identify and dissect the renal vessels in situ. The aorta and vena cava were incised longitudinally and patches of the aorta and vena cava were excised for the renal vessels. The kdn's were then removed and again flushed on the backtable. We have recently described this technique elsewhere [1].

HBD group. The procurement technique in HBD for singe or multiple organ procurement has been described by others [2] and also by us [3] and remains unchanged.

Recipient demographics

NON-HBD group. The 34 recipients all suffered from end-stage renal disease caused by glomerulonephritis in 17, polycystic kdn disease in 4, chronic pyelonephritis in 4, diabetic nephropathy in 3, Alport's syndrome in 2 and other chronic kdn affections in 4 patients.

HBD group. Of these 34 selected kdn transplant recipients, 12 suffered from glomerulonephritis, 10 from polycystic kdn disease, 3 from chronic pyelonephritis, 2 from Alport' syndrome and 7 from other chronic renal diseases.

Table 2 gives a summary and comparison of other relevant recipient data and pretransplant risk factors for both groups, such as recipient age, sex, primary graft or retransplant, dialysis time and type hemodialysis or continuous ambulatory peritoneal dialysis, number of HLA-A, -B, -DR mismatches and sensitization (highest preoperative percentage of antibodies). None of these data showed a statistically significant difference between the two recipient groups.

Postoperative treatment

For the HBD group (and for the 9 kdn in the NON-HBD group transplanted before 1986) our standard triple immunosuppressive therapy was used: prednisone (1 mg/kg per day tapered to 0 at 6 month), azathioprine (1 mg/kg per day, continuously) and cyclosporine 5 mg/kg per day intravenously for the first days and thereafter orally in doses depending on serum trough levels (desired range: 200–400 ng/ml). For the NON-HBD group, the prednisone and azathioprine regimen was identical but, in 1986, initial cyclosporine was replaced by the intravenous administration of antithymocyte globulin (ATG 3 mg/kg per day) until serum creatinine levels reached a normal range, but maximally for 14 days. Oral cyclosporine therapy was started in equal doses as in the HBD-group, overlapping about the last 2 days of ATG administration. In all other respects (thromboembolic and infection prophylaxis, monitoring of organ function, and so forth) both groups had the same postoperative mangement.

Table 1. Donor demographics and kidneys. Donor and graft characteristics such as need for catecholamines and type of preservation solutions used are expressed as frequencies, data such as age, diuresis during the last hour, serum creatinine level and cold ischemia time are given as average ± standarddeviation

	HBD	NON-HBD	
Donors *(n)*	34	19	
Age years	31.1 ± 14.4	33.9 ± 12.5	$P = ns$
Use of catecholamines	27 (79%)	16 (84%)	$P = ns$
Diuresis last hour ml/h	317.3 ± 468.2	100 ± 103.3	$P < 0.05$
Serum creatinine μmol/l	87.9 ± 20.3	133 ± 62	$P < 0.05$
Preservation UW/EC	14/20	10/9	$P = ns$
Cold ischemia time h	15.7 ± 7.4	17.3 ± 5.9	$P = ns$

UW, University of Wisconsin organ preservation solution; EC, Euro-Collins organ preservation solution

Table 2. Recipient demographics. Relevant recipient characteristics such as distribution of sex, type of preoperative dialysis and number of transplant (primary graft or retransplant) are expressed as frequencies; other pretransplant risk factors such as age, duration of pretransplant dialysis, number of HLA-A, -B, -DR mismatches and sensitization (maximal preoperative percentage of antibodies) are expressed as average ± standard deviation

	HBD	NON-HBD	
n	34	34	
Age years	46.2 ± 12.4	45.7 ± 13	$P = ns$
Sex f/m	13/21	13/21	$P = ns$
Primary graft/retransplant	27/7	26/8	$P = ns$
Dialysis type HD/CAPD	29/5	25/9	$P = ns$
Duration of dialysis month	51 ± 45	52 ± 45	$P = ns$
HLA mismatches A	1.2 ± 0.5	1.1 ± 0.6	$P = ns$
B	1.3 ± 0.6	1.3 ± 0.5	$P = ns$
DR	0.6 ± 0.5	0.9 ± 0.5	$P = ns$
Maximal preop antibody levels %	25.2 ± 29.1	25.6 ± 27.1	$P = ns$

HD, Hemodialysis; CAPD, continuous ambulatory peritoneal dialysis

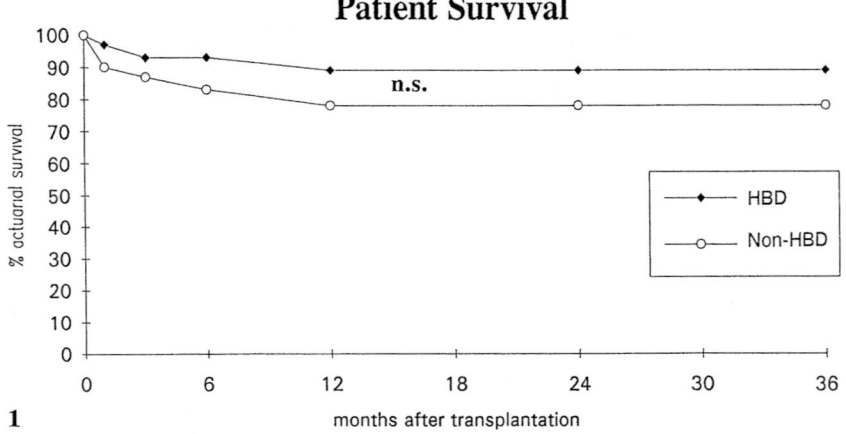

Fig. 1. Patient survival rates following kidney allotransplantation according to the origin of the grafts: kidneys from heartbeating donors [HBD] or non-heartbeating donors [NON-HBD]

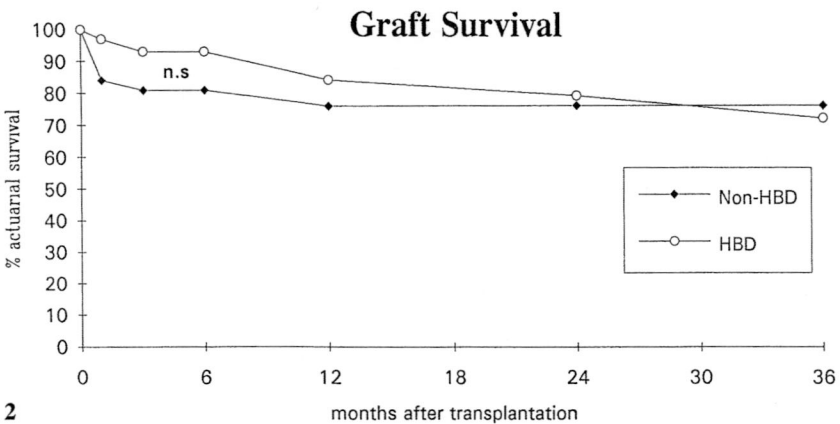

Fig. 2. Renal graft functional survival rates for kidneys from heartbeating donors [HBD] and from non-heartbeating donors [NON-HBD]

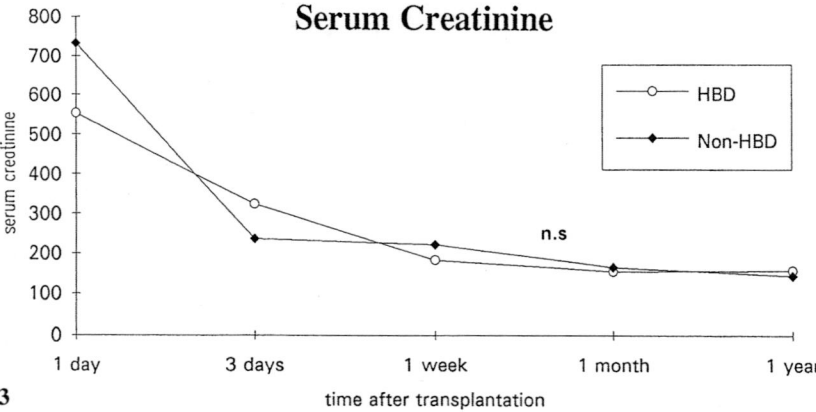

Fig. 3. Course of posttransplant serum creatinine levels in the early and late postoperative period (day 1 to 1 year) for kidneys from heartbeating donors [HBD] and from non-heartbeating donors [NON-HBD]. For days 1, 3 and 7, only creatinine values from patients that were not on dialysis during this time were taken

Statistics

Patient and graft survival rates were calculated by an actuarial method (Cutler-Ederer) on September 30, 1991, giving a minimum follow up of 1 month and a maximum of 77 months. Statistical significance (P-value < 0.05) was determined by the Student's t-test for comparison of means and the Chi-square test for comparison of proportions.

Results

The 1-year patient survival rate was 89.4% for the HBD group, and 78% for the NON-HBD group. The 1-year kdn transplant survival rate was 84.9% for the HBD group, and 76.1% for the NON-HBD group. Patient and

graft outcome for both groups are shown in Table 3 and depicted in Figs. 1 and 2. During the first posttransplant week 10 of 34 (29%) recipients in the HBD group and 17 of 34 (50%) recipients in the NON-HBD group needed dialysis support; diagnosis of acute tubular necrosis was assumed if clinical signs of acute rejection were absent and technical reasons were precluded. There was one case of primary non-function in the HBD group (3%) and three cases in the NON-HBD group (9%). The course of the serum creatinine levels in the early and late postoperative period for both groups is listed in Table 3 and depicted in Fig. 3. The comparison of all data showed no statistically significant differences between the two groups.

Major technical complications that needed surgical repair were four ureteric obstructions in the NON-HBD

Table 3. Results. Results such as incidence of temporary posttransplant dialysis support and occurrence of primary non-function are expressed as frequencies; postoperative serum creatinine levels are given as average ± standard deviation and patient and graft survival in percentages as calculated by actuarial method

	HBD	NON-HBD	
Temporary postoperative dialysis	10 (29%)	17 (50%)	P = ns
Primary non-function	1 (3%)	3 (9%)	P = ns
Creatinine µmol/l at 1 week	185 ± 113	223 ± 141	P = ns
Creatinine µmol/l at 1 month	154 ± 99.7	165 ± 101	P = ns
Creatinine µmol/l at 1 year	152 ± 92.5	147 ± 82.2	P = ns
1 year patient survival	89.4%	78%	P = ns
1 year graft survival	84.9%	76.1%	P = ns

group and three in the HBD group. There was one case of lymphocele in each group that needed surgical intervention.

Causes of graft failure or death

NON-HBD group. Of 34 transplanted kidneys in this group, 3 showed primary non-function; all 3 were retransplants and histological examination demonstrated acute vascular rejection; in two cases this was associated with haemolytic uremic syndrome. The same phenomenon (vascular rejection + haemolytic uremic syndrome) was observed in three more NON-HBD kidneys, two of which were retransplants; all had primary function, one graft failed at day 12, the other two recovered. Thus, 6 out of 34 kdn's (18%) in the NON-HBD group, 5 of which were retransplants, showed vascular rejection, 5 of them associated with haemolytic uremic syndrome (thrombotic microangiopathy); 2 of these 6 kdn's recovered, and 4 were lost (2 with primary non-function). One more graft failed from chronic rejection at 74 months. Two patients died with functioning grafts at 1 week and at 11 months from myocardial infarction and pneumonia respectively.

HBD group. Of 34 transplanted kidneys in this group, 1 showed primary non-function for unknown reasons. Three other grafts failed, one at 11 months due to recurrence of the original disease in the transplant (sclerosing glomerulonephritis), one at 19 months from chronic rejection and one at 31 months from undetermined reasons. Two patients in this group died with functioning grafts at 3 and 11 months from myocardial infarction and pneumonia respectively.

Discussion

To overcome the shortage of kdn's available for transplantation, we, along with other groups [4, 5], reactivated the concept of kdn retrieval from NON-HBD. However, at the beginning of this series we observed an increased incidence in the need for dialysis support during the first posttransplant week. Since it is known that delayed renal graft function due to acute tubular necrosis from preservation damage has a major imapct on the 1- and 5-year kdn graft survival [6], we tried some specific measures to improve the safety and success of this procedure.

For fear of increased risk of cyclosporine toxicity in kdn's from NON-HBD with inevitably prolonged warm ischemia time, we replaced the initial postoperative cyclosporine administration by ATG until serum creatinine levels reached a normal range (maximally 14 days). Since this modification in 1986, the need for temporary postoperative dialysis of kdn's from NON-HBD has been reduced from 89% (8/9) to 36% (9/25). However 18 of the 25 kdn with the new the immunosuppressive regimen were also preserved with UW solution, introduced to our program since 1989. It is not possible, in this study, to differentiate the impact of the two factors, but the clear improvement in results suggested that both measures are advantageous for kdn's from NON-HBD. Despite the potential benefit of UW, we intend to keep cold ischemia time for kdn's from NON-HBD below 24 h because the degree of preliminary damage from the uncertain duration of warm ischemia and from the administration of catecholamines is difficult to assess and further risks should be avoided. Provided that these precautions are respected, catecholamine administration (if not given over a prolonged period, and in exessive doses [7] or even cessation of diuresis are not contraindications for kdn retrieval from NON-HBD. It might be argued, that we could shorten warm ischmia time by the installation of peritoneal cooling or immediate insertion of an aortic catheter for kidney flush as proposed by others [8]; however, these manipulations outside the operating room don't seem to be essential and would not be ethically accepted by our hospital personnel.

The striking finding of this analysis was the fact that most of the kdn's in the NON-HBD group were not lost for technical reasons (e. g. preservation failure) but due to acute vascular rejection, mostly associated with haemolytic uremic syndrome. It has to be emphasized that five of six such reactions developed in retransplants; three cases never showed function of the graft (PNF), one lost function after 12 days and two recovered permanently. This phenomenon remains unexplained, but we speculate that endothelial lesions in the graft, caused by prolonged warm ischemia, might intensify endothelial antigenic presentation giving rise to acute vascular rejection and thrombotic microangiopathy. As long as this finding of acute vascular rejection associated with haemolytic uremic syndrome in retransplanted kdn's from NON-HBD is not clarified, we propose to use kdn's from this source for first transplants only. Furthermore, we see here another good reason to avoid cyclosporine in the early postoperative period because it is known that cyclosporine can aggravate thrombotic microangiopathy. It is worth noting that four of six cases with this kind of rejection still had initial cyclosporine immunosuppression according to our former protocol. Within the last 2 years the number of kdn's from NON-HBD increased significantly and actually constitutes about 25% of all kdn grafts in our program. The results in this study showed that good short- and long-term results can be achieved with kdn's from this source.

We concluded that organ procurement from NON-HBD is an adequate approach to an important cadaver donor source that in general is not efficiently used, but could significantly increase the number of kdn grafts in most transplant programs. Successful patient and graft survival rates can be achieved if limited cold ischemia time is guaranteed, and initial immunosuppression with cyclosporine avoided. Results might improve with routine use of advanced preservation solutions and if kdn's of this origin are used for primary transplants only. There seems to be an increased risk of vascular rejection associated with hemolytic uremic syndrome in retransplanted kidneys from NON-HBD and this phenomeon needs to be investigated.

References

1. Candinas D, Schlumpf R, Decurtins M, Largiadèr F. Die Nierenentnahme bei Spendern mit Kreislaufstillstand – Ein einfaches Verfahren, um den Mangel an gespendeten Nieren zu verringern. Schweiz Rundsch Med (submitted)

2. Starzl TE, Hakala T, Schaw BW Jr et al (1984) A flexible procedure for multiple cadaveric organ procurement. Surg Gynecol Obstet 158: 223–230

3. Dunn DL, Morel Ph, Schlumpf R, Mayoral JL, Gillingham KJ, Moudry-Munns KC, Krom RAF, Gruessner RWG, Payne WD, Sutherland DER, Najarian JS (1991) Evidence that combined procurement of pancreas and liver grafts does not affect transplant outcome. Transplantation 51: 150–157

4. Ruers TJM, Vroemen JPAM, Kootstra G (1986) Non-heart-beating donors: a successful contribution to organ procurement. Transplant Proc 18: 408–410

5. Kootstra G, Wijnen R, van Hooff JP, van Der Linden CJ (1991) Twenty percent more kidneys through a non-heart beating program. Transplant Proc 23: 910–911

6. Canafax DM, Torres A, Fryd DS, Heil JE, Strand MH, Ascher NL, Payne WD, Sutherland DER, Simons RL, Najarian JS (1986) Transplantation 41: 177–181

7. Whelchel JD, Diethelm AG, Phillips MG, Ryder WR, Schein LG (1986) The effect of high-dose dopamine in cadaver donor mangement on delayed graft function and graft survival following renal transplantation. Transplant Proc 18: 523–527

8. Garcia-Rinaldi R, Lefrak EA, Defore WW, Feldman L, Noon GP, Jachimczyk JA, DeBakey ME (1975) In situ preservation of cadaver kidneys for transplantation: laboratory observations and clincal application. Ann Surg 182: 576–584

Transplant Int (1992) 5 [Suppl 1]: S 429–S 432

TRANSPLANT
International
© Springer-Verlag 1992

A preliminary report of the HTK randomized multicenter study comparing kidney graft preservation with HTK and EuroCollins solutions

A. F. Groenewoud[1] **and J. Thorogood**[2] **for the HTK Study Group**

[1] Department of Surgery, Klinikum Rechts der Isar, München, FRG
[2] Eurotransplant, Leiden, The Netherlands

The main goal of transplantation is to restore good renal function and to improve the quality of life of thousands of dialysis patients, something which can only be achieved by providing them with well functioning grafts. Delayed renal allograft function is a serious problem. It is important to prevent this complication because it makes the diagnosis of acute rejection in the early postoperative period difficult, increases the necessity for diagnostic procedures, introduces dialysis treatments and prolongs hospital stay. The aetiology of delayed graft function (DGF) is multifactorial, and factors including donor management, technique used for organ procurement and preservation, age, anatomical variations in the graft, ischemia periods, use of cyclosporine A (CyA) or recipient immunological reactions have been implicated. Using different preservation solutions DGF rates vary from 30 % to 60 %. Recent clinical data have demonstrated better preservation and improved renal function posttransplant with HTK and University of Wisconsin (UW) solutions compared to EuroCollins solution. In a randomized multicenter study in collaboration with the Eurotransplant organ exchange organization, the efficacy of the HTK solution in renal transplantation was compared to EuroCollins and UW solutions in two parallel prospective randomized trials. The first preliminary results comparing HTK and EuroCollins solutions are reported here.

Key words: HTK solution – Kidney transplantation

Organization of the randomized trial

This randomized trial was organized in collaboration with Eurotransplant. This facilitated a uniform central policy for kidney graft allocation through HLA matching, standardized techniques and reagents for donor and recipient tissue typing and crossmatching. Randomized assignment

of the preservation solution for kidney donors and data collection were coordinated by Eurotransplant. The randomized multicenter trials started in July 1990 and the recruitment has progressed steadily since then. Our goal is to randomize 300 donors in each trial i.e. 300 donors in the HTK versus UW trial and 300 donors in the HTK versus EC trial. We need a large number transplants for an appropriate statistical analysis to detect a 10 % difference in delayed graft function (DGF) between HTK and the other solutions. In total, 14 centers are participating in the HTK versus UW preservation part of the trial and 26 in HTK versus EC.

With the efforts of many physicians and transplant coordinators, 529 donors have been randomized up to September 21st, 1991. The randomized donors and their transplants in the participating centers are presented in a Table 1, and the numbers of randomized donors and transplants are presented in Table 2. It is apparant that the number of transplants in the HTK versus EC trial is sufficient to fulfil our goal. Interim results based on all donors and those recipients for whom follow-up information has been returned are presented.

Clinical results

To date, complete information about 338 donors and 307 transplants at 1 month follow-up has been obtained and analyzed. The descriptive information of donor and recipient characteristics which could influence the delayed graft function, as presented in Table 3, show that the HTK and EuroCollins groups are comparable.

Delayed graft function (DGF) of the transplanted kidney was defined as the absence of life-sustaining renal function which required dialysis treatment on two or more occasions within the 1st week after transplantation. This definition of DGF included patients with initial non-functioning kidneys that recovered after dialysis treatment and patients with transplanted kidneys that did not recover and the patient returned to chronic dialysis treatment. The analysis of outcome, limited to the percentage of DGF with

---

Offprint requests to: A. F. Groenewoud, Department of Surgery, Klinikum Rechts der Isar, Ismaningerstraße 28, 8000 München 80, FRG

Table 1. Overview of the number of randomized donors and transplantations

Country Center	(Code)	Local HTK trial FUP-coordinator	Number of donors	Number of transplants
Austria				
Innsbruck	(IB)	Fetz/Steurer	9	8
Graz	(GA)[a]	Pogglitsch	0	9
Linz	(OE)[a]	Breitenfeller	0	4
Linz	(OL)	Kaiser	0	2
Vienna	(WM/WG)	Wamser	25	57
Belgium				
Antwerpen	(AN)	van Beeumen	5	5
Bruxelles	(BJ)	Amerycks	6	2
Bruxelles	(BR)	Kinnaert	3	18
Bruxelles	(LA)	Lecomte	4	16
Gent	(GE)	VanderVennet	0	7
Leuven	(LM)[a]	Roels	0	13
Liege	(LG)[a]	Delbouille	0	4
Germany				
Aachen	(AK)[a]	Homburg	0	4
Berlin	(BE)	Passfall	20	33
Berlin	(EB)	Rücker	0	6
Bonn	(BO)	Molitor	1	1
Bremen	(BM)	Grote	12	15
Düsseldorf	(DU)	Schäpers/Westhoff	30	40
Erlangen	(ER/NB)	Neumayer/Hüls	0	21
Essen	(ES)	Walz	19	38
Frankfurt	(FM)	Ernst	13	29
Freiburg	(FR)	Kirste	20	35
Göttingen	(GO)	Werner	6	13
Hamburg	(HG)[a]	Clausen	0	11
Hannover	(HO)	Gubernatis/Heigl	58	66
Hann Munden	(HM)	Schäfer	0	26
Heidelberg	(HB)	Beer	17	19
Homburg/Saar	(HS)	Riegel	0	1
Jena	(JE)	Börner	0	1
Kaiserslautern	(KS)	Nauth	8	15
Kiel	(KI)	Schütt	16	31
Köln Lindenthal	(KL)	Kerp	28	33
Köln Mehrheim	(KM)	Arns	11	23
Lübeck	(LU)	Kopmann	18	26
München	(MH)	Groenewoud	1	20
München	(ML)	Abendroth/Schneeberger	35	47
Münster	(MN)	Mauritz	32	62
Marburg	(MR)	Kuhlman	3	8
Mainz	(MZ)	Kreber	24	15
Mannheim	(MA)	Schnülle	0	5
Rostock	(RO)[a]	Hudemann	0	1
Stuttgart	(ST)	Ziech	11	16
Tübingen	(TU)	Fischer-Fröhlich	13	19
Ulm	(UL)	Grupp	2	7
Würzburg	(WZ)	Goetz	12	16
Luxembourg	(LX)	Duhoux	1	2
the Netherlands				
Amsterdam	(AB)	Oosterlee	18	24
Groningen	(GR)[a]	de Maar	0	18
Leiden	(LB)[a]	van der Woude	0	10
Maastricht	(MS)	Wijnen	8	14
Nijmegen	(NY)	Hoitsma	22	34
Rotterdam	(RD)[a]	Hendriks/Sietse	0	15
Utrecht	(UT)	Hené	9	8
Utrecht	(UW)	Donckerwolcke	0	3
Outside Eurotransplant			18	
		Total	520	994

[a] Not participating in the preservation part of the study

each solution used, is shown in Table 4. A clear-cut difference was observed in the incidence of DGF after transplantation when the treatment groups were compared, but final statistical comparisons await further follow-up. In the HTK group, 24 % (37/156) of the recipients had DGF of the transplanted kidney that required dialysis treatment compared to 37 % (56/151) in the EuroCollins group. No recovery of the kidney function with a return to chronic dialysis treatment was observed in 5 % (8/156) of the HTK group and in 3 % (5/156) of the EuroCollins group.

Serum creatinine levels were recorded daily for 1 month. Posttransplant serum creatinine levels decreased more rapidly in the HTK group than in the Euro-

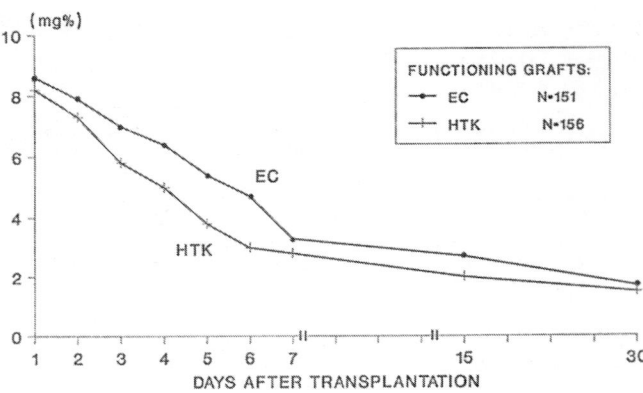

Fig. 1. Comparison of median serum creatinine decline. Eurotransplant Multicenter Study

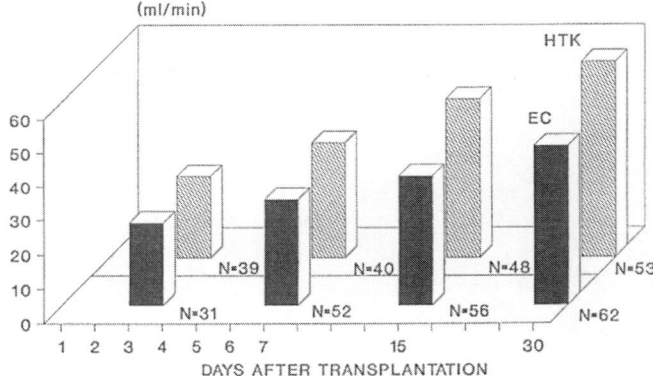

Fig. 2. Comparison of median creatinine clearance increase. Eurotransplant Multicenter Study

Collins group, as shown in Fig. 1. Creatinine clearances were documented on days 3, 7, and 14 and at one month. Higher creatinine clearances were observed at all times posttransplant in the HTK group compared with the EuroCollins group. Since not all centers calculate creatinine clearance values on a routine basis, this variable was obtained in a limited number of patients (Fig. 2).

Table 2. Overview of the number of donors and transplantations performed in each arm of the trial

Number of donors		Number of transplants	
HTK versus UW		HTK versus UW	
78	79	152	149
HTK versus EC		HTK versus UW	
181	182	352	341

Table 3. Characteristics of the kidney donor, transplant procedure and kidney recipient

	HTK solution		EC solution	
	(n)	%	(n)	%
Donor age (years)[a]	45		49	
Donor diagnosis				
– Multi trauma	(14/169)	8 %	(16/169)	9 %
– Trauma capitis	(32/169)	19 %	(50/169)	29 %
– Intracranial bleeding	(82/169)	49 %	(85/169)	50 %
– Others	(38/169)	23 %	(18/169)	12 %
Before donor nephrectomy				
– Resuscitation	(35/169)	21 %	(23/169)	14 %
– Hypotensive episodes	(100/169)	59 %	(96/169)	57 %
Donor drug treatment				
– Plasmaexpanders	(103/169)	62 %	(113/169)	68 %
– Bloodtransfusions	(59/169)	36 %	(59/169)	36 %
– Dopamine only	(152/169)	91 %	(153/169)	91 %
– Diuretics	(51/169)	31 %	(53/169)	31 %
Oliguria of the donor	(8/169)	8 %	(11/169)	10 %
Cold ischemia period (h)[a]	24		23	
Anastomisis time (min)[a]	33		33	
Recipient age (years)[a]	47		46	
Prior transplants				
– one or more	(21/156)	14 %	(130/151)	14 %

[a] Continous variables are shown as median values

Table 4. Kidney graft function after transplantation in both treatment groups

	HTK solution		EC solution	
	(n)	%	(n)	%
Initial graft function	(119/156)	76 %	(95/151)	63 %
Delayed graft function	(37/156)	24 %	(56/151)	37 %
– with recovery	(29/156)	19 %	(51/151)	34 %
– without recovery	(8/156)	5 %	(5/151)	3 %

Conclusions

This study reports the results of the randomized clinical comparison of two preservation solutions in postmortem renal transplantation. The most important preliminary finding in this study was that the incidence of DGF was reduced by 13 %, from 37 % in the EuroCollins group to 24 % in the HTK group, but these percentages do not necessarily reflect the final results. Improved renal function after transplantation was indicated by a rapid decrease in the serum creatinine levels in the HTK group compared to the EuroCollins group. Higher creatinine clearance values were also seen at all time periods posttransplant in the HTK group compared with the EuroCollins group.

We do not wish to prejudge the data of patients yet to be evaluated. A full analysis will be presented when sufficient follow-up information has been returned. We have, however, been able to demonstrate rapid recruitment and comparability of trial arms through international collaboration within Eurotransplant.

Acknowledgements. The results described in this trial are based upon the data of renal transplant recipients collected and submitted by the medical and administrative staffs collaborating with the Eurotransplant Foundation. The co-operation of the administrative staff and the medical students were of great value in the development of the HTK trial. The conduct of the trials was supported by an International Scientific Committee, in particular, we acknowledge G. Alexandre, H. J. Bretschneider, B. Buchholz, K. Dreikorn, F. Gubernatis, M. Hölscher, F. Isemer, G. Kootstra, R. Margreiter, Y. Vanrentergem, F. Mühlbacher, G. Persijn, J. Wilmink. Without the help of M. Kasterop-Kutz, the clinical data could not have been collected and stored in the computer for analysis.

Transplant Int (1992) 5 [Suppl 1]: S 433–S 434

TRANSPLANT
International
© Springer-Verlag 1992

The relationship between cause of death of the kidney donor and the presence of ischemic lesions in the kidney

A. T. J. Lavrijssen, H. G. Peltenburg, A. Tiebosch, F. H. M. Nieman, K. M. L. Leunissen, and J. P. van Hooff

Department of Nephrology, Department of Pathology, Methodology Section Directional Bureau, University Hospital Maastricht, Maastricht, The Netherlands

Chronic ischemic lesions in the donor kidney amplify the nephrotoxic effects of cyclosporine A [1]. With increasing age, the presence of chronic ischemic lesions in the kidney increases [2], and data concerning the fate of kidney grafts from older donors are conflicting [3–6]. Kidney from donors with an intracerebral bleed do less well compared to kidneys from other donors. Systematic data on the relationship between donor age, cause of death and severity of chronic ischemic lesions are lacking. This study was performed to investigate this relationship.

Key words: Age – Chronic ischemic lesions – Intracerebral beeding

Materials and methods

Biopsies of 156 consecutive cadaveric donor kidneys from patients, via Eurotransplant, reported to have died from intracerebral bleeding, subarachnoidal bleeding or trauma, were studied for the presence of pre-existing ischemic lesions. The biopsies were taken by a surgical procedure 1 h after reperfusion of the grafts.

The following items were scored blindly by one investigator on a semiquantitative scale (0–2): glomerulosclerosis, arteriosclerosis, interstitial fibrosis and mesangial proliferation. A score of 0 indicated no abnormal findings; a score of 2, severe abnormality. The individual scores were added (summation-score). Differences between the various groups were analyzed by the unpaired Student's t-test and a P-value of less than 0.05 was considered to be statistically significant. Multiple regression analysis was performed for the total group of biopsies with, as dependent variables, the individual scores and the summation-score. The predictive variables were donor age, cause of death of the donor and sex.

The patients reported to have died from subarachnoidal bleeding are included in the trauma group.

Offprint requests to: A. T. J. Lavrijssen, Department of Internal Medicine, University Hospital Maastricht, P. O. Box 5800, 6202 AZ Maastricht, The Netherlands

Results

The donor population consisted of 104 (66.7 %) males and 52 (33.3 %) females. In 119 (76.3 %) the cause of death was intracerebral bleeding; in 37 (23.7 %) a traumatic death or death due to subarachnoidal bleeding was reported. Of the males, 83 (79.8 %) died of intracerebral bleeding and 21 (20.2 %) of trauma. In the female group these figures were 36 (69.2 %) and 16 (30.8 %) respectively. These differences were not statistically significant. The mean age of the men was 30.9 years, and of the women, 37.8 years. The mean age of those donors dying of intracerebral bleeding was 46.0 years, and of those dying of trauma or subarachnoidal bleeding, it was 29.2 years. This difference reached statistical significance ($P < 0.01$).

The individual ischemic scores and the summation-score according to cause of death are reported in Table 1. The differences all reached statistical significance. This does not hold for the scores according to sex of the donor (Table 2). Regression analysis was done with the individual scores and the summation-score as dependent variables and the age of the donor, the cause of death and sex as predictive variables. In Table 3 the correlations between dependent and predictive variables are shown. In the trauma group the same pattern of significance was seen. In the intracerebral bleeding group only the correlations between age and vascular score, and age and summation-score were significant. It appeared that the predictive variables had significant correlations with all the dependent variables. When regression analysis was performed,

Table 1. Cause of death

		CVA	Trauma
Mean	age	46.0	29.2*
	glomerular score	0.95	0.32*
	vascular score	1.03	0.46*
	mesangial score	0.97	0.40*
	interstitial score	0.57	0.24*
	sum-score	3.51	1.42*

* $P < 0.01$

Table 2. Data according to sex

		Male	Female
Mean	age	30.9	37.8*
	glomerular score	0.44	0.52 ns
	vascular score	0.57	0.65 ns
	mesangial score	0.51	0.60 ns
	interstitial score	0.34	0.27 ns
	sum-score	1.86	2.04 ns

* $P < 0.01$

Table 3. Correlations

	Sex	Age	Cause of death
Sex	1		
Age	0.208*	1	
Cause of death	0.117	0.455*	1
Vascular score	0.065	0.418*	0.382*
Interstitial score	−0.059	0.389*	0.261*
Mesangial score	0.068	0.412*	0.402*
Glomerular score	0.050	0.460*	0.370*
Summation-score	0.043	0.522*	0.442*

* $P < 0.05$

the age of the donor had a more direct effect on the individual scores and the summation-score than the cause of death (glomerular score beta 0.367 vs 0.203, vascular score beta 0.308 vs 0.243, summation-score beta 0.455 vs 0.257). Only in the case of the mesangial score was the effect identical (beta 0.289 vs 0.270). The interstitial score was influenced more by sex than by cause of death.

Discussion and conclusion

The relative influence of donor age and cause of death on the presence of ischemic lesions in the donor kidney is a factor to be considered when accepting a particular patient as a donor. The occurence of an intracerebral bleed is related to the presence of hypertension, and there is a correlation between the presence of high blood pressure and certain ischemic lesions in the kidney [7]. However

the number of ischemic lesions increases with age, even in the absence of hypertension [8].

Our findings suggested that age is the main determinant for the development of ischemic lesions. So the fact that the patient who died of intracerebral bleeding had significantly more ischemic lesions could an be explained because they were older. However the data were collected retrospectively and the cause of death could not be verified. Because a subarachnoid bleed is usually due to a congenital abnormality of the vessel and is not associated with hypertension, these patients were included in the trauma group. Therefore, we could not exclude the possibility that some patients, reported as having died of intracerebral bleeding, in fact died of a subarachnoid bleed. A prospective study is necessary to exclude the possibility of this bias.

References

1. Leunissen KML, Bosman FT, Nieman FHM, Kootstra G, Vromen MAM, Noordzij TC, van Hooff JP (1989) Amplification of the nephrotoxic effect of cyclosporine by preexistent chronic histological lesions in the kidney. Transplantation 387: 590–593
2. Kappel B, Olsen S (1980) Cortical interstitial tissue and sclerosed glomeruli in the normal human kidney, related to age and sex. Virchows Arch Pathol Anat 387: 271
3. Hong JH, Shirani K, Arshad A, Parsa J, Malas A, Adamsons RJ, Butt KMH (1983) Influence of cadaver donor age on the succes of kidney transplants. Transplantation 32: 532–534
4. Foster MC, Wenham DW, Rowe PA, Blamey RW, Bishop MC, Burden RP, Morgan AG (1988) Use of older patients as cadaveric kidney donors. Br J Surg 75: 767–769
5. Rao KV, Ney AL (1988) Donor age does not affect the outcome of cadaver renal transplantation. Transplant Proc 20: 773
6. Roels L, Vanrentenghem Y, Waer M, Christiaens M, Gruwez J, Michielsen P (1990) The aging kidney donor: another answer to organ shortage? Transplant Proc 22: 368–370
7. Katafuchi R, Takebayashi S (1987) Morphometrical and functional correlations in benign nephrosclerosis. Clin Nephrol 28: 238–243
8. Tracy RE, Velez-Duran M, Heigle T, Oalmann MC (1988) Two variants of nephrosclerosis separately related to age and blood pressure. Am J Pathol 131: 270–282

Immunosuppression

Transplant Int (1992) 5 [Suppl 1]: S 437–S 439

TRANSPLANT
International
© Springer-Verlag 1992

High or low dose steroid therapy for acute renal transplant rejection after prophylactic OKT3 treatment: a prospective randomized study

D. De Backer[1], D. Abramowicz[1], M. Goldman[2], L. De Pauw[1], P. Viseur[1], J. L. Vanherweghem[1], P. Kinnaert[1], and P. Vereerstraeten[1]

Departments of [1] Nephrology and [2] Immunology, CUB Hôpital Erasme, Brussels, Belgium

Abstract. In this prospective randomized study, acute renal transplant rejections occurring in patients who received prophylactic OKT3 therapy were treated with either 3 pulses of 8 mg/kg methylprednisolone (MPS) in an alternate-day regimen (total dose 25 mg/kg in 1 week, H group, $n = 24$) or 5 daily pulses of 3 mg/kg MPS (total dose 17 mg/kg, L group, $n = 22$). Acute rejection was proven by biopsy in more than 85 % of cases in both groups. No difference was observed in rejection reversal (H 88 %, L 91 %), graft losses in the following 3 months (H 11 %, L 4 %) or the time evolution of the serum creatinine levels. The number (H 14, L 21) as well as the nature and severity of infections were similar in both groups. Only one death occurred in a patient who received OKT3 rescue therapy for corticoresistant rejections and developed Epstein-Barr virus (EBV)-related lymphoma. In conclusion, low dose MPS pulses appear as effective and safe as a higher dose to reverse acute rejection occurring after OKT3 prophylaxis. Thus, we favour the use of the low dose regimen in these patients.

Key words: Steroid therapy for rejection – Acute renal rejection – OKT3

Steroid pulses therapy has been the cornerstone of acute kidney graft rejection treatment for more than 3 decades [3, 5]. The optimal dose of steroids in patients who received polyclonal lymphocyte-specific antibodies (ALG), azathioprine (AZA), and cyclosporin A (CsA) as primary immunosuppression still remains a controversial issue [2, 6–8, 11, 13, 16]. Recently, it was found that primary immunosuppression with a 2-week course of prophylactic OKT3 resulted in a reduced incidence of early rejection episodes [4, 12, 15, 17]. More importantly, a significant long-term increase in kidney graft survival was observed in OKT3-treated recipients (Abramowicz et al., manu-

script submitted) as compared with those receiving a triple-drug regimen (CsA, AZA, prednisone). Although patient survival was similar in both groups, OKT3 prophylaxis was associated with an increased incidence of infectious episodes. It is therefore important to investigate the effectiveness in rejection reversal and the possible decrease in infectious complications of low steroid doses for acute rejection therapy in patients who received OKT3 prophylaxis as primary immunosuppression.

Patients and methods

All patients included in this study received a 2-week course of prophylactic OKT3, with AZA, prednisone and CsA being introduced on postoperative day 11. From July 1989 to November 1990, 45 episodes of acute renal graft rejection occurring in 38 patients (19 in each group) were randomly assigned to receive a methylprednisolone (MPS) dose of either 8 mg/kg · day, 3 times in an alternate-day regimen (high dose group) or 3 mg/kg daily over 5 consecutive days (low dose group). The 7 days' cumulative dose of MPS was 25 mg/kg in the high dose group and 17 mg/kg in the low dose group.

Both groups were identical as regards the age of the donors and recipients, cold and warm ischaemia times, number of human leucocyte antigen (HLA)-A, -B and -DR incompatibilities and the incidence and intensity of HLA-specific immunisation.

More than two-thirds of rejections occurred within 6 months after transplantation in both groups. Acute rejection was diagnosed

Table 1. Rejection episodes

	High dose ($n = 24$)	Low dose ($n = 22$)	P value
Corticosensitive	21 (88 %)	20 (91 %)	NS
Corticoresistant	3 (12 %)	2 (10 %)	NS
Rescued by OKT3	2 (8 %)	1 (5 %)	NS
ALG	–	1 (5 %)	NS
Graft losses after OKT3 course	1 (4 %)	–	NS
Re-rejection[a]	5 (24 %)	5 (25 %)	
Graft losses	2 (8 %)	2[b] (8 %)	

[a] Rejection occurring within 45 days after steroid pulses
[b] This patient died of a lymphoma after a second OKT3 course

Offprint requests to: P. Vereerstraeten, M.D., Nephrology Department, Route de Lennik 808, B-1070 Brussels, Belgium

Table 2. Creatinine evolution with treatment

| | Methylprednisolone dose | | | | | |
| | High | | Low | | P value | |
	Creatinine[a]	Day[b]	Creatinine	Day	Creatinine	Day
Rejection	3.1 ± 0.4	0	3.6 ± 0.7	0	NS	–
Peak	3.5 ± 0.4	1.8 ± 0.4	4.0 ± 0.7	1.5 ± 0.5	NS	NS
Nadir	1.7 ± 0.1	19.6 ± 1.8	1.6 ± 0.2	20.1 ± 1.6	NS	NS

[a] Serum creatinine, mg/dl (mean $\pm$ SEM)
[b] Mean $\pm$ SEM

when the serum creatinine level rose or failed to decrease in a recently transplanted patient without evidence of other causes of allograft dysfunction. Rejections were proven by biopsy in more than 85% of cases. The rejection was considered corticoresistant if the serum creatinine level continued to rise at the end of the MPS pulses. Some corticoresistant rejections were further treated with OKT3 or ALG according to clinical criteria. Infectious complications were recorded if they occurred within 3 months after steroid pulse therapy.

Results

Rejection episodes were corticosensitive in 90% of cases in both groups (Table 1). In these patients, the serum creatinine levels before treatment, at peak and at nadir were similar in both groups, as was the day of occurrence of peak and nadir (Table 2).

Corticoresistant rejections were successfully rescued by OKT3 or ALG (used in a patient immunized against OKT3) in 2 patients in both groups. One patient lost his graft from renal graft artery thrombosis after the second OKT3 injection given as rescue therapy (Table 1).

Re-rejection occurred within the next 45 days in about 20% of patients. Steroid pulses were effective in two-thirds. One patient who received OKT3 for re-rejection died of lymphoma.

Infections occurred within 3 months of steroid pulses in about 40% of cases (Table 3). Most were bacterial urinary tract infections, as well as benign herpetic and candida stomatitis.

The incidence of more severe infections [bacterial sepsis, lung infections due to cytomegalovirus (CMV) and aspergillosis and disseminated Epstein-Barr virus (EBV) infection] was similar in both groups.

Discussion

The main conclusion of this prospective randomized study is that acute kidney graft rejection occurring after OKT3 prophylaxis was very efficiently treated by low dose steroid pulses. The reversal rate, the evolution of renal function and the incidence of re-rejection were similar for both steroid doses. This is in agreement with all five previous randomized studies, which found no benefit in increasing the steroid dose [7, 8, 10, 11, 13].

Interestingly, the percentage of corticosensitive rejections in our patients who received OKT3 prophylaxis was substantially higher than the commonly observed 70% rate. This is in accordance with the results of our prospective randomized study demonstrating a higher proportion of cortico-sensitive rejections after prophylactic OKT3 as compared with CsA.

The small number of corticoresistant episodes could usually be rescued by a second OKT3 (or ALG) course. However, the dangers of giving multiple courses of OKT3 over short periods of time should be emphasized. Indeed, this strategy is associated with an unacceptable incidence of Epstein-Barr virus (EBV)-associated lymphomas [1,14].

Decreasing the steroid dose was not followed by a reduced incidence of infection. Infections were only recorded during the first 3 months following rejection. On the other hand, the difference between the 2 groups in the cumulative dose of corticosteroids was rather limited in the long term if only one episode of rejection was treated.

In conclusion, low dose MPS pulses appear as effective and safe as high dose pulses to reverse acute rejection occurring after OKT3 prophylaxis. We thus favour the use of the low dose regimen in these patients.

Table 3. Infectious episodes

	High dose ($n = 24$)	Low dose ($n = 22$)	P value
Number of rejection with infections	9 (38%)	10 (45%)	NS
Proportion infected per rejection episode	0.58	0.95[a]	$P < 0.05$
Number of infections	14	21	
Bacterial	10 (71%)	10 (48%)	NS
– With septicaemia	2 (14%)	1 (5%)	NS
Viral	3 (21%)	7 (33%)	NS
– HSV	2	4	NS
– CMV	1	2	NS
– EBV	0	1[b]	NS
Fungal			
– Oral candidosis	0	4 (19%)	NS
– Aspergillosis	1 (7%)	0	NS

[a] Seven infection episodes in a single patient
[b] Death from EBV-associated lymphoma
HSV, herpes simplex virus; CMV, cytomegalovirus; EBV, Epstein-Barr virus

References

1. Abramowicz D, Goldman M, De Pauw L, Doutrelepont JM, Kinnaert P, Vanherweghem JL, Vereerstraeten P (1991) Post-transplantation lymphoproliferative disorder and OKT3 (letter). N Engl J Med 324: 1438–1439

2. Alacron-Zurita A, Ladefoged J (1974) Treatment of acute allograft rejection with high dose of cortico-steroids. Kidney Ent 9: 351–354
3. Clarke AG, Salaman JR (1974) Methyl prednisolone in the treatment of renal transplant rejection. Clin Nephrol 2 (6): 230–234
4. Debure A, Chkoff N, Chatenoud L, Lacombe M, Campos H, Noel LH, Goldstein G, Bach JF, Kreis H (1988) One month prophylactic use of OKT3 in cadaver kidney transplant recipients. Transplantation 45: 546–553
5. Feduska NJ, Turcotte JG, Gikas PW, Bacon GE, Penner JA (1972) Reversal of renal allograft rejection with intravenous methylprednisolone "pulse" therapy. J Surg Res 12 (3): 208–215
6. Gray D, Shepherd H, Daar A, Oliver DO, Morris PJ (1978) Oral versus intravenous high-dose steroid treatment of renal allograft rejection: the big shot or not? Lancet T: 117–118
7. Kauffman HM, Stronstad SA, Sampson D, Stawicki AT (1979) Randomized steroid therapy of human kidney rejection. Transplant Proc 11: 36–38
8. Lui SF, Sweny P, Scoble JC, Varghese Z, Moorhead JF, Fernando OR (1989) Low-dose versus high-dose intravenous methylprednisolone therapy for acute renal allograft rejection in patients receiving cyclosporine therapy. Nephrol Dial Transplant 4: 387–389
9. Mussche MM, Ringoir SM, Lameire NN (1976) High intravenous dose of methylprednisolone for acute cadaveric renal allograft rejection. Nephron 16 (4): 287–291
10. Orta-Sibu N, Chantier C, Bewick M, Haycock G (1982) Comparison of high-dose intravenous methylprednisolone with low-dose oral prednisolone in acute renal allograft rejection in children. Br Med J [Clin Res] 285: 258–260
11. Park GD, Bartucci M, Smith MC (1984) High versus low-dose methylprednisolone for acute rejection episodes in renal transplantation. Nephron 36 (2): 80–83
12. Shield CF, Huches JD, Lemon JA (1988) Prophylactic OKT3 and cadaveric renal transplantation at a single center. Clin Transpl 2: 190–193
13. Stromstad SA, Kauffman HM, Sampson D, Stawicki AT (1978) Randomized steroid therapy of human kidney transplant rejection. Surg Forum 29: 376–377
14. Swinnen LJ, Costanzo-Nordin MR, Fisher SE, O'Sullivan EJ, Johnson MR, Meroux AL, Dizikes GJ, Pifarre R, Fisher RI (1990) Increased incidence of lymphoproliferative disorder after immunosuppression with the monoclonal antibody OKT3 in cardiac-transplant recipients. N Engl J Med 323: 1723–1728
15. Toussaint C, De Pauw L, Vereerstraeten P, Kinnaert P, Abramowicz D, Goldman M (1989) Possible nephrotoxicity of the prophylactic use of OKT3 monoclonal antibody after cadaveric renal transplantation. Transplantation 47: 524–526
16. Vicenti F, Amend W, Feduska NJ, Duca RM, Salvatierra O (1980) Improved outcome following renal transplantation with reduction in the immunosuppression therapy for rejection episodes. Am J Med (1): 107–112
17. Vigeral P, Chkoff N, Chatenoud L, Campos H, Lacombe M, Droz D, Goldstein G, Bach JF, Kreis H (1986) Prophylactic use of OKT3 monoclonal antibody in cadaver kidney recipients. Utilisation of OKT3 as the sole immunosuppression agent. Transplantation 41: 730–733

Transplant Int (1992) 5 [Suppl 1]: S 440–S 443

TRANSPLANT
International
© Springer-Verlag 1992

The risk of infection following OKT3 and antilymphocyte globulin treatment for renal transplant rejection: results of a single center prospectively randomized trial

U. J. Hesse[1], P. Wienand[1], C. Baldamus[2], M. Pollok[2], and H. Pichlmaier[1]

Departments of [1] Surgery and [2] Internal Medicine, University of Cologne, Cologne, Federal Republic of Germany

Abstract. Some 43 of 60 (72 %) renal allograft recipients who were prospectively randomized to receive either OKT3 monoclonal antibody ($n = 30$) or ALG (antilymphocyte globulin) polyclonal antibody ($n = 30$) for steroid-resistant rejection suffered from infection, 25 (83 %) following OKT3 and 18 (60 %) following ALG treatment ($P < 0.05$). Clinically evident herpes infection was most frequently seen (9 and 7, respectively), followed by pneumonia (6 and 1, respectively $P < 0.05$), urinary tract infection and wound infection (2 of each in both groups) fungal *(Candida)* and multibacterial infections. One patient died in each group due to cytomegalovirus (CMV) pneumonia, giving a mortality of 4.3 % in each group. Actuarial 1-year graft and patient survival rates were 80 % and 97 % in both groups, respectively. It is concluded that ALG and OKT3 are equally effective in renal allograft rejection resistant to steroid treatment, however, the risk of infection appears to be higher with OKT3.

Key words: Infection – OKT3 – Antilymphocyte globulin – Rejection

OKT3 monoclonal antibodies have heralded a new era in the treatment of organ transplant rejection. Although the relative advantages of OKT3 monoclonal antibodies in terms of graft survival in steroid-resistant renal allograft rejection has been well documented [4], the relative risk of serious life-threatening infections has not been detailed. Since polyclonal antibodies such as antilymphocyte globulin (ALG) have been used in the pre-OKT3 era as the sole antibody treatment for graft rejection, it was the purpose of this prospectively randomized trial to evaluate various factors associated with the incidence of infections following the treatment with antibodies when graft rejection did not respond to steroid administration.

Offprint requests to: PD. Dr. U.J. Hesse, Department of Surgery, University of Cologne, Joseph-Stelzmann-Str. 9, W-5000 Köln 41, Federal Republic of Germany

Patients and methods

Between 20 July 1987 and 26 June 1991 60 patients aged 41 ± 12 years (mean $\pm$ SD; range 17–65) were entered into the study and were followed for a minimum of 3 months up to 51 months. Eighteen (30 %) were female and 42 (70 %) were male. Two (3.4 %) had diabetes. One patient (1.6 %) received his graft from a mismatched related donor, and the rest (98.4 %) from a cadaver donor. Also, 59 patients (98.4 %) underwent transplantation for the first time, while one (1.6 %) underwent retransplantation. Half of these 60 patients were randomized to receive OKT3 monoclonal antibodies while the other half received ALG for steroid-resistant rejection.

In the OKT3 group 20 (66.6 %) patients were male and 10 (33.4 %) female; in the ALG group 22 were male (73.3 %) and 8 female (26.7 %). Each group had one diabetic patient. Both groups contained 29 patients with primary cadaver transplants. In the ALG group 1 patient had a secondary transplant, and in the OKT3 group 1 patient had a mismatched related graft. The age of the recipients, the presence or absence of diabetes, the number of transplants, the type of donors (cadaver or living related), the number of mismatches (A, B and DR) were statistically insignificantly different (Table 1).

Diagnosis of rejection. The patients only entered in the study had a clinical diagnosis of rejection, involving a rise in serum cratinine level over 0.3 mg/dl, decrease in diuresis of at least 500 ml/day, fever graft tenderness, and histological proof of rejection of the mononuclear interstitial cellular type.

Treatment of rejection. If a steroid bolus therapy of 0.5 g on 2–4 successive days did not lead to graft function improvement, the patients were randomized to receive either OKT3 or ALG for 10 days. Con-

Table 1. Patient demographics of the cohorts receiving OKT3 or antilymphocyte globulin (ALG) for steroid-resistant rejection

	ALG ($n = 30$)	OKT3 ($n = 30$)	P
Age (years)	40.9 ± 12.1	40.2 ± 12.8	n.s.
Sex (m/f)	22/8	20/10	n.s.
Diabetic	1	1	n.s.
HLA-A, -B mismatches	1.8 ± 1.0	1.8 ± 0.8	n.s.
DR mismatches	0.5 ± 0.6	0.7 ± 0.6	n.s.
first transplant	29	30	n.s.
Retransplant	1	0	n.s.
CAD/LRD	30/0	29/1	n.s.
Pres. time (h)	20 ± 5	20 ± 5	n.s.
Donor age (years)	41 ± 13	42 ± 15	n.s.

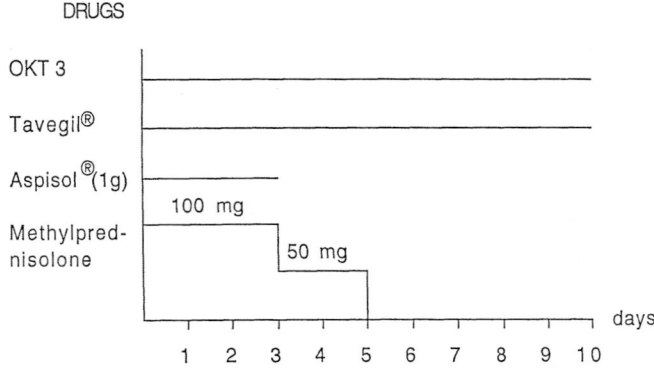

Fig. 1. Concurrent medication with OKT3 to prevent first-dose reactions

currently, the basic immunosuppression was continued with cyclosporin A (Sandoz), (up to 300–400 mg/ml TDX), azathioprine (Wellcome), and steroids as scheduled. The dosage of antilymphocyte globulin (Merieux) was 5 ml/10 kg body weight (maximum 30 ml/day) given via a central venous line. The dosage of OKT3 (Ortho) was 5 ml/day administered intravenously. In addition, methylprednisolone, 1 ampulla of Tavegil, and 1 g of Aspisol were given to the patients to prevent first-dose reactions (Fig. 1).

Basic immunosuppression. The induction and basic immunosuppression following transplantation were identical in all patients. ALG was administered for at least 7 days in a dosage of 5 ml/10 kg bodyweight with a maximum of 30 ml/kg daily. Cyclosporin A was given the first day postoperatively in a dose of 3 mg/kg intravenously and subsequently orally in a dose of 10 mg/kg daily and then reduced in steps as determined by TDX while trying to keep the level between 300 and 400 ng/ml. Prednisolone was given in a dose of 250 mg/day reduced in increments of 25 mg per day to 100 mg and then twice daily in 5-mg increments to a maintenance dose of 10 to 15 mg/day. Between 1 and 5 mg/kg azathioprine was given daily to the patients. For prophylaxis, a cephalosporin antibiotic was administered just prior to surgery. Every patient received a 3-day course of hyperimmunoglobulin 2 ml/kg body weight.

Diagnostic methods. All patients underwent chest roentgenograms on a regular basis (every 3–4 days). Sputum cultures were obtained, and if indicated, fiberoptic bronchoscopy with lavage or brushing was performed. The specimens were cultured and examined with special stains for bacteria, viruses, and fungi. A diagnosis of cytomegalic (CMV) inclusion disease was confirmed when the clinical picture was compatible and there was either serologic (a greater than four fold increase in complement fixing or indirect fluorescent antibody levels to CMV) and/or culture evidence of active CMV infection [5].

Treatment. Infections were treated with antibiotics, either empirically or according to sensitivity testing when cultures were available. Acyclovir was administered for CMV and herpes virus infections. Hyperimmunoglobulin was given to all patients with evidence of CMV infection.

Data retrieval. Each transplant patient completed a scheduled follow-up form at 1, 3 and 6 months following transplantation and every 6 months subsequently until 13 September 1991, loss of function, or death. Detailed information was collected for every week that a patient was hospitalized from the time of transplant until 13 September 1991, loss of function, or death. Computerized information included chest roentgenogram results, a code for infections, culture results, and clinical symptoms such as fever or white blood cell count, and causes of death.

Statistical evaluation. Fisher's exact test was used for comparing small groups of patients, and the χ^2 method was used for comparing larger groups. The graft survival rates were calculated by actuarial techniques. The P values were calculated over the entire period using Gehan's test [2]. In all tests the values were considered statistically significant when P was less than 0.05.

Results

The actuarial graft and patient survival rates are given in Fig. 2. There was no statistically significant difference in graft function or patient survival between those receiving OKT3 and those receiving ALG for steroid-resistant rejection.

Onset of treatment for rejections

The ALG treatement started a mean of 23.7 ± 15.7 days following transplantation, while OKT3 treatment was started 19.9 ± 13.2 days following transplantation. Each treatment was performed for 8.2 ± 1.8 and 9.1 ± 2.1 days, respectively. Neither difference was statistically significant (Table 2). A second rejection had to be treated in

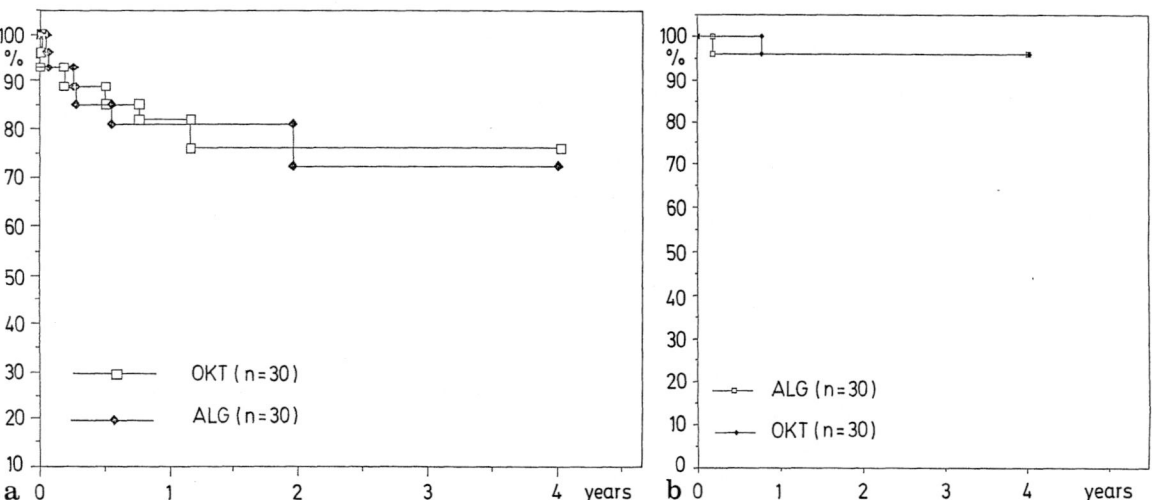

Fig. 2a, b. Actuarial graft (**a**) and patient (**b**) survival rates following OKT3 or ALG treatment for steroid-resistant rejection (P = n. s.)

Table 2. Onset and duration of primary rejection treatment

	ALG (days)	OKT3 (days)	P
Onset (mean ± SD)	21 ± 13	19 ± 9	n.s.
Range	6–61	7–74	n.s.
Duration (mean ± SD)	8.2 ± 1.8	9.1 ± 2.1	n.s.

Table 3. Character of first infection following OKT3 and ALG treatment for steroid-resistant rejection

	ALG (n = 30)	OKT3 (n = 30)	P
Pneumonia (CMV)	1 (1)	6 (4)	< 0.05
UTI	2	2	n.s.
Wound	2	2	n.s.
Meningitis	1	1	n.s.
Throat	2	2	n.s.
Sepsis (fungal)	0	1	n.s.
(virus)	7	9	n.s.
(bacteria)	3	2	n.s.
Total	18	25	< 0.05

CMV, cytomegalovirus

12 patients (40%) of the ALG group at a mean ± SD of 118 ± 82 days after transplantation (range 42–327). In the OKT3 group, 12 patients had to be retreated for rejection at a mean ± SD of 285 ± 396 days after transplantation (range 42–1240; Fig. 3). In each group, two patients had to be treated for a third rejection episode.

Incidence of infection

Out of these 60 patients, 43 (72%) contracted an infection requiring intensive antibiotic or chemotherapeutic therapy. Also, 12 (20%); 6 in each group) lost graft function due to causes unrelated to infection. The incidence of infection was 83.3% in the OKT3 group and 60% for the ALG group (P < 0.05).

The particular infections according to each group are listed in Table 3.

Ten (33%) patients in the OKT3 group had two episodes of infection 15 ± 17 and 17 ± 16 days (mean ± SD) following treatment. Only 3 patients (10%) in the ALG group suffered from a second infection (P vs OKT3 0.05) 21 ± 35 days and 9 ± 4.5 days, respectively (Fig. 4).

Discussion

This ongoing analysis of our prospectively randomized trial has been reported on several occasions [3, 7]. It is important to see that there are no statistically significant differences in patient or graft survival rates using both protocols for therapy, while the risk factors in the two groups were the same at the onset of the study. A very important finding of the study was that despite the use of ALG for induction therapy and prophylaxis of rejection, there was no disadvantage to reinstituting ALG for the treatment of rejection in terms of graft survival and incidence of infection. A low sensitization to ALG has been reported by

others [6] due to the polyclonal character of the serum. Since the 1-year graft survival rates are compatible in both groups, differences in morbidity become more important. There was a statistically lower incidence of infection, in particular of pneumonia, in the ALG group; however, the two patients who died of CMV pneumonia belonged one to each group. This might be due to the additional application of steroids which was administered to prevent first-dose reactions in the OKT3 group.

The course of each of the patients who died was complicated by one or more aggravating factors, while the patients in whom the pneumonia resolved experienced milder courses. Generally [1], there is an increased incidence of infection with rejection episodes and the ensuing treatment; however, according to our findings the incidence of infection was indeed higher with OKT3 than with ALG. We failed to find any particular predisposition for a specific etiologic microbe. CMV was the only viral pathogen (except for herpes virus), appearing by itself or in concert with other pathogens.

Thus, kidney recipients treated for steroid-resistant rejection can be subjected to ALG treatment without an in-

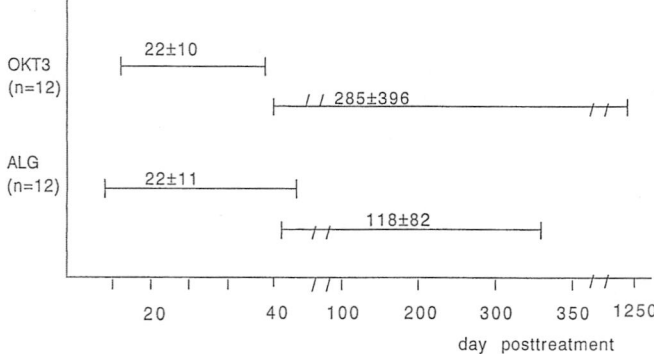

Fig. 3. Onset (mean ± SD) of primary and secondary rejection in patients with two rejection episodes

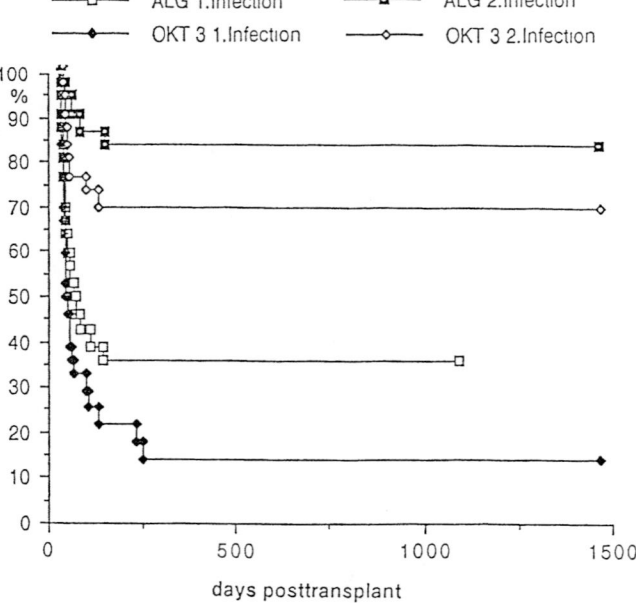

Fig. 4. Percentage of infection-free patients (primary and secondary) following ALG and OKT3 for steroid-resistant rejection

creased risk of infection and with similar graft survival rates when compared with OKT3 treatment, even if ALG is used as an induction therapy. This should allow us to reserve OKT3 for rescue occasions when steroids or a repeated course of polyclonal antibodies is unsuccessful in reversing rejection. The mortality was similar in patients receiving ALG or OKT3 treatment. There is certainly no evidence that ALG renders patients more susceptible to CMV infection than OKT3 treatment; in contrast, OKT3 treatment is accompanied by a higher incidence of CMV infection, which might be due to the increased amount of steroids given.

References

1. Bach MC, Acler JL, Beman P, et al. (1973) Influence of rejection therapy on fungal and noncardial infections in renal transplant recipients. Lancet I: 180–184
2. Gehan E (1965) A generalized Wilcoxon test comparing arbitrarily singly sesored samples. Biometrika 52: 203–223
3. Hesse UJ, Wienand P, Baldamus C, Arns W (1990) Preliminary results of a prospectively randomized trial of ALG versus OKT3 for steroid resistant rejection after renal transplantation in the early postoperative period. Transplant Proc 22: 2273–2274
4. Orthomulticenter transplant study group (1985) A randomized clinical trial of OKT3 monoclonal antibody for acute rejection of cadaveric transplant. N Engl J Med 313: 6
5. Peterson PK, Balfour HH, Marker SC, et al. (1980) Cytomegalovirus disease in renal allograft recipient: a prospective study of the clinical features, risk factors and impact on transplantation. Medicine 59: 283–300
6. Reis HJ, Hopt UT, Greger B, Schareck WD, Bockhoun H (1987) Antirejection treatment in kidney transplantation. Is there a proved rationale for the general use of monoclonal antibodies? Transpl Proc 19: 3565–3569
7. Wienand P, Hesse UJ, Kimming N, Baldamus C, Arns W (1989) Erste Ergebnisse einer prospektiv randomisierten Studie zur Verwendung von ALG bzw. OKT3 bei steroid-resistenten Abstoßungsreaktionen nach Nierentransplantation. Transplantationsmedizin 3: 52–56

Transplant Int (1992) 5 [Suppl 1]: S 444–S 447

TRANSPLANT
International
© Springer-Verlag 1992

Prophylactic use of the IL-2 receptor-specific monoclonal antibody LO-Tact-1 with cyclosporin A and steroids in renal transplantation

C. Hiesse[1], F. Kriaa[1], P. Alard[2], O. Lantz[2], J. Noury[3], H. Bensadoun[4], G. Benoit[4], B. Charpentier[1], D. Fries[1], and H. Bazin[5]

Departments of [1] Nephrology and [4] Urology, Hôpital de Bicêtre, Université Paris-Sud, Paris, France
[2] Laboratory of Cellular Immunology and Transplantation, ER 277 CNRS, Institut de Recherches Scientifiques sur le Cancer, Villejuif, France, [3] Innopharm, Boulogne-Billancourt, France, [5] Experimental Immunology Unit, Université Catholique de Louvain, Brussels, Belgium

Abstract. LO-Tact-1 is a rat anti-human monoclonal antibody which is directed to the 55-kD$_a$ α-chain of the interleukin 2 (IL2) receptor. We conducted a pilot trial in 15 first-time cadaveric renal transplant patients undergoing for immunosuppression a 14-day course of LO-Tact-1 (10 mg IV daily) together with cyclosporine, low dose steroids (0.5 mg/kg) and azathioprine. Results showed a good immunosuppressive effect, as measured by the similar incidence of acute rejection episodes (0.6 per patient) when compared with 20 patients treated during the same period with our standard quadruple prophylactic combination with higher initial doses of steroids (2 mg/kg) and antilymphocyte globulin (ALG) instead of LO-Tact-1 (0.4 per patient). At 2 years post-transplant, graft survival was 93%, and only 1 patient lost his kidney by rejection. No local or general adverse effect of antibody administration was encountered, and haematological changes remained of minor importance. Local bacterial infection was observed in 3 patients, but viral diseases (including cytomegalovirus, CMV) remained exceptional. In contrast, severe clinical CMV infections occurred in 3 patients (15%) treated by ALG. Nine of 15 patients developed rat-specific antibodies, but only 4 before the completion of LO-Tact-1 treatment, without any correlation with the further development of acute rejection. Patients who suffered rejection had lower LO-Tact-1 levels and higher soluble IL2 receptor levels during the period of infusion, suggesting the crucial importance of pharmacokinetic monitoring to adjust individual doses.

Key words: Interleukin 2 receptor – Monoclonal antibodies – Renal graft rejection

The prophylactic use of polyclonal anti-lymphocyte (ALG) or anti-thymocyte (ATG) globulins following

renal transplantation has become one of the most effective and safe strategies for managing renal transplant recipients during the immediate postoperative period [4, 6]. However, the more recent availability of monoclonal antibodies directed against targets on the T-lymphocyte membrane has enabled the clinical use of highly selective immunosuppression. Indeed, OKT3, a monoclonal antibody directed to the invariant CD3 component of the T-cell-receptor complex, is routinely employed, with a remarkable effect in preventing early rejection, but with the disadvantages of inducing severe and even life-threatening first-use reactions and being associated with an increased number of opportunistic infections [3, 13]. A more specific and less toxic kind of immunosuppression is to target only cells involved in the rejecting process which are expressing activation antigens. Among these antigens, interleukin 2 (IL2) receptor plays a crucial role by controlling the proliferative expansion of T lymphocytes. Several monoclonal antibodies specific for the low-affinity IL2 receptor have been produced and have demonstrated their ability to inhibit IL2 binding to its receptor. They have been shown to be effective in the prophylaxis of allograft rejection both in animal models [5] and in human transplantation [6, 7, 9]. We report herein the results of a pilot study conducted in 15 first time cadaver kidney transplants, treated for the prophylaxis of rejection with LO-Tact-1, a rat immunoglobulin (IgG2b) directed to the 55D$_a$ α-chain of the IL2 receptor, in combination with cyclosporine (CsA), low dose corticosteroids and azathioprine (AZA).

Materials and methods

Patient population. From May through August 1989, 15 study patients were elicited to receive a quadruple prophylactic regimen including LO-Tact-1 following their first renal transplantation. All patients who were transplanted in our unit during the week (from Monday to Wednesday) were included, in order to make easier the pre- and immediate post-transplant monitoring. During the same period, 20 patients who received their graft at the weekend (Saturday and Sunday) constituted the control group and received our

Offprint requests to: Dr. C. Hiesse, Service de Néphrologie, Hôpital de Bicêtre, 78, rue du Général Leclerc, 94275 Le Kremlin-Bicêtre Cedex, France

Table 1. Main patient and transplantation characteristics

	LO-Tact-1 ($n = 15$)	Control ($n = 20$)
Mean age (range)	49.5 y (35–63)	40.2 (21–65)
Sex ratio (male/female)	11/4	12/8
Immunized (PRA $> 80\%$)	8 (3)	8 (4)
Mean A-B mismatching	2.4 ± 0.2	2.4 ± 0.2
Mean DR mismatching	1.3 ± 0.2	0.9 ± 0.1
Cold ischaemia time (h)	31 ± 8.1	32 ± 7.5
Initial non-function	7 (47%)	11 (55%)

PRA, plasma renin activity

standard quadruple prophylactic immunosuppressive regimen with ALG. Although this pilot study was not randomized, no attempt was made to select the patients who received the monoclonal antibody, except that second transplants were excluded. The background characteristics of the patients and transplantation data are summarized in Table 1. Except for the mean age which was significantly higher in the study patients, there was no statistically significant difference between both groups with respect to the pre- and peritransplant variables.

Immunosuppressive regimens. Patients from the study group received LO-Tact-1 IV 10 mg daily for the first 14 days posttransplant. LO-Tact-1 is a rat anti-human monoclonal antibody of the IgG-2b isotype whic is directed to the 55-D$_a$ α-chain of the IL2 receptor. It was developed at the Experimental Immunology Unit of the University of Louvain, Medical School, Brussels, Belgium [15]. It was produced in vivo from ascitic fluids of LOU/C·IgK1b-OKA rats. Many carefully controlled purifications were performed to ensure the purity of the antibody, as well as to avoid harmful contaminants [10]. LO-Tact-1 competitively inhibits the high affinity binding of iodine-125 IL2 to activated T lymphocytes. A 50% inhibition of radio-labelled IL2 binding is observed at a concentration of $8 \times 10^{-9} M$ LO-Tact-1. The other immunosuppressive drugs included corticosteroids, a single bolus of 2 mg/kg methylprednisolone on day 0, then oral prednisone 0.5 mg/kg daily from day 1 to day 14, with subsequent doses being progressively reduced to a baseline of 10 mg/day at 1 month posttransplant. CsA was given IV on day 0 (4 mg/kg), then orally at 8 mg/kg, with the dose being further adjusted to whole blood trough levels (TDX; Abbott) and to the clinical events if acute nephrotoxic episodes occurred. AZA was introduced on day 45 at an initial dose of 1 mg/kg daily, eventually being reduced when the white blood cell (WBC) count had decreased under 4000/mm³.

Control patients received instead of monoclonal antibody a prophylactic course of polyclonal ALG (Lymphoglobuline; Merieux) 15 ml/day IV from day 1 to day 14 and a higher initial oral dose of prednisone: 2 mg/kg from day 1, reduced to 1 mg/kg at day 14, then to the baseline dose of 10 mg/day at 2 months posttransplant.

Histologically confirmed rejections were treated in both groups by IV methylprednisolone bolus for 6 days (10 mg/kg on day 1, then 5, 4, 3, 2 and 1 mg/kg). When rejections occurred later than the 14-day period of rejection prophylaxis, patients received an additional 7-day course of polyclonal ATG (Thymoglobuline; Merieux) 15 ml/day. Rejections that were resistand to a first anti-rejection therapy were treated by OKT3 monoclonal antibody 5 mg/day IV for 7 days.

Immunological monitoring. Serum samples were obtained preoperatively and every 2 days postoperatively until the 1 month after transplantation from patients receiving LO-Tact-1. The trough levels of LO-Tact-1 were retrospectively measured by enzyme-linked immunosorbent assay (ELISA), as described elsewhere [10]. LO-Tact-1-specific IgG and IgM antibodies were detected by another ELISA [10]. The serum concentration of the soluble IL2 receptor was measured twice weekly in patients of both groups. Whole blood samples were also collected in heparinized tubes for immunofluorescence flow cytometric analysis of different subsets of peripheral blood lymphocytes.

Statistical analysis. Actuarial graft survival and rejection probability curves were calculated by the Kaplan-Meier method and compared by log-rank test. The χ^2 and Student's t-test were used for other comparisons when appropriate.

Results

Graft and patient survival

No patient died who had received the quadruple therapy with LO-Tact-1 for the induction protocol. Among the 20 control ALG patients, 1 died at 4 months posttransplant from severe cytomegalovirus (CMV) infection. In the LO-Tact-1 group, the actuarial graft survival was 100% at 1 year and 93% at 2 years (Fig. 1). The only graft loss at 21 months posttransplant was due to chronic rejection. In the control group treated with ALG, graft survival was similar, 85% at 1 and 2 years. The causes of 2 graft losses in this group other than patient death were 1 immediate hyperacute rejection and 1 chronic rejection at 5 months.

Incidence of rejection and graft function

During the period of administration of LO-Tact-1, 2 patients had histologically proven acute rejection (13.3%), this incidence being similar in control patients (2/20, 10%). As shown in Fig. 2, the total number of rejections

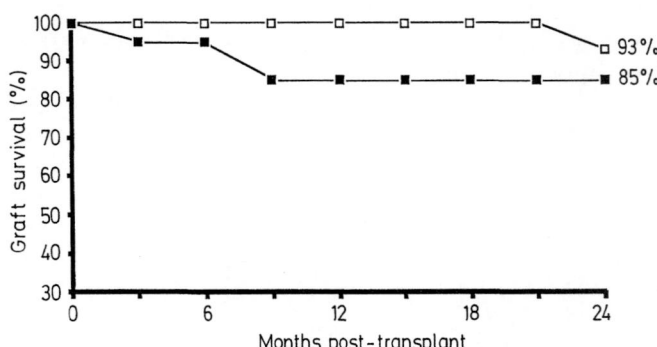

Fig. 1. Actuarial graft survival in 15 patients treated by LO-Tact-1 *(open squares)* and 20 control patients treated by antilymphocyte globulin (ALG; *(filled squares)*

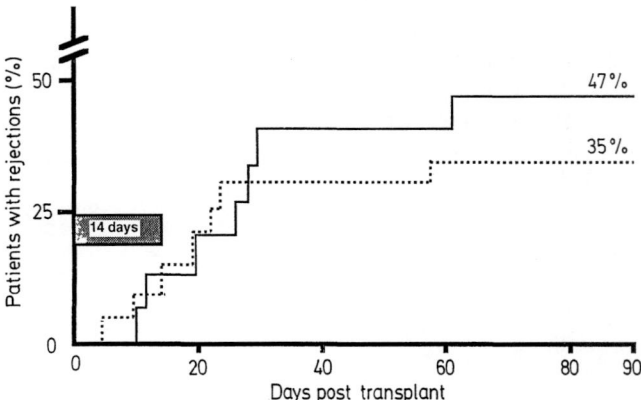

Fig. 2. Probability for rejection over the first 3 months posttransplant. *Solid line,* 15 LO-Tact-1 patients; *dashed line,* 20 control ALG patients

(9/15, 0.6 ± 0.19 per patient) recorded during the first 3 months posttransplant in 7 of the 15 study patients (47%) was comparable but slightly higher than in the control group: 8 rejections in 7 (0.4 ± 0.13 per patient) of the 20 patients (35%) treated by ALG. The time to the first rejection was also comparable in LO-Tact-1 patients (26.4 +/− 6.5 days) and in the control group (21.4 ± 6.3 days).

All acute rejection episodes were reversible in study patients, but 2 required a second anti-rejection treatment with OKT3. Chronic rejection was histologically documented in 3 patients at 2 years posttransplant. Similarly, one control patient of 7 experiencing rejection in this group required a second course with OKT3, but at 2 years, the incidence of chronic rejection was slightly higher than in the study patients: 6 of 18 patients who survived more than 3 months. At 2 years posttransplant, there was no difference between mean serum creatinine levels between study patients with functional grafts ($n = 14$; 147 ± 14 µmol/l) and control patients with functional kidneys ($n = 17$; 171 ± 26 µmol/l).

Infectious complications and tolerance

Only minor infections not directly related to immunosuppression were observed in LO-Tact-1 patients (2 urinary tract infections, and 2 local wound infections). Viral episodes remained exceptional in our group (1 local herpes simplex in a patient treated by OKT3). Comparatively, 3 CMV infections (including 1 lethal one) occurred in patients treated by ALG, this incidence of 15% being usual for patients treated by such a quadruple immunosuppressive regimen [6]. Considering the small number of patients entered in this study, no statistical conclusion was demonstrable.

After transplantation, a profound lymphopenia was observed in patients treated by polyclonal ALG, which persisted to the end of the 1 month posttransplant (total lymphocyte count per mm^3 2600 ± 460, 450 ± 120, 560 ± 220 and 900 ± 210 on days 0, 7, 14 and 28, respectively). In patients treated with LO-Tact-1, the total lymphocyte count dropped only moderately and remained significantly high ($P < 0.05$) from day 7 to day 28 (1900 ± 150, 1050 ± 100, 1530 ± 160 and 1540 ± 260 on days 0, 7, 14 and 28, respectively). Similarly, dramatic drops in CD3+, CD4+ and CD8 cell counts were observed in ALG patients, whereas only mild and transient decreases were observed during LO-Tact-1 treatment.

During the administration of LO-Tact-1, no major complication requiring the discontinuation of treatment was observed. In two patients, mild febrile episodes occurred, but with no evident relationship to the LO-Tact-1 infusion.

Immunological monitoring

Since the values of the LO-Tact-1 levels and information about the development of rat-specific antibodies were only retrospectively obtained, no attempt was made to adjust the dose to the trough levels or discontinuing treatment in immunized patients.

Nine study patients (60%) developed LO-Tact-1-specific IgG antibodies. In 4 (26.7%), these antibodies were detected during the 14-day period of LO-Tact-1 administration. There was no correlation between rejection and immunization: 3 of the 7 patients who experienced rejection developed LO-Tact-1-specific IgG (43%). IgM LO-Tact-1-specific IgM antibodies were detected in all patients before day 14, and as earlier as day 4 in 2 patients.

The mean trough levels of LO-Tact-1 increased progressively from 1.2 ± 1 µg/ml on day 2 to 2.2 ± 1 on day 4 and then remained stable throughout the LO-Tact-1 treatment (2.9 ± 2.5 µg/ml at day 14). There was no difference between the LO-Tact-1 mean levels in patients who developed LO-Tact-1-specific IgG and IgM antibodies and mean levels in patients developing only IgM. Importantly, there was a negative correlation between LO-Tact-1 trough levels and rejection: the group of 7 rejecting patients had significantly ($P < 0.05$) lower mean LO-Tact-1 levels from day 2 to day 7 (0.3, 1.3 and 1.2 µg/ml at days 2, 4 and 7, respectively) than patients who suffered no rejection episode during the 3-month posttransplant period (1.7, 2.7 and 2.4 µg/ml).

The plasma levels of the soluble IL2 receptor were significantly ($P < 0.05$) lower in LO-Tact-1 patients from day 2 (79 ± 16 pmol/ml) to day 17 (132 ± 35 pmol/ml) than in ALG patients (183 ± 24 and 240 ± 41 on days 2 and 17, respectively). There was no significant correlation between the soluble IL2 receptor plasma levels, anti-IgG immunization and the rejection episodes in patients treated with LO-Tact-1. Finally, the group of 7 patients who were treated for acute rejection had significantly lower soluble IL2 receptor levels from day 7 to day 14 posttransplant.

Discussion

The results of our pilot study conducted in 15 first-time cadaveric transplant patients suggest that an immunosuppressive prophylactic regimen including LO-Tact-1, a rat IL2 receptor-specific monoclonal antibody, is highly effective in preventing rejection. This effect is roughly similar to that obtained with a powerful quadruple prophylactic combination with polyclonal horse ALG, although we employed a fourfold lower (0.5 versus 2 mg/kg) initial dose of steroids. Moreover, despite the prolonged (14 days) serotherapy, we did not observed a significant number of opportunistic infections, and changes in the WBC and T-cell subsets remained transient and of minor importance. The local and general tolerance was excellent during LO-Tact-1 infusions. More than 2 years posttransplant, 12 patients (80%) had a normal renal function, and only 1 graft was lost by chronic rejection. Our results are similar to those reported by Soulillou et al. [12] with a different rat P55-specific monoclonal antibody (33b3.1), utilized in a different immunosuppressive regimen: higher initial doses of steroids, delayed introduction of CsA, and AZA given from day 1. Using another mouse receptor-specific IL2 monoclonal antibody (anti-Tac) in addition to a triple drug regimen (steroids, low dose CsA and AZA), Kirkman et al. [9] reported the efficacy of their antibody in preventing allograft rejection, but with a higher incidence of opportunistic infections, including lethal CMV infections, probably related to excessive immunosuppression. Both these large, randomized studies and our pilot trial are dealing with a clear effect of P55-specific monoclonal antibodies in the prophylaxis of rejection after renal transplantation. However, it should be pointed out that if monoclonal antibodies are able to produce comparable clinical results to old-fashioned drugs such as ALG, they do not seem to have a superior effect, and there was no clinical support for the in vitro demonstrated synergy between CsA and IL2-specific antibodies [14]. Moreover, when more refined criteria were used such as the rejection incidence during the antibody administration period [12] or the need for anti-rejection retreatment [9], as ALG had a nearly fully protective effect against rejection, but not the IL2 receptor-specific monoclonal antibody. The question is whether patients experiencing rejection under triple or quadruple therapy with P55-specific antibodies should be individualized as "immunologically high-risk" transplant recipients requiring heavy immunosuppressive protocols, or whether the relative lack of efficiency of IL2 receptor-specific monoclonal antibodies in some individuals is related to a pharmacokinetic interference such as an inadequate dose or the appearance of xenogeneic-specific antibodies inactivating the drug. Since the exact mechanisms by which IL2 receptor-specific monoclonal antibodies exert their action are still poorly understood, and probably vary between the different similarly available molecules, both explanations are advisable. If the lack of cytotoxicity of P55-specific antibodies can account for a relative lack of efficacy in some individuals, we can expect new strategies to improve antibody potency such the addition of a toxin molecule [8]. Another possibility is to attempt to reduce the immunogenicity of xenoantibodies. Recently, humanized anti-Tac has been injected into primates [5]. Results support the view that such chimeric monoclonal antibodies will avoid the immune response and improve its pharmacokinetic value. However, if our data deal with previous reports on the strong immunogenicity of IL2 receptor-specific rat [12] or murine [9] antibodies, it should be noticed that only four patients (27%) developed an IgG response by the end of the LO-Tact-1 administration. Moreover, the presence of LO-Tact-1-specific IgG did not correlate with low antibody trough levels nor with a further occurrence of allograft rejection and finally did not influence the graft outcome. On the other hand, we found that patients, who acutely rejected their graft had lower LO-Tact-1 levels and increased soluble IL2 receptor levels. Thus, close biological monitoring can provide helpful information during the administration of LO-Tact-1, since in a given patient a higher dose may be required to achieve efficient circulating and in situ concentrations.

In conclusion, the LO-Tact-1 anti-IL2 receptor monoclonal antibody administered in the prophylaxis of renal allograft rejection in combination with other conventional immunosuppressants was perfectly tolerated, did not induce severe infections related to overimmunosuppression and had a comparable effect in preventing rejection to the powerful quadruple combination CsA, AZA, high dose steroids, and polyclonal ALG. A randomised prospective study including a large number of patients is in progress in our centre, in order to confirm these preliminary results.

References

1. Bazin H, Cormont F, DeClercq L (1984) Rat monoclonal antibodies. II. A rapid and efficient method of purification from ascitic fluid or serum. J Immunol Methods 71: 9–14
2. Cantarovich D, Le Mauff B, Hourmant M, Giral M, Jacques Y, Soulillou JP (1989) Anti-interleukin 2 receptor monoclonal antibody in the treatment of ongoing acute rejection episode of human kidney graft. A pilot study. Transplantation 47: 452–457
3. Debure A, Chkoff N, Chatenoud L, Lacombe M, Campos H, Noel LH, Goldstein G, Bach JF, Kreis H (1988) One-month prophylactic use of OKT3 in cadaveric kidney transplant recipients. Transplantation 45: 546–555
4. Ferguson RM (1988) A multicenter experience with sequential ALG/cyclosporine therapy in renal transplantation. Clin Transplant 2: 285–294
5. Hakimi J, Chizzonite R, Luke DR, Familetti PC, Bailon P, Kondas JOA, Pilson RS, Ping-Lin, Weber DV, Spence C, Mondini LJ, Tsien W-H, Levin JL, Galatti VH, Korm L, Waldmann JA, Queen C, Benjamin WR (1991) Reduced immunogenicity and improved pharmacokinetics of humanized anti-Tac in cynomolgus monkeys. J Immunol 147: 1352–1359
6. Hiesse C, Freis D, Charpentier B, Neyrat N, Rieu P, Bellamy J, Benoit G (1987) Optimal results in cadaveric donor renal transplantation using prophylactic ALG, cyclosporine and prednisone. Transplant Proc 19: 3670–3671
7. Kirkman RL, Barret LV, Gaulton GN, Kelley V, Ythier A, Strom TB (1985) Administration of an anti-interleukin 2 receptor antibody prolongs cardiac allograft survival in mice. J Exp Med 162: 358–362
8. Kirkman RL, Bacha P, Barett LV, Forte S, Murphy JR, Strom TB (1989) Prolongation of cardiac allograft survival in murine recipients treated with a diphtheria toxin-related interleukin-2 fusion protein. Transplantation 47: 327–330
9. Kirman RL, Shapiro ME, Carpenter CB, McKay DB, Milford EL, Ramos EL, Tilney NL, Waldmann TA, Zimmerman CE, Strom TB (1991) A randomized prospective trial of anti-Tac monoclonal antibody in human renal transplantation. Transplantation 51: 107–113
10. Ravoet AM, Latinne D, Seghers J, Manouvriez P, Ninane J, De Bruyere M, Bazin H, Sokal G (1990) Methods for analysis of rat monoclonal antibodies directed against human leucocyte differentiation antigens. In: Bazin H (ed) Rat hybridomas and rat monoclonal antibodies. CRC Press, Boca Raton, pp 287–307
11. Soulillou JP, Peyronnet P, Le Mauff B, Hourmant M, Olive D, Mawas C, Delaage M, Hirn M, Jacques Y (1987) Prevention of rejection of kidney transplants by monoclonal antibody directed against interleukin 2. Lancet II: 1339–1342
12. Soulillou JP, Cantarovich D, Le Mauff B, Giral M, Robillard N, Hourmant M, Hirn M, Jacques Y (1990) Randomized controlled trial of a monoclonal antibody angainst the interleukin-2 receptor (33B3.1) as compared with rabbit antithymocyte globulin for prophylaxis against rejection of renal allografts. N Engl J Med 322: 1175–1182
13. Swinnen LJ, Costanzo-Nordin MR, Fisher SG, O'Sullivan J, Johnson MR, Heroux AL, Dizikes GJ, Pifarre R, Fisher R (1990) Increased incidence of lymphoproliferative disorder after immunosuppression with the monoclonal antibody OKT3 in cardiac-transplant recipients. N Engl J Med 323: 1723–1729
14. Tellides G, Dallman MJ, Morris PJ (1988) Synergistic interaction of cyclosporin A with interleukin 2 receptor monoclonal antibody therapy. Transplant Proc 20: 202–206
15. Xia H, Ravoet AM, Latinne D, Ninane J, De Bruyere M, Sokal G, Bazin H (1990) Rat monoclonal antibodies specific for human T lymphocytes. In: Bazin H (ed) Rat hybridomas and rat monoclonal antibodies. CRC Press, Boca Raton, pp 309–322

Transplant Int (1992) 5 [Suppl 1]: S 448–S 449

TRANSPLANT
International
© Springer-Verlag 1992

RS-61443: successful rescue therapy in refractory renal rejection

Hans W. Sollinger[1], Mark H. Deierhoi[2], Robert S. Kauffman[3], Arnold G. Diethelm[2], and Folkert O. Belzer[1]

[1] Department of Surgery, University of Wisconsin, Madison, Wisconsin, USA
[2] Department of Surgery, University of Alabama-Birmingham, Birmingham, Alabama, USA
[3] Syntex Research, Palo Alto, California, USA

Abstract. RS-61443, the morpholinoethyl ester of mycophenolic acid (mPA), is a potent, noncompetitive, reversible inhibitor of eucaryotic inosine monophosphate (IMP) dehydrogenases. Because of the importance of the guanosine and deoxyguanosine nucleotides in activating phosphoribosyl pyrophosphate (PRPP) synthesis and ribonucleotide reductase, respectively, it was postulated that depletion of GMP (and consequently GTP and GDP) would have antiproliferative effects on lymphocytes. Furthermore, since lymphocytes rely on de novo pruine synthesis whereas other cell types do not, antiproliferative effects produced in this way are more selective for lymphocytes than other cell types.

Key words: Rescue therapy – RS-61443 – Renal rejection

RS-61443, the morpholinoethyl ester of mycopherolic acid (MPA), synthesized by Dr. peter Nelson (Syntex Research), was found to have improved bioavailability as compared with MPA [1]. Previous investigations, primarily in the laboratory of Dr. Anthony Allison and Dr. Elsie Eugui (Syntex Research), demonstrated that the drug blocks the proliferative responses of T- and B-lymphocytes [2] and inhibits antibody formation [3] and the generation of cytotoxic T-cells. In vivo monotherapy with RS-61443 was shown to prolong the survival of heart allografts in rats [4] and islet allograft survival in mice [5]. When combined with low doses of cyclosporine A (5 mg/kg) and prednisone (0.1 mg/kg), RS-61443 significantly prolonged the survival of renal allografts in mongrel dogs [6]. Furthermore, RS-61443 has the ability to reverse ongoing acute allograft rejection in a rat heart allograft model [4]. Recent experiments in our laboratory have further demonstrated that a short course of RS-61443 at 80 mg/kg b.i.d. reversed acute ongoing acute renal allograft rejection in 14 out of 16 dogs [7]. Based on these experimental data, a clinical trial was initiated in an attempt to evaluate the efficacy of RS-61443 for the reversal of acute refractory renal allograft rejection and evaluate the safety and tolerance to this drug.

In order to qualify for entry into this study, patients had to have refractory renal allograft rejection followed by at least one course of high dose steroids and OKT3.

Patients and methods

Thirty patients who had undergone cadaver renal allografts followed by induction therapy with quadruple immunosuppression (MALG, cyclosporin A, prednisone, azathioprine) and 8 patients who had received live donor kidneys followed by triple immunosuppressive therapy (cyclosporin A, prednisone, azathioprine) were entered into the study. Study entry requirements included biopsy-proven, therapy-resistant renal allograft rejection after at least one course of high dose steroid bolus therapy and at least one course of OKT3 therapy.

Table 1 demonstrates the mean number of high dose steroid and OKT3 courses in patients enrolled into the study. RS-61443 therapy was initiated at a dose of 2000 mg/day and was increased to 3500 mg/day when tolerated. At the initiation of RS-61443 therapy, azathioprine was discontinued. At 28 days after the initiation of the RS-61443 rescue therapy, a follow-up renal biopsy was obtained in all patients.

Results

In the living related donor group 6 grafts (75 %) were successfully rescued, while in the cadaver group, 20 grafts (66 %) were rescued. The mean rescue rate in both groups was 68 %. Among patients successfully rescued, a significant improvement in renal function was demonstrated, as shown in Table 2.

Offprint requests to: Hans W. Sollinger, M.D., University of Wisconsin Hospital, H4/780 Clinical Science Center, 600 Highland Avenue, Madison, WI 53792, USA

Table 1. Study population

	Steroid courses ($\bar{x}$)	OKT3 courses ($\bar{x}$)
Live donor ($n = 8$)	3.3	1.5
Cadaver donor ($n = 30$)	2.8	1.1

Table 2. Improvement in renal function with RS-61443 rescue therapy

	Creatinine (mg %) ($\bar{x}$) Start of therapy	Creatinine (mg %) ($\bar{x}$) Now
Living donor	5.2 (2.7–10.3)	2.5 (1.4–4.2)
Cadaver donor	4.4 (2.3–11.2)	2.6 (1.0–4.0)

Table 3. Renal function after RS-61443 rescue therapy in comparison with initial creatinine level

	Creatinine > 5 mg %	Creatinine < 5 mg %
Rescue	6 (50%)	21 (81%)
Failure	6 (50%)	5 (19%)

Table 4. Side effects and complications

	No. of patients
Nausea/vomiting	4 (10%)
Diarrhea	4 (10%)
Cytomegalovirus (CMV)	3 (7.8%)
Leukopenia	2 (5%)
Loose stools	2 (5%)
CMV colitis	1 (2.5%)
Pancreatitis	1 (1.2%)
Hematuria	1 (1.2%)
Increased LFTs	1 (1.2%)

Successful rescue seemed to depend to a great degree on the serum creatinine level at which the patient was entered into the RS-61443 rescue protocol. As shwon in Table 3, 81% of the grafts were rescued when the patient was entered at a creatinine value below 5 mg %, while only 50% of the grafts were rescued when entered at a creatinine level above 5 mg %.

Significant side effects and complications of RS-61443 are listed in Table 4. Predominantly, the side effects related to the gastrointestinal system, such as nausea, vomiting, and diarrhea. Other complications such as cytomegalovirus (CMV) infection and leukopenia were associated with the therapy but could very well reflect the overall immunosuppressed state of the recipient, at least in part caused by prior antirejection therapy. In one patient, pancreatitis requiring discontinuation of RS-61443 seemed to have a clear relationship to the drug.

Discussion

This pilot rescue study demonstrated that RS-61443, even in therapy-resistant renal allograft rejection, has the ability to reverse or stabilize the rejection process. The failure or success of the rescue seems to depend largely on the degree of renal function at which therapy is initiated. In a few of the patients entered into this protocol, creatinine levels were above 9 mg %, and obviously the structural damage to the graft was irreparable at the time of initiation of rescue therapy. There were no life-threatening complications or major side effects, with the exception of gastrointestinal ones. The degree of nausea and vomiting, as well as diarrhea, may correlate with decreased absorption of the drug and may possibly explain the failure of the rescue therapy.

Of major interest in this study and the previous animal experiments in which ongoing acute allograft rejection was reversed is the possible mechanism by which an antiproliferative drug exerts this effect. For theoretical reasons, it seems unlikely that a drug which has solely antiproliferative effects is efficacious after clonal expansion of cytotoxic T-cells has already taken place. Therefore, an additional mechanism responsible for the rescue effect of RS-61443 is hypothesized. Recent data from the laboratory of Dr. Anthony Allison and Dr. Elsie Eugui provide a possible explanation (personal communication). In vitro studies have demonstrated that fucose and mannose are transferred through guanosine diphospho intermediates and dolicol phosphate. Mannose and fucose and their derivates are critical components of adhesion molecules. Allison and associates (unpublished observation) could demonstrate that in activated human peripheral blood lymphocytes, treatment with MPA significantly decreased the transfer of mannose to dolicol phosphate and to membrane glycoproteins, a process which is GDP-dependent.

In vitro studies show that one of the lymphocyte glycoproteins affected is VLA-4, the ligand for VCAM-1 on activated endothelial cells. Treatment of either B cells or IL-1-activated endothelial cells with MPA in therapeutically attainable doses decreased lymphocyte attachment, and when both cell types were treated with MPA, the attachment was further inhibited. If these findings can be extrapolated to the in vivo situation, treatment with MPA could decrease the recruitment of lymphocytes into sites of ongoing graft rejection and explain the rescue effects of RS-61443. At the current time, prospective, randomized trials are in progress to examine further the potential role of RS-61443 in the rescue therapy of therapy-resistant renal allograft rejections.

References

1. Lee WA, Gu L, Miksztal AR, Chu N, Leung K, Nelson PH (1990) Bioavailability improvement of mycophenolic acid through animo ester derivitization. Pharm Res 7: 161
2. Eugui EM, Mirkovich A, Allison AC (1991) Lymphocyte-selective antiproliferative and immunosuppressive effects of mycophenolic acid in mice. Scand J Immunol 33: 175
3. Eugui EM, Almquist S, Muller CD, Allison AC (1991) Lymphocyte-selective cytostatic and immunosuppressive effects of mycophenolic acid in vitro: role of deoxyguanosine nucleotide depletion. Scand J Immunol 33: 161
4. Morris RE, Hoyt EG, Murphy MP, Eugui EM, Allison AC (1990) Mycophenolic acid morpholinoethylester (RS-61443) is a new immunosuppressant that prevents and halts heart allograft rejection by selective inhibition of T- and B-cell purine synthesis. Transplant Proc 22: 1659
5. Hao L, Lafferty KJ, Allison AC, Eugui EM (1990) RS-61443 allows islet allografting and specific tolerance induction in adult mice. Transplant Proc 22: 1659
6. Platz KP, Sollinger HW, Hullett DA, Eckhoff DE, Eugui EM, Allison AC (1990) RS-61443, a new, potent immunosuppressive agent. Transplantation 51: 27
7. Platz KP, Bechstein WO, Eckhoff DE, Suzuki Y, Sollinger HW (1991) RS-61443 reverses acute allograft rejection in dogs. Surgery 110: 736

Transplant Int (1992) 5 [Suppl 1]: S 450–S 453

TRANSPLANT
International
© Springer-Verlag 1992

Lymphoproliferative disorders developing after transplantation and their relation to simian T-cell leukemia virus infection

H. P. J. D. Stevens[1, 2], L. Holterman[2], A. G. M. Haaksma[2], M. Jonker[2], and J. L. Heeney[2]

[1] Department of Plastic and Reconstructive Surgery, University Hospital Dijkzigt, Rotterdam,
[2] Department of Chronic and Infectious Diseases, Rijswijk, The Netherlands

Abstract. In this report the role of the HTLV-1-like simian T-cell leukemia virus (STLV) during the development of posttransplantation lymphoproliferative disorders (PTLPD) is described. To prevent rejection of an allogeneic transplant in 12 rhesus monkeys cyclosporin A (CyA), prednisone, and/or lymphocyte-specific monoclonal antibodies were used for immunosuppression. Seven monkeys died during the experiment between 22 and 179 days postoperatively. At autopsy in 4 monkeys PTLPD were found. In each case, STLV provirus was acquired during the experiment, either from the blood transfusions or allograft donors. Seroconversion of anti-STLV titers occurred in 3 monkeys. However, Southern blot analysis showed the presence of STLV provirus at the DNA level in all PTLP tissues. PTLPD morphology and phenotype varied significantly. In conclusion, for the first time the oncogenic potential of STLV is identified in a rhesus monkey transplantation model. Moreover, the importance of screening blood and organ donors for HTLV-1 must be emphasized.

Key words: Lymphoma – Immunosuppression – Transplantation – Simian/human T-cell leukemia virus (STLV, HTLV)

It has been reported that following clinical transplantation under cyclosporin A (CyA) and prednisone immunosuppression in man, lymphoproliferative disorders frequently develop [4]. Associations of the proliferative lymphoid lesions in transplant patients have been made with Epstein-Barr virus (EBV) [2] but, to our knowledge, never with HTLV-1. In primate species, HTLV-like viruses, designated simian T-cell leukemia viruses (STLV), occur with great frequency, especially in Old World primates. Studies revealed that more than 90 % se-

quence homology exists between these viruses, which have a marked similarity in genomic structure and morphology [12]. A spectrum of lymphoproliferative diseases has been described in a variety of STLV-infected non-human primates [11]. In this study, in *Macaca mulatta,* the role of STLV during the development of posttransplantation lymphoproliferative disorders (PTLPD) was investigated.

Materials and methods

Experimental design. To prevent rejection of allografts in 12 mature, outbred rhesus monkeys *(Macaca mulatta)* who had received a successfully transplanted allogeneic radial side of the hand, strong immunosuppressive therapy was administered [6]. In this respect, a daily maintenance dose of 25 mg/kg CyA was given, starting 1 day preoperatively. In addition, a high dose of steroids (Di-Adreson-$F_{aquosum}$ = DAF, 12 mg/kg daily) was administered for the first 3 postoperative days and the dosage tapered slowly until a maintenance dose of 1 mg/kg daily was reached after 12 days.

If rejection occurred and could be confirmed histologically, half of the affected allograft recipients were treated by increasing DAF to 12 mg/kg daily, followed by tapering of the DAF dose as described above. In the other monkeys, rejection was treated with a combination of 7 monoclonal antibodies (MAbs), administered as an (iv) bolus injection for a period of 10 days. MAbs were specific for CD3 + , CD4 + , CD8 + , and MHC class II-DR positive antigens and crossreactive with rhesus monkey lymphocytes. This cocktail of MAbs has a strong immunosuppressive potential [8].

Additionally, the effect of preoperative fully mismatched blood transfusions was tested. Six animals received three third party blood transfusions, consisting of 20 ml of fresh whole citrated blood from random donors, administered at biweekly intervals before transplantation. A combination of the aforementioned immunosuppressive treatments resulted in four different treatment groups I-IV with three monkeys per group (see Table 1).

Following successful surgery, 7 animals became terminally ill during the posttransplantion period. They were euthanized, and a complete autopsy was performed.

Histology and immunohistochemistry. The presence or absence of PTLP disorders was confirmed histologically and classified morphologically according to the NCI working formulation. For this purpose, tissue sections harvested at autopsy were fixed in buffered formalin and processed routinely for histology on hematoxylin and

Offprint requests to: J. L. Heeney, Department of Chronic and Infectious Diseases, ITRI-TNO, PO Box 5815, 2280 HV Rijswijk, The Netherlands

Table 1. Allograft recipients that died after transplantation of the radial side of the hand (rhesus monkey): anti-STLV titers in serum, immunosuppressive therapy administered, and cause of death

	Monkey	Anti-STLV titer	Protocol	Duration of basic immuno-suppressive therapy (days)[a]	Duration of antirejection therapy (days)	Cause of death
I	2799	+	MAbs	79	1×1^b	shock
	4023	sc	&	121	2×10	sepsis/PTLP disorder
	2988	sc	transf.	22	1×7^b	multicentric PTLP disorder
II	3439	lt	MAbs,	97	2×20	follicle center cell PTLP disorder
	3308	–	no transf.	179	–	multicentric PTLP disorder
III	2I	–	DAF &	29	1×8^b	sepsis
	3310	nt	transf.	85	–	sepsis
IV			DAF, no transf.			

[a] Daily maintenance doses of immunosuppression consisted of 25 mg/kg CyA and 1 mg/kg DAF

[b] The proposed duration of antirejection therapy (10 days for MAb therapy and 12 days for DAF therapy) was not completed

STLV, simian T-cell leukemia virus; PTLP disorder, posttransplantation lymphoproliferative disorder; cs, seroconversion; lt, low titer; nt, not tested; MAbs (in groups I & II), antirejection therapy consisted of a 10-day course of a combination of 7 monoclonal antibodies; transf. (in groups I & III), 3 third party blood transfusions were given to the recipient, preoperatively; DAF (in groups III & IV), antirejection therapy consisting of an increase in steroid treatment

azofloxine (H/A) stained sections. Parallel biopsy material was snap-frozen in liquid nitrogen-chilled isopentane and used for immunohistochemical studies. This technique and the semiquantitative method for scoring distribution and intensity of staining have been described previously [7]. A selection of MAbs was used to demonstrate expression of the following antigens: CD2, CD4, CD8, k-light chain, l-light chain, MHC class II antigens, and a proliferation-associated nuclear antigen. In control incubations, the primary antibody was omitted.

Serological assessment of HTLV-1-related virus infections. Serum samples to determine titers of STLV-specific antibodies were obtained (1) prior to preoperative third party blood transfusions, (2) following transfusions but before transplantation, and (3) several months posttransplantation. For the assessment of STLV-specific antibodies a commercially obtained HTLV-1 enzyme-linked immunoenzyme assay (ELISA; Du Pont de Nemours International S. A., Geneva) was used which had been demonstrated to be cross-reactive with STLV (J. L. Heeney, personal communication). To confirm further these ELISA results and the relatedness of these viruses to HTLV-1, various serum samples found to be ELISA-positive were tested for antigenic similarity on HTLV-1 Western blots and the results compared with serum from HTLV-1-infected patients.

Assessment of HTLV-1-like provirus infection at the DNA level. Remaining PTLP tissue was used to prepare DNA for Southern blot analysis. Probing of the DNA was done with $_{32}$P-labeled, 9 kb full length (minus the long termnal repeats) pCS-HTLV-1 clone (D. Derse, NCL, Frederick, Md.) or partial fragments consisting of the envelope or *tax* regions.

Statistical analysis. When appropriate, Fisher's exact-test, two sample t-test and log-rank test were performed for hypothesis testing. Differences were considered significant if $P < 0.05$.

Results

Findings at necropsy

Allograft survival times after transplantation of the radial side of the hand ranged from 21 to 179 days (Table 1). Detailed information on technical, immunological, and functional aspects of these experiments is described elsewhere [5, 6]. Unfortunately, 7 monkeys died during the experimental period.

In treatment group I (pretransplant blood transfusions and with MAbs antirejection therapy if indicated) 3 monkeys died, monkey #2799 due to an irreversible shock directly after the first administration of MAbs (79 days postoperatively); monkey #4023 due to sepsis, 10 days after onset of the second episode of antirejection treatment. In this monkey at autopsy, widespread lymphoproliferation was observed. Monkey #2988 died due to multicentric PTLP disorder 22 days after operation, its allograft being fully rejected despite 7 days of MAbs administration.

In group II (no pretransplant blood transfusions but with MAbs antirejection therapy if indicated), monkey #3439 died due to a malignant follicle center cell PTLP disorder, 22 days after onset of the second episode of rejection treatment with MAbs. Monkey #3308 died before rejection had occurred from a multicentric PTLP disorder 179 days postoperatively.

In group III (pretransplant blood transfusions and DAF antirejection treatment if indicated) monkey #2I died due to sepsis 29 days postoperatively, and monkey #3310 suffered from sepsis 85 days following transplantation.

In group IV (no pretransplant blood transfusions and DAF antirejection therapy if indicated), no monkeys died during experiment. However, it should be noted that allograft survival times in this group were shorter than in the other treatment groups, and thus they received immunosuppression therapy for a shorter period of time.

In the 4 monkeys which were found to have PTLP disorders, all lymphoproliferation was multicentric with variable morphologic characteristics ranging from a lymphoreticular to follicular center cell morphology.

Influence of immunosuppressive treatment and case history

The addition of MAbs therapy to baseline immunosuppression did not have a significant effect on the occurrence of death in general ($P > 0.05$, Fisher's exact test) [5].

Though the population treated was small, an enhanced predisposition to PTLP disorder development ($P = 0.03$, one-sided Fisher's exact test) was noted in monkeys which received MAb antirejection therapy, possibly as a consequency of additional, potent immunosuppression in addition to baseline therapy. Other factors in the case history of each animal like age, sex, CyA therapy whole blood trough levels, kidney donorship, and experimental low-dose radiation of the testis were examined for a possible correlation with PTLP disorder development but were found to be nonsignificant ($P > 0.05$, Fisher's exact test) [5].

Relevance of anti-STLV titers to PTLP disorder development

All animals were tested for the presence of anti-STLV antibodies before, during, and after the experiment. Four animals were seropositive before the experiment. Four animals acquired anti-STLV antibodies in the course of the experiment (Table 1). In each case of PTLP disorder development, the STLV provirus was acquired during the experimental period. This was clearly evident serologically in two of these animals, and a third which developed a low titer shortly before death.

Serologically, virus transmission could be traced to have come from STLV-positive monkeys, either by preoperative blood transfusions or by allograft donation through the demonstration of seroconversion for STLV titers in transplant recipients.

Animals which retrospectively had serologic evidence of STLV infection prior to the experiment ($n = 4$) did not develop PTLP disorders, suggesting that active STLV infection during immunosuppressive therapy was an important factor in PTLP disorder development.

Immunohistochemical staining of lymphoproliferative tissue

Frozen sections of lesions collected at necropsy were assessed for phenotypic characteristics. In each case the staining pattern varied and was frequently complicated by a mixed population of residual benign leukocytes. All cases stained strongly positively for the MHC class-II DR marker, and a small mixed population of light-chain-positive cells were frequently seen in each case. In the frozen tissues available to us to study, there were not enough sections of homogenous lymphoproliferative tissue to make a conclusive statement of the PTLP disorder phenotype.

Evidence of STLV infection at the DNA level

Southern blot analysis revealed that in all 4 monkeys with a PTLP disorder, STLV provirus was present. A common 5.4-kb band in the lymphoid tissue was present which hybridized with the full length HTLV-1 probe. Using partial HTLV-1 fragments as probes, it was confirmed that under conditions of high stringency the rhesus STLV had en-velope, polymerase, and *gag* regions which were highly homologous with HTLV-1. We were not able to demonstrate consistently hybridization of the Tax region of HTLV-1 with rhesus tumor DNA samples, suggesting that differences in this region exist at the molecular level.

Discussion

The incidence of lymphoma in normal healthy individuals infected with HTLV-1 is low. Less than 1% of HTLV-1-infected people are believed to develop cancer under normal conditons over an entire lifespan, although the virus transforms cells in vitro [3]. In this transplantation study, however, for the first time, the oncogenic potential of a HTLV-1-like virus in rhesus macaques is identified. Furthermore, several important problems are distinguished concerning the selection of transplantation donors and recipients and the immunosuppressive therapy used.

Four of 7 animals which died following allogeneic transplantation of the radial side of the hand developed lymphoproliferative disorders which contained STLV provirus at the DNA level. All 4 monkeys were seronegative before transplantation. In 2 of the 4 cases, it could be demonstrated serologically that STLV was acquired from the blood transfusions or organ donor. In another monkey, which did not receive any preoperative blood transfusion the graft came from a seronegative donor. These data suggest that infection was acquired during the period of intensive posttransplantation immunosuppressive therapy. Moreover, infection might also be possible via other routes than blood or an allograft. In this respect, it is interesting to note that monkeys in this study were housed 4 by 4 in separate cages in the same room during experiment.

If PTLP disorder development in this species infected with STLV is analogous to HTLV-1-associated lymphomas in man, then one would expect to identify a mature CD4 + T-cell phenotype [10]. However, the morphologic and phenotypic characteristics of these PTLP disorders in *Macaca mulatta* varied significantly. Results in this study therefore suggest that under these circumstances in rhesus monkeys STLV causes PTLP disorders of a more diverse cell type.

It has been reported that primary EBV infection carries a higher risk than reactivated infection in the development of PTLP disorders [2], but also anti-CD3 in itself does seem to precipitate lymphoid tumor development [9]. In our study, the finding that MAbs antirejection therapy showed an enhanced predisposition to PTLP disorder development ($P = 0.03$, one-sided Fisher's exact test) coincided with the fact that in each case of PTLP disorder development, STLV provirus was acquired during the experiment. This might indicate that two different mechanisms increased the chance of lymphoid proliferation, resulting in the variable morphologic characteristics of these disorders.

Furthermore, it should be noted that PTLP disorders in this study arose during high dose cyclosporin A treatment, which by itself can cause or permit tumor development in strongly immunosuppressive protocols [4]. Recently, it has been described that cyclosporin A acts through nuclear protiens involved in T-cell activation [1], some of which interact with the HTLV-1 *tax* gene, suggesting a mechanism by which T-cell cancer can develop.

This relationship between CyA and MAb (anti-CD3) therapy, HTLV-1 (STLV-1) infection, and PTLP disorder development in rhesus monkeys indicates the possible clinical risk of treating HTLV-1-infected patients with an immunosuppressive protocol which includes these drugs. Based on the findings in this transplantation model in *Macaca mulata,* the importance of screening blood or organ donors for HTLV-1 must be emphasized.

References

1. Emmel EA, Verwey CL, Durand DB, et al. (1989) Cyclosporin A specifically inhibits function of nuclear proteins involved in T cell activation. Science 246: 1617–1620
2. Ho M, Miller G, Atchison RW, et al. (1985) Epstein-Barr virus infection and DNA hybridization studies in post-transplant lymphoma and lymphoproliferative lesions: the role of primary infection. J Infect Dis 152: 876–886
3. Miyoshi I, Kubonishi I, Yoshimoto S, et al. (1981) Type C virus particles in a cord T cell line, derived by cocultivating normal human cord leukocytes and human leukemic T cells. Nature 294: 770–771
4. Nalesnik MA, et al. (1988) The pathology of posttransplant lymphoproliferative disorder occurring in the setting of cyclosporine A-prednisone immunosuppression. Am J Pathol 133 (1): 173–191
5. Stevens HPJD, Hovius SER, Heeney JL, Nierop PWM, Jonker M (1991) Immunological aspects and complications of composite tissue allografting for upper extremity reconstruction: a study in the rhesus monkey. Transpl Proc 23 (1): 623–625
6. Stevens HPJD, Hovius SER, Vuzevski VD, Nierop PWM van, Gotte M, Roche NA, Jonker M (1990) Immunological aspects of allogeneic partial hand transplantation in the rhesus monkey. Transpl Proc 22: 2006–2008
7. Stevens HPJD, Kwast TH van der, Timmermans A, et al. (1991) Monoclonal antibodies for immunohistochemical labelling of immunocompetent cells in frozen sections of rhesus monkey tissue. J Med Primat (in press)
8. Stevens HPJD, Roche N, Hovius SER, Jonker M (1990) In vivo immunosuppressive effects of monoclonal antibodies specific for CD3 + , CD4 + , CD8 + , and MHC class II positive cells. Transpl Proc 22: 1783–1784
9. Swinnen LJ, Costanzo-Nordin MR, Fisher SG, et al. (1990) Increased incidence of lymphoproliferative disorder after immunosuppression with the monoclonal antibody OKT3 in cardiac transplant recipients. N Engl J Med 323: 1723–1728
10. Takatsuki K, Uchiyama T, Ueshima Y, et al. (1982) Adult T-cell leukemia: proposal as a new disease and cytogenetic, phenotypic and functional studies of leukemic cells. Gann 28: 13–16
11. Tsujomoto H, Noda Y, Ishikawa KI, et al. (1987) Development of adult T-cell leukemia like disease in African green monkey associated with clonal integration of simian T-cell leukemia virus type I. Cancer Res 47: 269–274
12. Watanabe T, Seiri M, Hirayama Y, Yoshida M (1986) Human T-cell leukemia virus type 1 is a member of the African subtype of simian viruses (STLV). Virology 148 (2): 385–388

Transplant Int (1992) 5 [Suppl 1]: S 454–S 458

TRANSPLANT
International
© Springer-Verlag 1992

Toxicology of FK506 in the cynomolgus monkey: a clinical, biochemical, and histopathological study

R. M. H. Wijnen[1], B.-G. Ericzon[2], A. T. M. G. Tiebosch[3], W. A. Buurman[1], C. G. Groth[2], and G. Kootstra[1]

Departments of [1] Surgery and [3] Pathology, University Hospital Maastricht, Maastricht, The Netherlands
[2] Department of Transplantation Surgery, Karolinska Institute, Huddinge Hospital, Stockholm, Sweden

Abstract. We investigated clinical, biochemical, and histopathological parameters in FK506-treated cynomolgus monkeys. Eight monkeys given oral FK506, 1 ($n = 4$) or 10 ($n = 4$) mg/kg daily, survived the 90 days of treatment apparently in good health and without significant changes in biochemical and histopathological parameters, as did 2 control monkeys except one monkey on 10 mg/kg/day FK506 orally, who was found to have a malignant lymphoma. In contrast, monkeys given intramuscular FK506 1 mg/kg daily ($n = 4$) had to be sacrificed at day 20, 25, 32, and 47 because of severe illness. They showed abnormal biochemical parameters (increased serum urea and aspartate aminotransferase activity) and major histopathological changes in the kidney (mesangial cell proliferation and acute tubular necrosis), pancreas (depletion of beta cells), liver (steatosis), and heart (cardiomyopathy). Intramuscular administration of 1 mg/kg daily resulted in serum levels ranging from 10 to 15 ng/ml, while oral administration at a dose of 1 or 10 mg/kg daily resulted in equal or even higher serum levels (range 2–70 ng/ml). Thus, the height of the serum trough level of FK506 using the enzyme immunoassay is not related to the toxicity of FK506 in cynomolgus monkeys.

Key words: FK506 – Fujimycin – Toxicology – Pharmakinetics – Monkeys

FK506 is an immunosuppressive drug isolated from the fermentation of *Streptomyces tsukubaensis* [15]. It is a macrolide with a molecular weight of 822 D_a [29]. Although its working mechanism appears to be similar to that of cyclosporin A (CsA), the efficacy in vitro is compared by dose, about 100 times more potent [14]. The results from in vitro studies indicate that FK506 has a potent inhibitory activity on murine and human lymphocyte proliferative responses and on the generation of human cytotoxic cells [15, 17, 29]. In a variety of animal transplant models FK506 showed the prevention of allograft rejection [1, 9, 11, 13, 18–20, 23, 24, 27, 31–34, 36]. As far as side effects are concerned, early information indicates that these vary among different species. In rats, only a few pathologic effects of FK506 such as weight loss, thymic medullary atrophy (as with CsA), and dose-related elevations in nonfasting blood glucose levels have been reported [21]. Studies in 3 different groups of renal allografted dogs showed two major side effects: anorexia and vasculitis in various organs, particularly in the heart and the gastrointestinal tract [8, 24, 31]. In baboon kidney allograft recipients, anorexia, lethargy, and hyperglycemia have been reported [5]. In this study we investigated the clinical, biochemical, and histological parameters in FK506-treated nontransplanted cynomolgus monkeys, especially the dose, route of administration and serum levels of FK506 in relation to the side effects.

Materials and methods

Animals. Fourteen cynomolgus monkeys obtained from three different inbred colonies were used for the experiment. Previously these monkeys were involved in other behavioural studies or in programmes for the induction of antisera. Their estimated ages at the start of the study were 1.5–8 years, and their body weights ranged from 2 to 5 kg. The animals were kept in separate cages and fed with standard primate pellets (Hope Farm, Woerden, The Netherlands) and fresh fruit. They had ad libitum access to water.

Drug administration. FK506 was supplied by the Fujisawa Pharmaceutical Company, Osaka, Japan. For intramuscular use, the drug form, containing 27% of FK506 in mannitol and the surfactant HCD-60 (polyoxyl-60-hydrogenated castor oil), was suspended in normal saline solution to a concentration of 4 mg/ml. For oral use, a solid dispersion formulation (SDF) was used; FK506 was dispersed with hydroxypropyl methylcellulose, a water-soluble polymer, to give a content of 20% wt/wt [12]. The dose of FK506 given always refers to the dose of the mass of pure compound. The oral use of the placebo (control group) contained 100% of the water-soluble polymer. For the oral administration of FK506 and the placebo, the powder was rubbed onto the animals' favourite piece of fruit. Complete acceptance of the FK506 was monitored face to face.

Offprint requests to: R. M. H. Wijnen, M. D., Department of Surgery, Academical Hospital Maastricht, P.O. Box 5800, 6202 AZ Maastricht, The Netherlands

Table 1. Summary of clinical findings

| Treatment | Mortality | Morbidity | | Weight reduction[a] (mean) |
		Loss of appetite	Lethargy	
Placebo 1.0 mg/kg daily orally	0/2	−	−	4%
FK506 1.0 mg/kg daily intramuscularly	4/4	+	+	15%
FK506 1.0 mg/kg daily orally	0/4	−	−	4%
FK506 10.0 mg/kg daily orally	0/4	−	−	2%

[a] Mean weight reduction = (pretreatment body weight − body weight at 90 days or at sacrifice/pretreatment body weight) ×100%

Experimental design. The following groups were studied: 1 mg/kg placebo given orally onco a day (control group, $n = 2$), 1 mg/kg FK506 given intramuscularly (i.m.) once a day ($n = 4$), 1 mg/kg FK506 given orally once a day ($n = 4$), and 10 mg/jg FK506 given orally once a day ($n = 4$). A body weight reduction of more than 10% was taken as a sign of drug toxicity, and the dose was reduced to 50% of the initial value. After 90 days or when the animals became lethargic, the monkeys were sacrificed by a lethal dose of pentobarbital sodium given intravenously.

Clinical observations. Every day the monkeys were observed. Two times a week the animals were scored systematically for the following clinical observations: weight, appetite (none, mild, moderate, good), and activity (apathetic, slow, normal, hyperactive).

Biochemistry studies. Once a week fasting venous blood samples were taken for the measurement of potassium, sodium, chloride, calcium, serum urea nitrogen (SUN), creatinine (Cr), alkaline phosphatase (AF), γ-glutamyl transferase (GGT), aspartate aminotransferase (ASAT), alanine aminotransferase (ALAT), total bilirubin, amylase, lactodehydrogenase (LDH), fasting blood glucose, leukocytes, hemoglobin (Hb), and hematocrit (Hct).

Histology studies. A complete postmortem examination was performed in all animals with microscopical evaluation of necropsies of the liver, kidney, heart, lung, spleen, pancreas, small bowel, brain and paraaortic lymph nodes. Tissues were fixed in 10% neutral buffered formalin and were paraffin embedded. Sections of 4 μm thick were stained with H & E or with special techniques as indicated. All sections were examined blindly without knowledge of the treatment regimen. The histopathologic changes were graded on a 0–3 scale, recorded as normal (0), minimal (1), moderate (2), and severe (3).

Drug level monitoring. The 24-h trough serum level of FK506 was determined in weekly blood samples which were collected prior to the daily drug administration. The samples were centrifuged at room temperature and stored frozen at − 30°C until analysis. FK506 was extracted from the serum samples using Sep-Pak columns. The bound FK506 was eluted with methanol and evaporated to dryness under nitrogen at 37°C. The dried samples were analyzed by a modified enzyme immunoassay (EIA), in which a monoclonal antibody (Fujisawa, Osaka, Japan) directed against FK506 was used [3, 4, 28].

Results

Clinical studies

The monkeys given FK506 orally and the 2 placebo monkeys survived the 90 days of the experiment in apparently good health. They showed no clinical signs of side effects, and no significant body weight reduction was observed (Table 1). In contrast, all the monkeys treated with FK506 intramuscularly had to be sacrificed because of severe illness before the end of the experiment on days 20, 25, 32, and 47. From day 18 to 20 they developed a diminished appetite and signs of lethargy; two developed severe diarrhea during the last 3 days before sacrifice. Three of the four monkeys showed a body weight reduction of more than 10%, and accordingly protocol dosages were reduced to 0.5 mg/kg daily on days 14, 19, and 27. None of the animals showed clinical signs of infection.

Biochemistry findings

The biochemistry findings are summarized in Table 2. The most pronounced findings were found in the i.m.-treated animals. In these animals the SUN levels of monkeys MF2, MF3, and MF4 increased. The serum creatinine level of MF2 was elevated. GGT was increased after 90 days in MF3, and ASAT was increased in monkeys MF2 and MF3. One of the 4 monkeys on FK506 given intramuscularly, MF4, had an increased fasting B-glucose (from 2.8 to 11.1 mmol/l). The results concerning the influence of FK506 on glucose metabolism are described in detail elsewere [10]. The monkeys on orally given FK506, both the 1 mg/kg daily and the 10 mg/kg daily dosage, did not show significant changes of the biochemical parameters during the 90 days of the experiment. The other measured biochemical parameters did not show any significant changes.

FK506 levels in serum

The monkeys given the drug i.m. had after 1 week of daily treatment serum levels between 10 and 15 ng/ml. During the following weeks, the levels increased slowly in spite of dose reduction at days 14, 19, and 27. The serum levels in the animals given 1 mg/kg daily orally, ranged between 0.2 and 5.0 ng/ml, except for 3 peaks of 8 ng/ml in 1 monkey. The FK506 serum levels of the monkeys on 10 mg/kg oral dosage had levels ranging between 2.0 and 70 ng/ml. In none of these 4 monkeys were the serum trough levels stable; they differed from week to week and from monkey to monkey. Further details are described elsewere [35].

Table 2. Summary of biochemistry findings after FK506 administration (values at the beginning/end of the experiment)

Treatment	Monkey	Serum urea (mmol/l)	Serum creatinine (mmol/l)	GGT (mmol/l)	ASAT (mmol/l)
Placebo orally	MF5	7.9/ 6.5	76/ 81	48/ 44	40/ 27
	MF14	5.0/ 6.7	85/ 45	39/ 54	78/ 40
FK506 1 mg/kg daily intramuscularly	MF1	5.9/[a]	99/ [a]	45/ [a]	37/ [a]
	MF2	5.9/**73.2**	99/**335**	44/ 23	23/**256**
	MF3	8.4/**15.4**	98/ 79	46/**309**	43/ **98**
	MF4	5.6/**66.2**	84/108	41/ 28	49/ 45
FK506 1 mg/kg daily orally	MF6	6.6/ 7.7	97/ 85	40/ 43	51/ 23
	MF13	7.1/ 7.4	93/ 72	41/ 56	34/ 37
	MF57	9.6/ 8.5	72/ 58	129/116	61/ 51
	MF58	8.8/ 7.2	42/ 57	87/ 54	70/ 43
FK506 10 mg/kg daily orally	MF15	9.0/ 5.4	68/ 64	45/ 47	40/ 44
	MF16	6.4/ 5.6	84/113	48/ 45	44/ 51
	MF59	7.2/ 7.9	72/ 75	97/114	43/ 49
	MF60	8.6/10.3	59/ 80	77/ 52	46/ 42

[a] No reliable value available (MF1 died before sampling)

GGT, γ-glutamyl transferase; ASAT, aspartate aminotransferase

Table 3. Histopathology findings in monkeys given FK506 1 mg/kg daily intramuscularly

Monkey	Kidney	Pancreas	Liver	Heart	Lungs
MF1	Mesangial cell proliferation	Select B-cell depletion Amyloid deposition	Panlobular steatosis	normal	Interstitial pneumonia
MF2	Acute tubular necrosis	normal	normal	normal	Interstitial pneumonia
MF3	normal	normal	Panlobular steatosis	Cardiomyopathy	Peribronchitis
MF4	Mesangial cell proliferation	Select B-cell depletion Amyloid deposition	Panlobular steatosis	Cardiomyopathy	Peribronchitis

Histopathology studies

The histopathology findings are summarized in Table 3. The major changes were observed in animals given the drug i.m. The kidney revealed glomerular mesangial cell proliferation and an increase in the mesangial matrix, grade 2–3, in monkeys MF1 and MF4, while acute tubular necrosis was observed in MF2 only (Fig. 1a). Monkeys MF1 and MF4 showed hyalinization of the pancreatic islets characterized by deposition of amorphous eosinophilic material (Fig. 1b), positive for Congo red staining and with the characteristic birefringence after polarization, that is indicative of amyloid. On immunohistochemistry study using a polyclonal rabbit insulin-specific antibody, a selective depletion of insulin-producing beta cells was seen. The liver showed panlobular micro- and macrovesicular steatosis of hepatocytes, grade 2–3, in MF1, MF3, and MF4. Furthermore, MF3 and MF4 exhibited an upper gastrointestinal tract bleeding due to hemorrhagic gastritis.

Cardiomyopathy, characterized by a feathery degeneration of the cardiomyocytes with an influx of mononuclear leukocytes, was shown in MF3 and MF4 (Fig. 1c). In the lungs, signs of interstitial pneumonia were seen in monkeys MF1 and MF2, whereas in MF3 and MF4 peribronchial congestion could be observed.

The control animals and the animals given FK506 orally had similar and mild histopathological abnormalities. There was a slight increase in kidney mesangial cells and matrix grade 1 (MF13, MF15, and MF16) and centrilobular micro- and macrovesicular steatosis of hepatocytes grade 1 (MF13, MF15, MF16, and MF5). Pancreatic abnormalities, cardiomyopathy, or acute tubular necrosis was not observed.

Monkey MF15, who had been given FK506 10 mg/kg daily orally, was found to have a malignant lymphoma, a diffuse centroblastic form involving the paraaortic lymph nodes at sacrifice (day 90) (Fig. 1d).

All the monkeys given FK506, whether i.m. or orally, showed depletion of the germinal centers in the periarteriolar lymphocytic areas in the spleen. This was not observed in the monkeys receiving the carrier only (Fig. 2).

Discussion

Previous studies [5, 25, 30, 33] have shown contradictory results concerning the side-effects of FK506 in primates. In this study this controversy was reexamined with special reference to the dosage, route of administration, and serum levels of FK506 in cynomolgus monkeys.

Calne et al. reported that baboon kidney allograft recipients given FK506 at a dose of 0.5–1.0 mg/kg i.m. daily developed anorexia, lethargy, and hyperglycemia [5]. Todo et al. reported no major toxicity of FK506 when given orally, even at doses as high as 36 mg/kg daily to kidney allografted baboons [33]. Our results in nontransplanted cynomolgus monkeys are in accordance with these previous findings. Serious clinical, biochemical, and histological abnormalities were induced by the i.m. administration of FK506 1 mg/kg daily, while after oral dosage of even 10 mg/kg daily, no major side-effects besides some specific ones were observed.

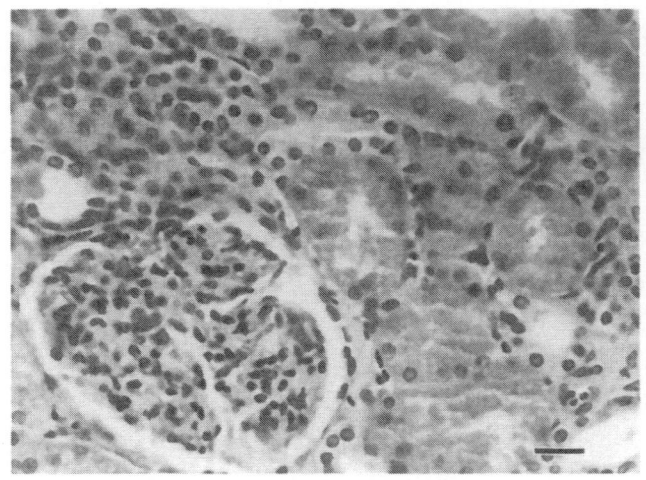

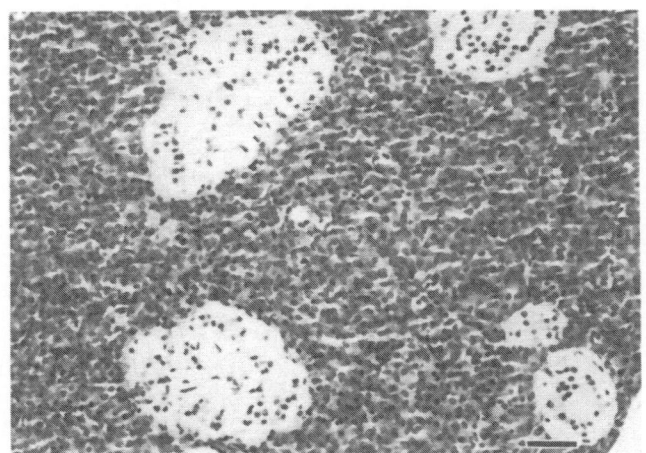

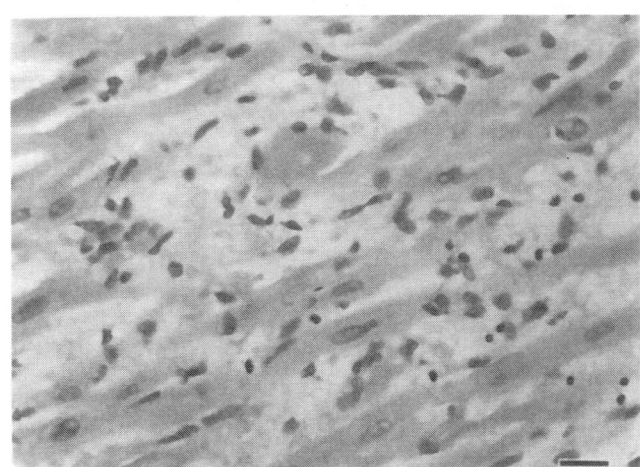

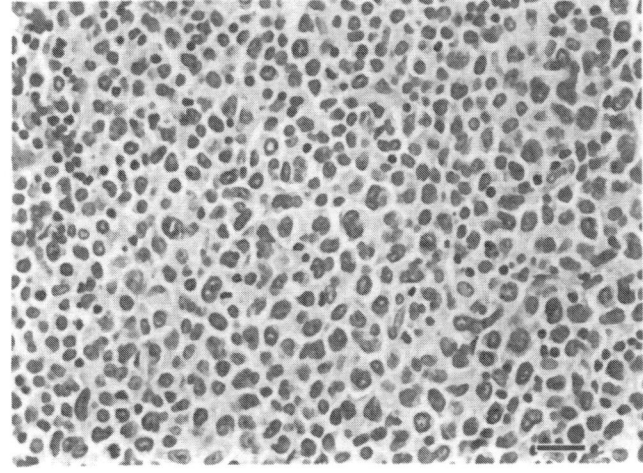

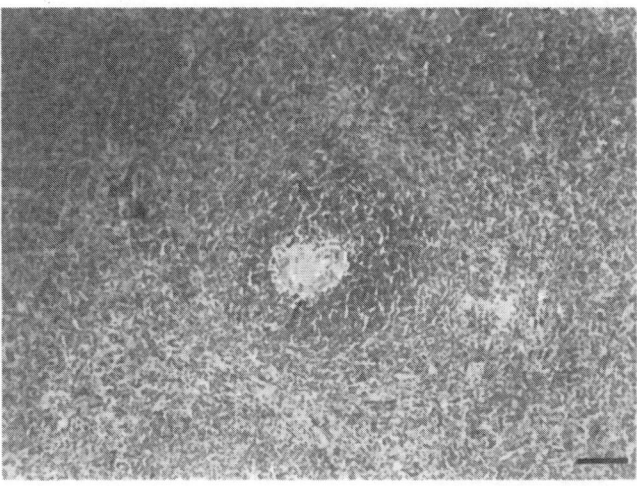

Fig. 2. Depletion of germinal centers in the periarteriolar lymphocytic areas in the spleen of monkey on orally given FK506. *Bar* indicates magnification in microns

The elevated SUN levels of MF3 and MF4 can be explained by the upper gastrointestinal tract bleeding due to hemorrhagic gastritis in these 2 monkeys. Nephrotoxicity was only seen in one of the i.m.-treated monkeys (MF2). Both the biochemical and the histopathological data showed these nephrotoxic changes. The fibrinoid necrosis of medium-sized arteries frequently observed in dogs in various organs, notably the heart and the gastrointestinal tract, was not noticed in any of our monkeys, indicating that monkeys do not become afflicted with this lesion. This is consistent with findings in other studies [5, 30, 33].

A diabetogenic effect in baboons has been described after i.m. administration of the drug and was thought to be due to peripheral insulin resistance [7]. The present study suggests, however, that there may be a direct toxic effect on the pancreatic islets, resulting in selective B-cell depletion, at least after i.m. administration of 1 mg/kg daily. After 3 month's oral administration of FK506 10 mg/kg daily, no direct histological or biochemical effect on the endocrine pancreas was found.

Thiru et al. has previously reported on one FK506-treated baboon which was found to have a malignant lymphoma [30], just as we saw in the animal receiving 10 mg/kg daily orally (FM15). It is well-known that lymphoproliferative disorders and lymphoid tumors occur with an increased frequency in the immunocompromised individual. A few patients treated with FK506 have also developed such lesions [22]. It remains to be seen, however, whether or not FK506 will cause any change in the frequency or the characteristics of transplant-associated lymphomas [2, 26].

One of our objectives was to look for a relation between FK506 serum level and toxicity. The height of the trough serum level using the EIA did not appear to be re-

Fig. 1a–d. Histopathological changes of monkeys treated with FK506 1 mg/kg daily intramuscularly: **a** acute tubular necrosis of the kidney (MF2), **b** hyalinization of pancreatic islets, **c** cardiomyopathy (MF3), **d** malignant lymphoma, diffuse centroblastic form after 90 days at 10 mg/kg daily orally (MF15). *Bar* indicates magnification in microns

lated to the toxicity in cynomolgus monkeys. The measuring of metabolites by the assay might explain the discrepancy observed between the serum levels and toxicity. Several studies indicate the importance of the liver in the metabolism of the drug, and in in vitro studies, metabolites have been found in human liver microsomes [6]. The first pass through the liver after oral treatment could lead to the formation of metabolites which are probably detected by the assay, and levels not related to toxicity will be measured. Another explanation could be the rapid accumulation of the unmetabolized FK506 in the tissues or extremely high peak levels of FK506 after parenteral administration, events which could both lead to tissue damage. Such high peak levels may lead to tissue damage without the trough levels being increased. Therefore, oral administration of the drug appears to be most important in order to avoid severe toxicity.

In conclusion, our results show that FK506 may cause severe side-effects when given i. m., while oral administration is well tolerated. No relation between toxicity and the drug serum levels was found using the EIA. Attempts should be made to elucidate the pharmacokinetics of FK506, with emphasis on the specific methods for detection of the original compound and eventual metabolites, of which some might be toxic and others nontoxic, eventually with species difference as well.

References

1. Arai K, Hotobuchi T, Miyahara H, et al. (1989) Limb allografts in rats immunosuppressed with FK506: I. Reversal of rejection and indefinite survival. Transplantation 48: 782
2. Barkholt L, Billing H, Juliusson G, Porwit A, Ericzon BG, Groth CG (1991) B-cell lymphoma in transplanted liver. Clinical, histological and radiological manifestations. Transplant Int 4: 8
3. Beysens AJ, Wijnen RMH, Beuman GH, Heijden J van der, As H van (1991) FK506: monitoring in plasma or in whole blood? Transplant Proc 23: 2745
4. Cadoff EM, Venkataramanan R, Krajack A, et al. (1990) Assay of FK506 in plasma. Transplant Proc 22: 50
5. Calne R, Collier DStJ, Thiru S (1987) Observations about FK506 in primates. Transplant Proc 19 [Suppl 6]: 63
6. Christians U, Kruse C, Kownatzki R, et al. (1991) Measurement of FK506 by HPLC and isolation and characterization of its metabolites. Transplant Proc 23: 940
7. Collier DStJ, Calne R, Thiru S, Friend PJ, Lim S, White DJG, Kohno H, Levickis J (1987) FK506 in experimental renal allografts. Transplant Proc 19:3975
8. Collier DStJ, Thiru S, Calne R (1987) Kidney transplantation in the dog receiving FK506. Transplant Proc 19 [Suppl 6]: 62
9. Ericzon BG, Kubota K, Groth CG, et al. (1990) Pancreaticoduodenal allotransplantation with FK506 in the cynomolgus monkey. Transplant Proc 22: 72
10. Ericzon B-G, Wijnen RMH, Kubota K, Kootstra G, Groth C-G (1992) FK-506 induced impairment of glucose metabolism in the primate: studies in pancreatic transplant recipients and in nontransplanted animals. Transplantation (in press)
11. Hoffman AL, Makowka L, Cai X, et al. (1990) The effect of FK506 on small intestine allotransplantation in the rat. Transplant Proc 22: 76
12. Honbo T, Kobayashi M, Hane K, Hata T, Ueda Y (1987) The oral dosage form of FK506. Transplant Proc 19 [Suppl 6]: 17
13. Inamura N, Nakahara K, Kino T, et al. (1988) Prolongation of skin allografts survival in rats by a novel immunosuppressive agent, FK506. Transplantation 45: 206
14. Kay JE, Moore AL, Doe SEA, Benzie CR, Schönbrunner R, Schmid FX, Halestrap AP (1990) The mechanism of action of FK506. Transplant Proc 22 [Suppl 1]: 96
15. Kino T, Hatanaka H, Hashimoto M, et al. (1987) FK506, a novel immunosuppressant isolated from a Streptomyces. I. Fermentation, isolation, and physiochemical and biological characteristics. J Antibiotics 40: 1249
16. Kino T, Hatanaka H, Miyata S, et al. (1987) FK506, a novel immunosuppressant isolated from a Streptomyces. II. Immunosuppressive effect of FK506 in vitro. J Antibiotics 40: 1256
17. Kino T, Inamura N, Sakai F, et al. (1987) Effect of FK506 on human mixed lymphocyte reaction in vitro. Transplant Proc 19 [Suppl 6]: 36
18. Lee P, Murase N, Todo S, Makowka L, Starzl T (1987) The immunosuppressive effect of FR 900506 in rats receiving heterotopic cardiac allografts. Surg Res Commun 1: 325
19. Mondon M, Gotoh M, Kanai T, et al. (1990) A potent immunosuppressive effect of FK506 in orthotopic liver transplantation in primates. Transplant Proc 22: 66
20. Morimoto T, Yamada T, Kobayashi S, et al. (1989) Pancreaticoduodenal allotransplantation with FK506 in the dog. Transplant Proc 21: 1074
21. Nalesnik MA, Todo S, Murase N, et al. (1987) Toxicology of FK506 in the Lewis rat. Transplant Proc 19 [Suppl 6]: 89
22. Nalesnik MA, Demetris AJ, Fung JJ, Starzl TE (1991) Lymphoproliferative disorders arising under immunosuppression with FK506: initial observations in a large transplant population. Transplant Proc 23: 1108
23. Ochai T, Nakajiama K, Nagata M, Hori S, Asano T, Isono K (1987) Studies of the induction and maintenance of long-term graft acceptance by treatment with FK506 in heterotopic cardiac allotransplantation in rats. Transplantation 44: 734
24. Ochiai T, Nagata M, Nakajima K, et al. (1989) Comparative studies of FK506 and cyclosporine in canine orthotopic hepatic allografts survival. Transplant Proc 21: 1066
25. Ohara K, Billington R, James RW, Dean GA, Nishiyama M, Noguchi H (1990) Toxicologic evaluation of FK506. Transplant Proc 22 [Suppl 1]: 83
26. Penn I (1987) Cancers following cyclosporine therapy. Transplantation 43: 32
27. Sato K, Yamagishi Y, Nakayama K, et al. (1989) Pancreaticoduodenal allotransplantation with cyclosporine and FK506. Transplant Proc 21: 1074
28. Tamura K, Kobayashi M, Hashimoto K, et al. (1987) A highly sensitive method to assay FK506 levels in plasma. Transplant Proc 19 [Suppl 6]: 23
29. Tanaka H, Huroda A, Marusawa H, et al. (1987) Structure of FK506: a novel immunosuppressant isolated from Streptomyces. J Am Chem Soc 109: 5031
30. Thiru S, Collier DStJ, Calne R (1987) Pathological studies in canine and baboon renal allograft recipients immunosuppressed with FK506. Transplant Proc 19: 98
31. Todo S, Demetris AJ, Ueda Y, et al. (1987) Canine kidney transplantation with FK506 alone or in combination with cyclosporine and steroids. Transplant Proc 14: 57
32. Todo S, Podesta L, Chapchap P, et al. (1987) Orthotopic liver transplantation in dogs receiving FK506. Transplant Proc 19 [Suppl 6]: 64
33. Todo S, Ueda Y, Demetris JA, et al. (1988) Immunosuppression of canine, monkey and baboon allografts by FK506 with special reference to synergism with other drugs, and to tolerance induction. Surgery 104: 239
34. Tsuchimoto S, Kusumoto K, Nakjima Y, et al. (1989) Orthotopic liver transplantation in rats receiving FK506. Transplant Proc 21: 1064
35. Wijnen RMH, Ericzon BG, Tiebosch ATGM, Beysens AJ, Groth CG, Kootstra G (1991) Toxicology of FK506 in the nonhuman primate, non-correlation with the serum levels. Transplant Proc 23: 3101
36. Yokota K, Takishima T, Sato K, et al. (1989) Comparative studies of FK506 and cyclosporine in canine orthotopic hepatic allografts survival. Transplant Proc 21: 1066

Transplant Int (1992) 5 [Suppl 1]: S 459

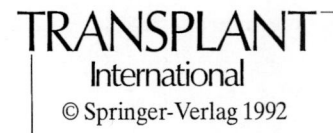

© Springer-Verlag 1992

CD4-specific monoclonal antibody can prolong cardiac allograft survival without T-cell depletion

C. R. Darby, P. J. Morris, and K. J. Wood

Nuffield Department of Surgery, John Radcliffe Hospital, Oxford, United Kingdom

Current immunosuppressive regimens for clinical transplantation are immunologically non-specific, are associated with acute and chronic toxic side-effects [1] and are unable to prevent chronic graft loss in a significant proportion of patients. Additionally, new and increasingly powerful drugs are being introduced to induce non-specific immunosuppression, and therefore this is likely to be followed by an increase in related complications such as the induction of cancers. Hence, there is a need for an alternative approach.

It has been shown that long-term survival of murine cardiac grafts can be induced by the monoclonal antibody YIS 191 that depletes CD4+T cells in vivo [2]. In this study, we have investigated the ability of a non-depleting antibody to produce better graft survival.

Key words: Immunosuppression – Monoclonal antibodies – YTS 191

Materials and methods

C3H/He mice were treated with 2 doses of either 25 µg of YTS 191 [3] (IgG2b) or 200 µg of KT6 [4] (IgG2a) intravenously (i. v.) on consecutive days, and lymph node single cell suspensions were assessed for the proportion of CD4+T cells present by flow cytometry. Adult C3H/He mice received heterotopic C57BL/10 heart transplants representing a H-2 and multiple minor antigen mismatch and were treated either with 25 µg of YIS 191 or increasing doses, from 25 to 200 µg, of KT6 i. v. on the day prior to and at the end of the transplant operation.

Results

Cellular depletion of CD4+ cells after treatment with YTS 191 was maximal by 3 days, when the animals were 87% depleted of CD4+ cells relative to naive mice. No

depletion occurred in animals treated with KT6 even at doses of 400 µg. In vivo, a 25-µg dose of depleting antibody YTS 191 given the day before and at the time of heart transplantation prolongs graft median survival time (mst) beyond 100 days. Grafts transplanted in animals receiving this same dose (2×25 µg) of KT6 were minimally prolonged ($n = 5$, mst 11.5 days) compared with untreated controls ($n = 6$, mst 8 days), but increasing doses of KT6 were progressively more immunosuppressive. When 2×200 µg of KT6 were used, marked prolongation of graft survival was obtained ($n = 9$, mst 58 days; versus controls $P = 0.0018$) and long-term survival in one-third.

Discussion

Perioperative treatment with the CD4+T-cell-depleting monoclonal antibody YTS 191 has been shown to induce immunosuppression and long-term graft survival in this transplant model. In humans, attempts to induce immunosuppression and tolerance by cellular depletion may be complicated by toxicity from cell lysis and a prolonged period of non-specific immunosuppression. A regimen involving only non-depleting CD4-specific antibody to induce immunosuppression and tolerance might avoid these complications and additionally should not be associated with the sequelae of T-cell activation as seen with T-cell receptor antibodies such as OKT3. Towards this aim we have shown that a simple non-depleting regimen targeting only the CD4+ subset of T-cells can be profoundly immunosuppressive and induce the long-term survival of vascularised grafts in a murine model.

References

1. Mahony JF, Sheil AGR (1987) In: Morris PJ (ed) Transplantation reviews, vol 1. Grune and Stratton, London, pp 47–58
2. Madsen JC, Peugh WN, Wood KJ, Morris PJ (1987) Transplantation 44 (6): 849–852
3. Cobbold SP, Jayasuriya A, Nash A, Prospero TD, Waldmann H (1984) Nature 312: 548–551
4. Tomonari K (1988) Eur J Immunol 18: 179–182

Offprint requests to: C. Darby, Nuffield Department of Surgery, John Radcliffe Hospital, Headington, Oxford OX39DU, United Kingdom

Transplant Int (1992) 5 [Suppl 1]: S 460–S 461

TRANSPLANT
International
© Springer-Verlag 1992

Prolongation of heart allograft survival in rats by interferon-specific antibodies and low dose cyclosporin A

J. Gugenheim[1], M. Tovey[2], M. Gigou[3], F. Crafa[1], B. Fabiani[4], M. Reynes[4], and H. Bismuth[4]

[1] Laboratoire de Recherches Chirurgicales et Service de Chirurgie Digestive, Hôpital Saint-Roch, Nice Cedex 1,
[2] Laboratory of Viral Oncology (UPR 274), CNRS, Villejuif,
[3] Unité de Chirurgie Hépato-Biliaire and
[4] Laboratoire d'Anatomie Pathologique, Hôpital Paul Brousse, Villejuif, France

Interferons (IFNs) are important cytokines which exhibit antiviral, antitumor, anticellular, as well as immunoregulatory activities [1]. Among these multiple activities, IFNs are potent inducers of MHC antigen expression of a great variety of cells [2–4], helper and maturation factors in B-cell antibody production [5], and macrophage function [6]. IFNs may therefore play a critical role in triggering antigen recognition and allograft rejection.

Cyclosporin A (CyA) is a potent immunosuppressor which selectively inhibits helper T-lymphocyte proliferation in response to alloantigen presentation [7, 8]. CyA has been reported to inhibit interleukin 2 and IFNγ production by helper T lymphocytes [9–11]. In addition, CyA may induce monocyte production of prostaglandin E2 [12], which then reduces MHC class II expression on endothelial cells, monocytes, and macrophages [13].

However, the clinical use of CyA is plagued by its toxic (in particular nephrotoxic) side-effects. These toxic effects are clearly dose-related. It may be very important to develop new products which can act synergistically with CyA to inhibit lymphokine production. The aim of this study was to investigate the effects of combined IFN-specific antibodies and low dose CyA on cardiac allografts in inbred strains of rats.

Key words: Immunosuppression – Cytokines – Interferons – Cyclosporine A

Material and methods

Adult male Lewis (Lew, RT1l) and brown Norway (BN, RT1n) rats weighing 200–250 g were purchased from CNSEAL (Orleans La Source, France). Rats were operated on under clean but not sterile conditions. Heterotopic intraabdominal heart transplantations were carried out according to the technique of Ono and Lindsey [14]. CyA (Sandimmune, Sandoz, Basel) was administered to rate by gavage via an orogastric tube. Polyclonal sheep antimouse IFNα/β, prepared

Offprint requests to: J. Gugenheim, Laboratoire de Recherches Chirurgicales et Service de Chirurgie Digestive, Hôpital Saint-Roch, 5 rue Pierre Dévoluy, F-06006 Nice Cedex 1, France

and purfied as described previously [15], had a neutralizing titer of 6.4×10^6 against 8 units of mouse IFNα/β when assayed on mouse L929 cells [16] and a titer of 2000 against 5 units of rat IFNα/β. Polyclonal sheep antirat IFNγ was a gift of H. Schellekens (Rijsnijk, The Netherlands) and had a neutralizing titer of 8000 against 16 units of rats IFNγ. These antibodies were administered intravenously via the dorsal penile vein. In the BN into LEW combination, heart allografts were performed, and 5 experimental groups of 10 rats each were constituted. In group 1, rats were treated by 0.5 ml of polyclonal sheep antirat IFNγ antibodies on days -4, -1, $+2$, $+5$, $+8$, and $+11$. Rats of group 2 were treated by 0.5 ml of polyclonal sheep antimouse IFNα/β antibodies on the same day schedule. In group 3, anti-IFNγ therapy was associated with low dose CyA (2.5 mg/kg body weight on day 0 and then every day). Group 4 consisted of rats treated only by CyA (2.5 mg/kg daily) and group 5, of heart allografts. The survival time of heart allografts was assessed by daily palpation. Rejection time was the moment of cessation of beating. At that time, the recipient was autopsied to detect technical complications. Heart allografts were excised and processed for conventional and immunohistochemical examination. A peroxidase-antiperoxidase method using mouse monoclonal antibodies to rat MHC antigens (F 16.4.4 for class I and MRC 0 $\times$ 17 for class II MHC Ag) was carried out as previously described [17]. Results were expressed as mean survival time ± standard error of the mean (MST ± SEM). Student's *t*-test was used for comparing the means of the different groups.

Results

In the BN into LEW combination of inbred rats (Table 1), the survival of heart allografts was significantly ($P < 0.05$) prolonged in rats of group 1 (treated by anti-INFγ antibodies; mean survival time, MST ± SEM = 9.7 ± 0.2 days), in rats of group 2 (treated by anti-IFNα/β antibodies; MST ± SEM = 8.0 ± 0.2 days), and in rats of group 4 (treated by low dose CyA; MST ± SEM = 9.4 ± 0.2 days) when compared with control heart allografts (group 5; MST ± SEM = 6.8 ± 0.7 days). The observed prolongation was more important when CyA was associated with anti-IFNγ antibodies (group 3; MST ± SEM = 14.6 ± 0.4 days). Immunohistochemical analysis of the control heart allograft revealed induction of the trexpression of MHC class I antigens on the myocardial cells. To the contrary, no expression was observed on the myocardium of anti-IFN-treated heart allografts.

Table 1. Rejection time of BN cardiac allografts into LEW recipients

Group	n	Graft survival (days)	MST ± SEM (days)
1 (Anti-IFNγ)	10	8, 9, 9, 10, 10, 10, 10, 10, 10, 11	9.7 ± 0.2[*]
2 (Anti-IFNα/β)	10	7, 7, 8, 8, 8, 8, 8, 8, 9, 9	8.0 ± 0.2[*]
3 (Anti-IFNγ + CyA)	10	12, 13, 14, 14, 15, 15, 15, 16, 16, 16	14.6 ± 0.4[**]
4 (CyA)	10	8, 9, 9, 9, 9, 9, 10, 10, 10, 11	9.4 ± 0.2[*]
5 (Control)	10	6, 6, 6, 7, 7, 7, 7, 7, 7, 8	6.8 ± 0.7[**]

[*] Difference between groups 1, 2, 4 significant ($P < 0.05$) and [**] between groups 3 and 5 significant ($P < 0.001$) BN, brown Norway rats; LEW, Lewis rats; MST, mean survival time

Discussion

IFNγ is mainly released by helper T lymphocytes upon activation by alloantigens and is a critical cytokine which is a potent inducer of MHC antigen expression on a great variety of cells [2–4] and an activator of monocyte-macrophage functions [6]. Previous studies have demonstrated that antibodies to IFNγ may delay allograft rejection [18, 19].

Our results confirm these studies and show that low dose CyA and antibodies to IFNγ may act synergistically to delay heart allograft rejection in the rat. In fact, CyA has been shown to inhibit lymphokine production [9–11] and in particular to reduce IFNγ production in mice [11] and in man [10]. In addition, CyA may reduce cytokine production by macrophages [20] and class II MHC Ag expression on macrophages [12, 13]. In our study, we observed the absence of the induction of expression of MHC class I antigens on rejected myocardial cells after treatment by antibodies to IFN. In conclusion, IFNγ-specific antibodies may represent an useful reagent to potentiate low dose CyA therapy, probably by MHC expression down-regulation.

References

1. Bloom BR (1980) Interferons and the immune system. Nature 284: 593–595
2. Heron I, Holland M, Berg K (1978) Enhanced expression of β₂ microglobulin and HLA antigens on human lymphoid cells by interferon. Proc Natl Acad Sci USA 77: 6215
3. Lindahl P, Gresser I, Leary L, Tovey MG (1976) Interferon treatment of mice: enhanced expression of histocompatibility antigens on lymphoid cells. Proc Natl Acad Sci USA 73: 1284
4. Skoskiewicz MJ, Colvin RB, Schneeberger EE, Russel PS (1985) Widespread and selective induction of major histocompatibility complex-determined antigens in vivo by γ interferon. J Exp Med 162: 1645
5. Sonnenfeld G, Mandel AD, Merigan TC (1978) Time and dosage, dependence of immunoenhancement by murine type II interferon preparations. Cell Immunol 40: 285–293
6. Rabinovitch M, Manejras RE, Rosso M, Abbey EE (1977) Increased spreading of macrophages from mice treated with interferon inducers. Cell Immunol 29: 86–95
7. Kupiec-Weglinski JW, Filho MA, Strom TB, Tilney NL (1984) Sparing of suppressor cells: a critical action of cyclosporine. Transplantation 38: 57
8. Shevach EM (1985) The effects of cyclosporine A on the immune system. Annu Rev Immunol 3: 397
9. Bishop GA, Hall BM (1988) Effects of immunosuppressive drugs on functions of activated T lymphocytes: cyclosporine inhibition of gamma interferon production in the presence of interleukin 2. Transplantation 45: 967
10. Kalman VK, Klimpel GR (1983) Cyclosporin inhibits the production of gamma interferon (IFNγ) but does not inhibit production of virus-induced IFNα/β. Cell Immunol 78: 122–129
11. Reem GH, Cook LA, Vilcek J (1983) Gamma interferon synthesis by human thymocytes and T lymphocytes inhibited by cyclosporin A. Science 221: 63–65
12. Whitler RL, Lindsey JA, Proctor KVW, Morisaki N, Cornwell DG (1985) Characteristics of cyclosporine induction of increased prostaglandins levels from human peripheral blood monocytes. Transplantation 38: 377
13. Snyder DS, Beller DI, Unanue ER (1982) Prostaglandins modulate macrophage Ia expression. Nature 299: 163
14. Ono K, Lindsey E (1969) Improved technique of heart transplantation in rats. J Thorac Cardiovasc Surg 57: 225
15. Gresser I, Morel-Maroger L, Chatelet F, et al. (1979) Delay in growth and the development of nephritis in rats treated with interferon preparations in the neonatal period. Am J Pathol 95: 329–346
16. Gresser I, Tovey MG, Bander MT, Maury C, Brouty-Boyé D (1976) Role of interferons in the pathogenesis of virus diseases in mice as demonstrated by the use of anti-interferon serum. J Exp Med 144: 1305–1315
17. Fabiani B, Astarcioglu I, Gugenheim J, et al. (1989) Expression of major histocompatibility complex antigens on vascular endothelium of spontaneously tolerated liver allografts. Transplant Proc 21: 407–408
18. Landolfo S, Cofano F, Giovarelli M, et al. (1985) Inhibition of interferon γ may suppress allograft reactivity by T lymphocytes in vitro and in vivo. Science 229: 176–179
19. Didlake RH, Kim EK, Sheehan K, Schreiber RD, Kahan BD (1988) Effect of combined anti-gamma interferon antibody and cyclosporine therapy on cardiac allograft survival in the rat. Transplantation 45: 222–223
20. Benson A, Ziegler H (1989) Macrophages as targets for inhibition by cyclosporine. Transplantation 47: 696

Transplant Int (1992) 5 [Suppl 1]: S 462–S 463

TRANSPLANT
International
© Springer-Verlag 1992

Effect of LS-2616 on the graft protection achieved by cyclosporin A, prednisolone, and 15-deoxyspergualin in heart-transplanted rats

A. Wanders, G. Gannedahl, B. Gerdin, and G. Tufveson

Departments of Urology, Surgery, and Pathology, University Hospital, Uppsala, Sweden

Abstract. The immunostimulator LS-2616 abolishes the effect of cyclosporin A in a rat cardiac transplantation model. The present paper compares the characteristics of rejection obtained under different immunosuppressive regimens with and without additional LS-2616 application in the same model. Cyclosporin A (CyA, 10 mg/kg daily), prednisolone (15 mg/kg daily), or 15-deoxyspergualin (2, 5, or 10 mg/kg daily), all given from the day of transplantation until day 9, protected the grafts during the treatment period. The addition of LS-2616 (160 mg/kg, day − 1 until stop) resulted in a total abrogation of the immunosuppressive effect of CyA and prednisolone. However, LS-2616 could only partially or not at all reverse the effect of 15-deoxyspergualine. These results show a certain drug selectivity of LS-2616 in promoting rejection of immunosuppressed allografts. Further studies with LS-2616 may be of benefit in evaluating the mode of action of different immunosuppressive compounds and, thus, contribute to finding more effective antirejection therapies.

Key words: Immunosuppression – Cyclosporine A – Prednisolone – 15-deoxyspergualin – LS-2616

The rejection of a allograft is an immune response in which the immune system acts detrimentally. This immune reaction can to a large extent be suppressed by immunomodulating compounds. Despite the impressive graft protective effectiveness of drugs like cyclosporin A (CyA), prednisolone, or 15-deoxyspergualin (15-DSG) in experimental transplantation models in rodents [5, 7], in man graft rejection does still occur in the presence of immunosuppressive therapy. This clinical experience suggests that alternative pathways might exist in activation of the immune system which cannot be blocked by these drugs.

We described earlier LS-2616 [3, 4] as an immunomodulating compound able to induce graft rejection in the presence of CyA [2, 7, 8]. This CyA-resistant pathway might reflect such an alternative activation of the immune system. Subsequently, we tested the nature of the effect of LS-2616 on the prolongation of graft survival brought about by prednisolone or 15-DSG. In the present paper, we report that LS-2616 abrogates the effect of CyA and prednisolone while it only partially reverses the effect of 15-DSG at low doses (2 and 5 mg/kg) and was without effect when combined with a high dose of 10 mg/kg.

Materials and methods

Cardiac allografts from male PVG donor rats were transplanted heterotopically to Wistar/Kyoto (Wi/Ky) recipients as described in detail elsewhere [8]. Rejection was defined as the absence of palpable contraction. LS-2616 (Linomide, Kabi Pharmacia, Sweden) was added to the drinking water. Treatment with a daily dose of 160 mg/kg started 1 day prior to transplantation and continued until the day of rejection.

Three different immunosuppressive protocols were used, all starting on the day of transplantation and maintained until day 9 after transplantation. (A) CyA (Sandimmune, Sandoz AG, Switzerland) was given orally in a daily dose of 10 mg/kg. (B) Prednisolone (Precortalone, Organon, The Netherlands) was given intraperitoneally at a dose of 15 mg/kg daily. (C) 15-DSG (Behringwerke AG, FRG) was given intraperitoneally at doses of 2, 5, or 10 mg/kg daily.

The Wilcoxon rank-sum test was used for the statistical analysis. The results are given as the median (and range) of the graft survival time. One cardiac graft recipient treated with 15-DSG 2 mg/kg daily which stopped 5 days after transplantation was excluded from the statistical analysis, since the pathohistological examination of this explanted heart showed no signs of necrosis and only a mild cellular infiltration within the intact normal heart muscle cells.

Results

The results are summarized in Table 1. No treatment (control) resulted in a graft survival time of 8 (8–9) days, which was not altered by LS-2616 treatment alone (median 8.5, range 7–11). Rats receiving CyA or prednisolone experienced graft survival of 19 (15–27) and 12 (9–15) days, respectively. The addition of LS-2616 to both treatment groups led to graft survival times identical to that of the un-

Offprint requests to: Alkwin Wanders, M.D., Ph.D., Department of Pathology, Uppsala University Hospital, S-751 85 Uppsala, Sweden

Table 1. Graft survival times of heart-transplanted rats receiving immunosuppression alone or combined with LS-2616

Treatment	Graft survival times (days)
None	8, 8, 8, 8, 8, 8, 9, 9, 9, 9, 9
LS-2616	7, 8, 8, 9, 10, 11
Prednisolone	9, 10, 10, 11, 13, 13, 14, 15
Prednisolone + LS-2616	8, 9, 9, 9, 9, 9[**]
Cyclosporine	15, 15, 16, 16, 17, 17, 18, 19, 19, 19, 20, 21, 21, 21, 22, 27, 27
Cyclosporine + LS-2616	8, 8, 8, 9, 9, 9[***]
15-DSG (2 mg/kg)	16, 17, 17, 18, 18, 20, 20, 27, 35
15-DSG (2 mg/kg) + LS-2616	6, 7, 9, 12, 13, 13, 13, 15, 17, 21[**]
15-DSG (5 mg/kg)	13, 15, 19, 20, 20, 31, 57, 98, >100, >100
15-DSG (5 mg/kg) + LS-2616	5, 9, 10, 13, 15, 17, 17, 18, 20, 21, 21, 29, 30, 30
15-DSG (10 mg/kg)	8, 18, 21, 21, 22, 23, 28, >100, >100, >100
15-DSG (10 mg/kg) + LS-2616	11, 21, 24, 26, 47, >100

15-DSG, 15-deoxy spergualin
[*] $P < 0.05$, [**] $P < 0.01$, [***] $P < 0.001$

treated group. Medication with 15-DSG resulted in a median graft survival of 18 (16–35) days in the group receiving a daily dose of 2 mg/kg, 25.5 (13 to >100) days in the 5 mg/kg group, and 22.5 (8 to >100) days in the 10 mg/kg group. The addition of LS-2616 here did not, in contrast to CyA and prednisolone, reverse the immunosuppressive effect of 15-DSG. LS-2616 only partially reversed the effect of a 2 mg/kg 15-DSG application, leading to a graft survival time of 13 (6–21) days. Three out of 10 animals rejected their heart during the treatment period with 15-DSG. In the group receiving 5 mg/kg one could see a slight and insignificant tendency towards a shortening of the graft survival time by the addition of LS-2616. Here, 2 out of 14 animals rejected their grafts in the presence of 15-DSG, and none of the LS-2616 plus 15-DSG-treated animals had grafts surviving longer than the 100 days observed in the animals given 15-DSG only. Recipients with the highest dose of 15-DSG 10 mg/kg in combination with LS-2616 had a comparable graft survival time to the animals receiving only 15-DSG.

Discussion

The results clearly indicate a certain drug-selective effect of LS-2616 on provoking rejection of rat cardiac allo-grafts. Both CyA and prednisolone totally lose their immunosuppressive potential upon the addition of LS-2616, whereas this was only observed to a considerably lesser extent or not at all in 15-DSG-treated animals.

The mode of action of LS-2616 is believed to be due not to an induction of interleukin 2 (IL-2) [6] but to a direct or indirect stimulation of already sensitized T-cell which are prevented from becoming cytotoxic by CyA [8]. The fact that LS-2616 was capable only to a minor extent of reversing the suppression of 15-DSG could find its explanation in the hypothesis that 15-DSG prohibits the sensitization of T-cell either by directly interacting with T-cell, like CyA, or by exerting its main effect on other cells of the immune system, e.g., macrophages [1]. Concerning the relevance of our findings, it is tempting to speculate that there are signals in man which lead to CyA- and prednisolone-resistant pathways of rejection crisis and, furthermore, that these signals might be identical with those provided or induced by LS-2616. Further studies in the LS-2616 model might lead to a better understanding of the mode of action of immunosuppressive compounds such as 15-DSG and thereby contribute to optimizing antirejection therapy by prohibiting CyA/prednisolone-resistant rejections.

References

1. Dickneite G, Schorlemmer HU, Sedlacek HH, Falck W, Ulrichts K, Müller-Ruckholtz W (1987) Suppression of macrophage function and prolongation of graft survival by the new guanidine-like structure, 15-deoxyspergualin. Transplant Proc 19: 1301–1304
2. Gerdin B, Wanders A, Tufveson G (1989) Rat cardiac allografts protected with cyclosporin A are rejected in the presence of LS-2616 (Linomide®). Transplant Proc 21: 853–855
3. Kalland T, Alm G, Ståhlhanske T (1985) Augmentation of mouse natural killer cell activity by LS-2616, a new immunomodulator. J Immunol 134: 3956–3961
4. Ståhlhanske T, Kalland T (1986) Effects of the novel immunomodulator LS-2616 on the delayed-type hypersensitivity reaction to *Bordetella pertussis* in the rat. Immunopharmacology 11: 87–92
5. Suzuki S, kanashiro M, Amemiya H (1987) Effect of a new immunosuppressant, 15-deoxyspergualin, on heterotopic rat heart transplantation, in comparison with cyclosporine. Transplantation 44: 483–487
6. Wanders A (1991) Drug modified rejection of rat cardiac allografts. Acta Universitatis Upsaliensis (dissertation) 298: 1–45
7. Wanders A, Larsson E, Gerdin B, Tufveson G (1989) Abolition of the effect of cyclosporine on rat cardiac allograft rejection by the new immunomodulator LS-2616 (Linomide). Transplantation 47: 216–217
8. Wanders A, Vogt P, Karlsson-Parra A, Wonigkeit K, Gerdin B, Tufveson G (1991) Evidence that LS-2616 (Linomide) causes acute rejection of rat cardiac allografts protected by cyclosporine but not of long-term surviving allografts. Transplantation 52: 234–238

Transplant Int (1992) 5 [Suppl 1]: S 464–S 469

TRANSPLANT
International
© Springer-Verlag 1992

A randomized pilot study of cyclosporin G in renal transplantation

S. Ohlman[1], A. Lindholm[1,2], H. Gäbel[1], H. Wilczek[1], G. Tydén[1], F. Reinholt[3], J. Säwe[2], and C.-G. Groth[1]

Departments of [1] Transplantation Surgery, [2] Clinical Pharmacology, and [3] Pathology, Huddinge Hospital, Karolinska Institute, Stockholm, Sweden

Abstract. Animal studies have suggested that the analogue cyclosporin G (CyG) may be less nephrotoxic than cyclosporin A (CyA). A pilot study was therefore performed in 10 primary cadaveric renal allograft recipients who were randomized to receive posttransplant immunosuppression with either CyA or CyG. The follow-up time was a minimum of 1 year. One graft was lost in each group. All patients in both groups experienced at least one acute rejection episode. Episodes of acute nephrotoxicity were observed in both groups. Renal function, as assessed by determinations of the serum creatinine level and chromium-ethylene diamine tetra-acetic acid (Cr-EDTA) clearance, did not differ between the two groups. Renal allograft biopsies showed a significantly higher degree of fibrosis in the CyG group than in the CyA group. All CyG-treated patients evidenced laboratory signs of acute liver toxicity, which was dose-dependent and reversible. Today, all CyG-treated patients have been switched to CyA. This study shows that immunosuppression after renal transplantation in man is possible with CyG; however, it does not seem to have any advantages over CyA.

Key words: Immunosuppression – Cyclosporin A – Cyclosporin G – Renal transplantation

---

Cyclosporin A (CyA) is presently the mainstay immunosuppressive agent [2–4, 6, 11, 21, 22, 31]. However, its nephrotoxic effect is a major concern [25, 27], and efforts have therefore been made to find a less nephrotoxic analogue. In 1982 Traber et al. [35] reported the discovery of Nva²-cyclosporine, also known as cyclosporin G (CyG). CyG differs from CyA only in being methylated on the second amino acid of the molecule, thereby changing α-aminobutyric acid to L-norvaline [34]. CyG has been shown to possess immunosuppressive and pharmacodynamic properties similar to those of CyA in vitro as well as

in animal models [18, 19]. Furthermore, some animal studies have suggested that CyG may be less nephrotoxic than CyA [5, 8, 12, 16, 19]. In view of these encouraging results, a small number of kidney transplant patients have received CyG for short periods [1, 20]. In this paper we report the results of a randomized pilot study comparing CyG with CyA as an immunosuppressant in renal transplant recipients.

Materials and methods

Patients. Ten patients receiving a cadaveric renal allograft were included in the study. Five patients were randomized to CyG and 5 to CyA. The exclusion criteria were insulin-dependent diabetes mellitus, retransplantation, T-cell panel reactive antibodies in current serum results, and a history of clinical liver disease or pathological liver values during the preceding 12 months. All patients aged 18–65 years who underwent transplantation between October 1989 and March 1990 and who met the criteria were asked whether they wished to participate in the study, and their informed consent was obtained. Only one patient refused to participate. The patient characteristics are summarized in Table 1. The follow-up time was 12–17 months. The study was approved by the local ethics committee and the Swedish Medical Board.

Immunosuppression. All patients received triple-drug immunosuppression with either CyG or CyA, azathioprine, and prednisolone. The standard oral solution of CyA (Sandimmun mixture, 100 mg/ml, Sandoz, Basel) or the standard intravenous preparation of CyA (Sandimmun in Cremophor EL) was used. CyG was supplied in identical vehicles. CyG and CyA were given orally twice daily from the day of transplantation in an initial dose of 10 mg/kg bw per day. The dose was then adjusted according to determinations of the 12-h cyclosporine trough concentrations. The recommended levels of CyA or CyG were 160–240 ng/ml during the 1st month after transplantation, 100–160 ng/ml during the 2nd and 3rd months, and 60–120 ng/ml thereafter. Azathioprine was given in a dose of 2 mg/kg bw per day during the 1st month and 1 mg/kg bw per day thereafter. Prednisolone was given in an initial dose of 100 mg/day and then reduced by 10 mg/day until day 9, when a dose of 20 mg/day was reached. The dose was then further reduced until a maintenance dose of 10 mg/day was reached at 3 months. During transplantation a single dose of 500 mg methylprednisolone was given intravenously (i. v.).

Offprint requests to: S. Ohlman, MD, Department of Transplantation Surgery, Huddinge Hospital, S-141 86 Huddinge, Sweden

Table 1. Patient characteristics

Treatment group	CyG	CyA
No. of patients	5	5
Mean age ± SD (years)	43 ± 5	52 ± 13
Sex M:F	3:2	3:2
End-stage renal disease		
Chronic glomerulonephritis	1	1
Pyelonephritis	2	2
Polycystic kidney disease	1	1
Reflux nephropathy	0	1
Nephrocalcinosis	1	0
Pretransplant blood transfusion		
0	3	3
≥ 1	2	2
Cold ischemia time (h)	13.4 ± 4.6	9.9 ± 8.1
Donor age ± SD (years)	60 ± 4	43 ± 17
Mismatches in HLA-A/B		
0	0	0
1	2	1
2	1	2
3	2	1
4	0	1
Mismatches in HLA-DR		
0	2	0
1	0	3
2	3	2

Cy, cyclosporine

Diagnosis of acute rejection and nephrotoxicity. Acute rejection episodes were diagnosed by clinical criteria in combination with positive findings from fine needle aspiration biopsies (FNAB) and/or core needle biopsies. Acute rejections were treated with i. v. pulses of methylprednisolone for 4 consecutive days (total dose 1.25 g). If this treatment was insufficient, antithymocyte globulin (ATG, Fresenius, FRG) was given i. v. for 7 days in a dose of 3 mg/kg bw.

Acute cyclosporine nephrotoxicity was assumed to exist if there was an increase in serum creatinine that had no other cause and the biopsy showed isometric vacuolization of the tubular epithelium.

Analyses. Whole blood sampling for analyses of the CyA and CyG levels was performed 10–12 h after dosing. Sampling was performed 3–5 times weekly until discharge, then twice weekly during the first 3 months and thereafter at each outpatient visit (once to twice monthly). The CyA was analyzed by specific monoclonal radioimmunoassay (RIA; Incstar Cyclotrac-SP). The intra- and interassay coefficients of variation for this method were 6.0% and 7.0%, respectively, and the limit of determination was 25 ng/ml. The CyG was analyzed by high performance liquid chromatography (HPLC), using a minor modification of the method described by Shibata et al. [29]. This assay had an intraassay coefficient varying from 3.1% to 7.0%. The interassay coefficient of variation was 7.2%. The limit of determination for this method was 20 ng/ml. In addition to cyclosporine trough level monitoring, frequent blood samples were taken during a 12-h dosage interval (0, 0.5, 1, 1.5, 2, 3, 4, 6, 8, 10, and 12 h after the dose) at 3 and 6 months after transplantation for calculation of the area under the concentration-versus-time curves (AUC) of CyG and A and the mean concentrations during the steady state. The AUC was calculated by the linear trapezoidal method.

Sampling for routine blood chemistry, hematology, and urine analyses was performed daily during hospitalization; additional investigations were performed twice weekly and once weekly from the time of discharge to month 3, twice monthly during months 4–6, and once monthly thereafter. The kidney function was monitored by se-

rial determinations of the serum creatinine levels and endogenous creatinine clearance. In addition, assessment of the glomerular filtration rate (GFR), using the chromium-ethylene diamine tetraacetic acid (EDTA) clearance method, was performed at 3 months after transplantation. When patients were switched from CyG to CyA, no further comparative evaluation of laboratory parameters was carried out.

Percutaneous transplant biopsies were performed at the time of transplantation and at 2–6 months after transplantation. All biopsies were fixed in 3% buffered formalin and embedded in paraffin by routine procedures. Sections were cut at 3 μm and stained with H & E, Ladewig's trichrome stain, and silver methenamine. Microscopy study of the biopsies was carried out without knowledge of the group to which the patient belonged. The relative volume (volume density) of the renal cortical interstitium was used as the main parameter for evaluating renal interstitial fibrosis, which is the usual finding in chronic cyclosporine nephrotoxicity [33]. In addition to this quantitative analysis, the following histological changes were semiquantitatively assessed on a 0–4 score scale: interstitial inflammation, arteriolar hyalinosis, arteriolar smooth muscle degeneration, arteriolar intimal swelling and thrombosis, arterial intimal fibrosis, arterial signs of chronic vascular rejection, and arterial signs of acute vascular rejection. The occurrence of glomerular changes and of significant interstitial edema was also recorded. The microscopical evaluation procedure has been described previously [38].

Biopsy data were analyzed by linear regression and one-way analysis of variance (ANOVA). For the difference between mean values, Student's *t*-test was used whenever applicable. A *P* value < 0.05 was considered to indicate a significant difference.

Results

Both preparations of cyclosporine were in general well tolerated. At the end of the follow-up period (1 year after transplantation), patient survival was 100% in both groups. In the CyG group one graft was lost 8 months after transplantation, due to rejection. In dhe CyA group one graft never functioned. When the graft was removed 1 month after transplantation, it showed severe signs of rejection. Thus, the graft survival was 80% in both groups at the end of the follow-up period.

Renal function, as expressed by the serum creatinine level and endogenous creatinine clearance, did not differ between the two groups during the first 2 months after transplantation (Table 2). Chromium-EDTA clearance at 3 months after transplantation did not differ between the CyG and the CyA groups (28.0 ± 10.6 ml/min and 28.3 ± 8.2 ml/min, respectively). Evaluation of the biopsy material showed no difference between the groups regarding fibrosis at the time of transplantation. In the follow-up biopsies, however, a statistically significant difference between the groups was found regarding the relative volume of the cortical interstitium. The mean interstitial volume was lower in the CyA-treated patients than in the CyG-treated group (33.5 ± 5.6 and 42.5 ± 3.4, respectively, $P < 0.05$) (Fig. 1). No statistically significant difference was found between any of the other parameters measured.

All patients in the study experienced at least one episode of rejection. The number of rejection episodes was 11 in the CyG group and 9 in the CyA group.

Two episodes of biopsy-verified acute cyclosporine nephrotoxicity were diagnosed in the CyA group and 1 in the CyG group.

Table 2. Blood chemistry results 2, 4, and 8 weeks after transplantation in the CyG- and in CyA-treated patients (reference limits for healthy subjects are given within parentheses)

	Two weeks		Four weeks		Eight weeks	
	CyG (n = 5)	CyA (n = 4)	CyG (n = 5)	CyA (n = 4)[a]	CyG (n = 3)[b]	CyA (n = 4)[a]
Creatinine clearance (ml/min) (85–145)	38.5 ± 4.9	44.7 ± 15.11	40.3 ± 7.0	36.3 ± 3.2	56.3 ± 6.7	37.7 ± 8.0
Serum creatinine (μmol/l) (< 120)	272.0 ± 110.7	179.8 ± 66.4	211.5 ± 32.2	289.8 ± 199.6	185.7 ± 14.2	178.0 ± 39.4
Serum urea (mmol/l) (3.0–7.5)	25.6 ± 11.3	12.5 ± 3.9	16.9 ± 5.8	23.3 ± 15.7	16.8 ± 3.0	15.4 ± 6.4
Serum bilirubin (μmol/l) (< 26)	30.8 ± 9.9	7.8 ± 1.6***	13.2 ± 4.2	13.7 ± 7.0	11.7 ± 4.9	9.7 ± 3.9
Serum ALAT (μkat/l)	1.6 ± 0.5	0.4 ± 0.3**	1.8 ± 1.9	0.3 ± 0.1	0.8 ± 0.7	0.3 ± 0.1
Serum ASAT (μkat/l) (< 0.7)	1.2 ± 0.7	0.3 ± 0.2*	0.6 ± 0.5	0.2 ± 0.1	0.4 ± 0.2	0.3 ± 0.1
Serum AP (μkat/l) (< 4.2)	2.6 ± 0.7	2.8 ± 1.1	4.0 ± 1.7	4.3 ± 0.9	3.4 ± 0.3	3.6 ± 1.0
Serum albumin (g/l) (35–46)	25.8 ± 2.1	27.3 ± 1.7	28.3 ± 5.1	29.3 ± 2.5	27.7 ± 2.9	31.0 ± 2.0
B-Hemoglobin (g/l) (115–165)	93.2 ± 17.2	90.6 ± 8.3	91.8 ± 15.4	95.8 ± 11.6	111.0 ± 11.1	119.8 ± 14.6

*** $P < 0.001$, ** $P < 0.005$, * $P < 0.02$
[a] One patient with a nonfunctioning graft posttransplant is excluded
[b] Two patients who switched to CyA therapy are excluded

ALAT, alanine aminotransferase; ASAT, aspartate aminotransferase; AP, alkaline phosphatase

The doses of CyG and CyA administered are shown in Fig. 2. During the first 2 months the trough levels of cyclosporine were higher than recommended in both groups (Fig. 2). Although the doses were significantly ($P < 0.05$) lower in the CyG group during the first 5 weeks, the trough levels were higher in this group at 2 weeks after transplantation. The doses of azathioprine and prednisolone did not differ between the two groups. The CyG trough concentration/dose ratio was higher than that in CyA-treated patients (intraindividual mean

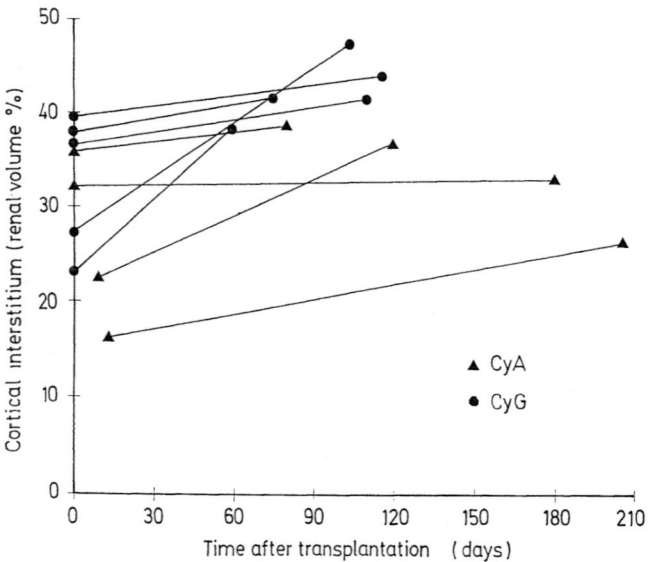

Fig. 1. Relationship between cortical interstitial volume and time interval between transplantation and biopsy in renal allograft biopsies from CyA- and CyG-treated patients with functioning grafts

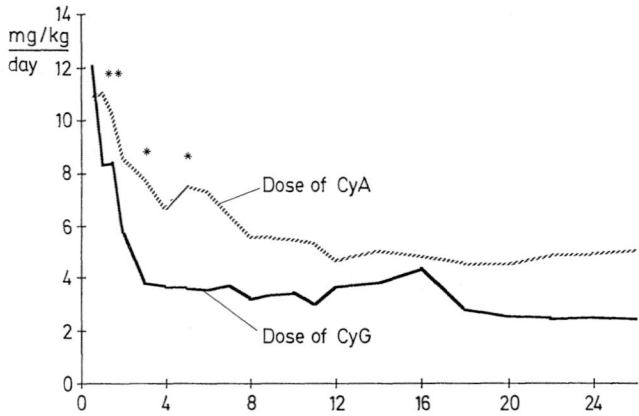

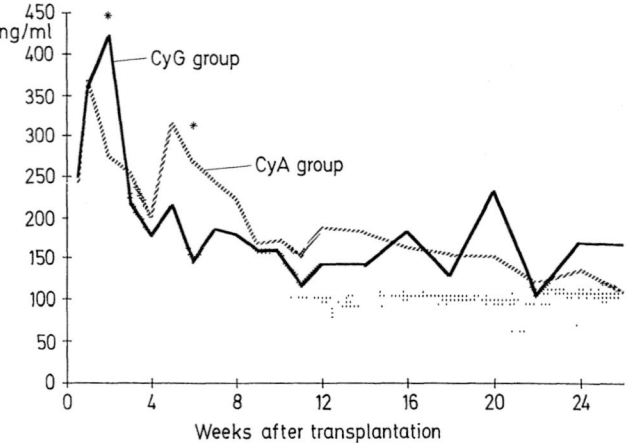

Fig. 2. Administered doses of CyA/CyG *(top)* and trough CyA/CyG concentrations *(bottom),* mean values. *Asterisks* indicate significant differences: * $P < 0.05$, ** $P < 0.01$ *(shaded areas* indicate intended levels)

0.79 ± 0.23 ng/ml·mg versus 0.53 ± 0.11 ng/ml·mg in the respective groups between 14 and 80 days after transplantation; $P < 0.05$), which would suggest that there is a difference in the pharmacokinetics of the drugs. However, the dose-adjusted 12-h AUCs at 3 and 6 months after transplantation did not differ between the groups. At 3 months the dose-adjusted AUCs were 1152, 627, and 680 ng·h/ml·mg in the CyG-treated patients and 809, 398, 872, and 497 ng·h/ml·mg in the CyA-treated patients (n.s.). Furthermore, the dose-adjusted 12-h AUCs at 6 months after transplantation did not differ significantly from those at 3 months in either group.

Marked signs of hepatotoxicity were observed in all patients in the CyG group (Table 2). Serum bilirubin, alanine and aspartate aminotransferase (ALAT, ASAT) activities were significantly higher in the CyG group during the 1st month after transplantation, but the serum alkaline phosphatase activity did not differ between the two groups (Fig. 3). The pathological liver chemistry in the CyG group was reversible after reduction of the CyG dose in all but 1 patient. In that patient, the liver enzymes normalized after switching to CyA. One patient in the CyG group suffered from severe headache during the weeks following transplantation and was also icteric at that time. Apart from hepatotoxicity, all other blood chemistry and hematology parameters were in the normal range and did not differ between the two groups during the first 2 months following transplantation (Table 2). No other adverse effects were recorded.

As study end-point it was decided that patients in the CyG group who had more than one rejection episode should be switched to CyA. This was the case in 3 patients who were switched to CyA after 1.5, 2, and 4.5 months of treatment. Another patient was switched to CyA therapy 3 months posttransplant, at his own request. Shortly after this, one patient experienced an acute rejection episode that was successfully treated. The concentrations of CyG and CyA before and after changing the preparation were adequate in this patient. Otherwise, no alterations in graft function were observed after switching from CyG to CyA. The single patient who remained on the study drug at the end of the follow-up period (1 year after transplantation) was given CyA 16 months after transplantation because it was decided to terminate the study. Before and after this, the patient has been doing well, with good and stable graft function.

Discussion

The immunosuppressive potential of CyG compared with CyA has been a matter of debate. The initial reports by Hiestand et al. [18, 19] implied that the immunosuppressive potencies were equivalent in the rat model (skin, heart, and kidney grafts). These findings were later supported by Grant et al. [14]. An identical immunosuppressive efficacy after liver transplantation in dogs was also reported [34]. In a similar type of canine model, Calne et al. suggested that CyG was more effective than CyA, but in that study the concentrations of CyG were higher than those of CyA [5]. Studies in rats undergoing heart

and lung transplantation, however, have suggested that CyG is less effective than CyA [28].

Conflicting reports have been presented regarding the pharmacological profile of CyG, as compared with that of CyA. Several groups have reported higher concentrations of CyG than of CyA when both drugs were given in equal doses. This finding was noted in both transplanted [5, 14, 34] and in nontransplanted animals [12, 16, 36]. It has been thought to be due to a lower clearance of CyG rather than to greater absorption from the gastrointestinal tract [15, 36]. However other studies indicate the attainment of equal CyG and CyA concentrations [7, 9, 17], or even lower concentrations of CyG [26], with equivalent dose administration. The general conclusion has been that there are both species [5] and strain [7, 9, 18, 19] differences in the absorption, metabolism, and excretion of the two cyclosporine analogues. Most of these analyses were performed with the polyclonal radioimmunoassay (RIA) method which gave a high cross-reactivity to drug metabolites. One possible explanation for the higher CyG levels found in most studies is that the CyG-induced hepatotoxicity reduces the clearance of metabolites and results in higher polyclonal RIA levels. Such an increased metabolite/parent compound ratio has been observed in CyA-treated patients with cholestasis or hepatic dysfunction after living transplantation [30, 39]. In a previous study in which CyG was administered to 6 nontransplanted patients with renal failure [37], the pharmacokinetics, as analysed by HPLC, were similar to those described for CyA in a corresponding patient population [13]. This finding suggests that the same dose strategies would apply for CyG use in man as those that have been established for CyA. In the present study, CyA and CyG levels were determined by specific monoclonal RIA and HPLC, respectively. Both of these levels were found to be higher than intended, in spite of the drug monitoring and frequent dose adjustments (Fig. 3). Furthermore, the concentration/dose ratio was somewhat higher for CyG than for CyA, although the AUCs in the two groups at one time did not differ. These data suggest that the pharmacokinetics of the two drugs may differ.

Hiestand and colleagues initially reported that CyG was neither nephrotoxic nor hepatotoxic in Wistar rats [18, 19]. In the same type of model, Faraci et al. [12] reported that CyG was less nephrotoxic than CyA, but more hepatotoxic. The lower nephrotoxicity in rats was also described by others [8, 16, 23]. In contrast, Duncan et al. [9, 10] reported that CyG shared the nephro- and hepatotoxic properties of CyA, at least in the high dose of 50 mg kg/bw per day, in Sprague-Dawley rats. By using a lower dose (25 mg kg/bw per day), Tejani et al. [32] observed less nephrotoxicity after CyG administration than after CyA in the same model. In the dog model, Calne et al. [5] suggested that CyG might be less nephrotoxic than CyA. Previous clinical experience is limited and consists of 12 patients who received CyG (initial dose 12 mg/kg daily) as primary therapy along with steroids for 3 months after transplantation [20]. The patients were then switched to other types of immunosuppression. The 1-year graft survival was 70%. In that study 6 patients showed clear signs of reversible hepatotoxicity. An addi-

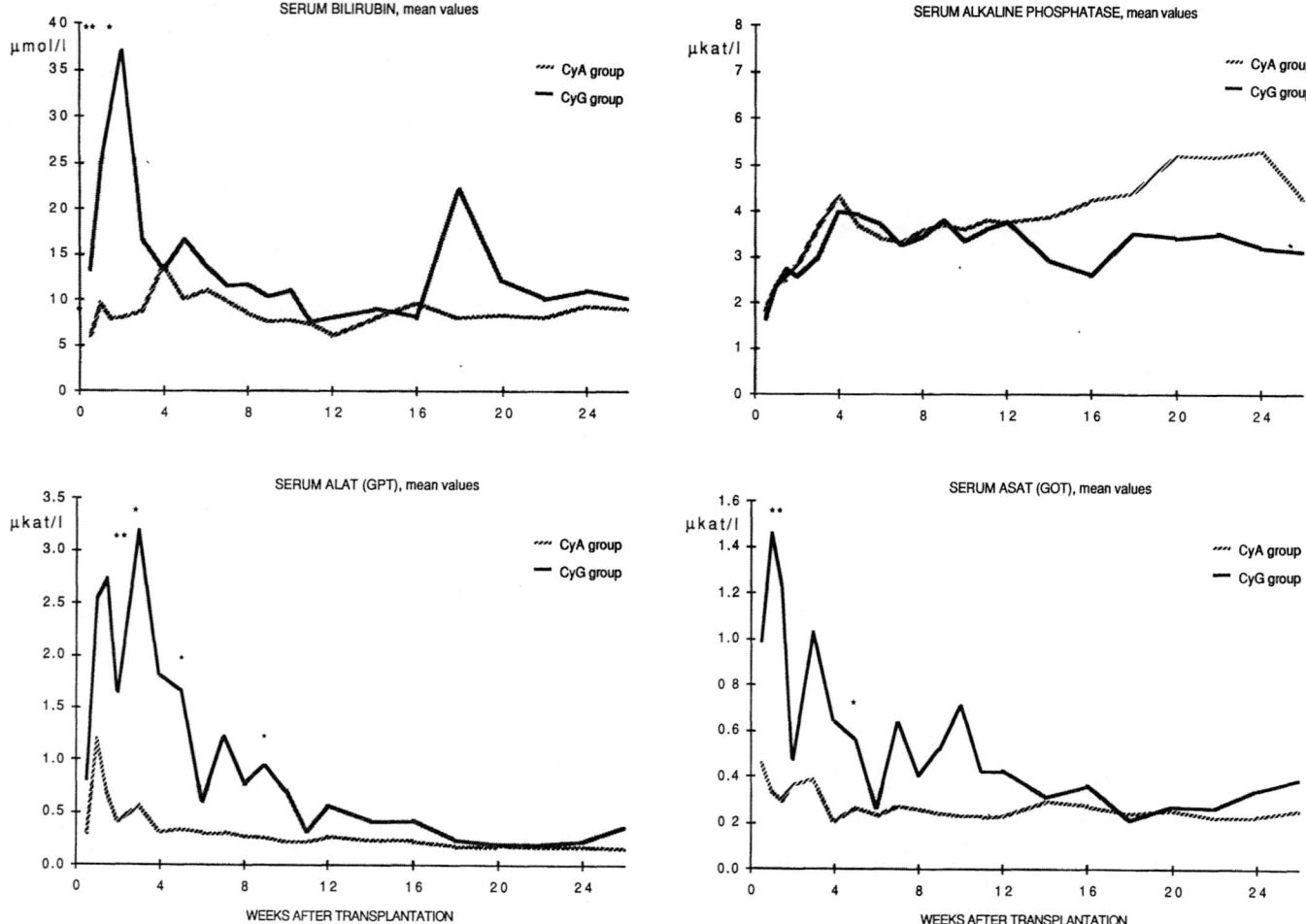

Fig. 3. The mean values of serum bilirubin, alkaline phosphatase, ALAT and ASAT in the CyA- and CyG-treated groups. *Asterisks* indicate significant differences: * $P < 0.05$, ** $P < 0.01$ (*shaded areas* indicate reference limits in healthy subjects)

tional 6 patients showed clear signs of reversible hepatotoxicity. An additional 6 patients with preexisting CyA-induced nephrotoxicity were converted to CyG for 6–12 months without any beneficial effect on renal function [1]. One of these patients experienced transient hyperbilirubinemia in conjunction with high whole blood CyG concentrations (1367 ng/ml, target concentration 250–600 ng/ml). In these studies the CyG doses were high and the CyG concentrations were much higher than intended.

In the present study we found that CyG like CyA can cause acute episodes of impaired renal function. The renal function, as expressed by laboratory parameters, did not differ between the two groups during the study period. In the follow-up biopsies we observed a significantly higher degree of fibrosis in the CyG group, but these data must be interpreted with caution because of the small number of patients. One must also take into account that 2 of the CyG patients had been switched to CyA 1 month prior to the follow-up biopsies. We found, however, that CyG was definitely more hepatotoxic than CyA. This hepatotoxicity was mainly observed during the first weeks after transplantation, when the dose given and the blood levels of CyG were highest. The pathological liver values normalized in all but 1 case when the dose of CyG was reduced.

In conclusion, we noted no clear advantages with the use of CyG as compared with CyA in renal transplantation. Its immunosuppressive properties were not superior to those of CyA, nor was there any indication that it was less nephrotoxic. CyG was, however, significantly more hepatotoxic than CyA. Our protocol allowed for the inclusion of more patients after the evalution of the first 10 patients. However, with the results obtained it was not thought justifiable to enter any additional patients.

Acknowledgments. We are grateful to Sandoz Pharma Ltd. for their support and for supplying the study drug. We thank Birgit Blom, R.N., for the meticulous collection of data and Britta Ekqvist for help with the analyses.

References

1. Beveridge T, Gugerli U, Huser B, Thiel G (1987) OG 37-325 tolerability/efficacy and first pilot studies in organ transplantation. Sandoz, Basel
2. Calne RY (1987) Cyclosporine in cadaveric renal transplantation: 5-year follow-up of a multicentre trial. Lancet 2: 506–507
3. Calne RY, Wood AJ (1985) Cyclosporin in cadaveric renal transplantation: 3-year follow-up of a European multicentre trial. Lancet 2: 549

4. Calne RY, White DJG, Thiru S (1978) Cyclosporivne A in patients receiving renal allografts from cadaver donors. Lancet II: 1323–1327

5. Calne RY, White DJG, Thiru S, Rolles K, Drakopoulos S, Jamieson NV (1985) Cyclosporin G: immunosuppressive effect in dogs with renal allografts. Lancet I: 1342

6. Canadian Multicenter Transplant Study Group (1983) A randomized clinical trial of cyclosporine in cadaveric renal transplantation. N Engl J Med 309: 809–815

7. Collier St J, Calne RY, White DJG, Winters S, Thiru S (1986) Blood levels and nephrotoxicity of cyclosporin A and G in rats. Lancet I: 216

8. Donatsch P, Ruffel D (1986) Effects of cyclosporine A and G on renal function. Experientia 42: 668

9. Duncan JI, Whiting PH, Simpson JG, Thomson A (1985) Nephrotoxicity of cyclosporin G in rats. Lancet II: 1004–1005

10. Duncan JI, Thomson AW, Simpson JG, Davidson RJL, Whiting PH (1986) A comparative toxicological study of cyclosporine and Nva²-cyclosporine in Sprague-Dawley rats. Transplantation 42: 395–399

11. European Multicentre Trial Group (1983) Cyclosporine in cadaveric renal transplantation: one-year follow-up of a multicentre trial. Lancet II: 986–989

12. Faraci M, Vigeant C, Yale JF (1988) Pharmacokinetic profile of cyclosporine A and G and their effects on cellular immunity and glucose tolerance in male and female Wistar rats. Transplantation 45: 617–621

13. Follath F, Wenk M, Vozeh S, Thiel G, Brunner F, Loertscher R, Lemaire M, Nussbaumer K, Niederberger W, Wood A (1983) Intravenous cyclosporine kinetics in renal failure. Clin Pharmacol Ther 34: 638–643

14. Grant D, Zhong R, Stiller C, Wallace C, Keown P, Duff J (1987) A comparison of cyclosporin A and Nva²-cyclosporine (cyclosporine G) in a rat allograft model. Transplantation 44: 9–12

15. Grant D, Freeman P, Keown P, Stiller C, Toman A, Blacker K (1987) Pharmacokinetic and pharmacodynamic profiles of cyclosporine and cyclosporine G in dogs. Transplant Proc 19: 3494–3495

16. Grant Hoyt E, Billingham ME, Maseh MA, Morris RE, Baldwin JC, Jamieson SW (1985) Assessment of cyclosporine G, a new immunosuppressant agent. Heart Transplant 4: 616

17. Hagberg RC, Hoyt EG, Billingham ME, Sibley RK, Starnes VA, Baldwin JC (1988) Comparison of cyclosporin A and G with and without azathioprine regarding immunosuppressive efficacy, toxicity and pharmacokinetics in Lewis rats. J Heart Transplant 7: 359–369

18. Hiestand PC, Gunn HC, Gale JM, Ryffel B, Borel JF (1985) Comparison of the pharmacological profiles of cyclosporine, (Nva²)-cyclosporine and (Val²)dihydrocyclosporine. Immunology 55: 249–255

19. Hiestand PC, Gunn H, Gale J, Siegl H, Ryffel B, Donatsch P, Borel JF (1985) The immunosuppressive profile of a new natural cyclosporine analogue: Nva²-cyclosporine. Transplant Proc 17: 1362–1364

20. Huser B, Landmann J, Mihatsch M, Bianchi L, Thiel G (1987) Clinical pilot study with cyclosporine G in kidney transplant recipients. Kidney Int 32: 431

21. Lundgren G, Groth C-G, Albrechtsen D, Brynger H, Flatmark A, Frödin L, Gäbel H, Husberg B, Klintmalm G, Maurer W, Persson H, Thorsby E (1986) HLA-matching and pretransplant blood transplantations in cadaveric renal transplantation – a changing picture with cyclosporine. Lancet II: 66–69

22. Lundgren G, Albrechtsen D, Brynger H, Flatmark A, Frödin I, Gäbel H, Persson H, Groth CG (1987) Improved early course after cadaveric renal transplantation by reducing the cyclosporine dose and adding azathioprine. Transplant Proc 19: 2074–2079

23. Masri MA, Naiem M, Pingle S, Daar AS (1988) Cyclosporine A versus cyclosporine G: a comparative study of survival, hepatotoxicity, nephrotoxicity and splenic atrophy in BALB/c mice. Transplant Int 1: 13–18

24. Myers BD (1986) Cyclosporine nephrotoxicity. Kidney Int 30: 964–974

25. Myers BD, Ross J, Newton, Luetscher J, Perlroth M (1984) Cyclosporine-associated chronic nephropathy. N Engl J Med 311: 699–705

26. Ogunnaike HO, Starkey TD, Baldwin JC, Porter KA, Billingham ME, Jamieson SW (1987) An assessment of Nva²-cyclosporine in primate cardiac transplantation. Transplantation 43: 13–17

27. Porter GA, Bennett WM (1986) Chronic cyclosporine-associated nephrotoxicity. Transplant Proc 18: 204–209

28. Prop J, Hoyt EG, Jamieson SW (1987) (Nva²)-cyclosporine – less potent than cyclosporin A in rats with lung and heart transplants. Transplantation 44: 5–8

29. Shibata N, Minoucki T, Hayashi Y, Ono T, Shimakawa H (1987) Qualitative determination of cyclosporin A in whole blood and plasma by high performance liquid chromatography. Res Commun Chem Path Pharmacol 57: 261–271

30. Sommerauer JF, Grant D, Freeman D, Mineault R, Duff J, Wall W (1989) Effect of cholestasis on cyclosporine metabolism in the pig. Transplant Proc 21: 835–836

31. Stiller CR (1984) Update for the Canadian multicenter trial of cyclosporine in renal allografts. N Engl J Med 310: 1464–1465

32. Tejani A, Lancman I, Pomrantz A, Khawar M, Chen C (1988) Nephrotoxicity of cyclosporine A and cyclosporine G in a rat model. Transplantation 45: 184–187

33. Thiru S, Mahler ER, Hamilton DV, Evans DB, Calne RY (1983) Tubular changes in renal transplant recipients on cyclosporine. Transplant Proc 15 [Suppl 1]: 2846–2851

34. Todo S, Porter KA, Kam I, Lynch S, Venkataramanan R, DeWolf A, Starzl TE (1986) Canine liver transplantation under Nva²-cyclosporine versus cyclosporine. Transplantation 41: 296–300

35. Traber R, Loosli HR, Hoffmann H, Kuhn M, Von Wartburg A (1982) Isolierung und Strukturermittlung der neuen cyclosporine E, F, G, H and I. Helv Chir Acta 65: 1655–1677

36. Venkataramanan R, Todo S, Zaghloul I, Lynch S, Kam I, Ptachinski RJ, Burckart GJ, Starzl TE (1987) Comparative pharmacokinetics of cyclosporine and Nva²-cyclosporine in dogs. Transplant Proc 19: 1265–1266

37. Wenk M, Bindschedler M, Costa E, Zuber M, Vozeh S, Thiel G, Abisch E, Keller HP, Beveridge T. Follath F (1988) Pharmacokinetics of cyclosporine G in patients with renal failure. Transplantation 45: 558–561

38. Wilczek H (1989) Renal allograft biopsy. Core and fine needle biopsy techniques for acute diagnosis and long-term follow-up. Academic thesis, Huddinge Hospital, Karolinska Institute, study III, pp 12–14

39. Wonigeit K, Kohlhaw K, Winkler M, Schaefer O, Pichlmayr R (1990) Cyclosporine monitoring in liver allograft recipients: two distinct patterns of blood level derangement associated with nephrotoxicity. Transplant Proc 22: 1305–1311

Transplant Int (1992) 5 [Suppl 1]: S 470–S 472

TRANSPLANT
International
© Springer-Verlag 1992

Long-term immunosuppression after liver transplantation: are steroids necessary?

R. T. A. Padbury, B. K. Gunson, B. Dousset, S. G. Hubscher, A. D. Mayer, J. A. C. Buckels, J. M. Neuberger, E. Elias, and P. McMaster

The Liver Unit, Queen Elizabeth Hospital, Edgbaston, Birmingham, United Kingdom

Abstract. Steroid therapy was withdrawn in 85 % of 152 orthotopic liver transplant recipients with grafts surviving for more than 3 months, and 87 % of these remained steroid-free. Steroid therapy was restarted in 8 % for reasons other than rejection. The most common was conversion of immunosuppression because of cyclosporine nephrotoxicity. The incidence of rejection after steroid withdrawal was low: 3.8 % for chronic rejection (CR) and 4.5 % for acute rejection. Only 3 grafts (1.9 %) were lost because of CR. No risk factors have been identified for the development of CR after steroid withdrawal, but a protective role for azathioprine has been suggested.

Key words: Immunosuppression – Steroids – Liver transplantation

Maintenance immunosuppression (IS) after orthotopic liver transplantation (OLT) in the cyclosporine (CyA) era has consisted of CyA in combination with prednisolone (PRED) or PRED and azathioprine (AZA). Long-term IS without steroids is not widely practised in liver transplant recipients.

Long-term IS without steroids is possible in approximately 30 %–50 % of kidney recipients [1–4]. Cessation of steroids at 3–6 months in patients with stable graft function has been achieved at the expense of higher rates of rejection, but with no difference in long-term patient or graft survival. In one randomised controlled trial, there was a significant reduction in the incidence of steroid-related complications in the patients who remained free of steroids [1].

It has been the policy of the Birmingham unit to taper the PRED dose down to withdrawal from the IS regimen by the end of the 3rd postoperative month. The aims of this study were to examine the rate of graft rejection in patients after cessation of PRED and to identify retrospectively risk factors for the development of chronic rejection (CR) in this cohort.

Materials and methods

Patients and grafts. There were 312 grafts in 271 adult (> 15 y) patients transplanted between Jan 1982 and June 1990 (M:F = 32 % : 68 %). A total of 197 (63 %) grafts in 177 patients (65 %) survived for more than 3 months and were therefore eligible for steroid withdrawal. PRED was stopped in 168 (85 %) of these grafts. Reasons for the non-withdrawal of PRED are given in Table 1.

In 14 grafts steroids were recommenced for reasons other than rejection (Table 2); it is the remaining 154 grafts in 152 patients (M:F = 31 % : 69 %; median age 48 years, range 16–68) that were studied (i.e. in patients in whom PRED had been stopped and was restarted only if a rejection episode occurred). In this group there were 143 first grafts, 10 second grafts, and 1 third graft.

Immunosuppression. There were 2 induction IS protocols used during this period, the details of which are given in Table 3. Episodes of acute rejection were treated with 200 mg p. o. prednisolone for 3 consecutive days and repeated if necessary for incomplete resolution.

Table 1. Reasons for non-withdrawal of steroids at 3 months after transplantation

	No. of patients
Early ductopoenic rejection	8
Poor condition and biliary complications	7
Previous graft loss (rejection)	3
Followed elsewhere	3
Miscellaneous	3
Unknown	3

Table 2. Reasons for recommencement of steroids

	No. of patients
CyA nephrotoxicity	6
CyA neurotoxicity	1
Musculoskeletal pain	4
Colitis	2
Other	1

CyA, cyclosporine A

Offprint requests to: R. T. A. Padbury, Liver Unit, Queen Elizabeth Hospital, Edgbaston, Birmingham B15 2TH, United Kingdom

Table 3. Immunosuppression protocols

	1982–1987 Double	Route of application	1987→ Triple
Induction			
Hydrocortisone	200 mg/day	p.o.	200 mg/day
Prednisolone	20 mg/day	p.o.	20 mg/day
CyA	2–5 mg/kg	i.v.	2 mg/kg
	10–15 mg/kg	p.o.	10 mg/kg
AZA			1–1.5 mg/kg
Prednisolone reduction	20 mg for weeks 1–3		
	15 mg for weeks 4–6		
	10 mg for weeks 7–9		
	5 mg for weeks 10–12		
	cease at week 12		
Maintenance	CyA alone		CyA alone or CyA + AZA

AZA, azathioprine

Table 4. Primary indications for orthotopic liver transplantation in study cohort

Primary diagnosis	Frequency	Chronic rejection
Primary biliary cirrhosis (PBC)	72[a]	1
Fulminant	23[a]	1
Primary sclerosing cholangitis	13	2[b,c]
Cryptogenic cirrhosis	13	
Tumours	12	2[b]
Metabolic	8	
Hepatitis B	6	
Autoimmune CAH	3	
Budd-Chiari syndrome	3	
Other	1	

[a] One patient had 2 grafts

[b] NS compared with PBC

[c] One patient had an incidental cholangiocarcinoma

Table 5. Influence of the severity of acute rejection

Acute rejection	Chronic rejection	No chronic rejection
None/mild, no treatment	2	31
Mild-moderate	4	75
Moderate-severe	0	35

For severe or recurrent episodes 1 g methylprednisolone i.v. was given. OKT3 was given if the rejection was steroid-resistant (that is, failure to respond to 2 courses of increased quantities of steroids).

PRED was stopped at 3 months or later if the graft function was not stable at this time (median 3 months, range 1–15). AZA, used as part of the triple therapy protocol from 1987 onwards, was stopped in some patients and continued in others at the discretion of the attending consultant (mean 3 months range 1–32; $n = 67$). In 57 grafts, the long-term IS regimen was CyA and AZA double therapy, and in the other 97, CyA monotherapy (induction IS: 30 CyA + PRED; 67 CyA + AZA + PRED). The CyA dose was adjusted to maintain whole blood levels between 100 and 250 ng/ml as measured by monoclonal whole blood radioimmunoassay.

Biopsies, follow-up, and rejection. Percutaneous biopsies were performed routinely 7 days post-OLT and as clinically indicated thereafter. Protocol biopsies were also performed during patient readmission for annual review.

Follow-up in these patients was continued until July 1991, giving a minimum potential follow-up of 12 months (actual follow-up mean 28 months, range 5–109). At 12 months or later biopsies were obtained in 137 grafts (mean 24 months, range 8–78). In 8 grafts the biopsies were either contraindicated or the patients refused, and in a further 9, death or graft loss occurred prior to 12 months.

Definitions of graft rejection were as follows:
Acute rejection (AR) histological features of acute cellular rejection with biochemical changes (bilirubin, aspartate aminotransferase, AST, and alkaline phosphatase, ALP). Episodes of AR were graded histologically as mild, moderate, or severe [5].

Chronic rejection, histological features of chronic or ductopoenic rejection [5] with biochemical changes.

Risk factors. The following risk factors for the development of CR were examined (comparisons by univariate analysis, χ^2 or Fisher's exact test; significance level $P = 0.01$): the primary indication for OLT, previous AR, previous OKT3 for steroid-resistant rejection, retransplantation, ABO blood group donor/recipient match, cytomegalovirus (CMV) infection, and maintenance CyA monotherapy versus CyA/AZA double therapy.

Results

Rejection

There were 13 episodes of rejection in 12 grafts (8%) after steroid withdrawal. Five grafts developed CR (mean 4.5 months, range 1–44 after PRED withdrawal), 6 grafts developed AR (mean 7 months, range 1 week–33 months), and 1 graft developed AR at 33 months, which resolved, but CR appeared 11 months later. This gives a CR and AR rate of 3.8% and 4.5%, respectively.

Steroids were restarted in 8 of these patients (5%) either permanently or until resolution of the rejection episode. Therefore, of the original 168 who ceased taking PRED, 146 (87%) remained steroid-free.

The AR resolved in all 7 grafts. Of the 6 grafts developing CR, 1 resolved, 2 were regrafted (1 of whom died), 1 is awaiting regraft, and 2 died, principally because of recurrent tumour, but with histological evidence of CR in postmortem sections of the liver. Thus, excluding these latter 2 patients, the incidence of graft loss due to rejection was 1.9% and patient loss, less than 1%.

Risk factors

The primary indications for OLT in the 154 grafts are listed in Table 4. In all, 121 grafts had an episode of treated AR prior to the cessation of PRED (Table 5). None of the grafts which had had a moderate/severe acute rejection developed CR after steroid withdrawal. Moreover, in 5 of these grafts, OKT3 had been used for steroid-resistant rejection. Similarly, CR did not occur in any of the 11 regrafts in this series, 5 of whom had been regrafted because of CR.

Five of the grafts with CR were from the set of 137 ABO blood group identical donor/recipient matches. CR developed in 1 of 4 with an ABO mismatch, and there was no CR in 11 with an ABO compatible match (NS).

A symptomatic cytomegalovirus (CMV) infection occurred in 15 patients. Two of these patients developed CR compared with 4 of the remaining 139 (NS).

CyA monotherapy was the IS regime in all 6 patients with CR versus none of the 57 on CyA and AZA double therapy ($P = 0.058$, NS).

Discussion

It is clear from this study that the cessation of steroid therapy is a safe undertaking in OLT recipients. The incidence of CR developing in grafts in this series (3.8 %) is identical to the incidence of CR developing after 3 months in patients maintained on 10–20 mg/day of PRED as reported by Klintmalm and associates [6]. Furthermore, the incidence of AR of 4.5 % in the present series compares favourably with an incidence of 7.7 % (8/104) occurring after 3 months in their patients. While these 2 groups of patients are not necessarily directly comparable, it is apparent that withdrawing steroids after 3 months, or when graft function is stable, does not lead to an increased rate of rejection.

This is in contrast to the experience with renal grafts. Rejection may occur in 24 %–47 % of renal recipients following steroid withdrawal [1, 2], although long-term patient and graft survival is not compromised. Moreover, successful steroid withdrawal may be achieved in a greater proportion of liver recipients. Some 56 % of renal recipients in whom steroid therapy was withdrawn remained steroid-free [3] (representing 43 % of all recipients with a primary functioning graft), whereas 87 % of the liver recipients in the present series did not require further steroids.

There were no definite risk factors identified for the development of CR after steroid withdrawal. A protective effect of AZA on ductopoenic rejection has been previously described by van Hoek et al. [7], and it is possible that the rejection rate may have been reduced if all patients had remained on CyA and AZA double therapy. However, because the rate of CR is low, further follow-up of these patients is required to determine whether or not there is a clinically significant difference.

It is noteworthy that a number of the risk factors examined may have been considered contraindications to steroid cessation. Grafts in which there had been a previously moderate to severe AR, steroid-resistant AR, and even regrafts, some of which were for CR, were not more susceptible to the development of CR after steroid withdrawal. We propose that the most important factor is stable graft function and that once this has been achieved, steroids may be successfully withdrawn in almost all patients.

References

1. Maiorca R, Cristinelli L, Brunori G, Setti G, Salerni B, De Nobili U, Mittempergher F (1988) Prospective controlled trial of steroid withdrawal after 6 months in renal transplant patients treated with cyclosporine. Transplant Proc 20: 121–125
2. Gulanikar AC, Belitsky P, MacDonald AS, Cohen A, Bitter-Suerman H (1991) Randomised controlled trial of steroids versus no steroids in stable cyclosporin-treated renal graft recipients. Transplant Proc 23: 990–991
3. Tamm M, Thiel G, Huser B, Brunner FP, Mihatsch M, Landmann J (1991) Cyclosporin monotherapy after kidney transplantation. Transplant Proc 23: 997–998
4. Griffin PJA, Salaman JR (1991) Long term results of cyclosporine monotherapy in kidney transplantation. Transplant Proc 23: 992–993
5. Hubscher SG, Buckels JAC, Elias E, McMaster P, Neuberger J (1991) Vanishing bile duct syndrome following liver transplantation – is it reversible? Transplantation 51: 1004–1010
6. Klintmalm GBG, Nery JR, Husberg BS, Gonwa TA, Tillery GW (1989) Rejection in liver transplantation. Hepatology 10: 978–985
Hoek B van, Wiesner RH, Ludwig J, Gores GJ, Moore B, Krom RAF (1991) Combination immunosuppression with azathioprine reduces the incidence of ductopoenic rejection and vanishing bile duct syndrome after liver transplantation. Transplant Proc 23: 1403–1405

Transplant Int (1992) 5 [Suppl 1]: S473–S475

TRANSPLANT
International
© Springer-Verlag 1992

Dosage of OKT3 independent of body weight: a mistake?

M. Bachofen[1], H. Gallati[2], I. Pracht[2], H. Bock[1], J. Landmann[1], and G. Thiel[1]

[1] Division of Nephrology, Departement of Internal Medicine and Surgery, University of Basel
[2] F. Hoffmann-La Roche Ltd., Basel Pharmacology Research, Basel, Switzerland

Abstract. Comparing OKT3 and antithymocyte globulin (ATG) in a prospective study, the dosage difference in regard to body weight (ATG: dependent on body weight/OKT3: independent) does not introduce any obvious source of mistake concerning clinical effectiveness or side effects. One explanation for the lack of influence of body weight may be the high effectiveness of 5 mg of OKT3, reaching a maximal effect even with lower plasma levels in heavier patients. We wonder, therefore, whether the OKT3 dosage could be lowered.

Key words: Immunosuppression – Monoclonal antibodies – OKT3 – Antithymocyte globulin

In renal transplantation OKT3 is administered independently of body weight in fixed doses of 5 or 10 mg/day [1–4] for initial prophylactic immunosuppression or treatment of severe, methylprednisolone-resistant rejection. This obviously contrasts with the usual regimen of antithymocyte and antilymphocyte globulins (ATG, ALG), which are both administered per kilogram of body weight [3]. Therefore, we wondered whether light-weight patients were relatively overdosed or obese patients underdosed with OKT3.

Materials and methods

A total of 71 renal transplanted patients received either OKT3 or ATG in a randomized study from 1990 till 1991. Murine orthoclone OKT3 (Cilag/Ortho) was given prophylactically as a 5 mg i. v. bolus intraoperatively and over the following 6 days in 36 patients (mean age 50.8 years, range 17–70). Intravenous rabbit ATG (Fresenius) was administered to the other 35 patients (mean age 49.7 years, range 18–82) at a dosage of 4 mg/kg daily for the same period of time as OKT3. Both groups received in addition azathioprine (2 mg/kg daily), methylprednisolone i. v. (1.0, 0.5 and 0.25 g on days 0, 1, and 2), prednisone orally (from day 3 at 5 mg/kg daily), and cyclosporine A (2 × 300 mg/day from day 4 on). The i. v. doses of methyl-prednisolone were given 1–4 h prior to the OKT3/ATG administration. In each patient the free OKT3/ATG trough plasma levels were measured 2 to 3 times during the 1 week after transplantation, using an enzyme-linked immunosorbent assay (ELISA) technique (sandwich principal in solid phase technique) with antimouse/antirabbit globulin antibodies. The same plasma samples were also screened for human antimouse antibodies (HAMA) and human antirabbit antibodies (HARA). One OKT3 patient developed HAMA on the 4th day, and his plasma values were therefore excluded from the calculation. HARA did not develop in ATG-treated patients during this early period.

To evaluate the biological effectivness of OKT3 or ATG we measured the level of CD3$^+$ cells (FACS). In order to estimate the clinical success rate we took the plasma creatinine values on days 7 and 28, the number of i. v. methylprednisolone pulses of 0.5 g given for rejection, and the OKT3/ATG retherapies needed for steroid-resistant rejection during the first 30 days after transplantation. Episodes of viral and fungal infections were counted and expressed as the total sum.

The effect of body weight was analyzed in two ways: (a) by plotting the individual data corresponding to their body weight or (b) by dividing both patient groups close to their median body weight (69.5 kg) into a heavy (> 70 kg) or a light subgroup (< 70 kg) and comparing their parameters (median of individual mean values). Thus, the 36 OKT3-treated patients were divided into 18 light patients (L-OKT3) with a median weight 60.9 kg and 18 heavy patients (H-OKT3), with a median weight of 78.3 kg. Correspondingly, the 35 ATG-treated patients were subdivided in 20 light patients (L-ATG) with a median weight of 63.7 kg and 15 heavy patients (H-ATG) with a median weight of 76.4 kg.

The results of all parameters were correlated with individual body weight and compared as well in all 4 subgroups. Statistical significance was calculated by using the regression of all correlations, the Mann-Whitney U-test, and the χ^2 test.

Results

By administering OKT3 in a fixed bolus the L-OKT3 patients received a 40 % higher dosage (0.089 mg/kg daily) than the H-OKT3 ones (0.063 mg/kg daily). This was not the case in the two ATG-treated subgroups, since the median dosage did not differ (3.8 mg/kg daily vs. 3.9 mg/kg daily). The hyperbolic relation between OKT3 dosage and body weight (formula: dose pro kg = 5 mg/patients' body weight) follows an almost linear course in the observed range (Fig. 1), whereas ATG-treated patients of all

Offprint requests to: M. Bachofen, Division of Nephrology, University of Basel, Switzerland

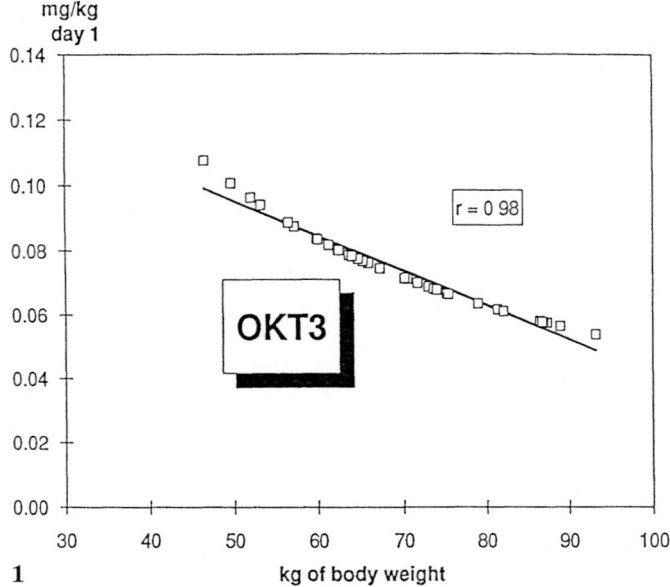

Fig. 1. Correlation of OKT3 dosage (mg/kg) and body weight ($n = 36$) on day 1 after kidney transplantation

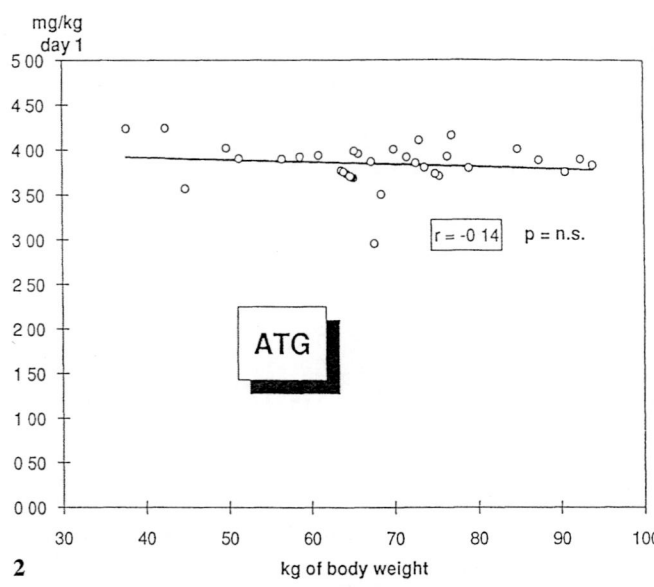

Fig. 2. Correlation of antithymocyte globulin (ATG) dosage (mg/kg) and body weight ($n = 35$) on day 1 after kidney transplantation

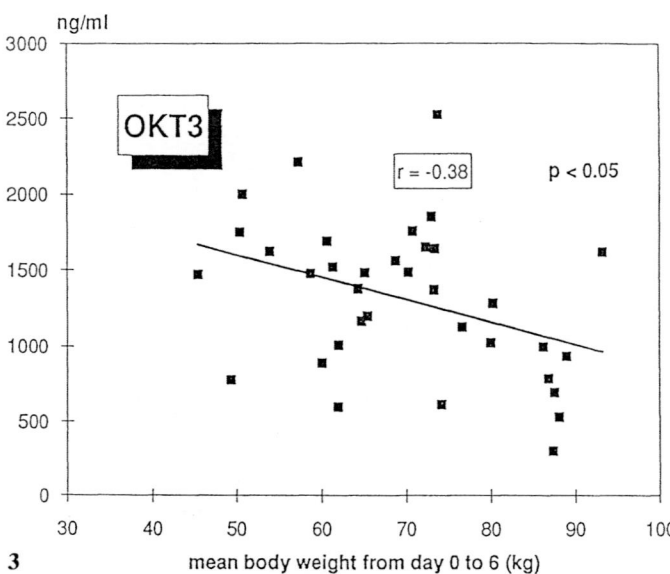

Fig. 3. Correlation of OKT3 mean plasma levels (day 0–6) and body weight

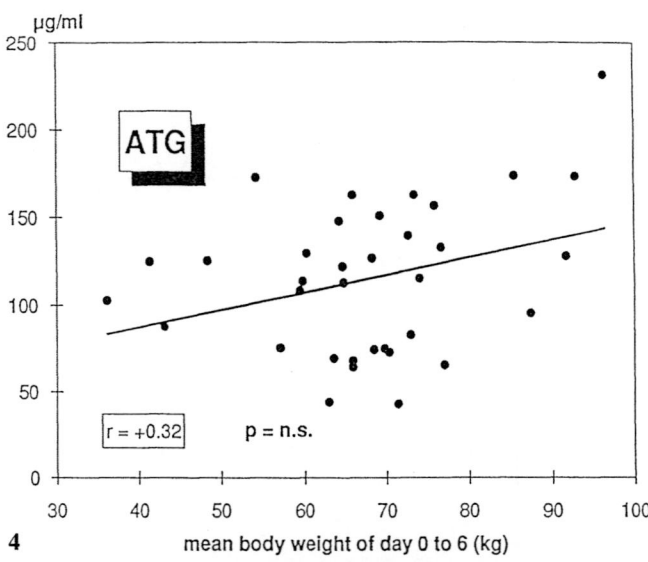

Fig. 4. Correlation of ATG mean plasma levels and body weight

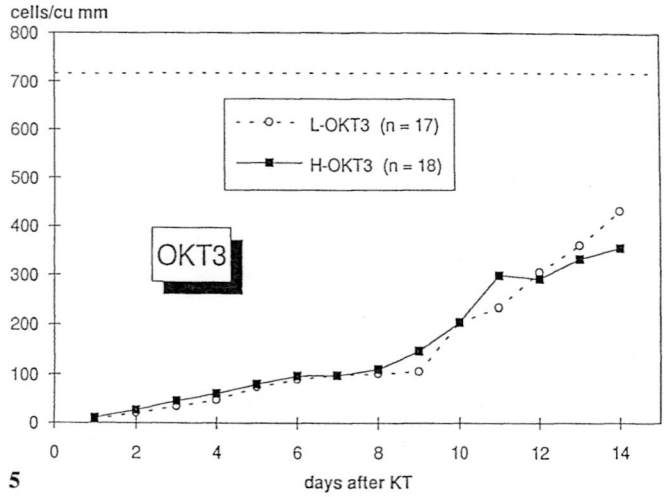

Fig. 5. Median of absolute CD3 count in OKT3-treated patients, below (L)/above (H) 70 kg in weight

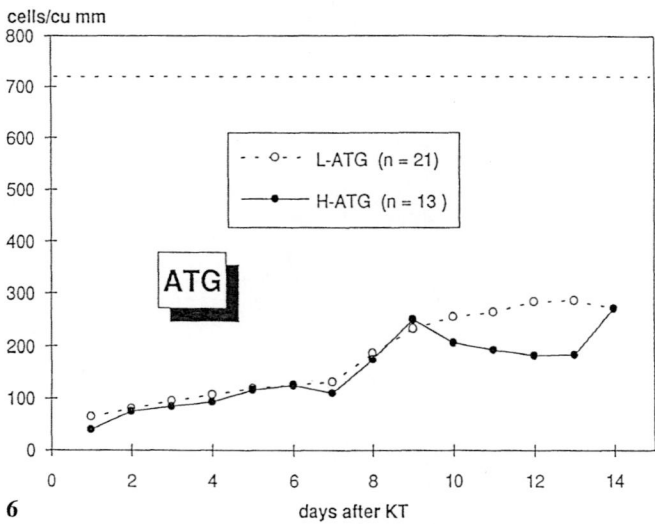

Fig. 6. Median of absolute CD3 count in ATG-treated patients, below (L)/above (H) 70 kg in weight

Table 1. Weight and plasma levels are indicated in median values of the individual mean (days 0–6)

Group	Weight (kg)	n	drug plasma level	Plasma creatinine level		CD3 count absolute (cells/µl)	Methylprednisolone pulses/ patient	OKT3/ATG retherapies	Viral and fungal infections
				Day 7 (µmol/l)	Day 28 (µmol/l)				
OKT3	< 70 (60.9)	18	1478 ng/ml	121	124	52	41/12	5	8
	> 70 (78.3)	18	1205 ng/ml	335	132	55	36/11	5	11
ATG	< 70 (63.7)	20	113 µg/ml	90	99	96	45/11	2	4
	> 70 (76.4)	15	128 µg/ml	124	122	96	27/9	2	3

Methylprednisolone pulses, retherapies, and infections were counted during the first 30 days after kidney transplantation

weight classes had a similar "per kilo dosage" ($r = -0.14$, n.s.) (Fig. 2). Small aberrations were due to the fact that the dosage was calculated with the initial weight and stayed so for the next 6 days independent of weight changes after operation.

As expected, OKT3 mean plasma levels of the first 7 days after kidney transplantation correlate significantly ($P < 0.05$) and inversely with the patients' mean body weight of the same period (Fig. 3). This was not the case in the ATG-treated patients (Fig. 4).

However, despite body weight-dependent blood level differences in OKT3 patients, the CD3-cell count was almost identical for the L-OKT3 and H-OKT3 patients over the first 2 weeks (Fig. 5). This was – not surprisingly – also the case for the L-ATG and H-ATG patients (Fig. 6). All other parameters for the clinical effectiveness of OKT3 (plasma creatinine level at days 7 and 28, number of methylprednisolone pulses, retherapies with OKT3) were not different in the L-OKT3 and H-OKT3 subgroups (Table 1), similar to the L-ATG and H-ATG subgroups.

Finally, the sum of episodes of viral and fungal infections showed no weight-related differences, i.e., was not different among all 4 subgroups.

For all mentioned parameters, correlations with individual body weight were calculated, but the regression analysis was found not to be significantly different in all of them (not shown), besides the OKT3 blood levels and body weight (Fig. 3) noted above.

Discussion

When two antilymphocytic substances like ATG or OKT3 are compared with regard to success in a clinical trial of renal transplantation, one might be disturbed by the fact that one substance is given in a weight-dependent dosage (ATG: 4 mg/kg daily) and the other independent of body weight (OKT3: 5 mg/day). This is particularly the case if the effective body weight among the patients ranges from 36 to 96 kg (ATG) and 45 to 93 kg (OKT3), as in our study. One may anticipate that OKT3 is more effective in lowering the CD3 counts or rejection rate in lighter than in heavier patients. The side effects of overdosage like viral or fungal infection may occur more frequently in light, relatively overdosed patients.

Our findings confirm only a weight-dependent difference in the average OKT3 plasma levels ($P < 0.05$) and – as expected – no such difference in the ATG-treated patients. For ATG there is even a tendency for the plasma concentrations to increase with body weight (n.s., Fig. 4). This might be explained by the higher proportion of adipose tissue in obese patients, which is associated with a relatively smaller volume of distribution of ATG.

The range of our mean OKT3 plasma levels is in agreement with the measurements of Chatenoud et al. [1] and Goldstein et al. [2], but higher than those of Todd and Brogden [4]. As far as we know, there are no published data on ATG Fresenius plasma levels, but our calculated levels with a factor difference of 100 for ATG look reasonable.

Measurements of OKT3 or ATG plasma levels by an ELISA technique have a common error source. The measured plasma level may not represent true free plasma levels of unbound substance; it can also comprise inactivated complexes with antimouse or antirabbit antibodies [1]. However, we tried to avoid this mistake by excluding the plasma samples from the calculation whenever the simultaneous search for HAMA or HARA was positive. Whether our measured plasma levels represent true "free plasma levels" of active OKT3 still remains unclear, since we failed to find a weight-dependent correlation with the CD3 counts. There was no weight dependency either for all parameterse of clinical relevance such as plasma creatinine level or the number of methylprednisolone pulses needed for the treatment of rejection. Another meaningful parameter for effectiveness is the number of retherapies with OKT3 or ATG for the rescue of steroid-resistant rejection. Again, there was no difference in the OKT3 patients above or below 70 kg of body weight. Viral and fungal infections were not increased in the light patients on OKT3 as compared with the heavy ones.

The number of patients in the two groups may be too small to evaluate properly significant differences correlated to body weight. We were even unable to show any trend in favour of body-weight dependency in the OKT3 patients, with the exception of the plasma levels.

References

1. Chatenoud L, Ferran C, Bach J-F (1990) In vivo use of OKT3: main issues for the monitoring of treated patients. Transplant Proc 22: 2605–2608
2. Goldstein G, Fuccello AJ, Norman DJ, Shield CF, Colvin RB, Cosimi AB (1986) OKT3 monoclonal antibody plasma levels during therapy and the subsequent development of host antibodies to OKT3. Transplantation 42: 507–510
3. Shield CF, Norman DJ, Marlett P, Fucello AJ, Goldstein G (1987) Comparison of antimouse and antihorse antibody production during the treatment of allograft rejection with OKT3 or antithymocyte globulin. Nephron 46: 48–51
4. Todd PA, Brogden RN (1989) Drugs focus on muromonab CD3. Reprint. Aids Press, Auckland

Transplant Int (1992) 5 [Suppl 1]: S476–S479

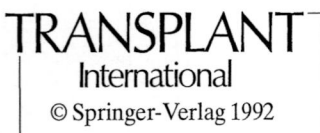

TRANSPLANT
International
© Springer-Verlag 1992

Polyclonal versus monoclonal rejection prophylaxis after heart transplantation: a randomised study

A. H. M. M. Balk, K. Meeter, M. L. Simoons, R. M. L. Brouwer, P. E. Zondervan, B. Mochtar, E. Bos, and W. Weimar

Thoraxcenter and Department of Internal Medicine I, University Hospital Rotterdam – Dijkzigt, Rotterdam, The Netherlands

Abstract. Recent studies comparing the effects of induction therapy with polyclonal antilymphocyte globulins (ALG) or with monoclonal T-cell-specific antibodies are not unanimous. Therefore, 55 heart recipients were allocated to either 7-day courses of polyclonal ALG ($n = 28$) or of monoclonal OKT3 ($n = 27$). Additionally, azathioprine and low dose steroids were given. There were no severe side effects after OKT3; the course of ALG, however, had to be discontinued in 20 patients because of extensive flares. No differences between the two groups were found in freedom from rejection or in the incidence of infection. The 1- and 2-year survival was 96% in both groups. Although monoclonal and polyclonal induction therapies are equally effective for rejection prophylaxis, OKT3 may be preferred because of a lack of important side effects. However, the fact that a shorter course of ALG is equally effective may be in favour of ALG.

Key words: Heart transplantation – Rejection prophylaxis – Polyclonal/monoclonal antibodies

Polyclonal antilymphocyte or antithymocyte globulins (ALG, ATG) as well as monoclonal antibodies against T cells have proved to be effective for reversing acute cardiac allograft rejection [5, 7, 10]. Subsequently, various protocols using these antibodies have been developed for rejection prophylaxis in heart transplant recipients [2, 11, 12, 19]. More recently, studies comparing the effects of polyclonal and monoclonal T-cell-specific antibodies have been reported [9, 13, 14, 17]. Their results, however, are not unanimous about the superiority of one antibody preparation with respect to another in terms of rejection prophylaxis, safety and infectious complications.

In an earlier, randomized, controlled study in heart transplant recipients, we demonstrated that OKT3 facili-

tates patient care by preventing renal failure in the immediate postoperative period but does not reduce the incidence of rejection when compared to cyclosporine given i. v. [2]. Polyclonal anti-T-cell prophylaxis may induce broader immunosuppression resulting in fewer rejection episodes but might also give rise to more infectious complications. The present study was undertaken to compare a polyclonal horse lymphocyte-specific immunoglobulin with monoclonal OKT3 with regard to rejection prophylaxis, safety and infectious complications.

Materials and methods

All consecutive heart transplant recipients between 1 August 1989 and 1 August 1991 were enrolled into the trial and were subsequently allocated to receive either OKT3 (Ortho Pharmaceutical, Raritan, N. J.) or ALG (horse lymphocyte-specific IgG2, Lymphoglobulin, Institut Merieux). OKT3 was started postoperatively in a dose of 5 mg/day, 1–2 h after arrival at the Intensive Care Unit while still on the ventilator, and continued for 7 days. Similarly, ALG was started 1–2 h after arrival at the Intensive Care Unit, in a dose of 425 lymphocytotoxic units (0.5 ml) per kilogram of bodyweight daily and continued for 7 days. In addition, azathioprine was administered postoperatively, 50 mg/day intravenously for 6 days, and prednisolone was given prior to the operation (20 mg) and 60 mg/day thereafter, in two divided doses, tapering down by 10 mg every 3 days to 20 mg/day and subsequently by 2.5 mg/week until the maintenance dose of 10 mg/day was reached at approximately 8 weeks postoperatively. Half of the daily corticosteroid dose was given shortly before the administration of OKT3 or ALG, in combination with 4 mg clemastine i. v., to alleviate side effects. Oral cyclosporine was initiated on postoperative day 5 in a dose of 8 mg/kg daily in two divided doses and adjusted to the plasma levels.

Cyclosporine levels were measured by specific ^{125}I-CSA radioimmunmoassay (Cyclotrac, Incstar, Stillwater, Minn.) to keep plasma 12 h trough levels between 80 and 120 ng/ml in the early postoperative period and between 50 and 100 ng/nl after 9–12 months.

The diagnosis of acute rejection was made by histological examination of endomyocardial biopsies and graded according to Billingham's criteria of none, mild, moderate and severe rejection [3]. For the diagnosis of moderate rejection, the coexistence of mononuclear infiltrates and myocyte necrosis was required.

Treatment of acute rejection was instituted in the case of moderate rejection and consisted of R(abbit)-ATG to keep T cells between

Offprint requests to: A. H. M. M. Balk, MD, Thoraxcenter, Bd 373, University Hospital Rotterdam – Dijkzigt, Dr. Molewaterplein 40, 3015 GD Rotterdam, The Netherlands

Table 1. Characteristics of the patients who received either monoclonal or polyclonal antibodies for rejection prophylaxis

Induction therapy		ALG	OKT3
Number of patients		28	27
Gender M/F		23/5	22/5
Recipient age (years, range)		45 (18–61)	48 (15–62)
Primary heart disease	CMP	16	14
	IHD	12	10
	VHD	–	3
Donor age (years, range)		26 (14–43)	24 (12–38)
CMV serostatus negative *(n)*		13	9
PRA (%, median, range)		0 (0–20)	0 (0–54)
Donor/recipient gender mismatch *(n)*		9	10
Mismatch HLA-A		1.3 ± 0.5	1.4 ± 0.7
HLA-B		1.6 ± 0.6	1.4 ± 0.6
HLA-A + B		2.9 ± 0.9	2.9 ± 1
HLA-DR		1.2 ± 0.5	1.3 ± 0.7
Mismatch HLA-A + B	0 *(n)*	1	0
	1 or 2	8	11
	>2	19	16
Mismatch HLA-DR	0 *(n)*	1	4
	1	20*	10*
	2	7	13

ALG, horse anti-lymphocyte IgG2; CMP, cardiomyopathy; IHD, ischemic heart disease; VHD, valvular heart disease; CMV, cytomegalovirus; PRA, panel reactive activity
* $P < 0.025$

0 and 150/mm³ for 14 days for the first episode of rejection, 1 g methylprednisolone i. v. on 3 consecutive days for the second episode and OKT3 5 mg/day for 10 days in case of ongoing rejection or an early third episode of rejection.

All cytomegalovirus (CMV) seronegative recipients received (CMV seronegative blood products and passive immunization with CMV-specific immunoglobulin (Cytotect, Biotest Pharma, Frankfurt, FRG) for 10 weeks, as reported before [15].

Infections were defined as symptomatic episodes with concurrent demonstration of the causative agent by culture or changes in serological status. CMV infection was defined by a rise of IgM antibodies, demonstration of immediate early antigen (IEA), or isolation of the virus from throat swabs or urine. CMV disease was defined as fever or signs of organ involvement in the presence of CMV infection.

Statistical analysis. Data are expressed as mean values ± 1 SD or medians as appropriate. The significance of differences between means was assessed by the 95% confidence interval. Comparisons of proportions are based on the χ^2 test. Log rank test was used to assess the differences in freedom from rejection. For survival analysis, the Kaplan Meier method was used.

Results

In all, 28 patients received ALG and 27 patients were treated with OKT3. Patient characteristics including the numbers of donor/recipient gender mismatches and numbers of mismatches for HLA-A and -B, as well as the current panel reactive activity (PRA) were similar in both groups, although there was some difference in HLA-DR mismatches (Table 1). All patients received at least one blood transfusion prior to transplantation. Crossmatches

of donor lymphocytes with recipient sera, performed in case of more than 5% PRA, were negative.

The scheduled 7-day course of ALG was discontinued in 20 out of 28 patients after 5 days (range 3–6) because of extensive flares. The development of pyrexia (mean highest temperature 39.1 °C) was not different from the fever in the patients from the other treatment group.

The full 7-day course of OKT3 could be completed in all 27 patients. Fever (mean maximal temperature 39.4 °C) occurred in all but 3 patients, a mild rash was noted in 4 patients and diarrhoea in 1 patient.

Median follow-up was 15 months (range 3–25). The 1- and 2-year graft and patient survival was 96% in the OKT3 as well as in the ALG group.

No difference was found in the mean number of acute rejection episodes per patient during follow-up. Actuarial freedom from rejection at 1, 3 and 12 months was 68%, 18% and 13% in the ALG group and 74%, 33% and 20% in the OKT3 group. These differences were not significant (Fig. 1). The numbers of acute rejection episodes per patient were also equally distributed among the two treatment groups: 5, 14, 5 and 3 (ALG) versus 4, 11, 6 and 7 (OKT3) patients with respectively 0, 1, 2 or more than 2 rejection episodes.

A total of 42 patients received 1 (29 patients), 2 (12 patients) or 3 (1 patient) additional courses of polyclonal or monoclonal antibodies after the inductional therapy for the treatment of rejection.

The mean numbers of infections per patient was 0.9 and 0.8 in the ALG and OKT3 groups, respectively. Bacterial infections occurred more frequently than viral infections. There was no difference in the occurrence of bacterial, parasitic and fungus infections between the two treatment groups. CMV disease and herpes zoster were the main virus-induced problems. Again, no difference in the occurrence of viral infections or disease between the ALG and OKT3 groups could be demonstrated (Table 2). In both treatment groups more, but not significantly different, bacterial infections and CMV disease or herpes

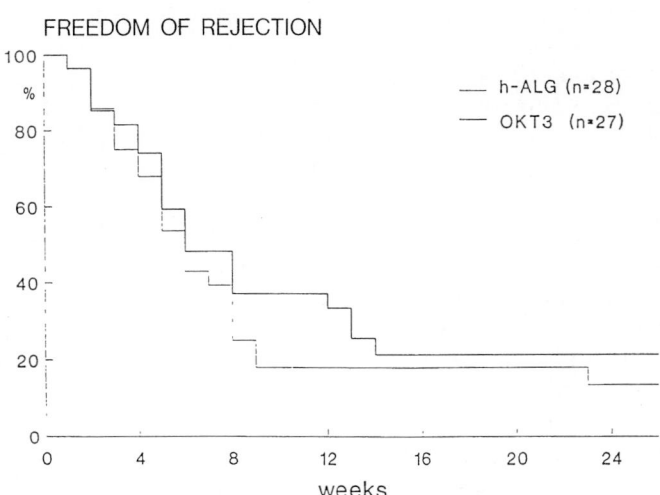

Fig. 1. Comparison of freedom from acute allograft rejection after induction therapy with ALG or OKT3 in 55 heart transplant recipients

Table 2. Infections after polyclonal or monoclonal T-cell-specific antibodies

Induction therapy	ALG	OKT3
All infections	26	23
Viral infections	9	6
CMV disease	4	2
Herpes zoster	3	1
Bacterial infections	15	14
Fungus infections (superficial *Candida*)	–	1
Parasitic infections	2	1
Pneumocystis carinii	2	–
Intestinal ascaris	–	1

zoster occurred in patients who received additional anti-T-cell therapy for rejection treatment compared with those without it. Bacterial infections occurred in 21 out of 41 patients with additional therapy versus 8 out of 14 patients without it and CMV disease or herpes zoster in 7 out of 41 patients with versus 3 out of 14 patients without additional anti-T-cell therapy.

Malignancies occurred in 1 patient from the ALG group and in 3 patients in the OKT3 group. The first patient, who received ALG for induction therapy, developed a squamous cell carcinoma of the external acoustic meatus 9 months after transplantation. The second patient died 18 weeks after transplantation from malignant lymphoma. After OKT3 induction therapy he had been treated with R(abbit)-ATG and a second course of OKT3 for intractable rejection. The third patient who received OKT3 initially was operated upon because of adenocarcinoma of the antrum, 7 months after transplantation. In the fourth patient a mucodermoid carcinoma of the palatum was noted, 12 days after transplantation.

Discussion

Although excellent short- and medium-term survival after heart transplantation can be achieved without the use of polyclonal or monoclonal anti-T-cell induction therapy [1], no efforts have been spared to develop an immunosuppressive regimen that would reduce the incidence of rejection as well as the complications of immunosuppression. In our centre the 2-year actuarial survival rates of 91% and 94% were achieved in heart transplant recipients, prior to this study, with and without OKT3 induction therapy, respectively [2]. The fact that OKT3 facilitated the immediate postoperative care, as the administration of cyclosporine could be avoided in the immediate postoperative period, but could not reduce the incidence of rejection made us embark on the present study, comparing the effects of polyclonal and monoclonal antibodies on cardiac allograft rejection. The graft and patient survival in both treatment groups was excellent. No superiority of one regimen over the other could be demonstrated with respect to freedom from rejection or time to detection of the first rejection.

The administration of ALG was hampered by fever and rapidly evolving, giant flares in 20 patients, necessitating premature discontinuation of the medication. No other complications were noted.

As in a previous study, almost all patients developed fever, but none experienced severe side-effects during or after the initial doses of OKT3 [2]. In contrast with the results of others, no haemodynamic deterioration or pulmonary oedema occurred. This may be explained by the fact that the first dose of OKT3 was given immediately postoperatively at the time the patients were still on the ventilator, while isoprenaline and dopamine were administered continuously [4, 8, 16, 18, 20]. Moreover, special care was taken to administer fluids in order to correct the drop of arterial blood pressure and right-sided filling-pressures resulting from the decrease in systemic arterial and venous vascular resistance.

Bacterial and viral infections occurred frequently and were associated with significant morbidity. No difference in the incidence of bacterial and viral infections was observed between the ALG and OKT3 groups despite the more selective action of OKT3. In earlier reports, there is no agreement about a difference in the incidence and nature of infections after monoconal and polyclonal antibodies [9, 13, 17]. However, comparison of the numbers of infections in patients who received additional anti-T-cell therapy with those in patients in whom the induction course was the only antibody therapy revealed that more bacterial as well as viral infections occurred in the patients who received additional antibodies. The difference was not significant.

Malignancy was the cause of death in one patient and appeared to have been treated effectively in two patients. The duration of follow-up is too short to appreciate the final effect of therapy. Although more malignancies occurred in the prophylactic OKT3 group, this difference was not significant. A longer follow-up will be necessary to confirm our earlier findings, in a larger group of patients, that malignancy is not associated with one specific antibody but with the total immunosuppressive load [6].

The data from this randomised trial indicate that polyclonal and monoclonal antibodies are equally effective for rejection prophylaxis after cardiac transplantation. OKT3 induction therapy may be preferred because of a lack of important side-effects. However, the fact that a shorter course of ALG (the scheduled course was discontinued early because of side-effects in the majority of patients). induces a similar freedom from rejection with subsequently similar incidences of the major complications of immunosuppressive therapy may be in favour of ALG.

References

1. Andreone PA, Olviari MT, Elick B, Arentzen CE, Sibley RK, Bolman RM, Simmons RL, Ring WS (1986) Reduction of infectious complications following heart transplantation with triple-drug immunotherapy. J Heart Transplant 5: 13–19
2. Balk AH, Simoons ML, Jutte NH, Brouer ML, Meeter K, Mochtar B, Weimar W (1990) Sequential OKT3 and cyclosporin after heart transplantation: a randomized study with single and cyclic OKT3. Clin Transplant 5: 301–305

3. Billingham ME (1981) Diagnosis of cardiac rejection by endomyocardial biopsy. Heart Transplant 1: 25

4. Breisblatt WM, Schulman DS, Stein K, Wolfe CJ, Whiteside T, Kormos R, Hardesty RL (1991) Hemodynamic response to OKT3 in orthotopic heart transplant recipients: evidence for reversible myocardial dysfunction. J Heart Lung Transplant 10: 359–365

5. Bristow MR, Renlund DG, Gilbert E, Lee HR, Gay WA, O'Connell JB (1988) Murine monoclonal CD-3 antibody in cardiac transplantation: anti-rejection treatment and preliminary results in a prospectively randomized trial for prophylaxis. Clin Transplant 2: 163–168

6. Brouwer RML, Balk AHMM, Weimar W (1991) OKT3 and the incidence of lymphoproliferative disorders after cardiac transplantation. N Engl J Med 324: 1437

7. Constanzo-Nordin MR, Silver MA, O'Connell JB, Pifarre R, Grady KL, Winter GI, Murdock DK, Sullivan HJ, Grieco JG, Scanlon PJ, Robinson JA (1987) Successful reversal of acute cardiac allograft rejection with OKT3 monoclonal antibody. Circulation 76 [Suppl V]: V 71–V 80

8. Cosimi AB (1987) OKT3: first dose safety and success. Nephron 46 [Suppl I]: 12–18

9. Frist WH, Merril WH, Eastburn TE, Atkinson JB, Stewart JR, Hammon JW, Bender HW (1990) Unique antithymocyte serum versus OKT3 for induction immunotherapy after heart transplantation. J Heart Transplant 9: 489–494

10. Gilbert EM, Dewitt ChM, Eiswirth CC, Renlund DG, Menlove RL, Freedman LA, Herrick CM, Gay WA, Bristow MR (1987) Treatment of refractory cardiac allograft rejection with OKT3 monoclonal antibody. Am J Med 82: 202

11. Gilbert E, Eiswirth CC, Renlund DG, Menlove RL, Dewitt CM, Freedman LA (1987) Use of orthoclone OKT3 monoclonal antibody in cardiac transplantation: early experience with rejection prophylaxis and treatment of refractory rejection. Transplant Proc 19: 45–53

12. Hegewald MG, O'Connell JB, Renlund DG, Lee HR, Burton NA, Karwande SV, Jones KW, Lassetter JE, Bristow MR (1989) OKT3 monoclonal antibody given for ten versus fourteen days as immunosuppressive prophylaxis in heart transplantation. J Heart Transplant 8: 303–310

13. Kirklin JK, Bourge RC, White-Williams C, Naftel DC, Thomas FT, Thomas JM, Phillips MG (1990) Prophylactic therapy for rejection after cardiac transplantation. A comparison of rabbit antithymocyte globulin and OKT3. J Thorac Cardiovasc Surg 99: 716–724

14. Menkis AH, Powell AM, Novick RJ, McKenzie FN, Kostuk WJ, Pflugfelder PW, Brown J, Rochon J, Chan I, Stiller C (1991) Prospective randomized trial of short term immunosuppressive prophylaxis using OKT3 or Minnesota equine ALG (abstr). J Heart Lung Transplant 10: 163

15. Metselaar HJ, Balk AHMM, Mochtar B, Rothbarth PH, Weimar W (1990) Prophylactic use of anti-CMV immunoglobuline in CMV seronegative heart transplant recipients. Chest 97: 396–399

16. Miller RA, Maloney DG, McKillop J, Levey R (1981) In-vivo effects of murine hybridoma monoclonal antibody in a patient with T cell leukemia. Blood 58: 78–86

17. Mundy J, Chang V, Keogh A, MacDonald P, Spratt P (1991) Prophylactic OKT3 versus equine antithymocyte globulin after heart transplantation: increased morbidity with OKT3 (abstr). J Heart Lung Transplant 10: 163

18. Orthomulticenter Transplant Study Group (1985) A randomized clinical trial of OKT3 monoclonal antibody for acute rejection of cadaveric renal transplants. N Engl J Med 313: 337–342

19. Starnes V, Oyer P, Stinson E, Dein J, Shumway N (1989) Prophylactic OKT3 used as induction therapy for heart transplantation. Circulation 80 [Suppl III]: 79–83

20. Stein KI, Landowski J, Kormos R, Armitage J (1989) The cardiopulmonary response to OKT3 in orthotopic cardiac transplant recipients. Chest 95: 817–821

Transplant Int (1992) 5 [Suppl 1]: S 480–S 481

TRANSPLANT
International
© Springer-Verlag 1992

Pregnancy in kidney recipients under cyclosporine

L. Berardinelli[1], **R. Dallatana**[1], **C. Beretta**[1], **M. Raiteri**[1], **G. Tonello**[1], **F. Quaglia**[2], **and A. Vegeto**[1]

[1] Department of Vascular Surgery and Kidney Transplantation, Policlinico University Hospital, Milan, Italy
[2] II Clinic Obstetric and Gynecologic, University of Milan, Milan, Italy

About 1 of every 50 women of child-bearing age who have a functioning kidney transplant become pregnant. Successful pregnancies following kidney allotransplantation with conventional immunosuppressive treatment are well described [8], and there is no evidence of abnormalities in the infants born. The use of cyclosporine (CSA) means new problems for the pregnant women and the fetus: the risk of congenital abnormalities, fetal growth retardation, hepato- and nephrotoxicity.

We report the experience of 16 pregnancies in 16 of our kidney transplant patients, of which 7 were treated with CSA.

Key words: Immunosuppression – Cyclosporine – Pregnancy

Materials and methods

From May 1969 to August 1991, 1438 kidney transplants were performed on 1355 patients; 471 of the 514 women were of child-bearing age. The kidney is usually located retroperitoneally, in the iliac fossa, using the recipient iliac vessels; an antireflux ureteroneocystostomy will have been preferably performed.

Nine patients were treated with conventional therapy at the mean dosage of 16 mg of prednisone every other day and 1.5 mg/kg daily of azathioprine.

From 1983, 7 patients have been treated with CSA at the mean dosage of 3 mg/kg daily.

Before their transplant, 13 patients presented with important alterations of their menses, and 5 of them had severe amenorrhea.

Menstrual patterns returned to normal within 6 months of the transplant in all patients.

The women become pregnant from 4 months to 11 years after transplantation. Eight women of this group were pregnant before the transplant but 5 aborted because of their uremic status. The clinical data of the 16 pregnant women on the basis of immunosuppressive therapy are reported in Table 1.

Six pregnancies started after an extensive evaluation of the patients' clinical situation by the physician. Good conditions for pregnancy included sufficient renal function (serum creatinine level less

than 2 mg% in patients treated with conventional therapy and 2.5 mg% in those treated with CSA), no sign of rejection, normal blood pressure values, no urinary tract dilatation, normal psychological status.

We checked the women monthly with ultrasonography examinations, serum determination of viral antibodies (cytomegalovirus (CMV), hepatitis B surface antigen, HbSAg, German measles) and other more routine examinations.

In case of fetal sufference we did amniocentesis.

Results

The immunosuppressive dosage was not modified throughout the pregnancy. The mean systolic pressure value was 140 mm Hg for the conventional therapy group and 125 mm Hg for the CSA group. Six women had a high blood pressure value during pregnancy. In 4 of them, there was preexisting hypertension.

Clinical signs of rejection were present in 2 women at the beginning of pregnancy that culminated in kidney failure 2 and 3 years after delivery. Other patients showed transient renal dysfunction between the 12th and 16th weeks. Generally mild variations in the creatinine levels were observed during pregnancy (Table 2).

Table 1. Clinical data of 16 women who became pregnant after transplantation on the basis of immunosuppressive therapy

	CsA therapy	Conventional therapy
No. of pregnant women	7	9
Kidney from living donor	–	4
Second transplant	–	1
Recipient's age at transplantation (years)[a]	27.5 ± 7.5	26.2 ± 5.4
Months of dialysis before transplantation[a]	52 ± 49.9	42.6 ± 34.5
Kidney placed in RIF (N^)	7	4
HBsAg positivity	3	2
Months between transplantation and pregnancy	36.2 ± 23.2	53.3 ± 40.3

[a] Mean ± SD
CsA, cyclosporine; HBsAg, hepatitis B surface antigen

Offprint requests to: L. Berardinelli, Department of Vascular Surgery and Kidney Transplantation, Policlinico University Hospital, Milan, Italy

Table 2. Creatinine levels in 14 pregnant women before, during, and after pregnancy on the basis of immunosuppressive therapy

	CsA therapy	Conventional therapy
Creatinine level before pregnancy	1.1 ± 0.3	1.3 ± 0.6
Creatinine level during pregnancy	1.08 ± 0.2	1.4 ± 0.6
Creatinine level after pregnancy	1.08 ± 0.19	1.5 ± 0.8

Mean values ± SD

Table 3. Clinical data of 15 children in relation to immunosuppressive therapy of the transplanted mothers[a]

	CsA therapy	Conventional therapy
Gestational period (weeks)	35.7 ± 2.2	35.0 ± 3.5
Birth weight (kg)	2.517 ± 0.444	2.797 ± 0.692
Apgar score	7 ± 0.8	7.8 ± 0.6

[a] We did not consider in this table the baby born preterm at the 23rd week

Four women (3 from the CSA group) developed hepatopathy or their condition worsened but returned to normal after delivery.

Five patients showed a HbSAg positivity during pregnancy without any clinical signs. Hepatitis B immunoglobulin was given to their babies within 12 h of birth, followed by hepatitis B vaccine. One women treated with conventional therapy developed gestational diabetes that required insulin therapy from the 25th week. Another patient treated with CSA had hyperglycemia which was well controlled by dieting.

Four cases of urinary tract infection had been observed, but only 1 was symptomatic. This patient had a vesicoureteral reflux that worsened during pregnancy, but no surgical treatment was necessary.

The hematocrit value went down in our group, but only 1 patient became severely anemia.

In all, 16 children were born, 8 of them preterm; 10 were boys and 6 girls. The mean gestational period was 35.7 ± 2.2 weeks for CSA-treated mothers and 34.7 ± 5.1 for the conventional groups, a course almost uneventful for the 16 mothers. All children are healthy except 1, from a patient affected by chronic rejection, who was born preterm at the 23rd week because of placenta rupture and died 3 days after delivery due to respiratory distress syndrome.

An elective cesarian section was decided for all patients. Eight children had a normal birth weight, in relation to the gestational period. Three weighed less than 2500 g, and 4 children had a weight over the 90th percentile. The baby born in the 23rd week weighed 600 g. Excluding this last baby, the mean birth weight was $2.703 \text{ kg} \pm 0.591$. The Apgar scores are shown in Table 3.

There were no major congenital abnormalities in the babies; one baby presented with small hemangiomas on the face and neck that regressed spontaneously. No bone abnormalities have been noted. The children are growing normally, remaining over the 20th percentile.

Bottle feeding was preferred for almost all of the babies.

Discussion

The risks of pregnancy undertaken by a kidney transplant patient are not increased either for the mother or for the baby by use of CSA for the immunosuppressive regimen, in according with other studies [3].

The abortion rate is related to the renal function [6].

An increase of acute reversible rejection after delivery has been noted [4, 5, 8].

We consider it unnecessary to increase the immunosuppressive regimen during pregnancy as other authors suggest [1].

Ultrasonography study is of primary importance to evaluate the course of fetal growth.

We agree with Cockburn's conclusions from a study of 51 pregnancies in 48 patients treated with CSA, in which he did not note any congenital anomalies in the babies nor damage to the mothers. CSA is often related to hypertension. The incidence of eclampsia could theoretically be higher than with conventional therapy, but in our group this was not noticed. However, the incidence of eclampsia is related to preexisting hypertension and/or renal impairment [6].

Our decision to perform cesarian sections on all the mothers was made in order to avoid trauma to the kidney during delivery.

Our incidence of 6.2% perinatal mortality is related to prematurity and is comparable with the incidence of 8% reported by Fine [6].

In 10 of our infants the birth weight appeared less than 2500 g, in according with other authors for either the CSA-treated [6] or the conventional group [7].

It is possible that the association of CSA and AZA could be dangerous for the synergic mutagenic effect of the two drugs [11].

Many problems are still to be cleared up about the use of CSA in pregnancy. The measurement of the whole blood CSA level may be an inappropriate measure of the free drug concentration during pregnancy because of the change in red cell volume [10].

Another problem is the higher concentration of CSA in the placenta related to the maternal or fetal blood [2].

It is better not to breast feed because of the high presence of drugs in the breast milk.

References

1. Biesenbach G, et al. (1989) Successful pregnancy in a rhesus incompatible cyclosporine-treated renal transplant recipient. Nephrol Dial Transpl 4: 511
2. Bourget P, et al. (1990) Transplacental passage of cyclosporine. Transplantation 49: 663
3. Cockburn I, et al. (1989) Present experience of cyclosporine in pregnancy. Transplant Proc 21: 3730
4. Davison J, Lindheimer (1982) Pregnancy in renal transplant recipients. J Reprod Med 27: 613
5. Davison J, Lind T, Lind P (1976) Planned pregnancy in a renal transplant recipients. Br J Obstet Gynecol 83: 518
6. Fine R (1982) Pregnancy in renal allograft recipients. Am J Nephrol 2: 117
7. Lau J, Scott J (1985) Pregnancy following renal transplantation. Clin Obstet Gynecol 28(2): 339
8. Penn I, Makowski E, Harris R (1980) Parenthood following renal and hepatic transplantation. Kidney Int 30: 397
9. Pujals JM, et al. (1989) Osseus malformation in baby born to a woman receiving cyclosporine. Lancet I: 667
10. Ross WB, et al. (1988) Transplantation 45: 1142
11. Zankl H, et al. (1987) Nephrol Dial Transpl 2: 467

Transplant Int (1992) 5 [Suppl 1]: S 482–S 483

TRANSPLANT
International
© Springer-Verlag 1992

Low-dose combination therapy of DUP-785 and RS-61443 prolongs cardiac allograft survival in rats

W. O. Bechstein*, Y. Suzuki, T. Kawamura, B. Jaffee, A. Allison, D. A. Hullett, and H. W. Sollinger

Department of Surgery, University of Wisconsin, Madison, Wisconsin, USA

The introduction of cyclosporine into the immunosuppressive armamentarium has revolutionized transplant surgery with significant improvements in graft survival. The apparent lack of effect of cyclosporine on humoral rejection mechanisms makes the search for other immunosuppressive agents desirable. Two anti-metabolites affecting nucleotide synthesis via different pathways have recently been evaluated for their immunosuppressive potential. DUP-785 (DUP), also known as brequinar sodium, reversibly inhibits de novo pyrimidine synthesis by blocking dihydro-orotate dehydrogenase, thus resulting in the delretion of critical precursors for RNA and DNA synthesis [2]. RS-61443, a morpholinoethyl ester of mycophenolic acid, reversibly and non-competitively blocks inosin monophosphate dehydrogenase, the key enzyme in purine de novo synthesis [10]. A possible additive effect of both drugs was investigated in the rat heart allograft model.

Key words: Immunosuppression – DUP-785 – RS-61443

Materials and methods

Heart grafts from male ACI (RT1[a]) rats were transplanted into male Lewis (LEW) (RT1[1]) rats in the heterotopic abdominal position using a modification of the technique described by Ono and Lindsey [9]. Syngeneic transplants between LEW rats served as controls. Drugs were applied by gavage, DUP 3 times weekly and RS daily. DUP was supplied in powder form as a gift from DuPont Merck, Wilmington, Del. RS was supplied as a gift from Syntex, Palo Alto, Calif. Graft function was monitored daily by abdominal palpation. Rejection was defined as the cessation of a palpable heart beat and confirmed by histology. Median graft survival between the groups was compared by the Mann-Whitney U-test. Recipients of syngeneic transplants were subjected to combination therapy with DUP and RS for a period of 30 days, whereafter they were sacrificed and any possible toxicity studied by histological evaluation of the lung, native and donor heart, stomach, small bowel, large bowel, kidney, pancreas, liver, and spleen specimens. Experimental groups included treatment with varying doses of DUP and RS alone or in combination (Table 1).

Results

Syngeneic transplants (group 0) survived for more than 100 days, whereas allogeneic transplants were rejected after a median of 6 days (group 1) (Table 1). Monotherapy with either DUP (3 or 6 mg/kg; groups 2, 3) or RS (10 mg/kg; group 4) in low doses led to a significant prolongation of graft survival; however, most transplants were rejected within 2 weeks. The addition of daily RS (10 mg/kg) to DUP (3 or 6 mg/kg, 3 times weekly; groups 5, 6) provided additional graft survival, and not only when compared with the control group; graft survival was significantly longer than in the respective groups treated by DUP alone (group 5 vs group 2, $P < 0.01$; group 6 vs. group 3 $P < 0.01$; Table 1).

Combination therapy with low doses of DUP and RS was well tolerated in all animals with no weight loss; ocasionally the animals would pass loose stools, but there was no frank diarrhea. Histological examination of tissue specimens in animals from the toxicity study who were sacrificed after 30 days of the combination therapy revealed no abnormalities except for 1 case each of slight gastric mucosal atrophy and some loss of large bowel mucosalepithelium in the DUP 6 mg/kg and RS 10 mg/kg combination therapy group.

Discussion

DUP-785 prevents cell proliferation by the inhibition of de novo pyrimidine biosynthesis [2]. It inhibits the development of delayed-type hypersensitivity to dinitrofluorobenzene (DNFB) in mice and prolongs heart, liver, and kidney allograft survival in the rat [3]. The effective

* *Present address:* Department of Surgery, University Clinic Rudolf Virchow, 1000 Berlin 65, Federal Republic of Germany

Offprint requests to: H. W. Sollinger, M. D., University of Wisconsin Hospital, H4/780 Clinical Science Center, 600 Highland Avenue, Madison, WI 53792, USA

Table 1. Experimental groups and results of rat heterotopic heart grafting and therapy with DUP or RS alone and in combination

Experimental groups (graft survival time, days)	Median graft survival (days)	P-value (vs. group 1)
0. Syngeneic (LEW-LEW) $n = 10$ (79, 101 × 5, 102 × 3, 113)	> 100	
A. Immunosuppression		
1. Allogeneic (ACI-LEW) $n = 10$ no treatment	6	
2. (6, 6, 6, 6, 6, 6, 7, 7, 7, 8) Allogeneic $n = 10$ DUP 3 mg/kg	9.5	< 0.01
3. (8, 8, 8, 9, 9, 10, 11, 12, 13, 21) Allogeneic $n = 6$ DUP 6 mg/kg	14.5	< 0.01
4. (12, 12, 14, 15, 15, 19) Allogeneic $n = 10$ RS 10 mg/kg	8	< 0.01
5. (6, 7, 7, 7, 8, 8, 8, 8, 8, 10) Allogeneic $n = 10$ DUP 3 mg/kg + RS 10 mg/kg (10, 11, 13, 13, 19, 19, 22, 33, 35,	19	< 0.001
6. > 100) Allogeneic $n = 9$ DUP 6 mg/kg + RS 10 mg/kg (19, 21, 23, 24, 26, 32, 34, 35, > 100)	26	< 0.001
B. Toxicity		
7. Syngeneic $n = 4$ (4 × 31 days) DUP 3 mg/kg + RS 10 mg/kg		
8. Syngeneic $n = 4$ (4 × 31 days) DUP 6 mg/kg + RS 10 mg/kg		

Group 3 vs 2, $P < 0.05$; group 5 vs. 2, $P < 0.01$; group 6 vs. 3, $P < 0.01$; group 6 vs. 5, $P = 0.1$

dose for prolonging rat heart allograft survival for more than 30 days is 12–24 mg/kg 3 times weekly [3].

RS-61443 also blocks the proliferative responses of T and B lymphocytes and inhibits antibody formation and the generation of cytotoxic T cells [1, 4, 5, 8]. Furthermore, it prevents the rejection of pancreatic islet allograts in adult mice [6]. The effective dose for the prevention of heart allograft rejection in rats has been shown to be 30–40 mg/kg daily [7].

Since both drugs affect nucleic acid metabolism, they show major effects in rapidly dividing cell populations. Higher doses of both drugs lead to gastrointestinal symptoms such as diarrhea and ultimately weight loss.

In this study, we examined the effects of a combination therapy of low doses of DUP and RS on rat heart allograft survival. The dosages of the respective agents were at least half of what had previously been reported as effective. Furthermore, it was investigated whether combination therapy was feasible in terms of toxicity. Combination therapy with low doses of DUP and RS was well tolerated in all animals, with no weight loss and only the occasional occurrence of loose stools. Minor histological signs of toxicity like mucosal atrophy in the gastrointestinal tract appeared in 2 of 4 animals after 30 days of combination therapy with DUP 6 mg/kg and RS 10 mg/kg.

Low doses of RS and DUP alone significantly prolonged allograft heart survival in rats, but a combination therapy of DUP and RS in low doses proved to be even more powerful in regard to graft survival without increased toxicity. There is at least an additive effect of both drugs; further studies to investigate this synergism between both drugs are currently in progress.

DUP inhibits the pathway of pyrimidine synthesis at a relatively early step, while RS interferes with purine de novo synthesis at a rather late stage. It may be hypothesized that treatment with DUP renders expanding lymphocyte populations more susceptible to the effects of RS treatment without any further increase in toxicity.

Acknowlegements: W.O. Bechstein received a research fellowship from the Deutsche Forschungsgemeinschaft, Bonn, FRG.

References

1. Burlingham WJ, Grailer AP, Hullett DA, Sollinger HW (1991) Inhibition of both MLC and in vitro IgG memory response to tetanus toxoid by RS-61443. Transplantation 51: 545–547
2. Chen SF, Ruben RL, Dexter DL (1986) Mechanism of action of the novel anticancer agent 6-fluoro-2-(2'-fluoro-1,1'-biphenyl-4-yl)-3-methyl-4-quinolinecarboxylic acid sodium salt (NSC 368390): inhibition of de novo pyrimidine nucleotide biosynthesis. Cancer Res 46: 5014
3. Cramer DV, Chapman FA, Jaffee BD, Jones EA, Knoop M, Hreha-Eiras G, Makowka L (1991) The effect of a new immunosuppressive drug, brequinar sodium, on heart, liver, and kidney allograft rejection in the rat. Transplantation (in press)
4. Eugui EM, Almquist SJ, Muller CD, Allison AC (1991) Lymphocyte-selective cytostatic and immunosuppressive effects of mycophenolic acid. Scand J Immunol 33: 161–173
5. Eugui EM, Mirkovich A, Allison AC (1991) Lymphocyte-selective antiproliferative and immunosuppressive effects of mycophenolic acid in mice. Scand J Immunol 33: 175–183
6. Hao L, Lafferty KJ, Allison AC, Eugui EM (1990) Rs-61443 allows islet allografting and specific tolerance induction in adult mice. Transplant Proc 22: 876–879
7. Morris RE, Hoyt EG, Murphy MP, Eugui EM, Allison AC (1990) Mycophenolic acid morpholinoethylester (RS-61443) is a new immunosuppressant that prevents and halts heart allograft rejection by selective inhibition of T- and B-cell purine synthesis. Transplant Proc 22: 1659–1662
8. Nelson PH, Eugui E, Wang CC, Allison AC (1990) Synthesis and immunosuppressive activity of some side-chain variants of mycophenolic acid. J Med Chem 33: 833–838
9. Ono K, Lindsey ES (1969) Improved technique of heart transplantation in rats. J Thorac Cardiovasc Surg 75: 225
10. Platz KP, Sollinger HW, Hullett DA, Eckhoff DE, Eugui EM, Allison AC (1991) RS-61443: a new, potent immunosuppressive agent. Transplantation 51: 27–31

Transplant Int (1992) 5 [Suppl 1]: S 484–S 486

TRANSPLANT
International
© Springer-Verlag 1992

Immunomodulation of dog islets using a cocktail of monoclonal antibodies

I. G. M. Brons[1], R. Champeney[1], S. P. Cobbold[2], H. S. Davies[1], H. Waldmann[2], and R. Y. Calne

Departments of [1] Surgery and [2] Pathology, University of Cambridge, Addenbrooke's Hospital, Cambridge, United Kingdom

Abstract. Islet allografts are particularly vulnerable to rejection, and current immunosuppressive agents are deleterious to their function. They are, however, highly suitable for 'immunomodulation', i.e., the removal or inactivation of passenger leukocytes to reduce their immunogenicity. For this purpose we have used 3 rat anti-dog monoclonal antibodies (Mabs) which are synergistic for leukocytolysis in the presence of autologous dog serum. Spleen cells or purified islets treated with these Mabs together with autologous serum were tested in mixed leukocyte and islet co-culture assays. The stimulatory properties of the Mab-pretreated splenocytes or islets were markedly reduced; moreover, the Mab cytolytic activity was shown to be confined to the leukocyte target cells and did not affect islet secretory function upon glucose stimulation. We conclude that this method of modifying the immunogenicity of dog islets could lead to successful islet grafting in vivo, allowing the reduction of conventional immunosuppression. Successful in vivo studies in this model, which are currently in progress, could have implications for clinical islet transplantation.

Key words: Islet transplantation – Dog model – Immunomodulation – Monoclonal antibodies

In our Department, a postmortem specimen of a transplanted, vascularized, duct-injected segmental pancreas graft was found to consist entirely of numerous, well-granulated islets 9 years after transplantation. The patient had been insulin-independent for over 9 years and died of a myocardial infarct during dialysis. She had rejected her simultaneously transplanted kidney graft 2 years after transplantation and was subsequently haemodialysed. This example of the survival and function of islets surrounded by totally fibrosed tissue, thus resembling a vascularized islet graft, has given us confidence in pursuing islet transplantation as an alternative therapy for insulin-dependent diabetes mellitus. However, compared with vascularized pancreas transplantation, rejection of islet tissue has been shown to be more difficult to prevent with the currently available immunosuppressive therapy [4].

One approach to this problem is to reduce the immunogeneicity of the islet graft by pretreatment with monoclonal antibodies (Mabs) directed towards passenger leukocytes, in particular dendritic cells and macrophages. The host immune response should then be diminished and therefore more easily immunosuppressed. In rodents such methods are well documented and can secure long-term survival of functional islet allografts [2]. However, these procedures must be proved effective in a large animal model before serious consideration can be given to clinical application. To this end we have developed rat anti-dog Mabs with selected properties for the immunomodulation of donor islet tissue prior to transplantation into diabetic recipients. In this report we describe in vitro studies of dog islet immunomodulation using 3 Mabs which, in contrast to most mouse Mabs, have the ability to fix autologous complement and lyse target cells.

Materials and methods

Monoclonal antibodies were produced by standard techniques and characterized by FACS analysis and a battery of in vitro functional assays. From a large number of rat anti-dog hybridoma supernatants we selected 3 Mabs (one IgG2a, two IgG2b) which synergise for the cytolysis of dog peripheral leukocytes (PBL) in the presence of autologous dog serum as the complement source. One of these Mabs binds to the CD45 leukocyte common antigen (LCA); the target molecules for the other two Mabs are currently being identified.

The binding of these Mabs to dog pancreas sections was visualized by standard immunohistochemical staining techniques using peroxide or alkaline phosphatase stains.

Islet isolation. Dog islets were isolated by static, intraductal collagenase digestion and purified over Ficoll gradients according to the

Offprint requests to: I. G. M. Brons, Department of Surgery, University of Cambridge, Addenbrooke's Hospital, Hills Road, Cambridge CB2 2QQ, United Kingdom

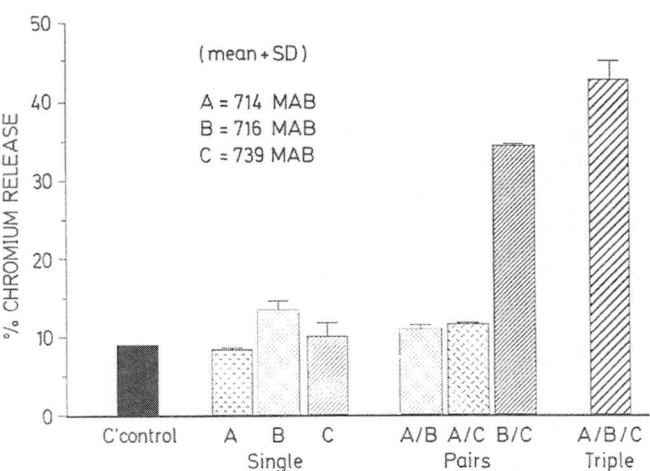

MIXING THE MABS INCREASES THEIR EFFECTIVENESS IN COMPLEMENT MEDIATED LYSIS OF DOG LEUKOCYTES

Fig. 1. Monoclonal antibodies (Mabs) were tested singly, in pairs or in triple cocktail for cytolytic activity using ^{51}Cr-labelled dog peripheral blood lymphocytes (PBL) and autologous dog serum as the source of complement. Cytolysis after 1.5 h at 37 °C was measured by chromium release expressed as percentage of total chromium in target cells

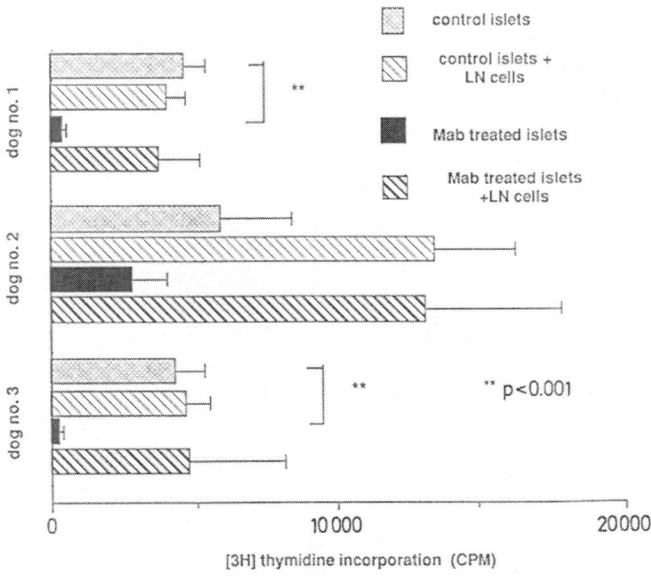

MAB PRETREATMENT OF FRESH DOG ISLETS REDUCES THEIR ABILITY TO STIMULATE ALLOGENEIC LEUKOCYTES IN VITRO

Fig. 2. Islets pretreated with mixed Mabs were co-cultured with allogeneic leukocytes in the mixed leukocyte islet co-culture (MLIC) assay. Proliferative responses were measured by titrated thymidine incorporation on day 7. Residual Mabs did not affect the responder population as seen by restored proliferation in cultures reconstituted with stimulator-type leukocytes

method of Warnock et al. [5]. Dithizone stain [3] was used for islet identification and assessment of purity. The viability was assessed by acridine orange/propidium iodide staining [1]. After overnight culture, dog islets with a purity of 60 %–90 % were incubated with Mab(s) together with autologous dog serum as the source of complement for 18 h at 37 °C and then washed extensively. Next, 30–50 irradiated (2000 rads), pretreated islets or pretreated splenocytes (1×10^5) were added to allogeneic dog lymphocytes (1×10^5) in the mixed lymphocyte islet co-culture (MLIC) assay or the mixed lymphocyte culture (MLC) assay, respectively.

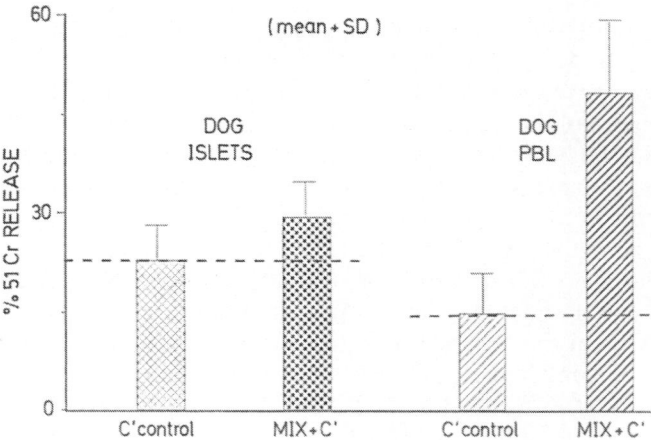

MIXED MABS ARE ONLY MARGINALLY LYTIC FOR DOG ISLETS COMPARED TO DOG PBL

Fig. 3. Lytic activity of mixed Mabs was tested on ^{51}Cr-labelled dog islets or ^{51}Cr-labelled dog PBL with autologous dog serum as the complement source. Cytolysis after 1.5 h was measured by ^{51}Cr release as percentage of total ^{51}Cr in target cells

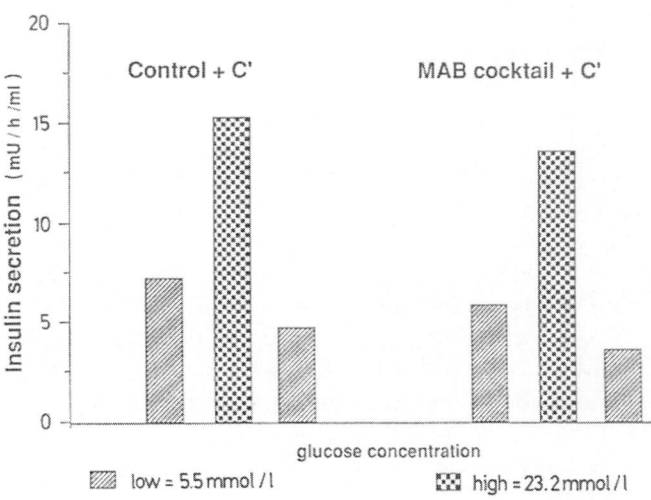

MAB PRETREATMENT OF DOG ISLETS DOES NOT IMPAIR THEIR *IN VITRO* INSULIN SECRETORY FUNCTION

Fig. 4. Islets pretreated with mixed Mabs were incubated with low and high glucose concentrations in a static glucose stimulation assay. Insulin secretion was measured by radioimmunoassay for dog insulin

Assay methods. Chronium-51 release assays were used to measure the cytolytic activity of Mabs on ^{51}Cr-labelled dog islets or peripheral blood leukocytes (PBL). The secretory function of islets after Mab pretreatment was tested by the standard static glucose stimulation assay as compared with untreated islets.

Results

The immunohistochemistry study of Mab binding to dog pancreas sections showed that none of the Mabs bound to the endocrine part of the islet. Two Mabs were found to bind to dendritic- and macrophage-type cells and passenger leukocytes distributed throughout the pancreas section. The cytolytic activity for dog PBL targets of Mabs used singly, in pairs and as a cocktail in the ^{51}Cr-release assay is shown in Fig. 1. Whereas single Mabs showed marginal cytolysis above the complement control level, one pair of Mabs and the mixture of all 3 Mabs gave substantial target cell lysis. This triple cocktail was therefore used to pretreat splenocytes, which were then tested in MLC assays. Results showed that the stimulatory capacity of splenocytes was greatly reduced by pretreatment with the Mab cocktail. Using Mab-pretreated dog islets as stimulators in the MLIC assay, similar results were obtained, as shown in Fig. 2 (three experiments shown). There was, however, a wide range of reduced proliferative responses, possibly related to islet purity and the use of unpurified Mab in the pretreatment procedure. The effect of Mab and complement pretreatment on islet cells and their function was measured by ^{51}Cr-release and by static glucose stimulation assays. The cytolytic activity of Mabs for islet targets was only marginally above the control level compared with PBL targets, in which a substantial isotope release was measured (Fig. 3). Figure 4 shows that the pretreatment had no discernible effect on insulin secretion, which was similar to that of control untreated islets.

Discussion

Successful application to a large animal species of methods developed in rodents for islet cell immunomodulation is a vital step before clinical application can be considered. The present work describes the preliminary in vitro assessment of the effectiveness of immunomodulation with Mabs and complement in mongrel dogs and holds promise for the in vivo studies in progress.

Though the mechanisms underlying the reduced proliferation in MLC and MLIC following Mab pretreatment of stimulator splenocytes or islets are not clear, several observations can be made:

1. It is unlikely that reduced proliferation results from Mab leakage from (thoroughly washed) treated islets. Thus, reconstitution of these cultures with small numbers of stimulator-type cells restored the normal proliferative responses (Fig. 2).

2. Intact complement seems to be needed for successful immunomodulation, suggesting that lysis of leukocytes is an important mechanism, although antibody-dependent cellular cytotoxicity (ADCC) may also be involved, particularly in vivo.

3. The ability of rat Mabs to utilise autologous dog serum for cytolysis avoids the use of heterologous complement sources which could prejudice islet function through the binding of xenoantibodies.

The variability of the MLIC results could be related to the use of supernatants as a source of Mabs and to the purity of different islet cell preparations. Undoubtedly, the methodology can be improved by using titrated mixtures of these Mabs, which are now available in purified form. Other Mabs are also being tested with the aim of improving the immunomodulation.

Conclusion

The results show clearly indicate that in vitro pretreatment of fresh dog islets with a cocktail of autologous complement-fixing Mabs can result in reduced immunogenicity in MLIC assays, which are an in vitro correlate to transplant rejection. Thus, if it is possible to reduce the immunogenicity of islet grafts, then low levels of conventional immunosuppression or therapy with rat anti-dog CD4 and CD8 Mabs may well allow prolonged survival and restoration of normoglycaemia in diabetic recipients. In vivo studies using a large animal model are currently in progress.

Acknowledgement. This work was in part supported by the Juvenile Diabetes Foundation International and the MRC programme grant (grant no. C2199). Dr. Brons is supported by a Wellcome Trust Postdoctoral Fellowship.

References

1. Bank HL (1987) Assessment of islet cell viability using fluorescent dyes. Diabetologia 30: 812
2. Faustman DL, Steinman RM, Gebel HM, Hauptfeld V, Davie JM, Lacy PE (1984) Prevention of rejection of murine islet allografts by pretreatment with anti-dendritic cell antibody. Proc Natl Acad Sci USA 81: 3864
3. Latif ZA, Noel J, Alejandro R (1988) A simple method of staining fresh and cultured islets. Transplantation 45: 827
4. Scharp DW, Lacy PE, Santiago JV, McCullough CS, Weide LG, Falqui L, Marchetti P, Gingerich RL, Jaffe AS, Cryer PE, Anderson CB, Flye MW (1990) Insulin independence after islet transplantation into type I diabetic patient. Diabetes 39: 515
5. Warnock GL, Cattral MS, Evans MG, Kneteman NM, Rajotte RV (1989) Mass isolation of pure canine islets. Transplant Proc 21 (2): 3371

Transplant Int (1992) 5 [Suppl 1]: S 487–S 489

TRANSPLANT
International
© Springer-Verlag 1992

Prolongation of murine thyroid allografts by interleukin 2 (DAB486)-toxin and RS-61443*

D. A. Hullett, A. S. Landry, D. E. Eckoff, J. C. Nichols, E. M. Eugui, A. C. Allison, and H. W. Sollinger

Department of Surgery, University of Wisconsin, Madison, Wisconsin, USA

Abstract. We evaluated the efficacy of interleukin 2 (DAB486)-toxin (IL-2-diphtheria toxin fusion protein; IL-2-toxin) in combination with RS-61443 to prolong murine thyroid allograft survival. B10.BR thyroid allografts were transplanted beneath the renal subcapsule in recipient (C57BL/10 mice and graft survival determined 21 days later. Treatment with IL-2-toxin (25 μg/day for 14 days) was unable to prolong graft survival significantly. RS-61443 treatment (21 days) achieved significant graft prolongation only at doses of 300 mg/kg daily or greater. When both drugs were used in combination (IL-2-toxin, 25 μg/day for 14 days RS-61443 200 mg/kg daily for 21 days), statistically significant ($P < 0.0001$) graft prolongation was obtained. Our results suggest that IL-2-toxin in combination with subtherapeutic RS-61443 levels significantly prolongs murine thyroid allograft survival. IL-2-toxin and RS-61443, because of their unique and complementary mechanisms, hold promise for more selective immunosuppression.

Key words: Immunosuppression – Interleukin 2 – RS-61443

RS-61443, a morpholinoethyl ester of mycophenolic acid (MPA), has been shown to be effective in prolonging canine kidney allograft [12] and murine islet allograft [5] survival. In vitro studies indicate not only inhibition of T-cell proliferation and cytotoxic T-cell generation, but also of B-cell proliferation and antibody secretion [2, 4].

Strom and colleagues have used recombinant DNA methodologies to replace genetically the eukaryotic cell receptor binding domain of diphtheria toxin with sequences encoding interleukin 2 (IL-2) [9, 10, 15]. Entry of IL-2 (DAB486)-toxin (IL-2-toxin) into the cell is via the high affinity IL-2 receptor [1]. IL-2-toxin treatment has been shown to produce marked immunosuppression of the murine delayed type hypersensitivity (DTH) response [8], be cytotoxic for activated human T helper and B cells [3], prolong murine islet allograft survival [11], and suppress an autoimmune response [7].

In this study we have determined the efficacy of IL-2-toxin and RS-61443 individually and in combination to prolong murine thyroid allograft survival. IL-2-toxin was not effective in prolonging allograft survival. Low dose RS-61443 therapy was marginally able to prolong graft survival. In contrast, combination therapy consisting of IL-2-toxin and low dose RS-61443 was effective in prolonging allograft survival.

Materials and methods

Mice. The Jackson Laboratory, Bar Harbor, provided B10.BR and C57BL/10 mice. All animals were maintained according to guidelines prepared by the Committee on Care and Use of Laboratory Animal Resources, National Research Council (DHEW publication no. 78–23, revised 1978).

Thyroid harvest and transplantation. Thyroid glands were removed from donor B10.BR mice, placed in minimal essential medium, and transplanted as previously described [6]. Thyroid graft function was determined 21 days posttranspslant. Briefly, recipient mice were injected with 0.5 μCi carrier-free Na^{125}I in saline (i. p.). Then 24 h later, the kidneys were removed and placed in saline buffered formalin. Incorporated counts were compared with background (counts incorporated into the nongrafted, right kidney), with a ratio ≥ 4.0 considered to be a functional, viable graft. Graft nonfunction due to rejection was confirmed by histology.

Histology. H & E stained sections (6 μ) were prepared. Histological scoring was determined by a blinded observer ($n = 3$): 0, no lymphocytic infiltrte; 1, small focal infiltrates; 2, moderate cellular infiltrates; 3, heavy cellular infiltrates; 4, heavy cellular infiltrates with graft destruction and necrosis.

Immunosuppression. RS-61443 was supplied in powdered form by Syntex (USA), Palo Alto. A suspension of Rs-61443 (20 mg/ml) in a carboxymethyl cellulose vehicle was prepared and stored at 4 °C. IL-2 toxin was provided by Seragen, Hopkinton, in lyophilized form and stored at −80 °C. Prior to administration, IL-2-toxin was reconstituted with TRIS buffered saline containing 0.1 % bovine serum albumin (BSA), aliquoted, and frozen (−20 °C) until use.

---

* This work was supported in part by NIH grant DK 41627-02

Offprint requests to: D. A. Hullett, Ph. D., University of Wisconsin Hospital and Clinics, 600 Highland Avenue, H4/749, CSC, Madison, WI 53792, USA

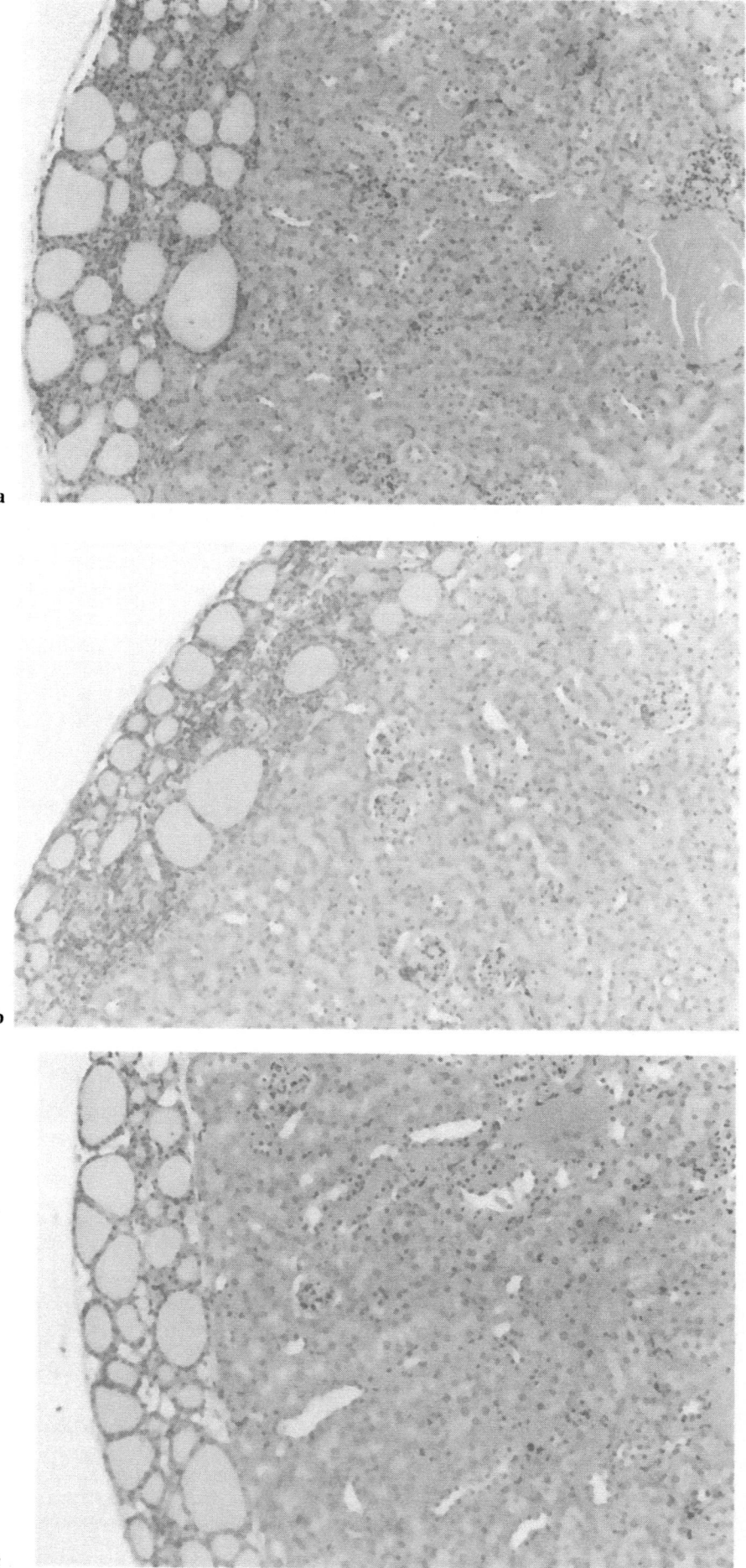

Fig. 1a–c. Combination IL-2-toxin and low dose RS-61443 therapy significantly improves murine thyroid allograft survival. **a** HVE of BIO.BR thyroid transplanted to BIO.Bl recipients; mean histological score 0.5. **b** HVE of C57BL/10 thyroid transplanted to BIO.BR receiving low dose (200 mg/kg) RS-61443 monotherapy; mean histological score 3.0. **c** HVE of C57BL/10 thyroid transplanted to BIO.BR receiving combination IL-2-toxin and RS-61443 therapy; mean histological score 1.5

Table 1. Combination therapy with RS-61443 and interleukin 2 (DAB486)-toxin prolongs murine thyroid allograft survival

Group	Recipient	Survival	Treatment[a]	Median[b] ^{125}I ratio	P value vs group 1	Histological score
1	B10.BR	21/22	–	18.8 ± 5.8		1
2	B10.BR	21/21	IL-2-toxin	12.5 ± 5.4	0.266	2
3	B10.BR	11/12	RS-61443	18.1 ± 5.1	0.666	1
4	B10.BR	7/7	RS-61443 plus IL-2-toxin	42.5 ± 11.7	0.272	2
5	C57BL/10	0/30	–	1.0 ± 0.09	0.0001	4
6	C57BL/10	9/34	IL-2-toxin	1.0 ± 1.01	0.0001	3
7	C57BL/10	20/31	RS-61443	6.9 ± 1.5	0.0001	4
8	C57BL/10	19/19	RS-61443 plus IL-2-toxin	25.2 ± 5.4	0.142	2

[a] Recipient animals were dosed with RS-61443 (200 mg/kg daily p.o.) for 21 days and/or IL-2-toxin for 14 days (25 µg/day s.c.)
[b] Graft function was determined at 21 days by ^{125}I incorporation.

The counts perminute (CPM) incorporated into the left, grafted kidney were compared with the CPM incorporated into the right, nongrafted kidney. A ratio ≥ 4.0 was considered a viable graft

Recipient mice were dosed with RS-61443 by oral gavage beginning on the day before transplantation and continuing until the conclusion of the experiment at day 21. IL-2-toxyin was administered at 25 µg/day subcutaneously for 14 days beginning on the day of transplantation.

Statistical analysis. Median graft incorporation ratios were compared by the Mann-Whitney test.

Results and discussion

RS-61443 significantly improved graft survival at doses of 300 mg/kg daily or greater (data not shown). However, a significant weight loss was noted in recipients, most likely due to the gastrointestinal toxicity [12]. This dose is considerably greater than that reported for muring islet allografts [5]. The difference could be due to the fact that islet allografts are less immunogenic than thyroid grafts or to the strain combination used. At lower RS-61443 doses (200 mg/kg daily; Table 1), graft prolongation was achieved in 64 % of recipients. Histological examination showed ongoing graft rejection and significant levels of lymphocyte infiltration (Fig. 1). This observation is also reflected in the median ^{125}I uptake ratio obtained for these grafts, indicating significant graft destruction and loss of functional viability (Table 1; 6.9 vs. 18.8 in controls). Significant weight loss did not occur at this dose.

IL-2-toxin alone failed to prolong thyroid allograft survival (Table 1). Again, this is in contrast to the results obtained with murine cardiac allografts. This difference may reflect immunogenicity differences between vascularized and nonvascularized grafts. The half life of IL-2-toxin in vivo is approximately 4.5 min (unpublished data). In a nonvascularized graft, sufficient amounts of IL-2-toxin may not be able to reach the graft to prevent rejection. In addition, activation of the T cell following IL-2 binding to its receptor requires approximately 18 h, while cell death following internalization of the diphtheria portion of the molecule requires 24 h [4–15]. Sufficient killing of activated T cells prior to the release of newly synthesized IL-2 may not occur, thus allowing newly synthesized IL-2 to compete effectively with IL-2-toxin [13, 14].

Eugui et al. [2] have shown that lymphocytes in the presence of RS-61443 express IL-2 receptors on their surface but are prevented from further differentiation and proliferation. Thus, activated T cells in the presence of RS-61443 are a ready target for IL-2-toxin therapy which requires the delivery of minimal amounts of toxin to the cytoplasm of the cell [13]. IL-2-toxin (25 µg/day) in combination with low dose RS-61443 (200 mg/kg daily) significantly prolonged thyroid allograft survival at 21 days (Table 1). When the median ^{125}I uptake ratios were compared, combination therapy resulted in significant improvement ($P > 0.0001$) and were comparable with those obtained in the synergic nontreated control group (Table 1). These results were confirmed by histology (Table 1; Fig. 1).

In this paper, we have demonstrated the immunosuppressive potential of IL-2-toxin and low dose RS-61443 combination therapy for prolonged murine thyroid allograft survival. The unique properties of these agents are complementary and together may provide a potent immunosuppressive therapy.

References

1. Bacha P, Williams DP, Waters C, Williams JM, Murphy JR, Strom TB (1988) J Exp Med 167: 612–622
2. Eugui EM, Mirkovich A, Allison AC (1991) Scand J Immunol 33: 146–183
3. Grailer AP, Nichols JC, Strom TB, Sollinger HW, Burlingham WJ (1991) Cell Immunol 132: 481–493
4. Grailer AP, Nichols JC, Hullett D, Sollinger HW, Burlingham WJ (1991) Transplant Proc 23: 314–315
5. Hao C, Lafferty KJ, Allison AC, Eugui EM (1990) Transplant Proc 22: 876–879
6. Hullett DA, Landry AS, Sollinger HW (1989) Transplantation 47: 24
7. Kelley VE, Gaulton GN, Hattorl M, Itegami H, Eisenbarth G, Strom TB (1988) J Immunol 140: 59–61
8. Kelly UE, Bacha P, Pankewycz O, Nichols JC, Murphy JR, Strom TB (1988) Proc Natl Acad Sci USA 85: 3980–3984
9. Lorberoum-Galski H, Fitzgerald D, Chandhary V, Adhya S, Pastan I (1988) Proc Natl Acad Sci USA 85: 1922–1926
10. Murphy JR, Kelley UE, Strom TB (1988) Am J Kidney Dis 11: 159–162
11. Pankewycz O, Mackie J, Hassarjian R, Murphy JR, Strom TB, Kelley UE (1989) Transplantation 47: 818–822
12. Platz KP, Eckoff DE, Hullett DA, Sollinger HW (1991) Transplantation 51: 27–31
13. Walz G, Zanker B, Murphy JR, Strom TB (1990) Transplantation 49: 198–201
14. Walz G, Zanker B, Brand K, Waters C, Genbauffe F, Zeldis JB, Murphy JR, Strom TB (1989) Proc Natl Acad Sci USA 85: 9486–9488
15. Williams DP, Parker K, Bacha P, Bishai W, Borowski M, Genbauffe F, Strom TB, Murphy JR (1987) Protein Eng 1: 493–498

Transplant Int (1992) 5 [Suppl 1]: S 490–S 493

TRANSPLANT
International
© Springer-Verlag 1992

The effects of nifedipine on cyclosporine nephrotoxicity in rats

C. J. Ferguson, C. von Ruhland, D. J. Parry-Jones, J. D. Williams, and J. R. Salaman

Department of Surgery and Institute for Nephrology, Cardiff Royal Infirmary, Cardiff, United Kingdom

Abstract. We have investigated the effect of nifedipine on cyclosporine nephrotoxicity in the Sprague-Dawley rat employing a repeatable, single-shot, isotopic technique of measuring the glomerular filtration rate (GFR) and effective renal plasma flow (ERPF). Groups of 10 rats received either cyclosporine 5 mg/kg daily or cremaphor with either nifedipine 0.5 mg/kg daily or its vehicle for 14 days. In the cyclosporine group the GFR ($P < 0.001$, paired t-test), ERPF and filtration fraction (FF) ($P < 0.01$) all fell significantly. The cyclosporine plus nifedipine group underwent an increase in the ERPF ($P < 0.01$), the GFR remained unchanged, and the FF fell significantly ($P < 0.0001$). In this model, nifedipine completely abolished the renal arteriolar vasospasm produced by cyclosporine. That the FF fell in the cyclosporine plus nifedipine-treated animals indicates that cyclosporine has an effect which is not mediated by arteriolar vasoconstriction. This action may be at the glomerular level and is resistant to calcium channel blockade.

Key words: Cyclosporine nephrotoxicity – Nifedipine – Calcium channel blockade – Renal haemodynamics

Cyclosporine remains the mainstay of clinical immunosuppression for both solid organ and bone marrow transplantation. The associated nephrotoxicity, however, has limited its clinical use and has imposed a narrow therapeutic window for clinicians. There is mounting evidence that long-term use of cyclosporine results in chronic renal damage in both renal allografts [7, 24] and in patients with functioning native kidneys [14, 15]. The future of cyclosporine may therefore heavily depend on the results of investigation of the nature of its nephrotoxic action and the development of therapeutic intervention strategies to limit this effect.

Mechanistically speaking, the organic calcium channel blocking group of drugs might counter cyclosporine nephrotoxicity. Most of the experimental evidence of a beneficial effect, however, has come from studies on animal models which poorly represent the clinical situation, in that the administration of cyclosporine was acute, and the animals underwent extensive surgical preparation in order to measure renal function. As a result, clinicians have generally remained unconvinced of their efficacy, and few routinely employ calcium channel blockers for this purpose.

We have developed a new rat model of cyclosporine nephrotoxicity which closely represents the clinical situation in terms of the dose of cyclosporine used, the decrement in renal function observed and the duration of administration of the drug. This study describes the effects of nifedipine on this model.

Materials and methods

Male Sprague-Dawley rats weighing 180–320 g were used. The animals were housed 5 per cage and were kept at a constant temperature of 21 °C with 12-h cycles of light and dark. They had free access to water and were fed on a standard diet (Pilsbury's modified rat and mouse breeding diet).

Technique of measurement. The method used to use to measure the glomerular filtration rate (GFR) and effective renal plasma flow (ERPF) was a single injection and single blood sample isotopic technique using chromium-51-labelled ethylene diamine tetra-acetic acid (^{51}Cr-EDTA) and iodine-125-labelled Hippuran (^{125}I-Hippuran) [4, 18, 21].

The animals were lightly anaesthetised in an ether chamber. Vascular access was obtained by puncture of the ventral tail vein with a 23 gauge butterfly needle. Providing there was good blood flow indicating that a clean puncture of the vessel had been obtained, the isotopes were injected. The isotopes were delivered in a volume of 0.4 ml 0.9 % NaCl, and the activity of each was approximately 0.5 becquerel. The animals were allowed to recover from the anaesthesia and re-anaesthetised 1 h later when 1–2 ml of blood was taken from the tail vein at a site distant from the injection site. The blood was anticoagulated with lithium heparin and the plasma separated. The dose of radioactivity administered, the specimens and the residual radioactivity in the syringe used for the injection were counted on a Scaler Timer ST7 scintillation counter (Nuclear Enterprises, Thorn EMI).

Offprint requests to: Mr. C. J. Ferguson, M. Ch. FRCS

Table 1. GFR, ERPF and FF before the institution of the various treatment regimens and after 14 days of treatment

Group	Day 1	Day 14
(A) Cyclosporine ($n = 8$)		
GFR (ml/min)	2.39 (0.4)	1.31 (0.33)[3']
ERPF (ml/min)	6.48 (0.66)	4.86 (0.78)[2']
FF	36.8 (4.67)	26.9 (4.7)[2]*
(B) Nifedipine and cyclosporine		
GFR (ml/min)	2.03 (0.28)	2.03 (0.26)
ERPF (ml/min)	5.14 (0.75)	5.87 (0.54)[1']
FF	39.5 (1.9)	34.5 (1.7)[4]
(C) Double vehicle		
GFR (ml/min)	2.24 (0.3)	2.51 (0.23)[1']
ERPF (ml/min)	5.72 (0.4)	6.35 (0.53)[2']
FF	39 (3.8)	39 (2.1)
(D) Nifedipine		2.12 (0.27)
GFR (ml/min)	2.02 (0.24)	5.71 (0.61)
ERPF (ml/(min)	5.51 (0.5)	37 (2.6)
FF	37 (2.1)	

[1'] $P < 0.05$, [2'] $P < 0.01$, [3'] $P < 0.001$, [4'] $P < 0.0001$, by paired t-test
Mean and SD
Cyclosporine (5 mg/kg daily) causes a marked reduction in all parameters. Nifedipine (0.5 mg/kg daily) administration with cyclosporine causes reversal of the effect of cyclosporine on the ERPF and significant amelioration of the effect on the GFR. The FF remains depressed despite nifedipine
Filtration fraction (FF) = GFR/ERPF × 100; GFR, glomerular filtration rate; ERPF, effective renal plasma flow

Calculation of renal haemodynamics. Assuming instantaneous mixing of the clearance substances in the intravascular compartment and excretion exclusively via the glomerulus, the clearance substances will disappear from the plasma in a monoexponential fashion. Thus, the logarithm of the concentration plotted against time will be a straight line.

The initial plasma concentrtion (P_0) can be calculated from the injected dose (I) and the volume of distribution (V) in the animal ($P0 = I/V$). From the line drawn between these points, the decay constant (k) can be calculated.

$$k = \ln(P_0/T_t)/t$$

$$Clearance = V \cdot k$$

$$Clearance = V \cdot \ln(P_0/P_t)/t$$

where t is the time from injection and
P_t the plasma concentration at time t.

V has already been calculated in the rat over a wide range of body weights for both ^{51}Cr-EDTA and ^{125}I-Hippuran. The published data have been employed in our calculations [4, 18].

Blood pressure. Systolic blood pressure was measured using a tail blood pressure cuff, a pulse sensor attached to a piezoelectric crystal and an automated electrosphygmomanometer (Narco Biosystems). The animals were lightly sedated using Hypnorm (fentanyl 3.15 g and fluanisone 0.1 mg). Each measurement was a mean of 3 estimations.

Cyclosporine 5 mg/kg daily dissolved in cremaphor (polyethoxylated castor oil) was administered by intraperitoneal injection at the same time every morning except for the day of measurement of GFR and ERPF.

Nifedipine 0.5 mg/kg · day was administered as a twice daily subcutaneous injection. Nifedipine was kindly supplied by Bayer U.K. (Newbury) in an injectable formulation.

Statistical methods. Data from other experiments using this model have shown a normal distribution for the parameters measured, therefore parametric statistical analysis was used. The paired t-test was employed to compare data within each group, and comparisons between groups have been made using the unpaired t-test.

Study plan. Measurement of GFR and ERPF was made before and after 14 days of administration of the various drug regimens. Weight and blood pressure measurement was carried out throughout the study.

There were 4 study groups according to treatment: (A) cyclosporine, (B) cyclosporine and nifedipine, (C) both vehicles and (D) nifedipine. Groups A and D also received the vehicle for the other agent.

Results

In the cyclosporine group A ($n = 8$) there was a significant fall in GFR ($P < 0.001$), ERPF ($P < 0.01$) and filtration fraction (FF) ($P < 0.01$) over the study period (Table 1).

In the nifedipine and cyclosporine group B, in contrast to group A, the addition of nifedipine prevented a fall in GFR. In addition, there was a significant rise in ERPF ($P < 0.05$). The relative difference in change in ERPF and GFR resulted in a fall in FF ($P < 0.0001$). This fall in FF (5.04 ± 2.06; mean and SD) was significantly less ($P < 0.02$, unpaired t-test) than that seen in group A (9.94 ± 5.3).

In the control, double vehicle group C there was a significant increase in both GFR ($P < 0.05$) and ERPF ($P < 0.01$) during the 14 day period of the study. The FF remained unchanged.

In the nifedipine group D, there were no significant changes in any of the renal functional parameters. The GFR and ERPF both rose slightly, and the FF remained unchanged.

When the results at day 14 of the study were compared between groups, there was no significant difference in the percentage change in GFR or ERPF for groups B, C and D (unpaired t-test) (Figs. 1–3).

Systolic blood pressure. There were not significant changes in blood pressure in any of the groups (Table 2).

Body weight. The animals in the group A gained significantly less weight than in the other groups ($P < 0.005$, unpaired t-test). Group B gained weight at an equivalent rate to the control animals.

Discussion

This study has clearly demonstrated that nifedipine has a beneficial effect on cyclosporine nephrotoxicity in the Sprague-Dawley rat. Using a dosage of both drugs equivalent to those used in clinical practice, nifedipine completely abolished the effect of cyclosporine on the ERPF and markedly reduced its influence on the GFR.

The increase in the ERPF seen in group B was of the same order as that which occurred with increasing body weight in the double vehicle group (C), indicating that the arteriolar vasoconstriction associated with cyclosporine did not occur during co-treatment with nifedipine.

In addition, the GFR in group B remained unchanged over the 14-day treatment period, and its percentage change did not differ between groups C and D. This demonstrates that nifedipine produced a significant amelioration of the effect of cyclosporine on the GFR. The consquence of the difference in change between these

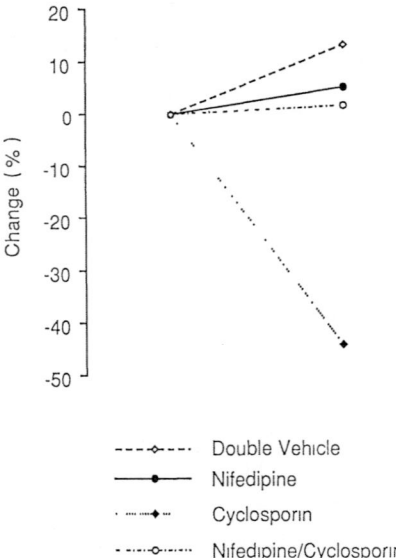

Fig. 1. Percentage change in GFR in each of the four groups. There was a significant fall in the cyclosporine-treated animals ($P < 0.001$, paired t-test) and a significant rise in the double vehicle group ($P < 0.05$, paired t-test), although when the percentage changes in GFR between the other three groups were compared, there was no significant difference between them

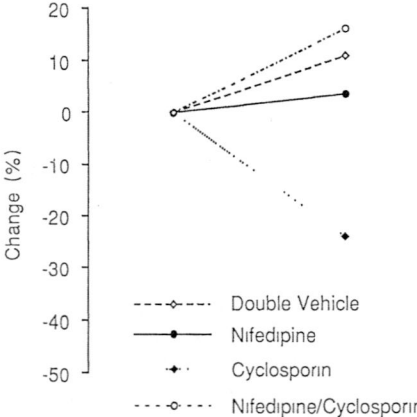

Fig. 2. Percentage change in ERPF in each of the groups. There was a significant fall in the cyclosporine-treated animals ($P < 0.01$, paired t-test) and a significant rise in the double vehicle and nifedipine/cyclosporine-treated gorups ($P < 0.01$ and 0.05, respectively, paired t-test)

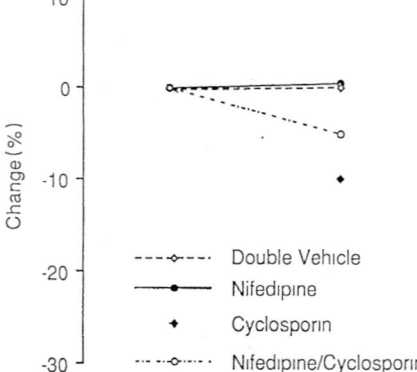

Fig. 3. Change in FF in each of the groups. There was a significant fall in both the cyclosporine-treated animals ($P < 0.01$, paired t-test) and the nifedipine/cyclosporine-treated group ($P < 0.0001$). The fall in FF in the cyclosporine-treated group was significantly larger than in the nifedipine/cyclosporine-treated group ($P < 0.05$, unpaired t-test)

Table 2. Systolic tail blood pressure for each group of rats before treatment and after 4 and 11 days of treatment. There were no significant changes in any of the groups showing that the changes observed in renal function were not a reflection of changes in systemic blood pressure

Group	Day 4	Day 11	Day 18
(A) Cyclosporine	133 (12)	136 (10.7)	131 (10.8)
(B) Nifedipine and cyclosporine	132 (6.3)	133 (10.9)	144 (16.8)
(C) Double vehicle	132 (23.5)	134 (14.8)	143 (20.2)
(D) Nifedipine	133 (16.4)	139 (17.3)	134 (14.6)

Treatment regimens instituted from day 7 to day 21 (mean and SD)
No significant differences by paired t-test

parameters was that the FF fell significantly, suggesting that arteriolar vasoconstriction is not the only mechanism by which cyclosporine is toxic to the renal microcirculation.

The mechanisms underlying the nephrotoxic effects of cyclosporine remain controversial and elusive. Cyclosporine nephrotoxicity is characterised by a reduction in the ERPF [8, 16, 22] and in the GFR [1, 5].

Current knowledge indicates that cyclosporine induces a reduction in renal plasma flow by causing constriction of the afferent glomerular arterioles. In a very elegant experiment using scanning electron micrographs of casts of the glomerular microcirculation, constriction of the afferent glomerular arterioles was demonstrated in Fischer rats which had received cyclosporine 50 mg/kg daily for 7 days [6]. The fall in GFR with cyclosporine may in part be a consequence of the afferent glomerular arteriolar constriction, which will cause a reduction in intraglomerular hydrostatic pressure.

The calcium channel blocking group of drugs are known to be potent renal vasodilators. They act via the voltage-sensitive calcium channels to reduce the calcium influx into the smooth muscle cell and thereby also the excitation-contraction coupling. It has been shown that these drugs are most active on the afferent glomerular arteriole [11], and this is the primary mechanism by which they could have a beneficial effect on cyclosporine toxicity.

Nifedipine was chosen for the present study as it is the only calcium channel blocking drug which has been shown not to interfere with the metabolism of cyclosporine [12, 23].

Recently, there has been some controversy as to whether cyclosporine causes a disturbance of glomerular filtration directly. Several groups of workers have demonstrated a reduction in the FF associated with cyclosporine in animal studies [3, 10, 17]. In human studies, a marked reduction in the FF in cardiac allograft recipients receiving cyclosporine was found [14], and in a study of 8 human volunteers receiving 4 mg/kg as an infusion over 6 h, a marked reduction in FF occurred [25].

Other workers appear to have found an opposite effect in animal [1, 19] and human [2] studies. In the rat studies that have not shown a decrease in FF, the renal functional parameters were measured after the acute administration of cyclosporine, and this may have influenced the results.

In our model, which closely represents the clinical situation, we have consistently shown a reduction in FF as a consequence of cyclosporine. As yet, there is no consensus, but overall it seems likely that cyclosporine does reduce the FF.

The most likely mechanism whereby cyclosporine could produce this fall in the FF is via contraction of the glomerular mesangial cells, resulting in a reduction in the surface area available for filtration within the glomerulus.

Using an isolated glomerular surface area model and cultured rat mesangial cells, cyclosporine has been shown to have a direct action on the contraction of these cells and to increase the contractile effect of other agents [13, 20]. This may be mediated via angiotensin II. It has been demonstrated in micropuncture studies that calcium channel blocking drugs reverse the effects of angiotensin II on the GFR and the ultrafiltration coefficient by preventing contraction of the glomerular mesangium [9].

That the FF remained reduced in the present study despite calcium channel blockade suggests that angiotensin II is not the sole mediator of the reduction in the FF in cyclosporine nephrotoxicity. This is in keeping with the in vitro studies which demonstrated that the mesangial cell contraction that occurred with cyclosporine was only partially reversed by verapamil and that it was more completely prevented by platelet activating factor antagonists [20].

The model of cyclosporine nephrotoxicity described here has several advantages over other models, particularly those which require surgical preparation of the animals in order to measure renal function. Our subjects undergo a minimum of stress and disruption to their physiological integrity. The ability to repeat the measurements in the same animals reduces the number of animals required as each acts as their own control, and the animals can be studied over a period of time that has relevance to the development of clinical cyclosporine nephrotoxicity. The techniques involved are also relatively easy to perform, resulting in a very low incidence of technical error.

In conclusion, it seems that the cyclosporine-induced vasoconstriction of the afferent glomerular arteriole is prevented by nifedipine; however, the effects of cyclosporine on the glomerular filtration are ameliorated, but not reversed. This may be cause cyclosporine has an action on the glomerular mesangium which is mediated by agents that are not countered by calcium channel blockade, possibly locally produced autocoids such as platelet activating factor or thromboxane A_2.

While the calcium channel blocking group of drugs do not offer a complete solution to cyclosporine nephrotoxicity, as demonstrated in this model, they do appear to provide useful therapy. It may be that this problem can be more completely solved by the use of calcium channel blockers in combination with other agents.

References

1. Barros EJG, Boim MA, Ajzen H, Ramos OL, Schor N (1987) Glomerular haemodynamics and hormonal participation on cyclosporine nephrotoxicity. Kidney Int 32: 19–25
2. Bentle JP, Boudreau RJ, Ferris TF, et al. (1987) Suppression of plasma renin by cyclosporine. Am J Med 83: 59
3. Besarab A, Harrel BE, Hirsch S, et al. (1987) Use of the isolated perfused kidney model to assess the acute pharmacological effects of cyclosporine and its vehicle, cremaphore EL. Transplantation 44(2): 195–201
4. Bryan CW, Jarchow RC, Maher JF (1972) Measurement of glomerular filtration rate in small animals without urine collection. J Lab Clin Med 80(6): 845–856
5. Dieperink H, Leyssac PP, Kemp E, et al. (1987) Nephrotoxicity of cyclosporin in humans: effects on glomerular filtration and tubular reabsorption rates. Eur J Clin Invest 17: 493–496
6. English J, Evan A, Houghton DC, Bennett WM (1987) Cyclosporine induced acute renal dysfunction in the rat. Transplantation 44(1): 135–141
7. Evans D (1989) Long term results of renal transplantation with cyclosporin. In: Cyclosporin. Five years on. The Medicine Group (UK), Oxford, pp 45–50
8. Humes HD, Jackson NM, O'Connor RP, et al. (1985) Pathogenic mechanisms of nephrotoxicity: insights into cyclosporine nephrotoxicity. Transplant Proc 17: 101–116
9. Ichikawa I, Miele JF, Brenner BM (1979) Reversal of renal cortical actions of angiotensin II by verapamil and manganese. Kidney. Int 16: 137–147
10. Jackson NM, Hsu C, Visscher GE, et al. (1987) Alterations in renal structure and function in a rat model of cyclosporine nephrotoxicity. J Pharmacol Exp Ther 242(2): 749–756
11. Loutzenhiser R, Epstein M (1989) Modification of the renal haemodynamic response to vasoconstrictors by calcium antagonists. J Clin Invest 83: 960–969
12. McMillen MA (1988) Cyclosporin: interactions that matter. Presc J 28(5): 136–139
13. Meyer-Lenhert H, Schrier RW (1988) Cyclosporine A enhances vasopressin induced Ca^{2+} mobilisation and contraction in mesangial cells. Kidney Int 34: 89–97
14. Myers BD, Ross J, Newton L, Luetscher J, Perlroth M (1984) Cyclosporine associated chronic nephropathy. N Engl J Med 311(11): 699–705
15. Myers BD, Sibley R, Newton L, et al. (1988) The long term course of cyclosporine associated chronic nephropathy. Kidney Int 33: 590–600
16. Paller MS, Murray BM (1985) Renal dysfunction in animal models of cyclosporine toxicity. Transplant Proc 17: 155–159
17. Pavao OF, Boim MA, Bregman R, et al. (1989) Effect of platelet activating factor antagonist on cyclosporine nephrotoxicity. Transplantation 47(4): 592–595
18. Provoost AP, Keijzer MH, Wolff ED, Molenaar JC (1983) Development of renal function in the rat. Renal Physiol 6: 1–9
19. Racusen LC, Kone BC, Solez K (1987) Early renal pathophysiology in an acute model of cyclosporine nephrotoxicity in rats. Renal Failure 10(1): 29–37
20. Rodriguez-Puyol D, Lamas S, Olivera A, et al. (1989) Actions of cyclosporin A on cultured rat mesangial cells. Kidney Int 35: 632–637
21. Ryffel B, Hiestand P, Foxwell B et al. (1986) Nephrotoxic and immunosuppressive potentials of cyclosporine metabolites in rats. Transplant Proc 16(6) [Suppl 5]: 41–45
22. Sullivan BA, Hak LJ, Finn WF (1985) Cyclosporine nephrotoxicity: studies in laboratory animals. Transplant Proc 17: 145–154
23. Tjia JF, Back DJ, Breckenridge AM (1989) Calcium channel antagonists and cyclosporine metabolism: in vitro studies with human liver microsomes. Br J Pharmacol 28: 362–365
24. Tufveson G, Brynger H, Broyer M, et al. (1989) Changes in graft function during second year post transplantation in patients on cyclosporine compared to conventional immunosuppression. Transplant Proc 21(1): 1532–1533
25. Weir MR, Klassen DK, Shen SY, et al. (1990) Acute effects of intravenous cyclosporine on blood pressure, renal haemodynamics and urine production of healthy humans. Transplantation 49: 41–47

Transplant Int (1992) 5 [Suppl 1]: S 494–S 496

TRANSPLANT
International
© Springer-Verlag 1992

Cyclosporine-induced insulin release in rats is related to an increase in plasma lipid levels

M. E. Ferrero, A. Marni, M. Parise, P. C. Salari, M. Corsi, and G. Gaja

Istituto di Patologia Generale, Università, and Centro di Studio sulla Patologia Cellulare del CNR, Milan, Italy

Abstract. We studied the modifications of plasma lipid levels induced by cyclosporine (CsA), streptozocin (STZ) or both drugs in rats. Male Wistar rats (RT1y) were administered i. p. with CsA or STZ or both at the dosage of 15 mg/kg daily for 8 days and were sacrificed on day 9. Total lipid, triglyceride and total cholesterol plasma levels were measured. The plasma total lipid content was significantly increased in CsA-treated and in CsA + STZ-treated rats with respect to controls (662 ± 29 and 632 ± 32, respectively, vs 472 ± 27 mg/dl). The triglyceride content was significantly higher in CsA-treated and in CsA + STZ-treated animals than in controls (137 ± 8.7 and 188 ± 14.1, respectively, vs 79 ± 7.7 mg/dl). The total cholesterol level was not significantly different in CsA- and STZ-treated rats with respect to controls. CsA-treated and STZ-treated rats concomitantly revealed a significant impairment of glucose tolerance. In fact, 150 min after orogastric administration of 350 mg glucose, glycaemia was significantly more elevated in treated animals than in controls. We conclude that the increase in lipid levels induced by CsA treatment could be related to drug-induced damage to the pancreas islets, as shown by the early insulin release and fatty tissue degeneration.

Key words: Cyclosporin A – Plasma lipids – Diabetic rats

A role for cyclosporine (CsA) in the pathogenesis of a hyperlipidaemic status in patients undergoing renal transplantation was recently proposed [10]. In fact, in stable kidney graft recipients with good transplant function, long-term immunosuppression with CsA and low-dose prednisolone was associated with higher serum lipid levels than therapy with azathioprine and prednisolone. Lipid abnormalities in renal transplant recipients treated with CsA have been observed 2 [8] and even 3 years [11] after transplantation. Since hyperlipidaemia represents an im-

portant atherogenic risk, the use of CsA theoretically could be limited in kidney-grafted patients in whom the previous uraemia [9] and treatment with antihypertensive drugs and steroids [1] can also accelerate atherosclerosis. A significant increase in the levels of plasma lipids has been observed in rats treated with CsA [6]. The use of fish oil (a lipid-reducing agent) as the CsA vehicle rather than olive oil induced an increase in the levels of plasma triglycerides but not of cholesterol in treated with CsA animals for 28 days [6].

In a previous study we demonstrated that CsA administration in rats treated with multiple low doses of diabetogenic streptozocin (STZ) precipitated the onset of diabetes [3]. We subsequently showed that CsA treatment increased in vitro insulin release from pancreatic beta cells [4]. Finally, we found that CsA potentiated the in vivo effect of STZ in impairing the insulin content of the rat pancreas [5].

In the present study we evaluated whether the CsA-induced insulin release was related to modifications of the plasma lipid levels and glucose tolerance. The bilirubin content was examined as an indicator of liver function. We also compared the effect of CsA alone with that of STZ alone and of the two drugs given together. STZ was administered in multiple low doses, thereby assuring the onset of an autoimmune diabetes which mimicked type I insulin-dependent diabetes mellitus in man [7].

Materials and methods

Animals and pharmacological treatment. Four groups, each containing 20 male Wistar rats (RT1y) weighing 250–300 g, were studied. Animals of the first group were untreated (controls). In the second group, CsA (a gift from Sandoz, Basel, Switzerland) was injected intraperitoneally (i. p.) at the dosage of 15 mg/kg daily for 8 days; the drug was mixed prior to the injection with Tween 80 and 96 % ethanol in physiological saline to achieve the final concentration of 2 mg/ml. The third group of rats was treated with multiple low doses of STZ (Upjohn, Kalamazoo, Mich., USA); the drug was dissolved in sterile 0.05 M sodium citrate buffer, pH 4.5, and injected i. p. within 5 min at the dosage of 15 mg/kg daily. The fourth group received

Offprint requests to: Dr. M. E. Ferrero, Istituto di Patologia Generale, Via Mangiagalli 31, I-20133 Milan, Italy

Table 1. Plasma content (in mg/dl) of total lipids, triglycerides, total cholesterol and bilirubin (total and direct) (mean ± SEM of 10 experiments) in rats after 8 days of treatment with cyclosporine (CsA), streptozocin (STZ) or both drugs (CsA + STZ) and in controls (C)

Treatment	Total lipids	Triglycerides	Total cholesterol	Bilirubin	
				Total	Direct
C	472 ± 27	79 ± 7.7	65 ± 2.6	0.17 ± 0.01	0.23 ± 0.04
CsA	662 ± 29*	137 ± 8.7*	69 ± 5.4	0.60 ± 0.06*	0.60 ± 0.08*
STZ	477 ± 61	77 ± 4.7	66 ± 4.6	0.22 ± 0.02	0.21 ± 0.03
CsA + STZ	632 ± 32*	188 ± 14.1*,+	54 ± 6.1	0.65 ± 0.06*	0.63 ± 0.07*

* $P < 0.01$ versus C, + $P < 0.05$ versus CsA

Table 2. Glycaemia values (in mg/dl) measured before and 150 min after orogastric administration of glucose (350 mg in 1 ml) to rats fasted for 18 h after being treated for 8 days with CsA, STZ or both drugs (CsA + STZ) and controls (C) (mean ± SEM of 10 experiments)

Treatment	Glucose administration	
	Before	After
C	65 ± 6.0	89 ± 3.8
CsA	86 ± 3.0*	128 ± 8.4**
STZ	101 ± 5.1**	134 ± 13.5*
CsA + STZ	128 ± 7.7**,+	177 ± 16.0**,+

* $P < 0.05$ versus C, ** $P < 0.01$ versus C, + $P < 0.05$ versus CsA and versus STZ

both CsA and STZ i. p. at the same dosages daily for 8 days. On day 9 following 18 h of fasting during the night with free access to water, 10 rats per group were exsanguinated at the aorta bifurcation level after brief ether anaesthesia. The blood was used for the biochemical assays. The remaining 10 rats were used for the glucose tolerance test.

Biochemical assays. The plasma triglyceride and cholesterol concentrations were determined by routine enzymatic methods (Boehringer, Mannheim, FRG). Lipids and bilirubin were measured by using colorimetric tests (Boehringer).

Glucose tolerance test. Following 8 days of pharmacological treatment, 10 rats were given orogastrically an aqueous glucose solution (350 mg in 1 ml) while under light ether anaesthesia and following 18 h of fasting. Glycaemia was evaluated before and 150 min after glucose administration. The blood glucose level was determined by using an enzymatic test (hexokinase/G6P dehydrogenase, Boehringer).

Statistical analysis. The results were expressed as mean ± SEM and subjected to variance analysis. Significance was assumed when P was < 0.05.

Results

Table 1 gives the plasma levels (mg/dl) of total lipids, triglycerides, total cholesterol and bilirubin (total and direct) in control rats and in those treated for 8 days with CsA, STZ, or CSA and STZ. The data represent the mean ± SEM of 10 experiments. Plasma levels of total lipids were significantly higher in CsA-treated rats than in controls. Treatment with STZ did not increase the total lipid levels with respect to controls, whereas the concomitant administration of both drugs did not seem to modify the effect due to CsA alone. Plasma levels of triglycerides were significantly more elevated in CsA-treated animals than in controls. Treatment with STZ

alone did not alter the plasma triglyceride content with respect to that of the controls, but concomitant treatment with STZ and CsA produced a significant increase compared with CsA treatment alone. CsA, STZ and CsA + STZ treatments did not determine a significant difference in plasma total cholesterol content, which appeared to be similar to that of the controls. The level of total bilirubin (which was all present as direct bilirubin) was significantly higher in CsA-treated and in CsA + STZ-treated rats than in the controls.

Table 2 gives the glycaemia values (mg/dl) of rats subjected to orogastric administration of 350 mg glucose in 1 ml. Blood glucose levels were studied before and 150 min after administration. Before glucose administration, the rats were fasted for 18 h, following 8 days of CsA, STZ or CsA + STZ treatment. The data represent the mean ± SEM of 10 experiments. Glycaemia levels in the CsA-treated rats were significantly more elevated than in the controls before glucose administration; hyperglycaemia was more evident in these rats than in the controls after administration. STZ-treated rats were significantly hyperglycaemic compared with the controls before glucose administration, and they maintained less evident but significantly more elevated glycaemia values than the controls after administration. CsA + STZ-treated rats, before and after glucose administration, presented significantly higher glycaemic levels than those of the controls; these levels were significantly more elevated than those of the CsA-treated and STZ-treated rats.

Figure 1 depicts the results of the glucose tolerance test in the pharmacologically treated rats. Treatment with CsA and with CsA + STZ significantly reduced, with respect to the controls, the glucose tolerance of the animals.

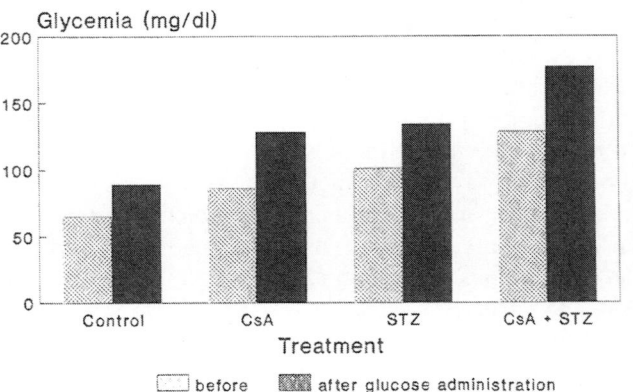

Fig. 1. Glucose tolerance test in rats after 8 days of pharmacological treatment. CsA Cyclosporin; STZ Streptozotocin

Discussion

In a previous study we demonstrated that the treatment of rats with CsA increased the release of insulin from the pancreas [5]. In fact, the total pancreatic insulin content was significantly lower (– 65 % of controls) in the CsA-treated rats and was related to a reduction of the total pancreatic protein content (– 31 % of control values). The effect was amplified by the concomitant treatment with CsA and STZ, and we presume that CsA has a direct toxic effect on the beta cells. Owing to the usefulness of CsA as an immunosuppressive drug in grafted patients and the modifications induced in the serum lipid content in stable renal transplant recipients [10], we believed it worthwhile to study the plasma content of total lipids, triglycerides and total cholesterol in the same experimental model we previously used [5].

In the present study we demonstrated that after 8 days of CsA treatment, the plasma total lipid levels significantly increased with respect to those of the controls. We also showed that the plasma triglyceride values were significantly more elevated in the CsA-treated animals than in the controls, whereas the cholesterol content did not vary.

We hypothesize that the early severe drop in the total pancreas insulin content of CsA-treated rats could be related to a mobilization of fatty acids from the adipose tissue. In fact, in STZ-treated rats, in which the total insulin pancreatic content was reduced to a lesser extent (– 26 % of controls) [5], the plasma triglyceride values were not significantly different from those of the controls. Moreover, in CsA + STZ-treated animals, in which the total pancreatic insulin content was dramatically reduced (– 80 % of controls) [5], the plasma triglyceride levels were significantly higher than in the controls and CsA-treated animals. During 8 days of treatment with CsA, the plasma cholesterol level did not appear to vary with respect to that of the controls. Since the increase in plasma cholesterol has also been demonstrated in 28-day treated animals [6], the modification in the plasma cholesterol content could be attributable to CsA treatment for more than 8 days. We agree that the increase in the lipid levels could have been due to a substantially altered hepatic synthesis of lipoprotein, as previously suggested [6]. In fact, in the present study we demonstrated an altered hepatic function at 8 days of treatment, as indicated by the roughly threefold increase in total bilirubin with respect to controls. In rats, the presence of only direct circulating bilirubin is indicative of severe hepatic liver alteration. It is also possible that the CsA treatment was responsible for the elevation of the plasma lipid levels through a reduction of the peripheral lipid catabolism, as observed in chronically uraemic rat models [9].

We previously revealed after CsA and CsA + STZ treatment a severe reduction in the pancreas protein content [5] associated with fatty tissue degeneration and hypoatrophy of the parenchyma. We concluded that the increase in lipid levels induced by CsA treatment could have been related to the fatty pancreas degeneration due to drug-induced damage to the islets. We believe that the beneficial effect obtained by CsA administration in diabetic patients with recent onset type I disease [2] deserves to be thoroughly evaluated. In fact, the usefulness of CsA treatment could be related to insulin release from undamaged beta cells in these patients. However, continuous drug administration could lead to significant and irreversible pancreas degeneration. Moreover, the subsequent drug-induced increase in the plasma lipid levels could favour the rise in diabetic metabolic disorders. The same considerations apply to diabetic patients who undergo pancreas transplantation.

With the experimental model of the present study, it was demonstrated that CsA significantly modified the plasma lipid levels more than the diabetogenic STZ. Our demonstration that CsA treatment significantly impaired the rat glucose tolerance capacity is in agreement with other results.

References

1. Chan MK, Varghese Z, Persaud JW, Fernando ON, Moorhead JF (1981) The role of multiple pharmacotherapy in the pathogenesis of hyperlipidemia after renal transplantation. Clin Nephrol 15: 309–313
2. Dupré J, Stiller CR, Gent M, Donner A, von Graffenreid B, Murphy G, Heinrichs D, Jenner MR, Keown PA, Laupacis A, Mahon J, Martell R, Rodger NW, Wolfe BW (1988) Effects of immunosuppression with cyclosporine in insulin-dependent diabetes mellitus of recent onset: the Canadian open study at 44 months. In: Kahan BD (ed) Cyclosporine. Grune & Stratton, Philadelphia, pp 184–192
3. Ferrero E, Marni A, Ferrero ME, Gaja G, Rugarli C (1985) Effect of cyclosporine and aminophylline on streptozotocin-incuded diabetes in rats. Immunol Lett 10: 183–187
4. Ferrero ME, Marni A, Gaja G (1989) Stimulation of insulin release from rat pancreatic islets induced by cyclosporine. Biochem Soc Trans 17: 351–352
5. Gaja G, Marni a, Ferrero ME (1990) Cyclosporine potentiates the in vivo effect of streptozotocin in impairing rat pancreas insulin content. Transplant Proc 22: 2250–2252
6. Jevnikar AM, Petric R, Holub BJ, Philbrick DJ, Clark WF (1988) Effect of cyclosporine on plasma lipids and modification with dietary fish oil. Transplantation 46: 722–725
7. Paik SG, Fleischer N, Shin SI (1980) Insulin-dependent diabetes mellitus induced by subdiabetogenic doses of streptozotocin: obligatory role of cell-mediated autoimmune processes. Proc Natl Acad Sci USA 77: 6129–6133
8. Raine AEG, Carter R, Mann JI, Morris PJ (1988) Adverse effect of cyclosporin on plasma cholesterol in renal transplant recipients. Nephrol Dial Transplant 3: 458–463
9. Roullet JB, Lacour B, Yvert JP, Prat JJ, Drueke T (1985) Factors of increase in serum triglyceride-rich lipoproteins in uremic rats. Kidney Int 27: 420–423
10. Schorn TF, Kliem V, Bojanovski M, Bojanovski D, Repp H, Bunzendahl H, Frei U (1991) Impact of long-term immunosuppression with cyclosporin A on serum lipide in stable renal transplant recipients. Transplant Int 4: 92–95
11. Vathsala A, Weimberg RB, Schoenberg L, Grevel J, Dunn J, Goldstein RA, Buren CT van, Lewis RM, Kahan BD (1989) Lipid abnormalities in renal transplant recipients treated with cyclosporine. Transplant Proc 21: 3670–3673

Transplant Int (1992) 5 [Suppl 1]: S 497–S 500

TRANSPLANT
International
© Springer-Verlag 1992

Cellular mechanisms: Induction of heart allograft survival in rats by 15-deoxyspergualin

H. Jiang[1], S. Takahara[1], M. Kyo[1], Y. Takano[1], H. Kameoka[1], Y. Kokado[1], M. Ishibashi[1], A. Okuyama[1], and T. Sonoda[2]

Departments of [1] Urology and [2] Organ Transplantation, Osaka University Medical School, Osaka, Japan

Abstract. Survival of ACI rat heart grafts in Lewis rat (LEW) recipients treated with a short course of 15-deoxyspergualin (DSG), in a dose of 5 mg/kg daily beginning from day 4 of grafting, was markedly prolonged, with a mean survival time of 29.8 ± 3.0 days. On day 20 after grafting, the cellular mechanism of inducing allograft survival after DSG treatment was analyzed by testing the activation of spleen cells in several assay systems. The results indicate that spleen cells from DSG-treated rats with surviving heart allografts show almost no proliferative response against donor strain stimulator cells in the mixed lymphocyte reaction (MLR) as compared with controls. Their cytotoxic activity was lower than that of spleen cells from rats with heart allograft rejection towards donor strain target cells. Adding various concentrations of spleen cells from DSG-treated LEW rats with surviving ACI heart allografts to the MLR when the responder cells from normal LEW rats were exposed to irradiated ACI or Wistar (third party) stimulator cells revealed a strong suppression, in a cell-dose-dependent manner. Moreover, the transfer of 2.0×10^8 spleen cells from DSG-treated LEW rats with surviving ACI heart allografts to an irradiated grafted host did not prolong the survival either of the ACI heart grafts or of the third party Wistar heart grafts. These results suggest that the proliferative response and cytotoxic activity are lowered and suppressor cells are induced by treatment with DSG, in rats with surviving allografts.

Key words: Immunosuppressive agent – Heart allograft survival – Rejection – Spleen cell

---

15-Deoxyspergualin, originally developed for its antibiotic and antitumor activity [4], has shown potential as a clinically valuable immunosuppressive agent. Several communications have reported that this agent has immunosuppressive activity against acute rejection in human renal transplantation [2]. In vitro experiments in human subjects have shown that the principle effect is an inhibition of the later phase of the mixed lymphocyte reaction (MLR), mainly by suppression of the expression of the interleukin 2 (IL2) receptors, and cytotoxic T-cell generation [10, 11]. Moreover, many studies in animals have demonstrated that DSG is an effective immunosuppressive agent, capable of inhibiting the immunoresponse in rat skin grafts, rat heterotopic heart transplantation, and dog renal transplantation [1, 5, 17]. These findings indicate that DSG may facilitate the prolongation of allograft survival and emphasize the need for further study of its mechanisms of action in the inhibition of allograft rejection in the rat model. In this present study, experiments were therefore designed to study the cellular mechanisms of allograft survival after a short course of DSG treatment.

Materials and methods

Animals. Male LEW rats (RT11) weighing 250–300 g were used as recipients. Male ACI rats (RT1a) weighing 150–200 g and Wistar rats (RT1e) weighing 150–200 g were used as donors and third party donors, respectively. The animals were obtained from commercial sources (LEW: Charles River, Japan; ACI: Hishino Experiment Animals, Japan; Wistar: SLC, Japan) and kept under specific-pathogen-free conditions in our animal facility.

Immunosuppression. 15-Deoxyspergualin was supplied by Nippon Kayaku Co. (Tokyo, Japan). The drug was dissolved in physiological saline and stored at $-70\,°C$ before use.

Heterotopic heart transplantation were performed using the modified technique of Ono and Lindsey [12]. Survival of the cardiac allograft was determined by daily palpation. Rejection was considered complete at the time of cessation of a palpable heartbeat and confirmed by histological examination.

Preparation of spleen cells. Lymphocytes were obtained from rat spleen. The spleen was isolated and minced, and the red cells were then lysed with buffered hypotonic TRIS-ammonium chloride (0.83 %, pH 7.21). Cells were washed twice with RPMI 1640 and then suspended in RPMI 1640 complete medium containing 10 %

Offprint requests to: S. Takahara, M.D., Department of Urology, Osaka University Hospital, Fukushima 1-1-50, Fukushima-ku, Osaka 553, Japan

Table 1. Effect of 15-deoxyspergualin (DSG) on heterotopically transplanted rat hearts

Experimental groups	Survival (days)	Mean ± SD	P value
No immunosuppressant (control, $n = 6$)	5, 6 (3), 7 (2)	6.1 ± 0.7	
DSG 5.0 mg/kg daily ($n = 8$)	26, 28, 30, 31, 34	29.8 ± 3.0	< 0.01

Table 2. Mixed lymphocyte reaction (MLR) response and cell-mediated lympholysis (CML) activity of spleen cells from DSG-treated LEW rat with surviving ACI heart graft on day 20 after grafting

MLR	Stimulator cells	Responder cells	cpm[a]
	LEW	LEW	11 901 ± 5204
	ACI	LEW	43 038 ± 4108
	ACI	DSG-treated LEW	14 207 ± 5151
CML	Effector Responder/stimulator	Target	Cytotoxicity (%)[b]
	LEW T R[c] ACI	ACI	20.2 ± 1.8
	LEW T S[d] ACI	ACI	5.7 ± 2.8

[a] Mean of three individual experiments

[b] CML activity was assessed at a 40:1 effector/target ratio

[c] Cells from LEW rat with rejected ACI heart graft

[d] Cells from DSG-treated LEW rat with surviving ACI heart graft

fetal calf serum (FCS), 30 mM HEPES, 2.5 mM L-glutamine, and 5 μg/ml gentamicin, in various concentrations of cells, for assay.

Mixed lymphocyte reaction. One-way MLR was performed, using spleen cells from DSG-treated LEW rats with surviving ACI heart grafts or from normal LEW rats as responder cells and ACI rats as stimulator cells. Responder cells (0.5×10^6 /ml were co-cultured with 2000-rad-irradiated stimulator cells (1.0×10^6/ml) in 96-well tissue culture plates in RPMI 1640 complete medium. The cells were incubated at 37°C in a humidified atmosphere of 5% CO_2 for 4 days and then treated with an 16–20 h tritiated-thymidine (^{3}H-Tde) pulse. The cells were harvested, and ^{3}H-TdR incorporation was measured by a liquid scintillation counter (Packard Tri Carb 4530). The percentage suppression was calculated using the formula:

$$\% \text{Suppression} = \left[1 - \frac{\text{cpm (experimental)} - \text{cpm (negative control)}}{\text{cpm (positive control)} - \text{cpm (negative control)}}\right] \times 100$$

Cell-mediated lympholysis. Spleen cells from DSG-treated LEW rats with surviving ACI heart grafts as responder cells were co-cultured with 2000-rad-irradiated normal ACI stimulator cells in RPMI 1640 complete medium at 37°C in a humidified atmosphere of 5% CO_2 for 6 days. Splenic responder cells from LEW rats with rejected ACI heart allografts were used as the control. After incubation, the cells were harvested and used as effector cells for CML. Target cells were prepared by culturing stimulator cells with 50 μg/ml concanavalin A (ConA) for 2 days. The 4.0×10^6/ml effector cells were cultured with 1.0×10^5/ml ^{51}Cr-labelled target cells for 4 h at 37°C in a humidified atmosphere of 5% CO_2. A fixed volume of supernatant was collected from each well after centrifugation at 1500 g for 10 min. The ^{51}Cr release was counted in a gamma-counter (Aloka, JDC-752). The percentage of cytotoxicity was calculated according to the following formula:

$$\% \text{Cytotoxicity} = \frac{\text{Experimental release} - \text{Spontaneous release}}{\text{Maximum release} - \text{Spontaneous release}} \times 100$$

Suppressor cell reactivity. Suppressor cell reactivity in the MLR was also assayed by adding 0.5×10^4, 1.0×10^4, and 2.0×10^4 spleen cells from DSG-treated LEW rats with surviving ACI grafts to the MLR

when responder cells from normal LEW rats were exposed to irradiated ACI or Wistar (third party) stimulator cells. In the control experiment, spleen cells from normal LEW rats were added.

Adoptive transfer by spleen cell. LEW rats were given 250 rads of whole body irradiation and, on the following day, grafted with ACI or Wistar (third party) hearts. On day 1 of grafting, they received an intravenous (i. v.) injection of 2.0×10^8 spleen cells. The spleen cells were obtained from DSG-treated LEW rats with surviving ACI grafts or normal LEW rats. Survival of the graft was the endpoint of this experiment.

Experimental design. Heart allografts were transplanted from ACI to LEW rats following 10 days of 5 mg/kg daily DSG treatment (from day 4 to day 13 after transplantation). On day 20 the spleen cells of LEW recipients with surviving ACI heart grafts, were used for testing activation by the following assays: (1) lymphocyte proliferative response, (2) cytotoxic T cell activity, (3) suppressor cell reactivity in the MLR, (4) adoptive transfer assay.

Statistical analysis: The statistical significance of the results was assessed by Student's *t*-test.

Results

Untreated allografted hearts (LEW/AIC, $n = 6$) were all rejected, with a mean survival time (MST) of 6.0 ± 0.7 days. However, the survival of ACI heart allografts in LEW recipients treated with 5 mg/kg daily of DSG for 10 days (from day 4 to day 13 postoperatively) was markedly prolonged, with graft MST of 29.8 ± 3.0 days (Table 1). The histopathological findings also demonstrated that severe hemorrhage, edema, and necrosis of myocardial muscle cells were present in the control, whereas rats treated with DSG showed only focal cellular infiltration among the myocytes on day 20 after grafting.

Mixed lymphocyte reaction

To test the proliferative response of spleen cells from DSG-treated LEW rats with surviving ACI heart grafts, spleen cells from DSG-treated recipients or normal LEW rats were used as responder cells, and normal ACI spleen cells were used as stimulator cells. The results are shown in Table 2. Responder cells from DSG-treated LEW recipients showed almost no proliferative response against ACI rat stimulator cells as compared with normal LEW responder cells.

CML activity

The cytotoxic activity of spleen cells from DSG-treated LEW rats with surviving ACI heart grafts on the donor strain target cell is shown in Table 2. The cytotoxic activity of spleen cells from LEW rats with rejected ACI heart grafts was taken as the control. The results showed that the mean cytotoxic activity was 20.20 ± 1.8% in spleen cells from untreated LEW rats with rejected allograft but was 5.70 ± 2.8% in spleen cells from the DSG-treated LEW recipients.

Table 3. Inhibition of MLR by adding spleen cells from DSG-treated rat with surviving ACI heart graft or normal LEW rat

MLR responder[a]/stimulator[b]	Cells added[c] (normal LEW rat) (n)	Inhibition (%)	Cells added[d] (DSG-treated LEW recipient rat) (n)	Inhibition (%)
LEW/ACI	0.5×10^4	-83.4 ± 28.0	0.5×10^4	34.5 ± 17.4
LEW/ACI	1.0×10^4	-101.0 ± 35.6	1.0×10^4	58.9 ± 16.8
LEW/ACI	2.0×10^4	-112.2 ± 64.3	2.0×10^4	86.2 ± 13.0
LEW/Wistar	0.5×10^4	-18.9 ± 32.0	0.5×10^4	22.8 ± 10.0
LEW/Wistar	1.0×10^4	-8.8 ± 17.6	1.0×10^4	50.2 ± 19.4
LEW/Wistar	2.0×10^4	-25.5 ± 28.1	2.0×10^4	76.0 ± 14.6

[a] Normal LEW spleen cells served as responder cells
[b] ACI or Wistar splenic stimulator cells
[c] Various concentrations of spleen cells obtained from normal LEW rat as control were added to MLR

[d] Various concentrations of spleen cells obtained from DSG-treated LEW rat with surviving ACI heart graft were added to MLR

Table 4. Survival of ACI and Wistar heart allografts in irradiated LEW rats after adoptive transfer of spleen cells from normal or DSG-treated LEW rats with surviving ACI heart grafts

Heart donor[a]	Cell transfer[b]		Graft survival (days [n])	Mean ± SD	P value
	Lymphocyte donor	No. of cells			
ACI	–	–	5, 6 (3), 7 (2)	6.1 ± 0.7	
ACI	Normal LEW	2.0×10^8	5, 6 (2), 7, 8	6.4 ± 1.1	NS
ACI	DSG-treated LEW with surviving ACI graft	2.0×10^8	5, 6, 7, 8, 10	7.2 ± 1.9	NS
Wistar	Normal LEW	2.0×10^8	14, 15 (2), 16, 17	15.4 ± 1.1	
Wistar	DSG-treated LEW with surviving ACI graft	2.0×10^8	14, 15 (2), 17, 18	15.8 ± 1.6	NS

[a] ACI or Wistar hearts heterotopically transplanted to 250-rad-X-irradiated LEW rats
[b] Spleen cells from normal or DSG-treated LEW rat with surviving

ACI heart graft transferred shortly to the unmodified LEW rat with ACI or Wistar heart graft on day 1 of grafting

Suppression of MLR

Studies were performed to assess the capacity of spleen cells obtained from DSG-treated recipients with surviving heart allografts to inhibit the MLR response. Spleen cells from normal LEW rats were used as responder cells and normal ACI or Wistar (third party) spleen cells were the stimulator cells. The results of experiments in which 0.5×10^4, 1.0×10^4, 2×10^4 of spleen cells obtained from DSG-treated LEW rats with surviving ACI heart grafts or from normal LEW rats were added to the MLR at the initiation of cultures are illustrated in Table 3. Spleen cells from DSG-treated rats markedly suppressed the MLR when the responder cells from normal LEW rats were exposed to irradiated ACI or Wistar (third party) stimulator cells. The addition of diluted cells to the MLR also resulted in cell-dose-dependent suppression. There were no significant differences in the suppressive rate between the donor strain and third party MLR. In contrast, when cells from the normal LEW rat were added, no inhibition was observed, in either the donor strain or the third party MLR response.

Effect of splee cell transfer

The alloreactivity of the spleen cells from DSG-treated LEW rats with surviving ACI heart grafts was further analyzed by adoptive cell transfer experiments. Control LEW rats undergoing irradiation alone or irradiation plus transfer of normal LEW spleen cells rejected their ACI grafts: the graft MST was 6.1 ± 2.1 days and 7.0 ± 2.1 days, re-

spectively and in the case of Wistar grafts (third party), the graft MST was 6.1 ± 1.1 days and 6.3 ± 1.2 days, respectively. The transfer of 2×10^8 spleen cells fro DSG-treated LEW rats with a surviving ACI graft did not significantly prolong the graft MST of the ACI or Wistar (third party) heart transplanted into irradiated LEW rats, although in 1 rt the graft survival was prolonged to 10 days after grafting (Table 4).

Discussion

It was confirmed in our experiments that a short course of DSG treatment at a dosage of 5 mg/kg daily from day 4 to day 14 posttransplantation, could inhibit the capacity of LEW rats to reject ACI heart grafts. This result strongly supports the clinical study result in renal transplantation by Amemiya et al. [2] that DSG is most effective in rescuing ongoing rejection.

With regard to the mechanism, we examined the MLR response and cytotoxic activity of spleen cells from DSG-treated LEW rats with surviving ACI heart grafts. The results showed that both the MLR response and CML activity were significantly decreased with spleen cells from the DSG-treated recipients. This effect strongly suggests that DSG could inhibit the lymphocyte response and cytotoxic T cell activity in the spleen in the rats with allografts and consequently allow the prolongation of allograft survival. These results coincide with our previous results in the human in vitro study of deoxymethylspergualin, which showed a suppression in the MLR and CML [10]. Moreover, our data also demonstrated that the CML response in the spleen cells of DSG-treated rats with surviving allografts is lower than in the spleen cells of rats with rejected allografts towards donor strain target cells. The findings indicate that the cytotoxic activity was most closely associated with allograft survival in the rat [9].

The mechanism of inducing allograft survival after a short course of DSG treatment was further studied by adding spleen cells to the MLR assay. The results show that the MLR in LEW spleen cells to donor party (ACI) and third party (Wistar) stimulator spleen cells were inhibited in a cell-dose-dependent manner. As various mechanisms of graft survival, such as the modulation of graft antigen expression [6, 14], depletion of clonally active cells following immunosuppression and exposure to the graft [7, 8], antigen/antibody blockade of effector cells [15, 16], activation of suppressor cells [3, 13], and production of suppressor humoral factor(s), have been postulated. Our results strongly suggest that DSG may fail to affect suppressor cells, and these cells may progressively develop and play a partial role in continuing allograft survival states. In addition, the inhibition of the MLR response between the donor and third party stimulator cells showed no significant difference on adding spleen cells from DSG-treated recipients. This indicates that the property of inhibition, on day 20 postgrafting, was a nonspecific suppression.

Studies to determine whether the spleen cells taken from DSG-treated rats with surviving allografts would be able to prolong the survival of the donor strain (ACI) or third party (Wistar) heart grafted into irradiated LEW rats showed that the spleen cells did not significantly prolong the graft MST of LEW recipients, either in the donor strain group or in the third party group, compared with the control group. The reasons for these results are not yet understood. We believe that the suppressive effect of spleen cells from DSG-treated rats with surviving allografts in the early phase may not be sufficient to control graft rejection.

In conclusion, the cellular mechanism of inducing heart allograft survival by DSG may mainly include (1) a decrease in lymphocyte response, (2) an inhibition of cytotoxic T cell acitivty, and (3) an induction of suppressor cells. Our next question is what is the role of humoral immunity in this rat model with DSG treatment.

References

1. Amemiya H, Suzuki s, Niiya S, Fukao K, Yamanaka N, Ito J (1989) A new immunosuppressive agent, 15-deoxyspergualin, in dog renal allografting. Transplant Proc 21: 3468–3470

2. Amemiya H, Sockeye S, Ota K, Takahashi K, Sonoda T, Ishibashi M, Amotio R, Koyama S, Dohi K, Fukuda Y, Fukao K (1990) A novel rescue drug, 15-deoxyspergualin, first clinical trials for recurrent graft rejection in renal recipients. Transplantation 49: 337–343

3. Dorsch SE, Roser B (1977) Recirculating, suprressor T-cells in transplantation tolerance. J Exp Med 145: 1144–1157

4. Dyuh D, Morris RE (1990) 15-deoxyspergualin is a more potent and effective immunosuppressant than cyclosporine but does not effectively suppress lymphoproliferation in vivo. Transplant Proc 23: 535–539

5. Fujii H, Takada T, Nemoto K, Abe F, Takeuchi T (1989) Stability and immunosuppressive activity of deoxyspergualin in comparison with deoxymethylspergualin. Tranplant Proc 221: 3471–3473

6. Hart DNJ, Winearls CG, Fabre JW (1980) Graft adaptation: studies on possible mechanisms in long-tern survival rat renal allografts. Transplantation 30: 73–80

7. Hutchinson IV (1980) Antigen-reactive cell opsonization (ARCO) and its role in antibody-mediated immune suppression. Immunol Rev 49: 167–197

8. Hutchinson IV, Zola H (1977) Antigen-reactive cell opsonization (ARCO): a mechanism of immunological enhancement. Transplantation 23: 464–469

9. Ito T, Stepkowski SM, Kahan BD (1990) Soluble antigen and cyclosporine-induced specific unresponsiveness in rats. Transplantation 49: 422–428

10. Jiang H, Takahara S, Takano Y, Machida M, Iwasaki A, Kokado Y, Kameoka H, Moutabarrik A, Ishibashi M, Sonoda T (1990) In vitro immunosuppressive effect of deoxymethylspergualin. Transplant Proc 22: 1633–1637

11. Jiang H, Takahara S, Kyo M, Kokado Y, Ishibashi M, Sonoda T (1992) Effect of FK-506 on heart allograft survival in the highly sensitized recipient rats as compared with ciclosporin and 15-deoxyspergualin. Eur Surg Res (in press)

12. Ono K, Lindsey ES (1969) Improved technique of heart transplantation in rats. J Thorac Cardiovasc Surg 57: 225–227

13. Pearce NW, Spinelli A, Gurley KE, Dorsch SE, Hall BM (1989) Mechanisms maintaining antibody-induced enhancement of allografts: II. Mediation of specific suppression by short lived CD4+ T cells. J Immunol 143: 499–506

14. Silvers WK, Kimura H, Desquenne-Clark L, Miyamoto M (1987) Some new perspectives on transplantation immunity and tolerance. Immunol Today 8: 117–122

15. Stuart FP, Fitch FW, Rowley DA, Biesecker JL, Hellstrom KE, Hellstrom I (1971) Presence of both cell-mediated immunity and serum blocking factors in rat renal allograft enhanced by passive immunization. Transplantation 12: 331–333

16. Stuart FP, Scolland DM, McKearn TJ, Fitch FW (1976) Cellular and humoral immunity after allogenic renal transplantation in rat V. Appearance of anti-idiotypic antibody and its relationship to cellular immunity after treatment with donor spleen cells and alloantibody. Transplantation 22: 455–466

17. Suzuki S, Kanashiro M, Amemiya H (1987) Effect of a new immunosuppressant, 15-deoxyspergualin, on heterotopic rat heart transplantation, in comparison with cyclosporine. Transplantation 44: 484–487

Transplant Int (1992) 5 [Suppl 1]: S 501–S 503

TRANSPLANT
International
© Springer-Verlag 1992

Control of humoral and cellular immunity-mediated accelerated heart allograft rejection in sensitized rats by low dose FK 506 and splenectomy

H. Jiang[1], S. Takahara[1], M. Kyo[1], Y. Takano[1], H. Kameoka[1], Y. Kokado[1], M. Ishibashi[1], A. Okuyama[1], and T. Sonoda[2]

Departments of [1] Urology and [2] Organ Transplantation, Osaka University Medical School, Osaka, Japan

Abstract. ACI heart grafts are rejected, at an accelerated pace, in Lewis (LEW) rats sensitized by donor-type blood admixed with immunoadjuvant (adjuvant complete Freund, ACF) 7 days earlier. In an in vitro study, the anti-ACI cytotoxic antibody titers in the serum increased from 1:4 in nonsensitized rats to 1:128 in sensitized rats; the spontaneous blastogenesis in spleen cells was higher in sensitized rats than in nonsensitized rats; spleen cells from sensitized rats showed a strong proliferative response against donor strain stimulator cells compared with the control; the cytotoxic T cell activity of spleen cells from sensitized rats was higher than that of spleen cells from nonsensitized rats. Treatment with low dose FK 506 in combination with splenectomy (Spx) synergistically prolonged the heart allograft survival in this sensitized rat model. In conclusion: (1) Both humoral and cellular responses against the donor antigen appear in the serum and in the spleen of rats sensitized by donor-type blood admixed with immunoadjuvant ACF. (2) A low dose of FK 506 together with Spx appears to control this sensitization through different mechanisms, resulting in a prolongation of heart allograft survival.

Key words: Heart allograft survival – Humoral and cellular immunity – FK 506 – Splenectomy

Control of allograft rejection in the sensitized recipient remains a challenge in both experimental and clinical transplantation [4]. In clinical studies, it has been shown that the various strategies used to overcome sensitization are mostly empirical. One major problem is the lack of understanding of the immunological mechanisms underlying the rejection of this type of transplant [3]. We have previously reported that the Lewis (LEW) rat, sensitized by donor-type blood admixed with immunoadjuvant (ad-

juvant complete Freund ACF), could reject an ACI heart allograft in an accelerated fashion and that FK 506 could significantly overcome this rejection, although the dose of FK 506 needed for such an effect was higher than that in the nonsensitized recipient rat [2].

Our present study was divided into two parts. In the first part, we tried to confirm that both humoral and cellular immunity play important roles in rejection in the sensitized recipient rat. In the second part, after having shown that both the humoral and cellular response could cause accelerated allograft rejection, we tested the effect of low dose FK 506 in combination with splenectomy (Spx) on heart allograft survival in this sensitized rat model.

Materials and methods

Animals. Male Lewis rats (RT11) weighing 200–250 g were used as recipients and male ACI rats (RT1a) weighing 150–200 g were used as donors. They were obtained from commercial sources (LEW: charles River, Japan; ACI: Hoshino Experiment Animals, Japan) and kept under specific pathogen-free conditions in our animal facility.

Donor-specific sensitization. One milliliter of donor-type blood admixed with 0.1 ml of the immunostimulating agent ACF was administered subcutaneously 7 days prior to heart transplantation and in the in vitro studies.

Preparation of spleen cells. Lymphocytes were obtained from the rat spleen. The spleen was isolated and minced, and the red cells were then lysed with buffered hypotonic TRIS-ammonium chloride (0.83%, pH 7.21). The cells were washed twice with PRMI 1640, then suspended in RPMI complete medium containing 10% fetal calf serum (FCS), 30 mM HEPES, 2.5 mM L-glutamine, and 5 µg/ml gentamicin, for the in vitro assay.

Complement-dependent cytotoxicity assay. Prior to transplantation, all LEW rats were tested for serum titers of anti-ACI cytotoxic antibodies by CDC assay, as previously described [8]. The cytotoxic antibody titer was read as positive when more than 50% of donor T lymphocytes were killed compared with the negative control.

Spontaneous blastogenesis assay. Spontaneous blastogenesis (SB) was performed in triplicate by adding 1 µCr of tritiated thymidine (^{3}H-TdR) to 100 µl of 1.0×10^6/ml spleen cells, obtained from non-

Offprint requests to: S. Takahara, M. D., Department of Urology, Osaka University Hospital, Fukushima 1-1-50, Fukushima-ku, Osaka 553, Japan

Table 1. Humoral and cellular immunity in nonsensitized or sensitized rats

Group	CDC[a]	SB[b] (cpm) ($n = 3$)	MLR[c] (cpm) ($n = 3$)	CML[d] (% killing) ($n = 3$)	Heart allograft survival[e] Length (days)	mean ± SD
Nonsensitized rats	1:4	5337 ± 1439	55659 ± 2012	0.39 ± 1.0	5, 6 (3), 7 (2)	6.1 ± 0.7
Sensitized rats	1:128	17229 ± 755	10278 ± 642	8.4 ± 1.8	2 (4), 3 (2), 4, 5	2.8 ± 1.1

[a] Serum titers of anti-ACI cytotoxic antibodies
[b] Spontaneous blastogenesis in spleen cells
[c] Spleen cells were used as responder cells and irradiated ACI spleen cells as stimulator cells
[d] Responder cells were cocultured with irradiated ACI stimulator

cells, which served as effector cells; target cells were prepared by culturing ACI spleen cells with concanavalin A for 2 days
[e] Nonsensitized and sensitized LEW rats were used as recipient and ACI rats as donor

sensitized or sensitized recipient rats. The mixture was incubated for 8 h at 37°C in a humidified atmosphere of 5% CO_2 in air. The cells were harvested onto glassfiber filter paper with an automatic harvester, and ³H-TdR incorporation was measured in a beta-scintillation counter (1205 Beta Plate).

Mixed lymphocyte reaction (MLR). One-way MLR was performed, using spleen cells from nonsensitized or sensitized LEW rats as responder cells and from ACI rats was stimulator cells. The 0.5×10^6/ml responder cells were co-cultured with 1.0×10^6/ml 2000-rad-irradiated stimulator cells in RPMI 1640 complete medium. The cells are incubated at 37°C in a humidified atmosphere of 5% CO_2 for 4 days and then treated with an 16–20-h tritiated thymidine pulse. The cells were harvested, and the ³H-TdR incorporation was measured as described.

Cell-mediated lympholysis (CML). Spleen cells from sensitized LEW rats as responder cells were co-cultured with 2000-rad-irradiated ACI stimulator cells in RPMI 1640 complete medium at 37°C in a humidified atmosphere of 5% CO_2 for 6 days. Splenic responder

cells from nonsensitized LEW rats were used as the control. After incubation, the cells were harvested and used as effector cells for CML. The target cells were prepared by culturing stimulator cells with 50 µg/ml concanavalin A (ConA) for 2 days. The 4.0×10^6/ml effector cells were cultured with 1.0×10^5/ml ⁵¹Cr-labeled target cells, for 4 h at 37°C in a humidified atmosphere of 5% CO_2. A fixed volume of supernatant was collected from each well after centrifugation of 1500 g for 10 min, and the ⁵¹Cr release was counted in a gamma-counter (Aloka. JDC-752). The percentage cytotoxicity was calculated according to the following formula:

$$\% \text{Cytotoxicity} = \frac{\text{Experimental release} - \text{Spontaneous release}}{\text{Maximum release} - \text{Spontaneous release}} \times 100$$

Heterotopic heart transplantation and splenectomy. Heart transplantation was performed using the modified technique of Ono and Lindsey [7]. The heart allograft survival was determined by daily palpation. Rejection was considered complete at the time of cessation of a palpable heartbeat and confirmed by histological examination. Spx was done at the time of grafting.

Immunosuppressive agent. FK 506 was supplied by Fujisawa Pharmaceutical (Osaka, Japan). The drug was dissolved in physiological saline and administered intramuscularly from day 0 to day 10 after transplantation.

Statistical analysis. The statistical significance of differences between the untreated and experimental groups was ascertained using Student's t-test.

Results

Humoral and cellular immunity

Table 1 illustrates the results of antibody titers, SB, MLR, CML, and heart allograft survival in nonsensitized or sensitized LEW rats on day 7 after immunization with donor-type blood admixed with immunoadjuvant ACF. The positive serum antibody titers increased from 1:4 in nonsensitized rats to 1:128 in sensitized rats. SB was the stable measure of the nonspecific immune status of the ungrafted animal. A significant difference was seen in this assay between nonsensitized and sensitized rats. In the MLR, responder cells from sensitized LEW rats showed a higher proliferative response against ACI rat stimulator cells compared with nonsensitized ones. The CML activity was 0.3 ± 1.0 % in spleen cells from nonsensitized LEW rats but 8.4 ± 1.8 % in spleen cells from sensitized ones. The average ACI heart graft survival in the nonsensitized LEW control group was 6.1 ± 0.7 days; however, sensitized LEW recipient rats showed a mean graft survival time of 2.8 ± 1.1 days. These results suggest that subcuta-

Fig. 1. Survival of heart allografts in sensitized recipient rats. ACI heart grafts were transplanted into sensitized LEW recipient rats. Splenectomy (Spx) was done at the time of grafting. FK 506 was administered intramuscularly from day 0 to day 10 after transplantation. A *P* value < 0.05 was considered to indicate significant difference between the untreated control group and the experimental group

neously injected donor-type blood admixed with immunoadjuvant ACF to the recipient rat 7 days prior to transplantation and in the in vitro assay could increase both humoral and cellular immunity against donor antigen, resulting in sensitization.

Effect of low dose FK 506 and Spx on heart allograft survival in sensitized rat

Graft survival results are shown in Fig. 1. Untreated controls showed rejection in 2.8 ± 1.1 days. FK 506 alone could significantly prolong ACI heart graft survival in the sensitized recipient rats in a dose-dependent manner. The lowest effective dose for overcoming sensitization was 1.0 gm/kg daily. Spx alone showed a prolongation of heart allograft survival to 4.2 ± 1.0 days on the average. On the other hand, the combinations of FK 506 0.1 mg/kg daily plus Spx and FK 506 0.32 mg/kg daily plus Spx prolonged heart allograft survival to 5.6 ± 1.3 days and 10.6 ± 2.1 days, respectively. These results indicate that the low dose of FK 506, in combination with Spx, could synergistically prolong the heart allograft survival in sensitized recipient rats.

Discussion

These studies demonstrate that the importance of both humoral and cellular responses against donor antigen which appear in the serum and spleen of rats sensitized by subcutaneously injected donor-type blood admixed with immunoadjuvant ACF. The role of humoral activity in sensitized recipients is emphasized by a progressive increase of serum CDC titers, and the cellular component is reflected by strong SB, MLR, and CML responses in the spleen. The appearance of these humoral and cellular responses are associated with a hyperacute-like rejection of donor heart allografts in the ACI to LEW rat combination [5, 6]. However, as the allografts in this experiment fail in 2.8 ± 1.1 days, the term accelerated rejection may be more suitable for this kind of allograft outcome.

The mechanisms of accelerated rejection, induced by donor-type blood admixed with immunoadjuvant ACF, are not clear, but it may be assumed that a strong histocompatibility mismatching in the rat combination and a strong stimulation of donor antigen with immunoadjuvant could cause (1) cytotoxic antibody formation and (2) nonspecific lymphocyte, T lymphocyte, and cytotoxic T lymphocyte activation in the recipient rat. These cytotoxic antibodies and activated lymphocytes may contribute to the accelerated allograft destruction in this sensitized rat model [1, 5, 6].

The data obtained in this study show that FK 506 could significantly prolong ACI heart graft survival in sensitized LEW recipient rats in a dose-dependent manner, with a dosage of 1.0 mg/kg daily, as compared with the control. However, the dosage of FK 506 needed for such an effect is higher than that in nonsensitized recipient rats. Spx could also prolong the heart allograft survival in this sensitized rat model, but it proved to be insufficient for sustaining a graft survival for more than 4.2 days. This may be due to the fact that the Spx can control the cytotoxic antibody production to a certain degree but failed to overcome another barrier, cell-mediated rejection, in the sensitized situation.

An important finding in the present study was that combined treatment with a low dose of FK 506 plus Spx could synergistically prolong the heart allograft survival in sensitized recipient rats. Although FK 506 by itself, at a high dose, could overcome sensitization, this can be considered toxic to the recipients. A combination of low dose FK 506 with Spx, as an adjunct therapy, appears to diminish the toxic effect of FK 506 and induce an synergistic effect of heart allograft survival in this sensitized rat model. These results indicate that the low dose of FK 506 combined with Spx could not only control the cytotoxic antibody formation but also overcome cellular immunity-mediated rejection, resulting in a 3.7-fold prolongation of heart allograft survival in sensitized recipient rats.

In conclusion, the accelerated rejection of a heart allograft in sensitized rats correlates with the host's humoral and cellular response. It can be controlled by a low dose of FK 506 together with Spx, through different effector mechanisms. This combination approach may become an effective strategy for overcoming sensitization in clinical transplantation.

References

1. Freiche JA, Lang J, Sedivy P, Touraine J (1990) Prolonged survival of renal transplants in nonimmunized and hyperimmunized rats receiving A platelet-activating factor antagonist. Transplantation 50: 8–13
2. Jiang H, Takahara S, Takano Y, Li D, Kyo M, Valdivia LA, Kokado Y, Ishibashi M, Sonoda T (1991) Effect of FK 506 on heart allograft survival in highly sensitized recipient rats in comparison with cyclosporine. Transplant Proc 23: 540–541
3. Jones MC, Propper DJ, Weber BK, Stewart KN, Catto GRD, Cunningham C (1991) Reduction of sensitization induced by blood transfusion in the rat by monoclonal antibodies. Transplantation 51: 681–685
4. Kupiec-Weglinski JW, Sablinski T, Hancock WW, Stefano RD, Mariani G, Mix CT, Tilney NL (1991) Modulation of accelerated rejection of cardiac allografts in sensitized rats by anti-interleukin 2 receptor monoclonal antibody and cyclosporine therapy. Transplantation 51: 300–305
5. Meiser BM, Morris RE (1991) The importance of the spleen for the immunosuppressive action of cyclosporine in transplantation. Transplantation 51: 690–696
6. Oluwole SF, Tezuka K, Wasfie T, Stegall MD, Reemtsma K, Hardy MA (1989) Humoral immunity in allograft rejection. Transplantation 48: 751–755
7. Ono K, Lindsey ES (1969) Improved technique of heart transplantation in rats. J Thorac Cardiovasc Surg 57: 225–227
8. Valdivia LA, Monden M, Gotoh M, Nakano Y, Tono T, Mori T (1990) Evidence that deoxyspergualin prevents sensitization and first-set cardiac xenograft rejection in rats by suppression of antibody formation. Transplantation 50: 132–136

Transplant Int (1992) 5 [Suppl 1]: S 504–S 505

TRANSPLANT
International
© Springer-Verlag 1992

Prevention of lethal graft-versus-host disease by monoclonal antibody treatment in vivo*

A. C. Knulst, G. J. M. Tibbe, C. Bril-Bazuin, and R. Benner

Department of Immunology, Erasmus University, Rotterdam, The Netherlands

Graft-versus-host disease (GVHD) is a major complication of allogeneic bone marrow transplantation (BMT). The disease is caused by mature T cells in the graft that recognize foreign antigens of the host and subsequently elicit an immune response to host tissues [1]. Although T-cell depletion of the graft strongly reduced the incidence and severity of GVHD, the overall survival of allogeneic BMT did not increase because of the increased rate of graft rejection and leukemic relapses [2]. New prophylactic and therapeutic approaches have to be developed to improve the outcome of allogeneic BMT. T-cell-specific monoclonal antibodies (mAb) administered in vivo to the allograft recipients seem to be promising in the prevention and treatment of lethal GVHD [3–5]. In this study we especially addressed the effect of in vivo treatment of recipients with anti-T-cell subset mAb in a murine model for acute GVHD. We also determined the long-term effects.

Key words: Bone marrow transplantation – Graft-versus-host disease – Monoclonal antibodies

Materials and methods

Mice. (C57BL/Ka × CBA/Rij)F1 (H-$2^{b/q}$) and BALB/c (H-2^d) mice were bred at the Department of Immunology of the Erasmus University. The mice were 12–18 weeks old at the start of the experiments. Mice were kept 2 per cage with access to acidified water and pelleted food ad libitum.

Induction of GVHD. Lethally irradiated (10 Gy) (C57BL × CBA)F1 recipients were intravenously (i.v.) injected with 10^7 BALB/c

* This study was supported by a grant from the Interuniversitary Institute for Radiation Pathology and Radiation Protection (IRS), Leiden, The Netherlands

Offprint requests to: A. C. Knulst, M. D., Department of Immunology, Erasmus University, P. O. Box 1738, 3000 DR Rotterdam, The Netherlands

spleen cells, 24 h after irradiation. Mice were examined daily for the development of signs of GVHD. Control mice that were injected with 10^7 syngeneic spleen cells survived > 250 days.

Antibodies. Purified rat anti-mouse mAb, anti-Thy-1 (YTS 154.7), anti-CD4 (YTS 191.5), and anti-CD8 (YTS 169.4), all of the IgG2b subclass, were purchased from Sera-lab, Sussex, U.K. Treatment with mAb was given within 4 h after irradiation.

Chimerism. To determine the degree of chimerism, peripheral blood cell samples were stained with fluorescein isothiocyanate (FITC) conjugated mouse anti-mouse H-$2K^d$ mAb (clone SF1-1.1) and mouse anti-mouse H-$2K^b$ mAb (clone AF6-88.5), which were purchased from Pharmingen, San Diego, Calif. Subsequently, the samples were analyzed using a flow cytofluorometer (FACScan, Becton Dickinson, Mountain View, Calif.).

Data analysis. Differences between groups were analyzed using the Wilcoxon-Mann Whitney statistic. Values of $P < 0.05$ were considered significant.

Results and discussion

We compared the effectiveness of mAb treatment given either by intravenous (i.v.), intraperitoneal (i.p.), or subcutaneous (s.c.) injection. To be able to detect minimal differences between these three routes of administration, we employed a dose of either 25 µg or 50 µg anti-Thy-1, which is suboptimal according to previous experiments [5]. In all three groups the higher dose resulted in a better survival rate than the lower dose. The survival of s.c.-injected mice was slightly but not significantly decreased in comparison with the i.v.- and i.p.-treated groups. This indicates that treatment via all above mentioned routes of administration is equally effective.

We further investigated the effect of anti-CD4 and anti-CD8 treatment as compared with the effect of anti-Thy-1. Earlier experiments showed that both anti-Thy-1 and anti-CD4 treatment decreased the morbidity and mortality of GVHD. A dose of 100 µg anti-Thy-1 resulted in 100% survival, whereas a similar dose of anti-CD4 was less effective. Anti-CD8 treatment did not decrease the

Table 1. Effect of anti-Thy-1, anti-CD4, and anti-CD8 monoclonal antibody treatment on the survival of mice after allogeneic spleen cell transplantation

Recipient strain	n	Donor	Treatment	Survival at day 30 (%)	Survival at day 60 (%)
Experiment 1					
(C57BL × CBA) F1	10	BALB/c	100 µg anti-Thy-1	100	100
(C57BL × CBA) F1	10	BALB/c	100 µg anti-CD4	60	30
(C57BL × CBA) F1	10	BALB/c	100 µg anti-CD8	0	0
(C57BL × CBA) F1	10	BALB/c	none	0	0
Experiment 2					
(C57BL × CBA) F1	8	BALB/c	100 µg anti-Thy-1	100	100
(C57BL × CBA) F1	8	BALB/c	200 µg anti-CD4	100	100
(C57BL × CBA) F1	8	BALB/c	200 µg anti-CD8	0	0
(C57BL × CBA) F1	6	BALB/c	none	16	16

(C57BL × CBA) F1 mice were lethally irradiated, treated with the indicated amount of mAb, and reconstituted with 10^7 BALB/c spleen cells. The percentage survival is given at days 30 and 60 after reconstitution

morbidity but appeared to postpone mortality [5]. This indicated a major role for CD4$^+$ T-cells, the role of CD8$^+$ T cells being less clear. To clarify the involvement of the CD4$^+$ and CD8$^+$ T-cell subset, we repeated the experiment with a dose of either 100 µg or 200 µg anti-CD4 and anti-CD8 mAb. The results are summarized in Table 1. Treatment with a dose of 100 µg of anti-Thy-1 or anti-CD4 improved the percentage survival, whereas treatment with a similar dose of anti-CD8 did not (experiment 1). Treatment with a double dose of anti-CD4 appeared to be as effective as treatment with 100 µg anti-Thy-1 and resulted in 100 % survival on day 60. However, even a dose of 200 µg anti-CD8 did not increase the survival at all (experiment 2). This is in harmony with the effect of mAb treatment on the development of clinical symptoms of GVHD. Symptoms of severe acute GVHD developed simultaneously in both the anti-CD8 (200 µg)-treated and the untreated group but were absent in the anti-Thy-1- and anti-CD4 (200 µg)-treated group. These data are consistent with our earlier observation that purified CD4$^+$ T cells were able to induce a lethal GVH reaction, whereas purified CD8$^+$ T cells could not. The discrepancy in the effect of anti-CD8 mAb as compared with previously reported data [5] might be explained by the fact that in the previous experiments the GVH reaction developed more slowly. CD8$^+$ T cells might play a role in chronic GVHD in this strain combination.

To exclude the possibility that the observed differences were due to a variable capacity of the mAb to eliminate the respective T-cell population in vivo, we analyzed the spleens from two mice of each group (experiment 2) for the presence of T-cell subsets 7 days after allogeneic reconstitution. It appeared that anti-CD8 mAb were even more effective than anti-CD4 mAb in eliminating their

target cell population in vivo. This means that the differences in effectiveness cannot be explained by a difference in the capacity to eliminate the respective target cells. Together, these data indicate a major role for the CD4$^+$ T-cell subset in the induction of acute lethal GVHD in this model.

We further determined the state of chimerism and tolerance of the mice that had become long-term stable chimeras. The total number of spleen cells appeared to be ± 50 % of normal. The percentages of B and T lymphocytes were within the normal range. Since > 99 % of the spleen cells as well as of the peripheral white blood cells reacted with the anti-H-2K^d mAb and < 1 % with the anti-H-2K^b mAb, the chimeric mice can be considered as complete chimeras. This was confirmed by the observation that spleen cells from these stable chimeras were able to induce a lethal GVH reaction in recipients syngeneic to the original host, but not in recipients syngeneic to the original donor. This also indicates that the state of tolerance in these long-term chimeras is not due to clonal deletion. Preliminary data suggest that the tolerance is maintained by a suppressive mechanism.

References

1. Korngold R, Sprent J (1987) Transplantation 44: 335
2. Champlin R (ed) (1990) Bone marrow transplantation. Kluwer, Dordrecht, p 9
3. Cobbold SP, Jayasuriya A, Nash A, Prospero TD, Waldmann H (1984) Nature 312: 548
4. Waldmann H (1989) Ann Rev Immunol 7: 407
5. Knulst AC, Bril-Bazuin C, Benner R (1991) Eur J Immunol 21: 103

Transplant Int (1992) 5 [Suppl 1]: S 506–S 510

TRANSPLANT
International
© Springer-Verlag 1992

Abdominal organ cluster transplantation in pigs and FK506*

N. Kobayashi, K. Sakagami, S. Takasu, T. Matsuno, and K. Orita

First Department of Surgery, Okayama University Medical School, Okayama, Japan

Abstract. Using a swine abdominal organ cluster transplantation model, we investigated the postoperative function and immunological reactions of a cluster graft and evaluated the immunosuppressive activity of FK506. The animals were divided into two groups. Group I ($n = 6$) served as controls, while in group II ($n = 6$) a daily dose of 0.1 mg/kg FK506 was given intramuscularly. Postoperative pancreatitis was the most important factor influencing the early outcome in both groups. In group I, the cause of late death was cachexia due to diabetes mellitus induced by pancreatic rejection. In group II, emaciation despite a well-functioning graft was the principal cause of late death. Histologically, in group I the grade of rejection in the pancreas was more severe than in the liver, and no sign of rejection was observed in group II. In conclusion, the pancreas suffered more severe rejection than the liver, and FK506 could significantly prevent cluster allograft rejection in this model.

Key words: Abdominal organ cluster transplantation – Postoperative pancreatitis – FK506 – Diabetes mellitus – pancreatic rejection

Since 1988, abdominal organ cluster transplantation (AOCTX) has been introduced into surgical practice to treat malignant tumors of the biliary tract, pancreas, or duodenum with secondary involvement of the liver [7]. AOCTX has created new surgical, physiological, and immunological problems which were not usually seen in the transplantation of a single organ. It is clear that the future development of AOCTX will depend upon more specific and less toxic forms of immunosuppression. FK506 (FK) is a recently developed agent with potent immunosup-

pressive activity, as shown by in vitro and vivo studies [2, 5]. In this study, we characterized the postoperative function and immunological reactions of a cluster graft and also evaluated the immunosuppressive activity of FK in swine AOCTX.

Materials and methods

Dulock-Jersy pigs and Large-White pigs weighing 20–25 kg were used as the donors and recipients, respectively.

Operative procedure. The transplantation procedure has been described in detail previously [3]. Briefly, the recipients underwent en bloc removal of the liver, pancreas, nearly all of the stomach, duodenum, and spleen under general anesthesia. The void upper abdomen was filled with an en bloc cluster graft consisting of the liver, pancreas, duodenum, spleen, and aortic conduit under venovenous bypass. Gastrointestinal reconstruction was performed by interposition of the duodenal graft between the recipient stomach and jejunum. Harvesting and transplantation procedures are shown in Fig. 1.

Experimental groups. Experimental animals were divided into two groups. Group I ($n = 6$) served as controls and underwent no special treatment. In group II ($n = 6$), a daily intramuscular injection of 0.1 mg/kg FK was commenced from the immediate postoperative period.

Biochemical and histopathological studies. Blood chemistry tests were performed regularly to monitor the function of the transplanted graft, including determinations of the serum total bilirubin (T. Bil), serum glutamic oxaloacetic transaminase (GOT), alkaline phosphatase (ALP), serum amylase (sAMY), and blood glucose. An autopsy was performed in each animal, and the cluster graft as well as other organs were histologically examined to determine the cause of death. Tissues were fixed with formalin and stained with H&E.

Statistical analysis. Differences between the mean values were assessed for significance by Student's unpaired t-test.

Results

As shown in Table 1, survival times ranged from 7 to 42 days in group I and from 7 to 112 days in group II. The

* This work was supported in part by grant no. 02454306 from Japanese Ministry of Education, Science and Culture

Offprint requests to: N. Kobayashi, M.D., First Department of Surgery, Okayama University Medical School, 2-5-1 Shikata-cho, Okayama 700, Japan

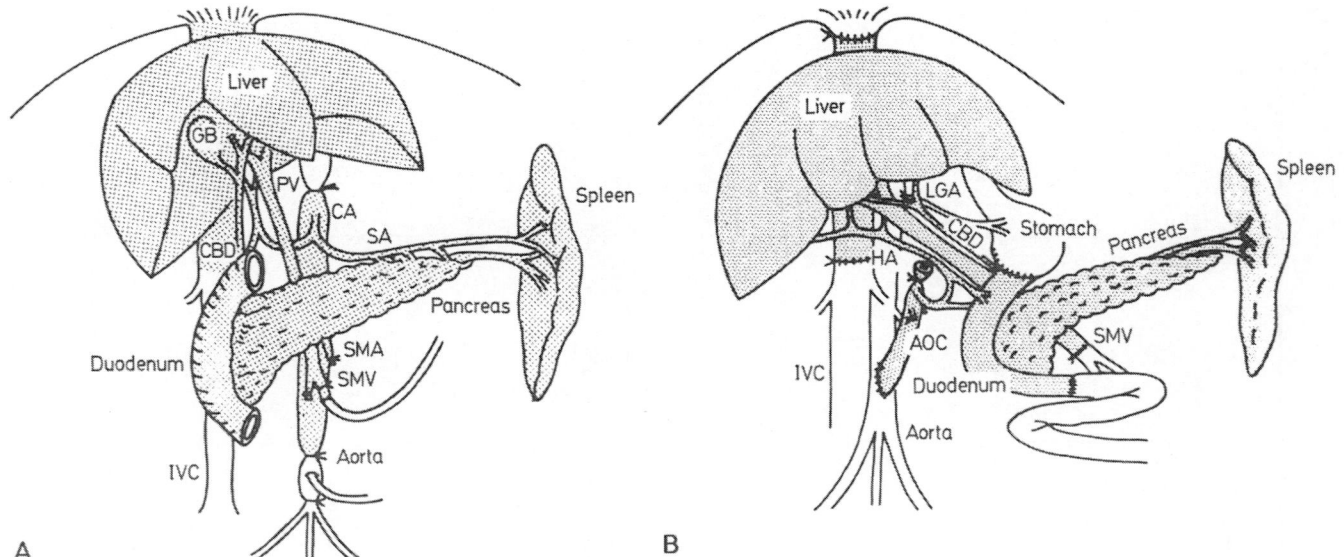

Fig. 1 A, B. The procedure for swine abdominal organ cluster transplantation (AOCTX). **A** Harvesting procedure, **B** transplantation procedure. The *shaded area* indicates the cluster graft. *AOC*, aortic conduit; *CA*, celiac artery; *CBD*, common bile duct; *HA*, hepatic artery; *IVC*, inferior vena cava; *LGA*, left gastric artery; *PV*, portal vein; *RRV*, right renal vein; *SA*, splenic artery; *SMA*, superior mesenteric artery; *SMV*, superior mesenteric vein

causes of early death in both groups were severe pancreatitis and complications following gastrointestinal reconstruction. In group I, the cause of late death was cachexia due to diabetes mellitus induced by pancreatic allograft rejection, and emaciation despite a well-functioning graft was the principal cause in group II.

In group I, in all animals, the T. Bil content increased rapidly on about day 4 after surgery, peaked on day 7 or 8, and gradually decreased thereafter. Furthermore, the GOT and ALP levels began to rise on about day 5. The sAMY level began to increase on day 6, while the blood glucose level began to rise on about day 10, and hyperglycemia persisted until death. In group II, the T. Bil value remained below 1.0 mg/dl throughout the postoperative course, and mild hyperglycemia was observed in only 1 pig (Fig. 2). In group I, the mean T. Bil level on day 7 was significantly higher than that in group II (3.55 ± 1.19 mg/dl vs. 0.32 ± 0.18 mg/dl; $P < 0.01$), and the mean blood glucose level on day 10 was significantly higher than in group II (317 ± 32 mg/dl vs. 176 ± 73 mg/dl; $P < 0.02$). Histopathologically, in group I the grade of rejection in the pancreas was more severe than in the liver (Fig. 3). No clinical sign of rejection was observed, and the reduction in histological evidence of rejection was dramatic in group II, as shown in Fig. 4. GVH reaction was not observed in any case.

Table 1. Summary of 12 pigs that survived for 7 days or more after AOCTX (mean ± SD)

Pig number	AHT (min)	TIT (min)	OPT (h)	Survival time (days)	Cause of death[a]
Group I (control group)					
1	41	101	5.5	7	Pancreatitis
2	36	93	5.8	10	Sacrificed
3	40	88	4.9	13	Pancreatitis
4	35	76	5.1	14	Pancreatitis/necrosis of the duodenal graft
5	43	107	5.9	41	Diabetes mellitus (rejection)
6	37	85	5.4	42	Diabetes mellitus (rejection)
Total	38.7 ± 3.1[b]	91.7 ± 11.2[b]	5.4 ± 0.4[b]		
Group II (FK506-treated group)					
1	42	101	5.4	7	Sacrificed
2	34	79	4.8	10	Sacrificed
3	38	89	5.1	10	Pancreatitis
4	40	102	5.5	10	Necrosis of the residual stomach
5	37	86	5.3	16	Pancreatitis
6	41	92	4.9	112	Emaciation
Total	38.6 ± 2.9[b]	91.5 ± 8.9[b]	5.2 ± 0.3[b]		

AHT, anhepatic time; TIT, total ischemic time; OPT, operation time
[a] Five out of 12 pigs (42%) died due to severe pancreatitis or pancreatic necrosis
[b] Group I vs. II, not significant

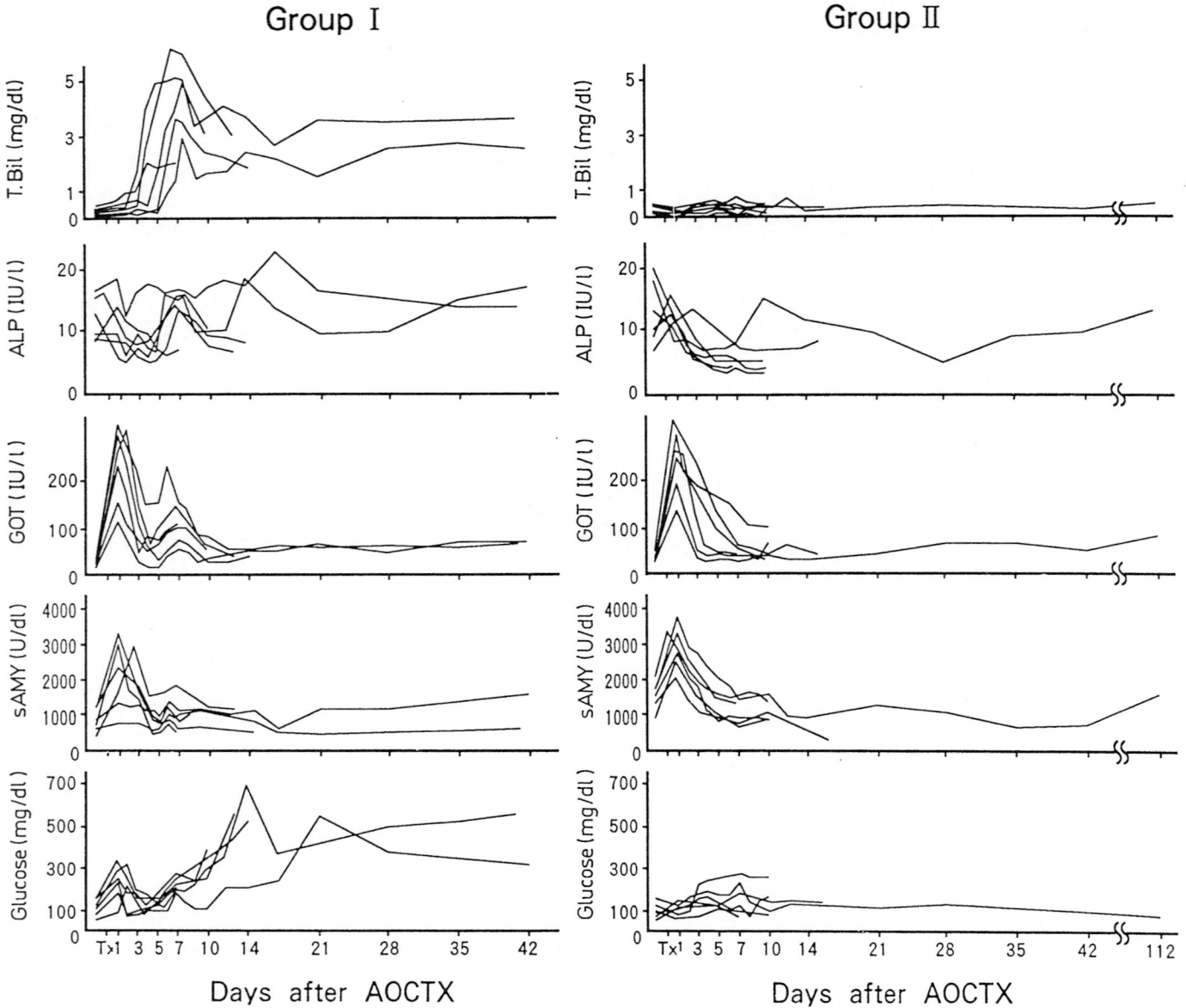

Fig. 2. Liver and pancreas function after AOCTX. The increases in serum bilirubin *(T. Bil)* level on day 5 and blood glucose on day 10 in group I were not observed in group II. *ALP,* alkaline phosphatase; *sAMY,* serum amylase; *GOT,* glutamic oxaloacetic transaminase

Discussion

In the postoperative course in our swine model, acute rejection could be detected in both the liver and pancreas. Acute rejection of the liver seemed mild and subsided without immunosuppressants and was equivalent to transient rejection.

However, acute rejection of the pancreas progressed to graft deterioration. The cause of late death was not hepatic failure but cachexia due to diabetes mellitus induced by pancreatic rejection. These findings suggest that there is a difference in severity between acute rejection of the liver and that of the pancreas. This may be explained by the fact that liver grafts are protected from rejection in comparison with grafts of other organs [1].

Postoperative pancreatitis was the most important factor influencing the early outcome of our swine AOCTX model as well as clinical AOCTX [8]. The prevention of postoperative pancreatitis seems to be extremely important for long-term AOCTX survival. Since marked mor-

bidity and mortality are associated with the transplanted pancreas, Tzakis et al. have proposed a modified cluster procedure with resection of the pancreas and intrahepatic islet allotransplantation. According to their report, all 10 patients demonstrated significant C-peptide production, and prolonged insulin independence was observed in 6 cases [9]. Recently, our group developed a new split-cluster transplantation technique in which the hepatic graft was located orthotopically and a pancreaticoduodenal graft with the spleen was transplanted auxiliarly with urinary bladder drainage to prevent lethal postoperative pancreatitis and to monitor exocrine pancreatic secretions [6].

There are some variations in the reconstruction procedure of the gastrointestinal tract in clinical AOCTX [4, 7]. In cases in which the proximal stomach was saved with an intact left gastric arterial supply, the duodenum was placed in continuity with the gastrointestinal tract so that ingested food passed through the duodenal graft. In this model, we used this simple physiological procedure for ga-

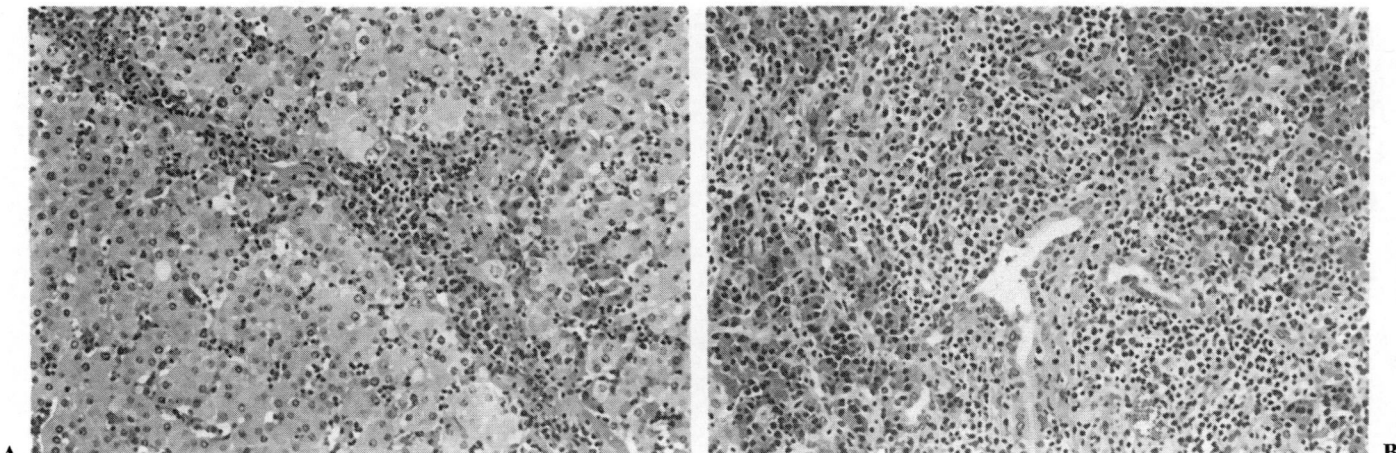

Fig. 3. A Liver and **B** pancreas from pig no. 6 (group I) on day 42 after AOCTX. The pancreas suffered more severe rejection than the liver

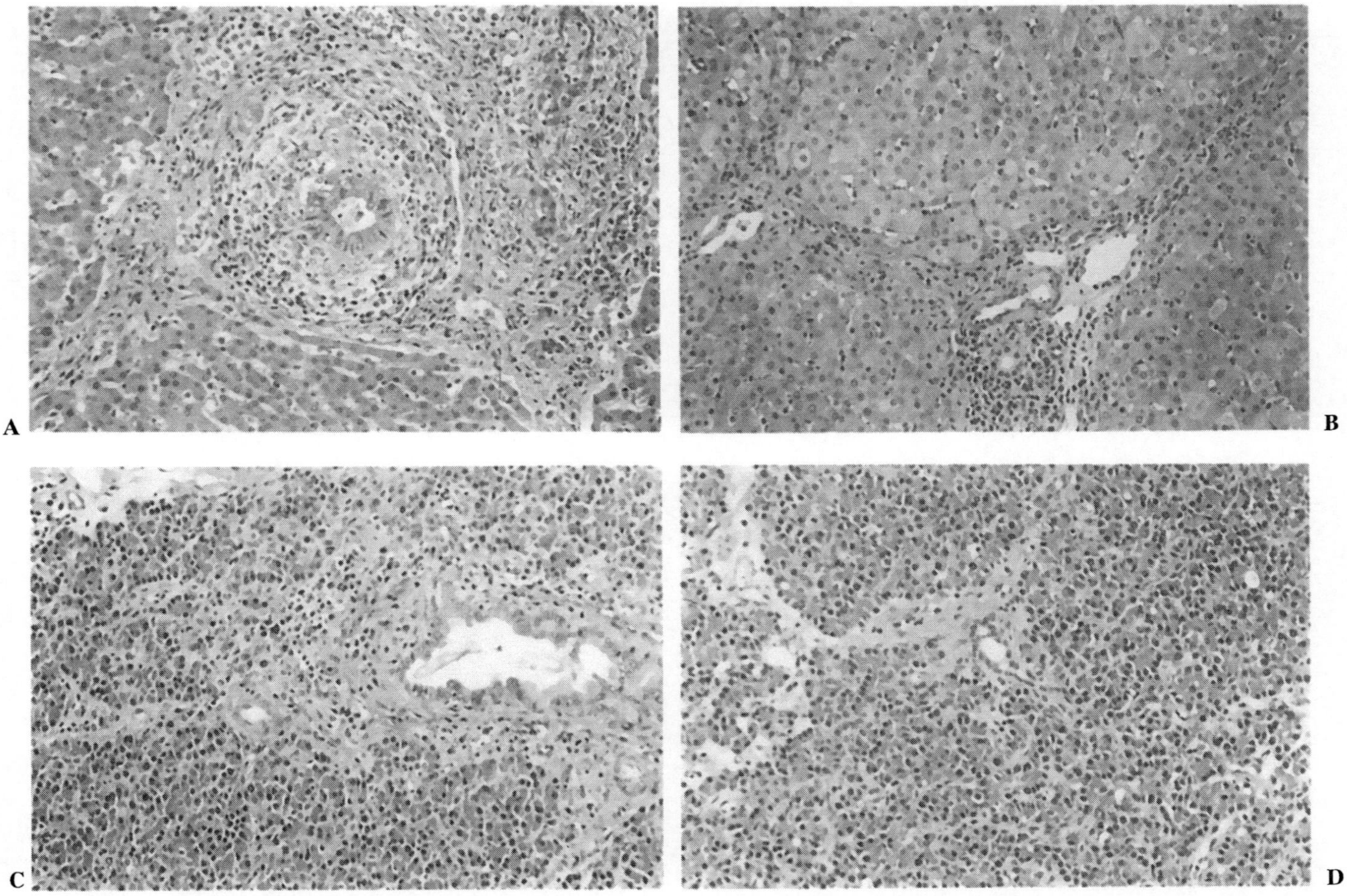

Fig. 4A–D. Hepatic allografts on day 7 after AOCTX in group I (**A**) and group II (**B**) and pancreatic allografts on day 10 in group I (**C**) and group II (**D**). In group I, each organ exhibited marked rejection in contrast with almost normal organs in group II

strointestinal reconstruction. However, the other cause of early death involved complications following gastrointestinal reconstruction, such as necrosis of the residual stomach.

This study clearly shows that FK is a potent immunosuppressive agent in swine AOCTX. Rejection of the transplanted cluster graft was effectively suppressed by daily intramuscular administration of 0.1 mg/kg FK. There are several reports concerning the major side ef-

fects of FK, such as nephrotoxicity and diabetogenesis. In this study, mild hyperglycemia due to generalized peritonitis was observed in only 1 pig, and the other animals were normoglycemic when administered with FK. Histologically, almost normal structures in pancreatic allografts were maintained in FK-treated pigs. According to the postmortem examinations, no side effects were observed except for emaciation, which may have been induced by long-term posttransplant administration of FK.

In conclusion, this study suggests that the pancreas suffers more severe rejection than the liver and that the prevention of postoperative pancreatitis is extremely important to obtain long-term survival in the swine AOCTX model. Daily intramuscular administration of 0.1 mg/kg FK can significantly prevent cluster allograft rejection.

Acknowledgments. We wish to express our sincere appreciation to Fujisawa Pharmaceutical, Osaka, Japan, for providing FK506.

References

1. Calne RY, Sells RA, Pena JR, Davis DR, Millard PR, Herbertson BM, Binns RM, Davis DAL (1969) Induction of immunological tolerance by porcine liver allografts. Nature 223: 472–476
2. Kino T, Hatanaka H, Miyata S, Inamura N, Nishiyama M, Yajima T, Goto T, Okuhara M, Kohsaka M, Aoki H, Ochiai T (1987) A novel immunosuppressant isolated from a *Streptomyces*. II. Immunosuppressive effect of FK-506 in vitro. J Antibiot (Tokyo) 40: 1256–1265
3. Kobayashi N, Sakagami K, Takasu S, Inagaki M, Hasuoka H, Yagi T, Onoda T, Matsuno T, Saito S, Kawamura T, Orita K (1991) Significance of pancreatic allograft rejection in swine abdominal organ cluster transplantation. Transplant Proc 23: 635–639
4. Mieles L, Todo S, Tzakis A, Starzl TE (1990) Treatment of upper abdominal malignancies with organ cluster procedures. Clin Transplant 4: 63–67
5. Ochiai T, Nagata M, Nakajima K, Suzuki T, Sakamoto K, Enomoto K, Gunji Y, Uematsu T, Goto T, Hori S, Kenmochi T, Nakagouri T, Asano T, Isono K, Hamaguchi K, Tsuchida H, Nakahara K, Inamura N, Goto T (1987) Studies of the effects of FK506 on renal allografting in the beagle dog. Transplantation 44: 729–733
6. Sakagami K, Kobayashi N, Nakagawa H, Saito S, Oiwa T, Orita K (1991) Experimental studies on a new splitting technique for simultaneous transplantation of liver/pancreas, duodenum and spleen in pigs: a preliminary report (in Japanese). Surg Therapy (in press)
7. Starzl TE, Todo S, Tzakis A, Podesta L, Mieles L, Demetris A, Teperman L, Selby R, Stevenson W, Stieber A, Gordon R, Iwatsuki S (1989) Abdominal organ cluster transplantation for the treatment of upper abdominal malignancies. Ann Surg 210: 374–386
8. Starzl TE, Todo S, Tzakis A, Alessiani M, Casavilla A, Abu-Elmagd K, Fung J (1991) The many faces of multivisceral transplantation. Surg Gynecol Obst 172: 335–344
9. Tzakis AG, Ricordi C, Alejandro R, Zeng Y, Fung J, Todo S, Demetris A, Mintz D, Starzl TE (1990) Pancreatic islet transplantation after abdominal exenteration and liver replacement. Lancet 336: 402–405

Transplant Int (1992) 5 [Suppl 1]: S 511–S 513

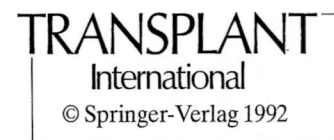

© Springer-Verlag 1992

Influence of hepatic dysfunction on cyclosporine metabolism in the pig

G. Mentha, C. Schopfer, L. Vadas, J. Belenger, P. Morel, F. Criado, and A. Rohner

Laboratory of Experimental Surgery, Departments of Surgery, Pharmacology, and Anesthesiology, University Hospital, Geneva, Switzerland

Abstract. Cyclosporine (CyA) is eliminated from the body via biliary excretion at a rate directly proportional to bile production and the functional status of the liver. Previous reports demonstrated that disturbances in the hepatic excretory function with a rise in the plasma bilirubin level are positively correlated with high blood concentrations of CyA and CyA plus metabolites (CyA + M). Less information is available about the blood concentrations of the CyA parental substance or CyA metabolites in the case of liver dysfunction when there was no elevation of serum bilirubin content. To answer this question, we compared the pharmacokinetic profile of CyA in a cholestatic and in a ischemic model in pigs. Our results show that in pigs receiving a single dose of CyA after liver ischemia, the blood concentrations of CyA and CyA + M are significantly increased independently of the serum bilirubin concentration, probably through a slow down of CyA metabolism by impairment of cytochrome P450 III A.

Key words: Cyclosporine metabolism – Liver dysfunction – Serum bilirubin

Cyclosporine (CyA) has been widely used in numerous transplantation protocols. This drug is extensively distributed in the body, as reflected by the large apparent volume of distribution. CyA is primarily metabolized in the liver through N-demethylation and mono- and dihydroxylation mediated by cytochrome P450 III A isoenzyme. Many metabolites of CyA have already been isolated, but none has an important immunosuppressive activity.

As the metabolism of CyA depends upon the activity of microsomal liver enzymes and its elimination upon the bile production [3, 5], the fact that some impairment of the liver function, a situation frequently encountered after orthotopic liver transplantation (OLT), induces large variations of the CyA blood concentrations is not surprising.

Because drug is liposoluble, it needs bile components in order to be absorbed from the upper small intestine after oral administration. Therefore, in the case of cholestatic icterus, very high blood concentrations of CyA and CyA metabolites can be expected when the drug is injected (i. v. route) and very low ones when it is orally administered.

The CyA parent drug can be measured by high performance liquid chromatography (HPLC) or by immunoassays RIA and fluorescence polarization immunoassay, FPIA based on a monoclonal antibody (MRIA) that only recognises the parental substance. The CyA metabolites are quantitated with the same immunoassays except that a polyclonal antibody (PRIA) is used which crossreacts with a number of metabolites plus the parental drug (CyA + M).

Previous reports showed a positive correlation between the serum bilirubin level, and impaired CyA and CyA + M excretion, as reflected in an elevation of the CyA PRIA/HPLC ratio [2, 4].

However, less information is actually available about whether or not liver cell damage, without a rise in the serum bilirubin level, is followed by the same variations of CyA and CyA + M blood level ratio.

To answer this question, we compared the pharmacokinetic profile of CyA in a cholestatic and in an ischemic liver model of pigs over 24 h after a single i. v. administration of CyA.

Pigs were chosen for this study because the interspecies differences between humans and pigs in cyclosporine disposition have been previously reported [1].

Materials and methods

Twelve pigs weighing between 25 and 35 kg were investigated. The pigs received a single i. v. dose of CyA (8 mg/kg). Blood samples were obtained before the injection and after 5, 15, 30, 60, 90, 120, 180, 240, 360, 540, 660, 780, 960, 1200, and 1440 min (24 h). Each pig was his own control. After a week, all pigs underwent surgery.

Under general anesthesia, exposition of the hepatoduodenal ligament was obtained through a midline incision. In the cholestatic

---

Offprint requests to: G. Mentha, M. D., Department of Surgery, University Hospital, CH-1211 Geneva 4, Switzerland

Table 1. Liver tests performed in the 3 groups

Liver tests	Control group	Gr A	Gr B
AST (U/l)	46 ± 12	157 ± 46	1211 ± 1113
ALT (U/l)	54 ± 16	61 ± 10	164 ± 69
GGT (U/l)	18 ± 4.75	38 ± 28	23 ± 12.67
ALP (U/l)	168 ± 47	310 ± 66	395 ± 121
BIL (μmol/l)	3.11 ± 0.3	63 ± 21	7.4 ± 4.6
PT (%)	87 ± 19	96 ± 6	67 ± 14

GrA, cholestatic group; GrB, ischemic group; AST, ALT, aspartate and alanine aminotransferases; GGT, γ-glutamyltransferase; ALP, alkaline phosphatase; BIC, bilirubin; PT, prothrombin time

group (A; $n = 6$), the common bile duct was distally ligated and divided. In the ischemic group (B; $n = 6$), the hepatoduodenal ligament was completely dissected and the hepatic artery ligated. At the end of the dissection, only the portal vein and the biliary tract, denuded, are conserved. Then, the falciform and the left and right triangular ligaments were divided. No drains were left in place.

At 48 h after surgery each pig received a second i. v. dose of CyA (8 mg/kg). Blood samples were obtained between 0 and 24 h, as indicated previously. Liver tests were performed before and 48 h after surgery.

Analytical methods. Both CyA and CyA + M were determined with commercial kits (Sandoz, Basel, Switzerland) of radioimmunoassay technique (MRIA and PRIA) and confirmed with FPIA (Abbott, Chicago, USA).

The PRIA/MRIA ratio, CyA half-life ($t_{1/2}\beta$; min), area under the curve (AUC; ng/ml · min), total clearance (tot CL; ml/min · kg), distribution volume (VD; ml/kg), and relation with liver tests were studied. Enzymes activities and serum bilirubin concentration were determined with a Technicon RA-1000 analyzer according to IFCC recommendations for alanine aminotransferase (ALT), aspartate aminotransferase (AST), γ-glutamyltransferase (GGT), alkaline phosphatase (ALP), and prothrombin time (PT).

Results

The serum bilirubin concentration was significantly higher in the cholestatic group than in the ischemic group or control group ($P < 0.01$). The ALT concentrations were significantly higher in the ischemic group than in the cholestatic group or control group ($P < 0.01$). Results are shown in Table 1.

In both groups A and B, the $t_{1/2}\beta$ of CyA and CyA + M, and the AUC increased and the tot CL decreased significantly compared with the control group ($P < 0.01$). The VD remained unchanged in the three groups (Table 2).

We found no difference between groups A and B except for the ratio of metabolites to total cyclosporine as a function of elapsed time [(AUC PRIA–AUC MRIA)/AUC PRIA], which is significantly more important in the cholestatic group.

Discussion

CyA is eliminated from the body via biliary excretion at a rate directly proportional to bile production and to the functional status of the liver [3]. The biliary concentration of CyA metabolites exceeds that of the parent drug, suggesting that most of the CyA is excreted in the bile [3, 5]. In clinical OLT, high levels of CyA expose the patient to the drug's side-effects and toxicity [2]. Conversely, a low

Table 2. Results of the CyA and CyA + M in the 3 groups

	CyA			CyA + M		
	Control	Gr A	Gr B	Control	Gr A	Gr B
$t_{1/2}\beta$	368 ± 31	634 ± 162	636 ± 110	373 ± 37	751 ± 60	740 ± 177
AUC	728 ± 110	1137 ± 428	1331 ± 659	842 ± 146	1176 ± 587	1700 ± 856
Tot CL	11.18 ± 1.87	7.64 ± 2.59	7.77 ± 4.93	9.71 ± 1.71	4.80 ± 1.57	6.29 ± 4.43
VD	5931 ± 1112	6619 ± 1361	6549 ± 279	5211 ± 1688	5175 ± 1688	5848 ± 2219

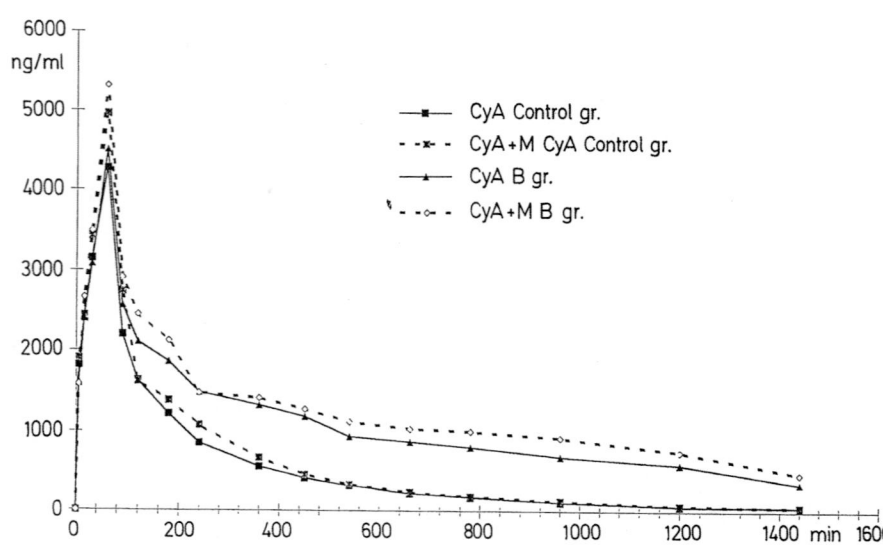

Fig. 1. Cyclosporine (CyA) and CyA + M (metabolites) blood concentrations (determined by radioimmunoassay) before and after liver desarterialization (group B)

concentration of the parental substance, even in the case of a high blood concentration of metabolites, expose the patient to rejection (metabolites have a undefined, but poor, immunosuppressive activity). It is thought that the accumulation of metabolites in the presence of liver dysfunction is due to impaired excretion. An increase in the plasma bilirubin level is known to be positively correlated with an increase of the ratio PRIA/MRIA [4].

The results of the present study show that in pigs receiving a single dose of CyA after liver ischemia, the blood concentrations of CyA and CyA + M are significantly increased (Fig. 1), although there is no elevation of serum bilirubin level (Table 1). A decrease in the CyA metabolism through dysfunction of the cytochrome P450 III A probably explains this increased CyA blood concentration. This fact indicates that in liver transplant patients, whatever the cause of the liver dysfunction and the plasma bilirubin level, careful monitoring of the CyA and CyA + M blood levels is mandatory.

In conclusion, this work supports the view that a sudden rise in the CyA levels in blood can take place independently of the serum bilirubin concentration.

Acknowledgments. We are tremendously grateful to M. A. Chiappe (Central Laboratory of Clinical Chemistry) for cyclosporine determinations and also to Sandoz and Abbott, Switzerland, for the gift of the reagents for cyclosporine determinations.

References

1. Frey BM, Sieber M, Mettler D, Gänger H, Frey FJ (1988) Marked interspecies differences between humans and pigs in cyclosporine and prednisolone disposition. Drug Metab Dispos 16: 285–289
2. Gunson BK, Jones SR, Maclean S, Neuberger J, McMaster P (1988) Is the new specific monoclonal radioimmunoassay for cyclosporine of value in liver transplantation? Transplant Proc 20: 323–329
3. Rodighiero V (1989) Therapeutic drug monitoring of cyclosporine. Practical applications and limitations. Clin Pharmacokinet 16: 23–37
4. Tredger JM, Steward CM, Williams R (1988) Blood cyclosporine concentrations in liver transplant recipients: assay method and influence of changed hepatic and renal function. Transplant Proc 20: 391–393
5. Venkataramanan R, Starzl TE, Yang S, Burckart GJ, Ptachcinski RJ, Shaw BW, Iwatsuki S, Thiel DH Van, Sanghvi A, Seltman H (1985) Biliary excretion of cyclosporine in liver transplant patients. Transplant Proc 17: 286–289

Transplant Int (1992) 5 [Suppl 1]: S 514–S 515

TRANSPLANT
International
© Springer-Verlag 1992

FK506 and rapamycin: differential sensitivity of human, baboon, cynomolgus monkey, dog and pig lymphocytes

S. Metcalfe, R. Svvennsen, and R. Y. Calne

Department of Surgery, Addenbrookes Hospital, Cambridge, United Kingdom

Abstract. It has recently been suggested that there are species differences in the sensitivity of T lymphocytes to the immunosuppressive effect of FK506 [3]. We explore this phenomenon further and compare FK506 with rapamycin in lymphocytes from dog, pig, baboon, cynomolgus monkey and man. We fond that the relative sensitivity of T cells to FK506 did not necessarily correlate with their sensitivity to rapamycin, further emphasising the different mode of action of each drug. The serum may alter results of dose-response curves, and thus autologous serum may introduce an uncontrolled variable when different species are being compared in vitro. We conclude that the differences in sensitivity of lymphocytes from various species to FK506 and rapamycin are independent of each other, and these differences are likely to reflect variation in the overall interactive pathways involved in T-cell mitogenesis.

Key words: Immunosuppression – FK506 – Rapamycin

The species differences in sensitivity to a given drug may result from intrinsic species differences between target cell types. Alternatively, the species differences in pharmacokinetics and metabolic pathways may result in the target cell being exposed to different concentrations of the active drug, giving an apparent, rather than real, difference in cellular sensitivity to the drug in vivo. Recent data suggest that baboon lymphocytes are relatively insensitive to the immunosuppressive effect of FK506, both in vitro and in vivo, when compared with those of rats, dogs and humans [3]. The implication that there are intrinsic species differences in the control of lymphocyte activation led us to explore this phenomenon further, and here we have compared FK506 with a second immunosuppressive macrolide, rapamycin, in vitro using five different large animal species. These drugs are known to act on either early (FK506) or late (rapamycin) pathways of lymphocyte activation [2, 5].

Materials and methods

Drugs. FK506 (kindly donated by Fujisawa Pharmaceuticals), and rapamycin (kindly donated by Wyeth Research Laboratories) were each prepared from stock solutions at 10^{-3} M in ethanol and stored at $+4°C$. Concanavalin A (conA; Sigma) was stored at 1 mg/ml in phosphate buffered saline (PBS) at $+4°C$.

Cells. Peripheral blood lymphocytes (PBL) were obtained from blood taken from the following: adult human volunteers, adult baboons (*Papio anubis,* kindly provided by Huntingdon Research Centre); adult cynomologous monkeys (*Macaca fascicularis,* kindly provided by Huntingdon Research Centre); outbred mongrel dogs; and pigs (Large White). Each species pair gave a good two-way mixed lymphocyte response (MLR). All PBL were preserved in liquid nitrogen using medium containing 50% autologous serum and 10% dimethyl sulphoxide (DMSO), at 10^7 cells/ml, until use. Autologous serum was collected from each blood sample and stored at $-20°C$ until use. Heat-inactivated fetal calf serum was obtained from Advanced Protein Products.

Cultures. Cells were washed and made up to 5×10^7 cells/ml in RPMI 1640. These were diluted tenfold into appropriate control or drug stocks for conA-activation experiments, with or without serum. DNA synthesis was measured at 2 days (conA) or 7 days (MLR). All detailed comparisons were made within a given experiment to avoid any variation due to the preparative procedure.

Results

In serum-free growth medium there were some differences in the order of sensitivity to both FK506 and to rapamycin between the different species. Moreover, the order of sensitivity to FK506 did not correspond to that for rapamycin, further emphasising the different modes of drug action (Table 1).

The use of serum in the culture medium could reduce the apparent drug sensitivity, presumably by sequestering drug molecules (Fig. 1a). Autologous serum could similarly cause a reduction in the dose-response curve. Thus, if autologous serum is to be used for the comparison of cells between species, then it would also be advisable to include experiments using a common source of serum (FCS), to

Offprint requests to: S. Metcalfe, Department of Surgery, Addenbrookes Hospital, Hills Road, Cambridge, United Kingdom

Table 1. FK506 and rapamycin: drug concentration resulting in 50% inhibition of mitogenesis in conA-stimulated peripheral blood lymphocytes (PBL) from dog, pig, cynomolgus monkey, baboon and man

Species	FK506 ($\times 10^{-10} M$)	Rapamycin ($\times 10^{-8} M$)
Dog	2	5
Pig	4^a	50
	$(1, 7)^b$	(10, 100)
Human	4	1
	(0.9, 4, 4, 20, 20)	(0.5, 1, 1)
Baboon	9	5
	(3, 3, 9, 12, 30)	(0.7, 0.9, 11, 11)
Cynomolgus monkey	20	8
	(11, 20, 20, 40)	(1, 1, 8, 10, 15)

[a] Median ID_{50} is given for repeat experiments
[b] Each experimental ID_{50} is shown to illustrate interexperimental variation

These experiments were in serum-free medium. Each species gave a stimulation index (SI) of 50 or more, with the exception of the dog, which responded poorly under serum-free conditions with a SI of 10. For this reason, the dog experiments were not repeated in this series, although other experimental series in the presence of serum (not shown) supported the relative data presented here

allow variation due autologous serum components to be identified. This will be especially relevant to drugs of high potency, such as FK506, where the molar concentration in culture is already low and thus particularly sensitive to sequestration by serum components.

When replicate experiments from conA-activated cultures (baboon, serum-free) were compared to an MLR, the dose-response curves were similar in their sensitivity to both FK506 and rapamycin (Fig. 1b). This supports the relevance of conA-activation studies for assessing these immunosuppressive drugs.

Discussion

Our data demonstrate some variation in the drug sensitivity between PBL from different species. Since these occur in serum-free experiments, this implies that the differences are at the cellular level and may relate to variations in the generation of activation signals between species. It is known that the activation pathway of lymphocytes is multifactorial and includes "cross-talk" between pathways [1, 4] and that the relative contribution of each pathway may differ between species. Any variation in the concentration of a putative target protein associated with a given pathway would result in a similar variation in the concentration of the drug required to reach immunosuppressive levels.

We were interested to note the differential order of sensitivities to FK506 compared with rapamycin. This indicates that any interspecies variation in cross-talk which culminates in activation (involving FK506-sensitive, early "activation genes" including c-*myc,* interleukin 2 and its receptor [2] is independent of the other interspecies variation which occurs later, that is in the rapamycin-sensitive signalling pathways for cell cycle progression (requiring further gene activation, including that of c-*myb* [1].

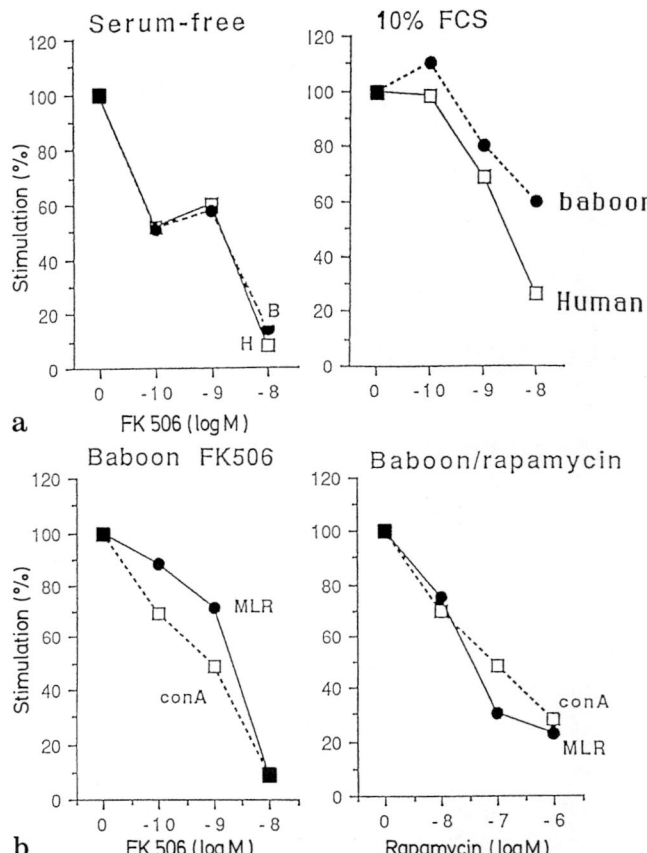

Fig. 1. a Dose-response curves to FK506 in concanavalin (conA)-stimulated cultures of baboon *(B)* or human *(H)* PBL in a single experiment. Cells and drugs were from respective common stocks, and the only variable was the presence or absence of 10% fetal calf serum (FCS). Control levels of DNA synthesis for baboon (human) were 24179 (37829) cpm under serum-free conditions and 81328 (46660) in 10% FCS. **b** FK506 and rapamycin. Dose-response curves for baboon PBL after 2 days of conA stimulation (in serum-free medium). This is the mean of the 5 experiments; in addition, a 7-day MLR (in 2% FCS) between the two baboons was measured. The MLR control gave 119903 cpm (background 2800), whilst the representative cpm for the conA control was 65106 cpm (background 439)

Acknowledgement. This work was funded by the British Medical Research Council.

References

1. Crabtree GR (1989) Contingent genetic regulatory events in T lymphocyte activation. Science 243: 355–361
2. Dumont FJ, Staruch MJ, Koprak SL, Melino MR, Segal NH (1990) Distinct mechanisms of suppression of murine T cell activation by the related macrolides FK506 and rapamycin. J Immunol 144: 1418
3. Eiras G, Imventarza O, Murase N, et al (1990) Species differences in sensitivity of T lymphocytes to immunosuppressive effects of FK506. Transplantation 49: 1170–1172
4. June CH, Ledbeter JA, Linsley PS, Thompson CB (1990) Role of the CD28 receptor in T cell activation. Immunol Today 11: 211–216
5. Metcalfe S, Milner J (1991) Evidence that FK506 and rapamycin block T cell activation at different sites relative to early reversible phosphorylation involving the protein phosphatases PP1 and PP2A. Transplantation 51: 1318–1320

Transplant Int (1992) 5 [Suppl 1]: S 516–S 520

TRANSPLANT
International
© Springer-Verlag 1992

Ex vivo perfusion of canine pancreaticoduodenal allografts using class-II-specific monoclonal antibody delays the onset of acute rejection*

K. Miyoshi, K. Sakagami, and K. Orita

First Department of Surgery, Okayama University Medical School, Okayama, Japan

Abstract. In the following study, we investigated whether ex vivo perfusion of canine pancreaticoduodenal allografts prior to transplantation using a class-II-specific monoclonal antibody (MoAb) OKIa1) could prevent acute rejection. Untreated grafts were rejected within 6 days after transplantation, and all of these recipients suffered severe hyperglycemia. In contrast, in recipients who received grafts which underwent ex vivo class-II-specific MoAb perfusion treatment, the mean urinary amylase levels were sustained significantly higher ($11\,733 \pm 4493$ vs. 3274 ± 2108 U/L on day 7, $P < 0.005$), and mean fasting blood glucose (FBG) levels remained within the normal range (13.4 ± 5.8 vs. 23.4 ± 3.9 mM on day 7, $P < 0.0005$). Low doses of cyclosporin A (CsA) were necessary in order to maintain lower FBG levels. Histopathology analysis on day 7 after transplantation showed that endotheliitis and necrosis were much less prominent in the MoAb-treated grafts. In the light of our results, we conclude that ex vivo perfusion of canine pancreaticoduodenal allografts using a class-II-specific MoAb is effective in delaying the onset of acute rejection, and low doses of CsA could extend this effect.

Key words: Pancreas transplantation – Class-II-specific monoclonal antibody – Immunomodulation – Dendritic cell

In pancreas transplantation, the most powerful stimulus for the initiation of acute rejection has been shown to come from interstitial dendritic cells (DCs), expressing large quantities of major histocompatibility complex (MHC) class II antigens. DCs are known to be present in the exocrine pancreas and circulate rapidly through the tissues to carry foreign antigens in a highly immunogenic form to the organized lymphatic tissues [8, 13, 14]. It has been suggested that inactivation of the DCs would result in the removal of the stimulating capacity of the allograft. Manipulation of allografts to modulate their antigenicity might be an attractive and potentially clinically applicable strategy as an alternative to current immunosuppression techniques. Pretreatment of the pancreas or islet allografts using class-II-specific monoclonal antibodies (MoAbs) was shown to result in prolongation of graft survival in rodent models [6, 9] but was ineffective in canine models [2, 15]. The following experiments were designed to determine whether or not ex vivo perfusion of canine pancreaticoduodenal allografts using class-II-specific MoAb could delay the onset of acute rejection. We also examined the effect of the combined use of cyclosporin A (CsA) at levels inadequate for normal grafts, since pretreatment with class-II-specific MoAb seems limited to the inhibition of acute rejection in a large animal model like a dog.

Materials and methods

Animals. Unrelated adult mongrel dogs of both sexes weighing 9–13 kg without infections were used in these experiments as the donors and recipients. All surgical procedures were performed under general anesthesia with ketamine hydrochloride (10 mg/kg i. m., Sankyo, Tokyo, Japan).

MoAb. OKIa1 (Ortho, Raritan, N.J.), a murine IgG2 antibody against human DR antigen complex, was used in this experiment. It has also been shown to crossreact with canine class II antigens [7].

Harvesting procedure for pancreaticoduodenal allografts. As shown in Fig. 1 A, the harvesting of the canine pancreaticoduodenal allografts was performed basically according to the method of Ekberg et al. [5]. Briefly, the whole pancreas and the duodenal segment were harvested together with a vascular pedicle comprising the portal vein and the aortic conduit with the celiac axis and the superior mesenteric artery (SMA). The common bile duct was divided where it approached the pancreas, and two or three hepatic branches originating from the common hepatic artery were divided. The pancreaticoduodenal artery along the duodenum was divided distal to the origin of the pancreaticoduodenal arcade to the SMA, and the arcade was preserved in its entirety. The distal part of the uncinate

Offprint requests to: K. Miyoshi, First Department of Surgery, Okayama University Medical School, 2-5-1 Shikata-cho, Okayama 700, Japan

* This work was supported in part by grant no. 02454306 from the Japanese Ministry of Education, Science, and Culture

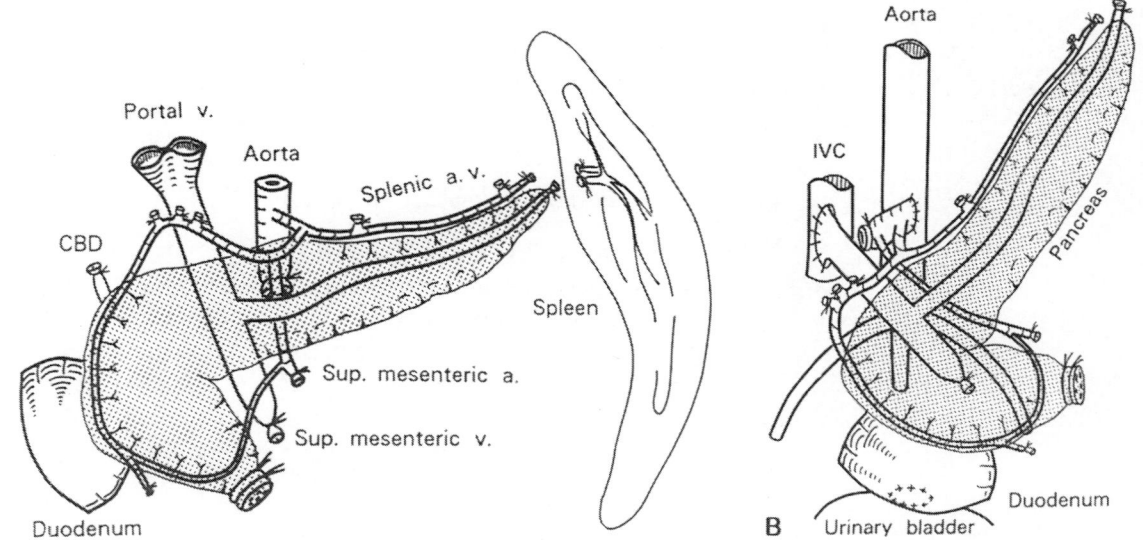

Fig. 1 A, B. Procedure for canine pancreaticoduodenal allotransplantation: harvesting (**A**) and transplantation (**B**). *CBD*, common bile duct; *IVC*, inferior vena cava

process that became ischemic was resected. The splenic artery and vein were divided distal to the pancreas, and the porta hepatis was divided up to its bifurcation at the hepatic hilum. After harvesting and perfusion with 300 ml Euro-Collins' solution (EC) at 4°C via the aortic conduit, the grafts were maintained in saline-ice slush at 4°C.

Transplantation procedure. As shown in Fig. 1 B, the portal vein was anastomosed end-to-side to the inferior vena cava, and the aortic conduit was anastomosed end-to-side to the aorta. The arterial supply of the allograft was based on the celiac axis and SMA. After revascularization, the closed duodenal segment was anastomosed side-to-side to the dome of the urinary bladder for exocrine drainage. Finally, the recipient pancreas and spleen was totally removed with preservation of the duodenum and its vasculature.

Experimental groups. Twenty dogs were divided into the following 4 groups. In group 1, 5 dogs received untreated grafts and were given no immunosuppressant. In group 2, 5 dogs received grafts after ex vivo perfusion with OKIa1 and were given no immunosuppressant. Following the perfusion with 250 ml of EC, the grafts were perfused with 50 ml of EC supplemented with 300 μg of OKIa1 and incubated for 90 min at 4°C. In group 3, 5 dogs received untreated grafts and were treated with subtherapeutic doses of CsA (Sandoz, Basel, Switzerland). CsA was started from the day of transplantation and maintained at a dose of 2.5 mg·kg^{-1}·day^{-1} intramuscularly. This treatment resulted in CsA trough levels of 100–200 ng/ml, which are inadequate to prevent canine islet allograft rejection [1]. In group 4, 5 dogs received grafts after ex vivo perfusion with OKIa1 and were treated with the same doses of CsA as group 3. Mean cold ischemic time was 126±23 min, and there was no significant difference among the 4 groups.

Immunoperoxidase technique. Biopsy specimens were obtained from the grafts before and after ex vivo perfusion and were examined to confirm whether the class-II-specific MoAb in the perfusate had combined with the class II antigens. The specimens were fixed using the AMeX method [11] and embedded in ordinary paraffin. Thin paraffin sections were deparaffinized with xylene and stained with the avidin-biotin-peroxidase technique. The sections were incubated with class-II-specific MoAb at 4°C overnight. This was followed by incubation with a biotinylated goat antimouse antibody (Biogenex, St Ramon, Calif.) for 60 min at 37°C and subsequently by incubation with avidin-biotin complex (Biogenex) for 60 min at 37°C. Diaminobenzidine tetrahydrochloride (0.025% solution, Sigma, St Louis, Mo.) was used as the chromogen.

Postoperative treatment and monitoring of graft function. In addition to the standard postoperative care, the following routines were observed: Some 300 mg gabexate mesilate (courtesy of Ono, Tokyo, Japan) was given intravenously on the day of transplantation, and adequate bicarbonate was given intravenously daily for 7 days. The exocrine pancreatic function was monitored by daily measurement of urinary amylase (UA) levels, and rejection was defined as UA <5000 U/l in two consecutive samples. Fasting blood glucose (FBG), serum amylase (SA), serum glutamic oxaloacetic transaminase (SGOT), and serum glutamic pyruvic transaminase (SGPT) levels were also monitored daily.

Open biopsies of the pancreas allografts in all recipients were taken on day 7 and examined by histopathology for the assessment of acute rejection.

Histopathology assessment. Biopsy specimens taken on day 7 were fixed in neutral-buffered formalin and embedded in paraffin. Multiple sections from each specimen were stained with H&E. Rejection features were defined according to the criteria of Carpenter et al. [4] as mixed neutrophilic and mononuclear cell infiltrates of pancreatic lobules, endotheliitis, thrombus, and coagulation necrosis. Each finding was graded as absent (−), mild (+), moderate (+ +), and severe (+ + +) for each specimen.

Statistical analysis. Differences between the mean values were assessed for significance by Student's unpaired *t*-test, with $P < 0.05$ considered significant.

Results

Immunostaining of the canine pancreas

In the specimens obtained before ex vivo perfusion with class-II-specific MoAb, a few cells expressing class II antigens were stained in the exocrine pancreas and within the parenchyma of the islets, as shown in Fig. 2 A. They were morphologically recognized as DCs. Class-II-specific MoAb did not react with parenchymal cells or with endothelial cells. After ex vivo perfusion with class-II-specific MoAb and incubation with biotinylated goat anti-mouse antibody, an almost similar number of cells was labeled, as shown in Fig. 2 B.

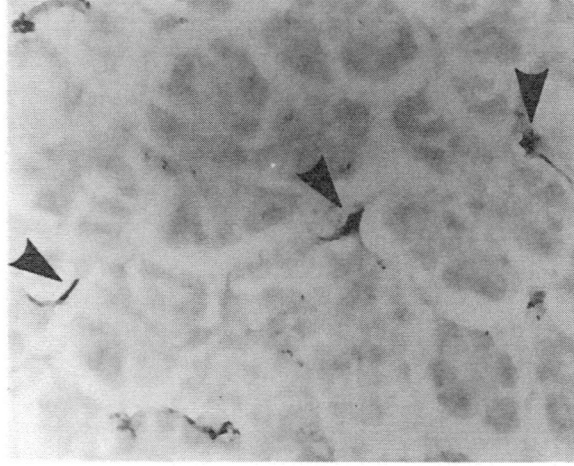

A

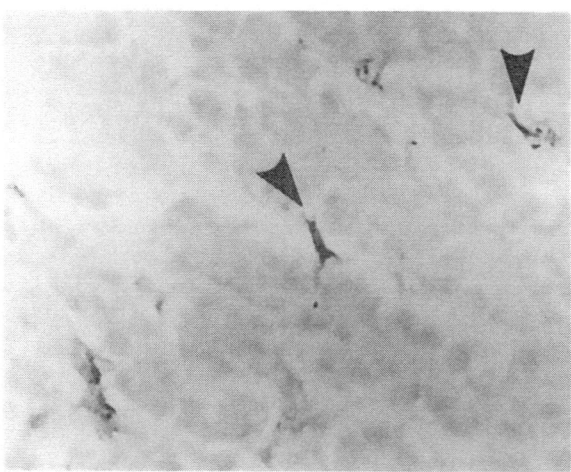

B

Fig. 2 A, B. Distribution of scattered class-II-positive cells showing dendritic morphology in the canine pancreas. Positive cells are present in the exocrine pancreas and within the parenchyma of the islets *(arrows)* (**A**). After ex vivo perfusion with class-II-specific monoclonal antibodies (MoAb), an almost similar number of cells was labeled *(arrows)* (**B**). Stained with the indirect immunoperoxidase technique and lightly counterstained with hematoxylin. × 800

Postoperative graft functions

Table 1 depicts the summary of graft function in the 4 groups during the 1st week after pancreaticoduodenal allotransplantation. The UA level in all successfully transplanted cases rose to over 10 000 U/L immediately after allotransplantation. In group 1, mean UA levels deteriorated progressively and fell below 5000 U/L on day 6. By contrast, in group 2, mean UA levels were sustained significantly higher for 7 days posttransplant ($11 733 \pm 4493$ vs. 3247 ± 2108 U/L on day 7, $n = 5$ in each group, $P < 0.005$). This significance was also seen between CsA-treated groups. All transplanted cases were normoglycemic (FBG < 14 mM) on the 1st postoperative day. In group 1, hyperglycemia occurred acutely on day 6 posttransplant. By contrast, in group 2, normoglycemia was sustained for at least 7 days after transplantation (13.4 ± 5.8 vs. 23.4 ± 3.9 mM on day 7, $n = 5$ in each group, $P < 0.0005$). The effect of CsA treatment in recipients was not significant but was helpful in maintaining the lower FBG levels.

SA levels were usually elevated on day 1, and SGOT and SGPT levels were maximized on day 1 or 2 posttransplant. They did not vary significantly in each study group (data not shown). Our protocol for CsA administration resulted in blood CsA trough levels of 100–200 ng/ml.

Histopathological findings

At the time of open biopsy on day 7, the anastomosis of either the aortic conduit or the porta hepatis was patent, and the duodenocystostomy was intact in all recipients. Table 2 depicts the comparison of histopathological findings in each group. All untreated grafts transplanted in nonimmunosuppressed recipients showed mild to severe mixed, predominantly mononuclear, cellular infiltration which was densest around the vascular tracts in the center of the lobules. Mild to severe endotheliitis and coagulation necrosis (arterial, venous, or both) was detected in all grafts. Thrombus formation was present in large vessels near the anastomosis in 2 of the 5 grafts. After ex vivo perfusion with class-II-specific MoAb, although a few grafts showed mild mixed cellular infiltrate, endotheliitis and thrombi were absent in all grafts. CsA treatment in recipients could, in part, suppress mixed cellular infiltration.

Discussion

It is well-known that MHC class II antigen-bearing cells possess an antigen presenting cell (APC) function, and they can stimulate T lymphocytes reactive to either antigen plus MHC or foreign MHC alone [10].

Several studies indicated that DCs are potentially important components of the rejection reaction and that the presence of DCs alone within the pancreas is sufficient for the initiation of pancreas allograft rejection. The results of our immunohistochemical studies provided evidence that class-II-specific MoAb could label the surface antigens of DCs in canine pancreas (recognized morphologically). This demonstrated that class-II-specific MoAb in the perfusate could permeate into the canine pancreas tissue and combine with MHC class II antigen epitopes on DCs during the incubation period (Fig. 2).

DCs appear to be as much as 10000-fold more potent than resting B cells [10]. DCs expressing large quantities of MHC class II antigen epitopes are known to be specialized to transport various antigens to the T area via blood or lymph. Migration to the lymphoid organ is suggested to be a more efficient means for DCs to select rare antigen-specific T cells from the recirculating pool in the early sensitization phase of an immune response [14]. Such observations on the function of DCs in the initiation of pancreas allograft rejection led several authors to attempt to modulate the antigenicity of DCs by treating the pancreas to be grafted rather than the recipient. The strategies of immunomodulation using class-II-specific MoAb in rodent pancreas transplantation models has succeeded in preventing acute rejection. Murine islets treated with DC-specific MoAb and complement were shown to survive for over 200 days [6]. Normothermic perfusion of rat pancreas allografts with class-II-specific MoAb using a perfusion circuit was demonstrated to pro-

Table 1. Summary of graft function in the 4 groups during 1st week after pancreaticoduodenal allotransplantation ($n = 5$ in each group)

	Before transplantation	Day 2	Day 6	Day 7
Urinary amylase (U/L)				
Group 1	44 ± 43	21932 ± 7040	3664 ± 3539	3274 ± 2108
Group 2	28 ± 16	36124 ± 9164	12586 ± 5673*	11733 ± 4493*
Group 3	30 ± 25	25572 ± 5444	5065 ± 2035	2044 ± 1181
Group 4	32 ± 12	23627 ± 8411	15451 ± 8716*	11689 ± 3777*
Fasting blood glucose (mM)				
Group 1	5.7 ± 0.4	7.8 ± 4.2	21.4 ± 4.1	23.4 ± 3.9
Group 2	4.8 ± 1.8	9.4 ± 4.8	12.9 ± 7.3*	13.4 ± 5.8*
Group 3	5.9 ± 1.6	6.3 ± 3.6	24.7 ± 7.8	27.3 ± 5.2
Group 4	5.2 ± 1.8	6.0 ± 2.2	7.6 ± 2.9*	9.2 ± 4.4*

* Data points where differences are significant ($P < 0.05$) vs. group 1 (control)

Table 2. Summary of histopathological findings in the 4 groups on day 7 after pancreaticoduodenal allotransplantation

Group	Ex vivo perfusion with OKIa1	Cyclosporin A	Dog no.	Rejection findings			
				Mixed cellular infiltrate[a]	Endotheliitis	Thrombus	Coagulation necrosis
1	No	None	1	+ +	+ +	–	+ +
			2	+	+	–	+
			3	+ + +	+ + +	+	+ +
			4	+	ND[b]	ND[b]	+ +
			5	+ +	ND[b]	+ +	+ + +
2	Yes	None	1	+	–	–	–
			2	+	–	–	–
			3	+	–	–	+
			4	+	–	–	–
			5	–	–	–	–
3	No	2.5 $mg \cdot kg^{-1} \cdot day^{-1}$	1	+ +	+	+ +	+ +
			2	+	+	+	–
			3	+	–	+	–
			4	+	–	+	+
			5	–	–	–	–
4	Yes	2.5 $mg \cdot kg^{-1} \cdot day^{-1}$	1	+	–	–	–
			2	+	–	–	–
			3	–	–	–	–
			4	–	–	–	–
			5	–	–	–	–

[a] Defined as mixed neutrophilic and mononuclear cell infiltrate
[b] Not diagnostic because of severe pancreatic necrosis

long graft survival significantly [9]. The mechanism of these beneficial effects with pretreatment using class-II-specific MoAb has been suggested: when DCs combine with MoAb, they would lose their APC function in pancreas allografts, and T-cell sensitization from alloantigens could not be carried out.

It is not yet known whether or not similar manipulations to modify allograft antigenicity are applicable to larger non-inbred mammals like dogs. There are few reports indicating the efficacy of treatment using class-II-specific MoAb in canine pancreas transplantation models. Treatment of freshly isolated canine islets with Ia-specific MoAbs and complement was reported to be inadequate to prevent acute rejection in outbred beagles [2]. Simple infusion of canine whole pancreas allografts with DC-specific MoAbs prior to transplantation was reported not to prolong graft survival [15].

Our results demonstrated that in recipients whose grafts received ex vivo perfusion using class-II-specific MoAb, the UA levels were sustained above 5000 U/L, and the FBG levels were maintained within 14 mM for 7 days posttransplant. By contrast, the function of untreated grafts was abrogated due to acute rejection by day 6 posttransplant. On days 6 and 7, the difference in the UA and FBG levels between the treated and untreated grafts was significant (Table 1). Histopathology analysis of the grafts on day 7 agreed with the above shifts in graft function. In the grafts undergoing ex vivo perfusion using class-II-specific MoAb, endotheliitis comprising cell swelling, mononuclear cell infiltrate, and basement membrane disruption [3] was not seen, and the results suggested that the tissue blood supply through the capillaries was sufficient when the open biopsy was performed (Table 2). Since it was reported that canine resting endothelial cells lack MHC class II antigens, we do not yet have a good explanation for the suppression of endotheliitis by our manipulation. Despite the failure to achieve prolongation of canine pancreas graft survival by other authors, our manipulation could delay the onset of acute rejection for a few days. It is known that DCs turn over fairly rapidly in the tissues, with a half-life on the order of 2 or 3 days [13], and that the degree of the expression of class II antigens in allografts increases dramatically after transplantation [12]. These facts explain the ability of our manipulation to inhibit the onset of acute rejection, which is limited in such a short period. Our results must have arisen because class-II-specific MoAb penetrated the pancreatic tissue sufficiently to interact with most of the DCs and its affinity to antigens was enough to reduce the antigenicity of the DCs. On the other hand, that the SA levels were not elevated suggests that the perfused class-II-specific MoAb did not induce parenchymal tissue damage in pancreas grafts. Similar changes in both SGOt and SGPT levels in the control group led to the conclusion that it also would not induce deterioration of liver function.

The relative strength of the rejection responses induced by pancreas allografts inactivated with DCs using class-II-specific MoAb is less than that induced by untreated allografts. This suggests that minimal immunosuppression at levels ineffective for untreated grafts would prevent acute rejection in DC-inactivated allografts. Successful prolongation of untreated canine islet allograft survival was demonstrated when serum CsA levels exceeded 400 ng/ml [1]. In the present study, subtherapeutic doses of CsA (blood CsA levels ranged from 100 to 200 ng/ml) could maintain the lower FBG levels and suppress, in part, mixed cellular infiltration to the grafts, but the difference was not significant.

In conclusion, we have described a new approach to reduce the antigenicity of canine pancreaticoduodenal allografts by ex vivo perfusion using class-II-specific MoAb prior to transplantation. This manipulation significantly delayed the onset of acute rejection. Additionally, subtherapeutic doses of CsA contributed to normoglycemia. Direct clinical application of this therapeutic approach is envisioned as an alternative to current nonspecific immunosuppression therapy, since no apparent side-effects in recipients were recognized during this study.

References

1. Alejandro R, Cutfield R, Shienvold FL, Latif Z, Mintz DH (1985) Successful long-term survival of pancreatic islet allografts in spontaneous or pancreatectomy-induced diabetes in dogs. Diabetes 37: 825–828

2. Alejandro R, Latif Z, Noel J, Shienvold FL, Mintz DH (1987) Effect of anti-Ia antibodies, culture and cyclosporin on prolongation of canine islet allograft survival. Diabetes 36: 269–273

3. Allen RDM, Grierson JM, Ekberg H, Hawthorne WJ, Williamson P, Deane SA, Champan JR, Stewart GJ, Little JM (1991) Longitudinal histopathologic assessment of rejection after bladder-drained canine pancreas allograft transplantation. Am J Pathol 138: 303–312

4. Carpenter HA, Barr D, Marsh CL, Miller AR, Perkins JD (1989) Sequential histopathologic changes in pancreaticoduodenal allograft rejection in dogs. Transplantation 48: 764–768

5. Ekberg H, Deane SA, Allen RDM, Hawthorne WJ, Williamson P, Grierson JM, Stewart GJ, Little JM (1988) Monitoring of canine pancreas allograft function with measurements of urinary amylase. Aust NZ J Surg 58: 583–586

6. Faustman DL, Steinman RM, Gebel HM, Hauptfeld V, Davie JM, Lacy PE (1984) Prevention of rejection of murine islet allografts by pretreatment with anti-dendritic cell antibody. Proc Natl Acad Sci USA 88: 3864–3868

7. Iwaki Y, Terasaki PI, Kinukawa T, Thai TH, Root T, Billing R (1983) Crossreactivity between human and canine Ia antigens using a mouse monoclonal antibody (CIA). Transplantation 36: 189–191

8. Lafferty KJ, Prowse SJ, Simenovic CJ (1983) Immunobiology of tissue transplantation, a return to the passenger leukocyte concept. Ann Rev Immunol 1: 143–173

9. Lloyd DM, Cotler SJ, Letai AG, Stuart FP, Thistlethwaite JR (1989) Pancreas-graft immunogenicity and pretreatment with anti-class II monoclonal antibodies. Diabetes 38: 104–108

10. Markmann J, Lo D, Naji A, Palmiter RD, Brinster RL, Heber-Katz E (1988) Antigen presenting function of class II MHC expressing pancreatic beta cells. Nature 336: 476–479

11. Sato Y, Mukai K, Watanabe S, Goto M, Shimosato Y (1986) the AMeX method, a simplified technique of tissue processing and paraffin embedding with improved preservation of antigens for immunostaining. Am J Pathol 125: 431–435

12. Settaf A, Milton AD, Spencer SC, Houssin D, Fabre JW (1988) Donor class I and class II major histocompatibility complex antigen expression following liver allografting in rejecting and nonrejecting rat strain combinations. Transplantation 46: 32–36

13. Spencer SC, Fabre JW (1990) Characterization of the tissue macrophage and the interstitial dendritic cell as distinct leukocytes normally resident in the connective tissue of rat heart. J Exp Med 171: 1841–1851

14. Steinman R, Inaba K (1989) Immunogenicity, role of dendritic cell. BioEssays 10: 145–151

15. Wilson TG, Hawthorne WJ, Jau H, Williamson P, Chapman JR, Grierson JM, Stewart GJ, Allen RDM, Little JM (1990) Pretreatment of canine whole pancreas allografts with monoclonal antibodies does not prolong graft survival. Transplantation Proc 22: 2163–2164

Transplant Int (1992) 5 [Suppl 1]: S 521–S 523

TRANSPLANT
International
© Springer-Verlag 1992

New immunosuppression with monoclonal antibody to intracellular adhesion molecule 1 (ICAM-1) in rat organ transplantation

M. Nozawa[1], I. Otsu[1], H. Kobayashi[2], T. Yamataka[2], T. Miyano[2], Y. Okumura[3], T. Tamatani[4], and M. Miyasaka[4]

[1] Department of Surgery, Meikai University, Saitama, Japan, Departments of [2] Pediatric Surgery and [3] Immunology, School of Medicine, Juntendo University, Tokyo, Japan [4] Department of Immunology, Tokyo Metropolitan Institute of Medical Science, Tokyo, Japan

Abstract. Inbred, male Lewis rats underwent heterotopic heart allografting from F344 donor rats, or streptozocin (STZ)-induced diabetic Lewis rats underwent pancreas allografting with bladder drainage from F344 or ACI donor rats. A monoclonal antibody (MoAb) to intracellular adhesion molecule 1 (ICAM-1) was given i. p. (1.0 mg/kg) for 10 days, and its immunosuppressive potency was evaluated. The mean survival time (MST) of the heart allografts was significantly prolonged in the MoAb-treated group. Both exocrine and endocrine MST of pancreas allografts were also prolonged by MoAb administration across the minor and major histocompatibility barriers. However, complete graft tolerance was not induced. Our study demonstrated that the MoAb to ICAM-1 alone can delay the allograft rejection in rat organ transplantation.

Key words: Heart and pancreas allotransplantations – Monoclonal antibody (MoAb) – Rat – Intracellular adhesion molecule 1 (ICAM-1)

Recently, an interruption of the attachment of lymphocytes to their targets via nonspecific accessory molecules, such as lymphocyte function antigen (LFA-1) or intercellular adhesion molecule 1 (ICAM-1) gained interest as a possible method to minimize rejection responses. At present, a monoclonal antibody (MoAb) to rat ICAM-1 is available [5]. The aim of this study was to investigate the immunosuppressive potency of a MoAb to ICAM-1 in in vivo experiments, i. e., rat heart and pancreas allotransplantations.

Materials and methods

Experiment 1. Male inbred Lewis rats (RT1l) underwent heterotopic heart allotransplantations (HTx) [4]. F344 rats (RT1l) were used as donors. These rats were divided into the following groups: (1) untreated HTx group ($n = 15$) and (2) ICAM-1-specific MoAb-treated HTx groups. Group 2 was further divided into 4 subgroups accord-

ing to the dosage and duration of MoAb administration: (2a) 0.2 mg/kg i. p. × 10 days ($n = 2$), (2b) 0.4 mg/kg i. p. × 5 days ($n = 2$), (2c) 0.4 mg/kg i. p. × 10 days ($n = 3$), (2d) 1.0 mg/kg i. p. × 10 days ($n = 15$). The MoAb was given from the 1st postoperative day in group 2. The graft survival was observed in each group.

Experiment 2. Male Lewis rats (RT1l), which were made diabetic by streptozocin i. v. injection (60 mg/kg), underwent pancreas allotransplantation (PTx) with bladder drainage [3]. Either F344 (RT1l) or ACI (RT1a) rats were used as donors. These rats were divided into the two groups: (1) untreated PTx group and (2) ICAM-1-specific MoAb-treated PTx group (1.0 mg/kg i. p. × 10 days). The ICAM-1-specific MoAb was given from the day of PTx. Each PTx rat was fed ad lib. in a metabolic cage. The blood sugar (BS) level and 24-h urinary amylase excretion were monitored daily. Furthermore, the groups whose grafts were harvested from ACI rats were subjected to biopsies of the grafted pancreas at day 5 after PTx for microscopic examinations (H&E staining).

In both experiments, statistical evaluations were done by Student's t-test or Cochran-Cox test, and the values were expressed as mean ± SE.

Results

In Experiment 1, the MST of the heart graft in the untreated group was 10 ± 1.5 days. The graft survival was not prolonged in subgroups 2a and 2b. When the MoAb was given at a dosage of 0.4 mg/kg for 10 days (group 2c), the

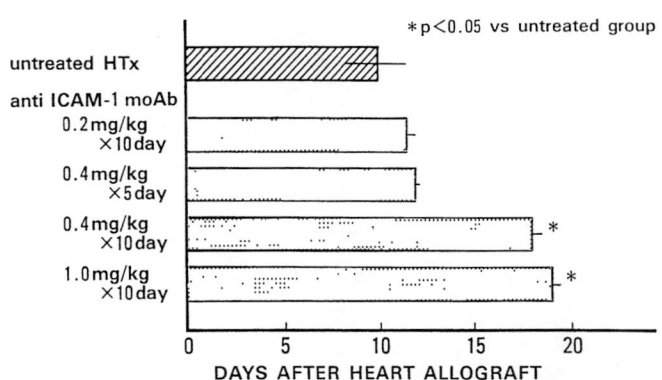

Fig. 1. Rat heart allograft survival with various dosage and duration of rat intercellular adhesion molecule 1 (ICAM-1)-specific monoclonal antibody (MoAb) administration (F344 to Lewis)

Offprint requests to: M. Nozawa, M. D., Department of Surgery, Meikai University, 1-1 Keyakidai, Sakado, Saitama 350-02, Japan

S 522

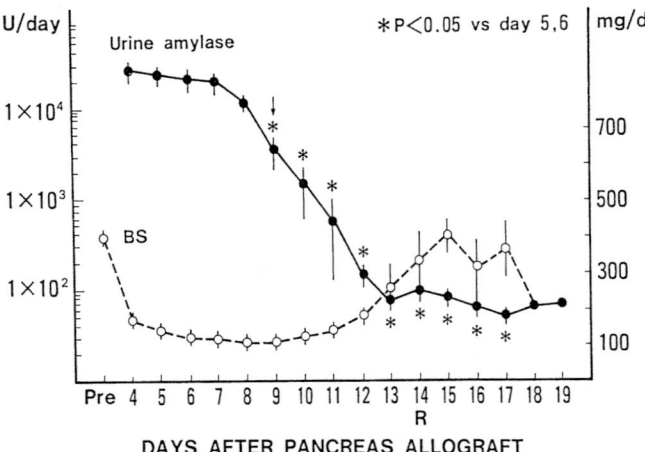

Fig. 2. The 24-h urine amylase and blood sugar *(BS)* changes in untreated pancreas allografted (PTx) rats (F344 to diabetic Lewis, *n* = 7). *Arrow,* rejection of exocrine function of graft pancreas; *R,* rejection of endocrine function

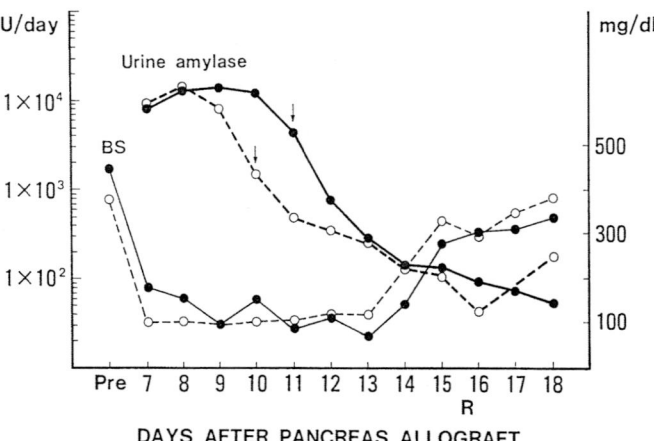

Fig. 3. The 24-h urine amylase and BS changes in PTx rats (F344 to diabetic Lewis) with ICAM-1-specific MoAb treatment (1.0 mg/kg for 10 days)

MST was 18.5 ± 0.5 days, which was significantly longer than the untreated group. When the MoAb was given at 1.0 mg/kg for 10 days (group 2d), the MST reached 19 ± 0.4 days (Fig. 1). The histology examination on day 5 after HTx revealed that the cell infiltration was less prominent, and the myocardial structures of the grafted heart were preserved in group 2d when compared with the untreated group.

In Experiment 2, in the F344 and Lewis combination, the 24-h urine amylase excretion decreased on day 9 after PTx, and the BS level increased to over 300 mg/dl on day 14 in the untreated group (Fig. 2). However, a drop in urine amylase excretion occurred either on day 10 or 11, and hyperglycemia appeared on day 15 or 16 in the MoAb-treated group (Fig. 3). When rejection of the exocrine function (a significant drop in urine amylase excretion) and endocrine function (hyperglycemia over 300 mg/dl) of the pancreas graft was observed in each PTx rat, the MST of these functions in the untreated group (*n* = 7) were 8.4 ± 0.3 days and 14.0 ± 0.6 days, respectively, whereas in the MoAb-treated group (*n* = 2), they were 10.5 ± 0.5 days and 15.5 ± 0.5 days, respectively.

In the combination of ACI to Lewis rats, the exocrine and endocrine MST of the pancreas graft in the untreated group (*n* = 5) were 6.2 ± 0.2 days and 7.5 ± 0.3 days, whereas those in the MoAb-treated group (*n* = 5) were 7.2 ± 0.4 days and 9.6 ± 0.2 days, respectively; the values were significantly longer than in the untreated group ($P < 0.05$). According to the microscopy examination of the graft on day 5, cellular infiltration was suppressed in the MoAb-treated group (Fig. 4).

Discussion

ICAM-1 is a 90-kD glycoprotein, expressed on the vascular endothelium, lymphocytes, macrophages and many other cells. The interaction of LFA-1 and ICAM-1 is re-

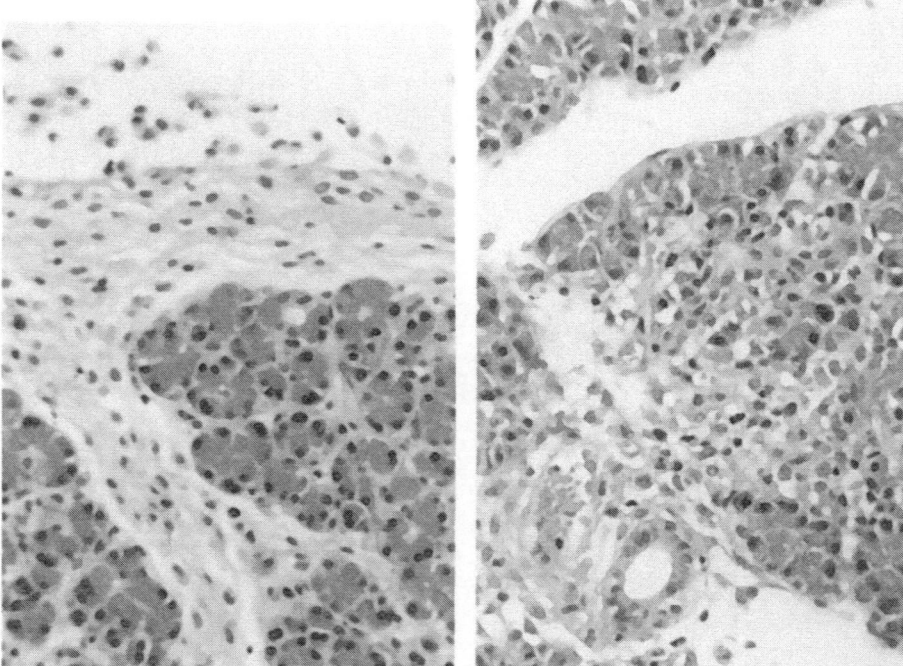

Fig. 4. Microscopy findings of pancreas allograft (ACI to diabetic Lewis rat) on day 5 after PTx (H&E, ×100). *Left,* untreated PTx rat; *right,* MoAb-treated PTx rat

quired for optimal T-cell function, which may play an important role in rejection responses. The MoAb to ICAM-1 has been used in large animal experiments [1, 2], but its immunosuppressive potency as a single agent in small animals has not been investigated. In our experiment, we administered rat ICAM-1-specific MoAb to the rats which underwent heterotopic heart or pancreas allografting and evaluated its immunosuppressive effects.

In rat heart allografts from F344 to Lewis, i. p. injection of more than 0.4 mg/kg of ICAM-1-specific MoAb for 10 days was necessary to achieve a significant prolongation of graft survival. When the MoAb was given at 1.0 mg/kg for 10 days, the MST was maximal.

Taking the result of the HTx into account, 1.0 mg/kg of ICAM-1-specific MoAb was given for 10 days after a rat pancreas allografting in order to obtain the maximum effect. In the F344 to Lewis combination, both exocrine and endocrine MST of the pancreas graft were longer in the MoAb-treated group than in the untreated group. We also examined the effect of the ICAM-1-specific MoAb across the major histocompatibility barriers. In the ACI to Lewis combination, both exocrine and endocrine MST of the pancreas graft were prolonged significantly in the MoAb-treated group when compared with those in the untreated group. Histological examination confirmed a suppression of cellular infiltration of the graft in the MoAb-treated group on the 5th postoperative day.

These results demonstrate that the ICAM-1-specific MoAb alone could prolong the graft survival in rat organ transplantations, probably through suppressing the initial rejection responses, across both minor and major histocompatibility barriers.

Acknowledgment. This study was supported in part by research grant no. 02857169 from the Ministry of Education, Japan.

References

1. Cosimi AB, Conti D, Delmonico FL, Preffer FI, Wee S, Rothlein R, Faanes R, Colvin RB (1990) In vivo effects of monoclonal antibody to ICAM-1 (CD54) in nonhuman primates with renal allografts. J Immunol 144: 4604–4612
2. Flavin T, Ivens K, Rothlein R, Faanes R, Clayberger C, Bilingham M, Starnes VA (1991) Monoclonal antibodies against intercellular adhesion molecule 1 prolong cardiac allograft survival in cynomolgus monkeys. Transplant Proc 23: 533–534
3. Nozawa M, Otsu I (1990) Experience in rat pancreas transplantation at Meikai University. Microsurgery 11: 145–151
4. Ono K, Lindsey ES (1969) Improved technique of heart transplantation in rats. J Thorac Cardiovasc Surg 57: 225–229
5. Tamatani T, Miyasaka M (1990) Identification of monoclonal antibodies reactive with the rat homolog of ICAM-1, and evidence for differential involvement of ICAM-1 in the adherence of resting versus activated lymphocytes to high endothelial cells. Int Immunol 2: 165–171

Transplant Int (1992) 5 [Suppl 1]: S 524–S 528

TRANSPLANT
International
© Springer-Verlag 1992

Japanese study of kidney transplantation:
1. Results of early phase II study

Japanese FK 506 Study Group

Abstract. For a 4-month period from July to October 1990, 37 primary renal transplant patients were enrolled in the early phase II study of FK 506. An i.v. dose of FK 506 0.075 mg/kg twice a day was administered initially, and then in oral dose of 0.15 mg/kg twice a day followed. Prednisolone was started at 1 mg/kg daily as an additioned drug. Some 32 live related donors with one-mismatched haplotype of HLA and 5 cadaveric donors underwent transplantation. All patients are alive, and all kidney allografts are functioning. A correlation between the trough level of FK 506 in whole blood and acute rejection or adverse events was retrospectively investigated. There was a significant correlation between the trough level in whole blood and acute rejection or renal impairment. In conclusion, the therapeutic dose of FK 506 should be adjusted by monitoring the trough level in whole blood, the range of which might be recommended to be 15–20 ng/ml during the early phase after transplantation.

Key words: FK 506 – Renal transplantation – Monitoring

FK 506 was introduced in liver transplantation in 1989 [1, 2, 6]. Only one preliminary pilot study in Pittsburgh on the prophylactic effect of FK 506 on kidney transplantation was reported in 1990 and 1991 [5, 7]. The results of an early phase II study of FK 506 on kidney transplantation performed by the Japanese Multicenter Study Group has recently been reported [3, 4]. The present paper focuses on the detection of an optimal therapeutic window of the FK 506 blood concentration in kidney transplantation evaluated, retrospectively, by monitoring the FK 506 trough level in whole blood of 36 enrolled renal transplant patients.

Offprint requests to: M. Ishibashi, M.D., Department of Urology, Osaka University Medical School, Fukushima 1-1-50, Fukushima-ku, Osaka 553, Japan

Materials and methods

Inclusion criteria. Excluded from the study were the following renal transplant recipients: (1) patients aged under 16 years old, (2) patients who had liver dysfunction as indicated by more than 1.6 mg/dl total bilirubin or twice or more glutamine-oxaloacetic transaminase (GOT) and glutamic-pyruvic transaminase (GPT) values than normal, (3) patients who had cardiac problems, with less than 60% of ejection fraction or an abnormal EKG, (4) patients who had pulmonary dysfunction of less than 70 mm Hg of PaO_2, (5) patients who had a history of pancreatitis or diabetic nephropathy, (6) patients who had a peptic ulcer, (7) patients who had a history of or currently had a malignant diesease, (8) patients who had infectious disease such as hepatitis B (HB) virus hepatitis or a carrier status of HB human immunodeficiency virus (HIV), or syphilis, (9) patients who had drug hypersensitivity or allergy, (10) patients who were pregnant or were expected to become pregnant, (11) patients who had undergone a previous kidney transplantation, (12) patients who had a minor mismatch for ABO blood group, (13) patients who had a positive T-cell crossmatch, (14) patients who received related, HLA identical or HLA nonidentical in 2-haplotype, sibling donor, or non-related living donor, (15) patients who did not consent to receive the FK 506 treatment.

Patients background. In all, 37 renal transplant patients were enrolled in this study. The mean age of the donors and recipients was 55.3 ± 7.6 and 31.6 ± 8.4, respectively. Some 31 received renal allograft from related, living, one HLA-haplotype mismatched donors, and 6 received them from cadaveric donors. One patient was excluded because of an unsuitable entry criteria (mismatch for ABO blood group). The PRA grade was 0% in 31 patients, less than 10% in 4, and undetectable in 1. The mean number of mismatched antigens of HLA-A, -B, and -DR were 1.8 ± 1.0.

Dosage of FK 506 and concomitant steroid. An initial dose of FK 506 0.15 mg/kg daily was administered intravenously over 4 h in 2 divided doses after revascularization, followed a few days later by 0.30 mg/kg orally divided info 2 doses. The daily dose of FK 506 was adjusted depending on the patients' clinical status or the severity of the acute rejection, with an upper limit (not to be exceeded) of 0.25 mg/kg twice a day. Prednisolone was used in combination with FK 506. On day 0 a bolus dose of 250 mg of methylprednisolone was administered, followed by 50 mg/day of prednisolone between days 1 and 6, 30 mg/day between days 7 and 13, 20 mg/day between days 14 and 20, 15 mg/day between days 21 and 27, and 10 mg/day from day 28 on.

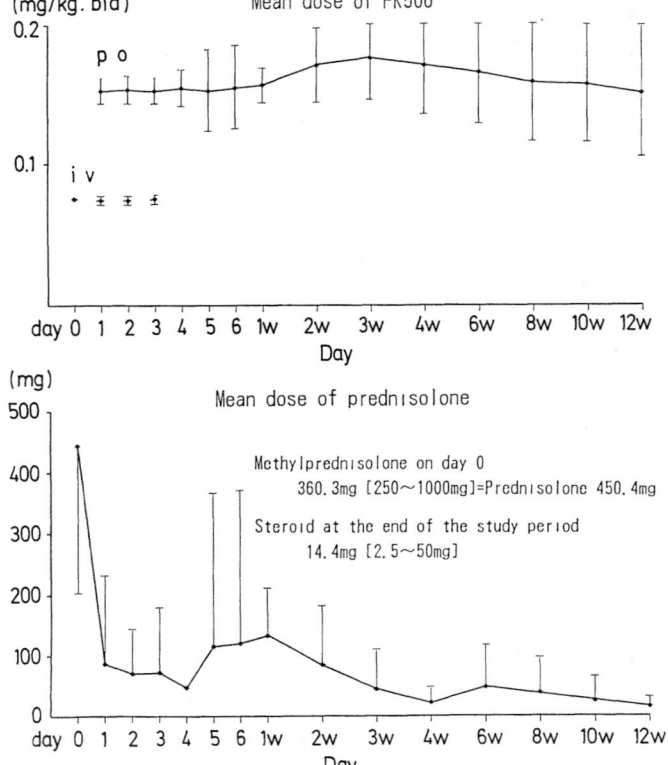

Fig. 1. Mean dose of FK 506 administered intravenously or orally and that of prednisolone administered including a bolus dose of methylprednisolone for 12 weeks of posttransplantation therapy in 36 enrolled transplant recipients

Monitoring of blood concentration. Trough levels of FK 506 in whole blood were monitored by the double sandwich enzyme-linked immunosorbent assay (ELISA). The procedure for the extraction of the blood sample was performed using dichloromethane.

Criteria of renal impairment. Renal impairment induced by FK 506 was diagnosed by a pathology study of a specimen taken by graft biopsy. The diagnosis was made from foamy vacuolization of proximal tubular cells, especially in the straight portion, calcification forming crystalloid in distal and/or proximal tubules, and a scanty vacuolization of the arteriolar wall.

Results

Mean dosage of FK 506 and prednisolone

The mean dosage of FK 506 in the transplant recipients enrolled during the first 3 months was calculated by their body weight every week (Fig. 1). The mean dosage of intravenous FK 506 during the first 3 days was 0.075 ± 0.002 mg/kg twice a day, and subsequently the oral dosage was about 0.16 ± 0.03 mg/kg twice a day up to 12 weeks. The increment of mean oral dosage of FK 506 in weeks 2–3 was explained by the relatively decreasing body weight after transplantation. On day 0, the mean dose of prednisolone was 442.6 ± 238.9 mg/day, and the dosage was increased twice at 1 and 6 weeks after transplantation. Steroid therapy was not withdrawn in any patient during the 12 weeks post-transplantation. The mean steroid dose at the end of the study period was 14.4 mg/day.

Patients and graft survival

At the end of the study, all 35 patients evaluated for efficacy were alive. All kidney allografts of the 23 patients who were able to continue taking FK 506 for 12 weeks and of the 12 patients who changed to another regimen owing to adverse effects or rejection were functioning 3 months after transplantation.

Monitoring of FK 506 blood concentration as related to rejection or adverse effects

To find an optimal blood concentration of FK 506 for kidney transplantation therapy, a correlation between its trough level in whole blood and episodes of rejection or adverse effects was investigated. Furthermore, to understand the drug monitoring of FK 506 in renal transplantation, a pharmacokinetics study was performed in 12 patients.

1. Pharmacokinetics of FK 506 in renal transplant patients: A pharmacokinetics study of the FK 506 whole blood concentration after either intravenous (10 patients) or oral (12 patients) administration was studied and reported in a previous paper [4]. All patients had normal liver function in the study. In brief, the mean $AUC_{(0-12h)}$ (area under the blood concentration-time curve) of i.v. administration of 0.075 mg/kg for 4 h, was 481 ± 129 (300–758) ng·h/ml and that of oral administration of 0.15 mg/kg was 249 ± 180 (95.1–743) ng·h/ml, for whole blood level. As shown in Fig. 2, variations in the absorption and excretion of all the FK 506 among the patients were noticed, while variations in the blood concentration on i.v. administration were minimal in patients with normal liver function except 1. Therefore, monitoring of the blood concentration of FK 506 should be strongly recommended, when administered orally, if there is a significant correlation between the trough level of FK 506 and clinical manifestations such as adverse events or onset of acute rejection.

2. Episodes of acute rejection and adverse events under the FK 506-prednisolone regimen:
Of the 35 patients, 26 rejection episodes were observed in 16 patients (45.7%, 1.63 episodes per patient). The incidence of steroid-resistant rejection of 26 rejection episodes was 30.8% (9 episodes). As shown in Fig. 3, there were two peaks of rejection episodes. The first one occurred between days 7 and 13, involving 8 episodes (22.9%) in the 35 patients treated with FK 506, but only 1 episode was steroid-resistant. The second peak occurred between days 28 and 55, and 9 episodes (28.1%) were noted in the 32 patients treated with FK 506, of which 4 were steroid-resistant.

Of the 36 patients enrolled, renal impairment (44.8%), abdominal distension (30.6%), cardiac symptoms (27.8%) such as chest pain, chest discomfort, palpitation, abnormal EKG, decreased ejection fraction, and tachycardia, hyperkalemia (27.8%), tremor (27.8%), and hyperglycemia (25.0%) were found. The incidence of three major adverse events, renal impairment, cardiac

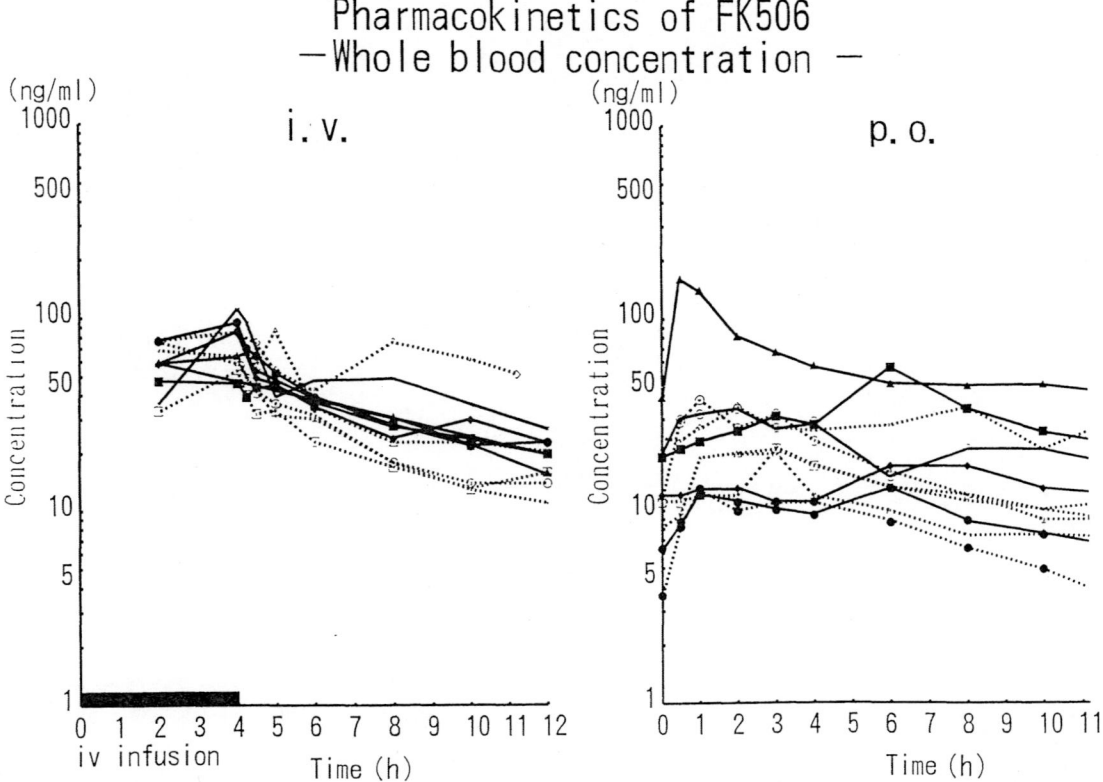

Pharmacokinetics of FK506
—Whole blood concentration —

Fig. 2. Pharmacokinetics study of FK 506 therapy in renal transplant recipients with normal liver function was done in 10 patients with a i.v. dose of 0.075 mg/kg of FK 506 in a 4-h infusion and in 12 patients with a p.o. dose of 0.15 mg/kg FK 506

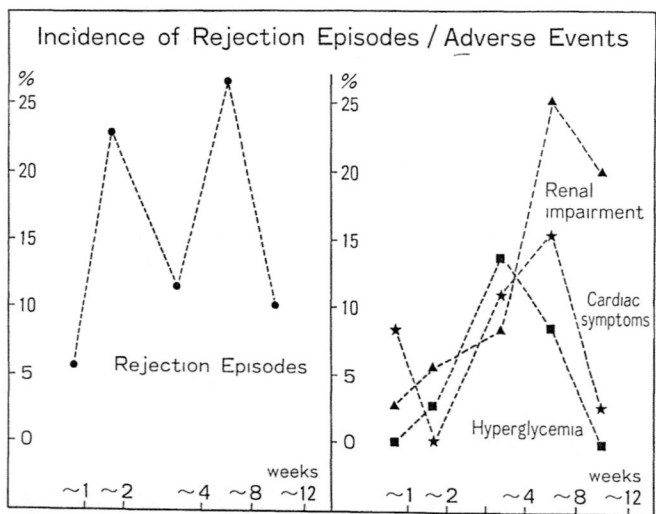

Fig. 3. Incidence of rejection episodes or adverse events in transplant patients under FK 506 administration. Incidence of episodes was calculated as follows: ratio of episodes observed to numbers of patients administered FK 506 at the time of diagnosis of the episodes

symptoms, and hyperglycemia, is shown in Fig. 3 and was seen to be high between weeks 3 and 10.

3. Correlation between FK 506 whole blood trough level and rejection or three major adverse events:
Figure 4 depicts a correlation between the FK 506 whole blood trough level and major clinical manifestations under FK 506 immunosuppression. As to rejection episodes, the background of patients with or without re-

jection was investigated (Table 1). There was no correlation between donor ages, HLA antigens mismatched, or total amount of prednisolone administered within 7 days. However, the trough level in whole blood during weeks 1–2 posttransplantation in patients with acute rejection was significantly lower than that in patients without acute rejection. As shown in Fig. 4, a significant difference between the mean trough level in whole blood in patients without rejection and that in patients with rejection was noticed. Therefore, the data implied that most of the rejection episodes appearing within 1–2 weeks (Fig. 3) were considered to be due to a suboptimal range of FK 506 blood concentration. The comparison between adverse events and FK 506 trough level in whole blood was made. Patients who had adverse events such as renal impairment, hyperglycemia, and cardiac symptoms always showed a higher trough level in whole blood, over 20 g/ml.

Conversion of FK 506-prednisolone
to conventional immunosuppression

Twelve patients (32.4%) converted from the FK 506-prednisolone regimen to another regimen. Nine of them discontinued using FK 506 because of rejection or adverse events. Figure 5 shows the reasons for the regimen change and the time that the FK 506 stopped or combined with another immunosuppressant. About 6–11 weeks posttransplantation, the FK 506-prednisolone regimen was changed frequently. The reasons for the regimen change were mainly rejection and renal impairment. Of the 9 pa-

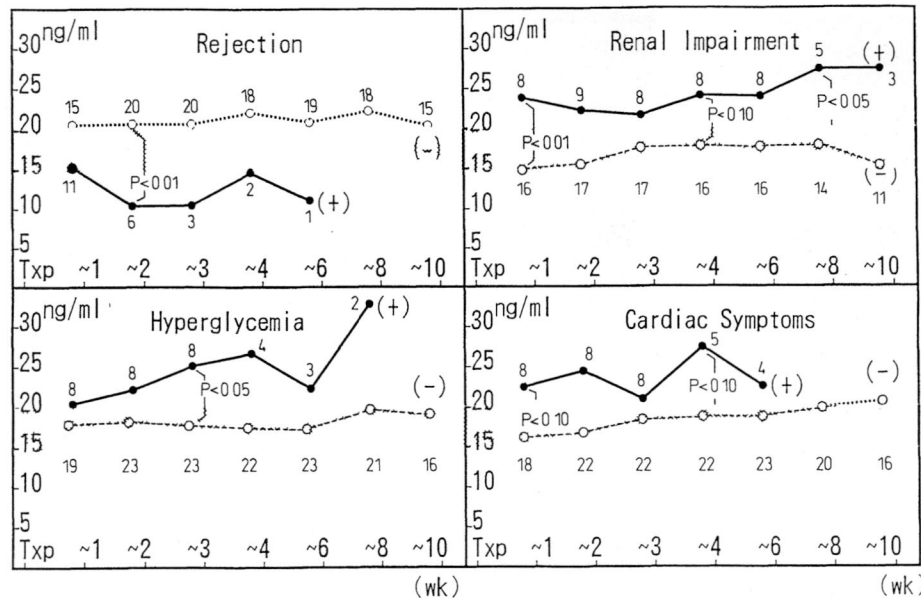

Fig. 4. A correlation between mean trough level of FK 506 in whole blood and clinical manifestations such as acute rejection, renal impairment, hyperglycemia, or cardiac symptoms. In the comparison of trough level at each episode observed, numbers of patients without episode (−) and with episode (+) are given. A statistical analysis between the two groups was performed by Student's t-test

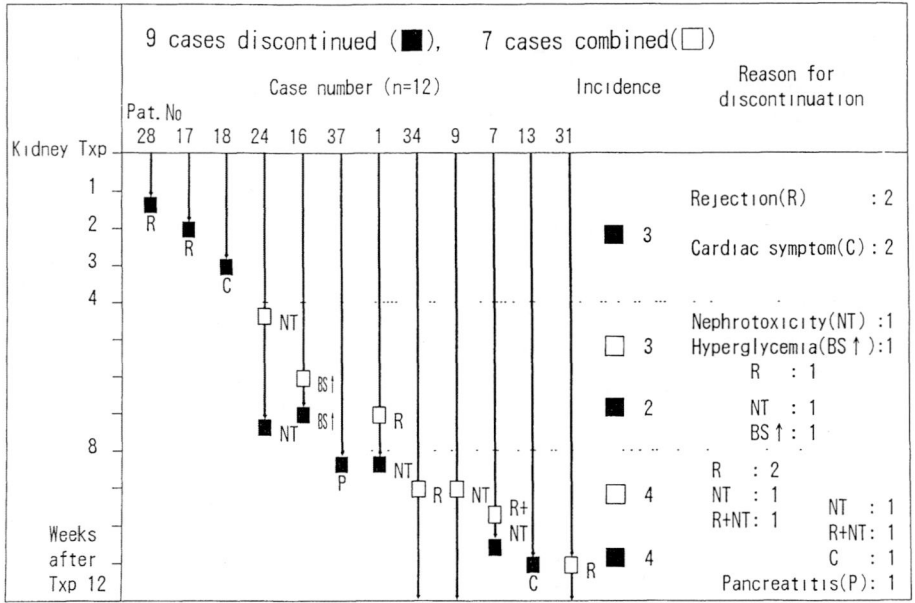

Fig. 5. Of the 36 cases evaluated, 12 (32.4 %) changed the FK 506-prednisolone regimen during the first 12 weeks post-transplantation

Table 1. Background of patients undergoing FK 506-prednisolone therapy

	Acute rejection		Significance
	With ($n = 16$)	Without ($n = 20$)	
Donor age	57.5 ± 8.1	53.4 ± 6.9	NS
HLA antigens mismatched			
A + B	1.3 ± 0.7	1.3 ± 0.9	NS
DR	0.5 ± 0.5	0.5 ± 0.5	NS
A + B + DR	1.8 ± 0.9	1.8 ± 1.1	NS
PRA grade (%)	8.6 ± 9.7	2.9 ± 7.2	NS
Total dosage of steroid (mg) (days 0~7)	840.0 ± 296.9	828.7 ± 189.4	NS
Trough level in whole blood (ng/ml) (1–2 weeks post-Tx)	11.6 ± 4.6 ($n = 8$)	20.6 ± 12.4 ($n = 20$)	$P < 0.01$

tients who discontinued, 5 stopped taking FK 506 for rejection or renal impairment (2 patients for rejection, 1 patient for rejection plus renal impairment, and 2 patients for renal impairment), and the remaining 4 patients discontinued because of other adverse events (2 patients for cardiac symptoms, 1 patient for hyperglycemia, and 1 patient for pancreatitis). Of the 7 patients receiving FK 506 with other immunosuppressants, 3 who were given FK 506 up to week 12 gave rejection or renal impairment as the reason for the regimen change.

Discussion

The Japanese FK 506 Study group has already reported the benefit of monitoring the FK 506 trough level in whole blood after kidney transplantation [4]. The monitoring of the FK 506 level in whole blood is superior to that in plasma and the reason is as follows:
1. Distribution of FK 506 in plasma is temperature-dependent
2. Concentration of FK 506 in plasma is markedly lower than in whole blood
3. Fluctuation of the FK 506 concentration is more prominent in plasma than in whole blood
4. FK 506 trough level in whole blood was well correlated with clinical manifestations including rejection episodes and adverse events.

The present early phase II study on kidney transplantation has confirmed the significantly important value of monitoring the FK 506 trough level in whole blood. With respect to acute rejection, the trough level in whole blood during weeks 1–2 posttransplantation was noticed to be a significant factor in the background of patients with or without rejection during the first 12 weeks posttransplantation. Although FK 506 has adverse effects such as renal impairment, hyperglycemia, or cardiac symptoms, its trough level in whole blood was significantly correlated with these adverse events. In addition to the obvious correlation between the trough level in whole blood and clinical manifestations such as rejection and adverse events, the pharmacokinetics study in kidney transplant patients without liver dysfunction has produced the useful information that there were variations in the trough level during FK 506 oral administration between individual transplant renal recipients, which indicates the importance of FK 506 monitoring.

The early phase II study was tentatively implied an optimal therapeutic dose of FK 506 in kidney transplantation therapy, and the range between 20 and 15 ng/ml for the trough level in whole blood during the first 3 months is recommended.

References

1. Fung JJ, Todo S, Jain A, McCauley J, Alessiani M, Scotti C, Starzl TE (1990) Conversion of liver allograft recipients with cyclosporine related complications from cyclosporine to FK 506. Transplant Proc 22: 6–12
2. Jain AB, Fung JJ, Todo S, Alessiani M, Takaya S, Abu-Elmagt K, Tzakis A, Starzl TE (1991) Incidence and treatment of rejection episodes in primary orthotopic liver transplantation under FK 506. Transplant Proc 23: 928–930
3. Japanese FK 506 Study Group (1991) Clinicopathological evaluation of kidney transplants in patients given a fixed dose of FK 506. Transplant Proc (in press)
4. Japanese FK 506 Study Group (1991) Japanese study of FK 506 on kidney transplantation: the benefit of minitoring the whole blood FK 506 concentration. Transplant Proc (in press)
5. Shapiro R, Jordan M, Fung J, McCauley J, Johnston J, Iwaki Y, Tzakis A, Hakara T, Todo S (1991) Kidney transplantation under FK 506 immunosuppression. Transplant Proc 23: 920–923
6. Starzl TE, Todo S, Fung J, Demetris AJ, Venkataramanan R, Jain A (1989) FK-506 for human liver, kidney and pancreas transplantation. Lancet II: 1000–1004
7. Starzl TE, Fung JJ, Jordan M, Shapiro R, Tzakis A, McCauley J, Johnston J, Iwaki Y, Jain A, Alessiani M, Todo S (1990) Kidney transplantation under FK 506. JAMA 264: 63–67

Transplant Int (1992) 5 [Suppl 1]: S 529–S 531

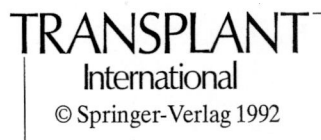

TRANSPLANT
International
© Springer-Verlag 1992

Subclinical impairment of distal renal acidification induced by low-dose cyclosporin A therapy

C. Quereda, C. Soria, N. Gallego, J. Sabater, M. Bermejo, J. Pascual, and J. Ortuño

Nephrology Department, Hospital Ramon y Cajal, Madrid, Spain

Abstract. Twenty-nine psoriasis patients on 5 mg/kg cy-closporin A (CyA) therapy were studied for 3 months using the furosemide test. Five of them (17 %) showed an abnormal renal acidification capacity after furosemide administration: The urinary pH did not sink under 5.3 after furosemide, while the ammonium and titrable acid levels were significantly low. There were no significant differences from controls regarding the serum potassium or fractional potassium excretion. Nevertheless, the transtubular potassium gradient was lower in patients with an abnormal furosemide test result. We conclude that some patients treated with a low dose CyA therapy developed an abnormality in the distal tubular acidification.

Key words: Immunosuppression – Cyclosporine A – Toxicity

Cyclosporine A (CyA) nephrotoxicity remains the greatest concern in the long-term use of the drug. Several toxic CyA-related effects in tubular function have been described in laboratory animals and in humans, including an impairment of the distal acidification capacity [1, 7, 9, 11]. Nevertheless, most of the clinical studies have been performed in patients with disorders which potentially may alter renal function, making the interpretation of results difficult. In this sense, psoriasis (Ps) patients treated with CyA constitute an excellent model for studying CyA nephrotoxicity [4, 5]. The aim of this work was to investigate the response of the renal tubular mechanisms of acidification to furosemide administration in a group of Ps patients treated with a low CyA dose by analysing its relationship with other renal function parameters.

Offprint requests to: Dr. C. Quereda, Servicio de Nefrologia, Hospital Ramon y Cajal, Cta de Colmenar Viejo, Km 9.2, E-28034 Madrid, Spain

Material and methods

After informed consent, 29 patients (18 males, 11 females) aged 19–59 years (mean 39.5) with severe Ps and normal basal renal function were treated with CyA. The initial dose was 5 mg/kg per day, which was continued for 3 months unless significant clinical side-effects appeared. Then, the drug was slowly tapered off over the next 3 months or stopped in the case of inefficacy. The renal function and electrolyte changes were evaluated monthly by the measurement of creatinine clearance and levels of serum and urine creatinine (Cr), urea, uric acid, sodium, potassium, chloride, total CO_2, magnesium, calcium and phosphate. The fractional excretion (FE) of Na, K and the transtubular K gradient (TTKG) were calculated. The blood CyA level was determined in each analytical control. The renal response to a furosemide test (FT) was performed at the end of the 3 treatment months. The results were compared with those obtained in 13 Ps patients who had not yet been treated with CyA and also with those of 19 Ps patients studied 1 month after stopping CyA treatment. The FT was performed in the morning, more than 12 h after the intake of the last CyA dose. Furosemide 80 mg was administered by the oral route, and new urine samples were then obtained hourly (1, 2, 3, and 4 h after administration) to determine the pH, acidification parameters, and electrolyte levels. The urinary pH was measured after voiding using a pHmeter. Titratable acid (TA) was determined by titration to pH 7.4a and ammonium (NH_4) using the Berthelo's reaction. Hydrogen excretion was calculated as: $[H+] = TA + NH_4$ and net acid excretion as $(NAE) = [H+]-CO_3H$. The analysis of variance for repeated measures and the paired-data Student's t-test were used in the statistical analysis. Data are presented as means and standard error of the mean (SEM); a P value of less than 0.05 was considered significant.

Results

Ps patients on CyA treatment had higher serum Cr (0.99 ± 0.03 vs 0.82 ± 0.12 mg/dl, $P < 0.01$), urea (35.9 ± 1.6 vs 29.8 ± 1.8 mg/dl; $P < 0.01$), and urate (5.73 ± 1.4 vs 4.59 mg/dl; $P < 0.05$) values than untreated Ps patients. Contrarily, serum magnesium (1.79 ± 0.03 vs 2.04 ± 0.04 mg/dl; $P < 0.01$) and total CO_2 (23.9 ± 0.37 vs 25.4 ± 0.59 mmol/l; $P < 0.05$) levels were lower. Patients studied after CyA withdrawal did not show any significant differences in any parameter as compared with the basal group. The FE Na, FE K and TTKG did not show any signficant differences among the 3 groups. Significant gly-

Table 1. Urinary response to furosemide in psoriasis patients

Group		Normal FT (n = 24)	Abnormal FT (n = 5)	Differences (P<)
U pH	b	5.59 ± 0.07	5.80 ± 0.21	n.s.
	p	4.64 ± 0.04	5.70 ± 0.26	0.01
U TA[a]	b	13.2 ± 0.84	8.83 ± 0.30	n.s.
	p	19.9 ± 1.01	13.50 ± 1.46	0.05
U NH₄[a]	b	23.9 ± 1.99	16.3 ± 2.00	n.s.
	p	38.9 ± 2.70	24.6 ± 4.03	0.05
U H⁺[a]	b	37.1 ± 2.20	26.0 ± 1.7	n.s.
	p	54.5 ± 3.09	36.5 ± 3.2	0.01
U CO₃H⁻[a]	b	3.01 ± 0.70	3.0 ± 1.7	n.s.
	p	46.70 ± 7.20	45.5 ± 6.8	n.s.
FE Na (%)	b	0.57 ± 0.08	1.07 ± 0.37	n.s.
	p	9.90 ± 2.29	8.3 ± 0.77	n.s.
EF K (%)	b	10.2 ± 1.0	11.1 ± 1.67	n.s.
	p	42.1 ± 5.8	37.3 ± 6.10	n.s.
TTKG	b	6.35 ± 0.42	4.07 ± 0.99	0.05
	p	7.94 ± 0.72	6.38 ± 1.52	n.s.

Mean ± standard error of the mean

[a] μmol/min · 100 ml FG

b, basal, prefurosemide; p, peak value postfurosemide; FT, furosemide test; U, urinary; FE, fractional excretion; TTKG, transtubular potassium gradient; TA, titratable acid

cosuria was absent in all cases. The mean lowest level of the postfurosemide urinary pH was higher in CyA-treated than in untreated patients (4.87 ± 0.09 vs 4.59 ± 0.03, $P < 0.05$). The peak postfurosemide urinary TA and NH₄ excretion were lower, although not significantly so. In 5 patients from the CyA-treated group (17%), the lowest postfurosemide urinary pH was always above 5.3, while in all untreated patients, pH values sank below 5.3. These 5 patients with an abnormal FT result did not show any significant differences when compared with those with a normal one as regards the CO₃H⁻ excretion. Nevertheless, the peak urinary NH₄, TA and NAE were significantly lower (Table 1). Total CO₂ concentration was also lower in patients with an abnormal FT results (22.1 ± 0.7 vs 24.6 ± 1.7 mmol/l, $P < 0.01$), while serum CR (1.2 ± 0.18 vs 0.95 ± 1.2 mg/dl, $P < 0.01$) and urea (47.2 ± 3.6 vs 35.7 ± 8 mg/dl, $P < 0.05$) levels were higher. Serum Na, K and urate levels were not significantly different. Basal or postfurosemide excretion of Na or K and the FE Na and FE K values were also similar. Nevertheless, the basal TTKG was lower in the group with an abnormal FT result (4.07 ± 0.99 vs 6.35 ± 0.42, $P < 0.05$). The blood CyA levels were similar in patients with a normal or abnormal FT result. Three of the patients with an abnormal FT result while on CyA therapy had normal PF test results 1 month after CyA withdrawal, but in 2 patients the abnormality continued, persisting in 1 of them for 3 months after stopping CyA treatment.

Discussion

Little is known about the potential renal damage induced by the prolonged use of low CyA doses or whether there is a threshold level of CyA dosage free of renal toxicity [2,

10]. We have studied the renal response to the FT in Ps patients treated with low CyA doses. This diuretic enhances Na⁺ reabsortion in excess of Cl⁻ in the cortical collecting tubule, thus creating a favourable lumen-negative electric gradient that facilitates the exit of K⁺ and H⁺ ions. The FT gives similar information to that provided by the infusion of sodium sulphate, but it is easier to perform and free of relevant secondary effects [8].

Five of our patients (17%) had an abnormal FT result. In these patients the postfurosemide urinary pH did not sink below 5.3 and a lower increase of NH₄, TA and NAE was seen than in patients with normal tests, but a similar CO₃H⁻ level, suggesting impairment of the distal mechanisms of acidification. The renal function was more extensively affected in these patients as shown by higher serum urea and Cr and lower total CO₂ values. Similar results have been found by Heering and Grabensee [7] in renal allograft patients treated with CyA: 23% of them showed an incomplete form of distal tubular acidosis with an inability of the sodium sulphate infusion to lower the urinary pH. Although the effects of CyA on the renin-angiotensin system are conflicting, hypoaldosteronism has been described as a cause of hyperkaliemic metabolic acidosis in transplant patients [1, 7, 9]. Nevertheless, this mechanism is unlikely in our patients: the impairment of renal function was minimal, significant hyperkaliemia was absent, and the basal and postfurosemide FE K values were normal. In addition, contrary to our cases, patients with hypoaldosteronism were able to lower their urinary pH by the stimulus of systemic acidosis or postfurosemide. In acute experiments in rats, Batlle et al. [4] observed a tubular impairment of acidification not mediated by renin-aldosterone abnormalities. In this model of CyA nephrotoxicity, diminished H⁺ secretion was associated with impaired distal K⁺ secretion when the treatment was prolonged for more than 8 days, suggesting a voltage-dependent type of distal renal tubular acidosis. However, on day 3 of therapy, the impairment of H⁺ secretion but not the abnormalities of K⁺ secretion could be demonstrated. The feature that is critical in the distinction of the two most common types of distal renal tubular acidosis (voltage-dependent or secretory) is the ability to secrete potassium. Our patients did not develop significant hyperkaliemia after CyA treatment, a finding also described by other authors using a similar dose schedule to ours [2, 3, 10]. The basal and postfurosemide urinary K excretion were also similar to those before CyA treatment and also similar in patients with a normal or abnormal FT result, suggesting that CyA induces an alteration in the H⁺-ATPase pump even using low doses for short periods of time.

Nevertheless, we cannot exclude a voltage-dependent mechanism to explain the impairment of acidification found in our study. Our patients with an abnormal FT result presented with a low basal TTKG, and the possibility exists that potassium alterations become more evident with time or when using other, more aggressive methods. Bantle et al. [3] were able to demonstrate a defect of potassium secretion of CyA-treated renal transplant recipients only after the administration of exogenous potassium chloride. Finally, it is possible that the FE K values in our patients with an abnormal FT result, although within the normal range, were inappropriately low in the presence of renal impairment.

We conclude that the FT discloses subtle alterations in distal acidification in low dose CyA-treated non-renal patients. Although these alterations are subclinical and seem to be reversible after drug withdrawal, we do not know whether they reflect structural anomalies which could become permanent and progressive with long-term treatment. The utility of the test in the early diagnosis of nephrotoxocity should be studied further.

References

1. Adu D, Turney J, Michel J, McMaster P (1983) Hyperkaliemia in ciclosporin-treated renal allograft recipients. Lancet II: 370–371
2. Balleta M, Libetta C, Fuiano G, Delfino M, Brunetti B, Ungaro B, Conte G (1991) Effects of a two-month treatment with low oral doses of cyclosporin on renal function. Nephrol Dial Transplant 6: 324–329
3. Bantle AP, Nath KA, Sutherland SER, Najarian JS, Ferris TT (1985) Effects of cyclosporine on the renin-angiotensin-aldosterone system and potassium excretion in renal recipients. Arch Intern Med 145: 505–508
4. Batlle DC, Gutterman C, Tarka J, Prasad R (1986) Effect of short-term cyclosporine A administration on urinary acidification. Clin Nephrol 25 [Suppl]: 62–69
5. Ellis CN, Fradin MS, Messana JM, Brown MD, Siegel MT, Howland A, Rocher LL, Wheeler S, Hamilton TA, Parish TG, Ellis-Madu M, Duell E, Annesley TM, Cooper KD, Voorhees JJ (1991) Cyclosporine for plaque-type psoriasis. N Engl J Med 324: 277–284
6. Gupta AK, Rocher LL, Schmaltz SP, Godfarb MT, Brown MD, Ellis CN, Voorhes JJ (1991) Short-term changes in renal function, blood pressure and electrolyte levels in patients receiving cyclosporine for dermatologic disorders. Arch Intern Med 151: 356–362
7. Heering P, Grabensee B (1991) Influence of ciclosporin A on renal tubular function after kidney transplantation. Nephron 59: 66–70
8. Kurtzman NA (1991) Disorders of distal acidification. Kidney Int 38: 720–727
9. Puschet JB, Greenbreg A, Holley J, McCauley J (1990) The spectrum of cyclosporin nephrotoxicity. Am J Nephrol 10: 296–309
10. Sabbatini M, De Nicola L, Ucello F, Conte RG, Dal Canton A, Andreucci VE (1990) Absence of acute nephrotoxicity with low doses of cyclosporin: experimental study in the rat. Nephrol Dial Transplant 5: 69–74
11. Stahl RAK, Kantz L, Maier B, Schollmeyer P (1986) Hyperchloremic metabolic acidosis with high serum potassium in renal transplant recipients: a cyclosporine A associated side effect. Clin Nephrol 25: 245–258

Transplant Int (1992) 5 [Suppl 1]: S532–S535

TRANSPLANT
International
© Springer-Verlag 1992

Cyclosporin A has no impact on alterations of the lipid profile after renal transplantation

J. Rosman[1], D. Evequoz[1], J. Landmann[2], and G. Thiel

Departments of [1] Internal Medicine, Division of Nephrology, and [2] Surgery, University Clinic of Basle, Basle, Switzerland

Abstract. The literature contains conflicting ideas regarding the role of cyclosporin A (CyA) in the induction of posttransplant dyslipidemia. The available studies contain small numbers of patients, especially on CyA monotherapy. We compared 65 patients on conventional azathioprine-prednisone therapy (AP) with 85 patients on CyA monotherapy, 19 on CyA-azathioprine therapy (CA), 20 on CyA-prednisone therapy (CP), and 52 on a triple therapy with CyA, azathioprine, and prednisone (CAP). From the results, it is concluded that patients on CyA monotherapy had lower serum cholesterol levels, with a lower high-density lipoprotein (HDL)-cholesterol level, probably due to the lower total cholesterol, compared with AP patients. From all groups, the CyA monotherapy group showed the most beneficial lipid profile. No additive negative influences of CyA when combined with other immunosuppressive drugs were noted. Thus, a correlation between derangements of the lipid profile and CyA therapy could not be confirmed. Further analysis of our data showed negative influences of antihypertensive treatment on lipid metabolism, particularly in the case of treatment with β-blockers or diuretics. It cannot be excluded that studies showing a negative influence of CyA therapy on lipid homeostasis were biased by secondary factors like antihypertensive therapy, which was often not taken into account.

Key words: Transplantation – Cyclosporin A – Lipids – Antihypertensive drugs – Insulin sensitivity – Immunosuppression

Modern immunosuppressive drugs, especially cyclosporin A (CyA), brought a radical improvement in the success rate of kidney transplantation. Graft survival after 1 year improved significantly [9–10]. The price paid for

this progress is the well-known side-effects of CyA [14], e.g., hypertension, hypertrichosis, gingival hyperplasia, and possible disturbances in lipid metabolism [6, 13]. Hypertension and alterations in lipoprotein metabolism are among the major cardiovascular risk factors [3]. Almost 40 % of renal recipient deaths are attributed to atherosclerotic cardiovascular disease [16].

Whereas prednisone negatively influences the lipid homeostasis [7], the role of CyA remains unclear. Most studies were carried out in small numbers of patients and are hampered by the fact that they were not controlled for blood pressure medication, a well-known cause of dyslipidemia [11]. Furthermore, there are no studies available with sufficient numbers of patients on CyA monotherapy. Most trials did not include lipoprotein analysis in their data, a necessary attribute to calculate the cardiovascular risk. A recent study demonstrated no harmful effect of CyA on cholesterol and triglyceride metabolism [12].

Since in the Renal Transplant Unit of Basle the ultimate goal is CyA monotherapy, we have the possibility to compare data derived from a large group of patients on CyA monotherapy with those on other immunosuppressive regimens.

Materials and methods

All patients that have undergone kidney transplantation come, apart from the usual follow-up, once a year for an intensive check-up to the transplantation center. As well as several clinical investigations, this includes blood samples taken in the morning after an overnight fast and before the morning dose of CyA for routine serum parameters and the estimation of the CyA level (parent drug level, monoclonal method, with normal range 75–200 ng/ml). On this occasion the lipid profiles are also analyzed: cholesterol and triglycerides by means of standard laboratory methods and the lipoproteins of cholesterol (high-density, low-density, HDL, LDL, and VLDL) by the ultracentrifuge method.

In all, 254 patients with stable renal function for at least 6 months and no change in medication for at least 6 months were enrolled in the study. Thirteen were excluded because of proteinuria exceeding 3 g/day or because they were on lipid-lowering drugs. Thus, 122 men and 119 women were available for the analysis. Data are expressed

Offprint requests to: Dr. J. Rosman, Chef de Clinique Néphrologie, Department of Internal Medicine, Division of Nephrology, CH-1011 Lausanne, Switzerland

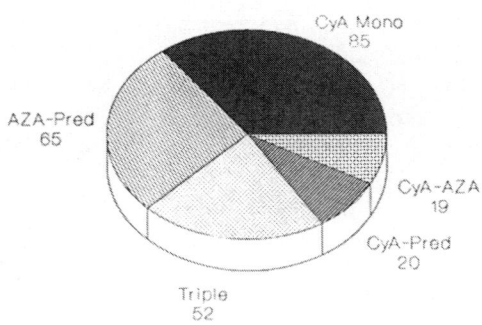

Fig. 1. Distribution of modalities of immunosuppressive therapy among the 241 patients included in the study

as medians since the underlying distribution of the data was not normal. Parameter-free testing by means of Wilcoxon and Mann-Whitney U-tests was applied.

Results

Five groups were created, depending on the modality of immunosuppression. The first one ($n = 65$) comprised all patients on the conventional combination therapy with azathioprine-prednisone (AP); the others were CyA monotherapy ($n = 85$) or combinations of CyA-prednisone (CP, $n = 20$), CyA-azathioprine (CA, $n = 19$), or triple therapy with CyA, azathioprine, and prednisone (CAP, $n = 52$) (Fig. 1).

The indications for the use of specific regimens will not be discussed here; it is worth mentioning that the CAP therapy was usually applied in the case of chronic rejection and that patients who were transplanted before the CyA era were maintained on their conventional therapy with AP if they had stable renal function.

As can be seen in Table 1, the AP group had the longest follow-up time, due to the aforementioned fact. There were no intergroup differences in age, body weight, and serum glucose level. If compared with the AP group, the serum creatinine level in the CP as well as in the CAP group was significantly higher, whereas the creatinine clearance was only significantly lower in the CAP group. This can be explained by the fact that the triple therapy

group is the one which posed major problems due to chronic rejection before the institution of this therapeutic modality. Proteinuria was significantly lower in the CyA monotherapy group. Here we have a positive selection of patients who were easy to maintain on CyA monotherapy. Blood pressure was well regulated in all groups. The CyA monotherapy group showed a tendency towards a higher systolic blood pressure (142 mm Hg vs. 132 mm Hg in the AP group). The diastolic blood pressure was equal in all groups and amounted to 82 mm Hg (median).

In Fig. 2, the respective values of total cholesterol and triglycerides in all groups are given. Compared with the conventionally treated AP group, only patients with CyA monotherapy had a significantly lower serum cholesterol level. There were complicated differences regarding the cholesterol lipoproteins, as shown in Fig. 3. Again compared with the Ap group, the HDL-C level was lower (probably because the total cholesterol value was also lower in this group), and the VLDL-C value was significantly higher in the CyA monotherapy group. The responses in the other groups were heterogeneous, but especially the HDL value was significantly lower than under AP treatment, except for the CP group.

Next, the entire cohort was divided into a group on treatment with prednisone-containing regimens ($n = 137$) and one without prednisone ($n = 104$). In Table 2, the results are given. It appears that patients on regimens without prednisone had significantly lower serum cholesterol values and a concomitantly lower HDL-C value.

The influence of diuretics (almost exclusively loop diuretics) and β-blockers (in this case atenolol) was studied separately, and the results are given in Table 3. Diuretics aggravate the lipid disturbances and lower the HDL-C level; atenolol raises the serum cholesterol as well as the LDL-C level.

The cardiovascular risk coefficient, LDL/HDL-C showed no significant differences in the groups with or without prednisone treatment, but significant derangement in the groups on diuretics or β-blockers (Table 4).

Discussion

Since disturbances in the lipid metabolism probably have an important impact on cardiovascular mortality, especially in a vulnerable group like patients with a grafted kidney, more attention should be paid to preventing

Table 1. Nonlipidemic parameters in the 5 groups

	AP ($n = 65$)	CyA mono ($n = 85$)	CyA-P ($n = 20$)	CyA-A ($n = 19$)	Triple ($n = 52$)
Years since transplant	9	4	5	4	4
Age (years)	46	52	51	46	46
Body weight (kg)	68	70	67	65	71
Serum creatinine (µmol/l)	102	110	134*	114	169**
Creatinine clearance (ml/min)	71	64	55	53	42**
Serum glucose (mmol/l)	5.3	5.6	5.3	5.5	5.7
CyA plasma level (ng/ml)	–	124	153	95	85
Proteinuria (g/24 h)	0.26	0.17*	0.20	0.16	0.44

AP, azathioprine-prednisone; CyA, cyclosporin A

* $P < 0.005$, ** $P < 0.0005$ vs. Al group

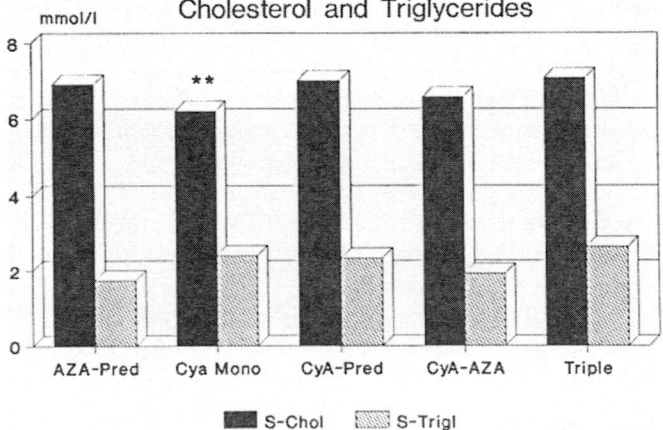

Fig. 2. Cholesterol and triglyceride values in the 5 different immunosuppressive regimen groups: $P < 0.01$ compared with conventional AP group

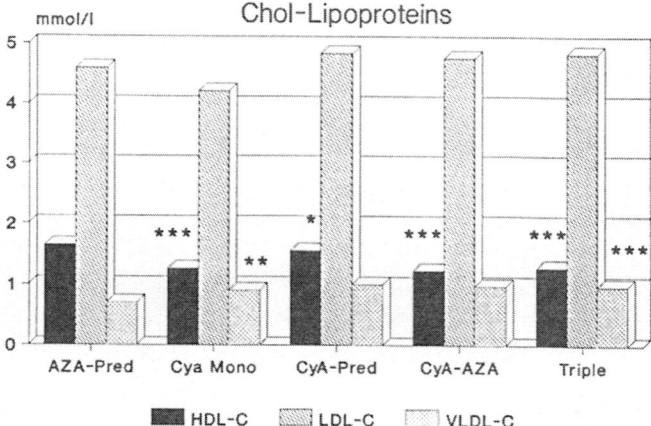

Fig. 3. Cholesterol-lipoprotein values in the 5 different immunosuppressive regimen groups: $P < 0.05, P < 0.01, P < 0.005$ compared with conventional AP group; HDL, high-density lipoprotein; LDL, low-density lipoprotein; VLDL, very low-density lipoprotein

potential risk factors, e. g., drugs that promote dyslipidemia.

Although some studies have shown a negative impact of CyA therapy on these risk profiles, the methodology of these studies should be reviewed critically. The study by Ballantyne et al. [1] showed in 36 patients with amyotrophic lateral sclerosis an increase of 21 % in the serum cholesterol level in the CyA group compared with placebo. However, the follow-up lasted only 6 months, and a wide scattering of cholesterol values was found in this small group of patients. Furthermore, there was no correlation between the CyA drug levels and serum cholesterol.

Fuhrer and Horber [6] found an independent hypercholesterolemic influence of CyA and postulated that prednisone and CyA together may have an additive negative impact on the serum cholesterol level. This conclusion, however, is to be criticized because there were no patients on CyA monotherapy to be analyzed separately. Lipoproteins and antihypertensive drugs were not taken into account.

There are also studies demonstrating that CyA is not a potential dyslipidemic agent [2, 12]. These studies also had the problem that they did not include patients on CyA monotherapy to be analyzed separately.

The study by Hodel et al. [8], performed prospectively, compared 16 patients on AP with 17 on CyA monotherapy. After a follow-up of 13–28 months, no difference in the lipid profiles were found.

Our study is the first with a large number of patients on CyA monotherapy. Compared with the other immunosuppressive regimens, the patients on this therapeutic modality had even better lipid profiles.

The impression of Fuhrer and Horber [6] that CyA, if added to an immunosuppressive regimen, aggravates lipid disturbances could not be confirmed, since the results of combination therapy like CP, CA, or even CAP did not differ consequently from those of the AP therapy.

More important seems to be the role of antihypertensive treatment, since we found a remarkable negative impact of diuretics and β-blockers on cholesterol and its lipo-

Table 2. The influence of prednisone-containing regimens on lipid profiles (values expressed as medians in mmol/l)

	With predni-sone ($n = 137$)	Without predni-sone ($n = 104$)	P value
Serum cholesterol	6.83	6.23	< 0.005
Serum triglycerides	2.22	2.04	N.S.
HDL-C	1.35	1.20	< 0.005
LDL-C	4.63	4.28	N.S.
VLDL-C	0.76	0.77	N.S.

Table 3. The influence antihypertensive agents on lipid profiles (values expressed as medians in mmol/l)

	With anti-hypertensive	Without anti-hypertensive	P value
Diuretics	($n = 20$)	($n = 54$)	< 0.01
Serum cholesterol	6.21	6.02	< 0.05
Serum triglycerides	2.24	1.82	< 0.01
HDL-C	1.17	1.44	N.S.
LDL-C	4.13	3.73	N.S.
VLDL-C	0.77	0.75	
β-Blockers	($n = 29$)	($n = 54$)	
Serum-cholesterol	6.56	6.02	< 0.001
Serum-triglycerides	3.91	1.82	< 0.001
HDL-C	1.19	1.44	< 0.01
LDL-C	4.11	3.73	N.S.
VLDL-C	0.76	0.75	N.S.

Table 4. Cardiovascular risk factor LDL/HDL cholesterol coefficient

Therapy mode	n	LDL/HDL	P value
CyA monotherapy	85	3.32	
With prednisone	134	3.32	N.S.
Without prednisone	104	3.32	
Diuretic monotherapy	20	3.42	
No antihypertensive agents	54	2.53	< 0.001
β-Blocker monotherapy	29	3.14	
No antihypertensive agents	54	2.53	< 0.01

proteins. Probably, an altered insulin sensitivity is the cause of these derangements [5].

Although the same effect has been shown to be due to CyA medication [15], the impact of steroid treatment after renal transplantation is probably quantitatively more important [4].

In conclusion, CyA seems to be a 'safe drug' in respect to lipid metabolism and, hence, cardiovascular risk factors. More attention should be paid to the drugs chosen for the treatment of hypertension in these patients. Recent meta-analysis showed that diuretics and β-blockers should be avoided, whereas calcium channel blockers and angiotension converting enzyme inhibitors have a neutral effect on lipid metabolism and may become the drugs of first choice [11]. To confirm this impression, prospective studies including all immunosuppressive regimens are needed.

References

1. Ballantyne CM, Podet EJ, Patsch WP, Harati Y, Appel V, Gotto AM, Young JB (1989) Effects of cyclosporine therapy on plasma lipoprotein levels. JAMA 262: 53–56
2. Bittar AE, Ratcliffe PJ, Richardson AJ, Raine AE, Jones L, Yudkin PL, Carter R, Mann JI, Morris PJ (1990) The prevalence of hyperlipidemia in renal transplant recipients. Associations with immunosuppressive and antihypertensive therapy. Transplantation 50: 987–992
3. Coronary Drug Project Research Group (1987) Natural history of myocardial infarction in the coronary drug project: long-term prognostic importance of serum lipid levels. Am J Cardiol 42: 489–498
4. Ekstrand A, Ahonen J, Groenhagen-Riska C, Groop L (1989) Mechanisms of insulin resistance after kidney transplantation. Transplantation 48: 563–568
5. Ferrari P, Rosman J, Weidmann P (1991) Antihypertensive agents, serum lipoproteins, and glucose metabolism. Am J Cardiol 67: 26B–35B
6. Fuhrer JA, Horber FF (1990) Additive effects of prednisone and cyclosporine-A therapy on serum cholesterol in renal transplant patients: effect of time interval after kidney transplantation and therapy with fibrates. J Am Soc Nephrol 1: 757
7. Ghosh P, Evans DB, Tomlinson SA, Calne RY (1973) Hyperlipidemia following renal transplantation. Transplantation 15: 521–525
8. Hodel K, Mordasini RC, Brunner FP, Thiel G (1986) Cyclosporin A und Hyperlipidaemie nach Nierentransplantation. Schweiz Med Wochenschr 116: 885–888
9. Johnson RWG (1986) Cyclosporine in cadaveric renal transplantation: three-year follow-up of a European multicentre trial. Transplant Proc 18: 1229–1233
10. Najarian JS (1988) Long term results at the University of Minnesota. Transplant Immunol 4 (4)
11. Rosman J, Weidmann P, Ferrari P (1990) Antihypertensive drugs and serum lipoproteins, J Drug Dev 3 [Suppl 1]: 129–139
12. Traindl O, Reading S, Franz M, Pohanka E, Pidlich J, Kovarik J (1991) Cyclosporin-A does not cause hyperlipidemia in kidney graft recipients. Clin Transplant 5: 265–267
13. Vathsala A, Weinberg RB, Schoenberg L, Grevel J, Dunn J, Goldstein RA, Buren CT van, Lewis RM, Kahan BD (1989) Lipid abnormalities in renal transplant recipients treated with cyclosporine. Transplantation 48: 37–43
14. Venkateswara Rao K, Andersen R (1988) Long-term results and complications in renal transplant recipients. Transplantation 45: 45–52
15. Wahlstrom HE, Lavelle-Jones M, Endres D, Akimoto R, Kolterman O, Moossa AR (1990) Inhibition of insulin release by cyclosporine and production of peripheral insulin resistance in the dog. Transplantation 49: 600–604
16. Wing AJ, Brunner FP, Brynger H, Jacobs C, Kramer P, Selwood NH, Gretz N (1984) Cardiovascular-related causes of death and the fate of patients with renovascular disease. Contrib Nephrol 41: 306–311

Transplant Int (1992) 5 [Suppl 1]: S 536–S 538

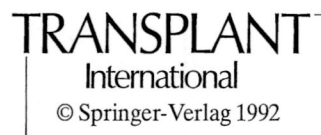

© Springer-Verlag 1992

Decrease of erythrocyte deformability in cyclosporine-treated renal transplant patients: correction with fish oil as well as corn oil

N. H. Schut, M. R. Hardeman, and J. M. Wilmink

Department of Internal Medicine, Renal Transplant Unit, Academic Medical Center, Amsterdam, The Netherlands

Abstract. Twenty-nine renal transplant recipients with good, stable transplant function were included in a double-blind cross-over study to investigate the effects of different immunosuppressive treatment modalities and also the effects of fish oil and corn oil supplementation on erythrocyte deformability. Ten patients were treated with cyclosporine (CyA) only, 10 patients with CyA and prednisolone, and 9 patients with azathioprine and prednisolone. Erythrocyte deformability, as measured by an ektacytometric technique, was significantly decreased in both CyA-treated groups compared with the azathioprine-prednisolone-treated group, and this decrease was corrected with fish oil and with corn oil. The cause and the clinical significance of less deformable erythrocytes due to CyA are not yet clear. However, less deformable erythrocytes could play a role in the genesis of the complications of CyA.

Key words: Cyclosporine – Erythrocyte deformability – Renal transplant recipients – Corn oil – Fish oil

---

Renal toxicity, hypertension, and arteriopathy are the well-known side-effects of cyclosporine (CyA) therapy. The mechanism of CyA toxicity is unknown but may involve rheological alterations, such as the impairment of erythrocyte deformability. It has been shown that a diet supplementation of fish oil can ameliorate the negative effects of CyA on kidney function and blood pressure [6]. Furthermore, erythrocyte deformability can be increased by fish oil in healthy subjects, in dialysis patients, and in renal transplant recipients [3, 10–12]. In one study, evidence was found that changes in the erythrocyte filterability were dependent on the use of CyA [11]. We therefore performed a study to evaluate whether erythrocyte deformability is changed in renal transplant recipients and whether any change is related to the use of different im-

munosuppressive treatment modalities. Furthermore, the effects of a supplementation of fish oil or corn oil on erythrocyte deformability were investigated.

Patients and methods

Twenty-nine renal transplant recipients who received cadaveric kidney allografts between 1979 and 1988 were included in this study. All patients had good, stable renal transplant function and no signs of rejection. Twenty patients were treated with CyA at a mean dosage of 3.0 ± 0.8 mg/kg body weight (mean $\pm$ SD), aiming at whole blood trough levels of between 75 and 150 µg/l. Ten of these patients were treated with CyA only, whilst 10 other patients received prednisolone (10 mg) in addition (CP). Nine patients were treated with azathioprine (100–150 mg daily) in combination with prednisolone (5–10 mg) (AP). The clinical characteristics of the three patient groups are shown in Table 1. In a double-blind, randomised, cross-over study, all patients were given fish oil or corn oil a day for a period of 4 months each. The capsules with fish oil contained 6 g fish oil (30% C 20:5 ω 3 – eicosapentaenoic acid and 20% C 22:6 ω 3 – docosahexaenoic acid), the capsules with corn oil contained 6 g corn oil (50% C 18:2 ω 6). The patients of all three groups were randomized to receive fish oil or corn oil for 4 months, and after the first 4 months the patients were given the alternative oil for another 4 months. The study design is shown in Fig. 1. Erythrocyte deformability was measured by an ektacytometric technique, using the laser-assisted optical rotational deformability meter [5]. With this device, a suspension of erythrocytes is submitted to a shear stress of 30 pascal,

Table 1. Characteristics of the study groups

	C	CP	AP
Number	10	10	9
Age (years)	53 ± 14	51 ± 14	53 ± 7
Male/female	4/6	9/1	5/4
Months post-transplantation	56 ± 17	28 ± 8	84 ± 29
GFR (ml/min)	57 ± 16	59 ± 16	65 ± 18
Cyclosporine dose (mg/kg)	2.8 ± 0.9	3.3 ± 0.7	

mean values $\pm$ SD

C, cyclosporine monotherapy group; CP, cyclosporine and prednisolone; AP, azathioprine and prednisolone; GFR, glomerular filtration rate

Offprint requests to: N. H. Schut, Department of Internal Medicine, Renal Transplant Unit, f 4-215 Academic Medical Center, 1105 AZ-Amsterdam, The Netherlands

design:
1. cohort study (cyclosporine vs. azathioprine)
2. prospective, double-blind, randomized, cross-over intervention study

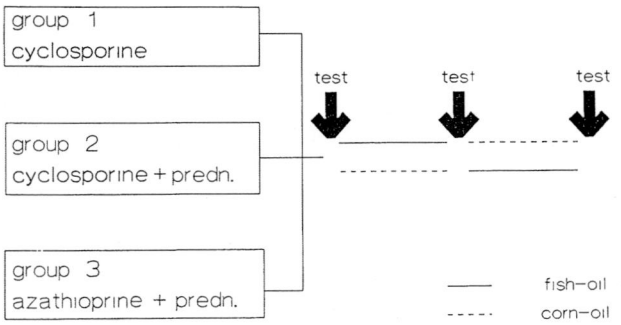

Fig. 1. Study design

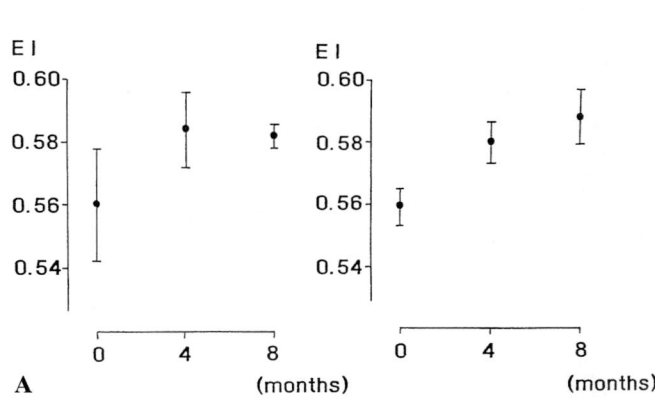

A

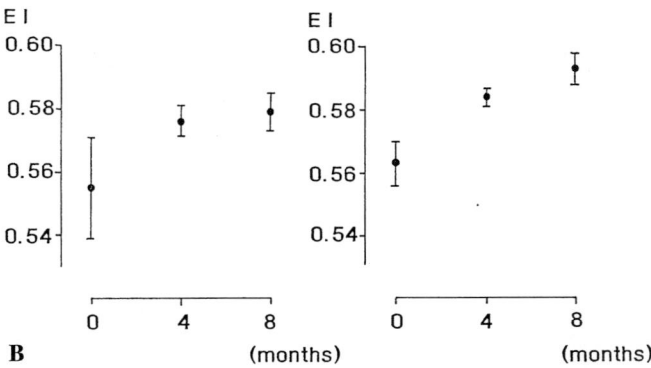

B

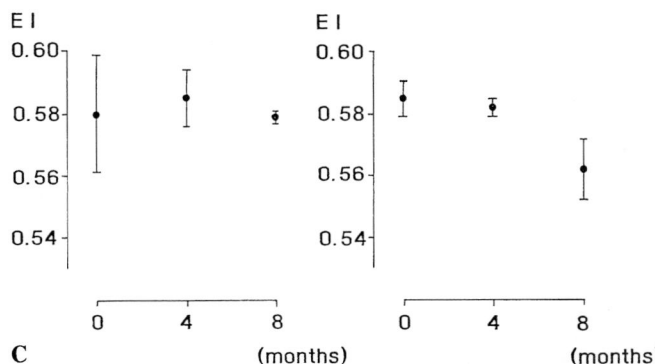

C

Fig. 2A–C. The results of the intervention with fish oil and corn oil on erythrocyte deformability in the 3 patient groups

generating an ellipsoid diffraction pattern. Using an ellipse-fit analysis, the long and the short axes of the Laser diffraction pattern are determined. The elongation index is the quotient of the difference between the long and the short axes divided by the sum of the long and the short axes. A lower elongation index means less deformable erythrocytes.

Results

The elongation index before intervention with fish oil or corn oil was normal in the AP group (0.583 ± 0.014) and significantly decreased in both CyA-treated groups (CyA 0.559 ± 0.014, CP 0.559 ± 0.014; CyA or CP versus AP $P < 0.005$ with Wilcoxon rank-sum W-test). During oil supplementation the elongation index increased in CyA- and CP-treated patients irrespective of the kind of oil (for each subgroup $P < 0.05$), but in the AP group the elongation index remained unaltered (subgroups after initial treatment for 4 months with fish oil: CyA 0.584 ± 0.012, CP 0.576 ± 0.005, AP 0.585 ± 0.009 and after corn oil: CyA 0.580 ± 0.007, CP 0.584 ± 0.005, AP 0.582 ± 0.009). After cross-over to the other oil, no further changes in the elongation index were observed (Fig. 2). The subgroup of AP patients who initially received corn oil and later on fish oil initially consisted of 4 patients, but after the fish oil supplementation, only 2 patients were available for follow-up study.

It is known that changes in the mean corpuscular volume (MCV) can contribute to changes in erythrocyte deformability. In these patient groups, however, changes in the MCV did not correlate with changes in erythrocyte deformability (Table 2).

Discussion

In this study we found a lower erythrocyte deformability in CyA-treated patients, which was also previously found with a different technique [11]. We concurred that supplementation with fish oil or corn oil corrected this abnormality. The reason for the lower erythrocyte deformability in CyA-treated renal transplant recipients is not clear. Changes in the MCV cannot explain this phenomenon; other possible explanations include changes in the viscoelastic properties of the red cell membrane or changes in the viscosity of the intracellular hemoglobin milieu [2]. A decrease of the arachidonic acid content of the erythrocyte has been reported in CyA-treated renal transplant recipients [8]. This may lead to a decrease in

Table 2. Changes in the mean corpuscular volume (MCV)

	Before oil	After 4 months	After 8 months
Group I (CyA)			
Fish oil – corn oil		92.5 ± 6.4	95.5 ± 2.6
Corn oil – fish oil		92.2 ± 7.2	98.2 ± 2.7
Group II (CP)			
Fish oil – corn oil	92.5 ± 8.2	93.8 ± 7.6	94.6 ± 2.7
Corn oil – fish oil	93.7 ± 4.6	87.9 ± 4.8	94.8 ± 6.6
Group III (AP)			
Fish oil – corn oil	101.4 ± 5.4	95.0 ± 4.1	101.9 ± 3.6
Corn oil – fish oil	97.7 ± 1.5	93.9 ± 7.6	103.2 ± 11.6

MCV in fl; mean ± SD

erythrocyte deformability due to either the lower arachidonic acid content in the membrane itself or a lack of substrate for prostacyclin. Some studies have indicated an increase in erythrocyte deformability during the administration of prostacyclin analogues [4, 7]. This, however, is controversial, because other studies described a similar or lower erythrocyte deformability after prostacyclin administration [1, 9]. The potential adverse effects of a lower erythrocyte deformability in CyA-treated patients need further investigation. A beneficial effect of fish oil on the adverse effects of CyA on renal function and blood pressure has been reported [6]. However, in this study this beneficial effect could only be shown for fish oil and not for corn oil.

Acknowledgments. We are grateful to Loes Clement, Ingrid Cuales, and Peter Goedhart for their excellent technical and practical assistance and to Anneke Cloos and Yvonne Robberse for typing this manuscript. This study was supported by grant no. 89-835 from the Dutch Kidney Foundation.

References

1. Belch JJF, Lowe GDO, Drummond MM, et al (1981) Prostacyclin reduces red cell deformability. Thromb Haemost 45 (2): 189
2. Bessis M, Mohandas N, Feo C (1980) Automated ektacytometry: a new method of measuring red cell deformability and red cell indices. Blood cells 6: 315–327
3. Cartwright IJ, Pockley AG, Galloway JH, et al (1985) The effects of dietary ω-3 polyunsaturated fatty acids on erythrocyte membrane phospholipids, erythrocyte deformability and blood viscosity in healthy volunteers. Atherosclerosis 55: 267–281
4. Dowd PM, Kovacs IB, Bland CJH, Kirby JTD (1981) Effects of prostaglandins I_2 and E_1 on red cell deformability in patients with Raynaud's phenomenon and systemic sclerosis. BMJ 283: 350
5. Hardeman MR, Bauersachs RM, Meiselman HJ (1988) RBC laser diffractometry and RBC aggregometry with a rotational viscometer: comparison with rheoscope and myrrene aggregometer. Clin Hemorrheol 8: 581–593
6. Homan van der Heide JJ, Bilo HJG, Tegzess AM, Donker AJM (1990) The effects of dietary supplementation with fish oil on renal function in cyclosporin-treated transplant recipients. Transplantation 49: 523–527
7. Maurin N (1986) Influence on platelet activity and red cell fluidity of epoprostenol and two stable prostacyclin analogues in vitro. Drug Res 36 II: 1180–1183
8. Phair PG, Powell HR, McCredie DA, et al (1989) Low red cell arachidonic acid in cyclosporine treated patients. Clin Nephrol 32: 57–61
9. Slott JH, Hall K, Clark DA, Stuart MJ (1982) Prostaglandin I_2 fails to influence red cell deformability. Prostaglandins Leukotrienes Med 8: 21–22
10. Terano T, Hirai A, Hamazaki T, et al (1983) Effect of oral administration of highly purified eicosapentaenoic acid on platelet function, blood viscosity and red cell deformability in healthy human subjects. Atherosclerosis 46: 321–331
11. Urukaze M, Hamazaki T, Kashiwabara H, et al (1989) Favourable effects of fish oil concentrate on risk factors for thrombosis in renal allograft recipients. Nephron 53: 102–109
12. Van Acker BAC, Bilo HJG, Popp-Snijders C, et al (1987) The effect of fish oil on lipid profile and viscosity of erythrocyte suspensions in CAPD patients. Nephrol Dial Transplant 2: 557–561

Transplant Int (1992) 5 [Suppl 1]: S 539–S 541

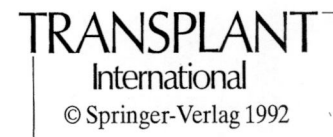

© Springer-Verlag 1992

Adjuvant treatment with ursodeoxycholic acid prevents acute rejection in rats receiving heart allografts

M. Olausson, L. Mjörnstedt, L. Wramner, H. Persson, I. Karlberg, and S. Friman

Department of Surgery (Transplant Unit), Sahlgrenska Hospital, University of Göteborg, Göteborg, Sweden

Abstract. Adjuvant treatment with ursodeoxycholic acid (UDCA) for liver-transplant recipients has been reported to reduce the frequency of acute rejection episodes. To explore this effect further, UDCA was given to rats in an experimental heart transplantation model, with or without concomitant immunosuppressive treatment with antihymocyte globulin (ATG). UDCA was administered orally 7 days before and 14 days after transplantation. Rats treated with UDCA alone or in combination with ATG were compared with untreated controls and ATG-treated recipients. Adjuvant treatment with UDCA was found to induce prolonged graft survival and increase the amount of transplant tolerance in rats. Serum levels of bilirubin and aminotransferases were not altered irrespective of the UDCA dose given. The results indicate that UDCA has an immunomodulatory capacity that might not be restricted to the liver, but also might apply to other transplanted organs as well.

Key words: Ursodeoxycholic acid – ATG – Rat-Heart transplant – Tolerance

---

Medication with hydropholic bile acid ursodeoxycholic acid (UDCA) has proven to be beneficial in cholestatic conditions, such as primary biliary cirrhosis, sclerosing cholangitis, biliary atresia and chronic hepatitis [1, 5, 14, 16]. It has also been shown to have a direct protective effect on hepatocytes both in vivo and in vitro [4, 6]. We have been using UDCA in our liver transplant program since 1989 and have observed that the recipients on adjuvant UDCA treatment had significantly fewer rejection episodes than historical controls [13]. The mechanism behind this beneficial effect of UDCA is not known.

To investigate the possible immunomodulatory effect of UDCA on organs other than the liver, UDCA was tested in an experimental transplantation rat model. The mechanism and effect of UDCA on tolerance induction were studied using UDCA alone or in combination with a potent immunosuppressive agent like ATG [9].

Materials and methods

Animals

Male inbred DA(RT1^a) rats, weighing 200–220 g, were used as recipients and female PVG/c(RT1^c) rats, weighing 110–130 g, as donors (Bantin and Kingman, Hull, UK).

Surgical technique

The rats were anesthetized intraperitoneally with 8% chloral hydrate in a dose corresponding to 3.5 ml/kg body weight. Heterotrophic heart grafts were done to the neck vessels using a nonsuture cuff technique [10]. Rejection was defined as loss of regular EKG activity.

ATG

ATG was prepared by immunization of rabbits with rat thymocytes [9]. The ATG was absorbed with rat erythrocytes to remove agglutinins and rat liver powder until free of liver and kidney-reacting antibodies, as determined by immunofluorescence. Finally, the cytotoxic titer against thymocytes was adjusted to 1:1024 with phosphate-buffered saline (PBS).

UDCA

Ursodeoxycholic acid (99% pure) and tauro-ursodeoxycholic acid (90% pure) were purchased from Sigma Chemicals, St. Louis, Mo. Unconjugated and conjugated UDCA were used in equal proportions, dissolved in PBS, and adjusted to a final concentration of 100 mg/ml. UDCA was administered orally in three different doses corresponding to 50, 100 and 200 mg/kg body weight. Since unconjugated UDCA is difficult to dissolve in PBS, the UDCA solution was vigorously shaken before administration.

Laboratory tests

Serum levels of alanine and aspartate aminotransferases (ALAT and ASAT), as well as bilirubin, were analyzed using a Reflotron (Kodak). Serum samples were collected before starting up UDCA treatment, on the day of transplantation, and 7 days post-transplantation.

Offprint requests to: Michael Olausson, M.D., Ph.D., Department of Surgery, Transplant Unit, Sahlgrenska sjukhuset, S-413 45 Göteborg, Sweden

S540

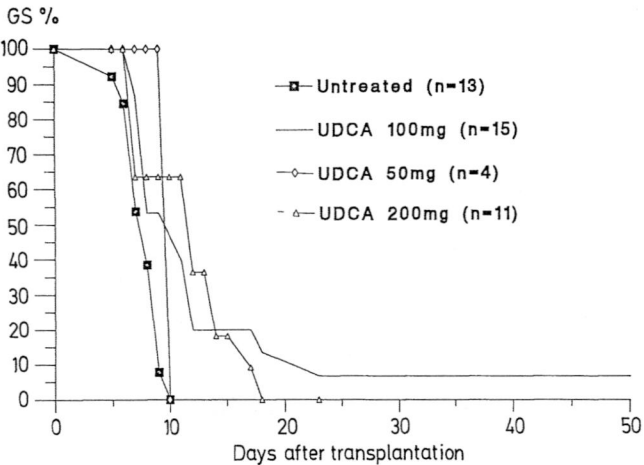

Fig. 1. Graft survival in rats with heart transplants treated with different doses of UDCA

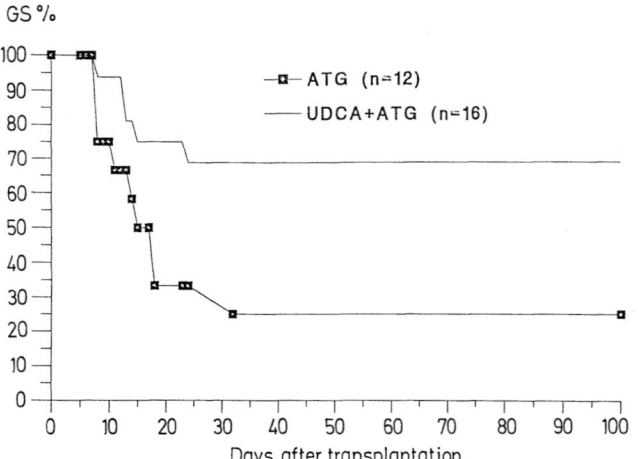

Fig. 2. Graft survival in rats with heart transplants treated with UDCA and ATG

Test protocol

The rats were divided into six groups and given the following treatment; I: 1 ml PBS 1 week prior to transplantation of an allogeneic graft. PBS treatment was continued until rejection was complete ($n = 13$). II: UDCA 100 mg/kg per day for 1 week prior and 2 weeks after transplantation ($n = 15$). III: As in group II and in addition 0.01 ml ATG intravenously (IV) 2 days before transplantation ($n = 16$). IV: 0.01 ml ATG IV 2 days before transplantation as the only treatment ($n = 12$). V: As in group II but 50 mg/kg per day of UDCA ($n = 4$). VI: As in group II but 200 mg/kg per day of UDCA ($n = 11$).

Statistical methods

The Wilcoxon rank sum nonparametric test for independent samples was used for analyses of statistical differences in graft survival between groups. Fisher's exact two-tailed test was used to compare differences in ratios of tolerant rats [3].

Results

UDCA alone improved graft survival significantly, irrespective of the dose tested, compared with untreated controls (Fig. 1). One of the 15 rats in the 100 mg UDCA

group did not reject the transplant during an observation time of > 100 days; the remaining rejected their grafts 2–23 days after transplantation ($P < 0.05$). The 200 mg UDCA-treated rats rejected all grafts 7–18 days post-transplantation ($P < 0.05$) and the 4 rats in the 50 mg UDCA group at day 10 ($P < 0.01$). Rats given UDCA in addition to ATG had a significantly better graft survival rate than rats treated with ATG alone ($P < 0.05$) and 68% of the grafts functioned over the long term compared to 25% in the group treated with ATG alone (Fig. 2). The proportion of tolerant rats in the combined UDCA and ATG group was higher than in the ATG-treated group, but the difference did not reach statistical significance ($P = 0.056$).

The different groups were also tested for variations in aminotransferases and bilirubin levels before and after UDCA treatment and transplantation. No statistical differences between groups given different doses of UDCA, with or without ATG, were registered before or after transplantation.

Discussion

Our study suggests that UDCA has an immunomodulatory effect in rat recipients of heart transplants and also confirms the clinical observations in liver-transplant recipients that there is a reduced frequency of acute rejection episodes the first year after transplantation [13]. The exact mechanism behind the immunomodulatory effect of UDCA is unknown, but Poupon and coworkers have shown that UDCA is capable of reducing class-I antigen expression on hepatocytes in patients with primary biliary cirrhosis [2]. In a more recent study from a German group, UDCA has similarly been shown to down-regulate class-I/II antigen expression on biliary duct cells [8]. Since HLA antigen expression in the liver is normally induced by cholestasis, a non-immunological improvement in the disease as a result of UDCA administration could indirectly reduce the up-regulation of HLA antigens [15]. A direct effect on hepatocytes and antigen expression could, on the other hand, also be one explanation for the reduced frequency of rejection episodes seen in liver transplant patients receiving adjuvant UDCA treatment [13].

UDCA administration to transplanted rats did not result in any pathological values of bilirubin or aminotransferases, even with a high dose of 200 mg/kg, which is in agreement with the data reported earlier on this bile acid, which has been described as being safe and atoxic in man [7]. In the experimental transplantation model used, ATG has earlier been shown to induce a tolerant state by a suppressor cell mechanism [11] rather than through reduced graft antigenicity, although this possibility could not be completely excluded [12]. Whether UDCA also acts directly on peripheral immunocompetent T cells, or via down-regulation of class-I/II antigens in the graft, or via some other unknown mechanism has not been clarified by our results. Our study suggests that the effect of UDCA treatment is not completely specific for liver transplants, and further studies are needed to elucidate the exact mechanism behind this effect on the immune system.

Acknowledgements. This study was supported by grants from the Medical Faculty of the University of Göteborg, The Professor L-E Gelin Memorial Foundation, Fresenius AG, Federal Republic of Germany, Svenska Läkaresällskapet, Göteborgs Kungl vetenskaps och vitterhets samhälle, Riksförbundet för Njursjuka. We thank Ms. Rovena Eriksson for skillful technical assistance.

References

1. O'Brien C, Senior JR, Batta AK (1989) Ursodeoxycholic acid treatment produces marked clinical and biochemical amelolioration of primary sclerosing cholangitis. Gastroenterology 96: A640

2. Calmus Y, Gane P, Rouger P, Poupon R (1990) Hepatic expression of class I and class II major histocompatibility complex molecules in primary biliary cirrhosis: effect of ursodeoxycholic acid. Hepatology 11: 12–15

3. Colton T (1974) Statistics in medicine, 1st edn, Little Brown and Company, Boston, Massachusettes

4. Galle PR, Theilmann L, Raedsch R, Otto G, Stiehl A (1990) Ursodeoxycholate reduces hepatotoxicity of bile salts in primary human hepatocytes. Hepatology 12: 486–491

5. Ghezzi C, Zuin M, Battezzati PM, Podda M (1987) Effects of ursodeoxycholate, taurine and ursodeoxycholate plus taurine on serum enzym levels in patients with chronic hepatitis. Hepatology 7: 1110

6. Heumann DM, Komito SF, Pandak WM, Hylemon PB, Vlahcevic ZR (1989) Tauroursodeoxycholic acid protects against cholestatic and hepatocytolytic toxicity of more hydrophobic bile salts. Gastroenterology 96: A607

7. Hoffman AF (1990) Bile acid hepatotoxicity and the rationale of UDCA therapy in chronic cholestatic liver disease: some hypotheses. In: Paumgartner G, Stiehl A, Barbara L, Roda E (eds) Kluwer Academic, Dordrecht, The Netherlands, pp 13–33

8. Leuschner U, Dieues HP, Güldütunana S, Birkenfeld G, Leuschner M (1990) Ursodeoxycholic acid (UDCA) influences immune parameters in patients with primary biliary cirrhosis (PBC). Hepatology 12: 957

9. Mjörnstedt L, Olausson M, Lindholm L, Brynger H (1984) Induction of longterm heart allograft survival in the rat by rabbit ATG. Int Arch Allergy Appl Immunol 74: 193–199

10. Olausson M, Mjörnstedt L, Lindholm L, Brynger H (1984) Nonsuture organ grafting to the neck vessels in rats. Acta Chir Scand 150: 463–467

11. Olausson M, Mjörnstedt L, Lindholm L, Brynger H (1984) Suppressor cells in the antihymocyte globulin induced transplantation tolerance in the adult rat. Int Arch Allergy Appl Immunol 75: 184

12. Olausson M, Mjörnstedt L, Wramner L, Lindholm L, Söderström T, Brynger H (1988) Characteristics of the induction phase of antithymocyte-globulin induced heart allograft tolerance in the rat. Int Arch Allergy Appl Immunol 86: 131

13. Persson H, Friman S, Scherste'n T, Svanvik J, Karlberg I (1990) Ursodeoxycholic acid for prevention of acute rejection in liver transplant recipients. Lancet 336: 52–53

14. Poupon R, Chretien Y, Poupon RE, Balter F, Calmus Y, Darnis F (1987) Is ursodeoxycholic acid an effective treatment for primary biliary cirrhosis? Lancet I: 834–836

15. Poupon RE, Balkau B, Eschwége E, Poupon R, UDCA-Study group (1991) A multicenter, controlled trial of ursodial for the treatment of primary biliary cirrhosis. The N Engl J Med 324: 1548–1554

16. Ullrich D, Rating D, Schröter W, Hanefeld F, Bircher J (1987) Treatment with ursodeoxycholic acid renders children with biliary atresia suitable for liver transplantation. Lancet II: 1324

Transplant Int (1992) 5 [Suppl 1]: S 542–S 543

TRANSPLANT
International
© Springer-Verlag 1992

RS-61443 reverses acute renal allograft rejection in dogs

K.-P. Platz[2], W. O. Bechstein[2], D. E. Eckhoff[1], D. A. Hullett[1], and H. W. Sollinger[1]

[1] Department of Surgery, University of Wisconsin School of Medicine, Madison, Wisconsin, USA
[2] Department of Surgery, Rudolf Virchow University Clinic, Berlin, Germany

Abstract. RS-61443 is a noncompetitive allosteric inhibitor of inosine monophosphate dehydrogenase. At blocks the proliferative response of T and B lymphocytes, prevents the generation of cytotoxic T cells, and inhibits antibody formation. This study was conducted to see whether or not RS-61443 can reverse acute renal allograft rejection in dogs. At was possible to reverse this process.

Key words: RS-61443 – Inosine monophosphate dehydrogenase – Renal allografts – Rejection – Reversing rejection

RS-61443, a morpholinoethyl ester and prodrug of mycophenolic acid (MPA) is a noncompetitive allosteric inhibitor of inosine monophosphate dehydrogenase. The drug blocks the proliferative response of T and B lymphocytes, prevents the generation of cytotoxic T cells [2], and inhibits antibody formation by selectively inhibiting the de novo pathway of guanosine nucleotide synthesis [1]. RS-61443 has been shown to prevent renal allograft rejection in dogs for more than 150 days when administered in combination with low-dose cyclosporine and prednisolone [4]. Morris et al. demonstrated that RS-61443 prevents rejection of cardiac allograft in rats, even if the start of treatment was delayed until 5 days after transplantion. This suggests that RS-61443 can reverse ongoing acute allograft rejection [4]. The purpose of this study was to test whether or not RS-61443 can reverse acute renal allograft rejection in dogs.

Materials and methods

Animals: Unrelated female mongrel dogs, weighing 20 to 25 kg, were used as donors and recipients. Anesthesia was introduced with 20 mg/kg of intravenous pentobarbital,

Offprint requests to: Hans W. Sollinger, Department of Surgery, University of Wisconsin School of Medicine, 600 Highland Avenue, Madison, WI 53792, USA

and halothane was used for maintenance. Donor kidneys were dissected out through a midline incision and flushed with 200 ml of ice-cold 0.9% saline solution containing 2000 units of heparine. After flushing, the kidney was immediately transplanted into the right iliac fossa of an unrelated recipient by routine techniques. Bilateral nephrectomy was performed after graft transplantation. Dogs were killed if the creatinine level exceeded 8 mg/dl, or if they were moribund. Autopsy was performed in all dogs.

Treatment schedule: Baseline immunosuppression consisted of 10 mg/kg RS-61443, cyclosporine (CyA) 5 mg/kg, and prednisolone 0.1 mg/kg, each given daily p.o. (this combination therapy had been shown to be unsuccessful in preventing acute allograft rejection in canine renal allografts). On the day of the diagnosis of rejection the dogs received an increased dose of RS-61443 p.o. for 3 consecutive days (80 mg/kg b.i.d.), also starting on the day rejection was diagnosed. After 3 days, upon completion of rejection treatment, baseline immuosuppression was increased to RS-61443 20 mg/kg. The dosages of CyA and prednisolone were not altered. If the serum creatinine rose > 3.0 mg/dl, CyA was discontinued to avoid nephrotoxicity. Rejection was defined as a 50% or greater increase in serum creatinine relative to the lowest observed creatinine level (Fig. 1). RS-61443 was supplied as powder by Syntex (USA) Inc. It was suspended in carboxymethylcellulose vehicle (100 mg/ml). Cyclosporine was supplied as a gift from Sandoz Pharmaceuticals, East Hannover, New Jersey, as a commercial solution. Prednisolone tablets were obtained from Upjohn Inc., Kalamazoo, Michigan. Before the initiation of rejection treatment, a percutaneous kidney biopsy was performed to confirm the diagnosis; these specimens were taken serially after the completion of rejection treatment.

Results

All animals experienced acute rejection. The diagnosis of rejection was made on day 7.5 ± 2.6 days. Serum creatinine on the day of diagnosis of rejection was

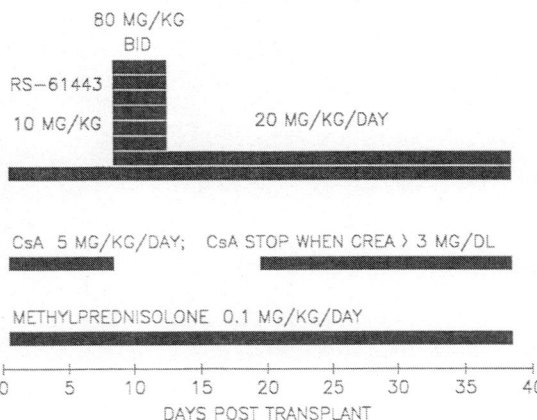

TREATMENT SCHEDULE DURING RS-61443 REVERSAL STUDY

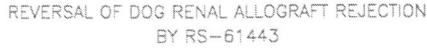

Fig. 1. Treatment of dog renal allograft rejection

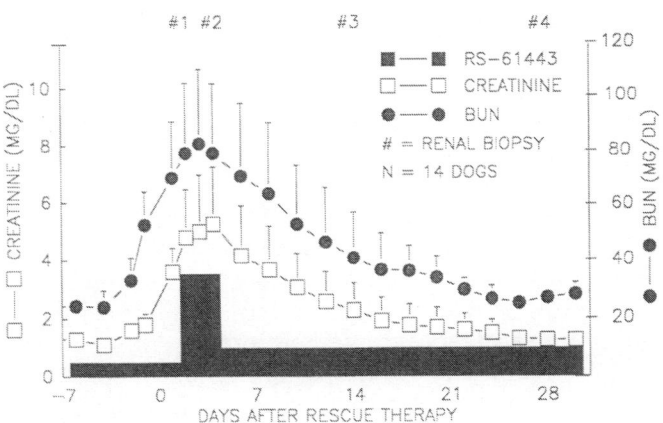

Fig. 2. Reversal of dog renal allograft rejection by RS-61443 (*n* = 14 dogs). Only in selected dogs were additional kidney biopsies performed at the intervals indicated (# 2, # 3)

3.6 ± 0.7 mg/dl. In 14 out of 16 dogs (87.5%), biopsy-proven acute cellular rejection could be successfully reversed by increasing the RS-61443 dosage to 80 mg/kg b.i.d.; however, it took up to 3 weeks after the diagnosis of rejection before serum creatinine and BUN returned to baseline levels (Fig. 2). Rejection treatment with increased doses of RS-61443 resulted in the development of severe, prolonged relative lymphopenia. Liver enzymes (AST, ALT) and alkaline phosphatase were slightly elevated. High-dose treatment with RS-61443 for 3 consecutive days was generally well tolerated. No weight loss or infectious complications occurred.

Discussion

RS-61443 had previously been shown to be effective in preventing kidney allograft rejection in dogs if used in combination with low-dose cyclosporine and prednisolone [4]. Reports of successful treatment of ongoing rejection of rat cardiac allografts [3] had prompted us to investigate the use of RS-61443 for reversal of kidney allograft rejection in dogs. Treatment with 80 mg/kg RS-61443 for established rejection of dog renal allograft could completely reverse rejection in 14 of 16 dogs (87.5%). In all of these 14 dogs, serum creatinine returned to baseline levels. High-dose treatment with RS-61443 for a period of 3 days was generally well tolerated in dogs. Intermittent loss of appetite and lassitude seemed to be related to the transient state of uremia. No weight loss or infectious complications occurred. Rejection treatment resulted in the development of severe, prolonged, relative lymphopenia. Liver enzymes (AST, ALT) and alkaline phosphatase were only slightly elevated, which are not necessarily signs of hepatotoxicity, but may rather be an indicator of mycophenolic acid effectiveness.

Acknowledgements. The support of Syntex Research, Palo Alto, California, is gratefully acknowledged. K.P.Platz and W.O.Bechstein received research fellowships from the Deutsche Forschungsgemeinschaft, Bonn, Germany.

References

1. Burlingham WJ, Grailer AP, Hullett DA, Sollinger HW (1991) Inhibition of both MLC and in vitro IgG memory response to tetanus toxoid by RS-61443. Transplantation 51: 545–547
2. Eugui EM, Almquist SJ, Muller CD, Allison AC (1991) Lymphocyte-selective antiproliferative and immunosuppressive effects of mycophenolic acid. Scand J Immunol 33: 161–173
3. Morris RE, Hoyt EG, Murphy MP, Eugui EM, Allison AC (1990) Mycophenolic acid morpholinoethylester (RS-61443) is a new immunosuppressant that prevents and halts heart allograft rejection by selective inhibition of T- and B-cell purine synthesis. Transplant Proc 22: 1659–1662
4. Platz KP, Sollinger HW, Hullett DA, Eckhoff DE, Eugui EM, Allison AC (1991) RS-61443: a new, potent immunosuppressive agent. Transplantation 51: 27–31

Transplant Int (1992) 5 [Suppl 1]: S 544–S 546

Gangliosides potentiate the immunosuppressive effects of cyclosporin A in rat skin allografts

G. Sconocchia[1], C. M. Ausiello[1], G. C. Spagnoli[1, 2], G. Sciortino[3], V. Filinger[3], F. Giudiceandrea[3], V. Cervelli[3], D. Adorno[1, 3], and C. U. Casciani[3]

[1] Istituto CNR "Tipizzazione Tissutale e Problemi della Dialisi", Roma, Italy
[2] Departments of Surgery and Research, University of Basel, Basel, Switzerland
[3] Cattedra di Clinica Chirurgica, II Universita' Tor Vergata, Roma, Italy

Abstract. In vitro gangliosides exert inhibitory effects on cellular immune responses, largely relying on an impairment of the IL-2/IL-2 receptor interaction. In a previous study we have demonstrated synergistic effects of gangliosides and cyclosporin A (CyA) in the inhibition of the generation of in vitro allospecific immune responses in humans. To evaluate the possibility of using these drugs in immunosuppressive therapy in organ transplantation, we investigated the effects of the combination of a gangliosides mixture (GAMIX) and suboptimal doses of CyA on rat skin allografts in vivo. Sprague-Dawley rats were implanted with skin grafts from Lewis rats and treated for 21 days by intraperitoneal administration of either GAMIX or CyA or a combination of the two drugs. Untreated, GAMIX-treated or CyA-treated rats rejected skin allografts. In contrast, when a combined GAMIX CyA treatment was administered, successful grafting could be obtained in 8 rats out of 10 tested. Cells derived from spleens on day 21 post graft were stimulated in vitro with PWM mitogen. We found that cells from transplanted rats, untreated or treated with low-dose CyA or GAMIX alone, showed comparable responses to PWM. Cells from rats treated with the combination of the two drugs were found to be virtually unresponsive to stimulation by PWM mitogen. Taken together, our results indicate that GAMIX potentiate in vivo and ex vivo immunosuppressive effects of low-dose CyA.

Key words: Cyclosporin A – Gangliosides – Immunosuppression – Skin allografts

The discovery and characterization of the pharmacological effects of cyclosporin A (CyA) has represented a major advance in the immunosuppressive treatment in clinical organ transplantation. CyA therapy reduced both number and severity of acute rejection episodes, thus markedly increasing the success rates in bone marrow, heart, pancreas, liver, and kidney transplants [2, 6, 9]. A major limitation in the clinical use of CyA, however, is represented by its toxicity [5, 6]. It is thus of interest to evaluate the possibility of potentiating the immunosuppressive effects of CyA by taking advantage of less toxic compounds.

Gangliosides are complex glycosphingolipids that have been reported to play a role in the control of cell proliferation and differentiation [1, 3] possibly related to an inhibition of protein kinase C activation by endogenous diacylglycerols [7], or mediated through the action of discrete ganglioside metabolites [4]. Furthermore, gangliosides have been shown by several authors, including ourselves, to exert immunosuppressive effects in vitro [8, 10, 12], largely due to an alteration in the binding of IL-2 to its receptors [10].

Considering the emerging clinical need for low-dose CyA immunosuppressive regimens, we previously investigated the synergic effects of these two drugs in in vitro inhibition of allostimulated cellular immune responses. We found that GAMIX, combined with low doses of CyA, can significantly potentiate the inhibitory effects of CyA on MLC and CTL generation. Furthermore, GAMIX and CyA efficiently synergize in inhibiting the production of IFN gamma induced in MLC [13].

In this study we sought to explore the possibility of combine gangliosides and suboptimal doses of CyA to obtain synergistic immunosuppression in rat skin allografts in vivo. We found that gangliosides potentiate the immunosuppression exerted by low doses of CyA both on skin rejections and on proliferative responses induced by mitogens in spleen lymphocytes from rats treated with the combined immunosuppressive therapy.

Materials and methods

Animals

Fortyh-three inbred strain Sprague-Dawley rats (Charles River, Italy) were used as recipients while inbred strain Lewis rats were used as skin graft donors. All animals

Offprint requests to: G. Sconocchia, Istituto CNR "Tipizzazione Tissutale e Problemi della Dialisi," c/o Ospedale S. Eugenio, Piazzale dell'Umanesimo, 10, I-00144 Roma, Italy

Table 1. Effects of CyA and GAMIX immunosuppressive therapy on skin allograft rejection*

Groups	Treatment	Skin rejections/no. rats
1	Skin autograft	0/5
2	Skin allograft	15/15
3	Skin allograft + CyA 2 mg/kg/day	0/5
4	Skin allograft + CyA 1 mg/kg/day	6/9
5	Skin allograft + CyA 0.5 mg/kg/day	13/14
6	Skin allograft + GAMIX 30 mg/kg/day	9/9
7	Skin allograft + GAMIX 30 mg/kg + CyA 1 mg/kg/day	1/5
8	Skin allograft + GAMIX 30 mg/kg + CyA 0.5 mg/kg/day	2/10

* $P < 0.001$, group 2 vs group 7; $P < 0.0001$, group 2 vs group 3 and group 8

were male with a mean age of 3–4 months and a mean weight of 300 g. The animals were maintained under standard laboratory conditions.

Surgical procedures

The rats were anesthetized intraperitoneally with ketamine, 30 mg/kg. The cervicodorsal area was prepared to obtain the graft or to implant it. A 2 cm^2 skin patch was removed by a full-thickness incision that included dermis and epidermis. The graft was then implanted and sutured in the cervicodorsal area of the recipient. Post-operatively the animals were kept in separate cages to avoid any possible damage to the graft.

Immunosuppressive treatment

Drugs. CyA (Sandoz, Basel, Switzerland) was dissolved in ethanol and further diluted in saline. CyA was injected intraperitoneally at doses ranging between 0.5 and 2 mg/kg per day. Bovine brain ganglioside mixture, here after referred to as GAMIX (Cronassial, FIDIA, Abano Terme, Italy), was composed as follows: GM1 21%, GD1a 40%, GD1b 16% and GT1b 19% weight/volume. GAMIX preparations were dissolved in saline and injected intraperitoneally at 30 mg/kg per day. Table 1 reports the experimental groups under study. The drugs were administered 5 days/week for a period of 3 weeks.

Proliferation studies. All rats were killed 21 days after the beginning of treatment and splenectomized. Spleen cells were resuspended at 1×10^6 in RPMI medium supplemented with glutamine (2 mM), 10% FCS and antibiotics (complete medium) and cultured in 96 flat-bottom microwell trays (Nunc, Denmark) in triplicate samples in the presence or absence of PWM (Sigma) for 3 days in humidified 5% CO_2 atmosphere. Proliferation was assessed by ^{3}H-thymidine incorporation following a 18-h pulse.

Statistical analysis. The significance of the differences of the means was analyzed by the one-tailed Student's t-test. The significance of the differences in skin rejections was analyzed by Fisher's exact test.

Results

Effects of CyA and GAMIX therapy on skin allograft rejection

Table 1 reports the data concerning the different groups of animals under study, the immunosuppressive treatments, the number of animals for each group, and the number of skin rejections recorded. In group 2 with no immunosuppressive therapy, group 5, treated with suboptimal doses of CyA, and group 6, treated with GAMIX alone, graft rejection was observed in all animals. The number of rejections was significantly ($P < 0.001$) lower in rats treated with CyA 2 mg/kg (group 3) or, more interestingly, in rats treated with GAMIX 30 mg/kg plus CyA 1 mg/kg (group 7) or GAMIX 30 mg/kg plus CyA 0.5 mg/kg (group 8).

Effects of CyA and GAMIX immunosuppressive therapy on mitogen induced spleen-cell proliferation

The effects of the combination of CyA and GAMIX were then studied on lymphocyte proliferation induced by PWM. Spleen cells from the different groups of animals under treatment were stimulated in vitro with an optimal dose of PWM (5 µg/ml). Table 2 shows the proliferation of spleen cells from group 2 – skin-recipient rats, group 5 – skin-recipient rats treated with CyA, group 6 – skin-recipient rats treated with GAMIX, or group 8 – skin-recipient rats treated with a combination of the two drugs. The data are reported as the mean of cpm ± SD values of spleen cell cultures from each rat (five animals in each group). Spleen cells from untreated or skin allografted animals showed an optimal proliferative response to PWM stimulation. Similarly, spleen cells from rats treated with CyA or GAMIX alone optimally proliferate following mitogen stimulation. In contrast, the proliferation of spleen cells from animals treated with a combination of CyA and GAMIX was significantly reduced compared to that of spleen cells from group 2 animals ($P < 0.03$). The proliferation induced by PWM was also significantly reduced ($P < 0.0001$) in spleen cells from rats treated simultaneously with CyA and GAMIX in comparison with spleen cells from animals treated with CyA alone.

Discussion

The data reported in this investigation indicate that gangliosides can augment in vivo the immunosuppression induced by low doses of CyA in skin-grafted rats. Indeed, in

Table 2. Effects of CyA and GAMIX immunosuppressive therapy on PWM-induced spleen-cell proliferation*

Groups	Treatment	^{3}H-Tdr incorporation (cpm × 10^{-3} ± SD)
	Untreated rats	40.4 ± 6.4
2	Skin allograft	42.2 ± 31.4
5	Skin allograft + CyA 0.5	27.3 ± 9.4
6	Skin allograft + GAMIX 30	35.5 ± 30.7
8	Skin allograft + GAMIX 30 + CyA 0.5	5.1 ± 6.8

* $P < 0.03$, group 2 vs group 8; $P < 0.001$, group 5 vs group 8

the group of rats treated with a combination of the two drugs, at the lowest dose of CyA used, a significant reduction in skin rejections could be observed. Moreover, spleen cells from animals treated with both drugs showed significantly decreased proliferative activity upon stimulation by PWM mitogen in vitro. These results are in accordance with our previous findings on the potentiation of immunosuppressive effects between CyA and GAMIX, in vitro, in the generation of allospecific immune response in man [13].

Still unclear is the nature of the mechanisms underlying this potentiation. As already reported [10, 12], gangliosides do not affect IL-2 production in vitro, in contrast to CyA, which exerts typical, dose-dependent, inhibitory effects. However, GAMIX can down-regulate IL-2 production in MLC performed in the presence of low doses of CyA. GAMIX does not influence Tac expression in MLC blasts, while again CyA shows dose-dependent inhibitory effects [13]. Considering the autocrine nature of IL-2 production [11], one suggestive hypothesis to explain the potentiation exerted by GAMIX on CyA-induced immunosuppression is that GAMIX might exert the immunosuppressive effects by inhibiting the interaction of IL-2 with its receptor [10] and thus prevent further IL-2 production. This mechanism might be of relevance in the presence of low-dose CyA, unable per se to efficiently inhibit IL-2 production.

It is also of interest that GAMIX alone, at the dose used, does not inhibit ex vivo the proliferation of spleen cells activated by PWM, thus suggesting that gangliosides are immunosuppressive in vivo only in combination with other drugs such as CyA.

In conclusion these findings might suggest a possible use of the association of CyA and GAMIX in immunosuppressive therapy in human transplantation. More information, however, is required on the in vivo renal and hepatotoxicity of this combined therapy, together with new insight into the molecular mechanisms of the immunosuppression exerted by CyA and GAMIX.

Acknowledgements. This work was supported in part by a FIDIA spa grant and by CNR grants, special projects "Biotecnologie e Biostrumentazioni," and "Applicazioni Cliniche della Ricerca Oncologica."

References

1. Bremer E, Schlessinger J, Hakomori SI (1986) Ganglioside-mediated modulation of cell growth. J Biol Chem 261: 2434–2440
2. Cohen DJ, Loertscher R, Rubin MF, Rubin MF, Tilney NL, Carpenter CB, Strom TB (1984) Cyclosporine: a new immunosuppressive agent for organ transplantation. Ann Intern Med 101: 667–681
3. Hakomori S (1981) Glycosphingolipids in cellular interaction, differentiation and oncogenesis. Ann Rev Biochem 50: 733–764
4. Hannun YA, Bell RM (1989) Functions of sphingolipids and sphingolipids breakdown products in cellular regulation. Science 243: 500–505
5. Kahan BD, Flechner SM, Lorber MI, Jensen C, Golden D, Van Buren CT (1986) Complications of cyclosporine therapy. World J Surg 10: 348–355
6. Kahan BD (1989) Cyclosporine. N Engl J Med 321: 1725–1738
7. Kreutter D, Kim JY, Goldenring JR, Rasmussen H, Ukomadu C, DeLorenzo RJ, Yu RK (1987) Regulation of protein kinase C activity by gangliosides. J Biol Chem 262: 1633–1637
8. Marcus DM (1984) A review of the immunogenic and immunomodulatory properties of glycosphingolipids. Mol Immunol 21: 1083–1091
9. Morris PJ (1984) The impact of cyclosporine on transplantation. Adv Surg 17: 99–115
10. Robb RJ (1986) The suppressive effects of gangliosides upon IL-2 dependent proliferation as a function of inhibition of IL-2 – receptor association. J Immunol 136: 971-976
11. Smith KA (1988) Interleukin-2: inception, impact, and implications. Science 240: 1169–1176
12. Spagnoli GC, Ausiello CM, Sconocchia G, Antonelli G, Amici C, Casciani CU (1990) Polymorphic effects of exogenous gangliosides on antigen-induced lymphoproliferation and generation of MHC unrestricted cell mediated cytotoxicity. Int J Immunopharmacol 7: 713–720
13. Spagnoli GC, Ausiello CM, Sconocchia G, Adorno D, Casciani CU (1991) Gangliosides potentiate cyclosporine A – induced suppression of allospecific immune responses. Transplant Proc 23: 342–345

Transplant Int (1992) 5 [Suppl 1]: S547–S551

TRANSPLANT
International
© Springer-Verlag 1992

Rescue therapy for acute rejection using 15-deoxyspergualin (DSG) in combination with superoxide dismutase (SOD) on cardiac allografts in rats*

S. Suzuki, M. Kanashiro, R. Hayashi, and H. Amemiya

Department of Surgical Research and Laboratory of Nuclear Magnetic Resonance, Research Institute, National Cardiovascular Center, Suita, Osaka, Japan

Abstract. This study was performed to investigate the effect of combination therapy using 15-deoxyspergualin (DSG) plus recombinant human superoxide dismutase (h-SOD) on acute graft rejection in heterotopic rat heart transplantation. DSG was intraperitoneally injected for 10 days at a dose of 5 mg/kg per day, and h-SOD (15,000 or 30,000 μm/kg per day) was continuously administered via external iliac vein for approximately 8 days with a mini-osmotic pump (Alzet model 2001). Administration of the drugs was started on the 4th day after grafting. The grafts treated with h-SOD alone survived slightly longer than the control allografts. The graft survival time was significantly prolonged in the groups treated with DSG alone or DSG plus h-SOD. A higher percentage of induction of immunological unresponsiveness was achieved in the group treated with DSG plus h-SOD at 30,000 μm/kg per day. The ratios of inorganic phosphate (Pi)/phosphocreatine (PCr) and PCr/ATP on the ^{31}P nuclear magnetic resonance spectrogram are useful parameters for assessing the graft injury associated with acute rejection. The ratio of Pi/PCr and that of PCr/ATP were found to increase and decrease, respectively, in proportion to the progress in rejection. In the animals treated with DSG alone, the Pi/PCr ratio was significantly increased from the 4th day, and PCr/ATP ratio decreased from 10th day after grafting. These parameters were not improved during the observation period. However, these parameters were significantly recovered in the animals treated with DSG and h-SOD in combination. Improvement of the parameters seemed to be related to SOD dosage.

These results clearly demonstrated that the oxygen free radical plays a toxic role in cardiac allografts with ongoing rejection and, therefore, the administration of h-SOD in combination with DSG can minimize the graft injury.

* This work was supported in part by the Japanese Ministry of Health and Welfare (Research Grant for Organ Replacement Technology, 2KO-1).

Offprint requests to: Seiichi Suzuki, Department of Surgical Research, National Cardiovascular Center, 5-Fujishiro-dai, Suita, Osaka 565, Japan.

Rejection response involves infiltration of inflammatory cells, i.e., lymphocytes, monocytes, and polymorphonuclear neutrophils (PMNs), at the graft site. There is much evidence that activated monocytes and PMNs can generate the oxygen free radical [10, 18, 26], which is toxic to biomolecules of the grafted organ. In addition, impairment of coronary flow and myocytic necrosis developed during acute rejection in non-immunosuppressed animals [6, 7, 27], although the coronary flow was not observed to decrease in the presence of mild or moderate rejection, which had occurred after a 4-day cessation of immunosuppression [5]. The disturbance of myocardial circulation and myocytic necrosis due to advanced rejection could contribute to myocardial acidosis. The acidosis in muscles may generate the oxygen free radicals through the cyclo-oxygenase pathway of arachidonic acid metabolism [25]. Therefore, a treatment for free radical in combination with direct inhibition of activated immunological cells will be potentially beneficial for the therapy of acute rejection. Kloc et al. [17B] have described a profound decrease in the activity of superoxide dismutase (SOD) in the heterotopically transplanted rat hearts on day 5 day after grafting, while glutathione peroxidase and catalase activities were little affected in the transplanted heart. This indicates that SOD is one of the primary tissue defence enzymes against graft rejection.

Thus, the following study was designed to verify the effect of combination therapy using a new immunosuppressant, 15-deoxyspergualin (DSG), with SOD on acute graft rejection in heterotopic rat heart transplantation. The bioenergetic status of the grafts after transplantation was serially evaluated by ^{31}P magnetic resonance imaging (MRI) spectroscopy.

Materials and methods

Animals

Inbred male ACI rats (RT-1^{av1}) and male WKAH rats (RT-1^k), weighing 200–250 g, were used as recipients and donors, respectively, for the heterotopic heart transplantation.

Drugs

15-Deoxyspergualin (DSG) and recombinant human cuprozinc SOD (h-SOD), both provided in powder forms by Nippon Kayaku Co. (Tokyo), were dissolved in physiological saline to therapeutic concentrations. DSG was daily injected i. p. to the recipients at a dose of 5 mg/kg for 10 days from the 4th day after grafting. h-SOD was continuously administered into the inferior vena cava of the recipients at a daily dose of 15,000 or 30,000 μm/kg with a mini-osmotic pump for approximately 8 days from the 4th day on after grafting.

Implantation of the mini-osmotic pump

A mini-osmotic pump (Alzet 2001, 200 μl of reservoir) with a polyethylene infusion tube (0.58 mm inside diameter and 90 mm long) was used for continuous administration of h-SOD. The reservoir and infusion tube of the pump were filled with h-SOD at experimental concentrations. The left iliac portion of the recipient was incised to expose the external iliac vein, and the infusion tube was inserted through this vein into the inferior vena cava. The pump was then subcutaneously implanted on the abdominal wall.

Heterotopic heart transplantation

The heterotopic, auxiliary cardiac grafts were placed in the neck of recipient rats by a modification of the method of Miller et al. [20], as previously reported [28, 31, 32]. Briefly, the pulmonary artery of the donor heart was anastomosed to the right external jugular vein of the recipient in a continuous end-to-side manner with 9-0 monofilament nylon suture, and the donor brachiocephalic artery was anastomosed to the recipient left common carotid artery in an end-to-end manner with continous 10-0 nylon suture. Finally, the aorta was flushed with saline and ligated distally with 3-0 silk suture. The day of grafting was regarded as day 0, and cardiac pulsation was assessed by daily palpation. The day of cardiac arrest was defined as the last day of graft survival. A graft that survived longer than 100 days was regarded as an indefinite survivor (recipients acquired immunological unresponsiveness).

^{31}P MRI spectroscopy

The ^{31}P MRI technique was applied to investigate in vivo energy metabolism of the graft in the period after transplantation. Details of the ^{31}P MRI method have been reported previously [20, 30, 31]. In brief, anesthetized recipient rats were fixed on a probe, and a four-turn, 13-mm-diameter surface coil was placed over the cervical allograft in direct contact with the skin. The recipient was then placed in a 6.34-Tesla, 89-mm vertical bore superconducting magnet (Oxford-270/89) operating with a JNM-

SMR 270 spectrometer. The coil was tuned to 270 mHz for ^{1}H and 109 mHz for ^{31}P. The magnetic field was scanned using the ^{1}H water signal from the tissue. ^{31}P MRT spectra were obtained with a 12-μs pulse width and 500 scans were made at 1.9-s intervals.

Experimental groups

The study was divided into five experiments: group 1, control receiving no drug; group 2, treated with h-SOD alone at a dose of 30,000 μm/kg per day; group 3, treated with DSG alone; group 4, treated with DSG plus h-SOD (15,000 μm/kg per day); group 5, treated with DSG plus _h-SOD (30,000 μm/kg per day).

Concentration of h-SOD

Separately from the above-mentioned experimental groups, five normal ACI rats were continuously injected with h-SOD at a dose of 30,000 μm/kg/day with a mini-osmotic pump. These animals were bled from the jugular vein on the day before h-SOD administration, and on days 2, 4 and 7 after administration. Plasma concentrations of h-SOD were determined by enzyme immunoassay using monoclonal antibody against h-SOD in accordance with the method of Adachi et al. [1].

Statistical analysis

The data obtained from each of the groups were expressed as mean ± SD. Intergroup differences in graft survival time were analyzed by generalized Wilcoxon's test and intergroup differences in ratios calculated from each phosphate areas on ^{31}P MRI spectra by the unpaired t-test.

Results

Graft survival (Table 1)

In the control allograft group (group 1), the graft survived for 9.2 ± 2.2 days ($n = 10$). The grafts in group 2 ($n = 10$) survived slightly but significantly $P < 0.01$) longer (12.0 ± 0.7 days) than in group 1. Compared with groups 1 and 2, graft survival time was significantly ($P < 0.01$) prolonged in group 3 ($n = 10$), group 4 ($n = 10$) and group 5 ($n = 10$). Indefinite graft survival was noted in two recipients in group 3, one in group 4 and four in group 5.

^{31}P MRI spectroscopy

As previously reported [20, 30, 31], the inorganic phosphate (Pi)/phosphocreatine (PCr) and PCr/ATP ratios on the ^{31}P MRI spectrogram were calculated from the peak areas. Only the peak of beta-phosphate of ATP was read as the ATP level since this peak contains only the signal from ATP. The mean values of Pi/PCr and PCr/ATP ratios were determined by 28 measurements using ^{31}P MRI spectroscopy in syngeneic grafts in the postoperative peri-

Table 1. Graft survival days in each experimental groups

Groups	DSG[a] (mg/kg)	h-SOD[b] (µm/kg)	Survival days	Significance	
				vs group 1	vs group 2
1 (n = 10)	0	0	9.2 ± 2.2		
2 (n = 10)	0	30,000	12.0 ± 0.7	P < 0.01	
3 (n = 10)	5	0	8, 10, 21, 21, 22, 23, 25, 26, > 100, > 100	P < 0.01	P < 0.01
4 (n = 10)	5	15,000	9, 16, 20, 20, 25, 25, 29, 30, 38, > 100	P < 0.01	P < 0.01
5 (n = 10)	5	30,000	7, 18, 20, 26, 26, 30, > 100, > 100, > 100, > 100	P < 0.01	P < 0.01

[a] DSG was intraperitoneally administered for 10 days from the 4th day after grafting.

[b] h-SOD was continuously administered for approximately 8 days, using the mini-osmotic pump (Alzey 2001), from the 4th day on after grafting

od from days 3–30 they were previously reported [30] to be 0.38 ± 0.11 and 1.88 ± 0.42, respectively. In all of the present groups, the Pi/PCr and PCr/ATP ratios on day 3 were not significantly different from those in the syngeneic grafts.

As shown in Fig. 1, an increase in the Pi/PCr ratio and a decrease in the PCr/ATP ratio were observed as time elapsed after grafting in both groups 1 and 2. The increase in the Pi/PCr ratio was observed earlier than the decrease in the PCr/ATP ratio. There were no significant daily differences in these ratios between groups.

In groups 3, the Pi/PCr ratio rapidly increased from the 4th day and PCr/ATP ratio gradually decreased from the 10th day after grafting. Although there were no significant daily differences in the ratios between groups 3

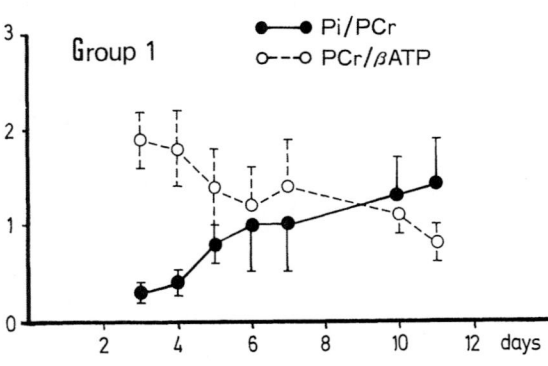

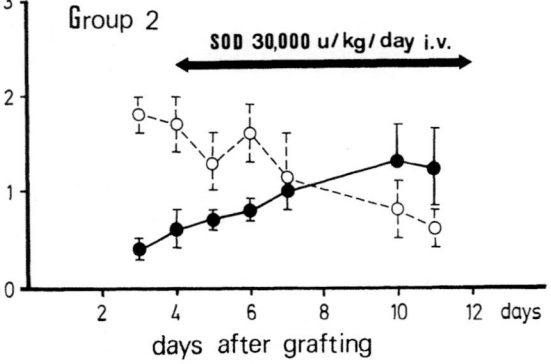

Fig. 1. Pi/PCr and PCr/ATP ratios in the control group (group 1) and in treated with h-SOD alone (group 2). h-SOD was continuously injected at a dose of 30,000 µm/kg per day via the external iliac vein with a mini-osmotic pump (Alzet model 2001) from the 4th day after grafting. In groups 1 and 2, Pi/PCr ratio increased and PCr/ATP ratio decreased in proportion to the progress in rejection. The increase in Pi/PCr ratio preceded the decrease in PCr/ATP ratio. There were no significant daily differences in these ratios between the two groups

and 4, these ratios tended to recover on day 17 in group 4 (Fig. 2). Furthermore, compared with group 3, Pi/PCr and PCr/ATP ratios in group 5 were significantly recovered from the 12th day and 14th day on, respectively (Fig. 2).

The Pi/PCr and PCr/ATP ratios from the grafts that survived for less than 19 days in groups 3–5 were excluded from the present analysis.

Concentrations of h-SOD in plasma

Figure 3 demonstrates the changes in the plasma concentration of h-SOD in rats continuously administered the enzyme with the mini-osmotic pump. It was clear that a constant plasma level of h-SOD was maintained by this administration method.

Discussion

Oxygen free radicals such as superoxide anion and its derivertives, hydrogen peroxide and hydroxyl radicals, mediate tissue injury during inflammation [9, 19, 24] and during reoxygeneration following myocardial ischemia [4, 8]. Abundant radicals may be generated at the graft site with ongoing rejection by activated macrophages and PMNs, as well as in the course of arachidonic acid metabolism. There is a defense system of intracellular enzymes, radical scavengers, to protect the tissue against oxygen toxicity [14]. However, it is postulated by Kloc et al. [17] that SOD activity may be decreased in rejecting allograft due to destruction of SOD in situ and/or to a decrease in SOD synthesis. Therefore, the graft with acute rejection must be attacked by both activated lymphocytes and the oxygen free radical.

The remarkable immunosuppressive effect of DSG has been confirmed in various organ transplantations using the mouse, rat, and dog [2, 11, 20, 21, 31, 35]. Furthermore, an indefinite graft survival was induced by short-term administration of DSG in allogeneic kidney [35], liver [12, 33], and heart [20, 31] transplantation in rats.

The immunological mechanism of action of DSG has not been well clarified. The production of IL-1 and IL-2 from macrophages and T cells, respectively, was not inhibited in DSG-treated rats [22]. The initiation of DSG treatment at the onset of acute rejection in rat heart trans-

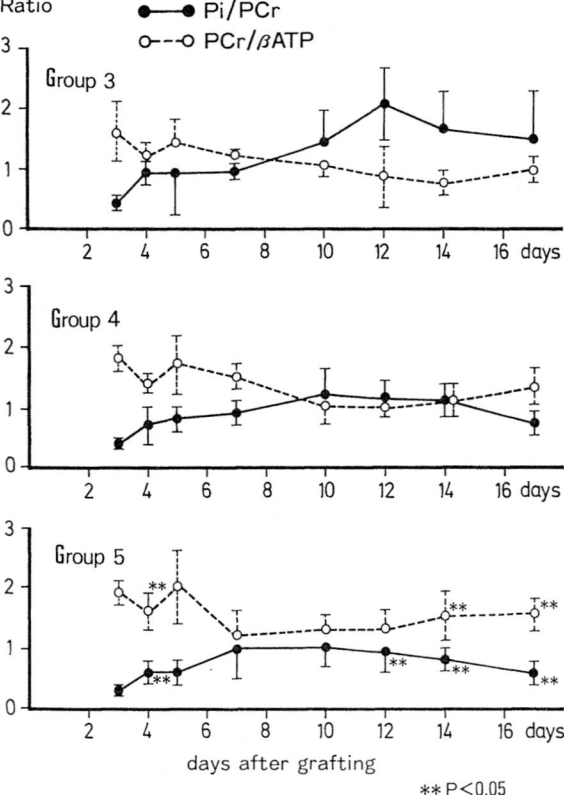

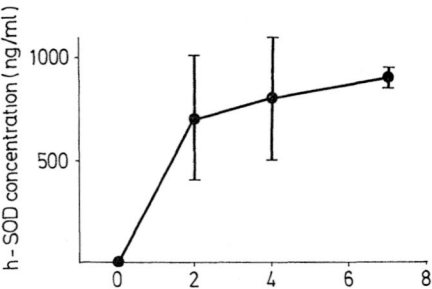

Fig. 3. Plasma concentration of h-SOD in rats continuously administered the enzyme with mini-osmotic pump. A constant plasma level of h-SOD was maintained in the h-SOD-infused rats

Fig. 2. Pi/PCr and PCr/ATP ratios in the allografts treated with DSG alone (group 3), DSG plus h-SOD at 15,000 μm/kg per day (group 4), and DSG plus h-SOD at 30,000 μm/kg per day (group 5). DSG was intraperitoneally injected for 10 days at a dose of 5 mg/kg per day from the 4th day. Continuous administration of h-SOD performed via the recipient external iliac vein with a mini-osmotic pump (Alzet 2001) from the 4th day after grafting. Statistical significance in group 3: Pi/PCr: $P < 0.01$, day 3 vs day 4, 5, 7, 10, 12, 14 and 17; PCr/ATP: NS, day 3 vs day 4, 5 and 7; $P < 0.05$, day 3 vs day 10 and 12; $P < 0.01$, day 3 vs day 14 and 17. Although there were no significant daily differences in the ratios between groups 3 and 4, these ratios tended to recover on the 17th day in group 4. Compared with group 3, the Pi/PCr and PCr/ATP ratios in group 5 were significantly recovered from the 12th day on and the 14th day, respectively. The significance of the daily ratios in groups 3–5 were: ** $P < 0.05$; others, NS

plantation induced higher degree of immunological unresponsiveness [31]. This indicates that the immunological mechanism of DSG action includes specific inhibition of expandes lymphocyte clones. Therefore, the drug may be used for the treatment of acute graft rejection. Indeed, DSG pulse therapy was highly effective on acute kidney rejection in canine transplantation [17A], as well as in clinical recipients [3, 29].

DSG has a significant rescue effect on acute rejection as mentioned above, although it seems to have no effect on the oxygen free radical. Therefore, combination therapy using DSG and SOD was considered to be highly effective for recovery from rejection. In the present study, the grafts treated with h-SOD alone survived slightly longer than the control allografts. In the groups treated with DSG alone or DSG plus h-SOD, the graft survival was significantly longer than the control allografts. Furthermore, a higher percentage of induction of immuno-

logical unresponsiveness was dose-dependently achieved with h-SOD in the DSG-treated groups.

The generation of oxygen free radical during acute rejection is different, in terms of duration, from that during reperfusion following myocardial ischemia; the former may last for several days, and the latter during the early phase of reperfusion [4]. Therefore, constant and long-lasting blood concentration of SOD should be necessary to protect the graft from free radicals during acute rejection. SOD is known to be rapidly cleared from the circulation. The circulatory half-life of this enzyme is less than 10 min [34]. Long-lasting derivatives of SOD have been prepared by coupling with polymers [15, 23, 24] or by entrapping with liposomes [16, 34]. In this study, we continuously administered native h-SOD, using the mini-osmotic pump, to maintain the constant circulating level of the enzyme. This method, in combination with DSG therapy, provided excellent protection from graft injury during acute rejection.

Previously, we reported [30] that Pi/PCr and PCr/ATP ratios on ^{31}P MRI spectrogram are useful parameters for assessing the metabolic dysfunction associated with acute graft rejection in heterotopically allografted hearts in rats. Fraser et al. [13] demonstrated that metabolic abnormality precedes functional or histological changes in allografts with ongoing rejection, and that an increase in the Pi/PCr ratio is seen earlier than a decrease in the PCr/ATP ratio. We also observed [20, 30, 31] that the onset of the increase in the Pi/PCr ratio indicates the early phase of graft rejection, and the PCr/ATP ratio decreases in proportion to the progress in rejection. The present study also demonstrated that the increase in the Pi/PCr ratio preceded the decrease of the PCr/ATP ratio. Although significant graft survival was obtained by the treatment with DSG alone, the highly increased Pi/PCr ratio from the 4th day and decreased PCr/ATP ratio from the 10th day, indicating severe graft injury, remained during the observation period. However, these parameters were significantly recovered in the animals treated with DSG and h-SOD in combination. Amelioration of the parameters seemed to be related to h-SOD dosage.

These results clearly demonstrated that the oxygen free radical plays a toxic role on cardiac allografts undergoing acute rejection and, therefore, the administration of h-SOD in combination with DSG minimized the tissue destruction. This is a novel and important finding that combination therapy using DSG and h-SOD is highly valuable for a smooth recovery from acute graft rejection.

References

1. Adachi T, Usami Y, Kishi T, Hirano K, Hayashi K (1988) An enzyme immunoassay for cuprozinc superoxide dismutase using monoclonal antibodies. J Immunol Method 109: 93–101

2. Amemiya H, Suzuki S, Niiya S, Fukao K, Yamanaka N, Ito J (1989) A new immunosuppressive agent, 15-deoxyspergualin, in dog renal allografting. Transplant Proc 21: 3468–3470

3. Amemiya H, Suzuki S. Ota K et al. (1990) A novel rescue drug, 15-deoxyspergualin. First clinical trials for recurrent graft rejection in renal recipients. Transplantation 49: 337–343

4. Arroyo CM, Kramer JH, Dickens BF, Weglicki WB (1987) Identification of free radicals in myocardial ischemia/reperfusion by spin trapping with nitrone DMPO. FEBS LET 221: 101–104

5. Bando K, Fraser CD, Chacko VP et al. (1991) Coronary blood flow does not decrease during allograft rejection in heterotopic heart transplants. J Heart Lung Transplant 10: 251–257

6. Bergsland J, Carr EA, Wright JW et al. (1985) Uptake of mycardial imaging agents by rejected hearts. J Heart Transplant 4: 536–540

7. Bergsland J, Hwang K, Driscoll R et al. (1989) Coronary blood flow and thallium 201 uptake in rejecting rat heart transplantation. J Heart Transplant 8: 147–153

8. Bosco PJ, Schweizer RT (1988) Use of oxygen radical scavenger on autografted pig kidney after warm ischemia and 48-hour perfusion preservation. Arch Surg 123: 601–604

9. Bulkley GB (1983) The role of oxygen free radicals in human disease processes. Surgery 94: 407–411

10. Colepicolo P, Camarero VCPC, Nicolas MT, Bassot JM, Karnovsky ML, Hastings JW (1990) A sensitive and specific assay for superoxide anion release by neutrophils or macrophages based on bioluminescence of polynoidin. Anal Biochem 184: 369–374

11. Dickneite G, Schorlemmer HU, Walter P, Sedlacek (1986) Graft survival in experimental transplantation could be prolonged by the action of the antitumoral drug 15-deoxyspergualin. Transplant Proc 18: 1295–1296

12. Engemann R, Gassel HJ, Lafrenz E, Stoffregen C, Thiede A, Hamelmann H (1987) Transplantation tolerance after short-term administration of 15-deoxyspergualin in orthotopic rat liver transplantation. Transplant Proc 19: 4241–4243

13. Fraser CD, Chacko VP, Jacobus WE et al. (1988) Metabolic changes preceding functional and morphologic indices of rejection in heterotopic cardiac allografts. Transplantation 46: 346–351

14. Fridovich I (1975) Superoxide dismutases. Ann Rev Biochem 44: 147–159

15. Fuertges F, Abuchowski A (1990) The clinical efficacy of poly(ethylene glycol)-modified proteins. J Control Release 11: 139–148

16. Imaizumi S, Woolworth V, Fishman RA, Chan PH (1990) Liposome-entrapped superoxide dismutase reduces cerebral infarction in cerebral ischemia in rats. Stroke 21: 1312–1317

17a. Itoh J, Takeuchi T, Suzuki S, Amemiya H (1988) Reversal of acute rejection episodes by deoxyspergualin (NKT-01) in dogs receiving renal allografts. J Antibiot (Tokyo) 41: 1503–1505

17b. Kloc M, Mailer K, Stepkowski S (1986) Superoxide dismutase decrease in cardiac transplants. Transplantation 41: 794–796

18. Makino R, Tanaka T, Iizuka T, Ishimura Y, Kanegasaki S (1986) Stoichiometric conversion of oxygen to superoxide anion during the respiratory burst in neutrophils. J Biol Chem 261: 11444–11447

19. McCord JM (1983) The superoxide free radical: Its biochemistry and pathophysiology. Surgery 94: 412–414

20. Miller JE, Tschoepe RL, Ziegler MM (1985) A new model of heterotopic rat heart transplantation with application for in vivo ^{31}P nuclear magnetic resonance spectroscopy. Transplantation 39: 555–558

21. Nemoto K, Hayashi M, Abe F (1987) Immunosuppressive activities of 15-deoxyspergualin in animals. J Antibiot (Tokyo) 40: 561–562

22. Nemoto K, Abe F, Nakamura T, Ishizuka M, Takeuchi T, Umezawa H (1987) Blastogenic responses and the release of interleukin 1 and 2 by spleen cells obtained from rat skin allograft recipients administered with 15-deoxyspergualin. J Antibiot (Tokyo) 40: 1062–1064

23. Noguchi K, Ojiri y, Kinjo N, Moromizato H, Nakasone J, Sakanashi M (1990) Effect of polyoxethylene-modified superoxide dismutase on recovery of myocardial dysfunction after coronary stenosis in dogs. Jpn J Pharmacol 54: 244–249

24. Oda T, Akaika T, Hamamoto T, Suzuki F, Hirano T, Maeda H (1989) Oxygen radicals in influenza-induced pathogenesis and treatment with pyran polymer-conjugated SOD. Science 244: 974–976

25. Okabe E, Kato Y, Kohno H, Hess ML, Ito H (1985) Inhibition by free radical scavengers and by cyclooygenase inhibitors of the effect of acidosis on calcium transport by masseter muscle sacroplasmic reticulum. Biochem Pharmacol 34: 961–968

26. Otamiri T (1989) Oxygen radical, lipid peroxidation, and neutrophil infiltration after small-intestinal ischemia and reperfusion. Surgery 105: 593–597

27. Salomon NW, Stinson EB, Griepp RB, Shumway NE (1987) Alterations in total and regional myocardial blood flow during acute rejection of orthotopic canine cardiac allografts. J Thorac Cardiovasc Surg 75: 542–547

28. Shimatani K, Suzuki S, Hayashi R, Amemiya H (1989) Prolongation of cardiac allograft survival in rats by recipient pretreatment with donor spleen cells and 15-deoxyspergualin. Transplantation 48: 865–867

29. Suzuki S, Hayashi R, Kenmochi T, Shimatani K, Fukuoka T, Amemiya H (1990) Clinical application of 15-deoxyspergualin for treatment of acute graft rejection following renal transplantation. Transplant Proc 22: 1615–1617

30. Suzuki S, Kanashiro M, Hayashi R, Kenmochi T, Fukuoka T, Amemiya H (1990) In vivo ^{31}P nuclear magnetic resonance findings on heterotopically allografted hearts in rats treated with a novel immunosuppressant, FK 506. Heart Vessels 5: 224–229

31. Suzuki S, Kanashiro M, Amemiya H (1987) Effect of a new immunosuppressant, 15-deoxyspergualin, on heterotopic rat heart transplantation, in comparison with cyclosporine. Transplantation 44: 483–487

32. Suzuki S, Kanashiro M, Watanabe H, Amemiya H (1988) Therapeutic effect of 15-deoxyspergualin on acute graft rejection detected by ^{31}P nuclear magnetic resonance spectroscopy and in vivo mechanisms of action in rat heart transplantation. Transplantation 46: 669–672

33. Thies JC, Walter PK, Zimmermann PA, Dickneite G, Sedlacek HH, Keller HE (1987) Prolongation of graft survival in allogeneic pancreas and liver transplantation by (−)15-deoxyspergualin. Eur Surg Res 19: 129–134

34. Turrens JF, Crapo JD, Freeman BA (1984) Protection against oxygen toxicity by intravenous injection of liposome-entrapped catalase and superoxide dismutase. J Clin Invest 73: 87–95

35. Walter P, Dickneite G, Feifel G, Thies J (1987) Deoxyspergualin induces tolerance in allogeneic kidney transplantation. Transplant Proc 19: 3980–3981

Transplant Int (1992) 5 [Suppl 1]: S 552–S 555

TRANSPLANT
International
© Springer-Verlag 1992

Japanese study of FK 506 on kidney transplantation: 2. Follow-up study of FK 506-treated patients

Japanese FK 506 Study Group

Abstract. Thirty-seven primary renal transplant patients were enrolled in the early phase II study on kidney transplantation. All grafts survived during the follow-up period. However, 10 of the 37 patients were changed from FK 506 to conventional drugs, and 3 were treated concomitantly with azathioprine (AZA) or mizoribine (MZR) in the 3-month period of observation. After 3 months posttransplantation, an additional 10 patients were treated continuously with AZA or MZR. In addition, 3 were converted from FK 506 to conventional drugs. No additional conversion was observed after 4 months. Trough level monitoring was effective enough to regulate the FK 506 dosage. Nephrotoxicity and hyperglycemia were associated with a high trough level of FK 506 (whole blood, > 20 ng/ml).

Key words: FK 506 – Renal transplantation – Clinical study – Follow-up study

Patients and methods

Exclusion criteria. The following patients were excluded: (1) under 16 years old, (2) liver dysfunction of more than 1.6 mg/dl of total bilirubin or twice or more higher glutamine-oxaloacetic (GOT) and glutamic-pyruvic (GPT) transaminase values than normal, (3) pulmonary dysfunction of less than 70 mm Hg of PaO_2, (4) cardiac problems with less than 60% of ejection fraction or abnormal ECG (6) peptic ulcer, (7) a history or present status of malignant carcinoma, (8) infectious disease including hepatitis B virus (HB) hepatitis, (9) drug hypersensitivity or allergy, (10) pregnant or expecting to become so, (11) a history of kidney transplantation, (12) a minor mismatch for ABO blood group, (13) positive T-cell crossmatch, (14) HLA identical or 2-haplotype mismatched living related donor, (15) did not consent to receive the FK 506 treatment.

Monitoring of blood concentration of FK 506. The trough level of FK 506 in the plasma and whole blood as measured by the double

Offprint requests to: S. Takahara, M.D., Department of Urology, Osaka University Medical School, 1-1-50 Fukushima, Fukushima-ku, Osaka 553, Japan

sandwich enzyme-linked immunosorbent assay (ELISA) were monitored. The extraction of the blood for the measurement of the drug concentration involves a liquid phase method using dichloromethane [5]. This method is different from the column extraction method which is available in the United States of America. The detection limit was 0.5 ng/ml in whole blood and 0.05 ng/ml in plasma. The intra- and interassay coefficients of variation were both less than 20%.

Nephrotoxicity was diagnosed from mainly histology observations. Briefly, a foomy vacuolization of the proximal tubular cells, especially in the straight portion, was the main criteria [6].

Trial design and statistical analysis. An early phase II study on kidney transplantation was performed as a multicenter open trial. After the observation period of 3 months, 26 of the 37 patients were still being maintained on FK 506 therapy.

The sign test was used in the analysis of dosage and blood levels. The Wilcoxon signed-rank test was used in the analysis of laboratory values.

Results

Characteristics of the study population

Table 1 lists the background characteristics of the patients. In all, 23 living related and 3 cadaveric cases were treated with FK 506 for more than 3 months after transplantation.

Table 1. Characteristics of the study population

			n
Donor	Living related		23
	Cadaveric		3
HLA	A + B + DR mismatched		1.7 ± 1.0
Direct crossmatch		(−)	26
PRA	T	(−)	25
($n = 25$)	B warm	(−)	24
		(+)	1
	B cold	(−)	23
		(+)	2

PRA, panel cell reactive antibody

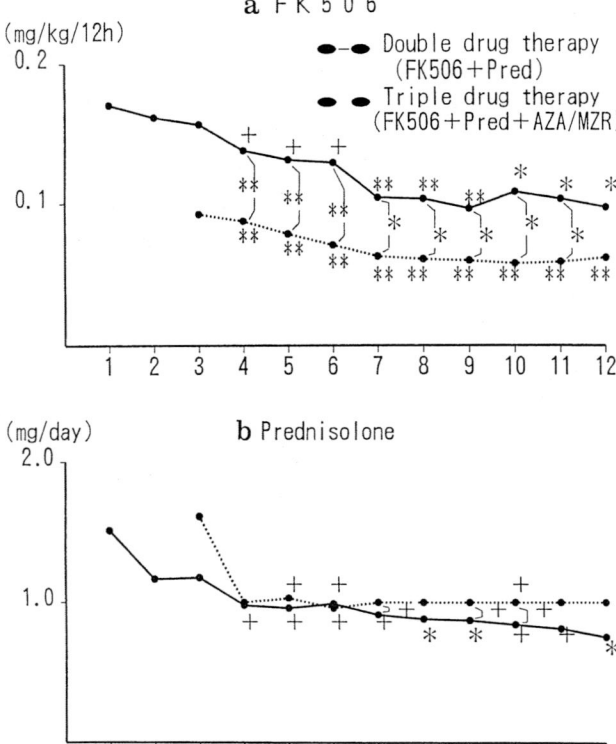

Fig. 1. Mean oral dosage of FK 506 and prednisolone (Pred)

The mean oral dosage of prednisolone in the triple drug therapy group was 16.1 ± 8.6 mg/day at 3 months, 9.6 ± 1.5 mg/day at 6 months, 10.0 ± 0.0 ng/day at 9 months, and 10.0 ± 0.0 mg/day at 12 months.

FK 506 trough levels

The FK 506 trough level in the whole blood was 15.4 ± 8.1 ng/ml at 3 months, 13.1 ± 6.5 ng/ml at 6 months, 11.4 ± 5.9 ng/ml at 9 months, and 9.3 ± 1.6 ng/ml at 12 months in the double drug therapy group Fig. 2 a). The trough level at 9 months was statistically significantly lower than that at 3 months ($P < 0.05$).

The FK 506 trough level in the plasma was 0.35 ± 0.16 ng/ml at 3 months, 0.26 ± 0.16 ng/ml at 6 months, 0.18 ± 0.11 ng/ml at 9 months, and 0.12 ± 0.15 ng/ml at 12 months in the double drug therapy group (Fig. 2 b). The trough levels were not stable during the follow-up period.

Graft survival and immunosuppressive protocol

All 26 grafts survived during the follow-up period (4–14 months after transplantation, average 332 ± 83 days).

At 3 months after transplantation, 23 of the 26 patients (88%) were treated only with FK 506 and prednisolone. AZA or MZR was administered to 3 patients in addition to FK 506 and prednisolone (Fig. 3).

Mean HLA-A, B, DR mismatches was 1.7 ± 1.0.

All direct crossmatches and panel cell reactive antibody (PRA) titers against T cells were negative, although the PRA against B warm cells was positive in 1 patient and against B cold cells, positive in 2 patients.

Dosage of FK 506 and prednisolone

The mean oral dosage of FK 506 in the double drug therapy group (FK 506 and prednisolone) was 0.16 ± 0.04 mg/kg b.i.d. at 3 months and thereafter was 0.13 ± 0.05 mg/kg at 6 months, 0.10 ± 0.05 mg/kg at 9 months, and 0.10 ± 0.05 mg/kg at 12 months (Fig. 1 a).

The mean oral dosage of FK 506 in the triple drug therapy group (FK 506, prednisolone, and azathioprine or mizoribine, AZA/MZR) was 0.09 ± 0.04 mg/kg b.i.d. at 3 months, 0.07 ± 0.03 mg/kg at 6 months, 0.06 ± 0.02 mg/kg at 9 months, and 0.06 ± 0.01 mg/kg at 12 months.

In the double drug therapy group, the dosage of FK 506 was decreased over 7 months. A statistically significant difference in the dosage was observed between 3 and 7–12 months ($P < 0.01$ or $P < 0.05$, respectively). A statistically significant difference in the dosage was observed between 3 and 4–12 months ($P < 0.01$) in the triple drug therapy group.

The mean oral dosage of prednisolone in the double drug therapy group was 11.8 ± 4.4 mg/day at 3 months, 9.9 ± 1.4 mg/day at 6 months, 8.7 ± 2.2 mg/day at 9 months, and 7.5 ± 3.6 mg/day at 12 months (Fig. 1 b).

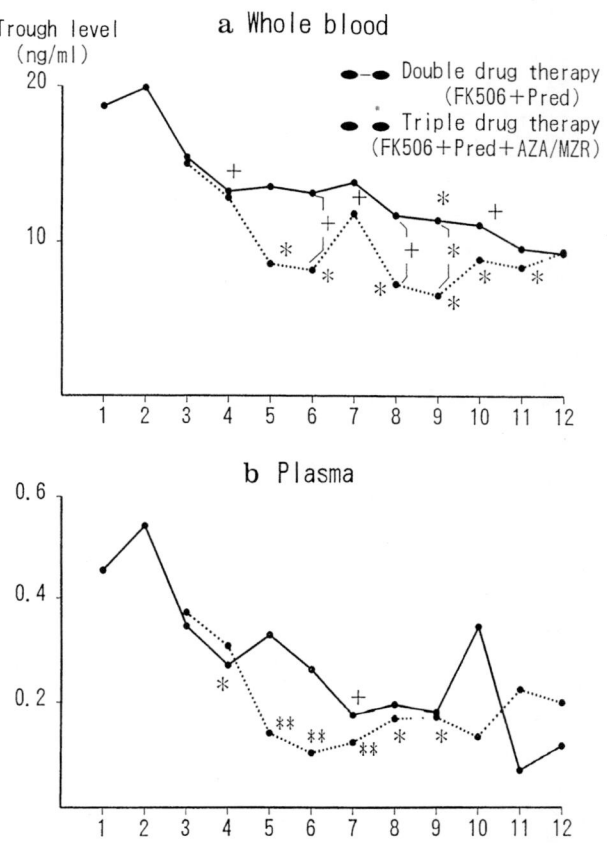

Mean oral dosage of FK506

Fig. 2. Mean FK 506 trough levels. AZA/MZR, azathioprine or mizoribine

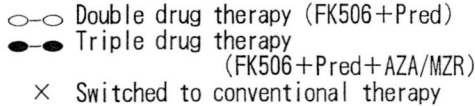

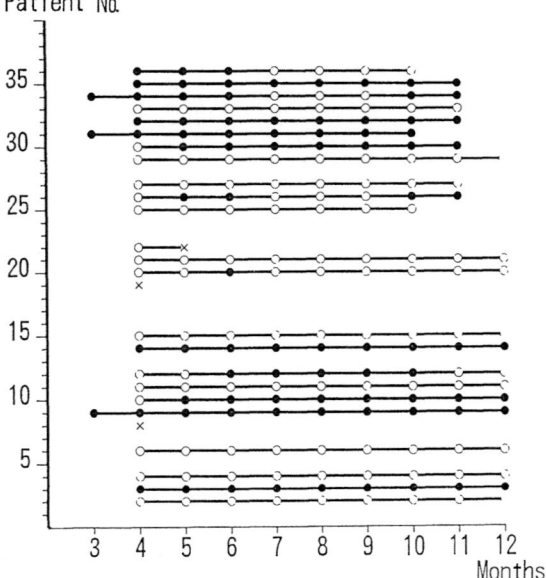

Fig.3. Immunosuppressant therapy in the follow-up period

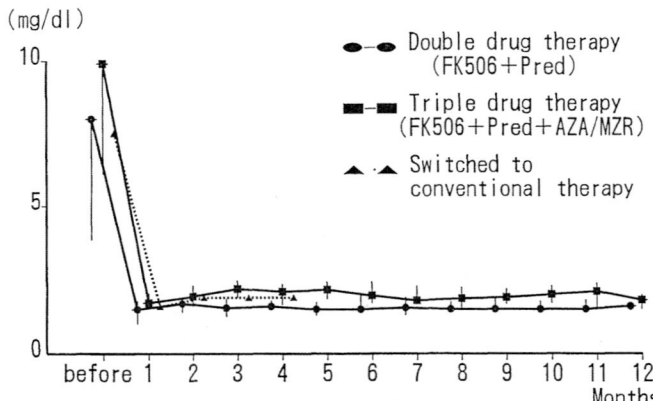

Fig.4. Median serum creatinine levels

Between 4 and 6 months, 10 other patients were transferred to the triple drug regimen group (rejection 3 cases, nephrotoxicity 6 cases, both 1 case) from the double drug group.

FK 506 was stopped, and the immunosuppressive protocol was changed to the protocols without FK 506 in the other 3 patients of the double drug therapy group (rejection 1 case, nephrotoxicity 2 cases). No further dropout case from FK 506 therapy was observed thereafter. Between 7 and 9 months, 14 of the 23 recipients were treated with FK 506 and prednisolone. The triple drug regimens of FK 506/AZA/prednisolone or FK 506/MZR/prednisolone were administered to the other 9 recipients.

More than 10 months after transplantation, 12 of the 23 recipients were treated with FK 506 and prednisolone. The triple drug regimens were administered to the other 11 recipients.

Rejection

Rejection was observed in 3 cases (4 episodes) in this follow-up period. Three cases were treated with bolus administration of methylprednisolone and/or by adding AZA or MRZ. In only 1 case was FK 506 stopped, and CyA and antilymphocyte immunoglobulin (ALG) were administered. All grafts recovered from their rejection episodes and kept to the previous serum creatinine levels.

Serum creatinine

The median serum creatinine level in the double drug therapy group was 1.6 mg/dl at 3 months, 1.5 mg/dl at 6 months, 1.5 mg/dl at 9 months and 1.6 mg/dl at 12 months (Fig.4). The median serum creatinine level in the triple drug therapy group was 2.2 mg/dl at 3 months, 2.0 mg/dl at 6 months, 1.9 mg/dl at 9 months, and 1.8 mg/dl at 12 months.

A statistically significant difference was observed between the two groups at 3 months ($P < 0.01$) and 6 months ($P < 0.05$).

Adverse events

No life-threatening adverse events were observed.

Insulin-dependent hyperglycemia occurred in 7 of the 26 cases (27%) within 3 months after transplantation (Fig.5a). However, insulin was required in only 5 of the 26 cases (19%) between 4 and 6 months, and 2 of 23 (9%) between 7 and 9 and 10 and 12 months.

Antihyperuricemic drugs were used in 3 of the 26 cases (12%) within 3 months, 5 of 26 (19%) between 4 and 6 months, 6 of 23 (26%) between 7 and 9 and 10 and 12 months (Fig.5b).

Antihyperkalemic drugs were administered to 8 of the 26 cases (13%) within 3 months, 2 of 26 (8%) between 4 and 6 months, and 1 of 23 (4%) between 7 and 9 months. No patient needed these drugs after 10 months (Fig.5c).

Antihypertension drugs were administered to 15 of the 26 cases (58%) within 3 months, 8 of 26 (31%) between 4 and 6 months, 8 of 23 cases (35%) between 7 and 12 months (Fig.5d). Therefore, no "de novo" hypertension was observed during the follow-up period.

No hepatotoxic episode was observed during the follow-up period.

In one case, mild chest pain was noted on day 154. Tachycardia was noted in another case on day 121. Nitroglycerin was administered temporarily, and the symptom disappeared.

Infections

Cytomegalovirus pneumonia was observed in 2 cases at 89 and 158 days posttransplant. Siagonanthitis was identified in another patient at 84 days posttransplant. All patients recovered after the administration of an antimicrobial agent or ganciclovir. In only 1 case was septicemia ob-

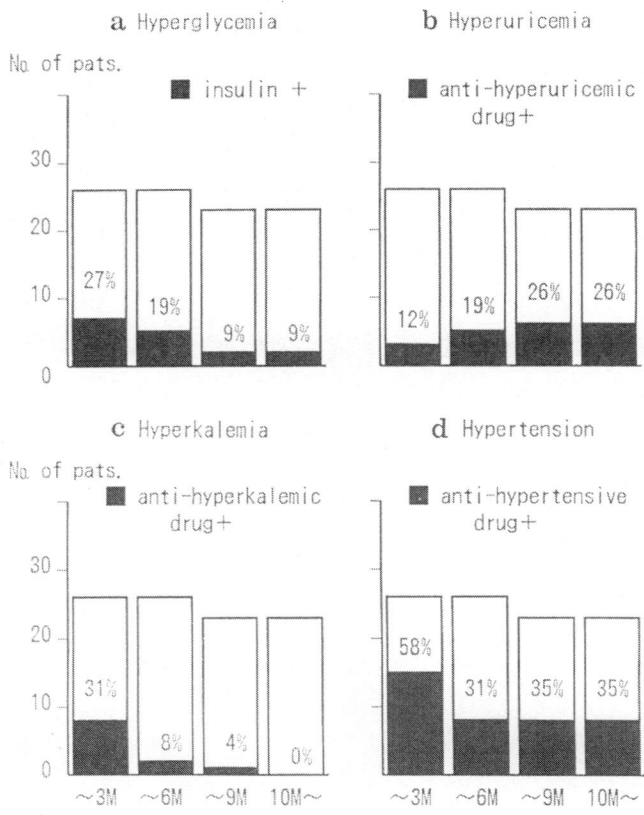

Fig. 5. Incidence of adverse events: **a** diabetes mellitus, **b** hyperuricemia, **c** hyperkalemia, **d** hypertension; *M*, months

served on day 314 posttransplant. This patient also recovered after the administration of antibiotics.

Discussion

This early phase II study produced several data on the efficacy, safety, and optimal therapeutic dose and blood level of FK 506 in patients undergoing kidney transplantation [4]. In particular, a higher reproducibility was indicated for the blood level monitoring by whole blood samples than for that by plasma samples. This new monitoring method was achieved by extracting with dichloromethane

[5]. Our recent blood level monitoring of FK 506 was only performed with whole blood samples. The therapeutic trough level in whole blood is suggested to be 10–15 ng/ml at 3–9 months and 10 ng/ml at 12 months in the double drug therapy group.

Although 3 patients were switched to another regimen without FK 506 at 3–5 months, all patients and grafts had survived. Almost all rejection and nephrotoxic episodes were reversible. No additional case of switching was identified thereafter.

In addition, the median serum creatinine level low remained low during the follow-up period in both double and triple drug therapy groups. Therefore, the trough level monitoring in whole blood was sufficient to monitor good graft function for a long period.

We also succeeded in reducing the dosage of prednisolone; in more than half of the cases, it was less than 10 mg/day at 4 months posttransplant. We could not find any major adverse events. Although infections were observed in 4 patients, recovery followed the administration of an antimicrobial agent or ganciclovir.

No hepatotoxicity occurred for more than 10 months, and the incidence of hypertension was very low. These merits have not been previously reported in CyA clinical studies [1–3].

Although hyperglycemia and hyperkalemia were observed in several cases, all these events were reversible.

In conclusion, this multicenter study of FK 506 therapy showed that a good graft function could be maintained for more than 10 months via monitoring the FK 506 trough level in whole blood.

References

1. Canadian Multicentre Transplant Study Group (1986) A randomized clinical trial of cyclosporine in cadaveric renal transplantation. N Engl J Med 314: 1219–1225
2. Chapman JR, Griffiths D, Harding NGL, Morris PJ (1985) Reversibility of cyclosporin nephrotoxicity after three months' treatment. Lancet I: 128–129
3. Hall BM, Tiller DJ, Hardie I Mahony J, Mathew T, Hatcher G, Mizch M, Thomson N, Shell R (1988) Comparison of three immunosuppressive regimens in cadaver renal transplantation: long term cyclosporine, short term cyclosporine followed by azathioprine and prednisolone, and azathioprine and prednisolone without cyclosporine. N Engl J Med 318: 1499–1507

Transplant Int (1992) 5 [Suppl 1]: S 556–S 558

Insensitivity to cyclosporine may explain the HLA-DRw6 recipient effect

S. Kudlacek, G. J. Zlabinger, E. Pohanka, G. Hamilton, A. Rosenmayr, and J. Kovarik

2nd Department of Medicine, Institute of Immunology, First Department of Surgery, Institute of Blood Group Serology, University of Vienna, Vienna, Austria

Abstract. Clinical as well as experimental studies have found an interindividual variability in the immunosuppressive effect of cyclosporine (CsA). In renal transplant patients treated with CsA and prednisolone alone, biopsy-verified rejections were significantly more frequent in DRw6-positive than in DRw6-negative graft recipients. The relative risk for developing a graft rejection independently of the CsA blood levels increased in HLA-DRw6-positive transplant patients. Although no statistical significance of the CsA levels within different DR phenotypes could be assessed, HLA-DR2-positive graft recipients with biopsy-verified rejection episodes had significantly lower CsA levels than DR2-negative patients ($P = 0.01$). Our results would indicate a very low CsA sensitivity of HLA-DRw6-positive graft recipients and might explain previous results describing an increased incidence of rejection and decreased graft survival rates in these patients.

Key words: Cyclosporine sensitivity – HLA-DRw6 phenotype – Kidney transplantation – Incidence of rejection

Studies of renal transplant patients who used cyclosporine (CsA) as part of their immunosuppressive regimen reported an overall increase in renal allograft survival rate of 15 % compared with conventional immunosuppression [9]. The selection of the appropriate CsA dose which produces immunosuppression but not toxicity is complicated by marked inter- and intraindividual variability in the drug pharmacokinetics [2, 6, 8]. Recently, we were able to demonstrate differences of in vitro sensitivity of mixed lymphocyte culture (MLC) to CsA among healthy individuals according to the HLA-DR phenotype of responder cells [12]. Based upon these results, the aim of the present study was to evaluate a possible genetic influence on CsA sensitivity in vivo.

Offprint requests to: Dr. G. Zlabinger, Institute of Immunology, Borschkegasse 8a, A-1090 Vienna, Austria

Patients and methods

We investigated 144 consecutive kidney transplant patients receiving baseline immunosuppression for a possible relationship of HLA-DR phenotype and CsA sensitivity. Some 22 patients were eliminated because of nonhistologically proven rejection episodes and infectious complications. The remaining 122 graft recipients were treated either with prednisolone and CsA ($n = 73$) or prophylactically with antithymocyte globulin (ATG) and/or OKT3; 31 patients received azathioprine in addition. Rejection episodes between days 5 and 13 after transplantation were observed in 70 patients and were proven histologically, whereas an uncomplicated follow-up was seen in 52 patients [13]. The patients were treated with CsA and corticosteroids, and rejection episodes were initially treated with 500 mg methylprednisolone for 3 days. The baseline immunosuppressive therapy consisted of CsA (5 mg/kg day intravenously for 3–4 days followed by oral administration) and methylprednisolone (200 mg at surgery, afterwards reduced to 15 or 10 mg/day). CsA levels were measured for dose adjustment in whole blood, using high-performance liquid chromatography (HPLC) as described previously in detail [3]. An average of the CsA blood levels from 4 consecutive days before starting antirejection therapy was calculated. As patients with and without rejection episodes received an identical immunosuppressive protocol, dosages were comparable in both groups.

HLA-A, -B, -C and -DR antigens were determined according to standardized serological methods. The NIH test was used for HLA-A, -B, -C typing and two-color fluorescence for HLA-DR typing. The rejection frequency in patients with different haplotypes was evaluated χ^2 analysis. Representative CsA levels in patients with and without rejection were correlated to the absence or presence of particular HLA haplotypes using a non-parametric analysis of variance (Kruskal-Wallis). Levels of significance were determined using two-tailed tests.

Results

To approach the matter of CsA sensitivity, we compared graft recipients receiving CsA and prednisolone by specific HLA-DR haplotype for the incidence of rejection episodes and found significantly ($P = 0.045$) more rejections in HLA-DRw6-positive (77 %, 20/26) than in DRw6-negative greft recipients (53 %, 25/47). We observed no statistical significance if transplant patients receiving additional immunotherapy, e.g., OKT3, ATG, azathioprine, were evaluated (Fig. 1).

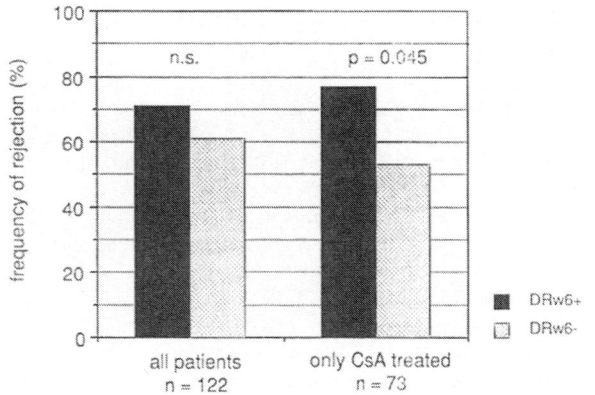

Fig. 1. Incidence of rejection (DRw6 + vs DRw6 −) according to HLA-DR haplotype and type of therapy (CsA, cyclosporine)

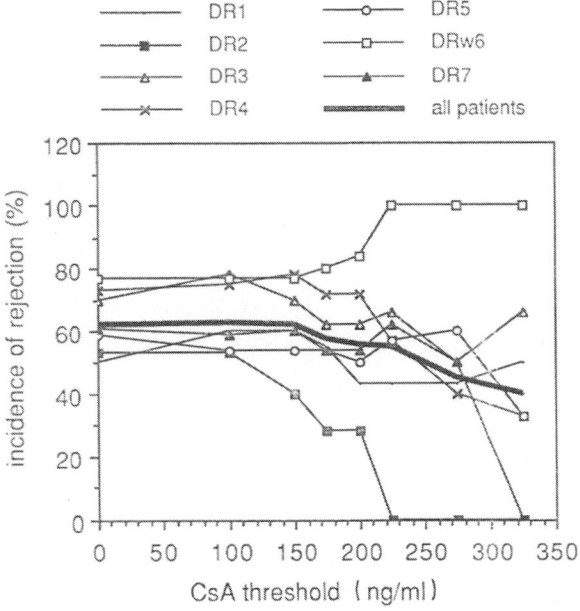

Fig. 2. Incidence of rejection according to HLA-DR haplotype and amount of CsA administered

Upon estimating the frequency of rejection with increasing CsA levels, we found that the relative risk for DRw6-positive graft recipients increased continuously because in this group the incidence of rejection was not influenced substantially by higher CsA levels, whereas in DRw6-negative graft recipients, rejections were less frequent at higher CsA levels (Fig. 2). In contrast, the relative risk for DR2-positive individuals of graft rejection decreased as a function of increasing CsA levels. No difference could be observed concerning the other class II haplotypes. Comparing patients with and without rejection, we found no significant difference in CsA dose between the groups (180 ± 85 ng/ml in rejection vs. 201 ± 91 ng/ml in uncomplicated courses). The mismatch of HLA phenotypes (A, B, DR) was significantly increased ($P = 0.015$) in patients with verified graft rejections (median 3; 0–4) compared with those with an uncomplicated posttransplant course (median 2; 0–4). Since the respective groups were matched similarly, the higher sensitivity of HLA-DR2-positive and the apparent insen-

sitivity of DRw6-positive patients could not be explained by differences in the degree of alloreactivity.

Discussion

To evaluate previous findings that the sensitivity to CsA in vitro might be correlated to the HLA-DR phenotype of the responding cell population in MLC, we investigated whether or not such a relationship could be confirmed in clinical practice [10, 12]. Variation in the immunosuppressive effect of CsA has been observed in transplanted patients [4–8]. Some graft recipients were reported to present with rejection episodes even at higher CsA levels, while others had excellent graft survival despite low CsA levels. An association with superior graft survival has been described for HLA-DR1-, -DR2-, or -DR3-positive patients [1, 9]. DRw6 has been associated with a high responsiveness to transplant antigens as evidenced by more frequent rejection episodes or low graft survival rates in these patients [1, 4, 5]. In the present in vivo study we tested an influence of the HLA-DR phenotype on CsA sensitivity in renal transplant recipients. CsA sensitivity in vivo was determined either by evaluating the rejection frequency in patients with a particular HLA phenotype or by comparing CsA levels within the rejecting or nonrejecting group in patients positive or negative for a particular haplotype. Our findings indicate that the rejection frequency in DRw6-positive patients could not be influenced by increased the CsA levels. Nevertheless, if transplant patients receiving OKT3, ATG, or azathioprine additionally were also evaluated, the DRw6 effect on the incidence of rejection could no longer be observed. DRw6-positive transplant patients who received their graft between 1982 and 1985 and whose immunosuppressive protocol was mainly based on CsA and prednisolone had significantly lower graft survival rates compared with DRw6-negative patients. In patients transplanted between 1986 and 1989 when other immunosuppressive agents (OKT3, ATG, azathioprine) were used more frequently, no such difference could be found (unpublished data). Previous results showed an increased rejection frequency in DRw6-positive patients with high dose prednisolone therapy. Additional ATG treatment improved the graft survival significantly [5]. These results are in good accordance with our findings that more aggressive immunosuppressive agents may overcome the DRw6 effect.

In conclusion, we have demonstrated that individual sensitivity to CsA in vivo might be linked to the class II histocompatibility antigens. At present, it cannot be concluded that CsA therapy should be discountinued in patients possibly insensitive to the drug; however, it might be helpful to use other immunosuppressive agents more frequently.

References

1. Cook D (1986) HLA-DR associated immune responsiveness. In: Terasaki P (ed) Clinical transplants. UCLA Tissue Typing Laboratory, Los Angeles, pp 247–256
2. Ferguson R, Canafax D, Sawchuck R, Simmons R (1986) Cyclosporine blood level monitoring: the early posttransplant period. Transplant Proc 28 (2) [Suppl 1]: 113–116

3. Hamilton G, Roth E, Wallisch E, Tichy F (1985) Semi-automated high performance liquid chromatographic determination of cyclosporine A in whole blood using one-step sample purification and column-switching. J Chromatogr 341: 411–419

4. Hendriks G, Schreuder G, Claas F, D'Amaro J, Persijn G, Cohen B, van Rood J (1983) HLA-DRw6 and renal allograft rejection. BMJ 286: 85–87

5. Hoitsma A, van Lier H, Reekers P, Koene R (1985) Treatment of acute rejection of cadaveric renal allografts with rabbit antithymocyte globulin: influence of blood transfusion and DRw6. Transplant Proc 1: 72–74

6. Kahan BD (1985) Individualization of cyclosporine therapy using pharmacokinetic and pharmacodynamic parameters. Transplantation 40: 457–476

7. Kahan BD, Grevel J (1988) Optimization of cyclosporine therapy in renal transplantation by a pharmacokinetic strategy. Transplantation 46: 631–644

8. Kasiske L, Hein-Duthoy K, Rao V, Awin M (1988) The relationship between cyclosporine pharmacokinetic parameters and subsequent acute rejection in renal transplant recipients. Transplantation 46: 716–722

9. Persijn G, D'Amaro G, De Lange P, Schreuder T, Thorogood J, Zantvoort F, Rood J van (1989) The effect of mismatching and sharing of HLA, B and DR antigens on kidney graft survival in eurotransplant 1982 to 1988. In: Terasaki (ed) Clinical transplant, UCLA Tissue Typing Laboratory, Los Angeles, p 237

10. Povlsen J, Rasmussen A, Madsen M, Lamm L (1990) Ciclosporine-induced immunosuppression in-vitro. Scand J Immunol 32: 45–51

11. Scorza R, Vanoli M Cigognini A, Fabio G, De Bernardi B, Zanussi C (1988) In vitro effects of cyclosporine A on allogenic and autologous lymphocyte stimulation: influence of HLA phenotypes. Transplant Proc 20 [Suppl 2]: 122–124

12. Zlabinger G, Pohanka E, Hajek-Rosenmayer A, Pavlicek E, Watschinger B, Traindl O, Kovarik J (1990) Influence of HLA pehnotypes on the inhibition of in vitro alloreactivity by cyclosporin A. Transplantation 50: 1038–1042

13. Zlabinger G, Ulrich W, Pecherstorfer M, Watschinger B, Traindl O, Meron G, Pohanka E, Wolfram J, Kovarik J (1989) Clinical experience with OKT3 monoclonal antibody for treatment of acute renal allograft rejection based on sequential histological evaluation. Clin Transplant 3: 215–222

Transplant Int (1992) 5 [Suppl 1]: S 559–S 560

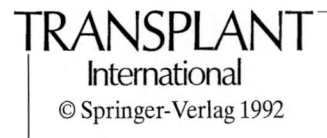

© Springer-Verlag 1992

An immunoglobulin-specific autoantibody occurring during alloimmunization suppresses the antibody response

P. Terness, C. Süsal, C. Baur, and G. Opelz

Department of Transplantation Immunology, Institute of Immunology, University of Heidelberg, Heidelberg, Federal Republic of Germany

Abstract. Our previous studies showed that a broadly reactive immunoglobulin G (IgG) anti-immunoglobulin (IgG-anti-Ig) autoantibody is induced during the immune response of LEW rats to BN blood cells. The present experiments analyze the immunoregulatory effect of this physiological autoantibody on antigen receptor-activated B cells in cell cultures. The results show that: (a) At 0.9 pg IgG-anti-Ig/10^6 B cells, an almost complete suppression of the antibody response is induced; we calculated that a few IgG-anti-Ig molecules are sufficient to suppress the antibody response of one B cell; (b) IgG-anti-Ig-induced B-cell suppression is dose-dependent; (c) IgG-anti-Ig suppresses B cells contained in their natural environment (mixed spleen cell population). These data demonstrate that the IgG-anti-Ig autoantibody is an extremely efficient regulatory molecule of the alloimmune response.

Key words: Immunoregulation – Antibody response – Alloimmunization

We have previously shown that an immunoglobulin G (IgG)-anti-immunoglobulin autoantibody (IgG-anti-Ig) appears in the serum of alloimmunized rats in addition to the donor-specific antibody [4]. Unlike antiidiotypes, this antibody recognizes a conserved domain of the IgG molecule. The current series of experiments addressed the question of whether this antibody has an immunoregulatory function.

Materials and methods

IgG-anti-Ig antibody. LEW rats were repeatedly transfused with 1 ml BN blood cells [5], and the sera of immunized animals with a high IgG-anti-Ig antibody titer were collected. The IgG fraction was separated by protein G chromatography and gel filtration, and anti-Ig was extracted by affinity chromatography on immunoglobulin-coupled sepharose [6].

B-cell separation. Mononuclear spleen cells (5×10^6) of LEW rats separated by density gradient centrifugation were incubated sequentially with 5 µl of mouse anti-rat lymphocyte monoclonal antibodies (Serotec, Oxford, UK) [against T cells, stem cells, plasma cells, Th cells, macrophages, Ts cells, cytotoxic T cells, natural killer (NK) cells], 6 µl goat F(ab′)2-anti-mouse IgG(Fc)-biotin, 3.7 µg avidin, 0.25 µl biotin-labelled magnetic ferrit-polyglucose particles and passed twice through a ferromagnetic separation column (Miltenyi Biotec, Bergisch-Gladbach, FRG).

Cell cultures. B cells (10^6 or mononuclear LEW spleen cells 2×10^6) were stimulated with 23 µg of goat F(ab′)2-anti-rat IgM and supernatant of concanavalin A (ConA)-activated LEW lymphocytes in serum-free medium as previously described [7]. Increasing amounts of affinity purified IgG-anti-Ig were added to the culture. Three days later, the antibody production of B cells was measured in a reverse plaque-forming cell assay (PFC/10^6 cells; $\bar{x} \pm SEM$) [6]. Stimulated cells served as the positive control (100% response) and unstimulated cells, as the negative control (0%).

Results

As increasing amounts of IgG-anti-Ig antibody were added to the culture, the B-cell response gradually decreased (Table 1). At 0.9 pg IgG/10^6 cells, an almost complete suppression was obtained. By increasing the antibody concentration further, the suppressive effect disappeared. IgG obtained from nonimmunized LEW rats ("irrelevant" control IgG) had no effect.

In the absence of T cells, B cells are more sensitive to IgG-induced suppression [3]. In vivo the B cells are part of a mixed cell population including T cells. To establish whether the regulatory antibody also suppresses B cells in their natural environment, spleen lymphocytes were cultured in the presence of suppressive antibody. As shown in Table 2, a similar dose-response curve as that obtained with purified B cells was obtained. The "irrelevant" control IgG had no effect.

Offprint requests to: P. Terness, Department of Transplantation Immunology, Institute of Immunology, University of Heidelberg, Im Neuenheimer Feld 305, W-6900 Heidelberg, Federal Republic of Germany

Table 1. Suppression of B cells by an affinity-purified IgG-anti-Ig autoantibody

Amount (pg IgG/10^6 cells)	B-cell response (%)	
	Irrelevant IgG (control)	IgG-anti-Ig
0.03	106	120
0.06	101	73
0.1	94	54
0.2	114	57 ± 17
0.5	102	48 ± 13
0.9	95	15 ± 15
1.9	107	39 ± 2
3.7	112	39 ± 0.7
7.5	114	40 ± 4
15	115	78 ± 17

Ig, immunoglobulin

Increasing amounts of "irrelevant" control LEW IgG or LEW IgG-anti-Ig were added to antigen receptor-activated purified B cells derived from LEW rats. The B cells' antibody production was determined in a reverse plaque-forming cell assay ($\bar{x} \pm$ SEM of PFC/10^6 cells) after 3 days of culture. The positive control consisted of stimulated B cells (6962 PFC/10^6 cells = 100%) and the negative control of unstimulated B cells (1088 PFC 10^6 cells = 0%). Maximum suppression was obtained at 0.9 pg IgG/10^6 cells

Table 2. Suppression of spleen lymphocytes by an affinity-purified IgG-anti-Ig autoantibody

Amount (pg IgG/10^6 cells)	B-cell response (%)	
	Irrelevant IgG (control)	IgG-anti-Ig
0.01	89	81 ± 7
0.02	94 ± 11	55 ± 6
0.05	98	26 ± 13
0.1	93 ± 5	10 ± 4
0.2	105 ± 9	7 ± 7
0.4	102 ± 2	25 ± 15
0.8	104 ± 11	25 ± 12
1.7	93 ± 7	54 ± 21
3.4	103 ± 5	94 ± 12

Increasing amounts of "irrelevant" control LEW IgG or LEW IgG-anti-Ig were added to antigen receptor-activated LEW spleen lymphocytes. After 3 days the antibody production was determined in a reverse plaque-forming cell assay ($\bar{x} \pm$ SEM of PFC/10^6 cells). The positive control consisted of stimulated cells (8189 PFC/10^6 cells = 100%) and the negative control of unstimulated cells (712 PFC/10^6 cells = 0%). Maximum suppression was obtained at 0.2 pg IgG/10^6 cells

Discussion

The IgG-anti-Ig produced during alloimmunization suppresses the B-cell response. The antibody is effective at extremely small concentrations. Based on the molecular weight of IgG and Avogadro's number, our results indicate that a few antibody molecules are sufficient to suppress the activity of one B cell.

We have reported previously that the mechanism of B-cell suppression by IgG-anti-Ig is Fc receptor-dependent [7]. Others have shown that heterologous Ig-specific anti-bodies crosslink the B cells' antigen receptor with its Fc receptor and that this crosslinking leads to an inactivating signal [2, 1]. In our test system, it is likely that the IgG-anti-Ig autoantibody induces suppression by the antigen receptor/Fc receptor crosslinking. It is known that anti-immunoglobulins have different affinities for the antigen receptor and the Fc receptor [9]. This provides an explanation for our finding that suppression is obtained only at a certain antibody concentration. Whereas an optimum concentration leads to co-crosslinking of the two receptors, higher concentrations may affect only one of the two receptors. An alternative explanation for the suppressive mechanism is the independent occupation of the Fc receptor (by IgG + anti-IgG immune complexes) and the antigen receptor (by its ligand) followed by their cocapping. The resulting sterical adherence of the two receptors leads to an inactivating signal [8].

Unlike our previous experiments [6] in which mitogen-stimulated B cells were studied, the current study analyzes the effect of IgG-anti-Ig on antigen receptor-activated B cells. In addition to this "physiological" B-cell activation, the relevance of our test system for the situation "in vivo" was increased by using antibody and lymphocytes derived from the same rat strain.

Our findings show that the IgG-anti-Ig antibody induced during the alloimmune response is a highly active, self-regulatory molecule of the immune system.

References

1. Bijsterbosch MK, Klaus GGB (1985) Crosslinking of surface immunoglobulin and Fc receptors on B lymphocytes inhibits stimulation of inositol phospholipid breakdown via the antigen receptors. J Exp Med 162: 1825–1836
2. Phillips N, Parker DC (1984) Cross-linking of B lymphocyte $FC\tau$ receptors and membrane immunoglobulin inhibits anti-immunoglobulin-induced blastogenesis. J Immunol 132: 627–632
3. Sinclair NRStC, Lees RK, Chan PL (1976) Interference with antibody-feedback by irradiation, thymus cells, the allogeneic effect, and serum factors. Adv Exp Med Biol 66: 623–633
4. Terness P, Süsal C, Opelz G (1989) IgG-anti-immunoglobulin induced by immunization with antibody-coated blood cells: mechanism for B-cell suppression? Transplant Proc 21: 153–155
5. Terness P, Schiffl R, Süsal C, Guo Z, Opelz G (1990) Long-lasting kidney graft survival after immunization with antibody-coated blood cells: mediation by immunosuppressive autoantibodies. Immunol Lett 26: 139–144
6. Terness P, Süsal C, Baur C, Guo Z, Opelz G (1990) A B-cell suppressive IgG-anti-immunoglobulin antibody induced by alloimmunization. Transplantation 50: 502–505
7. Terness P, Süsal C, Guo Z, Opelz G (1990) Fc-dependent suppression of in vitro B-cell response by IgG of alloimmunized rats. Transplant Proc 22: 1957–1959
8. Uher F, Dickler HB (1986) Cooperativity between B lymphocyte membrane molecules: independent ligand occupancy and cross-linking of antigen receptors and $Fc\tau$ receptors down-regulates B lymphocyte function. J Immunol 137: 3124–3129
9. Wofsy C, Goldstein B (1990) Cross-linking of $Fc\tau$ receptors and surface antibodies. Theory and application. J Immunol 145: 1814–1825

Transplant Int (1992) 5 [Suppl 1]: S 561–S 563

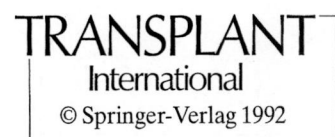

© Springer-Verlag 1992

Prevention of cardiac allograft rejection by FK506 and rapamycin: assessment by histology and nuclear magnetic resonance

B. Walpoth[1], J. Galdikas[1], A. Tschopp[1], F. Lazeyras[2], H. J. Altermatt[3], T. Schaffner[3], U. Althaus[1], M. Billingham[4], and R. Morris[5]

Departments of [1] Thoracic and Cardiovascular Surgery, [2] NMR Unit, and [3] Pathology, University of Berne, Berne, Switzerland,
Departments of [4] Pathology and [5] Cardiothoracic Surgery, Stanford University Medical Center, Stanford, California, USA

Abstract. We assessed the effect of FK506 and rapamycin (RPM) in a heterotopic abdominal rat heart transplant model using a major histocompatibility mismatch (DA to LEW). The end-point of our study was the histologic grading of rejection (Stanford) and ^{31}P magnetic resonance spectroscopy (MRS) at 1 week after transplantation. Two dosages of FK506 (2.0 and 8.0 mg/kg per os daily) and RPM (1.5 and 6.0 mg/kg intraperitoneally daily) were compared in allografts without and with cyclosporine (12.5 mg/kg per os daily) treatment. The results show: Weak heartbeat and full rejection at day 5 in all untreated allografts; severe rejection in groups on a low dose of FK506 and RPM; mild rejection in both high dose groups comparable to the results of the hearts treated with cyclosporine; MRS does not allow differentiation between no or mild forms of rejection. Energy-rich phosphates are near normal in the high dosage immunosuppression groups but show a significant reduction in the low dosage groups. We conclude that all three tested drugs can reduce the degree of rejection from severe (untreated allografts) to mild if given in an adequate dosage. MRS correlates well with the degree of histologic rejection but permits only the diagnosis of moderate or severe rejection.

Key words: Immunosuppression – Cardiac transplantation – Rejection – Magnetic resonance spectroscopy

---

Several serious side-effects have been reported in organ transplantations with various immunosuppressive regimes [1]. The need for life-long drug administration leads to irreversible adverse drug effects including conditions such as hypertension and renal failure or increased incidence of malignancies and consequences from corticosteroid treatment [2]. New immunosuppressive medication with fewer side-effects for long-term treatment or for use as a rescue drug for acute rejection have been proposed, such as FK506 [3, 4] and rapamycin (RPM) [5, 6].

We tested the drug efficacy and toxicity of FK506 and rapamycin in two different dosages and compared their immunosuppressive action with that of cyclosporine (CyA) in the heterotopic rat allotransplant model using a major histocompatibility mismatch (DA to LEW). Alterations of energy-rich phosphate compounds (^{31}P) were assessed in vivo by magnetic resonance spectroscopy (MRS) 1 week after transplantation, followed by euthanasia and histology evaluation.

Method

A major histocompatibility mismatch was used, DA/HAN (AV1) rats serving as donors (10–12 weeks old/200 g) and Lewis – LEW/HAN (RT1) rats as recipients (8–10 weeks old/250 g Hannover strains). For the group of isografts, Lewis rats served as donors and recipients. The classic heterotopic abdominal rat heart transplant model described by Ono and Lindsey was applied [7]. Donor hearts were flushed with ice-cold St. Thomas cardioplegic solution. Warm ischemia ranged between 30 and 35 min. Only well functioning hearts after the completion of transplantation were assigned in turn to a treatment group.

The following immunosuppressive drugs were used: FK506 (Fujisawa Pharmaceuticals Ltd., Osaka, Japan) was given per os by gavage at a dose of 2 mg/kg or (mg/kg pure drug). Rapamycin (RPM; Wyeth-Ayerst Research, Princeton, N. J.) was given by intraperitoneal injection at a dose of 1.5 mg/kg or 6 mg/kg. Both drugs were suspended after micronisation in carboxymethyl cellulose (CMC 0.2%, high viscosity) and further agitated in an ultrasonic bath before use. CyA (Sandoz Pharmaceuticals, Basel, Switzerland) was mixed in olive oil and given by gavage at a dose of 12.5 mg/kg. All drugs were given daily from postoperative day 1 until euthanasia (day 6 or 7).

Table 1 lists the different groups according to the immunosuppressive drug used and the respective dosage. All animals were assessed daily for their general condition, and the heartbeat of the abdominally transplanted heart was noted.

At the end point of our study (1 week), the animals were reanesthetised, and a median laparotomy was performed to allow in vivo MRS measurements. Each acquisition consisted of 512 FIDs (repetition time 2.0–2.4 s, spectral width ± 2000 Hz, resolution 4096 points) performed on a 2-T General Electric-CSI wide bore

Offprint requests to: Dr. B. Walpoth, Department of Thoracic and Cardiovascular Surgery, Inselspital, CH-3010 Berne, Switzerland

Table 1. Groups and number of animals listed according to immunosuppression and dosage after transplantation

Groups	POD	Dosage (mg/kg)	Number
Isografts (LEW-LEW)	10.5	–	6
Allografts (DA-LEW)	4.8	–	6
+ CyA	7.6	12.5	6
+ FK506 (low)	7.0	2	5
+ FK506 (high)	6.3	8	6
+ RPM (low)	6.0	1.5	5
+ RPM (high)	5.8	6	6

POD, mean postoperative day of examination; CyA, cyclosporine; RPM, rapamycin

magnet with a double tuned, 15-mm surface coil placed around the apex of the transplanted heart. Quantification of the spectroscopy scan was carried out using a Lorentzian curve-fitting procedure. MRS results are expressed as ratios between energy-rich phosphates such as phosphocreatine (PCr) or adenosine triphosphate (β-ATP) and inorganic phosphate (Pi). After the completion of MRS, the animals were euthanised and the hearts excised for histology evaluation (hematoxylin & eosin and Mason's trichrome stains). Five transverse sections of each heart were reviewed by two independent pathologists. The histologic evaluation of rejection was performed according to the classic Stanford grading system [8]: 0 = no signs of rejection, 1 = mild rejection with focal perivascular infiltrates, 2 = moderate rejection with additional focal myocyte necrosis, 3 = severe rejection with the above and focal hemorrhage.

Results

The efficacy of the tested immunosuppressive drugs was assessed by MRS alterations and the histologic degree of rejection at the end-point of our study. Table 2 summarises the results according to the different groups.

Graft survival and histology

All isografts survived well and showed a strong heartbeat up to euthanasia. The hearts did not reveal any signs of rejection histologically.

All untreated allografts survived well, but the transplanted heart showed a weak heartbeat or ceased to beat between days 5 and 6 and showed severe rejection on all histologic sections (grade 3).

Allografts treated with cyclosporine showed a strong heartbeat on day 7, and the animals tolerated the dosage of 12.5 mg/kg well. On histology the mean rejection score was 0.8, ranging from 0.4 to 1.0.

Animals treated with low dose FK506 had no adverse reaction to the drug but demonstrated a decreased heartbeat strength, with 1 heart out of 5 showing no function at day 7. The mean score of rejection was 2.4 (moderate to severe), ranging from 2 to 3.

In the high dose FK506 group all grafts showed a strong heartbeat, and histology revealed a mild degree of rejection (1.2) ranging from 0.5 to 1.5.

In the low dose RPM group all transplanted hearts either showed poor heartbeats or had ceased beating by 6 days after transplantation. Histologic analysis showed a mean grading of rejection of 2.8, ranging from 2.5 to 3.0.

In the high dose RPM group the heartbeats were strong, and the grafts looked normal. On histology the mean grading was 1.1 (mild rejection) with a range from 0.5 to 1.5.

Adverse reactions to immunosuppression

Except for 2 animals (1 FK506 high dose and 1 RPM high dose) showing symptoms consistent with drug toxicity (weight loss and lethargy despite a well-functioning transplanted heart), no lesion patterns indicative of drug toxicity were found upon histology examination of the animals' own heart, lungs, liver, kidneys, and pancreas. Only 1 animal in the FK506 high dose group receiving a daily dose of 10.5 mg/kg showed swollen kidneys and severe edema of most organs, probably a sign of drug toxicity.

Magnetic resonance spectroscopy

The assessment of energy metabolism by MRS is represented in Fig. 1 (spectrum from one animal) and by groups in Table 2; results are expressed as ratios between energy-rich phosphates and inorganic phosphate such as PCr/Pi or β-ATP/Pi. In isografts and in allografts with adequate immunosuppressive therapy, that is high doses of CyA, FK506, or RPM, no significant alterations in the phosphate metabolism could be detected (mild rejection on histology).

On the other hand, untreated allografts or allografts with insufficient immunosuppression (moderate to severe rejection) such as FK506 low dose or RPM low dose, the PCr/Pi and β-ATP/Pi ratios decreased significantly ($P < 0.05$) by 50% or more (Table 2).

Discussion

In our study we were able to show that relatively high doses of the three tested immunosuppressive drugs, i.e., CyA, FK506, and RPM, controlled the severe rejection that occurred in untreated allografts. Comparing our results with those published by R. Morris at Stanford

Table 2. Magnetic resonance spectroscopy (MRS) phosphate ratios and histologic degree of rejection according to groups

Groups	PCr/Pi	β-ATP/Pi	Rejection[a]
Isografts (LEW-LEW)	2.4 ± 0.9	1.1 ± 0.3	0
Allografts (DA-LEW)	1.6 ± 0.7	0.7 ± 0.5	3.0
+ CyA	2.3 ± 0.8	1.0 ± 0.2	0.8 ± 0.5
+ FK506 (low)	1.1 ± 0.1*	0.6 ± 0.2*	2.4 ± 0.8
+ FK506 (high)	2.3 ± 0.7	0.8 ± 0.4	1.2 ± 0.4
+ RPM (low)	1.0 ± 0.8*	0.5 ± 0.2*	0.8 ± 1.2
+ RPM (high)	1.9 ± 0.2	1.0 ± 0.1	1.1 ± 0.4

MRS result is expressed as ratios between energy-rich phosphates such as phosphocreatine (PCr) or adenosine triphosphate (β-ATP) and inorganic phosphate (Pi)

[a] Degree of rejection is based on the classic Stanford grading [ST] (0–3)

Results are expressed as mean values ± 1 SD. Significance by Student's t-test; * $P < 0.05$

Sequential 31P of an untreated rejecting heart

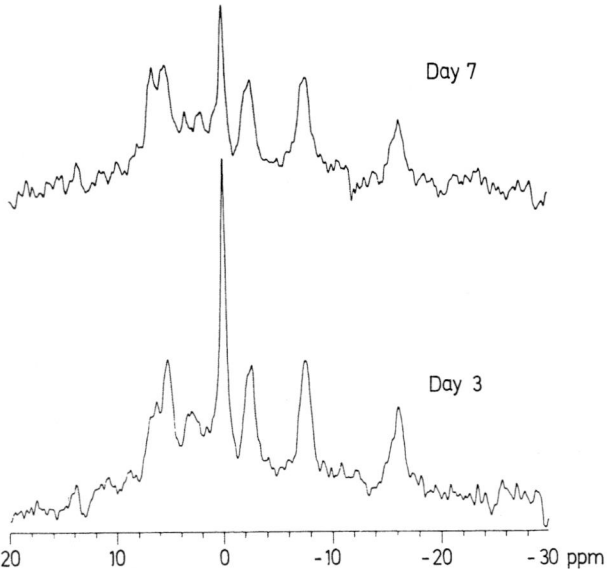

Fig. 1. Sequential ^{31}P MRS of an untreated rejecting heart. Peaks from left to right: phosphomonoester *(PME)*, inorganic phosphate *(Pi)*, phosphodiester *(PDE)*, phosphocreatine *(PCr)*, adenosine triphosphate $(\gamma, \alpha, \beta\text{-}ATP)$. Represented are a near normal ^{31}P spectrum 3 days after heterotopic transplantation *(lower panel)* and a severely altered spectrum of the same animal after 7 days *(upper panel)* with decreased PCr and ATP and increased PME and Pi (untreated allograft with severe histological rejection)

University using the same drug, it is noteworthy that he obtained a good level of immunosuppression with lower doses than we did [5, 9]. One possible explanation might be the different rat strains used. According to the literature and our own experience, the combination of DA to LEW rats seems to count among the strongest major histocompatibility mismatch models as reflected in our series by the cessation of heartbeat and full histologic rejection at day 5 to 6 in untreated allografts [10].

We purposefully set the end-point of our study at 1 week (most severe immune response) to assess the efficacy of immunosuppression [11]. As seen in Table 1, the mean postoperative day of the histologic examination varied only between days 6 and 7 for the treated allografts, whereas in the untreated allografts it was on average at 4.8 days due to the rapid deterioration of the graft (weak heartbeat). In contrast, isografts were doing well even at 10 days since in this group no immunological reaction occurred.

MRS findings correlated well with histologic grading in moderate or severe rejection, but MRS was not sensitive enough to differentiate between no and mild rejection. This might be due to the sparse and focal myocardial involvement seen in mild rejection.

The relatively good MRS results obtained in the untreated allografts are biased due to the early postoperative MRS assessment (4.8 versus 7 days in the other groups) necessary to perform in vivo MRS on beating hearts. Our MRS findings are less sensitive but comparable with the ones reported by Canby et al. [12] and Fraser et al. [13].

In conclusion, high doses of CyA, FK506, and RPM achieved adequate immunosuppression even in our strong major histocompatibility mismatch model, since none of the hearts showed more than mild (clinically not requiring treatment) or mild to moderate rejection at 1 week after transplantation. However, further investigations are needed to assess the possible toxic effects of FK506 and RPM at high dose levels. MRS findings confirm alterations in the phosphorous metabolism in moderately to severely rejecting hearts.

Acknowledgments. We would particularly like to thank the personnel of the central pharmacy who weighed and mixed the drugs for each animal under the expert guidance of Dr. Sonderegger. Our thanks go as well to Mr. Aebi from the Institute of Pathophysiology for taking good care of our animals and to Mrs. Binggeli from the Department of Pathology for preparing the histologic sections. This work was partly supported by the Stiftung zur Förderung der wissenschaftlichen Forschung an der Universität Bern.

References

1. Burdine J, Fischel RJ, Bolman RD (1990) Cardiac transplantation. Crit Care Clin 4: 927–945
2. Miller LW (1991) Long-term complications of cardiac transplantation. Prog Cardiovasc Dis 4: 229–82
3. Armitage JM, Kormos RL, Griffith BP, Hardesty RL, Fricker FJ, Stuart RS, Marrone GC, Todo S, Fung J, Starzle TE (1991) A clinical trial of FK506 as primary and rescue immunosuppression in cardiac transplantation. Transplant Proc 1: 1149–1152
4. Hildebrandt A, Meiser B, Human P, Reichenspurner H, Rose A, Odell J, Reichart B (1991) FK506 short- and long-term treatment after cardiac transplantation in nonhuman primates. Transplant Proc 1: 509–510
5. Morris RE (1991) Rapamycin: FK506's fraternal twin or distant cousin? Elsevier Science, London
6. Stepkowski SM, Chen H, Daloze P, Kahan BD (1991) Rapamycin, a potent immunosuppressive drug for vascularised heart, kidney, and small bowel transplantation in the rat. Transplantation 51: 22–26
7. Ono K, Lindsey ES (1969) Improved techniques of heart transplant in rats. J Thorac Cardiovasc Surg 57: 225–229
8. Billingham ME (1982) Diagnosis of cardiac rejection by endomyocardial biopsy. Heart Transplant 1: 25–30
9. Morris RE, Meiser BM (1989) Identification of a new pharmacologic action for an old compound. Med Sci Res 17: 609–610
10. Andrzejewski W, Brolsch C (1982) Postoperative reactions of rats after orthotopic liver transplantation: a model for the human response? A histological and biochemical study. Eur Surg Res 14: 428–439
11. DiSesa VJ, Masetti P, Diaco M, Schoen FJ, Marsh JD, Cohn LH (1991) The mechanism of heart failure caused by cardiac allograft rejection. J Thorac Cardiovasc Surg 101: 446–449
12. Canby RC, Evanochko WT, Barrett LV, Kirklin JK, McGriffin DC, Sakai TT, Brown ME, Foster RE, Reeves RC, Pohost GM (1987) Monitoring the bioenergetics of cardiac allograft rejection using in vivo P-31 nuclear magnetic spectroscopy. J Am Coll Cardiol 9: 1067–1074
13. Fraser CD Jr, Chacko VP, Jacobus WE, Soulen RL, Hutchins GM, Reitz BA, Baumgartner WA (1988) Metabolic changes preceding functional and morphologic indices of rejection in heterotopic cardiac allografts. Transplantation 46: 346–351

Transplant Int (1992) 5 [Suppl 1]: S 564–S 567

TRANSPLANT
International
© Springer-Verlag 1992

New morphological changes induced by FK506 in a short period in the rat kidney and the effect of superoxide dismutase and OKY-046 on THEM: the relationship of FK506 nephrotoxicity to lipid peroxidation and change in production of thromboxane A_2 in the kidney

K. Yamada[1], Y. Sugisaki[1], S. Suzuki[3], M. Akimoto[2], H. Amemiya[3], and N. Yamanaka[1]

Departments of [1] Pathology and [2] Urology, Nippon Medical School, [3] Department of Surgical Research, National Cardiovascular Center, Osaka, Japan

Abstract. Juxtaglomerular (JG) hyperplasia and tubular damage along with a decrease in the urine creatinine level induced by FK506 in rat kidney have already been reported in previous paper by us [6]. In this paper, we document the relationship of FK506 nephrotoxicity to the change in the production of thromboxane (Tx) A_2 and the lipid peroxidation of the cellular membrane in the rat kidney in order to clarify its morphogenesis. The urinary excretion of TxB_2 increased with FK506 administration even on day 1 ($P < 0.02$). Histologically, OKY-046 (thromboxane synthetase inhibitor) decreased tubular damage, although JG hyperplasia was not eradicated, while biochemically the excretion of TxB_2 decreased significantly ($P < 0.02$), and both the decrease in the urine creatinine level and the increase in the N-acetyl-β,D-glucosaminidase (NAG) index were relatively smaller. Although the FK506-induced morphological and biochemical changes could not be prevented by the continuous administration of superoxide dismutase (SOD) 30000 U/kg daily, the malondialdehyde content in renal tissue removed 1 h after FK506 administration had increased. These data suggest that FK506 nephrotoxicity is related to the change in the production of TxA_2 and lipid peroxidation of the cellular membrane. However, other mechanisms such as the involvement of sympathomimetic effects of FK506 and other vasoconstrictive factors cannot be rules out.

Key words: FK506 – Nephrotoxicity – JG hyperplasia – Thromboxane – Tubular damage – Vasoconstriction

FK506 is a potent immunosuppressive agent in vitro and in vivo in animals and shows great promise as a powerful means of inducing long-term allograft acceptance in the clinical setting [1–3]. However, there is a paucity of reports concerning morphological studies on nephrotoxicity, although some reports suggest that FK506 induces nephrotoxicity [4, 5]. In a previous paper, we reported that FK506

induced morphological changes [juxtaglomerular (JG) hyperplasia and tubular damage] in the rat kidney [6]. In this paper, we discuss the relationship of FK506 nephrotoxicity to the change in the production of thromboxane (Tx) A_2 and the lipid peroxidation of the cellular membrane in the rat kidney.

Materials and methods

In total, 33 8-week-old female SPF Wistar rats, purchased from a commercial breeder, were used. FK506 freezed-dry powder was supplied by Fujisawa Pharmaceutical, Osaka, Japan. It was dissolved in saline for intraperitoneal injection. OKY-046 (thromboxane synthetase inhibitor) was supplied by Ono Pharmaceutical, Osaka, Japan).

It was dissolved in water for oral administration. Recombinant human superoxide dismutase (SOD) was supplied by Nippon Kayaku, Osaka, Japan. It was dissolved in saline for intravenous administration.

Rats were randomly divided into 5 groups, with 4 rats each in groups 1, 2, and 3; 18 in group 4; and 3 in group 5. Animals in group 1 were given FK506 10 mg/kg daily intraperitoneally for 7 days. Animals in group 2 were given OKY 100 mg/kg daily orally in combination with FK506 10 mg/kg daily intraperitoneally for 7 days. Animals in group 3 were administered SOD 30000 U/kg daily continuously with an osmotic pump (ALZET; model 2001) in combination with FK506 10 mg/kg daily intraperitoneally for 7 days. The osmotic pump was set in the subcutaneous tissue and connected with the polyethylene catheter. The other side of the catheter was inserted into the left iliac vein, and its tip was kept in the inferior vena cava. In group 4, animals were administered intraperitoneally with FK506 10 mg/kg only once. As a control for group 4, group 5 animals were not given any drug. The first day of drug administration is classified hereafter as day 0.

Each kidney was removed 24 h after the last injection of FK506 for morphological examination in groups 1, 2, and 3; and 0.5, 1, 2, 4, 8, and 24 h after FK506 injection for measuring of malondialdehyde (MDA) content in group 4. The kidneys in group 5 animals were removed, too. For morphological examination, H & E, PAS (periodic acid Schiff), Masson trichrome and PAM (periodic acid methenamine silver) stains were employed, and some kidneys were examined under the electron microscope. Renal tissue for the measuring of MDA was frozen at −80°C. Urine samples over 24 h were collected on day 0 (from 24 h to just before the first administration of FK506), as well as on days 1, 3 and 7 to check the creatinine level, N-acetyl-β,D-glucosaminidase (NAG) activity, and TxB_2 content. The

Offprint requests to: K. Yamada, Department of Pathology, Nippon Medical School, 1-1-5 Sendagi, Bunkyo-ku, Tokyo 113, Japan

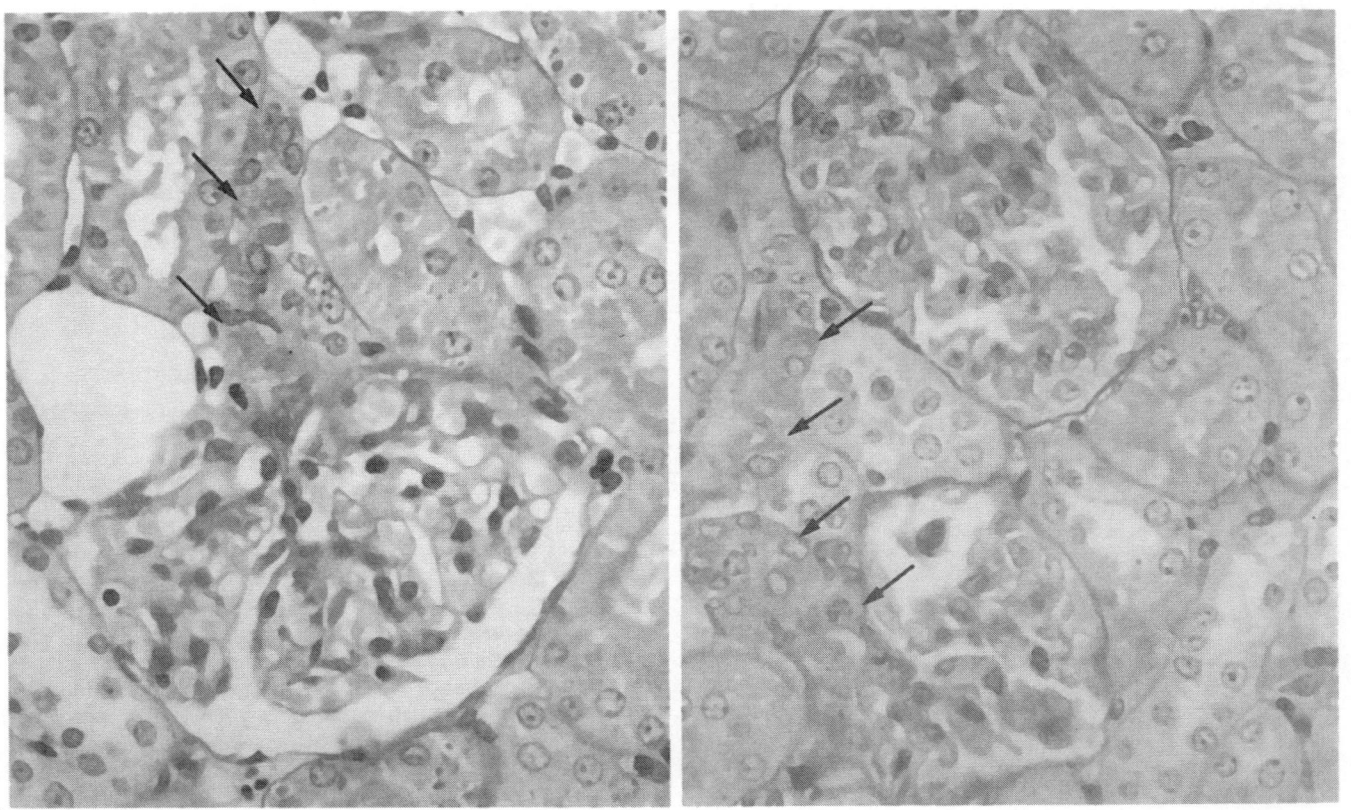

Fig. 1 A, B. Juxtaglomerular (JG) hyperplasia with a lot of renin granules in JG cell *(arrow)*. No significant differences between group 1 (**A**) and group 2 (**B**) (PAS, original magnification × 100)

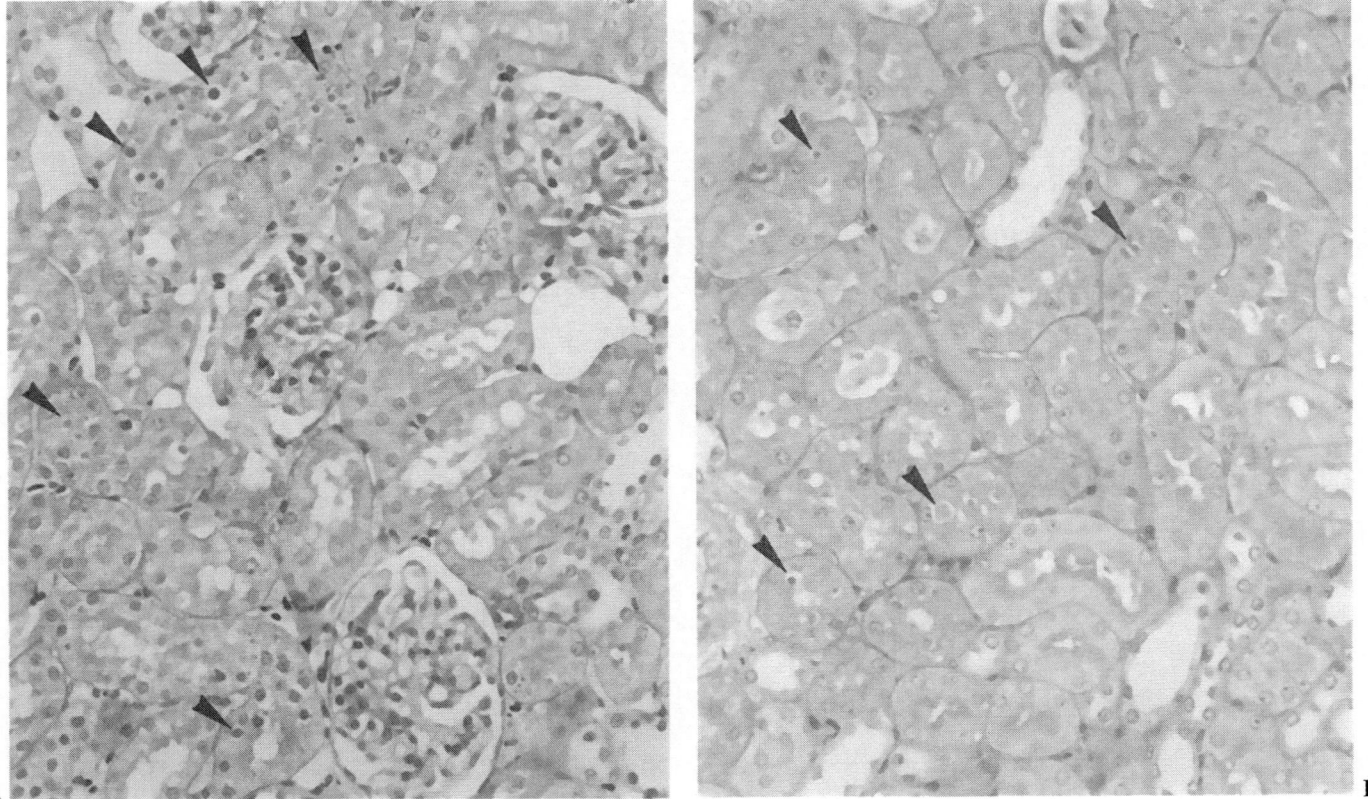

Fig. 2 A, B. PAS-stain positive large granules *(arrowheads)* in the proximal tubules prominent in group 1 (**A**), less prominent in group 2 (**B**) (PAS, original magnification × 50)

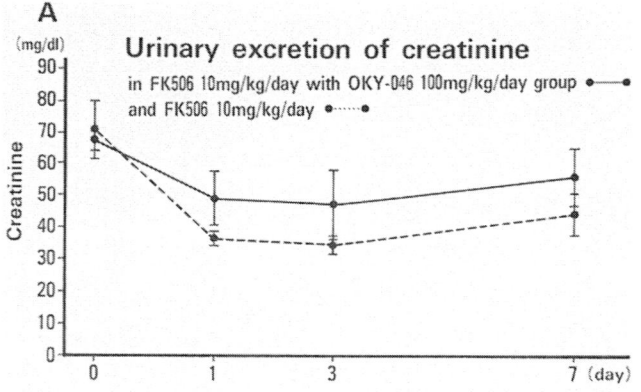

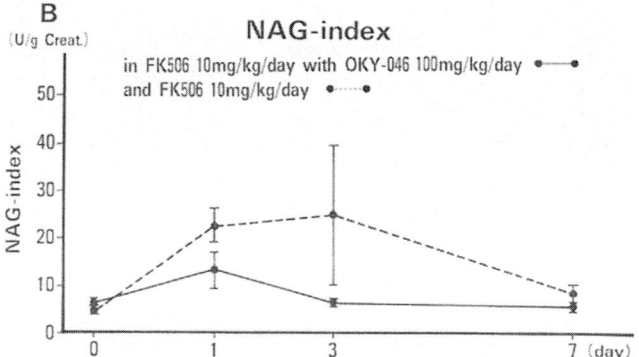

Fig. 3 A, B. Sequential changes of urine creatinine (**A**) and *N*-acetyl-β,D-glucosamini (NAG) index (**B**)

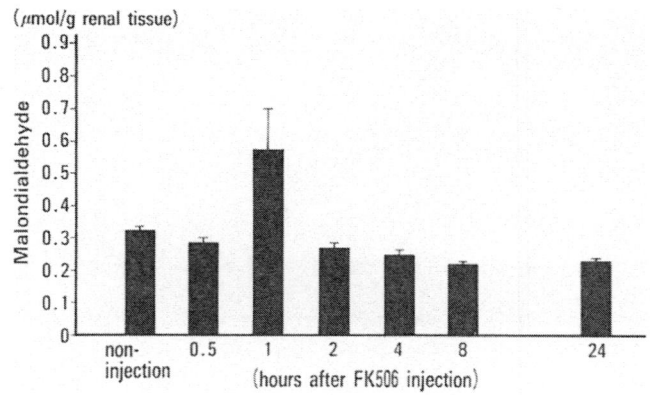

Fig. 5. Malondialdehyde content in renal tissue in groups 4 and 5

urine creatinine level was measured by colorimetry, and the NAG activity was measured by the alkali picrate method. TxB$_2$ was determined by radioimmunoassay (RIA). The concentration of FK506 in whole blood, i.e., the trough level, was determined by enzyme-linked immunosorbet assay (ELISA). In group 4, the MDA content in the kidneys removed at 0.5, 1, 2, 4, 8, and 24 h after FK506 administration was measured as a marker of lipid peroxidation of the cellular membrane by quantitating thiobarbiturate reactive substances (TRA-RS) and conjugated dienes by the methods of Ohkawa et al. and Suryanarayana and Recknagel, using high-performance liquid chromatography (HPLC). The MDA level was also checked in group 5, the control group.

Statistical analysis. Student's *t*-test was used for the statistical analysis of data for each group.

Results

Under morphological examination, juxtaglomerular (JG) hyperplasia and JG cell transformation as vascular change and PAS-positive large granules in the epithelial cells of the proximal tubules, especially at S1 and S2, as tubular damage were observed in group 1, as described in our previous paper [6] (Fig. 1 A, 2 A). In group 2, after the administration of both FK506 and OKY, PAS-positive large granules in the epithelial cells of the proximal tubules were less prominent and smaller in size compared with group 1 (Fig. 2 B). JG hyperplasia was almost the same as in group 1, although the expansion of the JG cell was slightly less prominent (Fig. 1 B). As for the biochemical data in group 1, the urinary excretion of creatinine declined significantly until day 3 ($P < 0.05$) (Fig. 3 A) and that of TxB$_2$ was significantly higher at days 1 ($P < 0.02$), 3, and 7 ($P < 0.05$) compared with preadministration values (Fig. 4 A). In group 2, the urinary excretion of TxB$_2$ was significantly low throughout the experimental period compared with the preadministration value ($P < 0.02$) (Fig. 4 B). Furthermore, both the decrease in the urine creatinine level and the increase in the NAG index during the experimental period were less than in group 1, although not critically so (Fig. 3 B). The urine creatinine level decreased by 37.5 % from day 0 to day 7 in group 1, while in group 2, it decreased by 16.1 % over the same period.

In group 3, histological changes induced by FK506 could not be prevented by the continuous administration

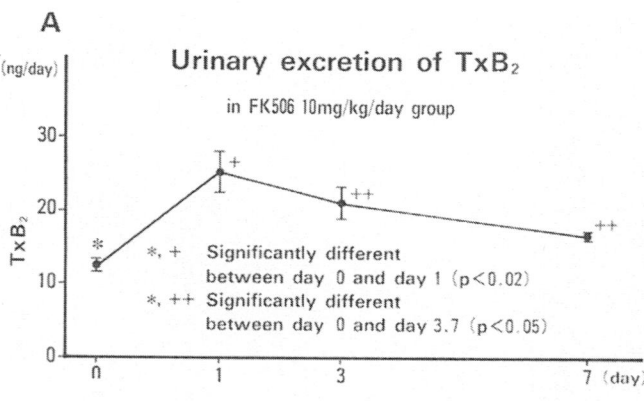

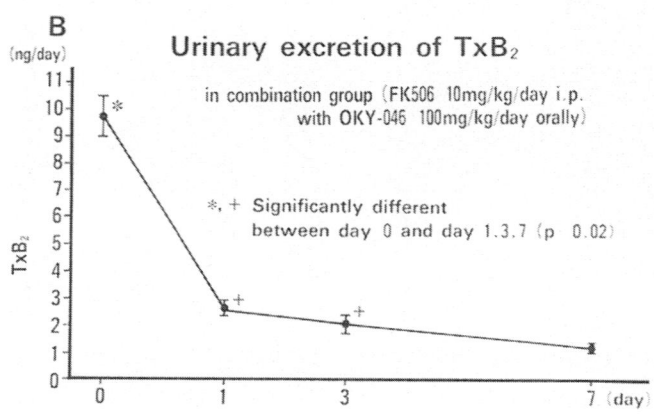

Fig. 4 A, B. Sequential changes sof urinary excretion of thromboxane (TxB$_2$) in group 1 (**A**) and Group 2 (**B**)

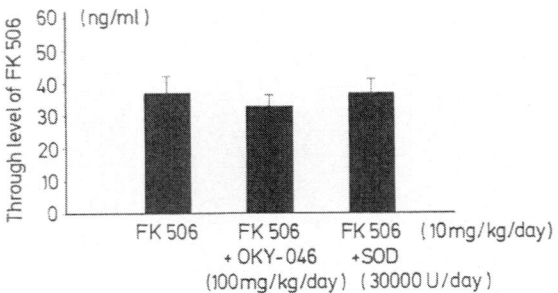

Fig. 6. Concentration of FK506 in whole blood, i.e., trough level, in groups 1, 2, and 3 on day 7 after injection. SOD, superoxide dismutase

of SOD 30000 U/kg daily; however, a relatively slight decrease in PAS-positive granules was observed. Although SOD was not effective, the MDA content in renal tissue removed 1 h after FK506 administration increased in group 4 compared with group 5 (Fig. 5). This rise is compatible with the peak level of FK506 concentration in whole blood (data not given here) when the aforementioned dosage of FK506 is administered intraperitoneally.

The concentration of FK506 in whole blood, i.e., the trough level, in groups 1, 2, and 3 was not significantly higher than in the clinical setting and was not significantly different in each group (Fig. 6).

Discussion

The present study suggests that the morphogenesis of nephrotoxicity induced by a daily intraperitoneal injection of FK506 even for a short period is related to both the change in the production of TxA_2 and the peroxidation of the cellular membrane in the rat kidney. FK506 induces vasoconstriction, especially proximal to the JGA. This vasoconstriction decreases the glomerular blood flow, which in turn causes JG hyperplasia as a compensatory reaction. This hypothesis is compatible with the biochemical data from group 1. The increase in the urinary excretion of TxB_2 even on day 1 suggests vasoconstriction in the renal vessels. Recent work by Benigni et al. [7] indicates that the urinary excretion of TxB_2 reflects the renal cell production of the TxA_2-strong vasoconstrictor, while an increased urinary excretion of 2,3-dinor-TxB_2 reflects TxA_2 synthesis by intrarenal platelets and macrophages. Furthermore, Petric et al. [8] demonstrated that a significant increase in the urinary TxB_2 excretion, along with a decrease in the renal blood flow, creatinine clearance, and urea clearance occurs in Sprague-Dayley rats treated with cyclosporin A. Hence, in our study, the increase in the urinary excretion of TxB_2 associated with FK506 administration in group 1 represents an increased production of TxA_2, specifically in the renal parenchyma. The decrease in the urine creatinine level is compatible with the decrease in the glomerular blood flow, and the increase in the urine creatinine level on day 7 may be a compensatory reaction caused by the decrease in the glomerular blood flow.

Although OKY could completely inhibit the increase in the urinary excretion of TxB_2 induced by FK506, morphological changes, especially in the JGA, could hardly be prevented. Therefore, other mechanisms like the involvement of sympathomimetic effects of FK506 and other vasoconstrictive factors causing the decrease in the glomerular blood flow cannot be ruled out. The rise of MDA in renal tissue 1 h after FK506 injection signifies damage to the cellular membrane, which would encourage the release of vasoconstrictive factors. TxA_2 is one of the strongest vasoconstrictors, and it is important to inhibit the stimulated synthesis of TxA_2 to prevent the vasoconstriction induced by FK506. For further confirmation of the relationship between vasoconstriction and peroxidation of the cellular membrane, experiments with an optimal dosage of SOD and other free radical scavengers and antagonists for vasoconstrictive factors are also necessary. The fact that the decrease in the urine creatinine level in group 2 was relatively less than that in group 1 indicates that the decrease in the number of PAS-positive large granules in the proximal tubules in group 2 might be related to the changes in the urine creatinine level caused by the change in the glomerular blood flow. If the glomerular blood flow decreases, a disturbance in the function of the tubular epithelial cell occurs. Our data on the daily morphological changes induced by FK506 suggests that the tubular damage changes with time and is related to the glomerular blood flow (manuscript in preparation). Hence, the decrease of the tubular damage in group 2 might be attributed to the slightly smaller decrease in the urine creatinine level compared with group 1.

Although the injection dose of FK506 might be thought too high, the trough level of FK506 in groups 1, 2, and 3 was not significantly higher than that in the clinical setting and was not significantly different in each group.

References

1. Goto T, Kino T, Hatanaka H, Nishiyama M, Okuhara M, Kohsaka M, Aoki H, Imanaka H (1987) Discovery of FK506, a novel immunosuppressant isolated from *Streptomyces tsukabaensis*. Transplant Proc 19 [Suppl 6]: 4–8
2. Ochiai T, Sakamoto K, Nagata M, Nakajima K, Goto T, Hori S, Kenmochi T, Nakagori T, Asano T, Isono K (1988) Studies on FK506 in experimental organ transplantation. Transplant Proc 20 [Suppl 1]: 209–214
3. Starzl T, Todo S, Fung J, Demetris A, Venkataramman R, Jain A (1989) FK506 for liver, kidney and pancreas transplantation. Lancet II: 1000–1004
4. Ochiai T, Sakamoto K, Gunji Y, Hamaguchi K, Isegawa N, Suzuki T, Shimada H, Hayashi H, Yasumoto A, Asano T, Isono K (1989) Effect of combination treatment with FK506 and cyclosporine on survival time and vascular changes in renal-allograft-recipient dog. Transplantation 48: 193–197
5. Kumano K, Wang G, Endo T, Kuwao S (1991) FK506 induced nephrotoxicity in rats. Transplant Proc 23: 512–515
6. Yamada K, Sugisaki Y, Akimoto M, Yamanaka N (1991) Short term FK506 induced morphological changes in rat kidney. Transplant Proc (in press)
7. Benigni A, Chiabrando C, Piccinelli A, Perico N, Gavinelli M, Furci L, Patino O, Abbate M, Bertani T, Remuzzi G (1988) Increased urinary excretion of thromboxane B_2 and 2,3-dinor-TxB_2 in cyclosporine A nephrotoxicity. Kidney Int 34: 164–174
8. Petric R, Freeman D, Wallace C (1988) Effect of cyclosporine on urinary prostanoid excretion, renal blood flow, and glomerulo-tubular function. Transplantation 45: 883

Immunology

Transplant Int (1992) 5 [Suppl 1]: S 571–S 577

TRANSPLANT
International
© Springer-Verlag 1992

Is tolerance a prospective for clinical research?

John W. Fabre

Division of Cell and Molecular Biology, The Institute of Child Health, 30 Guilford Street, London, WC1N 1EH, UK

Tolerance is an emotive issue in transplantation. It is the promised land for which we all strive and which we all hope we shall live to see. In such circumstances, tolerance must always be a prospective for clinical research! The question is, therefore, better posed in a more optimistic fashion and with a small act of faith: do we, in 1991, have that crucial combination of basic scientific knowledge and creative imagination to make it possible?

Key words: Tolerance induction – Non specific immunosuppression – T cells

Definitions and objectives

Tolerance can be most simply defined in operational terms as graft acceptance without the use of non-specific immunosuppressive agents. More precisely, it is donor-specific immunosuppression. The important thing to bear in mind is that the objective of introducing tolerance in the clinic is improved safety (e. g. fewer infections) and improved efficacy (i. e. fewer rejections). Of course, perfect safety and perfect efficacy is the ideal. But either improved safety alone or improved efficacy alone are honourable enough objectives in the shorter term. There are three broad possibilities with regard to clinical application:

1. Tolerance without any non-specific immunosuppression.
2. Tolerance with some non-specific immunosuppression, probably limited to the days, weeks or months after grafting. The objective here is to make a clinically useful reduction in the patient's burden of non-specific immunosuppression.
3. Tolerance with normal non-specific immunosuppression. The aim here is to improve efficacy.

Historical perspectives

The key discovery in the field was made in 1945 by Owen [1]. He observed that dizygotic cattle twins almost invariably have identical blood groups. Building on Lillie's earlier observation that cattle twins share vascular connections in utero by way of synchorial placentae [2], Owen proposed that the consequent exchange of haematopoietic precursors in foetal life resulted in the life-long acceptance of these foreign cells. He was, of course, absolutely correct and was able to demonstrate that the adult twins were stable haematopoietic chimaeras. It was on the foundation of Owen's observation that MacFarlane-Burnett proposed, in 1949, his brilliant clonal selection theory of immunity [3]. The seal was set on this phase of development of the field when Billingham et al. [4] reproduced in the laboratory what Owen had observed in nature. They induced the life-long acceptance of skin allografts in mice by the simple expedient of injecting donor haematopoietic cells during foetal life.

Although the experimental model of Billingham et al. [4] was of no immediate clinical relevance, the experiments were of great importance. The work of Owen and of Billingham et al. has demonstrated that the spectrum of antigens regarded as self is not a fixed and immutable characteristic, but an acquired characteristic subject to experimental and, therefore, potentially, therapeutic manipulation.

Preliminary points

There are three preliminary points which are useful to consider as a background to the more detailed discussion on tolerance.

1. The T-cell is the only important target
Although allograft rejection is a complex phenomenon involving many cell types and soluble factors, everything depends on the T-cell. If the T-cell is neutralised, nothing

Offprint requests to: John W. Fabre

happens. Therefore, the only target that needs to be considered for tolerance induction is the T-cell.

2. The thymic and peripheral compartments

A second and potentially very important point is that there exist two distinct T-cell compartments, and each needs to be considered separately for tolerance induction. These are the thymic and peripheral compartments. The peripheral compartment is the pool of mature T cells in the lymph nodes, blood, spleen and so on, which are present at the moment the vascular clamps are released and which are ready to attack the graft. Once sensitized, long-lived T cells with specificity for the graft can be generated. The thymic compartment continuously produces throughout our lives new T cells and seeds them into the peripheral compartment. There is no a priori reason why these new T cells should not have specificity for and be able to attack the graft. This generation of new T cells, although most marked in young persons, nevertheless persists throughout life.

3. Mechanisms of clonal T cell inactivation

There are believed to be three mechanisms:

(a) Clonal deletion. This involves destruction of the specifically reactive T-cell. Although clonal deletion is believed to occur mainly in the thymus [5], it has also been reported for peripheral T cells [6].

(b) Clonal anergy. This is a relatively new concept, and conveys the idea that the T cell is functionally inactivated, but not killed. It is believed to occur when T cells make contact with an antigen in the absence of costimulatory signals necessary for activation [7]. The anergic state is poorly understood. Although it is believed to occur mainly in the periphery, anergy might also be induced to some degree in the thymus [8].

(c) Clonal suppression. This is a familiar concept and implies the active suppression of a T cell clone by other T cells. Although the phenomenon is a real and powerful one, it is poorly understood [9].

Advances in basic science

Over the past 5 years there have been huge advances in our knowledge of two areas of basic immunology of immediate relevance to transplantation. These are the physiology of self tolerance and the nature of T-cell allorecognition in transplantation. These advances provide us with crucially important guide-lines for our objective of achieving tolerance in the clinic.

1. The physiology of self tolerance

Throughout our lives, T cell precursors from the bone marrow enter the thymus. These cells express neither CD4 or CD8 antigens nor any chains of the T cell receptor. They give rise to two types of T-cell, distinguished by the type of antigen receptor expressed [10]. A minor component become γδ T cells, which emigrate from the thymus and accumulate preferentially in the skin and mucosal surfaces. Although it is not yet certain, the available data suggest that γδ T cells do not play an important role in allo-recognition [11]. We can probably afford to ignore them in our discussion of tolerance, but we must not forget them entirely.

The major population of T cells has the αβT cell receptor, and in the course of its maturation it goes through two selection steps. Early in its development, the αβT cell co-expresses the CD4 and CD8 molecules and goes through a positive selection step by interacting with the epithelial cells of the thymus cortex. It is at this stage that the bias towards self (more precisely, towards the MHC molecules on the thymic epithelial cells), or the property of self MHC restriction, is acquired. Those T cells that have antigen receptors with too low an affinity for the MHC molecules on the thymic epithelium die by neglect. There then follows a negative selection step, where T cells with receptors having a high affinity for the MHC molecules on dendritic cells at the cortico-medullary junction die by a process called apoptosis. This is the clonal deletion which is responsible for much of self tolerance, and predicted in 1949 by MacFarlane Burnett [3]. Cells which survive this step become mature CD4 + or CD8 + positive αβT cells.

What is crucial to us as transplanters is that the dendritic cells responsible for the clonal deletion step are of bone marrow origin [12]. This was demonstrated many years before the role of these cells in clonal deletion had been established. It follows that in allogeneic haemato-poietic chimaeras, thymic tolerance towards donor al-loantigen will be brought about by the same powerful mechanisms which operate for self tolerance. This is the important message which the new knowledge on the physiology of self tolerance has to offer transplantation.

Donor bone marrow has been used in conjunction with ALS and other immunosuppressive agents for suppressing organ graft rejection experimentally for many years [13] and is currently being tested in a clinical trial in kidney graft recipients [14]. However, given the difficulty in establishing fully allogeneic haematopoietic chimaeras, it would seem very unlikely that the above protocols are in fact achieving chimaerism. The bone marrow might simply represent a source of donor antigen, such as that which would be present on any other source of donor cells.

2. T cell allorecognition

It is now well established that the T-cell does not recognise conventional antigens as intact 3-dimensional structures but only as peptides incorporated into self MHC molecules [15]. The outstanding exception to this general rule occurs in transplantation. T cells recognising allogeneic MHC molecules actually do recognise them as intact, 3-dimensional structures on the surface of the foreign cells. This is termed direct recognition. The precursor frequency of T cells responding in direct recognition is high, with estimates varying between 1% and 10% of all T cells in any individual being able to give proliferative responses to a foreign MHC haplotype [16]. Direct T cell recognition gives rise to strong primary immune responses, and it has been considered the major, if not the only, pathway for T cell recognition in transplantation.

Very little attention has been given to T cell recognition of graft antigens by the normal, physiological pathway, i.e. where the graft is treated simply as a source of foreign protein and the allogeneic MHC antigens (and other polymorphic proteins) are processed and presented on recipient antigen presenting cells (APC) [17–19]. Using synthetic peptides corresponding to polymorphic regions of donor MHC molecules [20] and isolated, denatured chains of donor MHC molecules [21] to prime graft recipients to indirect recognition without influencing direct recognition, we have recently obtained definitive proof that indirect allorecognition can play a significant role in allograft rejection.

3. An important implication of the recent advances

It is potentially of fundamental importance in tolerance induction that there exist these two quite distinct pathways for T cell recognition. For example, it is clear that thymic tolerance for direct recognition can occur only if there are living donor dendritic cells in the thymus, i.e. if there is donor haematopoietic chimaerism. It is otherwise quite impossible for the T cells to interact with the intact 3-dimensional form of donor MHC antigens in the thymus. By complete contrast, exposure to intraperitoneally injected ovalbumin peptides can result in deletion of specifically reactive T-cell clones in the thymus [22]. This suggests that peripheral exposure to histocompatibility antigens might result in thymic tolerance by clonal deletion for indirect allorecognition (irrespective of the effect on the peripheral lymphocyte pool).

An additional important consideration

When we consider the various approaches to tolerance induction, one additional theoretical point becomes very important. It concerns the susceptibility of the allograft to direct T-cell recognition at various times after transplantation. The dendritic cell is the major cell type for direct stimulation of T cells in vitro [23]. Whether or not other cell types have the capacity to stimulate direct recognition of unprimed T cells is somewhat controversial, the major argument being with the vascular endothelial cell [for discussion see 24]. However, most groups have found that MHC class II positive vascular endothelial cells, but not other cell types, do have the capacity to stimulate direct recognition in unprimed T cells, although the stimulation might not be as strong as with the dendritic cell.

These points are important for transplantation because allografts contain a special type of bone marrow derived dendritic cell, the interstitial dendritic cell [25], which is almost certainly the immunogenic passenger leucocyte. These cells are migratory, and 1 or 2 weeks after transplantation the donor interstitial dendritic cells in the graft have emigrated and been replaced by interstitial dendritic cells of recipient type [26]. It follows that the capacity of the graft to stimulate direct recognition will be much diminished or absent within 1 or 2 weeks after grafting, if the interstitial dendritic cell is the major cell type for stimulating direct T-cell recognition. If, however, the vascular endothelial cell also has this capacity, the graft retains the capacity to stimulate direct recognition throughout its life. This is because the vascular endothelial cell is an intergral component of the allograft and remains of donor type unless there has been much damage [27].

One of the major and most curious anomalies in transplantation might be explained on the above basis. It concerns the ease with which allografts are accepted in rodents, especially after very brief treatment with immunosuppression. I postulated some years ago that the species difference in expression of class II MHC antigens on vascular endothelial cells could be the crucial factor, the rat not normally expressing class II whilst in man many vascular endothelial cells normally do express class II antigens [28]. If our thinking is correct, this would leave rat allografts without the capacity to stimulate direct recognition after 1 or 2 weeks in the new host, whereas this capacity would be maintained indefinitely by human allografts [28].

Possible approaches to tolerance induction (Table 1)

Approach 1. Antibodies to CD4 molecules, cytokine receptors etc., aim to interrupt necessary costimulatory signals and thereby induce anergy. It should not be forgotten that this approach induces powerful non-specific immunosuppression, a fact which, surprisingly, is often overlooked.

Approach 2. This corresponds to the old definition of "active enhancement" and is the oldest approach to tolerance induction. Water soluble MHC molecules have long been seen as a potentially powerful approach for tolerance induction with low risk of sensitisation. Cells carrying donor MHC antigens but without costimulatory capacity (e.g. transfected fibroblasts) have been considered recently for the induction of anergy.

Approach 3. Selective irradiation of the organised lymphatic tissues appears to produce powerful non-specific suppression and might allow graft recipients in the longer term to stop all immunosuppressive medication [29].

Table 1. Possible approaches for tolerance induction

1. Antibodies to CD4 molecules, adhesion molecules, cytokines and cytokine receptors. Soluble competitors of these systems, e.g. soluble cytokine receptors

2. Donor antigen treatment
   (a) Water soluble MHC antigens
   (b) Cells expressing donor MHC antigens but lacking costimulatory capacity
   (c) Other forms, e.g. blood cells, spleen cells, liver membranes

3. Total lymphoid irradiation (TLI)

4. Passive enhancement, i.e., antibodies to donor MHC antigens

5. Toxins conjugated to IL-2 or to antibodies to the IL-2 receptor

6. Donor thymus graft

7. Donor haematopoietic chimaerism

However, TLI is a cumbersome technique, it produces long-term effects on the immune system and the results are not consistent.

Approach 4. The administration of antibodies to donor MHC antigens, known as passive enhancement, is probably effective by blocking donor interstitial dendritic cells [30], but is a weak form of immunosuppression with many problems in clinical application [31, 32].

Approach 5. The objective here is to destroy T cells which have been activated by graft antigens to express IL-2 receptors.

Approach 6. This is a superficially attractive idea since it implies that tolerance in the donor thymus will result in powerful tolerance to donor antigens. As we shall see this might not be the case.

Approach 7. The establishment of donor haematopoietic chimaerism is the most rigorous donor-specific treatment for organ transplantation.

Theoretical consideration of the various approaches to tolerance induction

In Table 2 and in the ensuing discussion I have tried to predict the effect on the thymic and peripheral T-cell compartments of some of the approaches listed in Table 1.

Table 2. Theoretical considerations concerning the effects of various protocols for tolerance induction

Treatment	Type of T-cell recognition	T-cell compartment	
		Thymus	Periphery
Cells without costimulatory capacity	Direct Indirect	No effect ? tolerance	Anergy ? sensitisation ? suppression
Antibodies to CD4 antigen	Direct Indirect	No effect (? tolerance)[a]	Anergy Anergy
Water soluble histocompatibility antigen	Direct Indirect	No effect ? tolerance	? No effect ? no effect ? sensitisation ? suppression
Donor lymphoid cells	Direct Indirect	No effect ? tolerance	? sensitisation ? suppression ? anergy ? sensitisation ? suppression
Donor thymus graft	Direct Indirect	? no effect ? anergy Tolerance	? sensitisation ? suppression ? sensitisation ? suppression
IL-2 toxin conjugates	Direct Indirect	No effect (? tolerance)[a]	Tolerance Tolerance
Donor haematopoietic chimaerism	Direct Indirect	Tolerance Tolerance[b]	(anergy)[b] (suppression)[b] (suppression)[b]

[a] The tolerance would be a consequence of antigen release from the accepted allograft, and not directly of the treatment
[b] Refers to situations with mixed haematopoietic chimaerism

1. Cells with donor MHC antigens but lacking costimulatory capacity

(a) Peripheral compartment. Assuming they work perfectly well (which is a major assumption) cells carrying donor MHC antigens but lacking costimulatory capacity should induce anergy for direct recognition in the peripheral T-cell compartment. However, as the antigens will be taken up and presented by recipient APC, the effect on indirect recognition in the peripheral pool is unpredictable. Either sensitisation or suppression could be generated, anergy not being possible since the antigen presentation is by professional APC. This approach, therefore is unlikely to be of value.

(b) Thymic compartment. From our preceding discussions, it is clear that there will be no effect at all on the production and release from the thymus of T cells with capacity for direct recognition of the graft. Therefore, once treatment is stopped, the newly released T cells with capacity for direct recognition should be able to attack the graft. Whether or not this will be a problem will depend on the capacity of the graft to stimulate direct recognition once the donor interstitial dendritic dells have emigrated, as previously discussed. In man, where grafts are likely to maintain the capacity for stimulating direct recognition in the long term, these newly emerging T cells are likely to represent a continuing and cumulative problem.

If there is sufficient access of administered donor antigen to the thymus, tolerance to the indirect recognition pathway is a possibility. Moreover, once the graft is accepted, release of antigen from the graft might by itself maintain tolerance for indirect recognition in the thymus. However, this is pure speculation at this stage.

2. Treatment with antibodies to CD4 antigen

(a) Peripheral compartment. Assuming antibodies to CD4 antigens work perfectly well, one would expect anergy for both direct and indirect recognition in the peripheral pool of T cells.

(b) Thymic compartment. There will not be any effect of antibodies to CD4 on direct allorecognition in the thymus, simply because there are no donor dendritic cells in the thymus. There will also probably not be any effect on tolerance to indirect recognition in the thymus. If anything, antibodies in CD4 antigens have been shown to interfere with self tolerance induction [33]. However, as discussed above, the presence of the graft and possibly access of donor antigens to the thymus might result in tolerance in the indirect pathway.

The problem in the clinical situation with the T cells for direct recognition newly emerging from the thymus would be as discussed in a preceding section. It is therefore unlikely that this approach will allow discontinuation of non-specific immunosuppression in man. It should really be seen as an adjunct to current therapy to improve efficacy.

3. Treatment with water soluble histocompatibility antigens

These have long been seen as a possible approach for potent induction of tolerance with minimal risk of sensitisation [34, 35]. In our hands, however, truly water soluble, monomeric class 1 MHC antigens have been without effect [36].

For an effective stimulatory interaction of a T-cell with an antigen, the antigen is required to be on a membrane, thereby allowing multiple interactions with the T-cell receptor, aided by accessory adhesion molecules. It is, therefore, hard to imagine that monomeric interactions with soluble, monomeric MHC molecules will occur to any significant degree. One would guess that water soluble MHC molecules will have no effect on direct recognition. With indirect recognition, suppression or sensitisation in the peripheral pool, as discussed for cells lacking costimulatory capacity, would be possible. The effects in the thymus would also be as for treatment with cells lacking costimulatory capacity.

Where water soluble MHC molecules have been shown to be effective for immunosuppression in rodent models or in in vitro systems, it is possible that contaminating aggregates might be responsible. Such aggregates are potentially dangerous in the clinical setting.

4. Treatment with allogeneic donor lymphoid cells

These have been shown to be a powerful approach for donor-specific immunosuppression in rodents. However, the results are never uniform, and the risk of unpredictable sensitisation makes this approach, and any other approach involving treatment with donor antigens (i.e. active enhancement), currently unacceptable for clinical application. However, from the theoretical point of view, the generation of powerful, donor specific suppression in the peripheral pool is very attractive. Not only would the peripheral pool be covered, but also any newly emerging T cells from the thymus. In the long-term this approach probably offers the only real hope of risk-free immunosuppression, but far too little is known about the factors that influence the immune response to antigen for it to be worth serious consideration at this stage.

Treatment with donor antigens sometimes induces alloantibodies to MHC antigens. These can be damaging but they can also suppress T cell immune responses, albeit indirectly. For example, in the rat, treatment with antibody to donor MHC antigens (passive enhancement) might be effective by inactivating donor interstitial dendritic cells [30].

5. Donor thymus grafts

This idea is superficially attractive and has been tried experimentally [37]. However, as the dendritic cells in the medulla of the donor thymus (once the dendritic cells resident at the time of grafting have emigrated) will be of recipient type, deletion of T cells directly reactive to donor MHC antigens will not occur. Nevertheless, as mentioned in a preceding section, the thymic epithelial cells probably can induce anergy [8] and this might be the mechanism operating in donor thymus grafts. The effect on peripheral T cells of donor thymus grafting might be that of any exposure to donor antigen.

6. IL-2 toxin conjugates

If optimally effective, i.e. if all of the potentially reactive T cells are activated during the course of treatment, this approach should result in deletion of all donor specific T cells in the peripheral pool. However, because there are no donor dendritic cells in the thymus, there will not be any effect on tolerance to direct recognition in the thymus.

7. Donor haematopoietic chimaerism

This is the only approach which will induce tolerance for direct recognition in the thymus, as it is the only approach which provides dendritic cells of donor type in the thymus medulla. If there is 100% donor haematopoietic chimaerism, this would have been achieved by a total destruction of the recipient's haematopoietic and immune systems. Questions of direct and indirect recognition of donor antigens in the periphery become irrelevant. However, the matter of indirect recognition in the thymus becomes both complicated and interesting. The developing donor T cells will have recipient MHC molecules as their restricting element since this is a characteristic acquired by interaction with and positive selection on the thymic epithelial cells. Therefore, indirect recognition should become irrelevant in this context.

With mixed donor and recipient haematopoietic chimaerism, some form of T cell inactivation must be operating in the periphery in both recipient-anti-donor and donor-anti-recipient directions. Since there would be abundant host and donor antigen in the thymus, tolerance for indirect recognition in both recipient-anti-donor and donor-anti-recipient directions would be likely.

Is tolerance, therefore, a prospective for clinical research? Let us look at the three clinical possibilities discussed at the beginning.

1. Tolerance without any recourse to non-specific immunosuppression

This is donor-specific immunosuppression that is as safe as a course of penicillin or vaccination against tetanus, i.e. achieved with minimal or no interference with the recipient's immune system. There is no known protocol whereby this could be achieved in the clinic at the present time. On theoretical grounds, as discussed in a preceding section, the induction of powerful peripheral suppression for direct and indirect recognition probably offers the only real hope of achieving this objective. A protocol involving treatment with donor antigen is probably how this will be achieved, but reliable production of peripheral suppression without the risk of sensitisation will require better understanding of the factors that influence the host response to antigen.

2. Tolerance with reduced non-specific immunosuppression

In practice, this means non-specific immunosuppression restricted to the weeks or months around the time of grafting. There are probably two approaches to achieve this: the use of total lymphoid irradiation (TLI) and the induction of donor haematopoietic chimaerism. TLI can induce powerful peripheral suppression, but is a cumbersome approach and has long-term effects on the immune system. The induction of donor haematopoietic chimaerism is currently a dangerous procedure and has long-term risks of malfunction of the immune system. However, if these problems can be solved or minimised, the implications for organ transplantation would be incalculable.

3. Tolerance to improve safety and/or efficacy in patients treated with normal courses of non-specific immunosuppression

The hopes here probably rest mainly with the use of humanised antibodies to CD4 and other adhesion and accessory molecules, and humanised antibodies to cytokines and cytokine receptors. While antibodies to CD4 antigens can result in tolerance without long-term immunosuppression in rodents [34] this is unlikely to be the case in man, as discussed earlier in this paper. Depleting donor organs of interstitial dendritic cells might also make an important contribution in reducing the strength of the rejection response that must be dealt with, but this depends on how important a contribution they make to the immunogenicity of human organs, as discussed in a preceding section.

Conclusion

The promised land is still beyond the horizon, so nobody knows how quickly or how slowly we shall reach it. I hope that this review has clarified some issues and focussed attention on the more promising paths, so that the wait might not be too long. Certainly, I think that today we have a clearer idea of where we stand and the magnitude of the problems that face us.

References

1. Owen RD (1945) Immunogenetic consequence of vascular anastomoses between bovine twins. Science 102: 400–401
2. Lillie FR (1916) The theory of the freemartin state. Science 43: 611–613
3. Burnet FM, Fenner F (1949) The production of antibodies, 2nd edn. Macmillan, p 76
4. Billingham RE, Brent L, Medawar PB (1953) Actively acquired tolerance of foreign cells. Nature 4379: 603–606
5. Marrack P, Lo D, Brinster R, Palmiter R, Burkly L, Flavell RH, Kapler J (1988) The effect of thymus environment on T cell development and tolerance. Cell 53: 627–634
6. Webb S, Morris C, Sprent J (1990) Extrathymic tolerance of mature T cells: clonal elimination as a consequence of immunity. Cell 63: 1249–1256
7. Mueller DL, Jenkins MK, Schwartz RH (1989) Clonal expansion versus functional clonal inactivation: a costimulatory signalling pathway determines the outcome of T cell antigen receptor occupancy. Annu Rev Immunol 7: 445–480
8. Ramsdell F, Lantz T, Fowlkes BJ (1989) A nondeletional mechanism of thymic self tolerance. Science 246: 1038–1041
9. Batchelor JR, Lombardi G, Lechler RI (1989) Speculations on the specificity of suppression. Immunol Today 10: 37–40
10. Nikolic-Zugic J (1991) Phenotypic and functional stages in the intrathymic development of $\alpha\beta$T cells. Immunol Today 12: 65–69
11. Hunig T, Tiefenthaler G, Lawetzky A, Kubo R, Schlipkoter E (1989) T-cell subpopulations expressing distinct forms of the TCR in normal, athymic and neonatally TCR $\alpha\beta$-suppressed rats. Cold Spring Harbour Symposia on Quantitative Biology 54: 61–68
12. Barclay AN, Mayohoffer G (1981) Bone marrow origin of Ia positive cells in the medullar of rat thymus. J Exp Med 153: 1666–1671
13. Monaco P, Wood ML (1970) Studies on heterologous antilymphocyte serum in mice. VII. Optimal cellular antigen for induction of immunologic tolerance with antilymphocyte serum. Transplant Proc 2: 489–496
14. Barber WH, Laskow DA, Deierhoi MH, Juilian BA, Curtis JJ, Diethelm AG (1989) Use of cryopreserved donor bone marrow in cadover kidney allograft recipient. Transplant Proc 21: 1787–1789
15. Berzofksy JA, Brett SJ, Streicher GZ, Takahashi H (1988) Antigen processing for presentation of T lymphocytes: function, mechanisms and implications for the T-cell repertoire. Immunol Rev 106: 5–31
16. Bevan MJ (1984) High determinant density may explain the phenomenon of alloreactivity. Immunol Today 5: 128–131
17. Butcher GW, Howard JC (1982) Genetic control of transplant rejection. Transplantation 34: 161–166
18. Lechler RI, Batchelor JR (1982) Restoration of immunogenicity to passenger cell-depleted kidney allografts by the addition of donor strain dendritic cells. J Exp Med 155: 31–41
19. Sherwood RA, Brent L, Rayfield LS (1986) Presentation of alloantigens by host cells. Eur J Immunol 16: 569–574
20. Fangmann J, Dalchau R, Fabre JW. The rejection of skin allografts by indirect recognition of donor class I MHC peptides. J Exp Med (Submitted)
21. Dalchau R, Fangmann J, Fabre JW. Allorecognition of isolated denatured chains of class I and class II MHC molecules. Eur J Immunol (In Press)
22. Murphy KM, Heimberger AB, Loh DY (1990) Induction by antigen of intrathymic apotosis of CD4$^+$, CD8$^+$, TCR^{10} thymocytes in vivo. Science 250: 1720–1723
23. Steinman RM, Witman MD (1978) Lymphoid dendritic cells are potent stimulators of the primary mixed leucocyte reaction in mice. Proc Natl Acad Sci USA 75: 5132–5136
24. Halttunen J (1990) Failure of rat kidney nephron components to induce allogeneic lymphocytes to proliferate in mixed lymphocyte kidney cell culture. Transplantation 50: 481–487
25. Hart DNJ, Fabre JW (1981) Demonstration and characterization of Ia positive dendritic cells in the interstitial connective tissues of rat heart and other tissues, but not brain. J Exp Med 154: 347–361
26. Milton AD, Spencer SC, Fabre JW (1986) The effects of cyclosporin A on the induction of donor class I and class II MHC antigens in heart and kidney allografts in the rat. Transplantation 42: 337–347

27. Hart DNJ, Fabre JW (1981) Localisation of MHC antigens in long-surviving rat renal allografts: probable implication of the passenger leucocyte in graft adaptation. Transplant Proc 13:95–99

28. Fabre JW (1982) The rat kidney allograft model: was it all too good to be true? Transplantation 34: 223–224

29. Slavin S (1987) Total lymphoid irradiation. Immunol Today 3: 88–92

30. Hart DNJ, Fabre JW (1982) The mechanism of induction of passive enhancement: evidence for an interaction of enhancing antibody with donor interstitial dendritic cells. Transplantation 33: 319–322

31. French ME, Batchelor JR (1972) Enhancement of renal allograft in rats and man. Transplant Rev 13: 115–141

32. Fabre JW (1982) Specific immunosuppression. In: PJ Morris (ed) Tissue Transplantation, Clinical Surgery International, vol. 8. Churchill Livingstone, Edinburgh, pp 80–94

33. MacDonald HR, Hengartner H, Pedrazzini T (1988) Intrathymic deletion of self-reactive cells prevented by neonatal anti-CD4 antibody treatment. Nature 335: 174–176

34. Medawar PB (1963) The use of antigenic tissue extracts to weaken the immune reaction against skin homografts in mice. Transplantation 1: 21–38

35. Reisfeld RA, Kahan BD (1971) Extraction and purification of soluble histocompatibility antigens. Transplant Rev 6: 81–112

36. Priestley CA, Dalchau R, Sawyer GJ, Fabre JW (1989) A detailed analysis of the potential of water soluble classical class I MHC molecules for the suppression of kidney allograft rejection and in vitro cytotoxic T cell responses. Transplantation 48: 1031–1038

37. Salaun J, Bandeira A, Khazaal I, Calman F, Coltbey M, Coutinho A, Le Douarin NM (1990) Thymic epithelium tolerizes for histocompatibility antigens. Science 247: 1471–1474

38. Cobbold SP, Martin G, Waldmann H (1990) The induction of skin graft tolerance in MHC mismatched or primed recipients: primed T cells can be tolerised in the periphery with anti CD4 and anti CD8 antibodies. Eur J Immunol 20: 2747–2755

Transplant Int (1992) 5 [Suppl 1]: S 578–S 579

TRANSPLANT
International
© Springer-Verlag 1992

Will chronic rejection ever respond to treatment?

Pekka Häyry and Ari Mennander

Transplantation Laboratory, IV Department of Surgery, University of Helsinki, Helsinki, Finland

In *acute* allograft rejection, the end-point is irreversible damage of the graft (microvascular) endothelium by inflammatory cells and antibodies, and thrombosis and necrosis of the graft. In *chronic* rejection a prime manifestation, common to all transplants, is persistant perivascular inflammation and concentric longitudinal allograft arteriosclerosis [1] affecting particularly the first and second order intragraft branches of transplant arteries (Table 1). Thus, to understand the molecular mechanism of chronic rejection, we should know how the immune inflammation regulates vascular smooth muscle cell (SMC) proliferation.

Key words: Chronic rejection – Allograft – Arteriosclerosis

Regulation of vascular smooth muscle cell proliferation

Vascular smooth muscle cells have two phenotypes, contractile phenotype relevant in adult organisms, and synthetic phenotype, relevant during embryogenesis. During arteriosclerosis, there is a gradual transition from the contractile to the synthetic phenotype [2], the phenotype that is capable to cell division.

In vitro studies have relevated a variety of molecules, including polypeptide mitogens (such as platelet-derived growth factor, insulin-like growth factor, epidermal growth factor, and fibroblast growth factor), interleukins (such as IL-1, and -6), vasoactive hormones (such as endothelin) and eicosanoids, which may induce vascular smooth muscle cell proliferation.

Aortic allografts: a model for transplant arteriosclerosis

In order to investigate which of these molecules may be operative in chronic vascular changes of an organ allograft, we have developed an in vivo model: aortic allo-

transplantation across histoincompatible rat strains [3]. Non-immunosuppressed allografts undergo an acute adventitial inflammatory episode after transplantation, with CD25 positive (blast) cells and oedema, which spontaneously subsides. This is followed by more a chronic type of inflammation in the adventitia, induction of smooth muscle cell proliferation in the media, focal fragmentation of the internal elastic lamina and appearance of proliferating smooth muscle cells in the intima. This process leads to concentric intimal thickening and gradual occlusion of the graft. Applications of proper antibody and immunofluorescence demonstrates increased expression of class II antigens in the allograft endothelium, and depositions of IgG and complement on the vascular wall. These alterations observed in aortic allografts, are virtually indistinguishable from those seen in human allograft vasculature during chronic rejection.

Role of eicosanoids

Out of the various regulatory molecules listed above and being possibly of significance in the induction of allograft arteriosclerosis, we have investigated the role of eicosanoids [4]. During the chronic stage there is an increased synthesis of thromboxane B2 in an aortic allograft which is lacking in syngeneic grafts, but only a small (compensatory?) increase in 6-keto-PGF1alpha and no change in LTB4. These observations are compatible with human studies, demonstrating increased levels of thromboxane in the urine of chronically-rejecting transplant recipients.

Modtification of allograft arteriosclerosis by extraneous factors

Of particular interest is whether and how this process may be modified by extraneous factors, particularly if the process is reversible; and what is the role of diet and the impact of CMV infection. Our preliminary studies indicate, so far, that retransplantation of an allograft back to the syngeneic host 1 month after transplantation, inhibited the progression of the intimal changes. On the other hand,

---

Offprint requests to: Dr. Pekka Häyry, Transplantation Laboratory, University of Helsinki, Haartmaninkatu 3, SF 00290 Helsinki, Finland; telefax: + 358-0-411 227

Table 1. Manifestations of chronic rejection in different organs

Heart[a]	Kidney[b]	Liver[c]
Inflammation	Inflammation	Inflammation
Arteriosclerosis	Arteriosclerosis	Arteriosclerosis
Fibrosis	BM thickening	Vanishing bile ducts &
	Glomerular sclerosis	portal arteries
	Tubular atrophy	Fibrosis
	Fibrosis	

[a] Rose and Uys, Pathology of graft atherosclerosis (chronic rejection), in Cooper and Novitsky, Transplantation and replacement of thoracic organs, Kluwer Academic Publ., Dordrecht 1990 [6]
[b] Croker and Salomon, Pathology of renal allograft, in Tisher and Brenner, Renal Pathology, L. B. Lippincott, Phila, 1989 [7]
[c] Oguma et al. Hepatology, 1989: 9: 204 [8]

transplantation to the allogeneic host definitely continued the process. Feeding the recipient rat with cholesterol and cholic acid induced hypercholesterolemia in the recipients, with increased levels of both VLDL and LDL, but with no change in HDL cholesterol. There was no alteration in the levels of triglycerides, either. This diet did not enhance the arteriosclerotic process in our animals, which might indicate that increased levels of cholesterol may not, per se, be enhancing to the process. It should be also noted that in man, a better correlation has usually been obtained between accelerated arteriosclerosis and triglycerides rather than with cholesterol.

Pharmacological interference with allograft arteriosclerosis

Drugs known to inhibit the immune response, such as cyclosporine (at the level of 5 mg/kg/day), azathioprine (2 mg/kg/day), or steroids (methyl prednisolone, 0.5 mg/kg/day), although anti-inflammatory for adventitial inflammation, did not inhibit allograft arteriosclerosis and the increase in intimal thickeness. In fact, at this dose level, the administration of CyA significantly enhances arteriosclerosis [5].

The separate application of two inhibitors for lipid mediators of inflammation, i. e., GR32191B (a thromboxane A2 receptor blocker), and WEB2170 (a PAF receptor blocker), significantly reduced the rate of smooth muscle proliferation in the allograft, but delayed the arteriosclerotic process by only 1–3 months (to be published). The application of BIM23401 (angiopeptin), a somatostatin analogue, also reduced the level of smooth muscle cell proliferation, but was able to delay the generation of arteriosclerosis by 3 months, at the most.

Discussion and conclusions

In order to understand chronic rejection, we should understand allograft arteriosclerosis. In particular, we should know how the immune inflammation regulates ar-

terial smooth muscle proliferation. Allograft arteriosclerosis seems to be under the control of the immune response, and may be reversible (at least) at very early stages post transplantation. In our hands, hypercholesterlemia did not enhance it, but we do not know the role of triglycerides. Conventional immunosuppressive drugs do not inhibit the process at levels capable of reducing the allograft immune response in the rat. In fact, cyclosporine may enhance it. Instead, the application of certain antagonists to lipid mediators of inflammation, or certain octapeptide analogues of somatostatin may inhibit the rate of proliferation of arterial smooth muscle cells and the induction of allograft arteriosclerosis.

We consider it likely that this condition will become treatable. Before the treatment format materializes one should, however, know in more detail the structure of the molecular cascade leading to smooth muscle cell proliferation in the allograft vascular wall. At present it is not possible to judge whether the treatment should be prophylactic, and directed particularly to the perioperative period (when the allograft seems to be most vulnerable to damage contributing to the process), or whether an effective treatment may be established when the process is already underway.

Acknowledgements. These studies were financed by grants from the Academy of Finland, the Sigrid Juselius Foundation, and the University of Helsinki, Helsinki, Finland.

References

1. Demetris AJ, Zerbe T, Banner B (1989) Morphology of solid organ allograft arteriopathy: identification of proliferating intimal cell populations. Transplant Proc 21: 3667–3669
2. Thyberg J, Hedin U, Sjölund M, Palmberg L, Bottger BA (1990) Regulation of differentiated properties and proliferation of arterial smooth muscle cells. Arteriosclerosis 10: 966–990
3. Mennander A, Tiisala S, Halttunen J, Yilmaz S, Paavonen T, Häyry P (1991) Chronic rejection in rat aortic allografts. An experimental model for transplant arteriosclerosis. Arteriosclerosis Thromb 11: 671–680
4. Mennander A, Tiisala S, Ustinov J, Paavonen T, Häyry P (1991) Chronic rejection of rat aortic allografts. III. Synthesis of the major eicosanoids by the vascular wall components, and the effect of inhibition of the thromboxane cascade. Submitted
5. Mennander A, Tiisala S, Paavonen T, Halttunen J, Häyry P (1991) Chronic rejection of rat aortic allografts. II. Administration of cyclosporine induces acclerated allograft arteriosclerosis. Transplant Int 4: 173–179
6. Rose AG, Uys CJ (1990) Pathology of graft atherosclerosis (chronic rejection). In: Cooper DKC, Novitsky D (eds) The Transplantation and replacement of thoracic organs. Kluwer Academic Publishers, Dordrecht, Boston, London, pp 161–182
7. Croker BC, Salomon DR (1989) Pathology of the renal allograft. In: Tisher CC, Brenner BM (eds) Renal Pathology. LB Lippincott, Philadelphia, pp 1518–1554
8. Oguma S, Belle S, Starzl TE, Demetris AJ (1989) A histometric analysis of chronically rejected human liver allografts: insights into the mechanisms of bile duct loss: direct immunologic and ischemic factors. Hepatology 9: 204–209

Transplant Int (1992) 5 [Suppl 1]: S 580–S 582

TRANSPLANT
International
© Springer-Verlag 1992

DNA typing: an important step forward?

Gerhard Opelz, Joannis Mytilineos, Sabine Scherer, Heather Dunckley, Jean Trejaut, Jeremy Chapman, Derek Middleton, David Savage, Gottfried Fischer, Jean-Denis Bignon, Jean-Claude Bensa, Ekkehard Albert, and Harriet Noreen, for the Collaborative Transplant Study

From the Transplant Immunology Laboratories at the Universities of Heidelberg, Sydney, Belfast, Vienna, Nantes, Grenoble, Munich, and Minneapolis
Department of Transplantation Immunology, Institute of Immunology, University of Heidelberg, Heidelberg, Germany

Abstract. In a collaborative project which was supported by 96 transplant centers, DNA typing of HLA-DR antigens was carried out on over 7,000 transplant donors and recipients at 8 participating laboratories. Approximately 25% of the individuals were found to have been typed incorrectly by serological means. An analysis of over 2,500 first cadaver kidney transplants showed a significant correlation of matching for the HLA-DR antigens in transplants where the serological typing was confirmed by DNA typing. In transplants where the serological typing was found to be incorrect, the analysis of serological HLA-DR mismatches resulted in no correlation with graft outcome whereas a significant correlation was found when the corrected DNA typed HLA-DR antigens were analyzed. Transplants which had been reported to the Collaborative Transplant Study based on serological typing as matched for HLA-A, -B, -DR or HLA-B, -DR were found to have a superior graft survival rate only if HLA-DR compatibility was confirmed by DNA typing.

Key words: DNA typing – Kidney transplantation – HLA matching

The application of DNA techniques allows a more accurate determination of HLA-DR alleles than the conventional serological technique [1, 2, 5, 7, 9]. We employed DNA typing to evaluate in a collaborative project the utility of this new technique for clinical histocompatibility matching. With the cooperation of 96 transplant centers, DNA typing of over 7,000 donors and recipients of kidney transplants was performed using the RFLP technique described by Bidwell et al. [1].

Offprint requests to: Gerhard Opelz, Department of Transplantation Immunology, Institute of Immunology, University of Heidelberg, Im Neuenheimer Feld 305, D-6900 Heidelberg, Germany

Materials and methods

Peripheral blood lymphocytes or spleen tissue from transplant recipients or donors was obtained at the transplant centers and frozen at $-20°$C. The cell material was shipped on dry ice to the study center at the University of Heidelberg where DNA was extracted by routine methods [4, 6]. Aliquots of DNA were distributed to the participating laboratories where DNA typing was performed. The laboratories were not aware which DNA samples belonged to recipients or donors. The typing results were reported to the study center for further analysis. The serological HLA typings obtained in the individual transplant centers' laboratories were used for comparison. Information on the transplants was collected within the framework of the Collaborative Transplant Study. Graft survival rates were computed by the Kaplan-Meier method. Statistical significance was estimated by log rank or weighted regression analysis [3]. The transplants were performed between 1988 and 1990. Only first transplants from cadaver donors were included in the analysis.

Results

Table 1 shows the rates of discrepancies between serology and DNA typing for the HLA antigens HLA-DR1 to HLA-DRw10. Serological typing errors were particularly frequent for "difficult" antigens, i. e. specificities for which monospecific serological reagents are difficult or im-

Table 1. Discrepancies RFLP versus serological HLA-DR typing (7265 individuals typed)

Allele	n	% Discrepancies
DR1	1532	14.5
DR2	2227	7.6
DR3	1829	8.4
DR4	2342	8.5
DR5	1839	14.2
DRw6	2237	32.0
DR7	1393	7.7
DRw8	510	27.8
DR9	15	33.3
DRw10	142	40.1

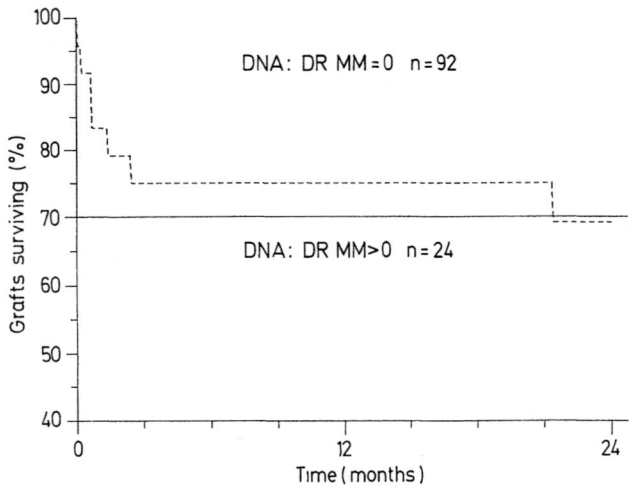

Fig. 1. Graft survival analysis of first cadaver kidney transplants that were reported, based on serological typing, to be HLA-A, -B, -DR compatible. Graft survival was significantly better if HLA-DR compatibility was confirmed by DNA typing as compared to grafts where DNA typing revealed an HLA-DR mismatch ($P < 0.02$)

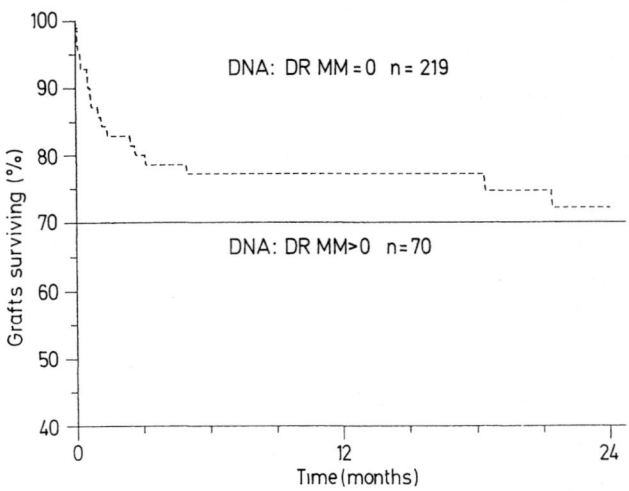

Fig. 2. Analysis of first cadaver transplants that were reported, based on serological typing, to be HLA-B, -DR compatible. Grafts in which HLA-DR compatibility was confirmed by DNA typing did significantly better than grafts with HLA-DR mismatches revealed by the DNA technique ($P < 0.01$)

possible to obtain. The error rate was approximately equivalent in recipient and donor typings.

The influence on the graft survival analysis of incorrect HLA-DR assignments based on serological typing is shown in Table 2. Whereas a significant effect of matching for HLA-DR was observed in transplants where both the recipient and donor typing were confirmed by the DNA technique, there was no correlation of matching with graft outcome when DNA typing revealed that the serological typing was incorrect. When the incorrectly typed transplants were analyzed according to the HLA-DR typings obtained by the DNA method, a significant correlation of HLA-DR matching with graft outcome became apparent.

We investigated the influence of incorrect HLA-DR assignment based on serological typing on the graft survival analysis of transplants that were reported to the Collaborative Transplant Study as matched for HLA-A, -B, and -DR. As shown in Fig. 1, transplants in which HLA-DR compatibility was confirmed by DNA typing had a significantly higher success rate than transplants in which DNA typing revealed HLA-DR mismatches ($P < 0.02$). In other words, even though all transplants had been con-

sidered "matched" based on serological HLA typing, only those in which the HLA-DR types were confirmed by the DNA technique had a superior graft outcome.

The analysis was extended to the "next best" match category, transplants matched for HLA-B, -DR (and mismatched for HLA-A). Even in this comparison, a significantly better graft survival rate was seen when the HLA-DR match was confirmed by DNA typing as compared to when DNA typing revealed an HLA-DR mismatch ($P < 0.01$) (Fig. 2).

Discussion

DNA typing provides a powerful tool for the exact determination of HLA-DR allels. Our results demonstrated that when the serological errors were corrected, the correlation of HLA matching with graft outcome was improved. The implications for clinical histocompatibility matching are obvious.

In the current project we used frozen cell material in a retrospective study to evaluate whether accurate DNA typing would be of benefit in the clinical setting. With the answer at hand, it will now be important to introduce DNA techniques for prospective typing and allocation of organs. The RFLP method used in this project is unsuitable for that purpose because it requires approximately 1 week to obtain results. For DNA typing to become competitive, the time requirement will have to be shortened to approximately that of serological typing (about 5 h). New DNA techniques, based on the use of the polymerase chain reaction (PCR) and hybridization with oligonucleotides appear to rapidly close the time gap. Typing with sequence-specific oligonucleotides or the PCR-RFLP technique reduces the time requirement to approximately 10 h [9, 10]. The newest and most exciting development in this regard is the allele-specific amplification method employing sequence-specific primers described by Olerup

Table 2. Effect of HLA-DR mismatches on graft survival; first cadaver transplants. Graft survival at 1 year (% ± SE)

Number of HLA-DR mismatches	Serology confirmed by DNA	Serology different from DNA	
		Analysis of serological mismatches	Analysis of DNA mismatches
0	84 ± 1 (n = 765)	82 ± 2 (n = 321)	87 ± 3 (n = 120)
1	82 ± 1 (n = 995)	80 ± 2 (n = 304)	81 ± 2 (n = 358)
2	78 ± 3 (n = 255)	81 ± 4 (n = 79)	78 ± 3 (n = 226)
P regression	0.02	ns	0.05

and Zetterquist [8]. This elegant technique allows the identification of HLA-DR alleles in approximately 3 h. It remains to be seen how soon this technique can be transferred from the research laboratory to the routine transplant laboratory setting. With a quick and accurate DNA technique at hand, the prospect for improved clinical histocompatibility matching appears good. If the rapid development in the DNA field during the last couple of years can be used as a guideline, improved matching and thus better transplant success rates should become reality in the foreseeable future.

Acknowledgement. We thank the centers participating in the Collaborative Transplant Study for their invaluable support. We also thank IBM Germany for providing computer hardware and software support for this project.

References

1. Bidwell JL, Bidwell EA, Savage DA, Middleton D, Klouda PT, Bradley BA (1988) A DNA-RFLP typing system that positively identifies serologically well-defined and ill-defined HLA-DR and DQ alleles, including DRw10. Transplantation 45: 640–646

2. Carlsson B, Wallin J, Böhme J, Möller E (1987) HLA-DR-DQ haplotypes defined by restriction fragment analysis. Hum Immunol 20: 95–113

3. Dunn OJ, Clark VA (eds) (1974) Applied statistics: analysis of variance and regression. Wiley, New York, p 236

4. Graham D (1978) The isolation high molecular weight DNA from whole organisms or large tissue masses. Ann Biochem 85: 609–613

5. Middleton D, Savage DA, Cullen C, Martin J (1988) Discrepancies in serological tissue typing revealed by DNA techniques. Transplant Int 1: 161–163

6. Miller ST, Dykes DD, Polesky HF (1988) A simple salting out procedure for extracting DNA from human nucleated cells. Nucleic Acids Res 16: 1215

7. Mytilineos J, Scherer S, Opelz G (1990) Comparison of RFLP-DR beta and serological HLA-DR typing in 1500 individuals. Transplantation 50: 870–873

8. Olerup O, Zetterquist H (1991) HLA-DRB1*01 subtyping by allele-specific PCR amplification: A sensitive, specific and rapid technique. Tissue Antigens 73: 197–204

9. Tiercy JM, Goumez C, Mach B, Jeannet M (1991) Application of HLA-DR oligotyping to 110 kidney transplant patients with doubtful serological typing. Transplantation 51: 1110–1114

10. Uryu N, Maeda M, Ota M, et al (1990) A simple and rapid method for HLA-DRβ and DQβ typing by digestion of PCR-amplified DNA with allele specific restriction endonucleases. Tissue Antigens 35: 20–31

Transplant Int (1992) 5 [Suppl 1]: S 583–S 586

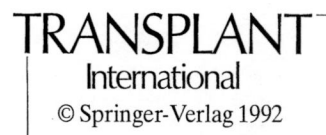

© Springer-Verlag 1992

The "rejection reaction" is not confined solely to the allograft

M. S. Graudenz and S. Thiru

Department of Pathology, University of Cambridge, Tennis Court Road, Cambridge CB2 1QP, UK

The rejection process refers primarily to the destruction of foreign tissues by host immune mechanisms. This process affects host lymphoid tissue profoundly and alters the migration patterns of lymphocytes in recipients of organ allografts [8]. It has been shown that specifically sensitized lymphocytes traffic both to and from the transplant [9, 10]. A considerable amount of knowledge has been gathered on the preferential migration pathways of lymphocytes through lymphoid and mucosa-associated lymphoid organs [1, 15]. The factors regulating lymphocyte migration through non-lymphoid tissue in normal conditions are not well known and even less well understood in the context of graft rejection.

In this article we described for the first time migration in a recipient non-lymphoid organ (heart) and it's potentially harmful effects in causing parenchymal damage during renal allograft rejection in the rat model. These lesions were detected during the process of developing a model of chronic renal allograft rejection. The pathogenesis of these cardiac lesions is not fully understood but possible mechanisms include upregulation of homing receptors/adhesion molecules, breakdown of peripheral tolerance and involvement of cross-reacting anti-endothelial antibodies.

Key words: Renal allograft rejection – Cardiac lesions – Pathogenesis

Materials and methods

Animals. Inbred male rats weighing 180 g to 300 g were used in all experiments, (Olac, Bicester, UK). PVG (RT1^c), AGUS (RT1^l), PVGRT1^u, PVGRT1^l, F344 (RT1^{lvl}) and (DA × PVG)F$_1$ were used as kidney donors; DA (RT1^{avl}), AO (RT1^u), LEWIS (RT1^l), PVG (RT1^c), PVGRT1^u, PVGRT1^l served as recipients.

Operative procedures. Orthotopic left kidney grafts were anastomosed end-to-end to the recipient's left renal vessels and an uretero-

Offprint requests to: Marcia Silveira Graudenz

ureteric anastomosis was performed using standard microvascular techniques. Seven days after transplantation the right kidney was removed and graft function was estimated by serial serum creatinine measurements. All animals that presented with evidence of localized or systemic infection at the post-mortems were excluded from this study.

Immunosuppression. Cyclosporin-A (CyA) (kind gift from Sandoz, Basel, Switzerland) dissolved in olive oil in an i.m. dose of 2.0, 3.5 and 5.0 mg/kg per day for 14 days post-transplant was administered to the recipient animals.

Histological examination. Full autopsies were performed on all animals that died during the post-operative period or that were culled due to development of graft insufficient. Graft insufficiency was defined as a level of serum creatinine double the normal control (40–50 umol/l). Samples of most tissues including lymphoid and various non-lymphoid organs were collected and routine haematoxilyn and special stains as required were performed.

Immunohistochemistry. Tissues obtained from autopsies were snap-frozen in liquid nitrogen. Five-micrometer-thick frozen sections were prepared and a two-step immunoperoxidase staining technique was used. The primary mouse anti-rat monoclonal antibodies were: OX-29 (leucocyte common antigen), OX-42 (macrophages and dendritic cells), OX-17 (anti-class II, Ia-E), OX-8 (T cytotoxic/suppressor), and W3/25 (T helper) from Serotec (Bicester, UK). The secondary antibody used was a sheep anti-mouse IgG horseradish conjugate (Amersham Int. Plc, UK).

Results

Histological and immunohistochemical characterization of the cardiac lesions. Postmortem findings showed that a great proportion of the rats that presented with rejection of the kidney graft at postmortem contained multiple foci of mononuclear cell infiltration in their own hearts. The cells were seen diffusely infiltrating the interstitium and also attacking and destroying isolated or bundles of myocardial fibres. In places of more advanced and extensive cell damage there were also foci of interstitial fibrosis with evidence of recent and old hemorrhage. In three cases acute fibrinoid necrosis of medium-sized arteries was present and two long-term survivor rats showed non-atherosclerotic intimal thickening of medium-sized ar-

Table 1. Table showing the experimental groups and the incidence of the cardiac lesions in those animals that presented with graft rejection at postmortem

Experimental groups	graft rejection	cardiac lesion
MHC + Minor mismatch with immunosuppression ($n = 104$)		
Acute rejection	31	26
Chronic rejection	20	15
MHC + Minor mismatch no immunosuppression ($n = 10$)		
Acute rejection	10	9
Minor mismatch alone no immunosuppression ($n = 46$)		
Acute rejection	3	3
Chronic rejection	2	2

Table 2. Table showing the development of the cardiac lesions after priming the recipients with splenic allogeneic cells

	Day after priming	Cardiac lesions
MHC + Minor	8	2/2[a]
Mismatch	15	5/6[b]
($RT1^c < - > RT1^u$)	22	2/2[b]
Minor Mismatch	8	2/2[a]
($RT1^u < - > RT1^u$)	15	2/2[b]
	22	1/1[a]

[a] Mild lesions
[b] Moderate lesions

teries. All these abnormalities were very similar to those seen in rejecting cardiac allografts.

Immunocytochemistry showed that the infiltrating cells were leukocyte common antigen and class II positive. The OX-42 monoclonal antibody stained a fair number of macrophages within the mononuclear cell infiltrate. The majority of the cells stained positively with W3/25 (CD4) and to a lesser extent with the anti-CD8 monoclonal antibody.

Incidence of the cardiac lesions. The cases were divided into two main experimental groups: the MHC plus Minor mismatch and the MHC-matched/Minor mismatch groups (see Table 1). Most of the recipients with MHC plus Minor mismatched grafts received CyA as immunosuppression and a smaller number taken as control did not receive any immunosuppression. To date of the 104 transplants in the MHC plus Minor group that received immunosuppression, 51 had evidence of rejection at postmortem and of these 41 developed the cardiac lesions described above. All animals in the MHC plus Minor mismatch group that did not receive CyA died of rejection and 9 out of 10 showed the cardiac lesions. In the MHC-matched/Minor mismatch group the majority of the animals survived beyond 150 days and to date only 5 died secondary to rejection. All these five cases presented rather extensive and florid myocardial cell damage. The cardiac

lesions have not been seen in the hearts of transplanted animals that did not show rejection of the allograft nor were they seen in normal non-transplanted controls.

When the rejection cases were divided into acute and chronic cases a high incidence of cardiac lesions was observed in both subgroups. These results point out the fact the this systemic organ damage can also occur in a chronic allograft rejection situation.

Is the cardiac lesion due to graft-versus host disease? Is it linked to the use of CyA? In order to address both questions in a single experiment kidneys obtained from 8 $(DA \times PVG)F_1$ were transplanted into 4 DA and 4 PVG parents without any post-transplant immunosuppression. In the F_1 to parent situation graft-versus-host cannot occur. All the DA and PVG recipients of $(DA \times PVG)F_1$ kidneys died of acute humoral and cellular rejection on day 8 after transplant and postmortem examinations showed the presence of cardiac lesions in all cases. In conclusion, neither graft-versus-host disease nor CyA are responsible for the development of the lesions present in the recipient's hearts.

The induction of the cardiac lesions in the recipient hearts is not specifically linked to renal allografts. Eight AO ($RT1^u$) male rats were primed intraperitoneally with 2×10^7 PVG ($RT1^c$) spleen cells (MHC plus Minor mismatch) and 5 PVGRT1^u male rats were primed with 2×10^7 AO spleen cells (MHC-matched/Minor mismatched) on day 0. Controls were injected with saline. The animals were culled on days 8, 15 and 22 after sensitization and full postmortems performed. Histological examination of recipients' hearts showed that the lesions were already present on day 8 being most intense on days 14 and 22 after allosensitization in the MHC plus Minor mismatch situation. (Table 2) Repeat experiments with MHC-matched/Minor mismatched allosensitization produced similar results with the exception that on day 22 the intensity of the lesions was already subsiding. Overall, the severity of cardiac lesions induced by allosensitization with spleen cells was always less than the ones observed in the context of renal allograft rejection.

There is a temporal relationship between acute graft rejection and the development of the cardiac lesions. Ten DA ($RT1^{av1}$) male recipients received PVG ($RT1^c$) kidney allografts and were left with the right kidney in situ to maintain renal function. No immunosuppression was administered in the post-operative period. Animals were sacrificed on days 3, 7, 10, 16 and 23 after transplantation and full post-mortems performed. The intensity of the cardiac lesions were analyzed and scored (+ = minimal, + + = mild, + + + = moderate, + + + + = severe) by two different pathologists independently. Figure 1 demonstrates the direct relationship between the peak of unmodified graft rejection around days 7 and 10 after transplantation paralleled by the development of moderately severe parenchymal destruction in the recipients hearts. Saline-injected controls did not develop the cardiac lesions.

Involvement of other non-lymphoid organs. The recipients' own right kidneys that were either removed on

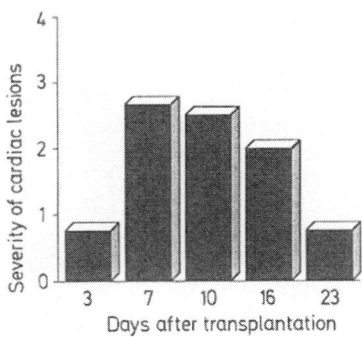

Fig. 1. Graph illustrating the temporal correlation between the intensity of the cardiac lesion and graft rejection

day 7 after transplantation or left in situ during the temporal relationship experiment were examined histologically. The findings included an increased mononuclear cell adhesion to vascular endothelium of veins, venules and peritubular capillaries. In places the cells were seen transmigrating the vessel wall and infiltrating the interstitium nearby. This latter finding, however, was infrequent and not accompanied by parenchymal damage. Preliminary observations in the recipients' lungs confirmed the presence of altered mononuclear cell trafficking, including increased leukocyte-endothelial cell adherence, transmigration and interstitial infiltration, very similar to the changes seen in rejecting lung allografts.

Discussion

The data presented in this paper suggested that the host response to allogeneic antigen was not confined to the allograft, and morphological abnormalities similar to rejection reaction could be seen in the host's own non-lymphoid organs. This response occurred in the context of both acute and chronic graft rejection and involved increased lymphocyte adherence and trafficking through a non-lymphoid organ, such as the recipient's own heart, with evidence of parenchymal damage. It was shown to be produced not only by the presence of a solid organ allograft like the kidney but also to a lesser extent by priming the recipient with allogeneic lymphocytes. The host response was seen in MHC plus non-MHC incompatibilities as well as in non-MHC disparities alone. Lastly, it was demonstrated that there was a temporal relationship between the peak of graft rejection and the development of the cardiac lesions.

The pathogenesis of these cardiac lesions is open to speculation. We showed that they were not due to graft-versus-host disease or Cyclosporin-A therapy. Other pathogenetic mechanisms that may be involved include upregulation of homing receptors/adhesion molecules secondary to the inflammatory response produced during graft rejection, breakdown of peripheral tolerance and the production of cross-reacting anti-endothelial antibodies.

Intense cellular reaction in host lymphoid tissues in response to untreated organ allografts has been previously reported [8]. However, our observation that recipient non-lymphoid organs, particularly the heart, could be involved during the process of graft rejection is unique. In lymphoid tissue, high endotheliac venules (HEV) cells lining the postcapillary venules control the nonrandom distribution of lymphocytes. The adhesion process between lymphocytes and HEV is mediated by lymphocyte homing receptors which show affinity for organ-specific endothelial ligands (vascular addressins) [3]. In non-lymphoid organs HEV are normally absent but ordinary endothelium can acquire HEV-like morphology and function when an inflammatory microenviroment is present [2]. Cytokines in chronic inflammatory sites can induce endothelial cells to develop HEV-like properties and promote lymphocyte-endothelial cell adhesion by enhancing the expression of organ-specific endothelial ligands. Lymphocytes bind to HEV in inflamed synovium via a recognition system that differs from homing receptors to lymphnode and mucosal HEV [1]. It is not known if the specificities observed are truly organ-specific or represent a general adhesive mechanism that is subject to regulation by inflammatory mediators. During acute renal allograft rejection the peritubular capillary endothelium obtains features similar to lymphnode HEV [10]. It has also been shown that the ligand responsible for the binding of lymphocytes to peritubular capillary is organ-specific and that the HEV in the kidney does not stain with a monoclonal antibody against rat lymphnode HEV. It seems that refined homing specificities allow the immune system to protect an organ from antigen-specific effector cells.

In addition to the tissue-specific homing receptor/ligand interaction it is now suggested that other families of adhesion molecules play an accessory role in lymphocyte-HEV adherence, in particular the integrins. They comprise the very late antigen (VLA) subfamily of integrins which function as receptors for extracellular matrix and the leukocyte integrins. There is some indication that extracellular matrix components have a co-mitogenic effect on T cells exposed to anti CD-3 antibody [13, 14]. Memory T cells express three to four times more VLA-4, VLA-5 and VLA-6 than do naive cells and bind more efficiently to fibronectin adn laminin [12]. Laminin has been shown to be a prominent heart cell surface protein [7]. It is possible that during the rejection reaction there is an enhanced expression of VLAs in circulating lymphocytes and this may promote transmigration of the lymphocyte with attachment to the surface laminin that normally surrounds both myocytes and capillaries in rat hearts [5]. It is possible that there may be cross-reactivity between glomerular basement membrane laminin and myocardial cell laminin.

The mechanisms of peripheral tolerance are not well understood. A general hypothesis is that whenever potentially self-reactive T cells in the periphery are isolated from their sources of "help" during antigen recognition these cells default to an anergic state [4]. If sufficient co-stimulation is provided, as in graft rejection, clonal anergy might be reversed and self-reactivity ensue. The pool of cytokines that are released during graft rejection could provide enough co-stimulatory factors to switch on anergic T cells in the periphery to respond to self tissues as if they were foreign. The production of cytokines upregulating the expression of MHC and adhesion molecules may lead to the generation of responses to other previously "cryptic" determinant regions in non-lymphoid organs such as the heart during a systemic inflammatory event [14]. Increased levels of ligand could activate low-affinity T cells and memory T cells thus contributing to broadening the autoimmune response. The persistence of the antigenic source, as in the case of a chronically rejecting organ graft, may help to perpetuate this reactivity in vivo. Finally, it is possible that anti-endothelial antibodies produced to graft vascular endothelium may cross-react with recipient endothelial cell antigens to produce vasculitic lesions in addition to increased lymphocyte adherence and transmigration.

Our observations of lymphocyte infiltration and parenchymal damage in the non-lymphoid organs of an allograft recipient have not been reported previously. However it was not surprising that the rejection reaction, which is an intense inflammatory event, did indeed produce such systemic effects. We intend to conduct further experiments on the migratory behaviour of lymphoid cells in recipients bearing rejecting grafts in order to clarify the possible pathogenetic mechanisms involved in this systemic reaction.

Acknowledgements. We wish to thank Margaret McLeish for her expert technical help and Stephen P. Cobbold for immunological advice. We also thank C.A.P.E.S. of the Ministry of Education, Brasil and the East Anglian Regional Health Authority for the support of this work.

References

1. Butcher EC (1986) The regulation of lymphocyte traffic. In: Current Topics in Microbiology and Immunology, vol 128. Springer-Verlag, Berlin, Heidelberg, New York, p 85
2. Chin Y, Falanga V, Streilein JW, Sackstein R (1988) Lymphocyte recognition of psoriatic endothelium: evidence for tissue-specific receptor/ligand interaction. J Invest Dermatol 91: 423
3. Chin Y, Sackstein R, Cai J (1991) Lymphocyte-homing receptors and preferential migration pathways. Proc Soc Exp Biol Med 196: 374
4. Cobbold S, Qin S, Waldmann H (1990) Reprogramming the immune system with monoclonal antibodies. Semin Immunol 2: 377
5. Contard F, Koteliansky V, Marotte F, Dubus I, Rappaport L, Samuel JL Specific alterations in the distribution of extracellular matrix components within rat myocardium during the development of pressure overload. Lab Invest 64: 65–75
6. Gammon G, Sercaz EE, Benichou G (1991) The dominant self and the cryptic self: shaping the autoreactive T-cell repertoire. Immunol Today 12: 193
7. Gulizia JM, Cunningham MW, McManus BM (1991) Immunoreactivity of anti-streptococcal monoclonal antibodies to human heart valves. Evidence for multiple cross-reactive epitopes. Am J Pathol 138: 258
8. Kupiec-Weglinsky JW, Tilney NL (1981) Migration patterns of lymphocytes from recipients of organ allografts. I. The unmodified host. Transplantation 32: 121
9. Kupiec-Weglinsky JW, Tilney NL (1989) Lymphocyte migration patterns in organ allograft recipients. Immunol Rev 108: 63
10. Nemlander A, Soots A, von Willebrand E, Husbers B, Hayry P (1982) Redistribution of rat renal allograft-responding leukocytes during rejection. II. Kinetics and specificity. J Exp Med 156: 1087
11. Renkonen R, Turunen JP, Rapola J, Häyry P (1990) Characterization of high endothelial-like properties of peritubular capillary endothelium during acute renal allograft rejection. Am J Pathol 137: 643
12. Shimizu Y, van Seventer GA, Horgan KJ, Shaw S (1990) Regulated expression and binding of three VLA (beta 1) integrin receptors on T cell. Nature 345: 250
13. Shimizu Y, van Seventer GA, Horgan KJ, Shaw S (1990) Co-stimulation of proliferative responses of resting CD4 + T cells by the interaction of VLA-4 and VLA-5 with fibronecting and VLA-6 with laminin. J Immunol 154: 59
14. Souza M, Tilney N, Kupiec-Weglinski JW (1991) Recognition of self within self: specific lymphocyte positioning and the extracellular matrix. Immunol Today 12: 262
15. Yednock TA, Rosen SD (1989) Lymphocyte homing. In: Advances in Immunology, vol 44. Academic Press, San Diego, California, p 313

Transplant Int (1992) 5 [Suppl 1]: S 587–S 588

TRANSPLANT
International
© Springer-Verlag 1992

Chronic rejection of rat aortic allografts: effect of inhibition of the thromboxane cascade

A. Mennander[1], J. Ustinov[1], T. Paavonen[1,2], A. Räisänen[1], and P. Häyry[1]

[1] Transplantation Laboratory, Fourth Department of Surgery and [2] Department of Pathology, University of Helsinki, Helsinki, Finland

Abstract. Non-immunosuppressed rat aortic allografts from DA (RT1^{av1}) to WF (RT1^u) strain develop, after a short reversible acute rejection episode, chronic arteriosclerotic changes in the vascular wall, which are indistinguishable from those seen in human allografts during chronic rejection [1]. Incubation of the aortic wall segments in vitro and immunochemical assays demonstrated that the allografts synthesized increased amounts of TxB2, but not 6-keto-PGF$_{1\alpha}$ or LTB4, compared to syngenic or normal aortas. The two major cellular components of the vascular wall, intima and adventitia, were incubated separately after microdissection. TxB2 was produced in the adventitia, whereas most of the 6-keto-PGF$_1\alpha$ was synthesized in the intima. Administration of a specific TxA2 receptor inhibitor to the recipient rat reduced significantly the proliferation of adventitial inflammatory cells and the intimal smooth muscle cells. Nevertheless, it only delayed but did not inhibit the overall sclerosis of the intima.

Key words: Chronic rejection – GR 32191B – Rat aortic transplants

Materials and methods

Aortic allografts were exchanged form DA (RT1^{av1}) to WF (RT1^u) strain, or for control, to DA strain. A group of rats was treated with a thromboxane A2 receptor inhibitor, GR 32191B, at the rate of 1.0 mg/kg per day. The recipients received a bolus of 250 mCi of ^{3}H-TdR by i. v. injection 3 h prior to sacrifice. The grafts were removed at various times, and were processed for histology, autoradiograms, immunohistochemistry or biochemical determinations [1].

Results and discussion

Morphologically, both types of grafts underwent an acute adventitial inflammatory episode, which subsided. The inflammation was more intense in the allografts, where the inflammatory cells also displayed the activation markers IL-2 receptor and Class II. The intima of the allograft, but not of syngeneic graft, developed an intimal proliferative lesions (arteriosclerosis) characteristic to chronic rejection. The cells in the media were lost in allografts, but preserved in syngeneic grafts.

The vascular wall components, adventitia (media lacking any nuclei) and intima were incubated either separately or together in vitro, and the prostanoids were quantitated by RIA. There was a significantly increased synthesis of TxB2 in the allografts, lacking in syngeneic grafts, but only a small increase in the synthesis of 6-keto-PGF$_{1\alpha}$ and no increase in the synthesis LTB4. The TxB2 synthesis occured mainly in the inflammatory component in the adventitia and 6-keto-PGF$_{1\alpha}$ synthesis in the intima.

Administration of a TxB2 receptor blocker, GR 32191B, did not inhibit the arteriosclerotic changes; nevertheless it delayed them for 1 month compared to the controls.

The incorporation of ^{3}H-TdR to proliferative adventitial and intimal cells was detected by autoradiography. These proliferative responses were significantly inhibited by the administration of GR 32191B. Since the adventitial cells were mainly LCA-positive white cells, and the intimal cells mainly α-smooth muscle actin positive smooth muscle cells, the administration of GR32191B was found to have an inhibitory effect on the proliferation on both of these cell types.

Taken together, the ^{3}H-TdR incorporation studies showed that the adventitial and the intimal proliferative responses were both downregulated by the administration of GR 32191B. Nevertheless, there was only a delay, but no definite inhibition of the generation of the arterio-

Offprint requests to: Ari Mennander, Transplantation Laboratory, University of Helsinki, Haartmaninkatu 3, SF 00290 Helsinki, Finland, Telefax: + 358-0-411227, Phone: + 358-0-434-6596

Grants: Supported by grants from the Academy of Finland, the Sigrid Juselius Foundation, the Finnish Cancer Society, the University of Helsinki, Helsinki, and Farmos Pharmaceuticals, Turku, Finland

sclerotic changes in the transplant as a consequence of the administration of GR 32191B. We concluded that lipid mediators of inflammation, particularly TxB2, were involved in the arteriosclerotic process of chronic rejection. However, this pathway, if blocked, may be bypassed by other, yet unidentified mediatory pathways.

Reference

1. Mennander A, Tiisala S, Halttunen J, Yilmaz S, Paavonen T, Häyry P (1990) Chronic Rejection in rat aortic allografts: an experimental model for transplant arteriosclerosis. Arteriosclerosis Thomb 11: 671–680

Transplant Int (1992) 5 [Suppl 1]: S 589–S 593

TRANSPLANT
International
© Springer-Verlag 1992

Factors involved in peripheral T cell tolerance: the extent of clonal deletion or clonal anergy depends on the age of the tolerized lymphocytes

L. M. Kuschnaroff[1], **K. De Belder**[2], **M. Vandeputte**[2] and **M. Waer**[2,3]

From the department of immunopathology, Rega Institute and Nephrology, University of Leuven, Belgium
This work was supported by the National Fund for Scientific Research of Belgium
[1] L. M. K. is a recipient of scholarship from CAPES, Brazil., [2] Rega Institute for Medical Research
[3] Department of Nephrology, University of Leuven, Belgium

Abstract. After injection of SEB (staphylococcus enterotoxin B), normal adult mice, or thymectomized irradiated mice (TX irr.) reconstituted with lymphocytes taken from normal adult mice became specifically tolerant of SEB. At the same time the percentage of $V\beta 8$ positive CD4 lymphocytes known to be responsive to SEB was almost 50% decreased, indicating that a high level of clonal deletion was realized. In contrast, mice with an exclusively old T cell compartment (old thymectomized mice, TX irr. mice reconstituted several months previously) became tolerant of SEB without deleting their $V\beta 8 +$ CD4 + cells, indicating that clonal anergy was the major mechanism in play in the induction of tolerance. Finally, TX irr. mice reconstituted with single positive thymocytes known to become recent thymic emigrants developed tolerance for SEB together with a high level (70%) of clonal deletion. Altogether these results indicated that the mechanism involved in peripheral tolerance depended on the age of the lymphocyte: very young lymphocytes underwent mainly clonal deletion whereas long lived lymphocytes underwent predominantly clonal anergy.

Key words: T cell tolerance – Clonal deletion – Clonal anergy

The mechanisms by which T lymphocytes become tolerant for self or foreign antigens have been extensively investigated in the recent years. Whereas the concept of active suppression is still controversial, the mechanisms of clonal deletion or clonal anergy are generally accepted as the major ones in T cell tolerance. The advent of superantigens, which are able to stimulate large fractions of T cells [2, 4, 5, 14], and the availability of monoclonal antibodies identifying the T cell receptors capable of reacting against these antigens [16, 20, 23] has made the discrimination between clonal deletion and clonal anergy very reliable. It is generally accepted that immature T cells are tolerized within the thymus. This process is called central tolerance and is realized mainly by clonal deletion [7, 10, 11, 15].

After their arrival in the periphery T cells have recently been shown to be susceptible to tolerance induction as well (called peripheral tolerance) [3, 6, 8, 19, 22]. However, the mechanisms involved in peripheral tolerance are still unclear and controversial. Some studies indicate that clonal anergy is the predominant type of peripheral T cell tolerance [6, 8, 18, 19], whereas other experiments – sometimes involving the same models – unequivocally show that clonal deletion can be achieved to a large extent in the periphery as well [22]. The present studies were undertaken to know more about the factors which determine whether a peripheral T cell undergoes tolerance induction through clonal deletion as apposed to clonal anergy. It was our hypothesis that recent thymic emigrants would still be susceptible to clonal deletion within the first days after their arrival in the periphery, whereas older (memory?) T cells would mainly undergo tolerogenic signals leading to clonal anergy.

To investigate this we created experimental models in which the peripheral T cell pool could be expected to be made up predominantly of old mature T cells or alternatively of a high proportion of recent thymic emigrants. Here we showed that in the former situation, tolerance was almost exclusively realized by clonal anergy, whereas a high level of clonal deletion was observed in the case of a T cell compartment consisting of a relatively important fraction of recent thymic emigrants.

Materials and methods

Animals. In all experiments BLAB/C (H-2^d) mice were used.

Neonatal thymectomy. Newborn mice, 1–3 days old were anesthetized by cooling, and thymectomy was performed through a sternotomy between the second and third ribs by vacuum suctioning of the thymus with a pipette.

Offprint requests to: M. Waer, Rega Institute for Medical Research, University of Leuven, Minderbroedersstraat 10, B-3000 Leuven, Belgium

Table 1. Effect of SEB priming on Vβ8 and Vβ6 receptor antigen expression and on the in vitro proliferative response of T lymphocytes

Groups	Percentage[d] of CD4 + lymphocytes expressing		Stimulation index:[e] after in vitro blastogenesis by	
	Vβ8 +	Vβ6 +	SEB	SEA
A. 2–4 month BALB/C ($N = 5$)	24 (15–29)	9[f]	284 (196–405)	308 (172–444)
B. 2–4 month BALB/C ($N = 3$)[a] primed with SEB	14 (9–17)	14[f]	11 (4–29)	206 (147–267)
C. LN reconstituted BALB/C[b] ($N = 2$)	21 (20–22)	ND	27 (3–52)	24 (2–47)
D. LN reconstituted BALB/C[c] primed SEB ($N = 2$)	12 (9–15)	ND	2 (2–3)	11 (3–20)

[a] SEB (33 µg) was injected 3 times within 1 week
[b] Lethally irradiated, thymectomized BALB/C mice, reconstituted with T cell depleted BM and lymph node cells from 2–4 month old BALB/C donors
[c] SEB (3×33 µg) was injected within 4 weeks after reconstitution

[d] Mean (range) are shown
[e] See materials and methods, means (range) are given
[f] Only one sample in group A and group B was examined on Vβ6 expression
ND = Not determined

Total body irradiation. Mice were exposed to irradiation using gamma rays from a 60-cobalt source (0.35 Gy per min) at a focus-skin-distance of 100 cm. A total dose of 8.5 Gy (850 Rad) was given.

Lymphohaematopoietic reconstitution after irradiation. Bone marrow (BM) cells were obtained from the femur of adult BALB/C mice. Subsequently, T cells were depleted from the BM by adding 50 µl of Thy 1.2 (Becton Dickinson, Mountain Vieuw, CA) for 30 min at 4 °C. Thereafter, the cells were washed twice and rabbit complement diluted 1/9 was added and incubated for another 45 min at 37 °C. Within one day of TBI, irradiated thymectomized mice received 20×10^6 T-depleted bone marrow cells together with either 50×10^6 single positive thymocytes obtained from 3–4 week old cortisone treated BALB/C mice in the first group, or in the second group, 60×10^6 peripheral T cells obtained from lymphnodes of 2–4 month old BALB/C mice

SEB injection: Staphylococcal enterotoxin B (SEB) was purchased from Sigma Chemical Company (St. Louis, Mo., USA). It was diluted and administered IP at a concentration of 33 to 100 µgr in 0.2 ml saline solution (phosphate-buffered saline). All in vitro tests were done 6–14 days after SEB injection.

Flow cytometry: One million splenocytes (passed through a nylon wool column) were stained for the expression of Vβ8 or Vβ6 positive T cell receptors using 20 µl mAbs obtained respectively from undiluted hybridoma culture supernatant from clones F23.1 [20] and F44-22-1 [16], followed by 50 µl fluoresceinated anti-mouse IgG (Fab) portion (Serotec, Oxford, England) for Vβ8 (F23.1) binding and 50 µl of rabbit anti-rat IgG (Fab) portion (Serotec, Oxford, England) for Vβ6 (F44-22-1) binding.

Double staining was done with an anti-mouse CD4 phycoerythrin conjugate (anti-L3T4, Becton Dickinson, Mountain View, Calif.) to measure the expression of Vβ receptors on CD4 positive cells only. Analysis was done using FACSTAR-PLUS (Becton Dickinson, Mountain View, Calif.) interfaced with a Hewlett Packard 300 computer. Cells were gated to exclude non viable ones.

Data are presented as percentage of positive cells after substraction of the number of cells stained with the fluorescent conjugate and irrelevant antibody.

Functional anergy to SEB. The responsiveness of lymphocytes and splenocytes in vitro was analyzed by measuring the stimulation index (SI) of lymphocytes after adding SEB (10 µg/ml), or staphylococcal enterotoxin A (SEA, 10 µg/ml, SERVA, Heidelberg, Germany) or phytoheamaglutinin (PHA, 72 µg/ml, Wellcome, England) into flat bottom micro-culture wells containing 5×10^5 cells in 0.2 ml RPMI 1640 medium supplemented with 20 % human AB serum. After 72 h of incubation, cells were pulsed with 1 µCi of ^{3}H-thymidine collected to a glass filter and counted 18 h later.

$$\text{SI:} \quad \frac{\text{cpm (cells + SEB)}}{\text{cpm (cells + medium)}}$$

The SI was calculated using the mean of quadriplucate counts per minute (cpm) samples measured by a scintillation counter:

Results

Injection of SEB into mice with an adult peripheral T cell compartment (2–4 month old) resulted in tolerance with a high level of clonal deletion (Table 1). BALB/C control (group A) mice, 2–4 months old, had a mean of 24 % of Vβ8-CD4 positive T lymphocytes in their spleen and reacted vigourously in vitro on stimulation with SEB (mean SI = 284). When a similar group of mice (group B) was injected with 100 µg of SEB IV one week before testing their lymphocytes became hyporeactive against SEB (SI = 11), and at the same time they deleted an important fraction of their Vβ8 + CD4 cells known to be reactive against SEB (decrease from 24 % to 14 %). These results were identical to those previously published by other groups [8, 9, 23]. The tolerance achieved after IV injection of SEB was specific for SEB as the reactivity against another stimulus (SEA) was not significantly decreased (SI of 206 as compared to 308 in uninjected mice). The somewhat decreased reactivity of SEB injected mice against SEA could be a consequence of the lymphokine release syndrome known to occur after super antigen injection [13, 14]. The deletion of lymphocytes after SEB injection was limited to those expressing a Vβ8 TCR known to be reactive against SEB, as the percentage of Vβ6 positive CD4 cells (which do not react to SEB) was not decreased by SEB injection (14 % in a SEB injected mouse as compared to 9 % in an uninjected animal).

Also BALB/C mice (group C) which were thymectomized, lethally irradiated, and reconstituted with T depleted BM cells and peripheral lymphocytes (spleen cells and lymphnode cells) obtained from 2–4 months old donors became specifically tolerant of SEB after IV SEB injection 1 week before. Indeed, the in vitro reaction to SEB was reduced to about 10 % of that observed in uninjected reconstituted mice (SI decreased from 27 to 2), whereas the reactivity against SEA remained considerable (SI decreased only from 24 to 11). Once again, SEB injection led to a significant deletion of Vβ8 + CD4 cells (decrease from 21 to 12 %).

Thus, in both situations – 2–4 month old unmanipulated mice, or irradiated, thymectomized mice recon-

Table 3. Effect of SEB priming on Vβ8 and Vβ6 receptor antigen expression and on proliferative response of T lymphocytes in "young" mice

Groups	Percentage[d] of CD4 + lymphocytes expressing		Stimulation index:[c] after in vitro blastogenesis by		
	Vβ8 +	Vβ6 +	SEB	SEA	PHA
A. 3 week old BALB/C (N = 2)	23 (21–26)	9 (9–10)	50 (23–78)	ND	288 (25–551)
B. 3 week old BALB/C primed with SEB (N = 2)	11 (10–12)	13 (12–15)	5 (2–7)	ND	64 (45–83)
C. 3 week old thymect BALB/C (N = 2)	15 (15–17)	6	4	ND	13
D. 3 week old thym. BALB/C primed with SEB (N = 3)	9 (8–14)	10	7 (3–14)	ND	26 (13–39)
E. thymocyte reconstituted[a] BALB/C (N = 3)	22 (19–25)	ND	59 (55–64)	48 (58–81)	ND
F. thymocytes reconstituted[b] primed with SEB (N = 2)	7 (5–10)	ND	4 (4–5)	36 (7–66)	ND

[a] Lethally irradiated, thymectomized BALB/C mice, reconstituted with T cell depleted BM and thymocytes from 3–4 month old BALB/C cortisone treated donors
[b] SEB (3 × 33 μg) was injected within 1 week after reconstitution
[c] See materials and methods
[d] Mean (range) was shown
ND = Not determined

Table 2. Effect of SEB priming on Vβ8 and Vβ6 receptor antigen expression and on proliferative response of T lymphocytes in "old" mice

Groups	Percentage[d] of CD4 + lymphocytes expressing		Stimulation index:[e] after in vitro blastogenesis by		
	Vβ8 +	Vβ6 +	SEB	SEA	PHA
A. 6–7 month BALB/C (N = 2)	28 (28–29)	10 (10–11)	552 (273–831)	ND	148 (84–212)
B. 6–7 month BALB/C (N = 2)[a] primed with SEB	24 (24–25)	9 (9–10)	6 (6–7)	ND	327 (133–522)
C. 6 month old thymect[b] (N = 2)	25 (24–25)	11	10 (51–152)	137	722
D. 6 month old thymect primed with SEB (N = 2)	25 (24–25)	6	2 (1–5)	35	895
E. TX-reconstituted with thymocytes primed with SEB[c] (N = 1)	30	ND	5	58	ND

[a] SEB (3 × 33 μg) was injected 10 days before the test
[b] Thymectomy was done within 2 days of birth
[c] Lethally irradiated, thymectomized BALB/C mouse reconstituted with thymocytes 2 months before SEB injection
[d] mean (range) are shown
[e] See materials and methods
ND = not determined

stituted with peripheral T cells from 2–4 month old mice – SEB injection induced specific tolerance, which seemed to be mediated to a significant extent by clonal deletion.

Injection of SEB into mice with an old peripheral T cell compartment resulted in specific tolerance but without significant clonal deletion (Table 2). In the next series of experiments we used various groups of mice whose peripheral T cell compartment would be expected to be composed mainly of long-lived T cells. The first groups (A and B) consisted of 6 months old mice. At that age it has been shown that the thymic export of T cells becomes extremely low [21] hence peripheral T cells consist mainly of old T cells. However, to exclude any thymic influence, old thymectomised mice (group C and D) were investigated as well. Finally, a thymectomized, lethally irradiated BM reconstituted mouse (E) was injected with single positive thymocytes, but was used in the experiments only 2 months after reconstitution and therefore could be considered as having a peripheral T cell pool of cells of at least 2 month old. As can be seen on Table 2, in all groups of mice SEB injection resulted in functional tolerance of

SEB (signifiant decrease of the SI of SEB induced blastogenesis to very low levels), but this time without any significant decrease of the number of Vβ8 + CD4 cells. Tolerance was specific, as the blastogenesis to another stimulus (PHA or SEA) was not consistently decreased. Also the number of irrelevant Vβ6 + CD4 cells was not significantly altered by the SEB injected (see group B and D). The overall conclusion of these experiments was, therefore, that in mice having a predominantly old T cell compartment SEB injection did lead to tolerance but without apparent clonal deletion.

Injection of SEB in mice with a predominantly young T cell compartment resulted in specific tolerance and clonal deletion of a high percentage of Vβ8 + CD4 cells. Three experimental situations were investigated where the peripheral T cell compartment could be considered as being composed mainly by young T cells. The first groups (A and B) consisted of 1 week old BALB/C mice. The following groups (C and D) were made up of 1 week old neonatally thymectomized mice to exclude thymic influence, and finally, in groups (E and F), lethally irradiated, thymectomized animals were reconstituted with single positive thymocytes (obtained from thymuses of cortisone treated animals) and injected 1 week later with SEB.

As shown on Table 3, in all situations SEB injection led to a high level of clonal deletion of Vβ8 + CD4 cells and this was most pronounced in group F (a decrease of Vβ8 + CD4 cells of about 70%). In this latter group the group of reconstituted mice could be expected to have the highest percentage of very young T cells, as they were reconstituted with single positive thymocytes, known to be the cells which migrate to the periphery. Once again, injection of SEB resulted in specific tolerance as the PHA or SEA stimulation indexes were not considerably influenced. Again the decrease of CD4 cells was not seen in the subpopulation of T cells bearing the irrelevant Vβ6 positive TCR.

Discussion

Recently, various experiments have indicated that peripheral T cell tolerance can be achieved. As far as the mechanisms are concerned, some authors find that clonal anergy is the major mechanism underlying peripheral T cell tolerance although they admit that the results can vary from animal to animal [18]. Other investigators [22] have shown that clonal deletion can also take place in the periphery. The present experiments were undertaken to solve this controversy. It was our hypothesis that T lymphocytes that only recently emigrated from the thymus would still be very susceptible to clonal deletion in the periphery, whereas those which persisted for a longer period would become resistant to deletion and would be tolerized without deletion, thus becoming anergic. We showed that in cases where the peripheral T cell pool would be expected to be composed of a high fraction of young lymphocytes, tolerance after SEB injection was specific and associated with a high level of clonal deletion (a decrease of about 50%) of the Vβ8 + CD4 cells known to be reactive against SEB. In contrast, in all three situations where the peripheral T cells could be expected to consist almost exclusively of long lived lymphocytes, tolerance was achieved without significant clonal deletion, and hence was due to clonal anergy.

We asked ourselves why young peripheral T cells are still susceptible to clonal deletion, and old T cells resistant to it. It is possible that young peripheral T cells contain a majority of virgin T cells, whereas old T cells should be mainly memory cells. Indeed, T cells probably die rapidly in the periphery if they do not see an appropriate antigen [12]. Memory T cells express more adhesion molecules, and therefore their contact with the antigen presenting cell (APC) must be different from that of virgin cells. The intensity of contact with the APC is known to be an important determinant in the type of tolerance (clonal deletion versus anergy) which is induced after a tolerogenic signal [1, 17]. Memory cells are also known to have lymphokine secretion profile other than that of virgin cells [1]. Interference with the lymphokine secretion profile of cells was has recently been shown to be an important factor in the induction of clonal deletion [1]. Therefore, the differences in the mechanisms underlying tolerance in virgin as opposed to memory T cells could be related to their constitutive lymphokine secretion profiles. We are presently trying to clarify these issues using mice reconstituted with T cells with either virgin or memory characteristics or by interfering with their specific lymphokine secretion patterns.

Acknowledgements. We thank O. Rutgeerts and C. Segers for their valuable technical assistance, and Dominique Brabants for preparation of the manuscript.

References

1. Akbar AN, Salmon M, Janossy G (1991) The synergy between naive and memory T cells during activation. Immunol Today 12: 184–188
2. Blackman M, Kappler J, Marrack P (1990) The role of the T cell receptor in positive and negative selection of developing T cells. Science 238: 1335–1393
3. Blackman MA, Finkel TH, Kappler J, Cambier J, Marrack P (1991) Altered antigen receptor signaling in anergic T cells from self-tolerant T-cell receptor β-chain transgenic mice. Proc Natl Acad Sci USA 88: 6682–6686
4. Buxser S, Vroegop S (1988) Staphylococcal enterotoxin B stimulation of BALB/C lymphocytes mitogenesis and potential relationship to the Mls response. J Immunogenet 15: 153–159
5. Janeway CA Jr, Yagi J, Conrad PJ, Katz ME, Jones B; Vroegop S, Buxser S (1989) T-cell responses to Mls to bacterial proteins that mimic its behavior. Immunol Rev 107: 61–88
6. Jones LA, Chin LT, Merriam GR, Nelson LM, Kruisbeck AM (1990) Failure of clonal deletion in neonatally thymectomized mice: tolerance is preserved through clonal anergy. J Exp Med 172: 1277–1285
7. Kappler JW, Staerz U, White J, Marrack PC (1988) Self-tolerance eliminates T cells specific for Mls-modified products of the major histocompatibility complex. Nature 332: 35–40
8. Kawabe Y, Ochi A (1990) Selective anergy of Vβ8 +, CD4 + T cells in staphylococcus enterotoxin B-primed mice. J Exp Med 172: 1065–1070
9. Kawabe Y, Ochi A (1991) Programmed cell death and extrathymic reduction of Vβ8 + CD4 + T cells in mice tolerant to Staphylococcus aureus enterotoxin B. Nature 349: 245–248
10. MacDonald HR, Schneider R, Lees RK, Howe RC, Acha-Orbea H, Festenstein H, Zinkernagel RM, Hengartner H (1988) T-cell receptor Vβ use predicts reactivity and tolerance to Mls^a-encoded antigens. Nature 332: 40–45
11. MacDonald HR, Pedrazzini T, Schneider R, Louis JA, Zinkernagel RM, Hengartner H (1988) Intrathymic elimination of Mls^a-reactive (Vβ6 +) cells during neonatal tolerance induction to Mls^a-encoded antigens. J Exp Med 167: 2005–2010
12. Mackay CR (1991) T-cell memory: the connection between function, phenotype and migration pathways. Immunol Today 12: 189–192
13. Marrack P, Kappler J (1990) The staphylococcal enterotoxins and their relatives. Science 248: 705–711
14. Marrack P, Blackman M, Kushnir E, Kappler J (1990) The toxicity of staphylococcal enterotoxin B in mice is mediated by T cells. J Exp Med 171: 455–464
15. Mazda O, Watanabe Y, Gyotoku J-I, Katsura Y (1991) Requirement of dendritic cells and B cells in the clonal deletion of Mls-reactive T cells in the thymus. J Exp Med 173: 539–547
16. Payne J, Huber BT, Cannon NA, Schneider R, Schilham MW, Acha-Orbea H, MacDonald HR, Hengartner H (1988) Two monoclonal rat antibodies with specificity for the β-chain variable region Vβ6 of the murine T-cell receptor. Proc Natl Acad Sci USA 85: 7695–7698

17. Pircher H, Hoffmann Rohrer U, Moskophidis D, Zinkernagel RM, Hengartner H (1991) Lower receptor avidity required for thymic clonal deletion than for effector T cell function. Nature 351: 482–485

18. Rammensee H-G, Krochewski R, Frangoulis B (1989) Clonal anergy induced in mature Vβ6 + T lymphocytes on immunizing Mls-1^b mice with Mls-1^a expressing cells. Nature 339: 541–544

19. Rellahan BL, Jones LA, Kruisbeek AM, Fry AM, Matis LA (1990) In vivo induction of anergy in peripheral Vβ8 + T cells by staphylococcal enterotoxin B. J Exp Med 172: 1091–1100

20. Staerz UD, Rammensee H-G, Benedetto JD, Bevan MJ (1985) Characterization of a murine monoclonal antibody specific for an allotypic determinant on T cell antigen receptor. J Immunol 134: 3994–4000

21. Stutman O (1986) Postthymic T-cell development. Immunol Rev 91: 159–194

22. Webb S, Morris C, Spreng J (1990) Extrathymic tolerance of mature T cells: clonal elimination as a consequence of immunity. Cell 63: 1249–1256

23. White J, Herman A, Pullen AM, Kubo R, Kappler JW, Marrack P (1989) The Vβ-specific superantigen staphylococcal enterotoxin B: stimulation of mature T cells and clonal deletion in neonatal mice. Cell 56: 27–35

Transplant Int (1992) 5 [Suppl 1]: S 594–S 595

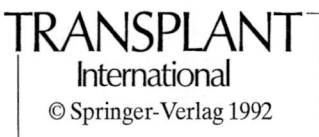

© Springer-Verlag 1992

Allo and auto crossmatches after transplantation

E. van den Berg-Loonen, R. Overhof, M. Tillemans, and H. van Hooff

Tissue Typing Laboratory, University Hospital Maastricht, P.O. Box 5800, 6202 AZ Maastricht, The Netherlands

The development of a positive donor-crossmatch after transplantation is usually seen as a bad prognostic sign with regard to graft survival. Since a number of positive post-transplant-crossmatches with the original donor in the absence of graft rejection was noticed in our center, we started a systematic investigation of donor-crossmatches after transplantation.

Key words: Kidney allografts – Crossmatches – Post-transplantation

Materials and methods

The development of T- and B-cell allo- and autoantibodies was investigated in 151 consecutive kidney allografts with a follow-up time of at least 1 year. Crossmatches were repeated with the original crossmatchsera as well as sera obtained after transplantation using frozen donor spleen cells and patients' peripheral blood lymphocytes. Crossmatches were performed using NIH and TCF techniques; DTT treatment was used to study the immunoglobulin class of the antibodies involved. Sera were collected at regular intervals and only patients with a minimum of three post-transplant sera were included in the study. The average number of post-transplant sera was six. Out of 151 patients, 100 had a negative donor crossmatch at the time of transplantation. Twenty-one grafts, performed with a positive T- and/or B-cell crossmatch due to autoantibodies, were excluded from the study, 19 patients had to be excluded for lack of material.

Results

After transplantation 60 patients formed neither allo- nor autoantibodies, 30 patients showed reactivity to donor B-cells but not T-cells and 20 patients developed antibodies

reactive with donor T-cells (Table 1). Graft survival in the different groups was 90%, 80% and 75% respectively. The presence of autoantibodies was investigated in the different groups. From 20 patients with a positive T-cell donor crossmatch, 10 were shown to possess auto-T-cell antibodies and 2 auto-B-cell antibodies. In 30 patients with a positive B-cell donor crossmatch, autoreactivity could be shown in 13. One year graft survival in patients with autoantibodies was 84% in contrast to 72% in the group without autoantibodies.

Since graft survival seems to be influenced by the formation of T-cell antibodies, we selected the patients with good 1 year graft survival and no rejections to see whether this group lacked antibody development. Out of 54 patients, 15 developed a positive donor crossmatch after transplantation (13 B-cell, 2 T-cell) (Table 2). Out of 39 patients

Table 1. Donor crossmatches after transplantation and autoantibodies

	Donor crossmatch		
	T – B –	T – B +	T + B +
Auto crossmatch			
T – B –	60 (6)	17 (4)	8 (3)
T – B +	0	13 (2)	2
T + B +	0	0	10 (2)
	60	30	20

(⊕) = Grafts lost within one year

Table 2. Donor crossmatches after transplantation and rejection

		Donor crossmatch		
	N	T – B –	T – B +	T + B +
No rejection treatment	54	39	13 (6)	2 (1)
Reversible rejection	39	15	11 (5)	13 (9)
Irreversible rejection or graft loss	17	6	6 (2)	5 (2)

(⊕) = Auto crossmatch positive

Offprint requests to: Ella van den Berg-Loonen

with reversible rejection, 24 became positive (11 B-cell, 13 T-cell) as well as 11 out of 17 patients with irreversible rejection or graft loss (6 B-cell, 5 T-cell). Of these positive donor crossmatches 50% were autocrossmatch positive.

All 7 patients who had been treated with OKT3 developed a positive donor-crossmatch after transplantation with strongly positive T + B + auto-crossmatches which reactivity could not be removed by DTT treatment. When the number of OKT3 treated patients was extended to 12, all of them (100%) showed a positive T-cell donor crossmatch after transplantation as compared to 3 out of 23 patients who received RATG as rejection treatment (13%). The sera of all treated patients were strongly cytotoxic as early as 24 h after the first administration of OKT3 and stayed positive until a maximum of 10 days after cessation of the therapy.

Conclusion

We concluded that the development of a positive T-cell donor crossmatch after transplantation influenced graft survival but was not necessarily a prediction of graft failure. A positive B-cell donor crossmatch did not seem to influence graft survival in patients with autoantibodies. Half of all positive donor crossmatches after transplantation were due to the development of autoantibodies. OKT3 caused strong cytotoxic activity of patient sera which could not be removed by DTT. Therefore sera collected during OKT3 treatment could not be used for crossmatching or antibody investigation.

Transplant Int (1992) 5 [Suppl 1]: S 596–S 598

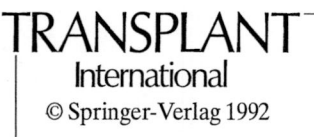
TRANSPLANT
International
© Springer-Verlag 1992

Remarkable correlation between increased HLA-DQ antigen positive monocytes and prognosis of renal transplantation

Y. Fukuda, T. Ishikawa, H. Yahata, S. Marubayashi, and K. Dohi

Second Department of Surgery, Hiroshima University School of Medicine, Hiroshima, Japan

Abstract. Since cyclosporin A (CsA), a widely used immunosuppressive drug, strongly suppresses interleukin-2 (IL-2) secretion, it is frequently difficult to estimate T lymphocyte activation in early acute rejection. We found that, when evaluated based on HLA-DQ antigen expression, monocyte activation in the peripheral blood of renal transplantation patients was a very sharp parameter in diagosing acute rejection. All of 16 episodes of early acute rejection, which were relatively easily suppressed by steroid pulse therapy, showed a sharp increase in the proportion of HLA-DQ antigen-positive monocytes (DQ^+mono) and a quick return of DQ^+mono to previous values, along with a fall in serum creatinine levels. Since, however, HLA-DR antigen-positive T lymphocytes (DR^+T) were markedly increased over a long period in episodes of therapy-resistant and chronic rejection, their prolonged high value was regarded as a parameter indicative of poor prognosis.

Key words: Immunological monitoring – HLA-DQ positive monocytes – Monocyte – HLA-DQ antigen

The immunological monitoring of acute rejection has often been carried out on activated T lymphocytes by means of expression of DR antigen [1] and interleukin-2 (IL-2) receptor [2] or by assay of lymphokines, such as IL-2 [3]. These parameters have frequently been reported as showing false negative results [4]. Cyclosporin A (CsA), currently a leading immunosuppressive drug, strongly suppresses T lymphocyte activation by blocking IL-2 seretion [5]. It is therefore surmised that because of this, T lymphocyte activation may not be clearly observed in early acute and mild rejection.

It has been reported that, although HLA-class I, HLA-DR and DP antigens are expressed in high density on the monocyte membrane, HLA-DQ antigen is expressed only in 10–40% of the monocytes in peripheral blood [6, 7]. Its expression has been confirmed as stimulated by interferon-γ [8].

Speculating that the HLA-DQ antigen might be used as a marker for activated monocytes, we investigated the kinetics of the HLA-DQ antigen of monocytes in the peripheral blood of renal transplantation patients. Apparent correlation was found between acute rejection and increaesd HLA-DQ antigen positive monocytes.

Patients and methods

Using 35 renal transplantation patients (32 living related donors and 3 cadaveric donors), surface markers of monocytes and lymphocytes in the peripheral blood were examined before, and 7, 14 and 28 days after transplantation. Examination was performed frequently when development of rejection was suspected. As immunosuppressive agents, cyclosporin A (CsA) and steroids were used in all patients. The same examination was also carried out in control groups of 25 healthy volunteers (11 males and 14 females, > 20 years old), 11 haemodialysis patients and 11 kidney transplant patients who had not experienced any problems for 1 year or longer after transplantation.

Surface markers investigated included CD3, CD8 and HLA-DR antigens for lymphocytes and HLA-DR and DQ antigens for monocytes, and were estimated by double-staining utilizing flowcytometry (FCM). Monoclonal antibodies used in staining were as follows:

1. Anti Leu4 + anti HLA-DR→activated T lymphocyte (DR^+T)
2. Anti Leu3a + anti Leu2a→T helper/suppressor ratio (H/S)
3. Anti LeuM3 + anti HLA-DR→HLA-DR$^+$monocyte (DR^+-mono)
4. Anti LeuM3 + anti Leu10→HLA-DQ$^+$monocyte (DQ^+mono)

Results

Values of surface markers in the control groups are shown in Table 1. DQ^+mono in the 25 healthy volunteers was 17.3% ±7.2%, with no significant difference according to sex or age (data not shown). In contrast, DR^+mono was 91.2% ±7.9%, which confirmed expression in the ma-

Offprint requests to: Yasuhiko Fukuda M.D., 2nd Department of Surgery, Hiroshima University School of Medicine, 1-2-3 Kasumi, Minami-Ku, Hiroshima, Japan 734

Table 1. FACS analysis of surface markers of lymphocytes and monocytes in control group. Results are expressed as mean ± SD

| | Healthy persons ($n = 25$) | Haemodialysis patients ($n = 11$) | |
		Before H.D.	After H.D.
DR⁺T (%)	9.2 ± 4.8	11.1 ± 5.4	7.8 ± 4.2
H/S	1.93 ± 0.68	1.98 ± 0.39	2.87 ± 0.75*
DR⁺mono (%)	91.2 ± 7.9	96.5 ± 3.0	97.6 ± 1.3
DQ⁺mono (%)	17.3 ± 7.2	28.4 ± 12.8	16.3 ± 7.3**

* $P < 0.001$; ** $P < 0.005$; as compared with before haemodialysis

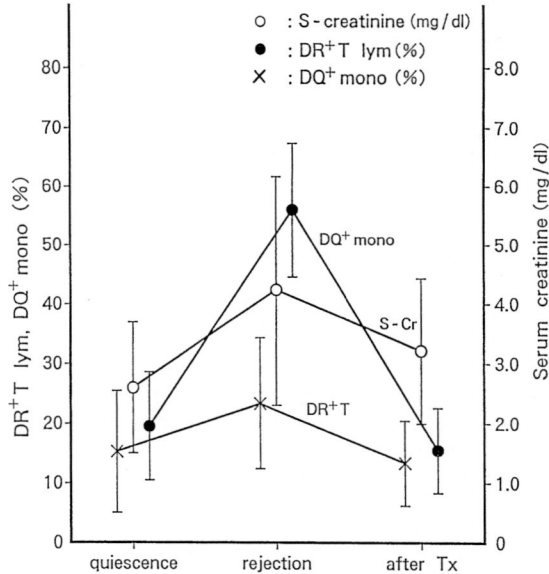

Fig. 1. Alteration of DQ⁺mono (x–x) and DR⁺T (●–●) in acute rejection of renal allograft recipients ($n = 16$)

jority of monocytes. In the haemodialysis patients, DQ⁺mono was 28.4% ± 12.8% before dialysis, which was higher than that in the healthy volunteers, and 16.3% ± 7.3% after dialysis. This should be taken into consideration when DQ⁺mono is measured in patients who need haemodialysis after renal transplantation.

Of the 35 renal transplantation patients who were prospectively monitored, 15 experienced no rejection. Table 2 shows data of DR⁺T and DQ⁺mono monitoring over time. DQ⁺mono showed a high value of 41.8% ± 27.0% before transplantation, which rapidly declined to 15.2% ± 11.1% and 13.0% ± 7.6% at 7 and 28 days after transplantation, respectively. In contrast, the mean value of DQ⁺mono in the 11 transplant patients who were incident free for 1 year or longer after transplantation was as low as 9.7% ± 4.5%. However, there was almost no change in DR⁺T. We, therefore, suggest that DQ⁺mono is a more accurate parameter.

There were 16 episodes of acute rejection which occurred within 3 months after transplantation and could be controlled by steroid pulse therapy, but DQ⁺mono quickly rose in all of them (Fig. 1). As serum creatinine levels were decreased with therapy, DQ⁺mono returned to previous values. In contrast, mean value of DR⁺T increased mildly when rejection occurred, and in 5 patients did not rise at all.

Interestingly, estimation of DQ⁺mono was also found to be a useful parameter for predicting the occurence of rejection (Table 3). When DQ⁺mono was 30% or more at 14 days after transplantation, acute rejection developed in 10 out of 13 patients (76.9%) within 3 months. When DQ⁺mono was less than 30% at 28 days after transplantation, acute rejection occurred in only 3 patients (16.7%). Such regular estimations of DQ⁺mono would appear to provide information useful for adjusting immunosuppressive therapy and setting a suitable date of discharge from hospital.

Ten episodes of intractable rejection resistant to steroid pulse therapy were experienced. Of note was a prolonged increase in DR⁺T, unresponsive to pulse therapy (Table 4). In contrast, DQ⁺mono decreased in response to therapy temporarily, despite lack of improvement in renal function. Intractable persistent rejection apparently showed a prolonged increase in activated T lymphocytes, which was presumably a sign of poor prognosis.

Deteriorated renal function due to CsA nephrotoxicity was confirmed by biopsy in 5 patients, their DQ⁺mono values remaining low (Table 5). DQ⁺mono did not increase at the time of viral infection in 2 patients. In 2 patients diagnosed by biopsy as having chronic rejection, DQ⁺mono showed low values, but DR⁺T was as high as 50% or more. Therefore, DQ⁺mono increase is assumed to be a phenomenon specific to acute rejection.

Discussion

Monocytes in the peripheral blood have been classified into 2 subsets depending on the presence of DQ⁺mono [6, 7]. It has been confirmed that DQ⁻mono are transformed into DQ⁺mono by treatment with interferon-γ [8, 9]. Therefore, it is assumed that they are derived from the same origin, and that their DQ antigen expression reflects

Table 2. Serial monitoring of DR⁺T and DQ⁺mono in renal allograft recipients ($n = 15$) who experienced no rejection. Results are expressed as mean ± SD. Pre-Tx analysis were done before the use of immunosuppressive drugs

| | Recipients | | | | Long-term surviving graft ($n = 11$) | Normal healthy group ($n = 25$) |
| | Stable graft function ($n = 15$) | | | | | |
	pre Tx	post Tx-7 days	14 days	28 days		
S-Cr (mg/dl)	10.9 ± 3.0	2.1 ± 1.6	1.6 ± 0.6	1.4 ± 0.5	1.4 ± 0.2	
DR⁺T lym (%)	8.7 ± 4.5	8.2 ± 6.6	8.3 ± 5.8	12.1 ± 8.3	11.5 ± 6.3	9.2 ± 4.8
DQ⁺mono (%)	41.8 ± 27.0	15.2 ± 11.1	15.0 ± 11.1	13.0 ± 7.6	9.7 ± 4.5	17.3 ± 7.2

Table 3. Correlation between incidence of acute rejection occurring within 3 months after renal transplantation and HLA-DQ$^+$mono in recipients ($n = 35$) on 14th and 28th post-operative days

HLA-DQ$^+$ monocytes	Incidence of acute rejection	
On 14th day after Tx		
≤ 30%	6/22 (27.3%)	$\chi^2 = 8.13$ ($P < 0.01$)
> 30%	10/13 (76.9%)	
On 28th day after Tx		
≤ 30%	3/18 (16.7%)	$\chi^2 = 12.58$ ($P < 0.01$)
> 30%	13/17 (76.5%)	

Table 4. Alteration of DR$^+$T and DQ$^+$mono in acute rejection of renal allograft recipients ($n = 10$) in whom anti-rejection therapy was not effective. Results are expressed as mean ± SD

	Quiescence	After anti-rejection Tx
S-Cr (mg/dl)	3.2 ± 1.0	4.6 ± 1.4
DR$^+$T lym (%)	24.7 ± 10.1	47.5 ± 7.6
DQ$^+$mono (%)	30.1 ± 14.4	13.6 ± 9.4

Table 5. Flowcytometric data of DR$^+$T and DQ$^+$mono in renal allograft recipients with CsA nephrotoxicity, viral infection and chronic rejection

		S-CR (mg/dl)	DR$^+$T (%)	DQ$^+$mono (%)
CyA nephrotoxicity	①	2.7	11.0	21.1
	②	2.6	16.3	5.1
	③	3.7	18.5	19.3
	④	3.9	15.2	7.3
	⑤	3.5	8.1	26.6
Viral infection	①	1.1	2.8	2.7
	②	1.4	8.6	8.8
Chronic rejection	①	4.0	67.9	24.6
	②	7.3	54.2	7.7

cellular maturation or activation. The strong correlation between acute rejection and DQ antigen expression, as shown by our data, corroborated the finding that the DQ antigen is a surface marker of activated monocytes.

It has been reported that DQ$^+$mono, when compared with DQ$^-$mono, possess very strong antigen presenting ability and strong stimulation activity in mixed lymphocyte cultures [10]. It is not known how DQ$^+$mono increase in rejection functions. Possibly, however, they not only increase antigen presenting ability but also the DQ$^+$mono may act as the direct effector cells on target organs.

As shown by our data, DQ$^+$mono, when compared with DR$^+$T, also increased by responding sharply to mild rejection. This indicated interferon-γ secretion from helper T lymphocytes in the early stage of rejection and in the state of insufficient immunosuppression. We suggest that monocytes might respond sharply to interferon-γ; therefore, it would appear that the indirect estimation of activated monocyte increase would be clinically more useful than the direct measurement of interferon-γ.

DR$^+$T may be a paramater of advanced rejection and not a very useful paramater for early detection. A prolonged increase in DR$^+$T was found in frequent and chronic rejection, which did not tend to decrease with pulse therapy. The authors therefore regard it as a paramater of poor prognosis.

1. Hayes JM, Valenzuela R, Novick AC, Steinmuller DR, Williams G (1987) Correlation between two-color flow cytometry quantitation of activated T cells and acute allograft rejection. Transplant Proc 19: 1605–1608
2. Ellis TM, Lee HM, Mohanakumar T (1981) Alteration in human regulatory T lymphocyte subpopulations after renal allografting. J Immunol 127: 2199–2203
3. Young-Fadok TM, Simpson MA, Madras PN, Dempsey RA, O'Connor K, Monaco AP (1991) Predictive value of pretransplant IL-2 levels in kidney transplantation. Transplant Proc 23: 1295–1296
4. Takahara S, Sakakibara I, Suzuki S, Amemiya H, Kokado Y (1989) Subpopulation of peripheral blood mononuclear cells are reliable for monitoring infiltrating mononuclear cells. Transplant Proc 21: 1846–1851
5. Borel JF (1990) Mechanism of action and rationale for cyclosporin A in psoriasis. Br J Dermatol 122: 5–10
6. Gonwa TA, Picker LJ, Raff HV, Goyert SM, Silver J, Stobo JD (1983) Antigen presenting capabilities of human monocytes correlate with their expression of HLA-DS, an Ia determinant distinct from HLA-DR. J Immunol 130: 706–711
7. Nunez G, Giles RC, Ball EJ, Hurley CK, Capra JD, Stastny P (1984) Expression of HLA-DR, MB, MT, and SB antigens on human mononuclear cells: identification of two phenotypically distinct monocyte populations. J Immunol 133: 1300–1306
8. Gonwa TA, Stobo JD (1984) Differential expression of Ia molecules by human monocytes. J Clin Invest 74: 859–866
9. Gonwa TA, Frost JP, Karr RW (1986) All human monocytes have the capability of expressing HLA-DQ and HLA-DP molecules upon stimulation with interferon-γ. J Immunol 137: 519–524
10. Nunez G, Ball EJ, Myers LK, Stastny P (1985) Allostimulating cells in man. Quantitative in the expression of HLA-DR and HLA-DQ molecules influences T-cell activation. Immunogenetics 22: 85–91

Transplant Int (1992) 5 [Suppl 1]: S 599–S 600

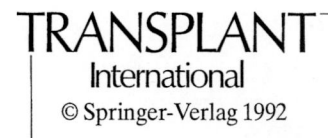

TRANSPLANT
International
© Springer-Verlag 1992

The influence of DR match of blood donor and recipient on the formation of T- and B-cell antibodies and on renal allograft outcome

J. P. van Hooff, and P. M. van den Berg-Loonen

Department of Internal Medicine, P.O. Box 5800, 6202 AZ, Maastricht, The Netherlands

It has been shown that patients transfused with one unit of blood mismatched for both HLA DR antigens have an increased rate of formation of cytotoxic leucocyte antibodies compared to patients who received blood which differs in only one DR antigen. In the same study it was found that DR sharing of the blood transfusion donor and patient improved results of kidney and heart transplantation. However, the data were mostly collected in a retrospective manner and came from various centres. Furthermore, no information was available on whether these antibodies were directed to B- or T-cells. Therefore, the influence of DR match of recipient and blood donor on the formation of T- and B-cell antibodies as well as on clinical course after kidney transplantation was studied prospectively in patients transplanted in one centre.

Key words: DR match – Blood donor and recipient – T- and B-cell antibodies – Kidney transplantation

Patients and methods

One unit of packed cells was given to 147 patients who had received neither a transfusion nor had been pregnant. Serum samples were collected at 2, 3 and 4 weeks. After 4 weeks, crossmatching was done with frozen cells from the blood transfusion donor and HLA typing of the blood transfusion donor was performed. When the crossmatch was negative (NIH), patients received another one or two units of blood ($n = 73$). Recently, this protocol was changed and patients received one unit of blood ($n = 74$). In the analysis only the results after one transfusion were included.

Crossmatches were performed according to the NIH and TCF techniques. DTT treatment was used to study the immunoglobulin class of the antibodies involved. All patients who received a renal allograft used cyclosporin-A and low dose prednisolone as immunosuppression. Antirejection treatment consisted of a 10 day course of rabbit ATG. Subsequent rejections were treated with 50–100 mg prednisolone on 3 alternate days. Rejection was diagnosed on clinical grounds and in most cases was confirmed by a biopsy.

Offprint requests to: J. P. van Hooff

Results

After one transfusion only 3 patients formed T-cell antibodies, while 29 patients formed B-cell antibodies (Table 1). There was no significant influence of DR match of the blood transfusion donor and recipient on the formation of either T- or B-cell antibodies (Table 1). In 9 of 21 patients with B-cell antibodies, auto-B-cell antibodies could be detected as well. If only those patients who formed allo-antibodies were analyzed, a significant influence ($P < 0.02$) of DR match of the blood transfusion donor and recipient on the formation of B-cell antibodies was present (Table 2). So far, 38 patients who received one unit of blood were transplanted (Table 3). No influence of DR match of the blood donor and recipient was present during the clinical course. In both groups no grafts were lost in the first 6 months due to immunological reasons. Moreover, the percentage of patients who were rejection free was comparable in both groups.

Discussion

In our study, only the formation of B-cell antibodies was influenced by the DR match of the blood donor and recipient and not the formation of cytotoxic T-cell antibodies. Our study is not completely comparable with the study of Lagaay [1] in the sense that we studied prospectively the formation of donor specific antibodies, while Lagaay analyzed retrospectively data on the development of antibodies against a random donor panel (NIH). It is unlikely

Table 1. The formation of antibodies and DR mismatch of blood donor and recipient

DR-mismatch N		T – B +	T + B +	Auto
0	17	1 (6%)	0	1
1	61	10 (16%)	3	6
2	69	18 (26%)	0	2

$P = NS$

Table 2. The formation of allo-antibodies and DR mismatch of blood donor and recipient

DR-mismatch	N	T − B +	T + B +
0	17	0	0
1	61	4 (7%)	3
2	69	16 (23%)	0

$P < 0.02$

Table 3. Kidney graft outcome and DR match of blood donor and recipient

DR mismatch	1	2
N	20	18
% Graft survival ($^1/_2$ year)	75	100
Non-immunological graft loss	5	0
Immunological graft loss	0	0
% Without rejection treatment	67	72

that this difference explains the lack of accordance of both studies. It is more likely that the different results are due to a different interpretation of serological results. This assumption is supported by the fact that Lagaay reported a higher sensitization grade in her study than we and others have found.

We could not confirm the beneficial effect of DR matching of the blood transfusion donor and patient on the clinical course. One could argue that the group was too small; but the groups studied by Lagaay [1] were not large. She studied 63 renal patients transplanted at various centres, and 20 heart patients transplanted in one centre.

There are, however, large differences between the two studies. Our renal patients were treated with cyclosporin and the renal patients of Lagaay received azathioprine and prednisone. Moreover, antirejection treatments differed some what. The matching procedure was completely different in both studies. Our patients received HLA A + B + DR matched kidneys, while in the study of Lagaay renal patients were selected on the basis of HLA A + B antigens and heart transplantations were not selected on the basis of either HLA loci.

Conclusion

After one transfusion, only 2 respectively 14% of renal patients formed allo-T and allo-B-cell antibodies. Only the formation of B-cell antibodies was influenced by the DR match of the blood transfusion donor and not the formation of T-cell antibodies. There was no significant influence of the DR match of the blood transfusion donor and patient on the clinical outcome of the kidney allograft.

References

1. Lagaay EL, Hennemann IPH, Ruigrok M, et al (1989) Effect of one-HLA-DR-antigen-matched and completely HLA-DR-mismatched blood transfusions on survival of heart and kidney allografts. N Engl J Med 321: 701
2. Opelz G, Graver B, Mickey MR, Terasaki PI (1981) Lymphocytotoxic antibody responses to transfusions in potential kidney transplant recipients. Transplantation 32: 177–183

Transplant Int (1992) 5 [Suppl 1]: S 601–S 603

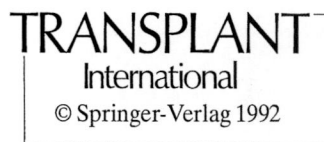

TRANSPLANT
International
© Springer-Verlag 1992

Success rate and impact of HLA matching on kidney graft survival in highly immunized recipients

G. Opelz for the Collaborative Transplant Study

Department of Transplantation Immunology, Institute of Immunology, University of Heidelberg, Im Neuenheimer Feld 305, D-6900 Heidelberg, Germany

Abstract. From 1985 to 1990, 225 highly immunized recipients were transplanted based on a program of serum exchange and priority allocation of kidneys to crossmatch negative recipients. The 1-year graft survival rate in first transplant recipients was 73% and in second transplant recipients, 71%. Recipients of third or fourth transplants had a 25% lower success rate. HLA matching exerted a significant influence on graft outcome. Twenty-five first or second grafts with zero mismatches for HLA-B,-DR had a 91% 1-year survival rate, in contrast to a 58% survival rate of 38 grafts with of three or four HLA-B,-DR mismatches (log rank $P < 0.001$).

Key words: Highly immunized recipients – HLA matching

The transplantation of highly immunized recipients continues to be a problem. Because the serum of these patients contains lymphocytotoxic antibodies that react against most potential donors, it is difficult to identify donors against whom the crossmatch test is negative. In 1985 we initiated a project aimed at identifying suitable donors for this special risk category of recipients. The current report is an extension of our previous publication in which we reported on the first 100 transplants. Since 1988, the number of patients who received transplants as a result of this project has more than doubled.

Patients and methods

A detailed description of the project's technical nature is provided in a previous publication [1]. Briefly, sera of highly immunized recipients (> 80% lymphocytotoxic panel reactivity in at least two consecutive recent screening) were collected every 2–3 months, added to tissue typing trays, and the trays were distributed to the participating transplant centers. Lymphocytes of potential kidney donors were added to the trays to identify patients with a negative crossmatch. A

Offprint requests to: Gerhard Opelz

second crossmatch was performed in the laboratory of the recipient center. Whereas the HLA match was disregarded during the initial 3 years, a recommendation was made in 1988 to transplant kidneys only if dondor and recipient shared at least one HLA antigen on each HLA locus (HLA-A,-B,-DR). The mean number of patients enrolled for each serum exchange "cycle" was 151 and the mean number of transplants performed during each cycle was eight.

The following centers participated in this project:
Aachen, Barcelona, Basel, Bern, Berlin-Friedrichshain, Brussels, Cologne, Düsseldorf, Essen, Frankfurt, Freiburg, Geneva, Gent, Gothenburg, Hannover, Heidelberg, Helsinki, Innsbruck, Kaiserslautern, Lausanne, Leuven, Lübeck, Lund-Malmö, Madrid, Marburg, Milan, Munich, Münster, Paris, Prague, Tübingen, Vienna, Warsaw, Zürich.

Graft survival rates were computed by actuarial methods. One transplant was excluded from the analysis because the repeat crossmatch in the recipient center was positive but the transplant operation had been completed without awaiting the crossmatch results. No other exclusions were made.

Results

Figure 1 demonstrates the overall graft survival rates for first, second, third, and fourth cadaver transplants. First and second grafts had a nearly identical success rate of approximately 70% at 1 year. This result was identical with the one reported 3 years ago for the first 100 patients [1]. The survival of a fifth transplant which is still functioning is not shown in Fig. 1.

The effect on graft survival of matching for HLA-A,-B antigens is shown in Fig. 2. Although a trend towards improved survival with better matching was noticeable, this was not statistically significant. Figure 3 shows the effect of matching for HLA-DR antigens. Whereas there was no difference in outcome between grafts with zero or one mismatch, grafts with two mismatches did significantly worse. The impact of matching for the combination of HLA-B and HLA-DR antigens is illustrated in Fig. 4. Graft outcome worsened as the number of mismatches increased.

We felt it was of interest, primarily because the "acceptable mismatch" program of Claas and van Rood is

S602

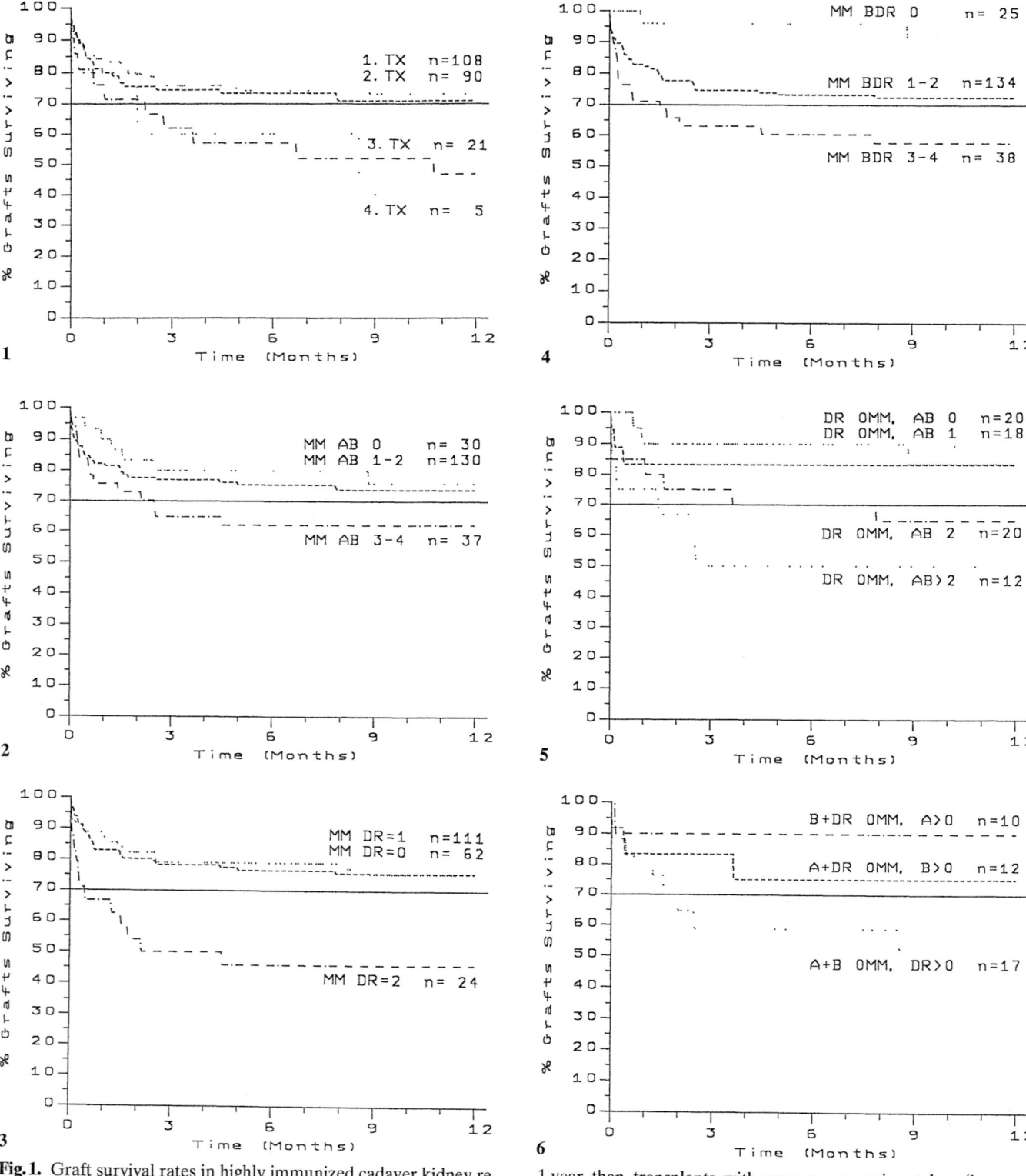

Fig. 1. Graft survival rates in highly immunized cadaver kidney recipients. First, second, third, and fourth transplants are plotted separately. The numbers of patients are indicated for each curve

Fig. 2. Influence of mismatches for HLA-A,-B antigens on graft survival (first and second grafts) in highly immunized recipients. The trend towards impaired survival with an increase in the number of mismatches is not statistically significant

Fig. 3. Impact of matching for HLA-DR antigens on graft survival (first and second grafts) in highly immunized recipients. Transplants with two HLA-DR mismatches had a 30% lower survival rate on

1 year than transplants with zero or one mismatches (log rank *P* < 0.001)

Fig. 4. Analysis of HLA-B and HLA-DR mismatches on graft survival (first and second grafts) in highly immunized recipients. The influence of matching was statistically significant (*P* regression < 0.01)

Fig. 5. Influence of mismatches for HLA-A and HLA-B antigens in HLA-DR matched transplants. Mismatches for HLA-A,-B appear to have a deleterious influence

Fig. 6. Attempt at comparing the strength of indivdiual HLA loci. When the two complementary loci were matched, HLA-DR antigens had the strongest influence on graft outcome

based on grafts with zero HLA-DR mismatches [2], to analyze the impact of HLA-A,-B mismatching in HLA-DR compatible transplants. As shown in Fig. 5, even though all transplants were done after two negative crossmatches, there was a deleterious influence of mismatching for HLA-A and -B antigens. Fig. 6 shows an attempt to compare the strength of mismatches at the HLA-A, HLA-B, or HLA-DR locus in situations where the other two loci were compatible. Although the numbers of patients studied were small, it appeared that mismatches for HLA-DR had the greatest impact followed by HLA-B, whereas HLA-A mismatches were not deleterious in the absence of HLA-B,-DR mismatches.

Discussion

It is impressive that the current results for first and second grafts were identical to those published for half the number of patients 3 years ago [1]. It appears that a stable 70 % 1-year success rate in highly immunized patients can be expected from this program. The success rate of third and fourth grafts was approximately 25 % lower.

The analysis of HLA matching clearly demonstrated that, in spite of the absence of crossmatch reactivity, matching did have an important influence in this patient population. The rationale that HLA-A,-B mismatches should not be deleterious if a highly sensitized recipient does not react against the mismatched antigens on donor cells in the crossmatch test apparently is flawed. It is important to note that even in the HLA-DR zero-mismatch group, HLA-A,-B mismatches increased the risk of failure.

It is important to point out that grafts with one HLA-DR mismatch had a success rate indistinguishable from that with a zero HLA-DR mismatch (Fig. 3). We do not feel that transplantation of highly sensitized patients should be limited to the zero HLA-DR mismatch group. Rather, we believe that our policy of avoiding two-antigen mismatches on each of the three loci is sensible, and that beyond that, the best possible match grade should be aimed for. There is a suggestion in our data that two mismatches for HLA-A can be accepted in the absence of HLA-B,-DR mismatches. However, because the number of transplants studied in this respect is very small, we must await further evidence before reaching a conclusion.

The results shown here for transplantation in highly sensitized recipients are gratifying. These patients have long been considered high risks and they experience prolonged waiting times. With good HLA matching, success rates indistinguishable from those in nonsensitized recipients can be obtained. We believe that the results shown here provide ample justification for the continuation of priority kidney allocation based on our serum exchange program.

Acknowledgements. We thank the staff at the participating transplant centers as well as the staff at Eurotransplant for their support. The excellent technical assistance of Martina Rausch, Michaela Kraft and Jaklin Inceoglu is gratefully acknowledged. This project was supported by a grant from Deutsche Stiftung Organtransplantation, Neu-Isenburg, Germany.

References

1. Opelz G for the Collaborative Transplant Study (1988) Priority allocation of cadaver kidneys to highly presensitized transplant recipients. Transplant Int 1: 2–5
2. Claas FHJ, De Waal LP, Beelen J, Reekers P, Berg-Loonen Pvd, de Gast E, D'Amaro J, Persijn GG, Zantvoort F, van Rood JJ (1989) Transplantation of highly sensitized patients on the basis of acceptable HLA-A and -B mismatches. In: Terasaki PI (ed) Clinical Transplants 1989. UCLA Tissue Typing Laboratory, Los Angeles, pp 185–190

Transplant Int (1992) 5 [Suppl 1]: S 604–S 605

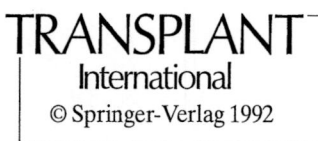

TRANSPLANT
International
© Springer-Verlag 1992

Flow cytometric crossmatching and outcome one year after renal transplantation

D. Talbot, B. K. Shenton, A. L. Givan, G. Cavanagh, G. Proud, and R. M. R. Taylor

Departments of Surgery and Tissue Typing, The Medical School, University of Newcastle upon Tyne.

Previous studies have shown that flow cytometric crossmatch assays can identify an at risk population in renal transplantation [1–5]. We used the assay for recipient selection for 1 year. Recipients with donor T cell directed IgG were excluded from transplantation and those with B cell directed IgG were treated with increased immunosuppression. The transplants performed over this period ($n = 126$) were compared with an earlier series ($n = 118$) in which flow cytometric crossmatch results did not influence patient management. The results were evaluated for mortality and graft outcome at 3 months and 1 year. In addition, postoperative complications and duration of hospital stay were also assessed.

Key words: Flow cytometric crossmatching – Renal transplantation – Recipient selection

Method

This has been described previously [6] and consisted essentially of incubating aliquots of 10^5 donor lymphocytes with recipient sera. After 15 min at 37 °C the cells were washed and then incubated with a combination of anti-IgG conjugated with fluorescein (Seratec) and either antileu 4 (T) or antileu 16 (B) conjugated with phycoerythrin (Becton Dickinson). After 15 min at 4 °C the cells were washed and analysed in a Facscan (Becton Dickinson). The intensity of 530 nm fluorescence of the 575 nm positive cells was compared with the fluorescence of standard AB0 sera as control. When the fluorescence of the test serum was greater than 2 standard deviations of the control it was considered positive.

Results

The current group was compared with the previous series for risk factors. Both groups were found to be identical for A/B match, ischaemic times, previous transplant history, panel reactivity, age, sex, and immunosuppressive regimes. The current series was found to have an im-

proved DR match in comparison to the retrospective series. The results at 3 months are summarised in Table 1. They showed a reduced complication rate with shorter primary non-function, fewer clinical rejection episodes and a shorter hospital stay. The mortality rate was similar between the groups but the graft success at 3 months was significantly higher in the current group using chi-square (94% versus 84.7%).

The effect of DR matching on the results at 1 year are shown in Fig. 1. The notable feature of this graph is that for each DR type, the graft success rate was better in the current series. This only reaches significant proportions in the DR 1 group using the Mantel Haenszel test ($P < 0.001$). The results at 1 year revealed a graft survival of 91.4% in the current group as opposed to 82.9% in the previous series, mortality excluded. This difference was significant if the graft survival curves were evaluated using the Mantel Haenszel test ($P < 0.001$) and was not lost if recipient mortality was also included.

Discussion

The different emphasis of DR match in the two groups illustrates the shortcomings of a retrospective control series as opposed to a prospective one. Both improved DR

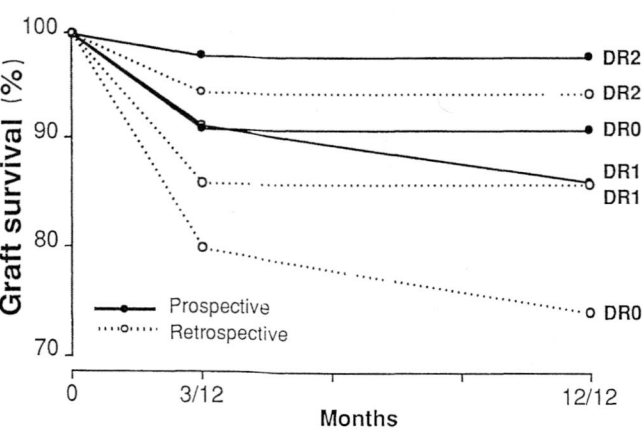

Fig. 1. Graft survival up to 1 year

Offprint requests to: David Talbot

Table 1. Results from retrospective and current series

Variable	Retrospective $n = 118$	Prospective $n = 126$	Probability
DR locus match	0.83 (1sd = 0.73)	1.32 (1sd = 0.63)	$P < 0.0001$ Mann Whitney U
FACS antibody (total)/%	22.0	13.4	NS
FACS antibody (T)/%	17.8	1.6	$P < 0.00001$ Fisher
Primary non function/days	12.6 (1sd = 20.6)	5.0 (1sd = 12.7)	$P < 0.0001$ Mann Whitney U
Rejection episodes	1.78 (1sd = 0.81)	1.05 (1sd = 0.99)	$P < 0.0001$ Mann Whitney U
Immunosuppression (types)	2.85 (1sd = 0.85)	2.91 (1sd = 0.98)	NS
ATG/OKT3/%	13.6	22.2	NS
Hospital stay/days	31.7 (1sd = 18.8)	17.6 (1sd = 7.6)	$P < 0.0001$ Student t test
3/12 Creatinine/μmol/l	154.8 (1sd = 57.6)	163.7 (1sd = 73.8)	NS
Death/%	5.1	5.6	NS
Failure/% (3 months)	15.3	6.0	$P = 0.037$ chi-square
Failure/% (1 year)	17.1	8.6	$P = 0.08$ chi-square

NS = Not significant

matching [7] and flow cytometric crossmatching are known to influence outcome and therefore both should be considered responsible for the excellent results.

In summary the current series of renal transplants had fewer complications and improved graft survival. Consequently the policy of improved DR matching and avoidance of positive T cell flow cytometric combinations is to be continued. In addition the use of increased immunosuppression for B cell flow cytometric combinations may also be advisable and will be evaluated further.

Acknowledgement. This work was sponsored by the Northern Counties Kidney Research Fund.

References

1. Garavoy MR, Rheinschmidt MA, Bigos M, et al. (1983) Transplant Proc 15: 1939
2. Thistlethwaite JR, Buckingham BS, Stuart JK, et al. (1986) Transplant Proc 18: 676
3. Cook DJ, Terasaki PI, Iwaki Y, et al. (1987) Clin Transplant 1: 253
4. Talbot D, Givan AL, Shenton BK, et al. (1989) Transplantation 47: 552
5. Talbot D, Givan AL, Shenton BK, et al. (1990) Transplantation 49: 809
6. Talbot D, Givan AL, Shenton B, et al. (1988) J Immunol Methods 112: 279
7. Thorogood J, van Houwelingen JC, van Rood JJ, et al. (1989) Transplantation 48: 231

TRANSPLANT
International
© Springer-Verlag 1992

Clinical relevance of soluble HLA and interaction of papain derived class I molecules with alloreactive CTL

N. Zavazava[1], **R. Hausmann**[1], **E. Kraatz**[2] and **W. Müller-Ruchholtz**[1]

[1] Institute of Immunology and [2] Department of Cardiovascular Surgery, University of Kiel, Kiel, Germany

Abstract. MHC class I and class II molecules are expressed in soluble form in the serum of both healthy and diseased individuals. Our aim was to investigate whether soluble class I (sHLA) levels in allograft patients correlate with their clinical status. Altogether, 20 renal and 30 cardiac graft recipients were examined. High levels of sHLA were measured at least 5 days preceding acute rejection episodes. Immune complexes between anti-HLA antibodies and sHLA were detected in a patient who died of a severe vascular rejection. In another study the interaction of papain-derived sHLA on alloreactive CTL in vitro was investigated. In a chromium-51-release cytotoxicity assay, 1,25 µg/ml of papain-digested class I molecules reduced CTL cytotoxicity to background levels. On the contrary, immobilized molecules triggered the release of serine esterase allospecifically. These data showed that the MHC molecule alone was a sufficient ligand for the interaction with alloreactive CTL.

Key words: Transplantation – Soluble HLA – Allo-antibodies – Inhibition – Alloreactive CTL – Serine esterase

Materials and methods

Patients. Venous blood was drawn from patients pre-transplant and at varying times thereafter, at which times biopsies were taken and examined histologically. Biopsies were staged according to Kemnitz et al. [1].

Quantitative Measurement of sHLA. sHLA were measured in a competitive ELISA assay as we have previously described [2].

Cytotoxic anti-HLA antibodies. Serum from patient RF was used in a cytotoxicity test using peripheral blood lymphocytes obtained from healthy blood donors. Sera were pre-diluted to 1:10 and 1:50 and used in a complement mediated cytotoxicity test. The test was performed on peripheral blood lymphocytes bearing the mismatched HLA-A3 and -B13. Sera were declared positive when they remained cytotoxic after pre-diluting to 1:10. The sera that re-

mained negative were incubated with immuno-magnetic beads coupled with the anti-class I antibody W6/32. The beads were separated and the sera retested for cytotoxic antibodies. The anti-HLA antibody index was used such that 5 represented > 95 % dead cells, 4 > 85 %, 3 > 75 %, 2 > 50 % and 1 < 50 %.

Generation of CTL. Alloreactive CTL were generated in vitro as we have previously described [3]. The stimulator and responder cells were selected such that CTL developed against HLA-A2.

CTL specificity and inhibition assays. The cytotoxicity of the alloreactive CTL was tested in a chromium release assay against PHA blasts, permanent tumor cell lines and EBV-transformed cell lines. To test the effect of sHLA, CTL were pre-incubated with varying concentrations of sHLA in 15 % AB serum at 37 °C for 30 min. Cells were harveted and washed 3 times in RPMI 1640 medium. Subsequently, cells were added to target cells which had been previously labelled with ^{51}chromium. The cells were incubated for 4 h before harvesting and measuring chromium release in a gamma counter.

Purification of papain-derived sHLA. Cell membranes were digested in papain, (Sigma, USA) at a concentration of 4 mg/ml as has been previously reported by Turner et al. [4]. The antibody PA2.1 (ATCC, USA), which binds HLA-A2 and -A28 was used to purify HLA-A2 polypeptides on affinity chromatography columns as we have previously reported [3]. The ME1 antibody (ATCC, USA) was used to purify HLA-B7 using the same procedure.

Serine esterase assay. The release of serine esterase was determined as has been previously reported by others [5].

Results

In our studies on the expression of sHLA in graft patients, we present a case report of a patient with vascular rejection. Patient RF maintained the cardiac graft for 29 days after which he rejected and died. During this period, there was no histological evidence of rejection on the biopsies examined. However, several peaks of sHLA elevation were noted as shown on Fig. 1. Retrospectively, we attempted to detect anti-allo antibodies. Three days post-transplant, cytotoxic antibodies against the mismatched HLA-A3 and -B13 could be identified. The antibodies gradually became less had completely disappeared by day 15. We depleted the negative sera of sHLA using immuno-magnetic beads to which the anti-class I antibody W6/32 was bound. These sera became positive for anti-

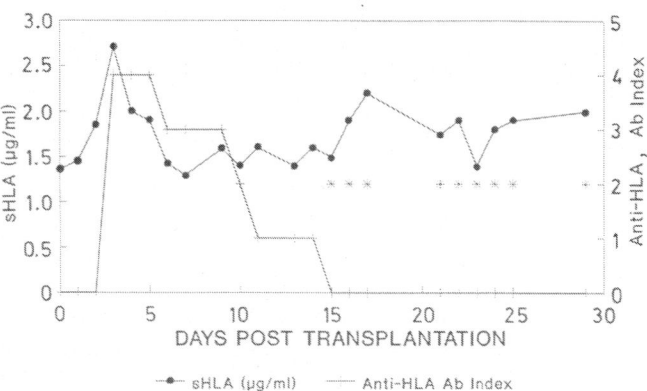

sHLA & anti-HLA Antibodies in a Cardiac Graft Recipient

— sHLA (µg/ml)   - - - Anti-HLA Ab Index

Fig. 1. sHLA (□) and cytotoxic anti-HLA antibodies (+) in a patient (RF) with vascular rejection. High increases of sHLA were noted soon after transplantation, between days 15 and 22 and between days 25 and 29. Anti-HLA antibodies were detectable only between days 3 and 15. Thereafter the sera were negative, but became positive (*) after sHLA depletion. The patient died of severe vascular rejection on day 29

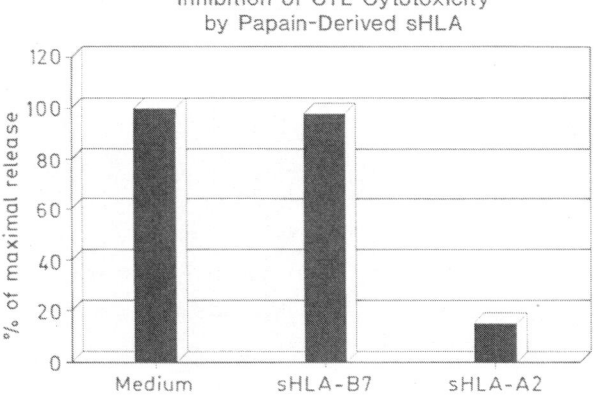

Inhibition of CTL Cytotoxicity by Papain-Derived sHLA

Fig. 2. Inhibition of CTL cytotoxicity by sHLA. CTL cytotoxicity was reduced to background levels by 1.25 µg/ml of papain-derived sHLA. Similar concentrations of sHLA-B7 were ineffective in abrogating CTL cytotoxicity

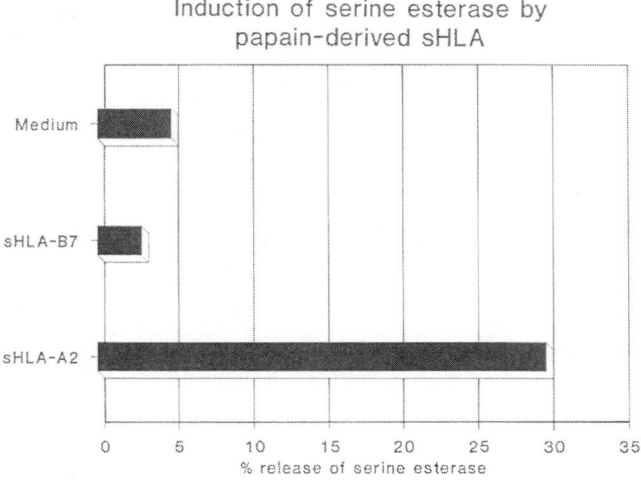

Induction of serine esterase by papain-derived sHLA

Fig. 3. sHLA triggered release of serine esterase by alloreactive CTL. The highest level of serine esterase was induced by the CTL by 0.15 µg/well HLA-A2 polypeptides. In the control experiment, HLA-B7 failed to trigger serine esterase release

HLA antibodies, as shown on Fig. 1, showing that antibodies had formed immune complexes with sHLA and could therefore not be detected in the cytotoxicity test. Post-mortem immunohistological examination of the graft showed deposition of complement factor C1q in the vascular bed (not shown). This finding was clear evidence of vascular rejection.

Patients who had acute rejection episodes expressed high sHLA levels at least 5 days preceeding histological evidence of rejection (not shown), confirming our previously published observations [6].

The CTL line generated was maintained in culture for several months. Only target cells that were HLA-A2 were lysed in the chromium-51 release assay. Over 98% of the cells were CD8[+].

In inhibition assays, CTL were pre-incubated with sHLA polypeptides before the chromium-51-release assays. CTL cytotoxicity was reduced to almost background levels by 1,25 µg/ml HLA-A2 (Fig. 2). Pre-incubation of the CTL with sHLA-B7 failed to influence CTL cytotoxicity. In a further attempt to investigate the molecular interaction of the CTL with the class I polypeptides, CTL were plated onto micro-titer plates which had been pre-coated with the polypeptides. The release of serine esterase into the supernatants was measured in an enzyme assay. Maximal release was measured at a concentration of 0.15 µg/well HLA-A2, whereas HLA-B7 polypeptides or culture medium failed to trigger the release of serine esterase (Fig. 3).

Discussion

In a previous report [6] we observed high elevations of sHLA during acute rejection episodes. In the present publication, we present a case report of a patient with vascular rejection who confirmed the earlier observations and showed that donor-derived sHLA form immune complexes with anti-HLA antibodies. Similar data have been reported by others [7, 8]. The formation of such complexes can potentially protect the graft from antibody-mediated tissue destruction. However, the possibility remains that they could increase the risks of graft rejection by sensitizing further the recipient. An important clinical point to consider is the fact that the presence of such complexes in pre-sensitized patients might lead to false negative cross-matches. Undetected antibodies in these patients could increase the chances of hyperacute rejection. Taken together, these data showed that sHLA measurement could be a useful indicator of rejection in graft patients and that they could play an important role in binding anti-allo antibodies. The inhibition studies suggested that sHLA are potential immunomodulators and could abrogate CTL cytotoxicity. The concentrations applied in these studies were reasonably low and allowed speculation on the in vivo clinical application of sHLA in inducing specific immunosuppression. Successful prolongation of graft survival using soluble class I molecules has been achieved in rats [9, 10]. These experiments demonstrated further that the interaction between sHLA and alloreactive CTL was allospecific, thus suggesting that the class I molecules reacted with the T cell receptor and either sterically blocked it or triggered a negative signal preventing further interaction with target cells. Whatever the mechanism was, monomeric class I molecules were sufficient ligands for alloreactive T cells.

In contrast to the inhibition assays, immobilized papain-derived sHLA were effective in triggering CTL degranulation to release serine esterase, a CTL specific enzyme. Since this interaction was allospecific, it again suggested a direct interaction of the polymorphic regions of the class I molecule with the T cell receptor. Similar experiments have been reported in a murine model, where the influence of intact class I molecules was investigated [5].

In conclusion, the data presented here showed that sHLA are important molecules in allo-transplantation and that they are potentially effective immunomodulators on their own without other accessory molecules. We are furthering these studies to elucidate the mechanisms involved in their expression in vivo and their physiological functions.

References

1. Kemnitz J, Cohnert T, Schäfers HJ, Helmke M, Wahlers T, Herrmann G, Schmidt RM, Haverich A (1987) A classification of cardiac allograft rejection. A modification of the classification by Billingham. Am J Surg Pathol 11: 503–515

2. Zavazava N, Westphal E, Müller-Ruchholtz W (1990) Characterization of soluble HLA molecules in sweat and quantitative HLA differences in serum of healthy individuals. J Immunogenet 17: 387–394

3. Zavazava N, Hausmann R, Müller-Ruchholtz W (1991) Inhibition of anti-HLA-B7 alloreactive CTL by affinity-purified soluble HLA. Transplantation 51: 838–842

4. Turner MJ, Cresswell P, Parham P, Strominger JL, Mann DL, Sanderson AR (1975) Purification of papain-solubilized histocompatibility antigens from a cultured human lymphoblastoidine, RPMI 4265. J Biol Chem 250: 4512–4519

5. Kane KP, Sherman LA, Mescher MF (1989) Molecular interactions required for triggering alloantigen-specific cytolytic T lymphocytes. J Immunol 142: 4153–4160

6. Zavazava N, Kraatz E, Gassel AM, Müller-Ruchholtz W (1991) Plasma MHC class I expression in cardiac graft patients: donor specific soluble antigen in a presensitized graft patient. Transplant Proc 23: 2258–2260

7. Siciu-Foca N, Reed E, D'Agati V, Ho E, Cohen DJ, Benvenisty AI, McCabe R, Brensilver JM, King DW, Hardy MA (1991) Soluble HLA antigens, anti-HLA antibodies, and antiidiotypic antibodies in the circulation of renal transplant recipients. Transplantation 51: 593–601

8. Siciu-Foca N, Reed E, Marboe C, Harris P, Xi YP, Yu-Kai S, Ho E, Rose E, Reemtsma K, King DW (1991) The role of anti-HLA antibodies in heart transplantation. Transplantation 51: 716–724

9. Sumimoto R, Kamada N (1990) Specific suppression of allograft rejection by soluble class I antigen and complexes with monoclonal antibody. Transplantation 50: 678–682

10. Ito T, Stepkowski M, Kahan BD (1990) Soluble antigen and cyclosporine induced specific unresponsiveness in rats. Transplantation 49: 422–428

Transplant Int (1992) 5 [Suppl 1]: S 609–S 612

TRANSPLANT
International
© Springer-Verlag 1992

Lack of correlation between IgG T-lymphocyte flow cytometric crossmatches with primary renal allograft outcome

P. R. Evans, A. C. Lane, C. M. Lambert, W. M. Reynolds, P. J. Wilson, K. R. Harris, M. Slapak, H. A. Lee and J. L. Smith

Wessex Immunology Service, Southampton University Hospitals, Tenovus Research Laboratories, Tremona Rd., Southampton, S09 4XY and Renal Unit, St. Mary's Hospital, Milton Rd., Portsmouth, P03 6AD, United Kingdom

Abstract. The flow cytometric crossmatch (FCXM) has been reported to be more sensitive and capable of detecting very low levels of antibodies than the normally used complement dependent cytotoxicity test. We studied both the two colour IgG T cell FCXM and CDC-XM in 146 renal allograft recipients, 111 primary and 35 regrafts, of which 26 % (29/111) of 1st and 20 % (7/35) of regrafts had a positive FCXM. There was no overall correlation between the FCXM results and early graft outcome in primary renal allografts. The FCXM did not appear to have any advantage over the CDC-XM in predicting graft outcome in unsensitized first grafts. In the small number of regrafts studied, a positive FCXM was associated with a higher degree of graft failure. FCXM can exhibit false negative results if sera are used solely neat although these prozone phenomena do not influence subsequent graft outcome.

Key words: Flow cytometry – Crossmatch – Renal transplantation – Antibodies – Prozone phenomenon

Following the introduction of pre-transplant crossmatching for recipients of renal allografts by complement dependent cytotoxicity (CDC) tests, the incidence of antibody mediated early graft failure, especially hyperacute rejection, fell dramatically [1]. However both hyperacute and accelerated acute rejections are still seen, even with a negative CDC crossmatch [7], and it has been suggested that a significant proportion of early failures including immediate graft non-function are due to undetected humoral rejection [8]. These findings have lead to attempts to either increase the sensitivity of current crossmatch techniques [9, 12, 15] or to search for alternative crossmatch target cells [3].

Offprint requests to: Mr. P. R. Evans, Wessex Immunology Service, Southampton University Hospitals, Tenovus Research Laboratory, Tremona Rd., Shirley, Southampton, Hampshire, S09 4XY, United Kingdom

The flow cytometric crossmatch (FCXM) is a very sensitive technique for measuring low levels of anti-donor antibodies which are not detectable by standard crossmatch techniques [2, 4]. The use of FCXM, however, in primary and secondary allograft recipients has been questioned as being too sensitive and not correlating with graft outcome [10]. Other reports have shown that positive FCXM is associated with an increased risk of rejection episodes especially in retransplant patients, allowing the identification of a high risk patient group which have a poor clinical course [2, 9, 12, 14].

In this report we examined the two colour IgG T-cell flow cytometric crossmatch (FCXM) in 146 renal allografts and identified a possible cause of false negative results if recipient sera are used solely undiluted. In addition we performed IgG B cell FCXM in 33 of these transplant recipients.

Patients and methods

Patients. A total of 146 cadaveric donor renal allografts in 143 patients (101 male and 42 female) transplanted between February 1987 and July 1991 were studied. Of these, 111 were first and 35 were regrafts (20 second, 10 third, 4 fourth and 1 fifth). Average age at transplant was 42.4 ± 14.4 years for male patients (range 19–75 years) and 41.2 ± 15.1 years for female patients (range 18–67 years). The mean number of HLA-A, -B and -DR antigen mismatches in the study group was 0.81 ± 0.69, 1.0 ± 0.68 and 0.73 ± 0.65 respectively. Of the patients studied 14.4 % (21/146) were beneficially matched according to the criteria of Gilks et al. [5].

Immunosuppression. Primary immunosuppressive therapy consisted of conventional azathioprine and prednisolone (4 cases), cyclosporin monotherapy or cyclosporin with prednisolone (15 cases), triple therapy with azathioprine (95 cases), triple therapy with mizoribine (9 cases), quadruple therapy comprising primary ATG/ALG tailoring onto triple therapy (21 cases), and two cases of primary graft failure.

Lymphocytotoxic assays. Donor lymphocytes were isolated from spleen or lymph node. Splenic lymphocytes were carbonyl iron-treated to remove phagocytic cells. Separated T and B lymphocytes

Table 1. Graft survival after first month post transplant in primary recipients

NIH CDC crossmatch		FACS crossmatch	
	Negative	Negative	Positive
	$N = 111$	$N = 82$	$N = 29$
>30 day survival	86% (95/111)	84% (69/82)	90% (26/29)
			N5 P = 0.2

Table 2. Graft survival after 1st month post transplant in retransplant recipients

NIH CDC crossmatch		FACS crossmatch	
	Negative	Negative	Positive
	$N = 35$	$N = 28$	$N = 7$
>30 day survival	86% (30/35)	89% (25/28)	71% (5/7)
			N5 P = 0.2

were obtained by neuraminidase-treated sheep red blood cell rosetting and lysis of sheep cells with ammonium chloride.

The extended NIH two-stage microlymphocytotoxicity test was performed. Recipient serum (1 μl) was added to a microtitre plate followed by 1 μl donor cells (2×10^6/ml) and incubated for 60 min at 22 °C. Then 5 μl rabbit complement (Biotest) was added, followed by further incubation for 120 min at 22 °C. The cytotoxicity test reactions were assessed by fluorescent microscopy, using acridine orange and ethidium bromide staining. The criterion for a positive test result was defined as a 5–10% or greater proportion of killed cells above background.

Panel reactive antibodies (% PRA). Recipient serum samples were routinely screened against a panel of at least 70 cells from 50 individuals; this panel comprised 20 isolated T and B cells, 20 peripheral blood lymphocytes and 10 chronic lymphocytic leukaemia cells. A serum was considered to have panel reactive antibodies if greater than 3% of the cell panel was positive. Unsensitized recipients were defined as having <10% PRA with a current serum sample at the time of transplant; 79.5% (116/146) patients were classified in this category. Sensitized patients were regarded as having >10% PRA with 20.5% (30 recipients) in this group and only 6 patients (4%) being highly sensitized, >85% PRA.

Flow cytometric crossmatch. Donor spleen cells were either isolated from fresh splenic material or retrieved from cyropreservation. Washed spleen cells were subsequently incubated at 37 °C for 30 min in RPMI 1640 at 10^7 cells/ml to ensure removal of any cytophilic immunoglobulin. Mean donor spleen cell viability was 78.0% ± 15.4 (range 40–100%) prior to use. Spleen cells were washed and resuspended in cold phosphate buffered saline (PBS), pH 7.2, containing 0.1% sodium azide, at 10^7 cells/ml. We added 100 μl cell suspension (10^6 cells) to a FACS sample tube, it was spun and the supernatant discarded; 100 μl recipient's serum was added to the cell pellet, cells resuspended, and incubated for 30 min at 22 °C.

In order to avoid possible false negative results due to 'prozone phenomena' patient sera were also tested at a 1:4 dilution in PBS. All tests included a positive control, consisting of a pool of 4 highly sensitized renal patient sera (>95% PRA) and a negative control, pooled human AB serum (minimum 6 individuals) that had been screened for the absence of erythrocyte antibodies, lymphocytotoxins and blocking activity in mixed lymphocyte cultures. Following the primary antibody incubation stage, the cells were washed 3 times in cold PBS/azide, the total wash volume being approximately 10 ml.

Subsequently, cells were pelleted and 20 μl FITC conjugated F(ab')₂ rabbit anti-human IgG (Dakopatts), diluted 1:10 in PBS was added, followed directly by either 5 μl R-phycoerythrin (PE) conjugated mouse monoclonal anti-human CD3 (Serotec) for T cells, or 5 μl PE-conjugated anti-CD19 (Dakopatts) for B cells; this was incubated for 30 min at 4 °C. Following a second wash cycle, cells were resuspended in 200 μl cold PBS/azide followed by the addition of 300 μl 0.5% paraformaldehyde in PBS. Cells were left at 4 °C prior to FACS analysis.

Data analysis. The labelled samples were analysed on a FACScan flow cytometer (Becton Dickinson) with a 15 mW argon Laser at 488 nM. Band pass filters of 530 nM and 585 nM were used for fluorescein and phycoerythrin fluorochromes respectively. Fluorescence detectors were on logarithmic amplifiers with 4 log decade scales. Forward angle (FSC) and side angle (SSC) light scatter profiles were collected and a lymphocyte gate constructed on the basis of these FSC/SSC characteristics. For T cell crossmatches, FITC staining was assessed for both CD3 + ve and CD3 – ve cells using histograms constructed for each group.

For B-cell crossmatches CD19 + ve and CD19 – ve histograms were used. In the initial phase of the study Consort 30 software was used for the analysis. In the later stages cells were analysed using Becton Dickinson Lysys 2 software. Median T cell or B cell fluorescence intensity was obtained for each histogram using geometric statistics, and the sample median (mean with Consort 30) then compared to both negative and positive controls.

A positive FACS crossmatch was defined as a shift in the median channel of fluorescence of >20 channels to the right of either the T cell peak (CD3) or B cell peak (CD19) in the patients sera compared with the human AB serum negative control [9].

Statistical analysis. Graft survivals were calculated using acturial life-table methods [6] over the first 90 days in cohorts of 5 days and at 1, 3, 6 and 12 months post transplant. Patients were followed for a minimum of one month and were included in the analysis irrespective of the cause of graft failure, including patient death with a functioning graft. Analysis of results were carried out using chi-square and Fisher's exact 2×2 contingency tables, t-tests and Mann-Whitney U-tests using the University of Southampton Faculty of Medicine MEDSTAT programme.

Results

All 146 renal allograft recipients had a negative NIH extended T cell crossmatch (Tables 1 and 2). One 1st graft recipient, 0.9% (1/111), had a positive B cell crossmatch due to an IgM non-HLA auto-antibody. The graft is currently surviving >11 months. In first graft recipients 26% (29/111) had a positive IgG T cell FCXM with 90% (26/29) surviving >30 days post transplant (Table 1). There was no statistically significant difference between 30 day graft survival in FCXM + and – groups (P = 0.2, Table 1). At 90 days post transplant the actuarial graft survival was 83% for T cell FCXM + compared to 79% for FCXM – recipients, P = 0.15 (Fig. 1). The 6 month and 1 year graft survivals were 83% and 78% for FCXM + recipients compared to 78% and 78% for FCXM-recipients respectively. On testing the recipient serum at neat and at a 1:4 dilution against donor spleen cells, 48% (14/29) of 1st graft recipients were shown to be Nt – and 1:4 +. This prozone phenomenon could have led to these grafts being regarded as FCXM negative giving false negative FCXM results if the patients serum had not been tested in dilution. However the presence of these T cell FCXM Nt –

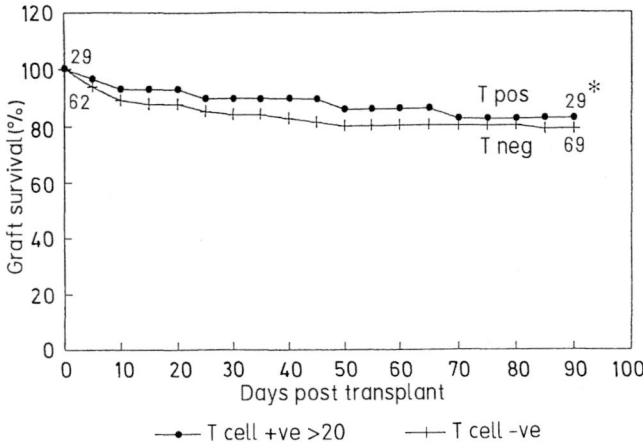

Fig. 1. IgG T cell FACS crossmatch: primary grafts. The *asterix* indicates the number of patients followed-up at each time interval

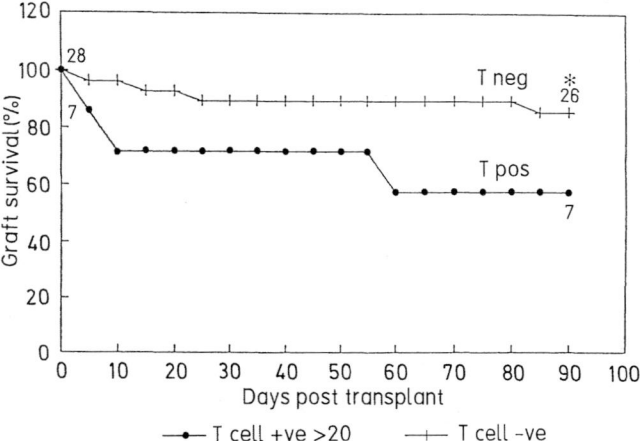

Fig. 2. IgG T cell FACS crossmatch: regrafts. The *asterix* indicates the number of patients followed-up at each time interval

1:4 + recipients did not alter the lack of correlation between T cell + recipients and graft outcome. Analysis of several patient parameters in first grafts revealed no statistical differences in HLA-A, -B, -DR locus mismatches, % peak and current PRA, % beneficially matched grafts, male:female ratio, the serum creatinine at 90 days and the number of rejection episodes post transplant in T cell FCXM + and FCXM − groups. However in the FCXM + grafts mean age at transplant was 48.8 ± 13.7 years compared to 42.3 ± 15.0 years in the FCXM − group ($P = 0.03$). The donor spleen cell viability also showed a significant difference, being $73.1\% \pm 15.6$ in the FCXM positive group compared to $80.3\% \pm 14.7$ in the FCXM negative group of patients ($P = 0.03$).

In the regraft recipients 20 % (7/35) had a positive T cell FCXM crossmatch with 71 % surviving > 30 days post transplant (Table 2). As with the first grafts there was no significant difference between 30 day graft survival in the FCXM + and − groups. At 90 days post transplant the actuarial graft survival was 57 % for T cell FCXM + compared to 85 % for T cell FCXM − recipients, $P = 0.28$ (Fig. 2). The number of FCXM positive regrafts of seven is too small to be of statistical significance, but the trend is towards graft failure in the FCXM + group. The 6 month and 1 year graft survivals were 57 % for FCXM + recip-

Table 3. Graft survival after 1st month post transplantion in 33 allograft recipients (23 1st and 10 regrafts)

NIH CDC crossmatch	FACS B-cell (CD19 +) crossmatch	
Negative	Negative	Positive
N = 33	N = 31	N = 2
> 30 day survival 94 % (31/33)	94 % (29/31)	100 % (2/2)
	N5 P = 0.9	

ients compared to 85 % and 73 % for FACS-recipients respectively. In the regraft patient group there were 29 % (2/7) prozone phenomena seen. Analysis of patient parameters as for first grafts (see above) revealed no significant differences between FCXM positive and negative groups. The IgG B cell FCXM was positive in 6 % (2/33) of patients studied (Table 3). There was insufficient data to examine the effect of B cell FCXM on graft outcome.

Discussion

The crossmatching of recipient sera and donor lymphocytes in order to avoid or reduce the incidence of antibody mediated rejection is still one of the major considerations prior to renal transplantation. It is arguably the most important role of tissue typing and histocompatibility laboratories. The incidence of hyperacute rejection, seen following the introduction of the CDC lymphocytotoxicity test as a pre-transplant crossmatching technique, fell from 10–12 % of all grafts in 1967 to less than 0.5 % in 1988 [1].

The criteria for, and the significance of, a positive crossmatch has been revised considerably. The current concensus about complement dependent cytotoxicity crossmatching is that a positive crossmatch on a current serum sample against donor T lymphocytes due to IgG HLA class I (A, B and C) alloantibodies is an absolute contraindication to transplantation [15].

The introduction of flow cytometric crossmatching to detect low levels of donor reactive antibodies [2, 4, 9, 11, 12, 14] has lead again to a reappraisal. In this study first grafts were successfully transplanted across a positive FXCM suggesting that renal transplantation can occur without hyperacute rejection even if low titer donor-reactive preformed antibodies are present. The incidence of false positive results in primary recipients was 27 % at 30 days post transplant (number of grafts FXCM + > 30 days/total number of grafts > 30 days). This suggests that the FXCM is over-sensitive and has a high rate of false-positive results not correlating with graft outcome. Similar findings have been reported by other groups [2, 11, 14].

One caveat to this is that in our study group 82 % (91/111) of primary graft recipients were unsensitised (< 10 % PRA). In primary allograft recipients FCXM appears to have no advantage over the NIH CDC crossmatch in predicting graft outcome (Table 1). Thus we feel that the prospective use of FXCM in primary allografts and denying a transplant on the basis of a positive FXCM is not warranted. In addition we were unable to identify groups of patients with a poor clinical course (high number of rejection episodes, serum creatinine at 90 days) as has been shown in other studies [11, 14]. With only 3 % (4/146) of allograft recipients receiving conventional azathioprine and prednisolone, the remainder having either CyA, CyA-Pred, Triple or Quadruple immunosuppressive therapy, the clinical relevance in the cyclosporin era and modern immunosuppressive regimen of detecting these low levels of weak donor reactive antibodies has to be re-evaluated [9, 11].

It has been suggested that FCXM should be confined solely to regraft patients [9, 12]. We had a limited number of grafts available to study (7 FCXM +) with no statistically significant difference between the FCXM positive and negative groups although there appeared to be a trend towards graft failure in the positive FCXM group. These findings require confirmation in a larger cohort of patients.

Acknowledgements. The authors are grateful to clinical colleagues at St. Mary's Hospital, Portsmouth for permission to include their patients in this study. We wish also to thank Mrs. Pauline Hutchins and Mrs. Win Whittaker for their expert secretarial assistance.

References

1. Cecka JM, Cho L (1988) Sensitization. In: Terasaki P (ed) Clinical Transplants 1988. UCLA Tissue Typing Laboratory, Los Angeles, pp 365–373
2. Cook DJ, Terasaki PI, Iwaki Y, Terashita GY, Lau M (1987) An approach to reducing early kidney transplant failure by flow cytometry crossmatching. Clin Transplant 1:253–256
3. Evans PR, Trickett LP, Gosney AR, Hodges E, Shires S, Wilson PJ, MacIver AG, Gardner B, Slapak M, Smith JL (1988) Detection of kidney reactive antibodies at crossmatch in renal transplant recipients. Transplantation 46:844–852
4. Garovoy MR, Rheinschmidt MA, Bigos M, Perkins H, Colombe B, Feduska N, Salvatierra O (1983) Flow cytometry analysis: a high technology crossmatch technique facilitating transplantation. Transplant Proc 15:1939–1944
5. Gilks WR, Bradley BA, Gore SM, Klouda PT (1987) Substantial benefit of tissue matching in renal transplantation. Transplantation 43:669–574
6. Harris KR, Digard N, Gosling DC, Tate DG, Campbell MJ, Gardner B, Sharman VL, Slapak M (1985) Azathioprine and cyclosporin: different tissue matching criteria needed? Lancet II:802–804
7. Ianhez L, Saldanha LB, Paula FJ, Neto DE, Sabbaga E, Arap S, Marin ML, Rosales C, Guilherme L, Rodrigues H, Kalil J (1989) Humoral rejection with negative crossmatches. Transplant Proc 21:720–721
8. Iwaki Y, Terasaki PI (1987) Primary non-function in human cadaver kidney transplantation: Evidence for hidden hyperacute rejection. Clin Transplant 1:125–131
9. Kerman RH, van Buren CT, Lewis RM, Devera V, Baghdahsarian V, Gerolami K, Kahan BA (1990) Improved graft survival for flow cytometry and antihuman globulin crossmatch-negative retransplant recipients. Transplantation 49:52–56
10. Johnson AH, Rossen RD, Butler WT (1972) Detection of alloantibodies using a sensitive antiglobulin microcytotoxicity test: identification of low levels of pre-formed antibodies in accelerated allograft rejection. Tissue Antigens 2:215–216
11. Lazda VA, Pollak R, Mozes MF, Jonasson O (1988) The relationship between flow cytometer crossmatch results and subsequent rejection episodes in cadaver renal allograft recipients. Transplantation 45:562–565
12. Mahoney RJ, Ault KA, Given SR, Adams RJ, Breggia AC, Paris PA, Palomaki GE, Hitchcox SA, White BW, Himmelfarb J, Leeber DA (1990) The flow cytometric crossmatch and early graft loss. Transplantation 49:527–535
13. Smith JA, Stark JH, Margolius LP, Botha JR, Thomson PD, Meyers AM, Myburgh JA (1991) The relevance of more sensitive ancillary crossmatch techniques in predicting early cadaver renal allograft outcome. Transplant Int 4:77–81
14. Talbot D, Givan AL, Shenton BK, Stratton A, Proud G, Taylor RMR (1989) The relevance of a more sensitive crossmatch assay to renal transplantation. Transplantation 47:552–555
15. Ting A (1989) Positive crossmatches – when is it safe to transplant? Transplant Int 2:2–7

Transplant Int (1992) 5 [Suppl 1]: S613–S616

TRANSPLANT
International
© Springer-Verlag 1992

Detection of latent human cytomegalovirus in organ tissue and the correlation with serological status

Y. J. Kraat[1], M. G. R. Hendrix[1], R. M. H. Wijnen[2], H. G. Peltenburg[3], J. P. van Hooff[3], J. L. M. C. Geelen[1], and C. A. Bruggeman[1]

Department of Med. Microbiology[1], Department of Surgery[2], and Department of Internal Medicine[3], Academic Hospital Maastricht, Maastricht, The Netherlands

Abstract. The presence of human cytomegalovirus (HCMV) genome in spleen tissue was studied by using DNA hybridization techniques in seropositive and seronegative organ donors without clinical or laboratory confirmed HCMV infection. The serum samples of these patients were screened by latex agglutination test (LA) and enzyme linked immuno sorbent assay (ELISA) for the presence of HCMV antibodies, and confirmed by immunoblotting technique (IB). For the detection of HCMV sequences in spleen tissue dot blot DNA hybridization (DBH) using probes derived from immediate-early and late regions (ES and BH fragment respectively) of the HCMV genome were used. Samples positive in DBH were further tested by in situ DNA hybridization (ISH) using the ES probe. The number of spleen tissue specimens positive for HCMV nucleic acids indicated that HCMV may be present in human beings, even without serological evidence.

Key words: Human cytomegalovirus – Latency – Hybridization – Antibodies

Human cytomegalovirus (HCMV), a member of the herpesvirus family, is an ubiquitous human viral pathogen. Infection with HCMV is usually asymptomatic in the immunocompetent host, but can result in a dramatic disease in immunosuppressed patients [15]. After primary infection the virus persists in the host as a chronic or latent infection, which can periodically reactivate to an active infection. HCMV is known to be transmitted through blood transfusions [1, 24] and transplanted organs [10, 33] which can result in a severe HCMV disease, especially in immunosuppressed and seronegative patients [3, 22]. Several studies indicate that in HCMV seropositive healthy individuals latent infection can be demonstrated by the presence of HCMV antigens. This is done by immunohistochemical techniques or by the detecting the presence of

HCMV genome by DNA techniques in smooth muscle cells of arteries and in different cell types of various organ tissues, including kidney, liver, lung and spleen [12–14, 21, 25, 32, 34]. The presence of HCMV specific antibodies as evidence of past or present infection is the most valuable indicator of a potentially infective donor [9, 20]. However, there is some doubt if all seronegative donors are really free from previous HCMV infection, with the possibility of the presence of a latent virus [8, 28, 29, 31].

This suggestion prompted us to analyze organ tissue derived from seronegative organ donors for the presence of HCMV genome in organ tissue. To detect HCMV nucleic acids in organ tissue in our study spleens were subjected to DNA hybridization techniques. Spleen tissue was used for several reasons: firstly, the availability of spleen tissue of organ donors, secondly, this tissue has been demonstrated to be a site of latency for HCMV [32] and for murine CMV [26], thirdly, the high density of cells in spleen tissue and fourthly, the immunocompetent function of this organ.

For these investigations spleen tissue from seronegative donors was first analyzed by dot blot DNA hybridization (DBH), followed by the more specific in situ DNA hybridization (ISH) of the DBH positive samples for localization of the latent virus. Spleen tissue from seropositive patients (kidney donors) known to contain latent HCMV in their arterial walls [12], served as a positive control group for all DNA hybridization techniques. For the detection of HCMV antibodies in the serum samples the latex agglutination test (LA), which is used in most laboratories, and the enzyme linked immuno sorbent assay (ELISA), were used [2, 11]. To confirm the HCMV antibody negative status of the patients the very sensitive immunoblotting technique described by Landini et al. [17] was performed.

Materials and methods

Selection of patients and specimens. Patients whose cause of death was a non-HCMV realted disease i. e. organ donors (trauma victums and patients whose cause of death was a sudden cardiac arrest), and whose spleen tissue (as routinely paraffine embedded) was available

---

Offprint requests to: Y. J. Kraat, Dept. of Med. Microbiology, Academic Hospital Maastricht, P. O. Box 5800, 6202 AZ Maastricht, The Netherlands

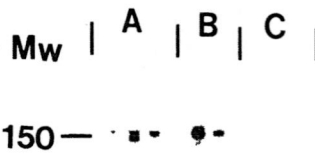

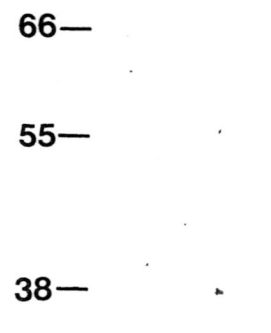

Fig. 1. Results from immunoblot detection of antibodies to HCMV proteins in sera of healthy persons.
(**A**) Three lanes of sera with only positive reaction for the 150 kD protein.
(**B**) Two lanes of sera with specific antibody reactivity for several proteins.
(**C**) Three lanes of sera without antibodies reacting to HCMV proteins

were included in this study. Patients suffering from immunosuppressive disease or undergoing immunosuppressive therapy were strictly excluded.

Latex agglutination (LA). The latex agglutination test (Becton Dickinson Microbiology Systems, Cockeysville, USA) was performed according to the instructions of the manufacturer. Undiluted serum samples were screened on a disposable card slide and allowed to agglutinate with the HCMV antigen coated latex particles.

Enzyme linked immuno sorbent assay (ELISA). The procedure for ELISA has been previously described [18, 19]. Briefly, antigen material was derived from HCMV (AD169 strain) infected human embryonal fibroblasts (HEF). The sera to be tested were diluted 1:200 and allowed to react with the antigens for 2 h at 37°C. Horse radish peroxidase-conjugated, goat polyclonal antihuman IgG (Institute Pasteur, Paris, France), diluted 1:1000 served as second antibody. The incubation with this conjugate was done for 2 h at 37°C. This was followed by adding substrate (o-phenylene diamine and hydrogenperoxidase) to the wells. The optical density at 492 nm was measured in a Titertek Multiscan by an ELISA reader (Flow Laboratories, Irvine, Scotland).

Immunoblotting technique (IB). The IB was performed essentially as described previously [7, 16]. Briefly, purified HCMV (AD169 strain) virons were subjected to sodium dodecyl sulfate polyacrylamide gel electroforesis (SDS-PAGE) and the separated polypeptides electrically transferred to nitrocellulose sheets (Schleicher and Schuell, Dassel, Germany). The human sera, routinely diluted 1:100, were incubated overnight at room temperature with the transferred proteins, followed by an incubation with rabbit antihuman IgG labelled with horse radish peroxidase (Dako, Glostrup, Denmark). The immune complexes were visualized by staining with 4-chloro-1-naphthol (Biorad, Richmond, California, USA). A serum specimen was considered positive for HCMV by immunoblotting if antibodies reactive to one or more of the major structural proteins having relative mobilities of 150, 82, 66, 55, 38 or 28 kiloDaltons (kD) were present.

DNA extraction. DNA was isolated as described previously [5]. Briefly, 5 tissue sections of 10 µm "thick" with an average surface of 1 cm² were deparaffinized by xylene followed by ethanol (96%) washes. Subsequently, the tissue was vacuum dried and digested overnight at 55°C in a mixture of 50 mM Tris (pH 8.5), 1 mM EDTA and 0.5% Tween 20 with 200 µg proteinkinase K in a final volume of 400 µl. To purify the DNA, a part of the lysate was added to guanidine thiocyanate-lysisbuffer (Fluka Chemie AG, Buchs, Switzer-

land) and diatom suspension (Sigma, St. Louis, USA). Finally, the nucleic acids were released from the diatoms in destilled water. The DNA concentration was determined spectophotometrically by measuring the extinction at 260 nm.

Dot blot hybridization (DBH). Aliquots of 5 µg cellular DNA were spotted on nitrocellulose filters (Amersham, Buckinghamshire, England). Hybridization was performed essentially as described previously [12]. To detect HCMV specific sequences the filters were hybridized with the major immediate early region of the HCMV genome (ES fragment) and the late region of the HCMV genome (BH fragment). The fragments were ^{32}P labelled in vitro by using a random primed DNA labelling kit (Boehringer, Mannheim, Germany). After hybridization the filters were washed under medium stringent conditions. The final wash-step was in 0.1 × SSC, 0.5% SDS for 45 min at 50°C. Hybridization was visualized by exposing the filters to a Kodak X-omat film (Eastman-Kodak Company, Rochester/New York, USA) for 4 days at −70°C.

In situ hybridization (ISH). For localization of the cell type(s) involved in a site for HCMV latency in spleen tissue the dot blot hybridization positive specimens were subjected to the specific ISH procedure with the ES fragment, derived from the immediate early HCMV genome. ISH was performed on 4 µm "thick" tissue sections as described previously [12]. For ISH the ES probe was labelled with biotin by incorporation of biotin-11-dUTP (Bethesda Research Laboratories) using a random primed hexanucleotide procedure (Boehringer, Mannheim, Germany). The hybrids were visualized by using the BLU gene ™kit (Bethesda Research Laboratories). The specificity of the probes was tested on DNA extracted from uninfected HEF monolayers and HEF monolayers infected with HCMV (AD169 strain). Other human herpes viruses (HSV, VZV, EBV, HHV-6) were used as controls.

Results

Selection of patients and specimens

As positive control 5 seropositive organ donors, with a mean age of 39 years, known to contain HCMV nucleic acid sequences in their arterial walls [13] were included in this study. Also included were 45 HCMV seronegative patients from whom splenic paraffine embedded tissue blocks were available. This group consisted of 24 men and 21 women, with a mean age of 49 years. Most patients were trauma victims (n = 26), while the other patients died of sudden cardiac arrest (n = 19).

Serology

A total number of 87 serum samples were screened by LA and ELISA for the detection of specific HCMV antibody. Using LA, 42 of 87 sera were positive and 45 of 87 serum samples were negative for antibodies to HCMV. Using ELISA, 41 of 87 sera were positive and 46 of 87 specimens were negative for HCMV antibodies. Sera from the positive control group gave positive reactions for specific HCMV antibodies using LA and ELISA. By immunoblotting, all seropositive control sera, as determined by LA as well by ELISA, reacted with the 150 kD HCMV structural polypeptide and some of them reacted with several HCMV structural proteins with the apparent molecular weight of 82, 66, 55, 38 and 28 kD. However, these reactions were of a lower intensity in comparison with the reaction with the 150 kD polypeptide, as demonstrated in Fig. 2. Of all the 45 LA and ELISA seronegative specimens, no reactivity was observed to any of the specific structural viral proteins.

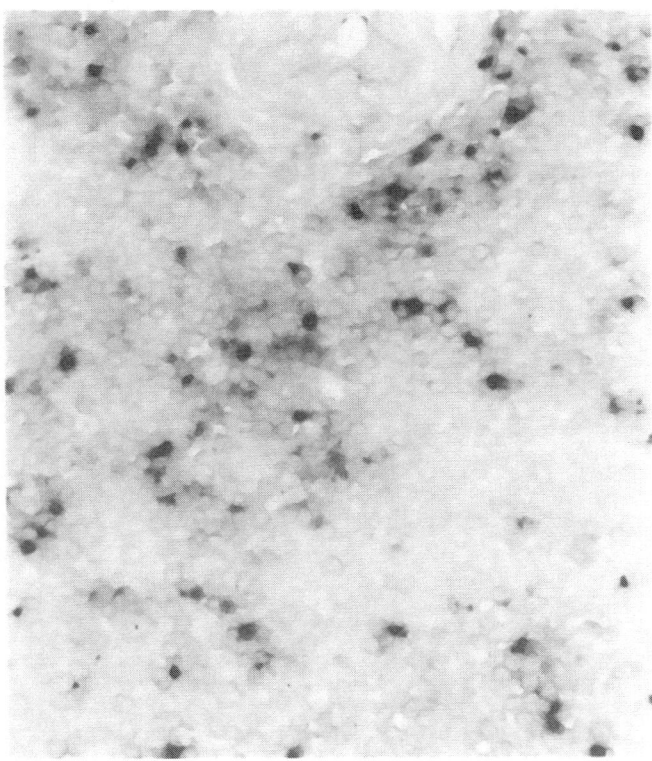

Fig. 2. HCMV DNA was detected in the nuclei of splenic red pulp cells of a section of a spleen from an organ donor. The slide was hybridized in situ with the HCMV subgenomic ES fragment labelled with biotin-11-dUTP. The *dark spots* represent the hybridization

Hybridization

Spleen tissue of the seronegative donors was tested for the presence of HCMV related sequences using DBH and ISH. Using DBH, 9 out of 45 (20 %) tested spleen specimens were positive for the presence of specific HCMV nucleic acids both with ES and BH fragment. Testing these 9 HCMV antibody seronegative spleen tissues by ISH with ES probe to determine the latent HCMV positive cells, in 7 out of these 9 (77.8 %) specimens a specific hybridization signal for the presence of HCMV was obtained in the nucleus of perifollicular red pulp cells (Fig. 2). This localization was in concordance with the ISH results of the seropositive control spleen specimens. Specimens positive by DNA hybridization techniques were randomly distributed over the seronegative patients. Of the control group 5 out of 5 spleen tissues gave positive result using DBH as well as ISH.

To exclude crossreactivity with cellular DNA or other human herpesviruses the ES and BH probe were tested on DNA extracted from infected HEF monolayers. No crossreactivity was observed, while DNA obtained from HCMV (AD169 strain) infected HEF always showed positive results.

Discussion

In this study we showed the presence of latent HCMV in splenic tissue in seropositive individuals. In the nucleus of the red pulp cells of the spleen HCMV positive ISH was found. This observation confirmed the results of other laboratories indicating that spleen tissue can be a site for latency of HCMV [32]. This localization is also in agreement with in vivo animal experiments; perifollicular red pulp cells are infected in acute infections [30] and are demonstrated to be a site for latency in CMV infected animals [26]. As has been shown in several other studies [6, 9, 11, 20], it is important to use a dependable serological assay for screening blood and organ donors to achieve a reduction of transmitted HCMV infection and HCMV disease in seronegative recipients at risk of primary infection. However, there is some debate about seronegative donors being free from previous HCMV infection and the possibility of presence of latent virus [10, 28, 29]. Using the DBH technique we found that in 9 out of the 45 (20 %) patients HCMV genome could be detected. The moderate number of HCMV seronegative normal individuals having HCMV nucleic acids detectable in the spleen tissue as demonstrated in this study could be explained by one of the following mechanisms. Firstly the HCMV antibodies could be absent in these patients due to some deficiency in antibody production to viral protein(s) [29]. Secondly, it is generally accepted that after HCMV infection, antibodies are developed and these antibodies persist throughout life. The question could be asked if this persistence is obtained by frequent (local) reactivation of the latent virus. If this is the fact than it is possible that without this reactivation the level of antibodies decline during life reaching an undetectable level (so called seronegativity) [23]. If this hypothesis is correct than seronegative patients could harbor latent HCMV in their organs. An explanation for this phenomenon is the suppression of viral expression due to an increased level of methylation of the viral genome [4, 27]. Thirdly, although the DNA probes used in this study were very specific for HCMV, the possibility of detecting an (unknown) (Herpes) virus with nucleic acid sequences in its genome similar to the immediate early and late regions of the HCMV genome exists.

Further investigations are needed to elucidate the presence of latent virus in seronegative humans and to detect factors leading to seronegativity due to suppression of the immune response in the immunocompetent host.

Acknowledgements. The authors wish to thank M. P. Landini for the invitation to learn and perform the immunoblotting technique in the laboratory of the Institute of Medical Microbiology, University of Bologna, St. Orsola General Hospital Bologna, Italy.

References

1. Adler SP (1983) Transfusion-associated CMV infection. Rev Infect Dis 5:977–993
2. Adler SP et al. (1985) Detection of Cytomegalovirus antibody with latexagglutination. J Clin Microbiol 22:68–70
3. Barkholt LM, Briczon BG, Ehrnst A, Forgren M, and Anderson JP (1990) Cytomegalovirus infections in liver transplant patients: incidence and outcome. Transplant Proc 22:235–237
4. Boom R, Geelen JL, Sol CJ, Minnaar RP and Noordaa J (1987) Resistance to de novo methylation of the Human Cytomegalovirus immediate early enhancer in a model for virus latency and reactivation in vitro. J Gen Virol 68:2839–2852

5. Boom R, Sol CJA, Salimans MMM, Jansen CL, Wertheim PME, Noordaa van der J (1990) Rapid and simple method for purification of nucleic acids. J Clin Microbiol 28:495–503

6. Bowden RA, Sayers M, Flournoy N, Newton N, Ranajii N, Thomas ED, Meyers JD (1986) CMV immunoglobulin and seronegative blood products to prevent primary CMV infection after marrow transplantation. N Engl J Med 314:1006–1010

7. Braun DK, Pereira L, Norrild B, Roizman B (1983) Application of denaturated, electrophoretically separated and immobilized lysates of Herpes simplex virus-infected cells for detection of monoclonal antibodies and for studies of the properties of viral proteins. J Virol 46:103–112

8. Brühmann A, Schmitz H (1991) High prevalence of antibodies to an epitope located on human Cytomegalovirus nucleocapsid particles in Abstract-book: "Third international cytomegalovirus Workshop", 11–14 June, Bologna, abstract number 62

9. Fox AS, Tolpin MD, Baker AL, Broelsch CE, Whittington PF, Jackson T, Thislethwaite JR, Stuart FP (1988) Seropositivity in liver transplant recipients as a predictor of CMV disease. J Infect Dis 157:383–385

10. Gleaves CA, Wendt SF, Dobbs DR, Meyers JD (1990) Evaluation of the CMV-CUBE assay for detecting CMV serologic status in marrow transplant patients and marrow donors. J Clin Microbiol 28:841–842

11. Gray JJ, Alvey B, Smith DJ, Wreghitt TG (1987) Evaluation of a commercial latex agglutination test for detecting antibodies to CMV in organ donors and transplant recipients. J Virol Methods 16:13–19

12. Hendrix MGR, Dormans PHJ, Kitselaar P, Bruggeman CA (1989) The presence of Cytomegalovirus nucleic acids in arterial walls of atherosclerotic and non-atherosclerotic patients. Am J Pathol 134:1151–1157

13. Hendrix MGR, Salimans MMM, Boven van CPA, Bruggeman CA (1990) High prevalence of latently present Cytomegalovirus in arterial wall of patients suffering form grade III atherosclerosis. Am J Pathol 136:23–28

14. Hendrix MGR, Daemen M, Bruggeman CA (1991) Cytomegalovirus nucleic acid distribution within the human vascular tree. Am J Pathol 138:563–567

15. Ho M (1982) Characteristics of Cytomegalovirus. In: Cytomegalovirus – Biology and Infection. Plenum Medical Book Co., New York, pp 9–32

16. Landini MP, Re MC, Mirolo G, Baldassarri M, La Placa M (1985) Human immune response to CMV structural polypeptides studied by immunoblotting. J Med Virol 17:303–311

17. Landini MP, Mirolo G, Coppolecchia P, Re MC, La Placa M (1986) Serum antibodies to individual CMV structural polypeptides in renal transplant recipients during viral infection. Microbiol Immunol 30:683–695

18. Loon van AM, Logt van der JTH, Veen van der J (1981) Enzyme linked immunosorbent assay for measurement of antibody against CMV and rubella virus in a single serum dilution. J Clin Pathol 34:665–669

19. Loon van AM, Heessen FWA, Logt van der JTH, Veen van der J (1981) Direct enzyme linked immunosorbent assay that uses peroxidase-labelled antiben for determination of immunoglobulin M antibody to CMV. J Clin Microbiol 13:416–422

20. McHugh TM, Savavant GH, Wilber JC, Stites PD (1985) Comparison of six methods for detection of antibody to cytomegalovirus. J Clin Microbiol 22:1014–1019

21. Melnick JL, Petrie BL, Dreesman GR, Burek J, McCollum CH, Debakey ME (1983) Cytomegalovirus antigen within human arterial smooth muscle cells. Lancet II:644–647

22. Metselaar HJ, Weimar W (1989) Cytomegalovirus infection and renal transplantation. J Antimicrob Chemother 23, [Suppl] E:37–47

23. Musiani M, Zerbini M, Zauli D, Cometti G, La Placa M (1988) Impairment of cytomegalovirus in host balance in elderly subjects. J Clin Pathol 41:722–724

24. Nelson JA, Gnann JW, Chazal P (1990) Regulation and Tissue-specific expression of Human Cytomegalovirus. In: Current topics on Microbiology and Immunology – Cytomegaloviruses. Springer-Verlag, Berlin, Heidelberg, 154:75–100

25. Petrie BL, Melnick JL, Adam E, Burek J, McCollum CH, Debakey ME (1987) Nucleic acid sequences of cytomegalovirus in cells cultured from human arteric tissue. J Infect Dis 155:158–159

26. Pomeroy C, Hilleren PJ, Jordan MC (1991) Latent murine Cytomegalovirus DNA in splenic stomal cells of mice. J Virol 65:3330–3334

27. Razin A, Cedar H (1991) DNA Methylation and Gene Expression. Microbiol Rev 55:451–458

28. Ronco P, Kadereit S, Michelson S, Mougenot B, Thibault Ph, Verroust P, Mignon F, Colimon R (1990) Polymerase chain reaction assay for the detection of cytomegalovirus genome in 22 kidney biopsies; a correlation with the serological status. Eur J Clin Invest 20:Abstracts part 2, number 17

29. Schrier RD, Nelson JA, Oldstone MBA (1985) Detection of Human Cytomegalovirus in periferal blood lymphocytes in a natural infection. Science 230:1048–1051

30. Stals FS, Bosman F, Boven van CPA, Bruggeman CA (1990) An animal model for therapeutic intervention studies.of CMV infection in the immunocompromised host. Arch Virol 114:91–107

31. Stanier P, Taylor DL, Kitchen AD, Wales N, Tryhorn Y, Tyms AS (1989) Persistence of Cytomegalovirus in mononuclear cells in periferal blood from blood donors. BMJ 299:897–898

32. Toorkey CB, Carrigan DR (1989) Immunohistochemical detection of an immediate early antigen of Human Cytomegalovirus in noral tissue. J Infect Dis 160:741–751

33. Wertheim PME, Buurman P, Geelen JLMC, Noordaa van der J (1983) Transmission of Cytomegalovirus by renal allograft demonstrated by restriction enzyme analysis. Lancet I:980–981

34. Yamashiroya HM, Ghosh L, Yang R, Robertson AL (1988) Herpes viridea in the coronary arteries and aorta of young trauma victims. Am J Pathol 130:71–79

Transplant Int (1992) 5 [Suppl 1]: S 617–S 620

Reactivity of renal transplant sera against a 17 kD mononuclear cell antigen

J. Neumann, M. Spadafora-Ferreira, A. C. Goldberg, R. Tuder, C. Macaubas, E. Sabbaga, and J. Kalil

Laboratory of Transplantation Immunology Heart Institute and Renal Transplant Unit – Division of Urology Faculty of Medicine University of Sao Paulo, Brazil

In recent years, studies have shown that non-HLA antigens can be involved in renal graft rejection [1]. The so called minor antigens have been found to be expressed on a variety of cells, including endothelial cells [2]. With the aim of understanding better the role of minor antigens in graft rejection, we undertook a Western blot screening of sera from patients waiting for or having received grafts from living-related or cadaveric donors. In this study we described the reactivity of these sera against a 17 kD antigen with expression in many different cell types.

Key words: Mononuclear cell antigen – Renal transplant sera

Methods

Forty-seven sera were studied, comprising sera from 20 patients on a waiting list for their first kidney transplant. 18 kidney transplanted patients, 6 heart transplant recipients and 3 patients who had received platelet transfusions. Of the total, 29 had high and 18 had low PRA (panel reactive antibodies).

Western blots were made according to Towbin et al. [3]. Lysates equivalent to 1×10^6 cells were loaded onto each gel slot, and separated in 5 to 15 % gradients SDS-PAGE gels run under reducing conditions. The electrophoresed proteins were transferred to nitrocellulose filters overnight and incubated with the sera diuluted 1/40. The reactions were developed with anti-human IgG linked to peroxidase or alkaline phosphatase. Lysates were prepared from the following: T and B nylon wool-purified lymphocytes, Petri dish-adhered monocytes, blood platelets and erythrocytes, cultured fibroblasts from cell line (MRC-5), cultured endothelial cells from umbilical cord vein and liver, heart and kidney biopsies.

Specific antibodies to the 17 kD antigen were obtained by elution of the nitrocellulose filter after incubation with serum AT. The antibody elution protocol was performed according to Tovey and Baldo [4] and consisted of incubating a 0.5 mm wide strip of the filter containing the antigen and the antibody with 0.1 M Glycine, pH 2.8, for 2 min followed by brief centrifugation and neutralization with 1 M

Offprint requests to: Jorge Neumann, MD, Laboratorio de Imunologia de Transplantes, Faculdade de Medicina – USP, Av. Dr. Arnaldo 455 3° andar sala 33, 01246 – Sao Paulo, Brazil

Tris buffer, pH 7.6. The eluted antibody was incubated with the CEM T cell line, followed by incubation with Protein A-Gold conjugate. The cells were processed for electron microscopy without any further staining.

In another set of experiments, mononuclear cell lysates on Western blot strips were submitted to sodium metaperiodate treatment at two molar concentrations: 10 and 100 mM. The blots were incubated in the dark, with one or other of the metaperiodate solutions for 10 min, followed by incubation with serum and color development. The 10 mM solution was used to oxidize and remove sialic acid residues from the proteins and the 100 mM eliminated galactose and other simple sugars.

Results

1. Reactivity pattern

Sera from forty-seven patients waiting for or having received kidneys from living-related or cadaveric donors were submitted to Western blotting against mononuclear lysates from normal individuals. The sera were classified as high (greater than 50 % Panel Reactive Antibodies PRA) or low (under 20 % PRA) according to panel reactivity. The number of transfusions received by the individuals in each group varied greatly. In other words, high PRA sera from moderately-transfused patients as well as sera with low PRA from individuals with multiple transfusions were included for analysis. Positive reactions to a protein with an apparent molecular weight of 17 kD were frequent and usually of high intensity. The results are shown in Table 1 and Fig. 1. An increased frequency in

Table 1. Recognition of the 17 kD protein by 47 patients' sera. High (29) and low (18) PRA sera were tested. In both groups part of the sera recognized the specific-bound band by Western blot, although high PRA sera were more frequently reactive

	Panel reactivity	
	High (n)%	Low (n)%
17 kD +	(13) 68.4	(6) 31.6
17 kD −	(16) 57.1	(12) 42.9

A B C D E F G H I J K L M N

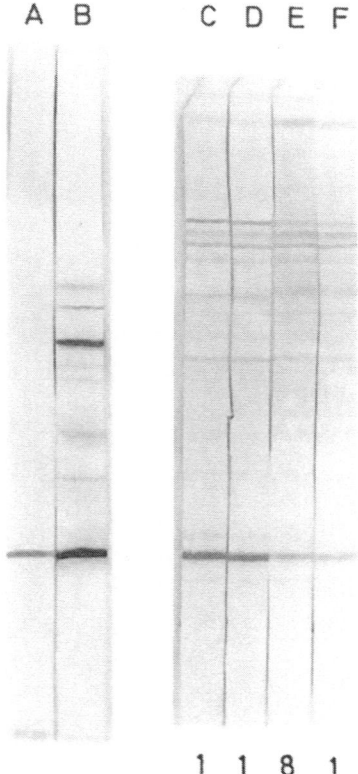

Fig. 1. Western blot using peripheral blood lymphocyte lysates as blotted antigen. From A to K: sera from transplanted kidney patients. Seven of the 11 sera were positive for the 17 kD antigen *(arrow)*. Lanes L and M are sera from normal controls. Lane N shows total PBL lysate

A B C D E F

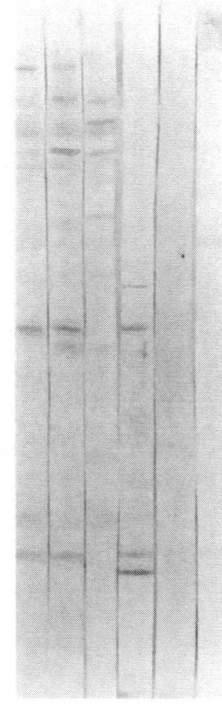

Fig. 3. Testing for heart recipient reactivity and for autoimmunity. In lanes A and B, sera of kidney recipients were tested against normal donors. In lane C the serum was from a heart transplant recipient, negative to the 17 kD antigen. Lanes D, E and F show an auto-Western experiment. In lane D, serum 1 reacts positively against cells from patient 2. In lane E, serum and cells are from patient 2 and reaction is negative and, in lane F, serum from patient 2 tests positive against third-party PBL

A B   C D E F

1 1 8 1

Fig. 2. Western blot with mono and multi-reactivity (A and B) and platelet absorption experiments (C to F). Lane A is a kidney recipient (AT) tested against normal PBL, showing monoreactivity compared to B where a multireactivity was observed. Lanes C and D showed reactivity before and after platelet absorption. Lanes E and F showed elimination of cytotoxicity after platelet absorption (8 to 1) with no change in reactivity to the 17 kD antigen

Six serum samples from heart-transplanted patients, followed for over a year, were negative for the 17 kD antigen. These patients had not received any transfusion prior to grafting, according to the heart transplant protocol established at our Institution. However, the number of transfusions received did not correlate with percentage of positivity of sera to the 17 kD antigen in the high and low groups. Additionally, three patients who received platelet-rich transfusions exhibited the antibody against the 17 kD antigen on mononuclear cells. Finally, there was no correlation between the presence of the anti-17 kD antibody and AB0 blood groups of the patients.

Platelet-absorbed sera did not change their reactivity to the 17 kD antigen (Fig. 2). Besides, serum samples collected on different dates from the same patient (three different patients), with high and low reactivity always exhibited the same pattern and level of reaction irrespective of the PRA level.

2. Nature of the anti-17 kD antibody

Reaction on Western blots was consistently developed with anti-IgG conjugates. Thus, in accordance with the nature of the antibody, cytotoxicity assays against mononuclear cells were performed simultaneously using unabsorbed and platelet-absorbed sera. Reactivity to the 17 kD antigen was never removed, even when absorption led to loss of the cytotoxicity, thus indicating that this antigen was not involved in cytotoxic processes (Fig. 2). Reactivity to the 17 kD antigen was unchanged after treatment with two molar concentrations of sodium metaperiodate (data not shown), indicating that the antibody was directed against the protein structure and not the glycosilation residues.

the high PRA group, though not statistically significant, was observed. In addition, comparison of graft survival rates in transplanted patients showed a slight increase in positivity to the 17 kD antigen of 84% (10/12) in the group of patients who lost their transplanted kidney, compared to 66% (4/6) in the group of patients with good outcome.

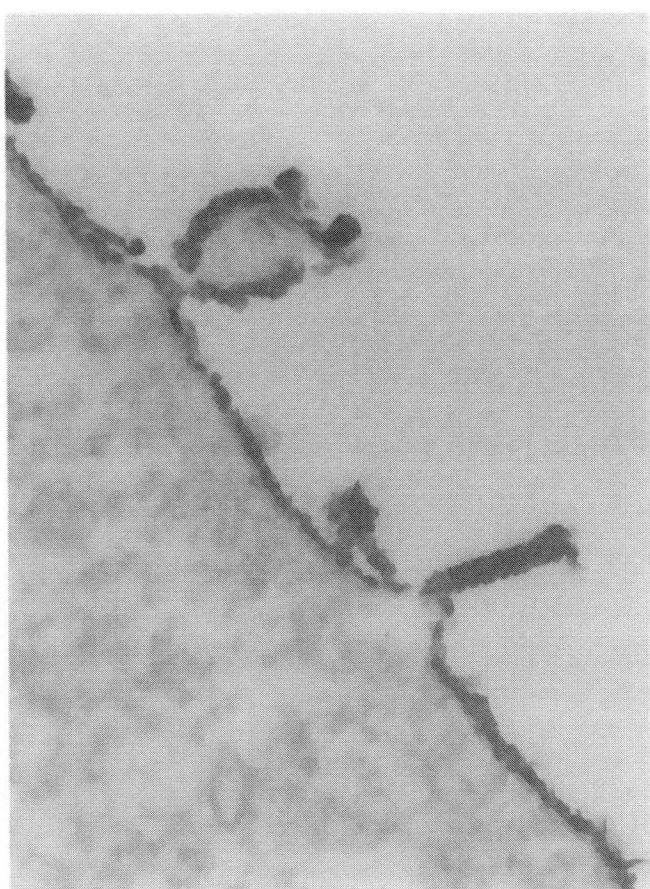

Fig. 4. Electron microscopy of CEM T cell line. Specific antibodies to the 17 kD antigen were eluted after reacting with the band on nitrocellulose filters. After incubation with fixed CEM T cells, reactivity was developed with colloidal gold conjugated second antibody

3. Expression of the 17 kD antigen

Sera from four positive patients were submitted to an auto-Western blot and were shown to be negative (see Fig. 3). In order to confirm the presence of this antigen on the cell membrane, specific antibodies were eluted from the nitocellulose filter and were incubated with the CEM

Table 2. Cell distribution of the 17 kD antigen. Erythrocytes and liver cells were the only negative cells tested so far

Type of cell	Presence of 17 kD antigen
T lymphocytes	+
T lymphocytes, activated	+[a]
B lymphocytes	+
Monocytes	+
Endothelial cells	+
Kidney	+
Heart	+
Liver	−
Platelets	+ / −
Fibroblasts	+
Erythrocytes	−

[a] T lymphocytes, fresh and cultured for 3 days in the presence of phytohemagglutinin, were analyzed simultaneously showing no change in intensity of band staining

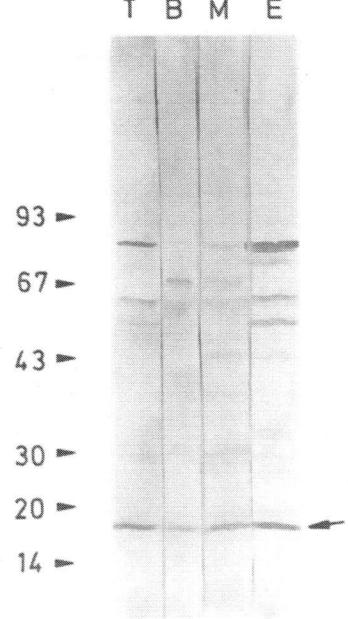

Fig. 5. Western blot with different cell types from the same donor. Serum from a renal transplant recipient was tested against T and B lymphocytes, monocytes and endothelial cells from the same umbilical cord. The *arrow* points out the 17 kD antigen

T cell line. Incubation with protein A – gold conjugate followed and the resulting reaction was observed with an electron microscope. The photomicrographs showed a linear staining on the cell membrane, even in finger-like protusions of the cytoplasm. No intracellular structures were stained (see Fig. 4).

Finally, sera with strong positive reactivity were analyzed by Western blotting against several types of cells. In one experiment serum was incubated with lysates from T and B lymphocytes, monocytes and umbilical vein endothelial cells from the same donor. Reactivity was equivalent in the four types of cells as shown in Fig. 5. Table 2 shows the results obtained with cells from several different tissues.

Discussion

In order to identify new cell antigens recognized by transplant recipient sera, we studied the reactivity of selected sera against cell lysates by Western blotting. In the course of this screening, an antigen of 17 kD was identified and recognized by 19 of 47 sera tested (40%). The reactivity was elicited by allostimulation since non-transfused nontransplanted donors do not react with this band. Blood transfusion seems to be the most common way of immunization, high PRA individuals presenting with the antibody more frequently. It is not an autoantibody since positive sera repeatedly do not recognize the antigen on autologous cells. Nevertheless, a putative polymorphism of the system was not assessed so far and further analyses are needed. Electron microscopic immuno-staining with protein A showed uniform distribution of the antigen on the surface of the CEM T cell line. Paradoxically, antibodies to the 17 kD protein did not cause complement-dependent cell lysis.

The distribution of this molecule was widespread, being found on T and B lymphocytes, monocytes, endothelial cells, fibroblasts and possibly platelets, as well as diverse tissues such as kidney and heart. However, it was not present on erythrocytes, excluding the possibility of a blood type antigen.

Although we were unable to show correlation with graft rejection, reactivity with the 17 kD band is most frequently present in graft rejecting recipients.

We do not know the origin of this antigen. An analogy may be drawn with the Ly-6 family of surface antigens [5]. This family comprehends surface antigens of low molecular weight (12–18 kD), which exhibit a certain degree of polymorphism and are expressed on several types of cells. As in our case, a function for these molecules has not been found.

References

1. Kalil J, Guilherme L, Neumann J, Rosales C, Marin M, Saldanha L, Chocair PR, Ianhez LE, Sabbaga E (1989) Humoral rejection in two HLA identical living-related dodnor kidney transplants. Transplant Proc 21: 711–713
2. Cerilli J, Jesseph JE, Miller AC (1972) The significance of antivascular endothelium antibody in renal transplantation. Surg Gynecol Obstet 155: 246
3. Towbin H, Staehelin T, Gordon J (1979) Electrophoretic transfer of proteins from polyacrylamide gels to nitrocellulose sheets: Procedure and some aplications. Proc Natl Acad Sci USA 76: 4350–4354
4. Tovey ER, Baldo BA (1989) Specialised Aspects of Protein Blotting. In: BA Baldo, ER Tovey, NSW St. Leonards (eds) Protein Blotting: Methodology, Research and Diagnostic Applications. Karger, Basel, pp 43–46
5. Shevach EM, Korty PE (1989) Ly-6: a multigene family in search of a function. Immunol Today 10: 195–200

Transplant Int (1992) 5 [Suppl 1]: S 621–S 624

TRANSPLANT
International
© Springer-Verlag 1992

Strength of HLA-A, HLA-B, and HLA-DR mismatches in relation to short- and long-term kidney graft survival

G. Opelz for the Collaborative Transplant Study

Department of Transplantation Immunology, Institute of Immunology, University of Heidelberg, Im Neuenheimer Feld 305, D-6900 Heidelberg, Germany

Abstract. The separate influence of HLA-A, HLA-B, and HLA-DR mismatches on short- and long-term kidney graft survival was analyzed in a series of over 40,000 recipients of first cadaver kidney transplants. As expected, during the early posttransplant period, HLA-DR mismatches had a stronger influence on graft survival than HLA-B mismatches, and HLA-A mismatches had a very small influence. Surprisingly, during the period from 6 months to 5 years post transplantation, all three HLA loci had approximately the same influence. When the graft survival computation was started at 100 % at 6 months, the difference between grafts with zero or two mismatches at the end of 5 years was 6 %, regardless of whether HLA-A, HLA-B, or HLA-DR antigens were analyzed. The influence of the three loci was additive so that the survival rate difference between transplants with zero or six mismatches for HLA-A, -B, -DR was 17 % at 5 years. We concluded that, although the HLA-A locus exerts only a weak influence during the early posttransplant course, its influence on long-term survival is comparable to that of HLA-B and HLA-DR. In order to obtain optimal long-term survival, all three loci must be considered in the donor-recipient matching procedure.

Key words: Strength of HLA mismatches – Long-term graft survival.

It has been recognized for many years that HLA-DR mismatches have a stronger influence on graft survival than HLA-B mismatches, and that HLA-A mismatches have the smallest impact. Understandably, kidney sharing organizations have adopted policies whereby compatibility for HLA-DR was given greater weight than that for HLA-B, and HLA-A was considered even less important. Re-

cently, Thorogood et al. have shown that, whereas this hierarchy was applicable to the first 5 months post transplantation, only the HLA-B locus had a significant impact on graft survival during the period from 5 months to 3 years [1]. The HLA-A locus appeared to have no significant influence on either short-term or long-term survival, suggesting that HLA-A could be ignored in the matching procedure. We report here on an analysis of over 40,000 primary transplants in cyclosporine-treated recipients. The results lead us to argue that HLA-A mismatches should not be ignored.

Methods

The transplants were reported to the Collaborative Transplant Study by 297 transplant centers in 41 countries. HLA typings were performed at the individual centers' tissue typing laboratories and reported to the study center for analysis. The distinction of HLA antigen "splits" and "broad antigens" has been published previously [2]. Graft survival rates were computed by the Kaplan-Meier method. Statistical significance was estimated by weighted regression analysis [3]. Only first transplants were analyzed and the immunosuppressive protocol of all patients included cyclosporine. The transplants were performed from 1982 to 1990. No exclusions of any types of failures were made.

Results

Figure 1 demonstrates the importance of separating transplants which were typed for HLA-A,-B antigen "splits" from those that were typed merely for the "broad" antigen specificities. "Splits" are the best defined specificities. Among transplants typed for "broad" specificities, a correlation of antigen matching with graft outcome was not apparent. Therefore, we restricted all subsequent analysis steps to transplants in which both the recipient and donor were typed for antigen "splits".

The well known hierarchy of importance with respect to their influence on early graft survival is illustrated for the HLA-A, HLA-B, and HLA-DR loci in Figs. 2–4. Dur-

Offprint requests to: Gerhard Opelz

HLA-A+B MISMATCHES

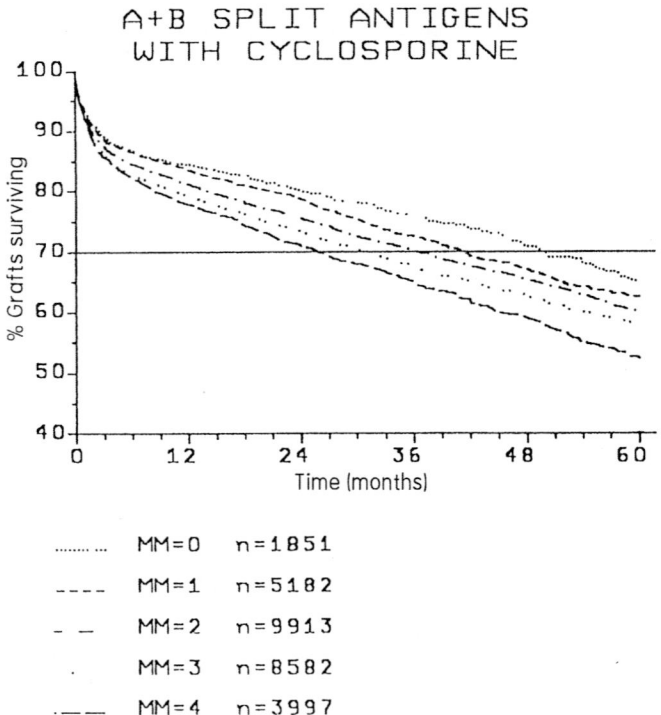

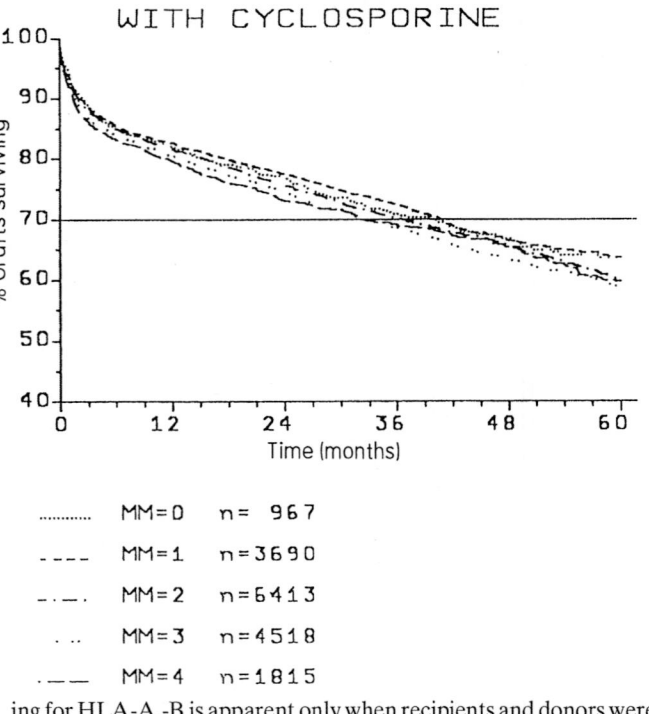

Fig. 1. Influence of HLA-A and HLA-B antigen mismatches on the survival rate of first cadaver kidney transplants. All patients were immunosuppressed with cyclosporine. A strong influence of match-ing for HLA-A,-B is apparent only when recipients and donors were typed for "split antigens" (*left* half of figure) and not when typing was performed for "broad" antigens (*right* half of figure)

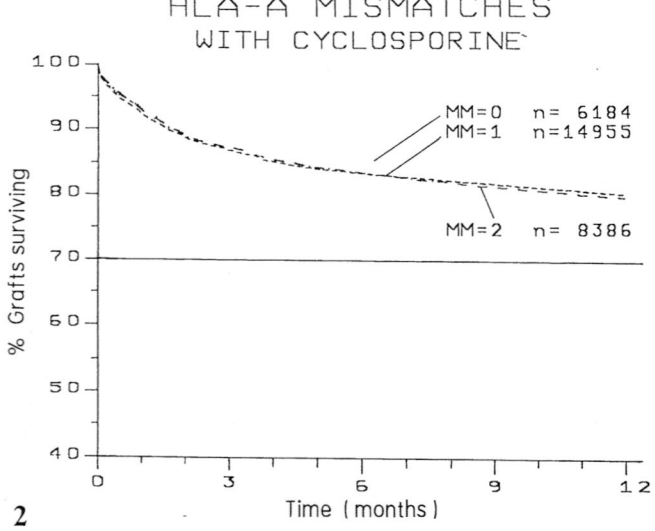

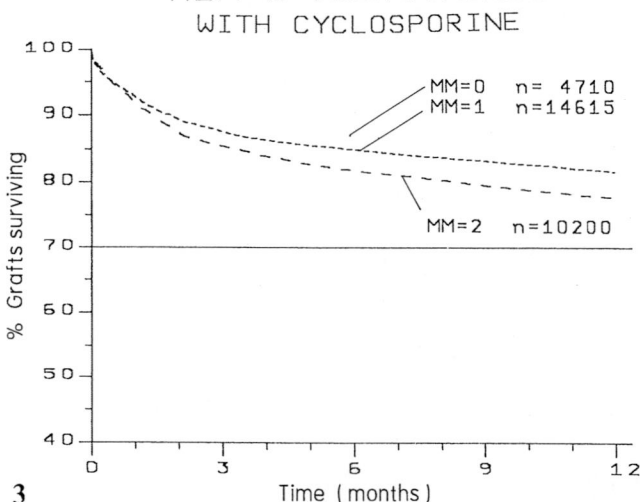

Fig. 2. Effect of HLA-A mismatches on first cadaver transplant survival. During the 1st year, the effet of the HLA-A locus was small, although statistically significant (*P* regression = 0.001). Numbers of mismatched antigens and numbers of patients studied are indicated at ends of curves

Fig. 3. Influence of HLA-B mismatches on first cadaver transplant survival. HLA-B mismatches had a stronger influence than mismatches for HLA-A (compare Fig. 2). Statistical significance: *P* regression < 0.0001

ing the 1st post-transplant year, the influence of the HLA-A locus was barely noticeable. HLA-DR had the strongest impact.

Quite different was our assessment for the period following the first 6 months after transplantation. At the end of 5 years, each of the three loci contributed approximately 6 percentage points to the graft survival rate (Figs. 5–7). We thus did not confirm the report by Thoro-

good that it is only the HLA-B locus that influences long-term graft outcome. In our experience, all three loci were of approximately equal influence. Moreover, the individual influences were apparently additive as shown in Fig. 8. Starting from a 100% rate at 6 months, all three loci together contributed to a 17% difference in graft survival at 5 years between transplants with zero or six mismatches.

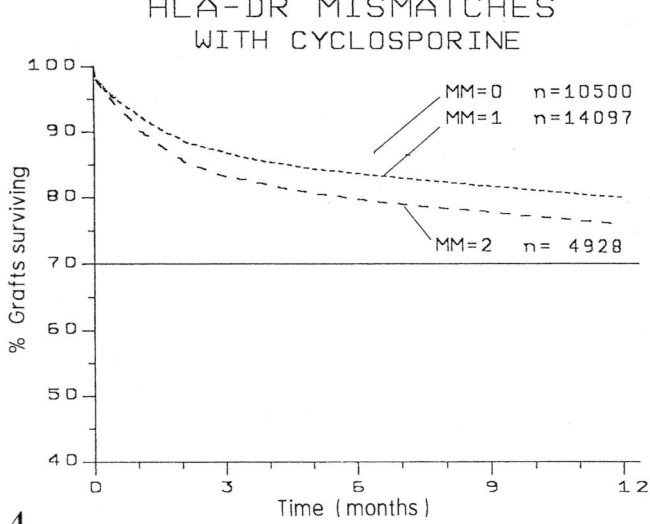

Fig. 4. Influence of HLA-DR antigens on graft survival. DR locus mismatches had a slightly stronger influence during the 1st year than HLA-B mismatches (compare Fig. 3). Statistical significance: *P* regression < 0.0001

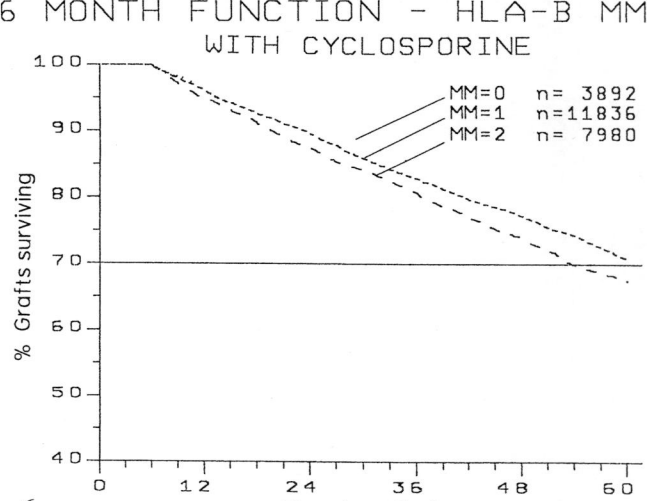

Fig. 6. Influence of HLA-B antigen mismatches during the period from 6 months to 5 years. The effect was comparable to that of HLA-A mismatches (see Fig. 5). At 5 years: *P* regression < 0.0001

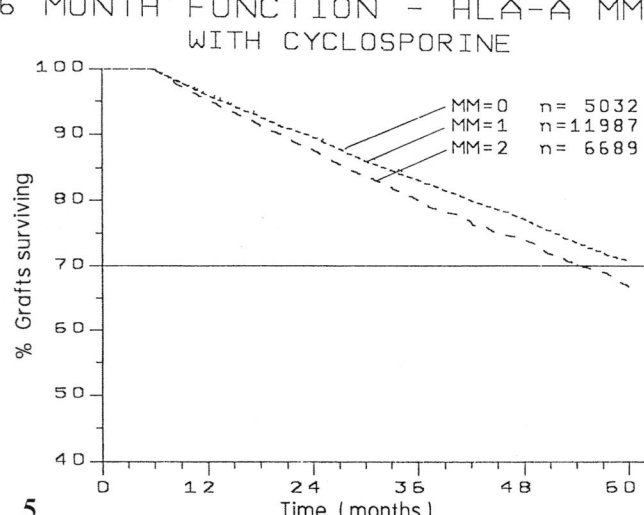

Fig. 5. Influence of mismatches for HLA-A antigens during the period from 6 months to 5 years post transplantation. All transplants analyzed had a functioning graft at 6 months. First cadaver transplants in patients on immunosuppression including cyclosporine were analyzed. At 5 years: *P* regression < 0.0001

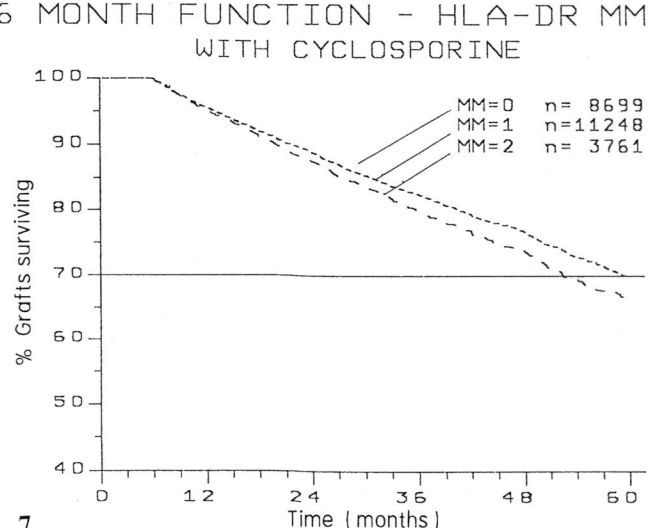

Fig. 7. Influence of HLA-DR mismatches during the period from 6 months to 5 years. The influence was equivalent to that shown for HLA-A and HLA-B in the two previous figures. At 5 years, *P* regression < 0.0001

We concluded that it would be a mistake to ignore the HLA-A locus in the matching procedure because of its long-term impact. For an optimal matching effect to be realized, all three loci must be considered. This was also demonstrated in the computation of long-term half-life risks for the period beyond 6 months. The combined impact of HLA-A,-B,-DR resulted in a difference from a half-life time of 11.8 years for zero-mismatch grafts to 6.6 years for six-mismatch transplants (Fig. 9). If the HLA-A locus was left out, the half-life time for HLA-B,-DR zero-mismatch transplants was 10.6 years and that for four-mismatch grafts was 7.1 years. Thus, including the HLA-A locus improved the power of resolution.

Discussion

Our results demonstrated that whereas there is a hierarchy of a decreasing influence during the early posttransplant period from HLA-DR to HLA-B to HLA-A, no such distinction could be made for the period from 6 months to 5 years. Our assessment did not agree with that by Thorogood et al., possibly because we restricted our analysis to transplants typed for HLA-A and HLA-B "split antigens" and due to the larger number of patients studied and the longer follow up.

In practical terms, for the purpose of organ allocation, this still means that greater weight should be attached to the HLA-DR and HLA-B loci than to HLA-A, simply be-

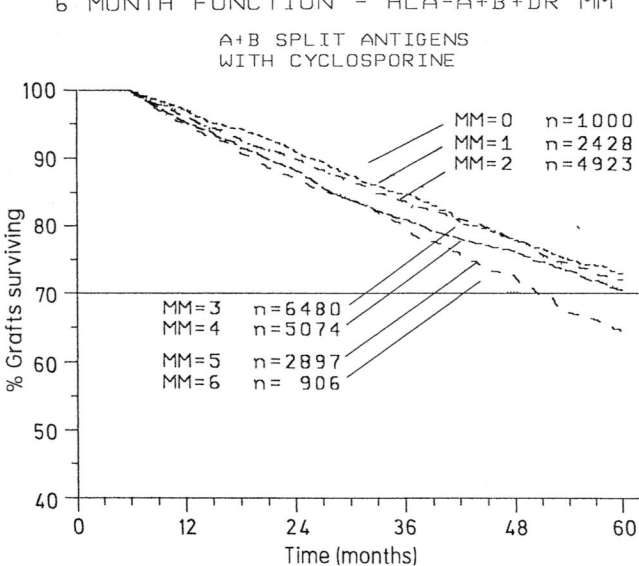

6 MONTH FUNCTION - HLA-A+B+DR MM

A+B SPLIT ANTIGENS
WITH CYCLOSPORINE

MM=0 n=1000
MM=1 n=2428
MM=2 n=4923

MM=3 n=6480
MM=4 n=5074
MM=5 n=2897
MM=6 n= 906

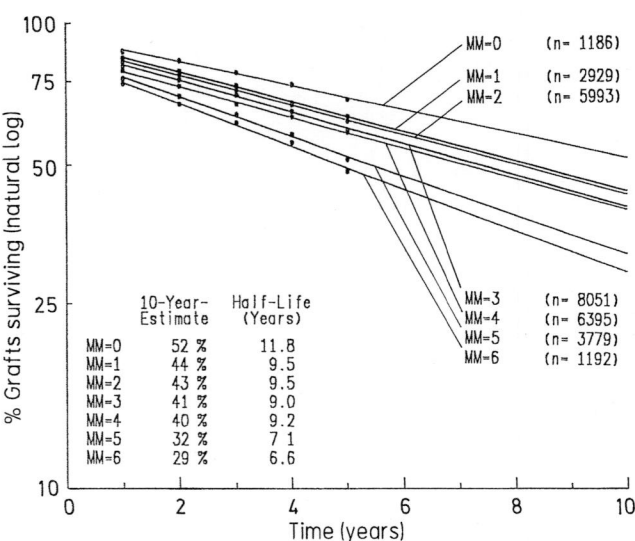

MM=0 (n- 1186)
MM=1 (n- 2929)
MM=2 (n- 5993)

MM=3 (n- 8051)
MM=4 (n- 6395)
MM=5 (n- 3779)
MM=6 (n- 1192)

	10-Year-Estimate	Half-Life (Years)
MM=0	52 %	11.8
MM=1	44 %	9.5
MM=2	43 %	9.5
MM=3	41 %	9.0
MM=4	40 %	9.2
MM=5	32 %	7 1
MM=6	29 %	6.6

Fig. 8. Combined effect of HLA-A,-B,-DR mismatches on graft survival during the period from 6 months to 5 years. First cadaver transplant recipients on cyclosporine immunosuppression were analyzed. The individual effects of the three loci were additive. Whereas the difference between zero and two mismatches for each individual locus was 6% at 5 years, all three loci together resulted in a 17% difference at 5 years. P regression < 0.0001

Fig. 9. Half-life computation for the period from 1 year to 5 years. First cadaver kidney transplants in cyclosporine-treated patients were analyzed. The combined impact of HLA-A,-B,-DR locus mismatches on the long-term attrition rate is shown. The individual influence of each of the three HLA loci was similar during this period

cause a greater early impact influences not only the early but also the late outcome. However, the results demonstrated that, when an optimal long-term graft outcome is aimed for, the HLA-A locus cannot be ignored.

Acknowledgements. The generous support of the centers participating in the Collaborative Transplant Study is gratefully acknowledged. We thank IBM Germany for providing computer hardware and software for these studies.

References

1. Thorogood J, Persijn GG, Schreuder GMTh, D'Amaro J, Zantvoort F, van Houwelingen JC, van Rood JJ (1990) The effect of HLA matching on kidney graft survival in separate posttransplantation intervals. Transplantation 50: 146–150
2. Opelz G for the Collaborative Transplant Study (1988) Importance of HLA antigen splits for kidney transplant matching. Lancet II: 61–64
3. Dunn OJ, Clark VA (eds) (1974) Applied statistics: analysis of variance and regression Wiley, New York, p 236

Transplant Int (1992) 5 [Suppl 1]: S 625–S 626

TRANSPLANT
International
© Springer-Verlag 1992

Pretransplant serum IgG-anti-F(ab')$_{2\gamma}$ activity and kidney graft outcome: comparison of results obtained at two centers

C. Süsal[1], J. Groth[2], H.-H. Oberg[1], P. Terness[1], G. May[3], G. Staehler[4], and G. Opelz[4]

[1] Department of Transplantation Immunology, Institute of Immunology, University of Heidelberg, Im Neuenheimer Feld 305, D-6900 Heidelberg, Germany
[2] Department of Experimental Organ Transplantation, Humboldt University School of Medizin, Berlin, Germany
[3] Department of Urology, Friedrichshain Hospital, Berlin, Germany
[4] Department of Urology, Surgical Clinic, University of Heidelberg, Heidelberg, Germany

Anti-IgG autoantibodies are reported to possess immunoregulatory properties [1, 2]. In the present study, we investigated the effect of pretransplant serum IgG-anti-F(ab')$_{2\gamma}$ autoantibody activity on kidney graft outcome in recipients from two transplant centers.

Key words: Kidney transplantation – Autoantibodies – JgG-anti-F activity.

Materials and methods

Pretransplant sera of 215 kidney graft recipients from Heidelberg and 474 recipients from the Berlin Friedrichshain center were tested retrospectively for IgG-anti-F(ab')$_{2\gamma}$ activity. All patients from Heidelberg and 330 patients from Berlin had a 1-year follow up. The patients were separated into those with excellent graft function (creatinine < 130 µmol/l), good graft function (creatinine 130–260 µmol/l), mediocer graft function (creatinine 260–400 µmol/l), poor graft function but no chronic dialysis (creatinine > 400 µmol/l), and graft failure. Evaluation of graft function was registered at 3, 6, and 12 months after transplantation.

For the determination of IgG-anti-F(ab')$_{2\gamma}$ activity, 96-well microtiter plates (Nunc, Roskilde) were coated at 37 °C for 16 h with 0.5 µg/well of human IgG,F(ab')$_2$ fragments (Dianova, Hamburg, Germany). The plates were washed and uncoated sites were blocked with 50 µl of 1 % BAS-PBS solution at 37 °C for 3 h. We added 50 µl of 1:128 diluted test serum to the F(ab')$_{2\gamma}$-coated wells. PBS-Tween 0.05 % was used as washing buffer and p-nitro-phenyl phosphate disodium solution (Sigma, St. Louis, Mo.) as substrate. Incubation steps with sera or antibodies were performed at 22 °C for 1 h. After each step the plates were washed four times with washing buffer. The reaction was developed with 50 µl of an alkaline phosphatase-conjugated goat antibody specific for IgG,Fc (Dianova, working dilution 1:5000). The results are expressed as mean optical density (OD) ± SEM read at 405 nm using an MR 700 Microplate Reader (Dynatech, Chantill Y, Va.). Statistical analysis was performed using the rank-sum test of Wilcoxon.

Results

The results were concordant at the two centers. A significant association was found between pretransplant IgG-anti-F(ab')$_{2\gamma}$ activity and 3-month (Table 1) and 1-year (Table 2) kidney graft outcome. When all patients were analyzed, IgG-anti-F(ab')$_{2\gamma}$ activity in pretransplant sera of recipients with graft failure or poor graft function (creatinine > 400 µmol/l) at 3 month was significantly lower than the activity in recipients with a 3-month serum creatinine of < 130 µmol/l ($P = 0.0085$). A particularly high IgG-anti-F(ab')$_{2\gamma}$ activity was found in patients with immediately functioning grafts and a 3-month creatinine of < 130 µmol/l ($P < 0.0001$, as compared to patients with graft failure or poor graft function). Patients with 3-month creatinines of 130–260 µmol/l or 260–400 µmol/l had intermediate IgG-anti-F(ab')$_{2\gamma}$ activities (compared to patients with immediately functioning grafts and creatinine

Table 1. Pretransplant IgG-anti-F(ab')$_{2\gamma}$ activity and early 3-month graft function

Recipients from the Heidelberg and Berlin Friedrichshain transplant centers were separated into groups according to their 3-month serum creatinines. The highest IgG-anti-F(ab')$_{2\gamma}$ activity (mean ± SEM) was found in patients with immediately functioning grafts and a 3-month serum creatinine of < 130 µmol/l

Serum creatinine (µmol/l)	IgG-anti-F(ab')$_{2\gamma}$ Serum activity		
	Heidelberg	Berlin	All patients
< 130 and immediate function	1297 ± 102 $n = 64$	1390 ± 78 $n = 81$	1330 ± 62 $n = 145$
< 130	1152 ± 65 $n = 141$	1175 ± 51 $n = 162$	1168 ± 40* $n = 303$
130–260	1197 ± 181 $n = 31$	1032 ± 46 $n = 201$	1063 ± 48 $n = 232$
260–400	738 ± 208 $n = 7$	1046 ± 94 $n = 35$	991 ± 86 $n = 42$
> 400 or graft failure	934 ± 106 $n = 36$	1014 ± 81 $n = 76$	987 ± 65* $n = 112$

* Excellent graft function versus poor graft function or graft failure, $P = 0.0085$

Offprint requests to: C. Süsal

Table 2. Pretransplant IgG-anti-F(ab')$_{2\gamma}$ activity and 1-year kidney graft outcome

Recipients from the Heidelberg and Berlin Friedrichshain centers were separated into groups according to their 1-year serum creatinine levels. The highest IgG-anti-F(ab')$_{2\gamma}$ activity (mean $\pm$ SEM) was found in patients with immediately functioning grafts and a 1-year serum creatinine of < 130 µmol/l

Serum creatinine (µmol/l)	IgG-anti-F(ab')$_{2}\gamma$ Serum activity		
	Heidelberg	Berlin	All patients
< 130 and immediate function	1271 ± 108 $n = 60$	1350 ± 89 $n = 44$	1310 ± 72 $n = 104$
< 130	1166 ± 70 $n = 123$	1145 ± 60 $n = 104$	1157 ± 47* $n = 227$
130–260	1146 ± 174 $n = 31$	986 ± 51 $n = 112$	1018 ± 55 $n = 143$
260–400	971 ± 245 $n = 8$	967 ± 99 $n = 26$	971 ± 93 $n = 34$
> 400 or graft failure	886 ± 98 $n = 48$	971 ± 74 $n = 88$	934 ± 58* $n = 136$

* Excellent graft function versus poor graft function or graft failure, $P = 0.0009$

< 130 µmol/l at 1 year: $P = 0.0001$ and 0.0012, respectively) (Table 1).

The association between IgG-anti-F(ab')$_{2\gamma}$ activity and kidney graft outcome was evident even more clearly at 1 year. As shown in Table 2, a high IgG-anti-F(ab')$_{2\gamma}$ activity was found in recipients who had a serum creatinine of < 130 µmol/l at 1 year. The IgG-anti-F(ab')$_{2\gamma}$ activity in patients with immediately functioning grafts and a 1-year creatinine of < 130 µmol/l was significantly higher than that in recipients with a creatinine of 130–260 µmol/l, 260–400 µmol/l, or in recipients with graft failure or poor function (creatinine > 400 µmol/l) at 1 year ($P < 0.0003$, 0.0051, and $P < 0.0001$, respectively).

Discussion

The results described here are an extension of our previous finding that anti-F(ab')$_{2\gamma}$ antibodies of athe IgG isotype are associated with good kidney graft outcome [3], both with respect to early and 1-year graft function. The results were in agreement with data published by Chia et al. [4], however, they did not agree with a recent study published by the same group in which they could not confirm their previous finding [5].

The protective effect of IgG-anti-F(ab')$_{2\gamma}$ antibodies on graft survival may be due to their antiidiotypic activity as suggested by Nasu et al. [6], or to negative Fc$_\gamma$ signaling induced by IgG-immune complexes [7, 8]. It is unknown whether the antigenic sequence recognized by IgG-anti-F(ab')$_{2\gamma}$ is in the constant or variable region of IgG. Evidence exists for both alternatives [6, 9]. We believe that anti-immunoglobulin antibodies of different isotypes and different specificities with diverse and even counteracting effects exist.

Acknowledgements. We wish to acknowledge the excellent technical assistance of Cima Farahmandi, Sibylle Braun, and Angela Edelmann. This work was supported by a grant from the Transplantationszentrum Heidelberg.

References

1. Parker DC (1980) Induction and suppression of polyclonal antibody responses by anti-Ig reagents and antigen-nonspecific helper factors: a comparison of the effects of anti-Fab, anti-IgM, and anti-IgD on murine B cells. Immunol Rev 52: 115–139
2. Terness P, Süsal C, Baur C, Opelz G (1990) A B-cell suppressive IgG-anti-immunoglobulin antibody induced by alloimmunization. Transplantation 50: 502–505
3. Süsal C, Guo Z, Terness P, Opelz G (1990) Role of anti-IgG autoantibodies in kidney transplantation. Immunol Lett 26: 121–125
4. Chia D, Horimi T, Terasaki PI, Hermes M (1982) Association of anti-Fab and anti-IgG antibodies with high kidney transplant survival. Transplant Proc 14: 322–324
5. Feduska NJ Jr, Chia D, Terasaki PI, Sugich L (1991) Effect of anti-Fab antibodies on renal allografts. Transplant Proc 23: 1277–1278
6. Nasu H, Chia DS, Knutson DW, Barnett EV (1980) Naturally occuring human antibodies to the F(ab')$_2$ portion of IgG. Clin Exp Immunol 42: 378–386
7. Bijsterbosch MK, Klaus GGB (1985) Crosslinking of surface immunoglobulin and Fc receptors on B lymphocytes inhibits stimulation of inositol phospholipid breakdown via the antigen receptors. J Exp Med 162: 1825–1836
8. Uher F, Lamers MC, Dickler HB (1985) Antigen-antibody complexes bound to B-lymphocyte Fc$_\gamma$ receptors regulate B-lymphocyte differentiation. Cell Immunol 95: 368–379
9. Wolfe LD, Abruzzo JL, Heimer R (1984) Specificity of IgM antibodies to pooled human F(ab')$_2$ fragments. Immunol Commun 13: 15–27

Transplant Int (1992) 5 [Suppl 1]: S 627–S 628

TRANSPLANT
International
© Springer-Verlag 1992

The impact of ischemic lesions in the donor kidney, donor age, recipient age and HLA (A, B, C, DR, DQ) matching on clinical course after kidney grafting

M. H. L. Christiaans[1], H. G. Peltenburg[1], F. H. M. Niemann[1], G. Kootstra[2], A. T. J. Lavrijssen[1], P. M. van den Berg-Loonen[3], A. Tiebosch[4], K. M. L. Leunissen[1], and J. P. van Hooff[1]

[1] Department of Internal Medicine, [2] Surgery, [3] Tissue Typing and [4] Pathology, University Hospital Maastricht, Maastricht, The Netherlands

It is generally accepted that HLA matching improves graft survival [1]. However, there is no consensus on whether this improvement is reflected on daily clinical course. Clinical course after renal transplantation depends on many factors, such as donor age, recipient age, ischemic score in the kidney [2], and HLA matching [3]. The relative contribution of these factors is unknown. Because management of the recipients in the various centers differs considerably, only a single centre study would reveal the relative contribution of all these factors. Therefore, in our centre we studied the influence of these parameters on the clinical course after renal allografting.

Key words: Kidney transplantation – Ischemic lesions – Donor age – Recipient age – HLA matching

Patients and methods

We included in our study 169 transfused consecutive recipients of a renal allograft with a follow-up of at least 1 year, transplanted between December 1983 and August 1990 under the auspices of Eurotransplant. All patients were given cyclosporine and low dose prednisolone as basic immunosuppression. Antirejection treatment consisted of a 10 day course of rabbit ATG. Subsequent rejections were treated with 500–1000 mg methylprednisolone on 3 alternative days. The recipient characteristics were as follows: mean age 45 years (range 16–72 years, 29 % > 55 years), 77 % first transplant, 17 % second, gender: male 67 %. The donor characteristics were as follows: mean age 35 years (range 1–69 years, 32 % > 45 years, 14 % > 55 years), mean ischemic score 1.9 (range 0–8, 0 = 36 %, 1 or 2 = 32 %, others = 32 %), mean CIT 30.5 h (sd 8.48).

The following parameters were studied: 1 year graft and patient survival, 1 year creatinine clearance, the occurrence of an acute rejection (within 6 months of grafting), duration of hospitalization, need for dialysis, and duration of dialysis dependency. Rejection was diagnosed on clinical grounds and in most instances was confirmed

Offprint requests to: J. P. van Hooff, Department of Internal Medicine, University Hospital Maastricht, PO Box 5800, 6202 AZ Maastricht, The Netherlands

by a biopsy. Statistical analysis was performed with SPSS/PC + (version 3.1) using ANOVA, paired t-test and multiple regression.

Results

The 1 year patient and graft was survival 94 % and 79 % respectively. Of the predictors (donor age, recipient age, ischaemic score and HLA A, B, C, DR and DQ matching), only donor age over 45 years influenced graft survival significantly: donor > 45 years 69 % graft survival, donor ≤ 45 years 83 % graft survival. There was a highly significant influence of various HLA matches on the occurrence of an acute rejection (Table I) e. g. only 1 out of 22 (5 %) HLA A + B + DR identical grafts needed antirejection treatment. No influence of rejection frequency could be shown for HLA A, B, A + B or C matching. Recipients *without* an acute rejection ($n = 121$) had a significantly shorter duration of hospitalization than recipients

Table I. Influence of HLA matching on the occurrence of acute rejection

Number of mismatches		n	%	acute rejection
DR	= 0	102	30	$P < 0.01$
	> 0	94	47	
DQ	= 0	134	34	$P < 0.02$
	> 0	51	55	
B + DR	= 0	34	18	$P < 0.05$
	= 1	67	40	
	≥ 2	94	44	
B + DQ	= 0	34	18	$P < 0.02$
	= 1	92	42	
	≥ 2	59	42	
A + B + DR	= 0	22	5	$P < 0.001$
	= 1	46	52	
	≥ 2	127	39	ns
A + B + DQ	= 0	21	5	$P < 0.001$
	= 1	47	51	
	≥ 2	127	38	ns

with an acute rejection ($n = 75$): 26.4 versus 35.7 days, $P = 0.000$. However, there was no difference between these groups in creatinine clearance (49.6 versus 50.9 ml/min) and in graft survival (82% versus 74%).

None of the predictors had a correlation with need for dialysis or duration of dialysis dependency. In recipients with a functioning kidney graft at 1 year the ischemic score in the donor kidney correlated with the duration of hospitalization (ANOVA $P = 0.005$). In multiple regression, only the ischemic score correlated with the duration of hospitalization (hospital stay = $25.0 + 1.56 \times$ ischemic score, beta = 0.24, $P = 0.006$). The 1 year creatinine clearance correlated with donor age and recipient age, but not with ischemic score nor with HLA matching (Creatinine clearance = $85.4 - 0.457 \times$ donor age $- 0.362 \times$ recipient age; multiple r = -0.43, $P = 0.000$; donor age r = -0.29, $P = 0.002$; recipient age r = -0.18, $P = 0.03$).

Discussion and conclusion

1) Of the factors studied only donor age influenced graft survival. Recipients of a kidney from a donor > 45 years had a significantly lower 1 year graft survival compared to recipients of a kidney from a donor ≤ 45 years.

2) By matching for HLA A + B + DR the occurrence of acute rejection could be decreased to 5%. The same held for matching for HLA A + B + DQ. Because of the high linkage disequilibrium between HLA DR and HLA DQ and the small number of recipients, no prediction could be made about the relative contribution of both loci.

3) Less acute rejection would be of great benefit for the recipient. This was reflected in a significant shorter duration of hospitalization (9 days) for recipients without an acute rejection compared to recipients with an acute rejection.

4) A high ischemic score in the donor kidney resulted in a significantly longer duration of hospitalization.

5) Creatinine clearance at 1 year after grafting was influenced by donor and recipient age, but not by the occurrence of acute rejection, HLA matching or by the ischemic score.

References

1. Opelz G, Schwarz V, Engelmann A, Bach D, Wilk M, Keppel E (1991) Long-term impact of HLA matching on kidney graft survival in cyclosporine-treated recipients. Transplant Proc 23: 373–375
2. Leunissen KML, Bosman FT, Nieman FHM, Kootstra G, Vromen MAM, Noordzij TC, van Hooff JP (1989) Amplification of the nephrotoxic effect of cyclosporine by preexistent chronic histological lesions in the kidney. Transplantation 48:590–593
3. van Hooff JP, van Hooff-Eykenboom YEA, Kalff MW, de Graeff J, van Rood JJ (1979) Kidney graft survival, clinical course, and HLA-A, B and D matching in 208 patients transplanted in one center. Transplant Proc 11:1291–1292

Transplant Int (1992) 5 [Suppl 1]: S 629–S 630

TRANSPLANT
International
© Springer-Verlag 1992

Non specific increased expression of class I major histocompatibility complex (MHC) antigens on rat liver grafts

J. Gugenheim[1], L. Amorosa[1], B. Fabiani[2], I. Astarcioglu[3], M. Gigou[3], F. Crafa[1], M. Reynes[2], H. Bismuth[3]

[1] Laboratoire de Recherches Chirurgicales et Service de Chirurgie Digestive, Hôpital Saint-Roch, B. P. 319 06006 Nice Cedex
[2] Laboratoire d'anatomie Pathologique, [3] Unité de Chirurgie Hépatobiliaire, Hôpital Paul Brousse, 94800 Villejuif, France

Major histocompatibility complex (MHC) antigens play a major role in the rejection reaction and their increased expression may increase the host response to the foreign graft [1]. Several clinical [2–5] and experimental studies [6, 7] have demonstrated increased expression of MHC antigens on the different cell components of liver allografts during rejection. However modified expression of MHC antigens may also occur in certain liver diseases [8–10], after cholestasis [11] or on a regenerating liver [11]. In this experimental study in inbred rats, we compared the expression of MHC antigens on liver cells during rejection and non-immunological situations (cholestasis, cytolysis, regeneration).

Key words: MHC antigens – BN rats – Rejection

Animals and methods

Rats. Inbred rats of the following strains were purchased from CNSEAL (Orleans La Source, France): Brown Norway (BN) (RT1[n]), DA (RT1[a]).

Experimental protocol

There were seven groups of BN rats in this study. In group 1, liver from DA donors were grafted into BN recipient rats and biopsies were carried out on days 5, 8 and at time of death. In group 2, liver isografts were carried out in BN rats and biopsies were performed at days 5, 10 and 15. In group 3, cholestasis was induced by bile duct ligation and rats were sacrified 21 days later. In group 4, cytolysis was induced by the injection of galactosamine and rats were sacrified 48 h later. In group 5, normothermic ischemia was induced by a 90 min occlusion of the portal pedicle and rats were sacrified 30 days later. Group 6 consisted of BN rats with a 70 % hepatectomy, sacrificed 48 h later. Group 7 consisted of control BN rats.

Offprint requests to: J. Gugenheim, Laboratoire de Recherches Chirurgicales et Service de Chirurgie Digestive, Hôpital Saint-Roch, B. P. 319 06006 Nice Cedex

Surgical procedures

Liver transplantation. Orthotopic liver transplantation was performed using cuff techniques for the portal vein, infrahepatic vena cava and biliary anastomoses, as described by Kamada [13]. Ischemia times were in the range of 20–30 min.

Induction of cholestasis. Biliary obstruction was induced by a double ligation of the common bile duct with a non-resorbable suture (7-0 silk). The common bile duct was then transected between the ligatures to prevent recanalization. After closure of the abdominal incision, rats were allowed to recover. Rats were killed 21 days post-ligation.

Ischemic-induced cytolysis. A temporary normothermic ischemia of the liver was induced as follows: the hepatic pedicle was occluded for 90 min with a microvessel clip. Rats were sacrificed 30 days after the end of the occlusion.

Galactosamine-induced cytolysis. Rats were given galactosamine 1.2 mg per kg body weight intraperitoneally. Rats were sacrificed 48 hours later.

Study of regenerating liver after partial hepatectomy. Fast growth of the liver was provoked by the removal of two-thirds of the total liver mass, according to the method described by Higgins and Anderson [14]. Animals were sacrificed 48 h later.

Histological and immunohistological studies

Hematoxylin-eosin stain and Masson trichrome were used for conventional histological examination. For immunohistological studies, a peroxydase antiperoxydase method using mouse monoclonal antibodies to rat MHC antigens (MRC OX27 for class I and MRC OX 17 for class II AG) was carried out as described by Fabiani et al. [7].

Results

Expression of class I MHC antigens (Table 1)

In control livers, there was no detectable class I antigen on the hepatocytes. Positive staining was seen on sinusoidal lining cells and was not modified in experimental groups.

Table 1. Expression of class I MHC antigens on rat hepatocytes

Groups	Grades of staining				
	n	0	+	+	+ + +
1. Allografts	5	0	0	3	2
2. Isografts	5	1	4	0	0
3. Bile duct ligation	5	0	0	3	2
4. Galactosamine cytolysis	5	0	0	1	4
5. Ischemic cytolysis	5	0	0	1	4
6. 70 % hepatectomy	5	2	3	0	0
7. Control	5	5	0	0	0

In the isografts, weak (+) class I induction on hepatocytes and biliary cells was noted on days 5, 10 and 15. In DA to BN allografts, strong (+ +) induction of class I Ag was seen on hepatocytes on days 5, 8 and at time of death. A similar induction was seen in rats with cholestasis. A very strong (+ + +), induction of class I Ag was noted in rats with galactosamine and ischemic-induced cytolysis.

Expression of class II MHC antigens

No expression of class II antigens was seen on hepatocytes in any of the specimens studied. Induction of expression of class II antigens was seen only on biliary epithelium and on sinusoidal cells after liver allografting (group 1).

Discussion

In this study, we did not observe any expression of class I antigens on the hepatocytes of normal non-transplanted livers. This result is in line with several experimental [15] and clinical [16] studies, but the possibility that there is a low level of expression below the limit of sensitivity of the immunodetection method cannot be excluded.

This study demonstrated the induction of expression of MHC class I antigens on hepatocyte membranes during rejection of liver allografts. Isografts also became class I positive, though to a lesser extent than allografts. A massive induction of class I antigens was observed after cholestasis, galactosamine-induced or ischemic cytolysis. Alternatively, class II induction on biliary epithelium and sinusoidal cells appeared to be specific for allograft rejection. Induction of class I antigens on tissue that was previously class I negative may have some important consequences for T cell cytotoxicity. It is known that class I expression is necessary for cytotoxic T cells to recognize and lyse virally-infected cells [1] or tissues bearing alloantigens [17]. Increased hepatocyte MHC class I antigen expression may increase susceptibility of hepatocytes to lysis by cytotoxic T lymphocytes [1]. This may explain the significantly higher incidence of rejection observed after severe preservation injury [18]. In fact cholestasis, ischemic and toxic cell damage, and regeneration are frequently present after liver grafting. All these conditions may contribute to an increased sensitivity of liver allografts to rejection.

References

1. Zinkernagel RM, Doherty PC (1979) MHC cytotoxic T cells: studies on the biological role of polymorphic transplantation antigens determining T cell restriction-specificity, function and responsiveness. Adv Immunol 27:51
2. Demetris AJ, Lasky S, van Thiel DH, Starzl TE, Whiteside T (1985) Induction of DR/IA antigens in human liver allografts: an histocytochemical and clinopathologic analysis of twenty failed grafts. Transplantation 40:504–509
3. So SKS, Platt JL, Ascher NL, Snover DC (1987) Increased expression of class I major histocompatibility complex antigens on hepatocytes in rejecting human liver allografts. Transplantation 43:79–85
4. Gugenheim J, Rouger P, Gane P, Capron-Laudereau M, Reynes M, Bismuth H (1987) Expression of blood group antigens including HLA markers on human liver allografts. Transplant Proc 19:223–225
5. Rouger P, Gugenheim J, Gane P, et al. (1990) Distribution of the MHC antigens after liver transplantation: relationship with biochemical and histological parameters. Clin Exp Immunol 80:404
6. Settaf A, Milton AD, Spencer SC, Houssin D, Fabre JW (1988) Donor class I and class II major histocompatibility antigen expression following liver allografting in rejecting and non-rejecting rat strain combinations. Transplantation 46:32–40
7. Fabiani B, Astarcioglu I, Gugenheim J, Tricottet V, Bismuth H, Reynes M (1989) Expression of major histocompatibility complex antigens on vascular endothelium of spontaneously tolerated liver allografts. Transplant Proc 21:407–408
8. Fukusato T, Gerber MA, Thung SN, Ferrone S, Schaffner F (1986) Expression of HLA class I antigens on hepatocytes in liver diseases. AM J Pathol 123:264
9. Ballardini G, Bianchi FB, Doniach D, Mirakian R, Pisi E, Bottazzo GF (1984) Aberrant expression of HLA-DR antigens on bile duct epithelium in primary biliary cirrhosis: relevance to pathogenesis. Lancet I:1009
10. Barbatis C, Woods J, Morton JA, Fleming KA, Mc Michael A, Mc Gee JOD (1981) Immunohistochemical analysis of HLA (A, B, C) antigens in liver disease using a monoclonal antibody. Gut 22:985–991
11. Innes GK, Nagafuchi Y, Fuller BJ, Hobbs KEF (1988) Increased expression of major histocompatibility antigens in the liver as a result of cholestasis. Transplantation 45:749–752
12. Jonjic S, Radosevic Stasic B, Cuk M, Jonjic N, Rukavina D (1987) Class II antigen induction in the regenerating liver of rats after partial hepatectomy. Transplantation 44:165–168
13. Kamada N, Calne RY (1979) Orthotopic liver transplantation in the rat: technique using cuff for portal vein anastomosis and biliary drainage. Transplantation 28:47
14. Higgins GM, Anderson RM (1931) Experimental pathology of the liver. Arch Pathol 12:1986
15. Lautenschlager I, Hayry L (1981) Expression of the major histocompatibility complex antigens on different liver cellular components in rat and man. Scand J Immunol 14:421
16. Franco A, Barnaba V, Natalio, Balsano C, Musca A, Balsano F (1988) Expression of class I and class II major histocompatibility complex antigens on human hepatocytes. Hepatology 8:449–454
17. Mc Michael AJ, Ting A, Zweevink HF, Askonas BA (1977) HLA restriction of cell mediated lysis of influenza virus infected human cells. Nature 270:524
18. Howard TK, Klintmalm GBG, Cofer JB et al. (1990) The influence of preservation injury on rejection in the hepatic transplant recipient. Transplantation 45:103

Transplant Int (1992) 5 [Suppl 1]: S 631–S 635

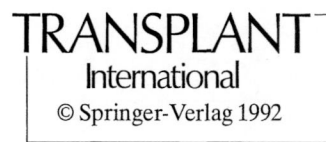

© Springer-Verlag 1992

Intraoperative cytokines production during orthotopic liver transplantation

J. Pirenne, F. Noizat-Pirenne, D. De Groote, Y. Vrindts, M. Lopez, R. Gathy, P. Damas, M. Meurisse, N. Jacquet, P. Honoré, and P. Franchimont

Departments of Surgery, Transplantation, and Anesthesiology, and Laboratory of Radioimmunology, University of Liège, CHU Sart Tilman, 4000 Liège, Belgium. Medgenix Diagnostics, 6220 Fleurus, Belgium

Abstract. In summary, we established that a significant production of the monokines interleukin-6, tumor necrosis factor apha, and interleukin-1 occurred during orthotopic liver transplantation whereas the lymphokines interferon gamma and interleukin-2 were not detected. Levels of interleukin-6 reached their maximum values before and especially at the end of the anhepatic phase. They remained high after the anhepatic phase, i. e. after reperfusion of the new livers. Tumor necrosis factor alpha and interleukin-1 reached their maximum values after the anhepatic phase. Not only were interleukin-6, tumor necrosis factor apha, and interleukin-1 present in the serum but they could also be detected in the bile produced by these new livers. Mechanisms of monokine production during orthotopic liver transplantation is multifactorial in origin and further studies will have to evaluate the relative contribution of the various factors involved. The possibility of an association between peroperative monokines and transplant outcome and their potential clinical implication will have to be elucidated.

Key words: Cytokines – Interleukin-1 beta – Interleukin-6 – Tumor necrosis factor alpha – Liver transplantation

The liver plays a pivotal role in the cytokine network; cytokines act on the liver, liver cells produce cytokines, and the liver is a major clearance organ for circulating cytokines [1]. Orthotopic liver transplantation (OLTx) is a major abdominal surgical procedure in which a diseased liver is removed and a new liver is transplanted. Operative induced tissue injury, endotoxinemia, and kupffer cell activation after liver graft reperfusion are various conditions encountered during OLTx [2, 9, 11, 14]. Since each of these conditions has been shown to stimulate cytokine synthesis, OLTx should thus be accompanied by a significant production of cytokines. Moreover, the absence of

hepatic clearance during hepatectomy and during the anhepatic phase is likely to interfere with cytokine elimination [1]. OLTx should thus impose a considerable impact on both cytokine production and metabolism.

The aims of this study were twofold. The first was to determine peroperative cytokine production during OLTx by measuring cytokines in the serum during the different phases of OLTx. The second was to assess whether cytokines could be detected in the bile produced by the new liver.

Materials and methods

Patients. This study included 7 recipients of hepatic allografts. Indications for OLTx were as follows: hepatocellular carcinoma, $n = 2$, primary graft nonfunction, $n = 2$, alcoholic cirrhosis, $n = 1$, secondary biliary cirrhosis, $n = 1$, and posthepatitic cirrhosis, $n = 1$.

OLTx. The principles of OLTx were removal of the diseased liver and placement of the graft followed by circulation reestablishment and biliary tract reconstruction. During hepatectomy and placement of the graft, a venovenous bypass was routinely used.

Collection of serum samples and bile. Serum samples of systemic venous blood were collected preoperatively in the right atrium through a swan ganz catheter immediately before the anhepatic phase (< AP), at the end of anhepatic phase (AP), after reperfusion of the transplanted liver (> AP), and at day 1 posttransplant. Bile was recovered from the transplanted liver > AP, and at day 1 posttransplant.

Cytokine immunoassays. The cytokines interleukin-1 beta (IL-1), interleukin-6 (IL-6), and tumor necrosis factor alpha (TNF) were measured in the serum and bile of all patients. Moreover, the lymphokines interleukin-2 (IL-2) and gamma interferon (IF) were measured in four patients. These cytokines were measured by using specific commercially available immunoassays from Medgenix Diagnostics (Medgenix Diagnostics, Fleurus, Belgium). The methods used, type of tracer sensitivity, precision, reproducibility, and accuracy are described in Table 1.

By performing recovery tests, we established in an earlier study that cytokines can be detected in the bile, using similar immunoassays (Cytokines measurement in the bile, manuscript in preparation).

Offprint requests to: Jacques Pirenne, M. D., M. S., CHU Sart Tilman, 4000 Liège, Belgium

Table 1. Characteristics of cytokine immunoassays

Cytokine	Type of assay	Tracer[a]	Sensitivity	Precision	Reproducibility	Accuracy	Int. Std. origin	Correspondence weight/units
IL-1	IRMA 1 step	Mab-I^{125}	4 pg/ml	3.2%	7.2%	98%	MRC:86/552	1 ng/150 IU
IL-6	IRMA 2 steps	Mab-I^{125}	5 pg/ml	5.6%	7.5%	89%	MRC:88/514	1 pg/0.25 IU
TNF	IRMA 1 step	Mab-I^{125}	5 pg/ml	6%	7%	101%	MRC:87/650	1 pg/24 mIU
IL-2	RIA sequential saturation	Mab-I^{125}	0.5 U/ml	8%	11%	82%	BRMP:ISDP 841	100 pg/1 IU
IF	IRMA 1 step	Mab-I^{125}	0.2 U/ml	3.8%	9.9%	97%	NIH:Gg 23/901/530	50 pg/1 IU

IRMA, Immunoradiometric assay. 1 step, standards or samples + tracer incubated together. 2 steps, standards or samples incubated in a first step; washing and incubation of the tracer in a second stepRIA, classical radioimmunoassay
[a] By a modification of the chloramine T method

Table 2. Preoperative values as compared with control values. Control sera were obtained from normal healthy volunteers

	Control Values	Preoperative values
IL-1 (pg/ml)	< 15 ($n = 40$)	Range: 0–3 Mean: 0.5
IL-6 (pg/ml)	0 ($n = 49$) 3–8.5 ($n = 29$) 24 ($n = 1$) 72 ($n = 1$)	Range: 0–205 Mean: 78
TNF (pg/ml)	3–20 ($n = 72$) O ($n = 8$)	Range: 7–30 Mean: 20

Results

A. Preoperative values of IL-6, TNF, and IL-1

Preoperative values of IL-6 and TNF were increased as compared with a group of 80 normal healthy volunteers (Table 2). Preoperative values of IL-1 were not increased as compared with 40 normal sera.

B. Peroperative production of monokines IL-6, TNF, and IL-1

Serum. Peroperative production of monokines IL-6, IL-1, and TNF are shown in Fig. 1 a–c. These three monokines were elevated during OLTx as compared to preoperative values. IL-6 reached its maximal value at the end of AP. IL-6, however, was already elevated before AP and continued to display high levels after AP, i. e. after reperfusion of the new liver. TNF reached its maximal values after AP, i. e. after reperfusion of the new liver. IL-1 had a production pattern similar to TNF with maximum values reached after AP, i. e. after reperfusion of the new liver. The levels reached, however, were low. The levels reached by all these three monokines had returned to preoperative values by day 1 posttransplant.

Bile. High levels of IL-6, TNF, and low levels of IL-1 were detected in the bile produced by the new livers (Fig. 2 a–c).

Except for IL-1, biliary levels of these cytokines had significantly decreased by day 1 posttransplant.

C. Perioperative production of IL-2 and IF

IL 2 and IF were not detected in serum in bile during OLTx.

Discussion

There were high serum levels of the cytokines IL-6, and TNF, and low serum levels of IL-1 during OLTx. IL-6, TNF, and IL-1 were also detected in the bile produced by the newly transplanted liver. We believe that this cytokine production was triggered by intraoperative events occurring *during* OLTx procedure as these cytokines reached their maximal value during OLTx and subsequently returned to preoperative values by day 1 posttransplant. A similar observation has already been made by Tono et al. who found a transient but significant elevation of IL-6 in the bile soon after OLTx in rats [13]. The lymphokines IL-2 and IF were detected in the serum in the bile during OLTx. This demonstrated that the cytokine production we observed reflected merely a major stimulation of monokine synthesis by monocytes/macrophages in the absence of lymphocyte activation and detectable lymphokine production at this early stage of recipient immune activation.

At present, there is evidence supporting four possible mechanisms of monokine production during OLTx. These involve the stimulation of cytokine production by (1) tissue trauma, (2) endotoxinemia, (3) lack of hepatic clearance, and (4) kuppfer cell activation. Tissue trauma induced by surgery can lead to monokine synthesis which in turn can initiate the acute phase response that is generally observed after surgical operations [11]. The significance of both monokine production and acute phase response have been shown to correlate with the significance of the surgical operation. Since OLTx is a major abdominal surgical procedure, it should trigger considerable monokine production. Endotoxinemia has been shown to

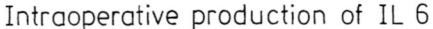
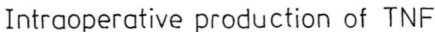
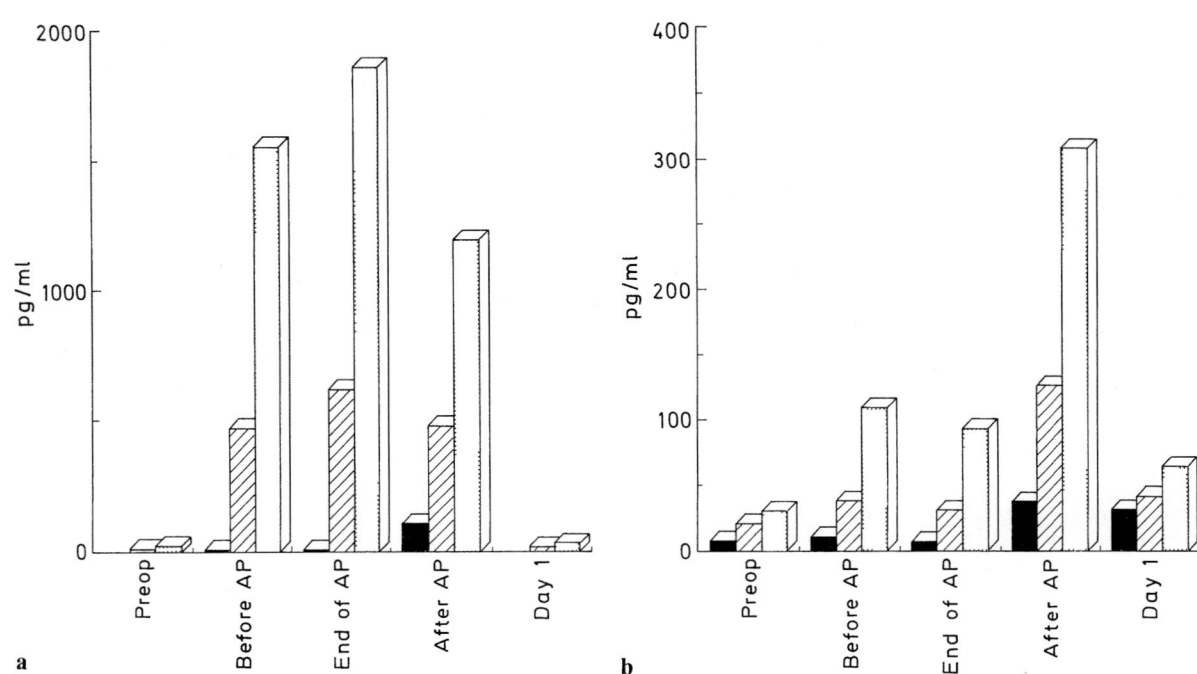

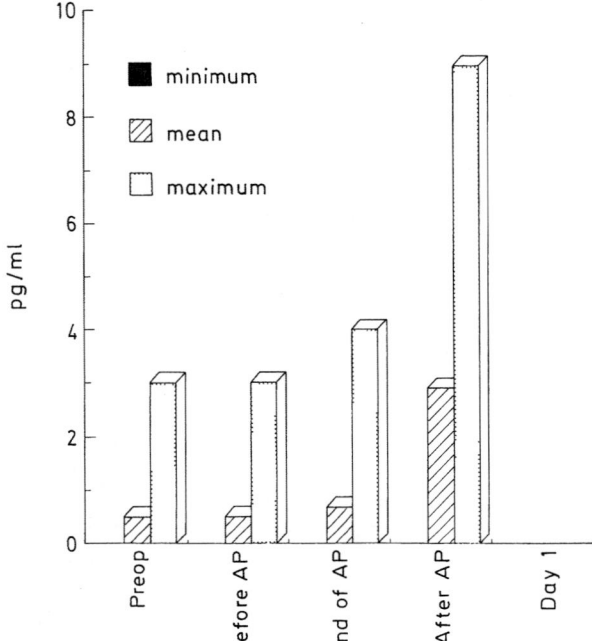

Fig. 1 a–c. Peroperative production of **a** IL-6, **b** TNF, and **c** IL-1

occur during OLTx, especially at the end of AP [9, 10, 14]. Monokines are among the various biologically active substances that are released following monocyte exposure to endotoxin. Thus, endotoxinemia would explain, at least partly, the high levels of monokines that we observed during OLTx, in particular IL-6 whose serum levels reached their maximal value at the end of AP.

A third hypothesis needs to be taken into account. The liver is the principal clearance organ of circulating cytokines [1]. Hepatic clearance is obviously absent during AP, and is already severely compromised before AP due to both surgical manipulation of the diseased recipient liver and to the presence of the venovenous bypass that we rou-

tinely use. Lack of hepatic clearance might account for impaired cytokine elimination and the increased serum levels that are observed before the new liver is functioning. Again, this would be, true mainly for IL-6 whose levels reached their maximum value before and especially at the end of AP. Reduction of hepatic clearance in patients with liver failure might also account for the observation that preoperative serum levels of IL-6 and TNF are increased when compared to normal values [1].

Maximum levels of the monokines IL-1 and particularly TNF were detected after AP, i.e. by the time the newly transplanted livers were revascularized. Interestingly, these monokines were present in the bile produced

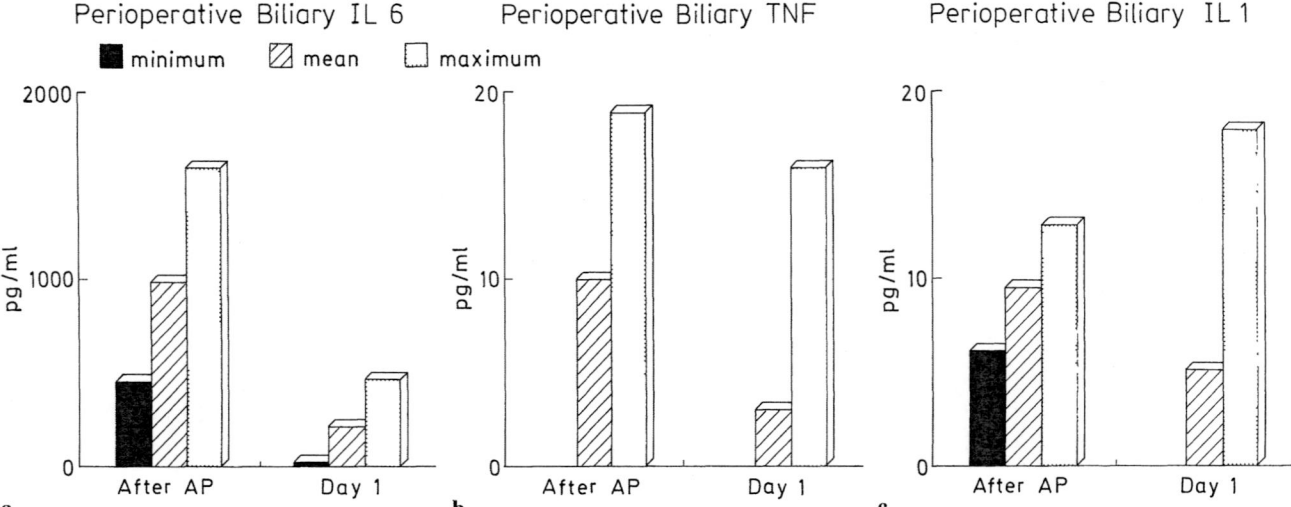

Fig. 2a–c. Peroperative biliary **a** IL-6, **b** TNF, and **c** IL-1

by the transplanted livers. Based on these two findings, it is attractive to speculate that the new livers might be a major source of monokine synthesis. This fourth hypothesis is substantiated by several published observations. Kupffer cells are biologically capable of producing large amounts of IL-1, IL-6, and TNF when activated [6]. Caldwell-Kenkel et al. have demonstrated that activation of Kupffer cells occurs after increasing periods of cold ischemic storage and reperfusion of rat livers [2]. Rao et al. have shown that reperfusion following cold preservation not only results in significant activation of Kupffer cells but also in the subsequent release of IL-1 and TNF [12]. Finally, Colletti et al. have demonstrated that TNF is released following hepatic ischemia and reperfusion in a rat model [3, 4].

Although the appearance of IL-1 was demonstrated in serum and bile, this cytokine did not reach as high levels as IL-6 and TNF. A discrepancy between the levels of TNF and IL-1 has already been shown in other pathological circumstances such as sepsis [5]. Coproduction of an IL-1 inhibitor, or presence of the soluble form of the IL-1 receptor might neutralize IL-1 and explain our inability to detect IL-1 in circumstances in which this cytokine is likely to be produced.

High levels of endotoxin at the end of AP have been shown, more than any other factor, to have more serious prognostic implications in terms of graft failure, difficulty of convalescence, and ultimate outcome [9, 10, 14]. Given the fact that endotoxin is a major stimulus for monokine release, it is possible that the effects of endotoxinemia could be mediated, at least partly, by the liberation of cytokines. The monokines IL-6, TNF, and IL-1 exert important effects on hepatocyte metabolism [1]. Increased levels of cytokines during OLTx might thus have important implications with regards to function of the new liver and particularly to the pathophysiology of liver graft dys- and non-function. Because of the positive effect of TNF on cell membrane MHC expression, and on intercellular adhesion molecule expression, these observations might also be significant in terms of graft immunogenicity and pre-

disposition to the rejection process. Interestingly, it has been shown by Howard et al. that preservation injury results in a significantly higher incidence of rejection [8]. The hypothesis that this vulnerability to rejection might be mediated through the effect of cytokines is substantiated by a recent observation that intraoperative elevation of TNF seems to precede early postoperative rejection [7]. OLTx still has a significant peroperative morbidity and mortality [14]. Problems such as coagulopathy, cardiovascular collapse, renal failure, and respiratory insufficiency are still observed. These problems have been attributed, at least partly, to endotoxin [14]. It is possible, however, that high levels of the cytokines IL-6, TNF, and IL-1 would explain better some of these peroperative and early postoperative pathophysiological changes that are currently observed in the course of OLTx and that can jeopardize or even preclude transplant success. For example, TNF has been shown to be directly involved in the development of a severe pulmonary injury following hepatic ischemia and reperfusion [3, 4]. Overall then, peroperative assessment of monokines might be a useful prognostic premonitor in predicting short and long term outcome after OLTx. In order to assess a possible correlation between peroperative monokine production and both graft and patient outcome, we are now conducting a prospective long-term analysis including a larger number of patients.

In summary, we established that a significant production of the monokines IL-6, TNF, and IL-1 occurred during OLTx whereas the lymphokines IF and IL-2 were not detected. Levels of IL-6 reached their maximum values before and especially at the end of AP. They remained high after AP. TNF and IL-1 reached their maximal values after AP, i.e. after reperfusion of the new livers. The mechanisms of monokine production during OLTx are multifactorial in nature and further studies are needed to evaluate the relative contribution of the various factors involved. The possibility of an association between peroperative monokine levels and transplant outcome and their potential clinical implication will have to be elucidated.

References

1. Andus T, Bauer J, Gerok W (1991) Effects of cytokines on the liver. Hepatology 13:364–375
2. Caldwell-Kenkel JC, Currin RT, Tanaka Y, Thurman RG, Lemasters JJ (1990) Kupffer cell activation and endothelial cell damage after storage of rat livers: effects of reperfusion. Hepatology 13:83–95
3. Colletti LM, Remick DG, Burtch GD, Kunkel SL, Strieter RM, Campbell DA (1990) Role of tumor necrosis factor-alpha in the pathophysiologic alterations after hepatic ischemia/reperfusion injury in the rat. J Clin Invest 85:1936–1943
4. Colletti LM, Burtch GD, Remick DG, Kunkel SL, Strieter RM, Guice KS, Oldham KT, Campbell DA (1990) The production of tumor necrosis factor alpha and the development of a pulmonary capillary injury following hepatic ischemia/reperfusion. Transplantation 49:268–272
5. Damas P, Reuter A, Gysen P, Demonty J, Lamy M, Franchimont P (1989) Tumor necrosis factor and interleukin-1 serum levels during severe sepsis in humans. Critical care. Medicine 17:975–978
6. Decker K (1990) Biologically active products of stimulated liver macrophages (Kupffer Cells). Eur J Biochem 192:245–261
7. Fugger R, Hamilton G, Steininger R, Mirza D, Schulz F, Muhlbacher F (1991) Intraoperative estimation of endotoxin, TNF and IL-6 in orthotopic liver transplantation and their relation to rejection and postoperative infection. Transplantation 52:302–306
8. Howard TK, Klintmalm GBG, Cofer JB, Husberg BS, Goldstein RM, Gonwa TA (1990) The Influence of preservation injury on rejection in the hepatic transplant recipient. Transplantation 49:103–107
9. Miyata T, Todo S, Imventarza O, Ueda Y, Furukawa H, Starzl TE (1989) Endogenous endotoxemia during orthotopic liver transplantation in dogs. Transplant Proc 21: 3861–3862
10. Miyata T, Todo S, Selby R, Yokoyama I, Tzakis A, Starzl TE (1989) Endotoxaemia, pulmonary complications, and thrombocytopenia in liver transplantation. Lancet I:189–191
11. Nishimoto N, Yoshizaki K, Tagoh H, Monden M, Kishimoto S, Hirano T, Kishimoto T (1989) Elevation of serum interleukin 6 prior to acute phase proteins on the inflammation by surgical operation. Clin Immunol Immunopathol 50:399–401
12. Rao PN, Liu T, Snyder JT, Platt JL, Starzl TE (1991) Reperfusion injury following cold ischemia activates rat liver Kupffer cells. Transplant Proc 23:666–669
13. Tono T, Monden M, Yoshizaki K, Valdivia LA, Nakano Y, Gotoh M, Ohzato H, Doki Y, Ogata A, Kishimoto T, Mori T (1991) Interleukin 6 levels in bile following liver transplantation. Transplant Proc 23:630–631
14. Yokoyama I, Todo S, Miyata T, Selby R, Tzakis AG, Starzl TE (1989) Endotoxemia and human liver transplantation. Transplant Proc 21:3833–3841

Transplant Int (1992) 5 [Suppl 1]: S 636–S 638

TRANSPLANT
International
© Springer-Verlag 1992

Studies on the participation of different T cell subsets in rat liver allograft rejection

Comparison of liver with heart graft

R. Sumimoto, H. Kimura, A. Yamaguchi, and N. Kamada

Department of Experimental Surgery, National Children's Medical Research Center, 3-35-31, Taishido, Setagaya-ku, Tokyo, 154 Japan

Abstract. In this study, we investigated which subsets of rat T cells (CD8 + vs. CD4 +) are involved in the rejection of liver allografts by the in vivo administration of monoclonal antibody (OX-8 or OX-38, and W3/25 MAb) into thymectomized recipient Lewis (RTI^l) rats prior to DA (RTI^a) liver transplantation. We also compared the results of allograft survival of liver and heart transplants under the same experimental conditions. In order to deplete either CD8 + T cells or CD4 + T cells from recipient animals, 0.4 ml of OX-8 (ascitic form) or a 0.8 ml cocktail of MAb W3/25 and OX-38 (0.4 ml each) was injected into thymectomized recipient rats, respectively. Untreated Lewis rats consistently rejected donor DA liver grafts between 9 and 11 days ($n = 7$, 9.8 days ± 1.1 days). In contrast, anti-CD8 MAb pretreatment extended the survival times of DA liver grafts for up to 40 days ($n = 5$, 26.8 days ± 8.4 days). Furthermore, survival of DA liver grafts was significantly prolonged in Lewis rats that had been pretreated with anti-CD4 MAb ($n = 7$, 35.6 days ± 17.9 days). Two out of seven recipient animals survived for more than 60 days. For heart transplantation, untreated Lewis rats rejected DA heart grafts between 6 and 8 days after operation ($n = 6$, 6.5 days ± 1.2 days). Anti-CD4 MAb treatment prolonged heart graft survival for more than 60 days in all cases ($n = 3$, > 60 days). However, there was virtually no effect of anti-CD8 MAb treatment on heart graft survival ($n = 4$, 7.0 days ± 0.9 days). These results suggested that when whole MHC disparity prevailed between donor and recipient, both subsets of T cells were required for the rejection of liver allografts and that class II reactive T cells predominantly mediated liver graft rejection. Furthermore, CD8 + T cells played a differential role in the rejection of rat liver and heart allograft.

Key words: Allograft rejection – CD4 + /CD8 + T cell – Rat liver graft

It has been well established that allograft rejection is primarily mediated by T cells [11]. The relative role of CD4 + T cells and CD8 + T cells in allograft rejection depends partly upon the MHC disparity between donor and recipient [14] and partly upon whether the CD8 + T cells need help from the CD4 + T cells [1] but it is not yet fully determined. Experiments using either the adoptive transfer system or in vivo administration of MAb specific for T cell subsets show that CD4 + T cells play a central and essential role in mediating the allograft rejection while CD8 + T cells do not. If CD8 + T cells do play a role in graft rejection, it is a specialized one.

Liver allografts, in particular strain combinations of inbred rats and pigs, are not rejected but induce a state of donor specific transplantation tolerance [7]. Liver also has a potent regenerative capacity, and it has been shown that liver secretes an immunosuppressive moiety, "soluble class I MHC antigen" into the blood circulation [12]. These observations differ from those of other organ grafts such as heart and kidney, and tissue grafts such as skin and islet. It is, therefore, in our interest to study the participation of each T cell subset in liver allograft rejection. We also compared the results of allograft survival in liver and heart transplants.

Materials and methods

Rats. Inbred strains of male Lewis (RTI^l) and DA (RTI^a) rats weighing 160–260 g were purchased from CLEA Ltd., Japan.

Organ transplantation. Orthotopic liver transplantation was performed as we have described in an earlier study [8]. Reconstruction of the hepatic artery was not performed. No blood transfusion was administered. Autopsy was done on all rats after death, and the livers were subjected to microscopic examination. Heterotopic heart transplantation was performed in the right neck of the recipient animal according to the modified methods originally described by Heron [4]. Grafts were inspected and palpated daily, and rejection was defined by cessation of beating of the graft and confirmed histologically in all cases.

Thymectomy. Adult thymectomy of the recipient Lewis rats was performed 2 weeks prior to heart and liver transplantation according to the standard procedures [5].

Offprint requests to: Ryo Sumimoto, M. D., 2nd Department of Surgery, School of Medicine, Hiroshima University 1-2-3, Kasumi, Minami-ku, Hiroshima, 730 Japan

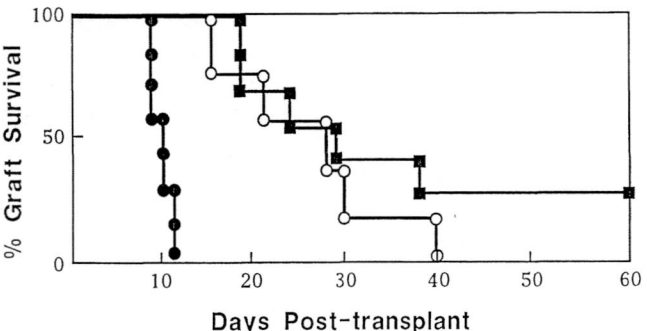

Fig. 1. Survival times of Lewis rats transplanted with DA liver grafts. Untreated Lewis rats (●), anti-CD4 MAb therapy and thymectomy (■), anti-CD8 MAb therapy and thymectomy (○)

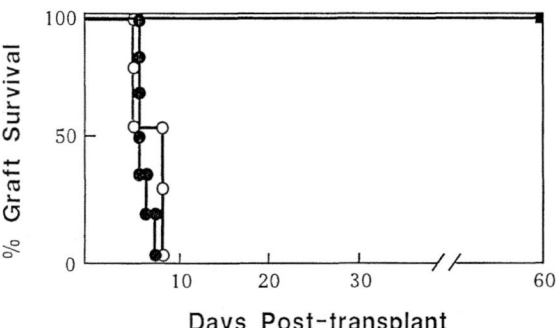

Fig. 2. Survival times of DA heart grafts in Lewis recipient rats. Untreated Lewis rats (●), anti-CD4 MAb therapy and thymectomy (■), anti-CD8 MAb therapy and thymectomy (○)

Flow cytometry (FACS) analysis. Peripheral blood obtained from the tail vein was diluted 1:3 in phosphate-buffered saline containing heparin, and the mononuclear cells were recovered from Ficoll/Hypaque gradient centrifugation. For a single color analysis, the cell suspensions were divided into two aliquots, one for staining with a saturating amount of monoclonal antibody and the other without primary antibody. After incubation on ice for 30 min, the cell suspension was washed and binding of the primary antibody was revealed by affinity-purified FITC-conjugated F(ab')2 rabbit anti-mouse Ig antibodies (heavy chain and light chain specific) purchased from Southern Biotechnology Association (Birmingham, Ala.). The latter exhibits some cross-reactivity with rat Ig, but this was minimized by passing the antibody through a Sepharose 4B (Pharmacia Fine Chemicals, Piscataway, N.J.) column cross-linked with rat IgG. For two-color analysis, phycoerythrin-tagged OX 19 (PF-OX19) and FITC-tagged OX 8 or OX-35 (FITC-OX8 or FITC-OX35) were used for direct staining. Using EPICS, 10^5 cells were analyzed.

Statistical analysis. The significance of differences in graft survival between control and treatment groups was assessed by the generalized Wilcoxon test.

Monoclonal antibodies. MAbs used in this study were W3/25, OX-35 and OX-38 for anti-CD4, and OX-8 for anti-CD8. These MAbs were generously provided to us by A. F. Williams and D. W. Mason (Oxford). PE-OX 19 (anti-CD5), FITC-OX 8 and FITC-OX 35 were obtained from Serotec (Kidlington, England).

Depletion of CD8 positive T cells and CD4 positive T cells in vivo. In order to deplete CD8 + T cells from recipient animals, 0.4 ml of OX-8 MAb (ascetic form) was dissolved in 2.0 ml saline and sterilized by passing through a membrane filter (0.45 μm pore size) and injected intravenously into thymectomized Lewis rats 3 days prior to organ transplantation. For the depletion of CD4 + T cells, 0.8 ml cocktail of MAbs W3/25 and OX-38 (0.4 ml each) was diluted 1:1 with saline

and 1.6 ml of this was injected into recipient animals 3 days before organ transplantation.

Results

Survival times of DA liver and heart graft in Lewis recipient are shown in Figs. 1 and 2. We prepared donor liver grafts from DA rats and employed Lewis rats as recipients. Major rejection of the liver graft occurred in this combination, unlike the DA into PVG (RTI^c) combination where the liver grafts are often tolerated in the allogeneic recipients without immunosuppressive reagents. Indeed, untreated Lewis rats rejected donor DA liver grafts and died consistently between 9 and 11 days. Survival of DA liver grafts was significantly prolonged in anti-CD8 MAb treated rats with simultaneous thymectomy (26.8 days ± 8.4 days) ($P < 0.001$). The administration of anti-CD4 MAb to thymectomized Lewis recipients caused marked prolongation of DA liver allografts; two out of seven animals survived for more than 60 days. This effect was significantly better than that of anti-CD8 MAb treatment ($P < 0.05$).

Untreated Lewis rats rejected DA heart grafts between 6 and 8 days after operation ($n = 6$, 6.5 days ± 1.2 days). Anti-CD4 MAb treatment prolonged heart graft survival for up to 60 days in all cases ($n = 3$). However, there was virtually no effect of anti-CD8 MAb treatment on heart graft survival ($n = 4$, 7.0 days ± 0.9 days).

FACS analysis of peripheral blood from the recipient Lewis rats treated with anti-CD8 MAb revealed profound reduction of OX 19 + and OX-8 + T cells which are believed to contain class I restricted killer T cells (15.2% ± 2.3% before treatment and 0.2% ± 0.03% at 24 h after treatment). In contrast, elimination of CD4 + T cells by anti-CD4 MAb was incomplete (58.7% ± 4.42% before treatment and 24.4% ± 5.18% at 24 h after treatment).

Discussion

In vitro studies demonstrate that the CD4 + helper T cells are class II MHC reactive T cells, the CD8 + cytotoxic T cells are class I MHC reactive T cells, and naive class I reactive CD8 + T cells cannot be activated without help from activated CD4 + T cells in most strains. These studies indicate that CD4 + T cells may play a dominant role in allograft rejection, and suppression of CD4 + cell function by anti-CD4 MAb and/or matching for class II MHC may result in effective inhibition of rejection. On the other hand, in particular strains of mice such as B6 [10] and high responder rats such as Lewis and W/F [9], CD8 + T cells can be activated and can effect rejection independent of help from CD4 + cells. In these situations, anti-CD4 MAb therapy and/or matching for class II have limited use. Thus, the relative roles of CD4 + and CD8 + T cells in mediating allograft rejection are dependent upon whether CD8 + T cells are provided help by CD4 + T cells.

In our study, heart graft rejection was completely suppressed by anti-CD4 MAb therapy. All heart grafts survived over 60 days with no evidence of rejection. This result was consistent with the results of Herbert [3] and Ilano [6], who have demonstrated that CD4 + T cells play an essential role in cardiac rejection by using in vivo administration of OX-35 and/or OX-38 to the recipient of neonatal or vascularized heart grafts. Also in agreement with the results of Herbert and Ilano, the rejection of liver allografts in our study was markedly delayed by anti-CD4 MAb therapy. Thus, anti-CD4 MAb treatment was an effective regimen for the prolongation of heart and liver allograft survival, suggesting that CD4 + T cells participate predominantly in allograft (both heart and liver) rejection. In contrast, anti-CD8 MAb therapy had no effect on heart graft survival. All heart grafts were rejected in the same time period as the control group despite complete depletion of CD8 + T cells. This was, however, in sharp contrast to the results of liver allografts. The depletion of CD8 + T cells from the recipient caused marked prolongation of the liver graft survival.

In our study, the strain combination studied used DA rats as donors and high responder Lewis rats as recipients differing at class I and class II MHC and non-MHC loci. Thus, the differences in efficacy of anti-CD8 MAb could be attributed to graft factors alone. Why CD8 + T cells played a differential role in the rejection of liver and heart allograft was not clear. One explanation could be the difference in the susceptibility of the allografts to the immune response. That is, an RTI^a heart graft in a high responder RTI^l recipient may be principally rejected through an antibody-mediated pathway rather than a cell-mediated pathway. It has been shown that the CD4 + T cell alone is sufficient to reject a graft either independently or in collaboration with other cells. It can provide help for B cells to generate alloantibody against graft antigen. This is seen especially in high responder RTI^u recipients of RTIA^a class I disparate kidney grafts. RTI^u recipients rejected class I disparate kidney grafts not by CD8 + T cytotoxic T cell but by alloantibody, and this alloantibody can be transferred to cyclosporin-treated RTI^u recipients to restore their ability to reject an RTIA^a graft in an antigen specific manner [2].

The other difference could be in the immunogenicity of the organ graft. It has been shown that liver is richer in class I MHC antigen than other organs, and that liver secretes a soluble class I antigen into the blood circulation. The serum of Lewis (RTI^l) rats that had received DA (RTI^a) livers shows a high titer of RTIA^a class I activity which includes not only soluble form (Mw: 38–40 Kd) class I antigen but an aggregated form or cell membrane fraction (Mw: > 200 Kd). The latter are believed to be the products of destruction of liver tissue by immune attack [13]. This class I activity, however, was not detected in the serum of Lewis rats of a DA heart (unpublished data). Therefore, it may well offer the hypothesis that these ma-

terials may stimulate CD8 + T cells and, subsequently, recruit them to participate in liver graft rejection.

In conclusion, survival of heart and liver allografts was significantly prolonged by the in vivo administration of anti-CD4 MAb to thymectomized recipients prior to organ transplantation. Profound and sustained elimination of CD8 + T cells by the combined therapy of MAb administration with thymectomy led to a marked prolongation of liver graft survival but did not affect the survival of heart allograft. These results suggest that CD4 + T cells played a central and essential role in liver and heart allograft rejection, and that CD8 + T cells also played an essential role in liver graft rejection, but not in heart allograft rejection. For the clinical application of monoclonal antibody, we should take into account organ specificity in selecting an effective MAb.

References

1. Engleman EG, Benike CJ, Grumet FC, Evans RL (1981) Activation of human T lymphocyte subsets: helper and suppressor/cytotoxic T cells recognize and respond to distinct histocompatibility antigens. J Immunol 127: 2124
2. Gracie JA, Bolton EM, Porteous C, Bradley JA (1990) T cell requirements for the rejection of renal allografts bearing an isolated class I MHC disparity. J Exp Med 172: 1547–1557
3. Herbert J, Roser B (1988) Strategies of monoclonal antibody therapy that induce permanent tolerance of organ transplants. Transplantation 46: 128S–134S
4. Heron I (1971) A technique for accessory cervical heart transplantation in rabbits and rats. Acta Pathol Microbiol Scand 79: 366
5. Howard JC (1972) The life-span and recirculation of marrow-derived small lymphocytes from the rat thoracic duct. J Exp Med 135: 185
6. Ilano AL, McConnel MV, Gurley KE, Spinelli A, Pearce NW, Hall B (1989) Cellular basis of allograft rejection in vivo: V. Examination of the mechanisms responsible for the differing efficacy of monoclonal antibody to CD4 + T cell subsets in low and high-responder rat strains. J Immunol 143: 2828–2836
7. Kamada N (1985) The immunology of experimental liver transplantation in the rat. Immunology 55: 369
8. Kamada N, Calne RY (1983) A surgical experience with five hundred and thirty-five transplant in the rat. Surgery 93: 64–69
9. McConnel M, Hall BM (1989) Comparison of CD4 and CD8 cell reactivity in high and low responder combinations in the rat. Transplant Proc 21: 3294–3295
10. Sprent J, Schaefer M, Lo D, Korngold R (1986) Properties of purified T cell subsets. II. In vitro responses to class I versus class II H-2 differences. J Exp Med 163: 998–1011
11. Sprent J, Webb S (1987) Function and specificity of T cell subsets in the mouse. Adv Immunol 41: 39
12. Sumimoto R, Kamada N (1990) Specific suppression of allograft rejection by soluble class I antigen and complexes with monoclonal antibody. Transplantation 50: 678–682
13. Sumimoto R, Shinomiya T (1991) Examination of serum class I antigen in liver-transplanted rats. Clin Exp Immunol 85: 114–120
14. Swain S (1983) T cell subsets and the recognition of MHC class. Immunol Rev 74: 129

Transplant Int (1992) 5 [Suppl 1]: S 639–S 644

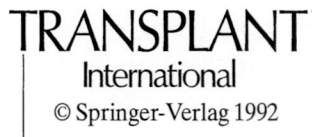

© Springer-Verlag 1992

Chronic renal allograft rejection: the significance of non-MHC alloantigens

A. Duijvestijn, L. Vlek, L. Duistermaat, H. van Rie, and P. van Breda Vriesman

Department of Immunology, University of Limburg, Maastricht, The Netherlands

Abstract. We studied the role of polymorphic endothelial antigens other than MHC in antibody-mediated chronic renal allograft rejection in two models. In the first model, donor Lewis rat kidneys were transplanted into BN recipients that had been made tolerant for donor class I antigens at the B cell (antibody) level. In this setting Lewis kidney grafts were chronically rejected with stable renal function but increasing proteinuria (> 100 mg/24 h). Rejected graft tissue showed mononuclear cell infiltration and the presence of glomerular vasculonecrotic lesions with fibrinoid material, associated with IgG and IgM deposition, but with absent or weak C3 binding. Graft endothelium showed no expression of MHC class II antigens. Serum antibodies were not reactive with donor class I antigens, but did react with endothelial non-MHC alloantigens. In the second model, more direct information on the role of endothelial non-MHC alloantigens in renal allograft rejection was obtained by transplanting Lewis 1 N kidneys into unmodified BN recipients (MHC-matched transplants). Here, similar to the first model, the animals developed severe proteinuria with stable renal function. Histopathological examination showed mononuclear cell infiltration and deposition of IgM and IgG along the glomerular vasculature, but this time in the presence of strong C3 reactivity. However, glomerular vasculonecrotic lesions with intense fibrin deposition were not observed. The data showed that although clinically the two kidney transplantation models used gave similar chronic rejection phenomena, histopathologically some striking differences were observed in the glomeruli. The precise mechanisms effecting chronic rejection of the grafts is still a puzzle. However, immune reactivity against graft (endothelial) non-MHC antigens may play a significant role.

Key words: Renal allograft – Chronic rejection – Non-MHC – Endothelial cells

Offprint requests to: Adrian M. Duijvestijn, Ph. D., Dept. of Immunology, University of Limburg, P. O. Box 616, 6200 MD Maastricht, The Netherlands

Clinically, chronic renal allograft rejection is still a problem. Despite improved HLA matching and immune suppression strategies, kidney grafts can be subjected to rejection several months or years after transplantation [1–3]. The mechanisms that are involved in chronic rejection puzzel (transplantation) scientists from various disciplines, and have led to scientific research from fields such as immunology, pharmacology, and hemostasis and thrombosis. The vascular endothelium is a major target of immune reactivity in vascular organ transplants such as the kidney. Endothelial cells express high levels of class I major histcompatibility complex (MHC) antigens [4–7], and they can be induced to express class II antigens by cytokines released in local immune reactivity [8–10]. However, in closely matched transplants, MHC antigens cannot be considered major targets in the process of rejection A contribution to rejection in such closely-matched transplants seems to be delivered by non-MHC alloantigens expressed by graft cells, and, in particular, those expressed by endothelial cells [11–13]. If graft endothelial non-MHC antigens are indeed targets in chronic rejection, one may expect various degrees of vasculonecrotic lesions, dependent not only on the type (humoral or cellular) and intensity of the immune response, but also on the type and local constitution of the blood vessels involved (e. g., arterial or venous, small or large vessels). In this study we compared two rat models of renal transplantation with clinical phenomena of chronic rejection in which major involvement of (endothelial) non-MHC alloantigens could be expected. Histopathological and serological studies were executed to determine the immunological mechanisms related to chronic rejection of non-MHC mismatched kidney grafts. In the first model Lewis kidneys were transplanted into BN recipients that had been made tolerant to Lewis erythrocytes (Lew-E). These Lew-E tolerant BN rats were unable to make an antibody response to Lewis class I antigens [14, 15]. As a result, these BN recipients chronically rejected the Lewis allografts (survival > 40 days), clinically showing increasing proteinuria, but stable renal function (serum urea levels < 200 mg/100 ml). In the second model, kidneys from

CHRONIC RENAL ALLOGRAFT REJECTION

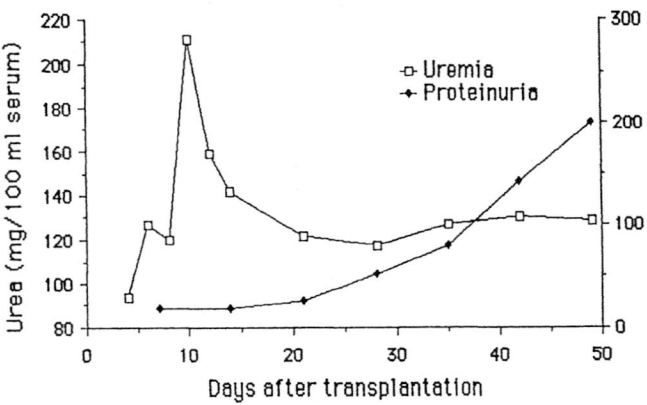

Fig. 1. Serum urea and urine protein levels in Lew-E tolerant BN recipients after grafting of Lewis kidneys (average values; $n = 7$)

Lewis IN congenic rats were transplanted into BN recipients. Here, the renal grafts that only differed from the recipient in non-MHC antigens were chronically rejected with similar clinical signs as the previous model, e.g. increasing proteinuria, stable renal function and a survival of more than 40 days. Histopathological and immunohistochemical analysis of rejected grafts, and analysis of recipient serum was carried out to study local immunological reactivity and antibody reactivity with donor endothelial cells respectively. The data showed that in both models clinical rejection of the kidney grafts was attended with histological rejection showing glomerular and interstitial lesions with mononuclear cell infiltration and antibody deposition in the renal vasculature. Serological studies demonstrated antibody reactivity with endothelial cells. Although glomerular lesions in both models were not similar, we suggest that (endothelial) non-MHC alloantigens played an important role in the development of (humoral) immune reactants against the graft, eventually leading to rejection.

Materials and methods

Experimental animals and surgery. Lewis (RT1^l) and Brown Norway (BN; RT1^n) rats were obtained from the Central Animal Facility of the University of Limburg. Only male rats were used. The animals were maintained under SPF conditions until use and had free access to food and water. Lewis IN (RT1^n) and BN.1L (RT1^l) were from the Central Institute for Laboratory Animal Breeding in Hannover, Germany. Donors and recipients of renal grafts were between 10 and 12 weeks of age. LEW erythrocyte (LEW-E) donor rats were 12–20 weeks old.

Kidneys were perfused via the abdominal aorta with 100 ml cold Collins solution, containing 2 % bovine serum albumen, using 40 cm hydrostatic pressure. The kidneys were then transplanted into bilaterally nephrectomized BN recipients using standard techniques [16].

Induction of tolerance to LEW class I MHC antigens. BN recipients were, unless indicated as unmodified, intravenously infused with high doses of Lewis erythrocytes (LEW-E) to induce B cell (antibody) tolerance to Lewis class I MHC antigens [14, 17]; 0.5–1.0 10^{10} LEW-E were infused at 6, 4 and 2 weeks before transplantation. Details of erythrocyte purification and infusion have been described previously by Majoor et al. [14]. Prior to transplantation the serum of the BN recipients was measured for LEW-E hemagglutinating anti-

bodies. Only animals in which hemagglutinating antibodies were absent were used as graft recipients.

(Immuno)histology. Animals were perfused with cold saline via the left heart ventricle. Grafts were removed and slices of the tissue were snap frozen in isopentane and stored at -70 °C until use. Another piece of graft tissue was fixed in 4 % formalin and processed for paraffin embedding. Paraffin sections (2–4 mm thick) were routinely stained with silvermethenamine and counterstained with hematoxylin and eosin (HE). Heart tissue used for serum staining was removed, snap frozen and used for frozen sections.

For immunohistochemistry, 4–6 μm thick frozen sections were cut, acetone-fixed for 10 min and air dried for at least 60 min using a fan. Sections were stained with antibodies using a 2 step immunoperoxidase technique as previously described by Duijvestijn et al. [18]. Briefly, sections were incubated with the first antibody for 60 min and were then washed in PBS. Next, the sections were incubated with the second step reagent, a horse radish peroxidase (HRP) conjugated rabbit-anti-mouse Ig or a HRP-conjugated goat-anti-rabbit Ig (DAKO, Denmark). To block cross-reactivity with rat Ig in the sections, 2 % normal rat serum was added to the conjugates. For staining of heart sections, sera diluted 1/80 were used. The second stage antibody was a HRP-conugated rabbit-anti-rat Ig (DAKO, Denmark). After washing, the sections were incubated with a di-amino-benzidine solution containing 0.02 % H$_2$O$_2$ for 10 min. Subsequently, the sections were rinsed, counter-stained (not for heart sections) with hematoxylin, dehydrated, and covered with Entallan (Merck, Germany). Immunofluorescence staining with FITC-conjugated antibodies was performed on non-fixed frozen sections. Sections were covered with 50 % glycerol in PBS and examined under epifluorescent light.

Antibodies used were W3/13 (pan T-cel marker), OX-6 (recognizes MHC class II antigens), and OX-18 (anti MHC class I antigens), donated by A. Williams (Oxford, England), EDI (monocyte/macrophage marker) donated by C. Dijkstra (Amsterdam, The Netherlands), MARM (anti IgM), and MARGI, 2a, 2b, 2c (anti IgG subsets) obtained from Sanbio (The Netherlands), anti C3 (recognizes complement component 3) donated by M. Daha (Leiden, The Netherlands) and RECA-1 (anti-endothelial cell antigen) from our laboratory.

Results

Clinical parameters in chronic renal allograft rejection

In both rat models used to study rejection mechanisms, and in particular the involvement of non-MHC alloantigens, recipient protein and urea levels in urine and serum were measured after kidney transplantation. When Lewis kidneys were transplanted in Lew-E tolerant recipients ($n = 7$), a transient rejection crisis was frequently observed around day 10, as measured by increasing serum urea levels. No proteinuria was measured at that time. However, from week 3 on, while urea levels remained stable, a slowly increasing proteinuria occurred in all animals, reaching avarage levels of more than 200 mg/24 h around day 50 (Fig. 1). Recipients suffering from proteinuria had severe weight loss, were in a poor clinical condition and were sacrificed between 6 and 12 weeks after transplantation. By this time they had developed severe proteinuria. The pattern of clinical data of Lewis 1N renal grafts rejected in unmodified BN recipients ($n = 4$) was similar. Proteinuria developed later, around week 5 or 6, but also reached levels of more than 200 mg/24 h and led to severe weight loss. Although in the 1st days after transplantation serum urea

Table 1. (Immuno)histology of chronic kidney rejection

	Antibody	Kidney graft of Lewis → Lew-E tolerant BN	Kidney graft of Lewis 1N → BN
Mononuclear cell in intration/margination	na (HE)	+	+
T cells	W3/13	+	+
Monocytes/macrophages	ED-1	+	+
Class I expression	OX-18	diffuse	diffuse
Class II expression in tubules	OX-6	some tubules	some tubules
Class II expression on endothelium	OX-6	–	–
Glomerular vasculonecrotic lesions with fibrin deposition	na (HE)	+	–
IgM deposition	MARM	glomerular capillaries (sometimes mesangial)	glomerular capillaries
IgG deposition	MARG (1, 2a, 2b, 2c)	entire renal vasculature	entire renal vasculature
C3	anti C3	– (–/+) in glomeruli	+ in glomeruli

na, not applicable
HE, hematoxylin/eosin staining

levels in some animals were rather high, levels stabilized after the 1st week, seldomly exceeding 200 mg/100 ml. In contrast to the first model, a transient rejection episode with increasing urea levels around day 10 was not observed.

Histopathology and immunohistochemistry (Table 1)

Similarities between the two models of chronic renal allograft rejection. Renal allografts were studied in a late stage of chronic rejection (about 7 to 10 weeks after transplantation), when the recipients had severe proteinuria, but stable renal function. In both models of chronic rejection, interstitial mononuclear infiltrates and marginating mononuclear leukocytes in glomeruli and peritubular capillaries were observed. Infiltrating and marginating cells consisted predominantly of monocytes/macrophages (ED-1 positive) and T cells (W3/13 positive). In the interstitial infiltrates B cells and plasma cells (IgM or IgG positive) were also present, whereas neutrophils were only occasionally observed. Class II expression (OX-6) was seen on marginating leukocytes present in glomerular and peritubular capillaries, and in interstitial infiltrates. In addition, the epithelial cells of some tubules, especially those in the vicinity of interstitial infiltrates expressed class II MHC antigens. No class II expression was seen on vascular endothelium of peritubular and glomerular capillaries or other renal blood vessels. Immunostaining for IgM and

IgG (subclasses 1, 2a, 2b, 2c) in chronically rejected renal grafts showed, in addition to stained B and plasma cells, selective deposition along the renal vasculature. All IgG subclasses were present in the renal vessels, including glomerular and peritubular capillaries. Figure 2 A shows a staining pattern representative of all IgG subclasses of Lewis kidneys rejected by Lew-E tolerant BN recipients. A similar staining pattern was obtained for Lewis 1N kidneys rejected by unmodified BN recipients. In both models of chronic renal allograft rejection IgM deposition was detected selectively in the glomerular vasculature and sometimes in a few large blood vessels; no IgM was detected in the peritubular capillaries. Control syngeneic transplantations showed no graft pathology.

Discrepancies between the two models of chronic renal allograft rejection. A striking difference between the two models was the type of glomerular lesions in the individual models. Undoubtedly the glomerular lesions were related to the proteinuria developed by the recipients. In the Lewis renal grafts rejected by Lew-E modified BN recipients, the glomeruli were irregular in morphology, were frequently large with swollen endothelium and showed vasculonecrotic lesions with eosinophilic fibrinoid material deposited in variable intensities (Fig. 2 B). In the Lewis 1N renal grafts no such glomerular vasculonecrotic lesion with fibrinoid necrosis was observed, although swollen glomerular endothelium and mononuclear leukocytes were seen in most glomeruli (Fig. 3 A). Complement C3 deposition was studied in the rejected kidneys, and absent or only weak C3 staining was observed in the glomeruli of Lewis grafts in Lew-E tolerant BN recipients, whereas strong granular C3 staining was observed along the glomerular capillaries of Lewis 1N grafts in unmodified BN recipients (Fig. 3 B).

Reactivity of serum antibodies with non-MHC endothelial cell antigens

Serum was collected from renal allograft recipients in a late stage of chronic rejection when the animals had severe proteinuria, but stable renal function. Immunostaining with sera diluted 1/80 from BN recipients of both chronic rejection models clearly showed reactivity with Lewis heart endothelial cells, but not with heart muscle cells. No reactivity was seen with BN endothelial cells. Serum staining patterns in Lewis hearts were similar to immunostaining with RECA-1, a monoclonal antibody specific for rat endothelial cells [19]. Due to background problems, and perhaps endothelial low density antigen expression, kidney sections could not be used for the detection of anti-endothelial cell reactivity of serum antibodies. Because recipients of Lewis renal transplants were antibody-tolerant for Lew-E and therefore also for class I, serum reactivity with heart endothelial cells, which did not express class II antigens, was most likely directed against endothelial non-MHC antigens. Also the serum antibodies from BN recipients of Lewis 1N kidneys must have been directed against endothelial non-MHC antigens, because both graft and recipient were MHC haplotype-

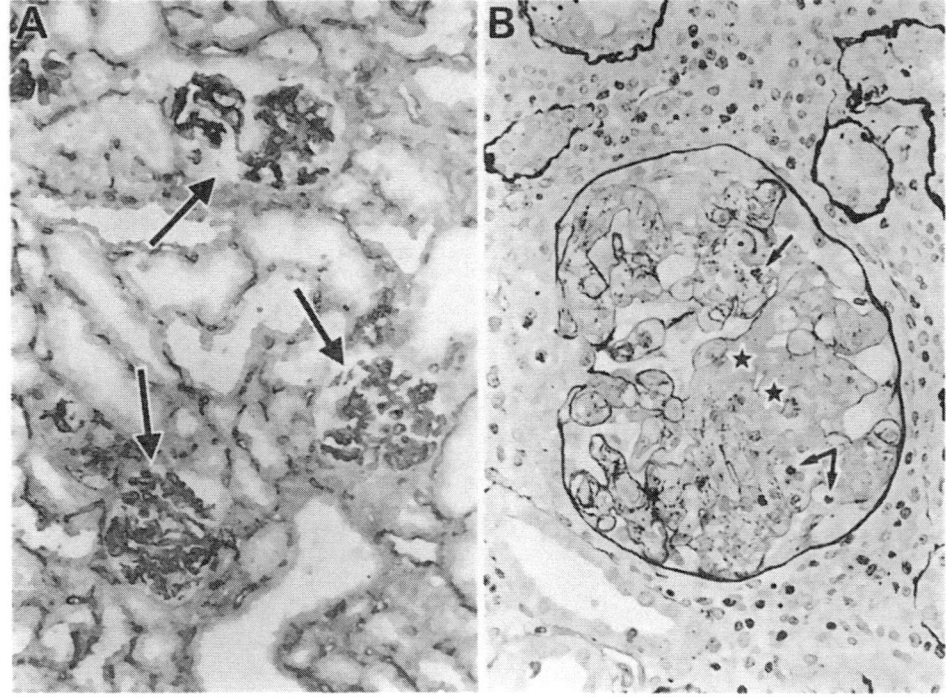

Fig. 2 A, B. Chronically rejected Lewis kidney in Lew-E tolerant BN recipient. **A** Immunoperoxidase staining for deposited IgG2c with antibody MARG2c. Note deposition along glomerular *(arrows)* and peritubular capillaries. × 200.
B HE/silver staining shows glomeruli with vasculonecrotic lesions with fibrin deposition *(asterisks)*. Note marginated mononuclear leukocytes in the glomerulus *(arrows)*, and the presence of interstitial infiltrate. × 500

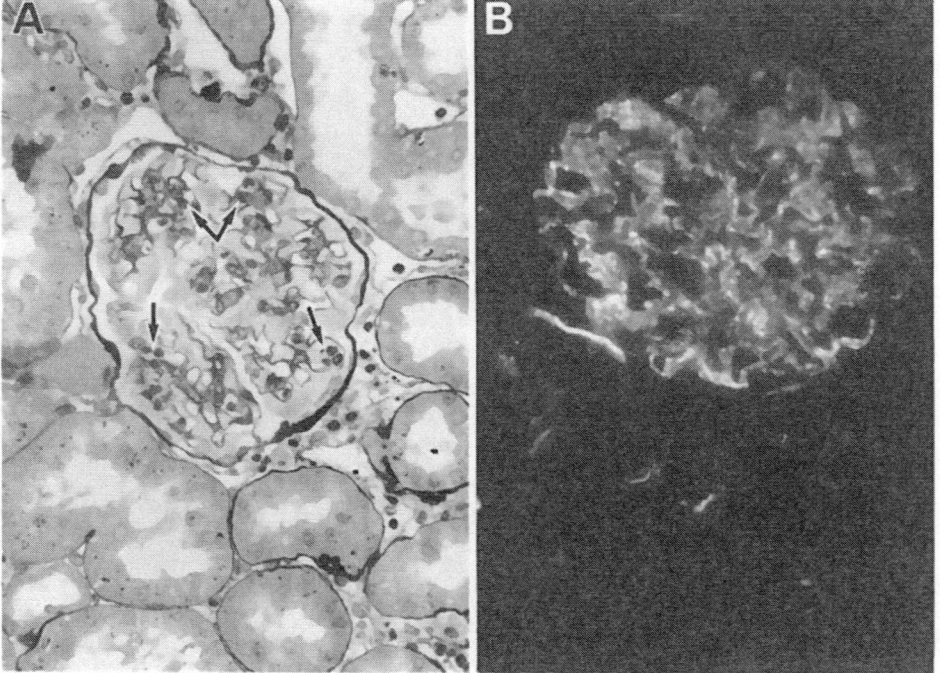

Fig. 3 A, B. Chronically rejected Lewis 1N kidney in unmodified BN recipient. **A** HE/silver staining shows absence of vasculonecrotic lesions with fibrin deposition in the glomeruli. Note glomerular mononuclear cell margination *(arrows)* and the presence of interstitial infiltrate. × 500.
B Fluorescent staining using anti-C3 antibodies shows deposited C3 in glomeruli. Note the granular staining along the glomerular capillaries. × 500

matched. Because staining for class I in heart sections also gave a staining pattern similar to RECA-1 (data not shown) the sera were tested on heart sections from Lewis 1N (carrying the BN MHC type) and BN 1L (carrying the Lewis MHC type) congenic strains, to ascertain that reactivity was with endothelial non-MHC antigens and not with MHC antigens. Sera from recipients in both transplantation models did not react with BN.1L endothelial cells (which excludes reactivity with Lewis MHC class I antigens), but did react with Lewis 1N endothelial cells, demonstrating that reactivity was indeed with non-MHC

antigens on endothelial cells (Table 2). Control BN sera, or sera from control transplantations showed no reactivity with heart endothelial cells.

Discussion

We studied two models of chronic renal allograft rejection in the rat. Keeping in mind that, (1) endothelial cells in vascularized allografts can be considered a first and major target in rejection, and that, (2) endothelial cells are po-

Table 2. Reactivity of recipient serum antibodies in chronic rejection

Recipient	Graft	No. of transplantations tested	Serum staining[b] with heart endothelium of:			
			Lewis[c]	BN[d]	Lewis 1N[e]	BN.1L[f]
Lew-E tolerant BN	Lewis kidney	5	+	−	+	−
Unmodified BN	Lewis 1N	3	+[a]	−	+[a]	−

[a] One recipient, which was sacrificed 24 days after transplantation showed only weak staining of endothelium

[b] Frozen heart sections were stained with 1/80 diluted recipient serum using the immunoperoxidase technique

[c] MHC RT1[l], [d] MHC RT1[n], [e] MHC RT1[n], [f] MHC RT1[l]

tent responders to various cytokines released in local immune reactivity, we emphasized the role of vascular endothelial cells in this study. Since in mismatched grafts the MHC disparity leads to acute rejection, our models of chronic rejection were based on a partial MHC-tolerance of the recipient, or on non-MHC mismatch only. In the first model, the BN recipient had been made antibody (B cell) tolerant to donor erythrocytes, and therefore to donor class I antigens (rat erythrocytes are class I positive), leading to chronic renal graft rejection. Apparently, antibodies to graft class I antigens, which are highly expressed by endothelial cells, play a significant role in acute rejection. We observed intense interstitial mononuclear (monocytic and lymphocytic) cell infiltration and margination in peritubular and glomerular capillaries. Apparently, high cellular reactivity in these grafts is involved in the rejection process. We have suggested in a previous study, based on the lymphocyte profile and the moderate tubular damage, that this local immune reactivity is involved in regulatory (e.g. B cell help) rather than cytotoxic activity [20]. Because in the present study chronic rejection was clinically manifested by proteinuria in the presence of good renal functioning, we suspected glomerular lesions of playing a major role in the rejection process. The glomerular vasculonecrotic lesions that we observed with intravascular coagulation and deposition of IgM and the various IgG subclasses suggested that the lesions are most likely brought about by an antibody mediated mechanism. The fact that none or only weak C3 deposition in the glomeruli was detected suggested that glomerular thrombotic mechanisms leading to occlusion and glomerular lesions, may be due to glomerular endothelial cell activation (possibly with induced procoagulant activity) rather than antibody-mediated endothelial disruption. Also, other studies refer to the presence of noncytotoxic anti-endothelial cell antibodies in chronic rejection [12]. The vasculonecrotic lesion occurred selectively in the glomeruli and not in the renal blood vessels, for example the peritubular capillaries, where IgG was also found to be deposited along the vessel wall. This suggested that in the glomeruli it may be the combination of IgM and IgG deposition, probably supported by effects of locally released cytokines, that triggered the (endothelial) thrombotic mechanisms [20, 21]. With respect to the reactivity of the deposited immunoglobulins, our date showed

that they were not directed to graft endothelial MHC class II antigens, which were not expressed on the renal endothelium, nor to class I antigens because the recipient was antibody tolerant to graft class I antigens. The reactivity of the recipient sera with Lewis 1N but not BN.1L heart endothelial cells demonstrated that the serum antibodies, and thus most likely also antibodies deposited in the graft, reacted with graft endothelial non-MHC antigens. The data from our second model of chronic renal allograft rejection (Lewis 1N → unmodified BN) showed a similar clinical condition, and also similar immune reactivity in the graft, demonstrated by cellular infiltration and vascular IgM and IgG deposition, as the first model. However, major differences were found in the glomeruli. Glomerular vasculonecrotic lesions with intense fibrin deposition were absent, and strong glomerular C3 deposition was observed. This suggested that although the clinical data of chronic rejection were similar in the two models, the actual mechanism leading to glomerular protein leakage may have been different. Most likely, the C3 deposition was related to direct vascular damage and loss of the integrity of the glomerular filtration unit (viz. the layer of endothelial cells, glomerular basal membrane, and epithelial cells). Serum antibody reactivity with endothelial cell non-MHC antigens was also demonstrated in this model. The selective deposition of IgM in the glomeruli and not in other renal vessels in both models may indicate that we were dealing with locally formed or preformed and trapped immune complexes. To understand further the mechanism(s) responsible for the development of proteinuria during rejection, precise information on the localization of glomerular immunoglobulins and/or immunoglobulin-antigen complexes is essential, and, therefore, currently under investigation in our laboratory. In agreement with other authors [22–25], we concluded that, although different mechanisms may effect proteinuria in chronic kidney rejection, in this study non-MHC alloantigens on vascular endothelial cells played a significant role in chronic rejection of MHC-matched or partly (class II) mismatched renal allografts.

Acknowledgement. We thank Francine Teng-Vangrootloon for excellent secretarial support.

References

1. van Rood JJ (1987) Prospective HLA typing is helpful in cadaveric renal transplantation. Transplant Proc 19: 139

2. Gilks WR, Bradley BA, Gore SM, Klouda PT (1987) Substantial benefits of tissue matching in renal transplantation. Transplantation 43: 669

3. Opelz G (1985) Correlation of HLA matching with kidney graft survival in patients with or without cyclosporin treatment. Transplantation 40: 240

4. Paul LC, Baldwin III WM, van Es LA (1985) Vascular endothelial alloantigens in renal transplantation. Transplantation 40: 117

5. Häyry P, von Willebrand E, Anderson LC (1980) Expression of HLA-ABC and DR locus antigens on human kidney, endothelial, tubular and glomerular cells. Scand J Immunol 11: 303

6. Baldwin WM III, Claas FHJ, van Rood JJ, van Es LA (1984) Antigenic composition of human renal vascular endothelium assessed by kidney perfusion. Tissue Antigens 23: 256

7. Williams KA, Hart DNJ, Fabre JW, Morris PJ (1980) Distribution and quantitation of HLA-ABC and DR (Ia) antigens on human kidney and other tissues. Transplantation 29: 274
8. Colson YL, Markus BH, Zeevi A, Duquesnoy RJ (1988) Interactions between endothelial cells and alloreactive T cells involved in allograft immunity. Transplant Proc 20: 273
9. Pober JS, Collins T, Gimbrone MA Jr, Libby P, Reiss CS (1986) Inducible expression of class II major histocompatibility complex antigens and the immunogenicity of vascular endothelium. Transplantation 41: 141
10. Pober JS, Gimbrone MA JR, Cotran RS et al (1983) Ia expression by vascular endothelium is inducible by activated T cells and by human gamma-interferon. J Exp Med 157: 1339
11. Blankert JJ, Muizert Y, van Es LA, Paul LC (1987) Immunogenicity of the non-MHC-encoded endothelial antigen EAG-1 in various tissues in the rat. Transplantation 43: 736
12. Joyce S, Flye MW, Mohanakumar T (1988) Characterization of kidney cell-specific, non-major histocompatibility complex alloantigen using antibodies eluted from rejected human renal allografts. Transplantation 46: 362
13. Gilks WR, Gore SM, Bradley BA (1990) Renal transplantation rejection. Transplantation 50: 141
14. Majoor GD, van de Gaar MJWH, Vlek LFM, van Breda Vriesman PJC (1981) The role of antibody in rat renal allograft rejection. Transplantation 31: 369
15. Majoor GD, van Breda Vriesman PJC (1986) Requirement for both MHC and non-MHC antigens residing on the same erythrocyte for donor erythrocyte-mediated prolongation of rat renal allograft survival. Transplantation 41: 92
16. van Schilfgaarde R, Hermans P, Terpstra JL, van Breda Vriesman PJC (1980) Role of passenger lymphocytes in the rejection of renal and cardiac allografts in the rat. Transplantation 29: 209
17. Majoor GD, van de Gaar MJWH, van Breda Vriesman PJC, Günther E (1981) Rat erythrocytes elicit antibody formation against RT1.A region-determined antigens in allogeneic recipients. Immunology 43: 467
18. Duijvestijn AM, Kerkhove M, Bargatze RF, Butcher EC (1987) Lymphoid tissue- and inflammation-specific endothelial cell differentiation defined by monoclonal antibodies. J Immunol 138: 713
19. Duijvestijn AM, van Goor H, Klatter F, Majoor GD, van Bussel E, van Breda Vriesman PJC (in press) RECA-1, a pan endothelial cell-specific monoclonal antibody. Lab Invest
20. van Breda Vriesman PJC, Vlek LFM, Duistermaat L, Duijvestijn AM (1990) Endothelial target cell dependent, differing patterns of chronic vascular renal allograft rejection in the rat. Transplant Proc 22: 2519
21. Duijvestijn AM, van Breda Vriesman PJC (1991) Chronic renal allograft rejection: selective involvement of the glomerular endothelium in humoral immune reactivity and intravascular coagulation. Transplantation 52: 195
22. Paul LC, van Es LA, Fleuren G (1979) Demonstration of transplantation antigens on the endothelium of peritubular capillaries in renal allografts by the immunoperoxidase method. Transplantation 28: 72
23. Cerilli J, Brasile L, Galouzis T, DeFrancis ME (1981) Clinical significance of antimonocyt antibody in kidney transplant recipients. Transplantation 32: 495
24. Paul LC, Busch GJ, Paradysz JM, Carpenter CB (1983) Definition, genetics and possible significance of a newly defined endothelial antigen in the rat. Transplantation 36: 533
25. Cerilli J, Brasile L, Clarke J, Galouzis J (1985) The vascular endothelial cell-specific antigen system: three years experience in monocyte crossmatching. Transplant Proc 17: 567

Transplant Int (1992) 5 [Suppl 1]: S645–S647

TRANSPLANT
International
© Springer-Verlag 1992

Lysis of heart endothelial cells from donor origin by cardiac graft infiltrating cells

N. H. P. M. Jutte[1], M. H. van Batenburg[1], C. R. Daane[1], P. Heijse[1], L. M. B. Vaessen[1], A. H. H. M. Balk[2], B. Mochtar[2], F. H. J. Claas[3] and W. Weimar[1]

[1] Departments of Internal Medicine I and [2] Thorax Center, Erasmus University Rotterdam/Academic Hospital Rotterdam, Dijkzigt, Rotterdam and [3] Immunohaematology and Bloodbank, Academic Hospital Leiden, Leiden, The Netherlands

Abstract. Endothelial cells may be involved in the acute rejection of allografts. In the present study, graft infiltrating lymphoid cell lines were propagated from a heart graft at the time of histological diagnosis of rejection. The cell lines containing CD8+ cells lysed donor-derived BLCL and endothelial cells (EC) but not third party BLCL or random EC, suggesting that HLA antigens were recognized. The cell lines containing CD4+ cells only did not lyse any target cells. The lysis of EC without preincubation with gamma interferon (gIFN) indicated that the HLA antigens recognized were class I antigens. These results suggested that lysis of donor EC may be one of the mechanisms involved in rejection.

Key words: Endothelial cells – Graft infiltrating cells – Allograft – Acute rejection – Cell mediated lysis – HLA antigens

Apart from HLA antigens, human endothelial cells (EC) bear antigens specific for the EC-monocyte system [10]. It has been suggested that antigens unique for EC, which are not assessed by screening using monocytes, can give rise to antibodies that cause renal [2] or cardiac [1, 3] allograft rejection. In addition, it has been shown for canine EC [5, 6] and for human fetal EC [4, 11] that these cells can be targets for cell mediated lysis in vitro. Both HLA antigens and EC specific antigens may play a role in the mechanism of EC destruction.

In previous studies we have shown that heart graft infiltrating cells (GIC) can specifically lyse cells of donor origin [9]. In these experiments we used T cell lymphoblasts or EBV transformed B cell lines (BLCL) carrying donor antigens as targets. However, in vivo, the cells that are initially encountered by the immune competent cells from the recipient blood are donor EC. Therefore, the

reactivity against EC and in particular donor-EC-specific reactions might be relevant for the study of the process of rejection.

We succeeded n isolating EC from a redundant piece of donor heart. We used these cells to investigate their role in cellular rejection. In the present study we described the lytic capacity of cells infiltrating the donor heart at the time of diagnosis of rejection against EC from this heart. The reactivity was compared with the lysis of other target cells by these GIC.

Materials and methods

Patient. A male patient (HLA type: A2, A11, B15 (62), B35, DR4) received a heart graft (HLA type: A1, A19 (29), B8, B12 (44), DR3, DRw52) at 46 years of age. After prophylactic immunosuppression with OKT3 for 6 days his maintenance therapy was cyclosporin A and low dose steroids. At 36 days posttransplant an endomyocardial biopsy (EMB) showed myocytolysis and the patient was treated for rejection. A concurrently taken EMB was cultured in RPMI 1640 Dutch Modification containing 10% human serum, 10% lymphocult (Biotest) and 0.5% phytohaemagglutinin in the presence of a feeder cell mixture of 10^4 random peripheral blood cells and 10^3 third party BLCL in round bottom 96 well plates. Cells growing from the EMB for 6–7 and 8–9 days after the start of the culture were harvested and plated in 96 well plates. After 49 days of culture the wells were screened for phenotype and cytotoxicity and 8 wells were propagated further and tested for cytotoxicity against EC.

Isolation of EC. EC were isolated from a piece of donor heart trimmed during surgery, and from a random piece of blood vessel left after bypass surgery, according to the method described by Klein-Soyer and Cazenave [8]. In short, the vessel was opened lengthwise with a scissors. The EC sides of the tissues were rinsed with phosphate buffered saline containing calcium and magnesium and were scraped with a scalpel blade. The scalpel was rinsed in culture medium (RPMI 1640:M199 1:1 containing 12.5 mM Hepes and 30% inactivated human serum). The cell suspension was plated in Primaria dishes (Falcon). The medium was changed twice a week and 100 U/ml recombinant gamma interferon (gIFN) (Genzyme, Boston, Mass.) was added 3 days before use of the EC, unless stated otherwise.

The phenotype of the GIC, BLCL or EC was determined according to standard methods [9] on the FACScan using conjugated monoclonal antibodies leu 4 (CD3), leu 2 (CD8), and leu 3 (CD4) (Becton Dickinson) for the GIC and B1.1G6 (anti β2 microglobulin)

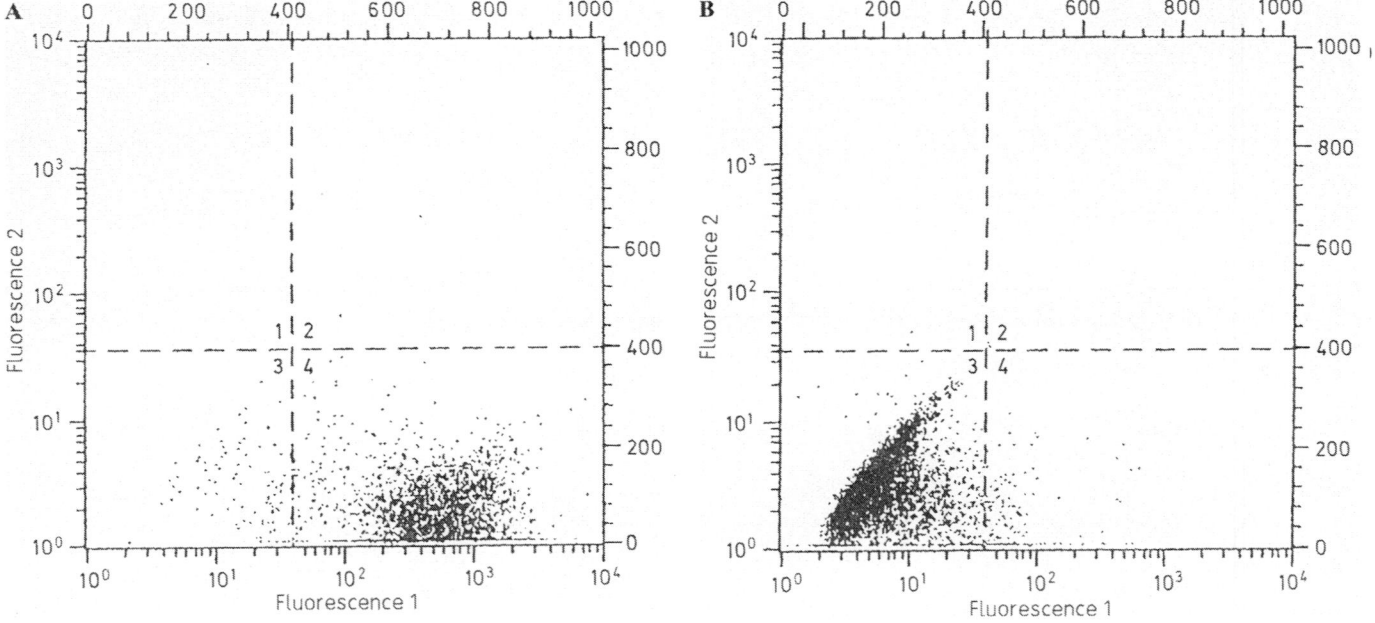

Fig. 1. A Cultured donor heart derived EC or **B** random fibroblasts stained with FITC conjugated Ulex Europaeus lectin after trypsinization

plus goat-anti-mouse FITC and anti-HLA DR-FITC for HLA class I and class II antigen measurements respectively. FITC-labeled Ulex Europaeus lectin was used as a marker for EC [7] (Fig. 1). FITC labeled factor VIII was used to stain EC on cytospots.

The cytotoxicity of the GIC was measured by a 4 h ^{51}Cr release test according to standard methods. Target EC were detached by trypsin EDTA (0.05 %/0.02 %) in PBS without calcium and magnesium and used in the cell suspension.

Results and discussion

After culture in plain medium, EC carried HLA class I antigens but not HLA class II antigens. The addition of gIFN to the cultures induced the expression of HLA class II antigens and slightly increased the expression of HLA class I antigens as measured by FACScan analysis (Table 1). This increase was time dependent and reached maximal values not later than 3 days after the addition of 50 U gIFN/ml. After culture in the presence of gIFN the intensity of expression of HLA antigens on EC was comparable to that on BLCL (Table 1).

T cell lines derived from the heart at the time of diagnosis of rejection and consisting of more than 90 % CD8$^+$ cells,

lysed both donor BLCL and donor EC (Table 2). Third party BLCL and a random EC line were not lysed. This differential pattern of lysis, in addition to the observation that in a previous test these cell lines did not lyse K562, suggested that HLA antigens present both on BLCL and EC were recognized. The lysis of EC cultured without gIFN, which were shown not to express HLA class II antigens, indicated that the HLA antigens recognized are class I antigens. CD4$^+$ cell lines did not lyse any target cells. The specificity of the reaction will have to be confirmed by blocking studies. We must not exclude the possibility that EC specific antigens as well as HLA antigens are recognized by GIC. We obtained comparable results for three EMB from two other heart transplant recipients i. e. cells cultured from the EMB could lyse both donor derived B cells and donor derived heart EC (results not shown).

It has been shown previously that EC can be targets for cell mediated lysis by peripheral blood cells after an activation phase in vitro [4–6]. The present study showed that

Table 1. Expression of HLA class I and class II antigens on EC in comparison with BLCL

	Class I		Class II	
	positive cells (%)	median fluorescence	positive cells (%)	median fluorescence
BLCL				
Donor	91	586	91	661
3rd party	98	555	98	712
EC				
Donor − IFN	80	445	0	0
Donor + IFN^a	90	622	72	500
Random − IFN	80	492	0	0
Random + IFN^a	87	636	82	549

^{a} 100 U/ml gIFN was present for 3 days of culture

Table 2. Cell mediated lysis of donor derived BLCL and EC by GIC propagated from an EMB taken at the time of diagnosis of acute rejection

	Specific lysis (%)^a							
Phenotype	> 90 % CD8$^+$ cells					mix	100 % CD4$^+$	
Cell line	1	2	3	4	5	6	7	8
BLCL								
Donor	100	96	76	88	58	87	1	0
3rd party	0	2	5	3	1	2	0	2
EC								
Donor − gIFN	47	42	7^c	30	21	43	9	2
Donor + gIFN^b	61	52	34	73	68	100	0	5
Random − gIFN	4	9	6	0	5	0	0	2
Random + gIFN^b	4	2	2	4	0	1	3	3

^{a} Effector target ratio 20:1
^{b} 100 U/ml gIFN was present for 3 days of culture
^{c} Ratio 40:1 19 % specific lysis

allograft infiltrating cells activated in vivo can lyse the EC from the specific allograft donor, indicating a role for lysis of EC in the process of rejection.

Acknowledgement. This work was supported by grant 87-049 of the Dutch Heart Foundation.

References

1. Brasile L, Zerbe T, Rabin B, Clarke J, Abrams A, Cerilli J (1985) Identification of the antibody to vascular endothelial cells in patients undergoing cardiac transplantation. Transplantation 40: 672–675
2. Cerilli J, Clarke J, Doolin T, Cerilli G, Brasile L (1988) The significance of a donor-specific vessel crossmatch in renal transplantation. Transplantation 46: 359–361
3. Cerilli J, Brasile L, Clarke J, Zorbee T, Griffen M, Rabin B (1988) Vascular endothelial cell-specific antibody in the pathogenesis of early cardiac allograft rejection. Transplant Proc 20: 775–777
4. Clayberger C, Uyehara T, Hardy B, Eaton J, Karasek M, Krensky AM (1985) Target specificity and cell surface structures involved in the human cytolytic T lymphocyte response to endothelial cells. J Immunol 135: 12–18
5. Groenewegen G, Buurman WA, van der Linden CJ, Jeunhomme GMAA, Kootstra G (1983) Cellular cytotoxicity against canine endothelial cells analysis of determinants recognized by CTL. Tissue Antigens 21: 114–128
6. Groenewegen G, Buurman WA, van der Linden CJ, Jeunhomme GMAA, Kootstra G (1985) Cell mediated cytotoxicity patterns of cloned cytotoxic T lymphocytes. Cytotoxicity directed against lymphoblasts, monocytes and endothelial cells. Transplantation 39: 657–660
7. Holthöfer H, Virtanen I, Kariniemi AL, Hormia M, Linder E, Miettinen A (1982) Ulex Europaeus I lectin as a marker for vascular endothelium in human tissues. Lab Invest 47: 60–66
8. Klein-Soyer C, Cazenave JP (1986) Culture de cellules endothéliales vasculaires humaines. In: Sultan Y, Fischer AM (eds) Progrès en hématologie. Doin editeurs, Paris, pp 83–93
9. Ouwehand AJ, Vaessen LMB, Baan CC, Jutte NHPM, Balk AHMM, Essed CE, Bos E, Claas FHJ, Weimar W (1991) Alloreactive lymphoid infiltrates in human heart transplants. Loss of class II-directed cytotoxicity more than 3 months after transplantation. Human Immunology 30: 50–59
10. Paul LC, Carpenter CB (1980) Antibodies against renal endothelial alloantigens. Transplant Proc 12 [Suppl 1]: 43–48
11. Pober JS, Collins T, Gimbrone MA, Cotran RS, Gitlin JD, Fiers W, Clayberger C, Krensky AM, Burakoff SJ, Reiss CS (1983) Lymphocytes recognize human vascular endothelial and dermal fibroblast Ia antigens induced by recombinant immune interferon. Nature 305: 726–729

Transplant Int (1992) 5 [Suppl 1]: S648–S650

TRANSPLANT
International
© Springer-Verlag 1992

Expression of human decay accelerating factor or membrane cofactor protein genes on mouse cells inhibits lysis by human complement

D. J. G. White, T. Oglesby, M. K. Liszewski, I. Tedja, D. Hourcade, M.-W. Wang, L. Wright, J. Wallwork, and J. P. Atkinson

From the Clinical School of Medicine, University of Cambridge Addenbrooke's Hospital, Hills Rd., Cambridge CB2 2QQ, and The Howard Hughes Medical Institute at Washington University, St. Louis, MO, USA

Abstract. Mouse cells expressing the human complement regulatory proteins decay accelerating factor (DAF) or membrane cofactor protein (MCP) were produced both by hybridoma technology and by transfection with the appropriate cDNAs. The expression of either or both of these products protected the mouse cell from lysis by human (though not rabbit) complement in the presence of naturally occurring human anti-mouse antibody. This effect could be abrogated by the addition of monoclonal antibody against DAF or MCP. These data suggested that the production of animals transgenic for human complement regulatory proteins should in principle be similarly protected from hyperacute xenograft rejection.

Key words: Decay accelerating factor – Membrane cofactor – Mouse cells

Vascular grafts transplanted between distantly related species are hyperacutely rejected minutes after revascularisation. Numerous investigations have demonstrated that complement is critically involved in this process [13, 14] although the precise mechanisms by which this occurs are poorly understood. Platt et al. [15] have demonstrated that pig endothelium can be activated as assessed by the release of hipuran sulphate by the fixation of C3b via the classical pathway. Forty and coworkers [5] have demonstrated that platelet thrombus formation induced by classical pathway activation of complement causes rapid failure of rabbit hearts perfused with human blood. However both he [4] and others [8, 11, 18] have also demonstrated a role for the alternate pathway of complement in hyperacute xenograft rejection. The enzymatic cleavage of C3 by the C3 convertases is a key step in complement-mediated destruction via both pathways and is regulated b a family of proteins termed the regulators of complement activation (RCA) [16]. This family includes serum proteins (factor H and C4 binding protein), receptors (CR1 and CR2), and membrane bound proteins [decay accelerating factor (DAF) and membrane cofactor protein (MCP)]. Since DAF and MCP are believed to protect autologous tissue from endogenous complement activation [12], we sought to determine whether these human proteins could protect discordant mammalian cells from human complement-mediated destruction.

Materials and methods

Human/mouse cell hybrids generated by fusion of human EBV transformed B cells with the non-secreting mouse myeloma X63–AG8.653 [9] were screened for the presence of human chromosome 1. This was performed by hybridization with oligonucleotide primers specific for human chromosome 1 following PCR amplification of DNA extracted from cell lines. Both upstream (5′-CCACAGGT-GTAACATTCTGT-3′) and downstream (5′-GAGATAGTGT-GATCTGAGGC-3′) primers were from the sequence of human antithrombin II (AT3) gene [22]. A human/mouse hybridoma, B10, (which secretes human anti-tetanus antibody, N. Hughes-Jones personal communication) retained human chromosome 1. An EBV transformed human tonsilar B cell line, T5 and a mouse/mouse hybridoma, DB3 (also produced by fusion with X63-Ag8.653; [21]) were used as negative and positive controls respectively.

Chromium release assay was performed as previously described [3]. Complement was absorbed at +4°C with mouse spleen cells (2 mls/spleen) to remove lytic naturally occurring anti-mouse antibodies. Human or pig serum was used as a source of naturally occurring antibodies and was heat inactivated at 56°C for 30 min. Monoclonal antibodies were added to labelled cells immediately prior to the start of the assay at 10 µg/ml.

Mouse fibroblasts were transfected with DAF and MCP cDNAs subcloned in the forward orientation into the EcoR1 site of the expression vector pHBapr-1-neo [6]. An additional construct, in which the MCP sequences were cloned into the expression vector in the reverse orientation, was isolated and used as a control. Cloned cDNA for DAF and MCP were obtained and characterized as previously described [1, 10]. Plasmid DNA was prepared using the pZ523 kit (5′-3′ Inc West Chester, Pa. USA). NIH 3T3 cells were transfected utilizing lipofectin (Bethesda Research Laboratories, Gaithersburg, Md. USA) and then cultured for 2 days in DME supplemented with 10% horse serum following which geneticin (Gibco Grand Island NY USA) was added to the medium at an active concentration of 0.5 mg/ml. Cells were subsequently maintained in this medium. DAF transfectants were further selected by fluorescence activated cell sorting (EPIC 75, Coulter Corp, Hialea, Fla. USA).

Offprint requests to: D. J. G. White

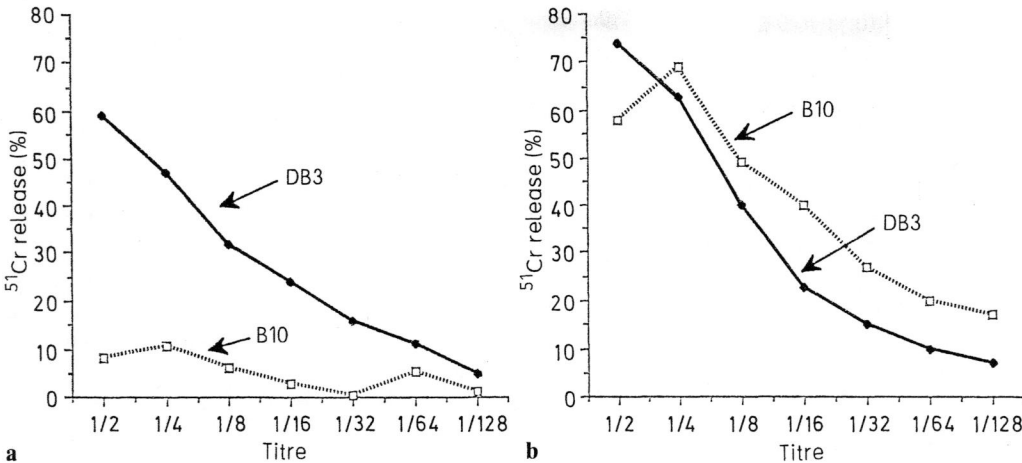

Fig. 1. Shows a comparison between the ability of **a** human and **b** rabbit complement, in the presence of "naturally occurring" human anti-mouse antibody, to lyse either a mouse/human hybrid, B10 possessing human chromosome 1 and expressing human DAF or a mouse/mouse hybrid control, DB3

Results

FACS analysis using the monoclonal antibodies 1A10 [17] and E4.3 [20] showed that the selected human/mouse hybrid, B10, expressed both human DAF and MCP as did the human tonsilar cell line T5. The mouse/mouse hybrid did not express these RCA products. Figure 1a shows that naturally occurring human anti-mouse antibodies and human complement were able to lyse DB3, the mouse/mouse hybridoma, but not B10, the human/mouse hybridoma. Both cell types were killed by rabbit complement (Fig. 1 b). T5 exposed to pig anti-human antibodies was lysed in the presence of rabbit complement but not human complement (data not shown).

Cell lines transfected with the DAF or MCP constructs were isolated and shown by FACS analysis to be expressing DAF or MCP. The MCP transfectant (unsorted) expressed approximately 1×106 copies per cell (in the range of a malignant epithelial cell line [19]) while the

DAF transfectant (sorted twice) expressed approximately 30 000 copies per cell, similar to a normal peripheral nucleated cell. The cytoprotective effect of transfecting the individual genes for DAF or MCP was tested by treating all three cell lines (the two expressing cell lines and the control transfected in the reverse orientation) with human complement and naturally occurring human anti-mouse antibodies. The mouse fibroblasts expressing human DAF (Fig. 2a) or MCP (Fig. 2b) were almost completely protected from lysis by human complement while the reverse MCP control line was lysed. Appropriate controls demonstrated that this cell lysis was complement mediated. The protective effect was abrogated by the addition of monoclonal antibodies against DAF (IC6 [2]) or MCP (GB24 [7]) to the appropriate assay. A nonspecific monoclonal served as a control in these assays.

Discussion

A precise understanding of the steps of the complement reaction that participate in hyperacute xenograft rejection will be needed to design appropriate strategies for therapeutic intervention. This paper describes experiments demonstrating the complement regulatory activity of human DAF and MCP on the surface of hybrid and transfected mouse cells. These data also provide a demonstra-

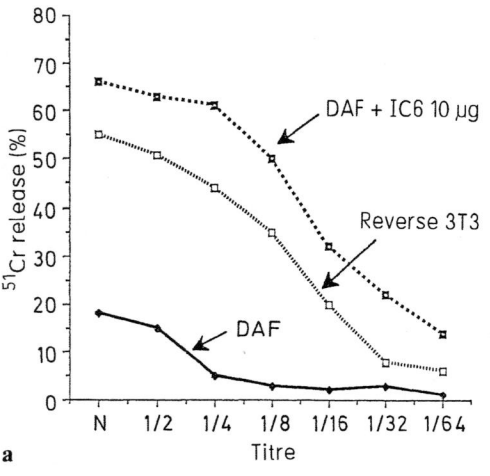

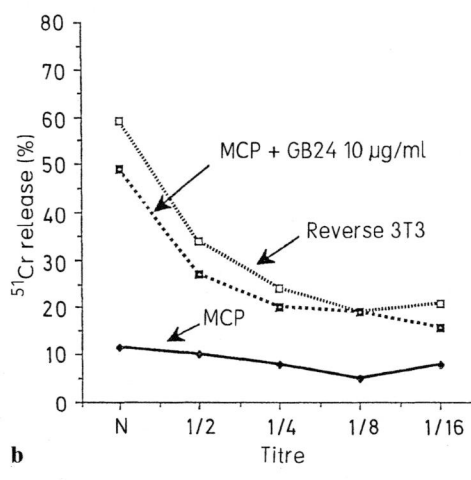

Fig. 2 a, b. The cytoprotective effect of transfecting a mouse fibroblast cell line (3T3 NIH) with **a** MCP or **b** DAF. Controls are the transfected cell line blocked with monoclonal antibody against the expressed product and 3T3 cell line transfected with the MCP gene in the reverse orientation *(Reverse)*

tion of cytoprotection from complement by genetic manipulation of the target cell. The assay used is in many respects analogous to the mechanisms involved in hyperacute xenograft rejection. Recently Yannoutsos and co-workers produced mice transgenic for human DAF (manuscript in preparation). The production of such transgenic animals expressing human complement regulatory products such as DAF and MCP at appropriate levels, should, in principle, permit organs derived from such animals to be transplanted into man without hyperacute rejection. What subsequent immune damage such an organ xenograft might suffer is not known.

Acknowledgements. We thank N.Hughes-Jones, M.Davitz and N.K.Spurr for the gift of reagents, also A.Williams, C.Milstein and J.Bogaerde for helpfull discussions. This work was supported by The Howard Hughes foundation and Imutran Ltd.

References

1. Caras IW, Davitz MA, Rhee L, Weddell G, Martin DWJ, Nussenzweig V (1987) Cloning of decay-accelerating factor suggests novel use of splicing to generate two proteins. Nature 325: 545–549

2. Cho S-W, Oglesby TJ, Hsi BL, Adams EM, Atkinson JP (1991) Characterization of three monoclonal antibodies to membrane cofactor protein (MCP) of the complement system and quantification of MCP by radioassay. Clin Exp Immunol 83: 257–261

3. Davies HS, Taylor JE, White DJG, Binns RM (1978) Major transplantation antigens of pig kidney and liver-comparison between whole organs and their parenchymal constituents. Transplantation 25: 290–295

4. Forty J, Carey N, White DJG, Wallwork J (1991) Hyperacute rejection of rabbit hearts by human blood is mediated by the alternative pathway of complement. Transplant Proc. In press

5. Forty I, Watson CJ, Carey N, White DJG, Wallwork J (1991) Perfusion of rabbit hearts with human blood results in immediate graft thrombosis which is temporally distinct from hyperacute rejection. Transplant Proc. In press

6. Fuhlbrigge RC, Fine SM, Unanue ER, Chaplin DD (1988) Expression of membrane interleukin 1 by fibroblasts transfected with murine interleukin 1 cDNA. Proc Natl Acad Sci USA 85: 5649–5653

7. Fujita T, Kamato T, Tamura N (1985) Characterization of functional properties of C4 binding protein by monoclonal antibodies. J Immunol 134: 3320–3324

8. Johnston PS, Lim SML, Wang MW, Wright L, White DJG (1991) Hyperacute rejection of xenografts in the complete absence of antibody. Transplant Proc 23: 877–879

9. Kearney JF, Radbruch A, Liesegang B, Rajewesky K (1979) A new mouse myeloma cell line that has lost immunoglobulin expression but permits the construction of antibody secreting hybrid cell lines. J Immunol 123: 1548–1550

10. Lublin DM, Liszewski MK, Post TW, Arce MA, Le-Beau MM, Rebentisch MB, Lemons LS, Seya T, Atkinson JP (1988) Molecular cloning and chromosomal localization of human membrane cofactor protein (MCP). Evidence for inclusion in the multigene family of complement-regulatory proteins. J Exp Med 168: 181–194

11. Miyagawa S, Hirose H, Shirakura R, Naka Y, Nakata S, Kawashima Y, Seya T, Matsumoto M, Uenaka A, Kitamura H (1988) The mechanism of discordant xenograft rejection. Transplantation 46: 825–830

12. Nose M, Katoh M, Okada N, Kyogoku M, Okada H (1990) Tissue distribution of HRF20, a novel factor preventing the membrane attack of homologous complement, and its predominant expression on endothelial cells in vivo. Immunology 70: 145–149

13. Paul LC (1991) Mechanism of humoral xenograft rejection. In: Cooper DKC, Kemp E, Reemtsma K, White DSG (eds) Xenografting. The transplantation of organs and tissues between species. Springer-Verlag, Berlin, pp 47–79

14. Perper RJ, Najarian JS (1966) Experimental renal heterotransplantation in widely divergent species. Transplantation 4: 377–381

15. Platt JL, Vercellotti GM, Dalmasso AP, Matas AJ, Bolman RM, Najarian JS, Bach FH (1990) Transplantation of discordant xenografts: a review of progress. Immunol Today 11: 450–456

16. Rey-Campos J, Rubinstein P, Rodriguez-de-Cordoba S (1988) A physical map of the human regulator of complement activation gene cluster linking the complement genes CR1, CR2, DAF, and C4BP. J Exp Med 167: 664–669

17. Rodriguez de Cordoba S, Dykman TR, Ginsberg-Fellner F, Ercilla G, Aqua M, Atkinson JP, Rubenstein P (1984) Evidence for linkage between loci coding for the binding protein for the forth component of complement (C4Bp) and for the C3b/C4b receptor. Proc Natl Acad Sci USA 81: 7890–7892

18. Schilling A, Land W, Pratschke E, Brendel W (1976) Dominant role of complement in the hyperacute xenograft rejection reaction. Surg Gynecol Obstet 142: 29–35

19. Sparrow RL, McKenzie IFC (1983) Hu Ly-m5: a unique antigen physically associated with HLA molecules. Hum Immunol 7: 1–15

20. Weis JH, Morton CC, Bruns GAP, Weis JJ, Klickstein LB, Wong WW, Fearon DT (1987). J Immunol 138: 312–315

21. Wright LJ, Feinstein A, Heap RB, Saunders JC, Bennett RC, Wang MW (1982) Progesterone monoclonal antibody blocks pregnancy in mice. Nature 295: 415–417

22. Wu S, Seino S, Bell GI (1989) Human anti-thrombin II (AT3) gene length polymorphism revealed by the polymerase chain reaction. Nucleic Acids Res 17: 6433–6437

Transplant Int (1992) 5 [Suppl 1]: S 651–S 652

TRANSPLANT
International
© Springer-Verlag 1992

TNF staining of graft biopsy in renal transplantation

A. Aikawa[1], P. J. McLaughlin[2], H. S. Davies[2], P. M. Johnson[2], I. McDicken[3], A. Bakran[1], and R. A. Sells[1]

[1] Renal Transplant Unit, Royal Liverpool Hospital, Liverpool, UK
[2] Department of Immunology, [3] Department of Pathology, The University of Liverpool, Liverpool, UK

Tumour Necrosis Factor (TNF) is a cytokine which may be found in patients' plasma and urine in association with acute rejection in renal transplantation [1]. TNF is produced mainly by macrophage/monocytes and activated lymphocytes and its release in acute rejection may damage the nephron leading to renal dysfunction. However localization of TNF in renal grafts has not yet been demonstrated. We investigated TNF localization in renal graft tissue and the association with acute rejection compared with non-immunological events (cyclosporine toxicity and acute tubular necrosis) in graft biopsy.

Key words: Tumor necrosis factor – Renal transplantation – Graft biopsy

Materials and methods

We used 50 graft biopsy specimens from 44 renal transplant patients in this study.

TNF staining (immunoperoxidase method: ABC-HRP)
1. Deparaffinise with xylene 5 mins.
Absolute ethanol 2 changes, 3 mins each.
95 % ethanol 2 changes, 3 min each.
Rinse in distilled water.
Wash in PBS.
2. Trypsinise with 1 % trypsin for 20 mins.
Wash in PBS. Tap off.
3. Block with 10 % non-immune rabbit serum for 10 min.
4. Incubate with mouse primary antihuman TNFα monoclonal antibody (J1D9) 60 min at 37 °C
Wash with PBS.
5. Incubate with biotinylated second antibody (anti-mouse) 5 min at room temperature.
Wash with PBS.
6. Incubate with enzyme conjugate 5 min at room temperature.
Wash with PBS.
7. Incubate with substrate chromogen mixture 5 min at room temperature.

Offprint requests to: P.J. McLaughlin, Department of Immunology, The University of Liverpool, Prescot street, Liverpool, L7 8XP, UK

Wash with distilled water.
8. Counterstain with haematoxylin 3 min at room temperature.
Wash well with tap water.
9. Mount section using dehydrate + mount with DPX.

Results

Localization of TNF staining in the nephron

Staining was observed mainly in cells of the distal tubules and Henle's loop. The staining pattern was cytoplasmic or luminal in them and occasionally patchy in proximal tubular cells less strongly. Occasionally, lymphoid cells (mainly small lymphocytes but some macrophages) were stained. No staining was observed in the vascular endothelium or the glomerular mesangial cells (Table 1, Figs. 1 and 2).

Association with graft status

No staining was observed in the donor kidneys before transplantation. TNF was observed mainly in the distal tubules in acute rejection episodes. During chronic vascular rejection TNF was found in half of the biopsies, whereas in primary non-function or cyclosporine toxicity, TNF was not a usual feature (Table 2).

Discussion

TNF was observed mainly in distal tubular cells and Henle's loop in graft biopsy specimens of acute rejection. This characteristic staining pattern reflects that Tamm-

Table 1. Localization of TNF in renal graft biopsies

Glomerulus	Proximal tubular cells	Distal tubular cells Henle's loop	Vascular endothelium
–	±	+	–

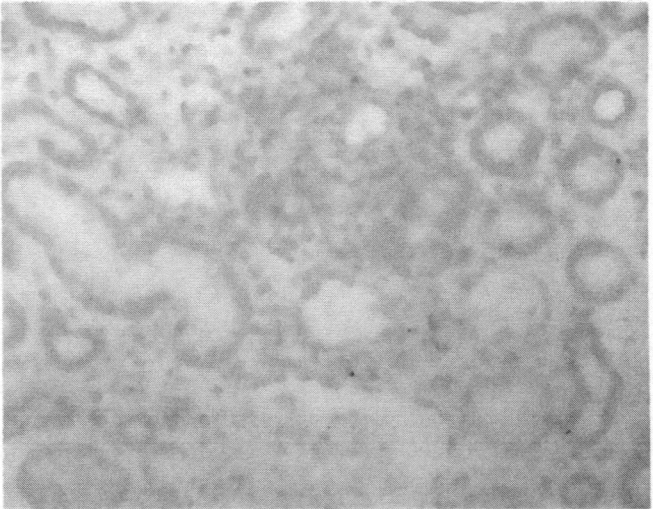

Fig. 1. Acute rejection. TNF was stained mainly in destal tubules. Proximal tubules were stained less strongly and patchy. Some infiltrated lymphoid cells were stained. No staining was observed in glomerulus

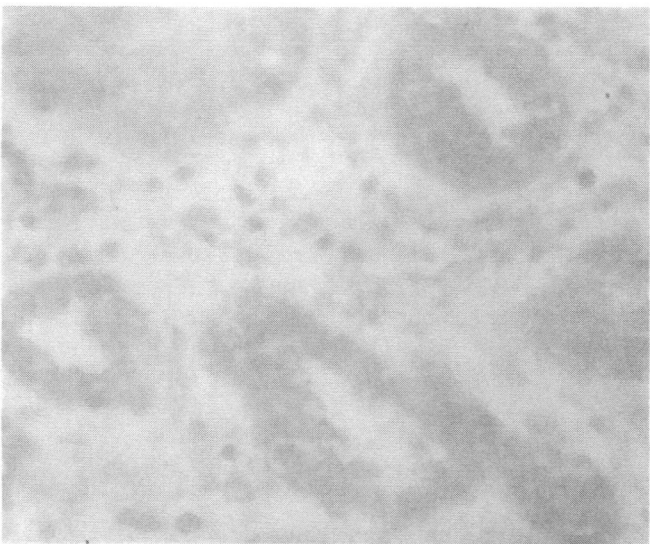

Fig. 2. Acute rejection. The staining pattern of distal tubular cells was cytoplasmic. Some infiltrated lymphoid cells were stained.

Horsfall glycoprotein (THG) which tends to ligand with TNF, is localized particularly in the distal tubular cells and collecting ducts. TNF may be produced by activated mac-

Table 2. TNF staining in various graft status

Donor's kidney	AR	CVR	Primary non-function	CyA Toxicity
0/5 (0%)	17/23 (74%)	7/14 (50%)	2/6 (33%)	0/2 (0%)

AR, Acute rejection; CVR, chronic vascular rejection; CyA, cyclosporine

rophage/monocyte and lymphocytes in acute rejection and in the case of severe acute rejection, some infiltrating cells were strongly stained [2]. Staining of TNF might indicate the severity of acute rejection and the active phase of the rejection process even in chronic vascular rejection.

TNF staining is never observed in donor kidney biopsies before grafting and rarely observed in non-immunological events (cyclosporine toxicity or acute tubular necrosis in primary non-functioning graft). TNF staining might be of value in differentiating between these non-immunological events and active rejection.

Summary

TNF staining was not observed in the glomerulus, the vascular endothelium, and the distal tubules stained better than proxymal tubles. TNF staining occurred more frequently in acute rejection compaired with non-immunological events.

Conclusion

The pattern of TNF staining in renal graft biopsy may be of value in the understanding of the action of TNF in acute rejection and may differentiate between active rejection and non-immunological events.

References

1. McLaughlin PJ, Aikawa A, Davies HM, Ward RG, Bakran A, Sells RA, Johnson PM (1991) Evaluation of sequential plasma and urinary tumour necrosis factor alpha levels in renal allograft recipients. Transplantation 51: 1225
2. Noronha IL, Hartley B, Eberlein-Gonska M, Cameron JS, Wardherr R (1991) Expression of Tumor Necrosis Factor (TNF), Interferon-gamma (INF-γ) and Interleukin 2 (IL-2R) in renal allograft biopsies. 5th Congress European Society for Organ Transplantation, Book of Abstracts, p 61

Transplant Int (1992) 5 [Suppl 1]: S 653–S 658

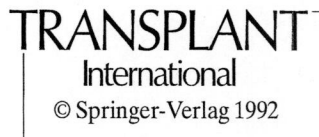

TRANSPLANT
International
© Springer-Verlag 1992

Analysis of suppressor T cells induced by donor-specific transfusion (DST): establishment of a human T cell hybridoma producing an antigen-nonspecific suppressor factor

T. Fujiwara, K. Sakagami, S. Kusaka, M. Uda, and K. Orita

First Department of Surgery, Okayama University Medical School, 2-5-1 Shikata-cho, Okayama 700, Japan

Abstract. Formation of suppressor T cells (Ts) induced by donor-specific transfusion (DST) is one of the most commonly suggested mechanisms for the beneficial effect of DST. In this study, we established a human T cell hybridoma derived from the peripheral blood lymphocytes (PBL) of a DST-treated patient, which produced an antigen-nonspecific suppressor factor. Post-DST PBL were fused with an azaguanine-resistant mutant of a human T cell leukemia cell line, CCRF-CEM^{AG}. After selection and cloning, we established one clone producing the mixed lymphocyte reaction (MLR) inhibitory factor (C524: 18 %–43 % suppression). Suppressive activity of the supernatant obtained from C524 after activation by PHA was highly augmented (64 %–88 % MLR suppression). This factor inhibited MLR dose-dependently in an antigen-nonspecific and HLA non-restricted manner. These results indicated that Ts clones could be generated in patients receiving DST and that the immunoregulatory factors produced by activated clones may play a role in the prolongation of renal allograft survival.

Key words: Donor-specific transfusion – Renal transplantation – Suppressor T cells – Donor-specific transfusion – T cell hybridoma – Suppressor T cells

The beneficial effect of donor specific transfusion (DST) on the survival of one-haplotype-identical living-related transplants is well-established [12], but the mechanisms responsible for the DST effect remain obscure. In our laboratory we have been investigating the mechanisms of the DST effect in human renal transplantation by examining the induction of antiidiotypic antibodies and suppressor T cells (Ts) to inhibit donor-specific primary mixed lymphocyte reaction (MLR) after DST. Previously, our studies have shown that DST can induce antiidiotypic antibodies and/or Ts and the induction of these cells and

antibodies correlates well with the reduction of rejection episodes and with better graft survival [4, 9, 13]. Recently, we have reported the establishment of a human-mouse hybridoma [7] and human T cell hybridoma [5, 6] derived from patients preconditioned with DST, both of which secreted donor-specific MLR inhibiting factors. The human-mouse hybridoma produced IgG antibody reacting with the T cell antigen-specific receptors. The supernatant of the T cell hybridoma cocultured with donor cells inhibited donor-specific MLR in a dose-dependent manner when added during the early phase of MLR.

In this study, to explore immunoregulatory factors produced by DST-induced Ts, we established a novel T cell hybridoma (termed C524) propagated from peripheral blood lymphocytes (PBL) of a patient receiving DST. The culture supernatant of C524 (C524, CS) inhibited MLR in an antigen-nonspecific and HLA non-restricted manner. Interestingly, the culture supernatant of C524, after activation by PHA-P for 3 days (PHA-activated C524, CS), showed a marked inhibitory effect on MLR in the same manner as C524, CS. PHA-activated C524, CS did not affect the kinetics of MLR and showed its suppressive effect only when added early in the culture.

Materials and methods

DST protocol and human subjects. A patient was transfused on three occasions with 200 ml of fresh whole blood from the same donor at 2-week intervals. To prevent sensitization, azathioprine was given orally at a dose of 150 mg/day on the day before and on each day of DST [4]. The recipient's PBL, collected pre-DST and post-DST, were cryopreserved in liquid nitrogen until use. PBL of three healthy volunteers from our laboratory staff were used as a control. Serological HLA-phenotyping of the recipient, donor and all volunteers was performed using a standard antibody-dependent microcytotoxicity test. The recipient (EK) was HLA-A –; B35, w48; C w3; DR 4,7 and the donor (TK) was HLA-A 2, 31; B w48, w42; C –; DR 2,4. The healthy volunteers' HLA-phenotypes were as follows: TF (HLA-A 24, –; B44, w62; C w4; DR 5,7; DQ w6); MU (HLA-A24, w3; B w57 –; C w1, w3; DR w14, w52; DQ w2); SK (HLA-A2,3; B44, w48; C –; DR w15, w12; DQ w6).

Offprint requests to: Takuzo Fujiwara

Table 1. Inhibition of MLR by hybridoma supernatant

Responder[b]	Stimulator[b]	^{3}H-Thymidine incorporation (cpm)		
		Control (medium only)	Supernatant[a]	
			C524 (% suppression)	CEM (% suppression)
EK	TK	15331.7 ± 859.7	11257.0 ± 497.9* (26.5)	17145.7 ± 1648.8 (−12.1)
EK	TF	9533.5 ± 532.5	7055.7 ± 370.8* (26.0)	8330.3 ± 999.3 (12.6)
EK	SK	6641.7 ± 832.7	3748.3 ± 704.0** (43.6)	7859.6 ± 703.7 (−18.3)
TF	TK	31677.6 ± 2126.7	18137.5 ± 138.6* (42.6)	31381.8 ± 2992.5 (0.9)
MU	TK	27793.3 ± 1432.3	22796.5 ± 895.5** (18.0)	30803.7 ± 1654.6 (−10.8)
SK	TK	11322.2 ± 1041.8	9156.8 ± 620.8*** (19.1)	15320.7 ± 1538.9** (−35.3)
TF	MU	39745.1 ± 3258.8	22606.6 ± 883.8* (43.1)	35906.7 ± 1598.3 (9.7)
TF	SK	38161.7 ± 2415.6	26285.6 ± 1857.7** (31.1)	36440.3 ± 1937.3 (4.5)

[a] Fifty microliters of culture supernatant was added to the mixture (150 μl) of responder cells and stimulator cells
[b] HLA-typing of responder, stimulator cells were described iin Materials and methods section. EK is the recipient, FK is the donor and the others (TF, MU and SK) are controls
* $P < 0.001$ ** $P < 0.01$ *** $P < 0.05$

Table 2. Inhibition of MLR by PHA-activated C524 supernatant

Responder[b]	Stimulator[b]	3H-Thymidine incorporation (cpm)		
		Control (medium only)	Supernatant[a]	
			PHA-activated C524 (% suppression)	PHA-activated CEM (% suppression)
EK	TK	16978.2 ± 1240.3	6166.7 ± 258.2* (63.7)	17564.0 ± 1462.3 (−3.5)
EK	TF	8134.7 ± 1358.5	2928.7 ± 199.9* (64.0)	6236.1 ± 518.0 (23.3)
EK	MU	17251.6 ± 1694.9	3535.2 ± 160.6* (79.5)	15063.4 ± 2466.3 (12.7)
EK	SK	10446.0 ± 975.6	3494.2 ± 161.6* (66.5)	9994.2 ± 1041.0 (4.3)
TF	TK	27303.2 ± 1454.3	3748.8 ± 393.4* (86.3)	26692.6 ± 2256.3 (2.2)
MU	TK	13591.2 ± 1545.6	2507.3 ± 445.2* (81.6)	15276.8 ± 1286.3 (−12.4)
SK	TK	22323.4 ± 2200.4	4199.0 ± 123.2* (81.2)	20730.6 ± 828.5 (7.1)
TF	MU	20011.5 ± 2028.9	5095.1 ± 560.1* (74.5)	18252.4 ± 2241.5 (8.8)
TF	SK	29924.7 ± 3494.5	3600.6 ± 47.6* (88.0)	25822.6 ± 679.7 (13.7)

[a] Fifty microliters of PHA-activated C524 or CEM supernatant was added to the mixture (150 μl) of responder cells and stimulator cells
[b] EK is the recipient, FK is the donor, and the others are controls.
Their HLA-typings were described in Materials and methods section
* $P < 0.001$

Cell fusion. PBL were isolated from heparinized venous blood by Ficoll-Conray density gradient centrifugation. Freshly prepared post-DST PBL were stimulated with mitomycin C (MMC)-treated donor PBL for 3 days. These allostimulated post-DST PBL were then hybridized with an azaguanine-resistant mutant of a human leukemic T-cell line, CCRF-CEM^{AG}, provided by DR Minowada (Hayashibara Biochemical Laboratories Inc., Okayama, Japan), in the presence of polyethylene glycol (m. w. 1450 BRL) according to a slightly modified technique of Okada et al. [11]. Fused cells were cultured overnight in a 24-well tissue plate (Falcon 3047; Becton Dickinson Labware, Oxnard, Calif.) in RPMI 1640 medium (GIBCO Laboratories, Grand Island, N.Y.) supplemented with

10% heat-activated fetal calf serum (FCS). The culture medium was then replaced with hypoxanthine, aminopterin, and thymidine (HAT) medium. After 2 weeks, the HAT medium was replaced by RPMI 1640 medium containing 10% FCS, hypoxanthine, and thymidine for 1 week, and then the medium was switched to maintenance culture medium (RPMI 1640 medium plus 10% FCS without selection components). Supernatant fluids from cultures were filtrated through a 0.2 μm membrane and assayed for their suppressive activity in donor-specific primary MLR. Selected hybridomas were cloned using a limiting dilution method, and supernatant fluids were again tested for suppressive activity.

Inhibition of MLR by hybridoma supernatant. MLR was prepared in quaduplicate in 96-well, round-bottomed microculture plates in a final volume of 200 μl in RPMI 1640 HEPES medium (GIBCO) supplemented with 10% FCS. Were added 50 μl culture supernatants or control fluids to the mixture (150 μl) of 5×10^4 responder cells and 5×10^4 MMC-treated stimulator cells. Cultures were incubated for 5 days, pulsed with ³H-thymidine (1 μCi/well) for 24 h, and harvested on glass fiber paper. Incorporation of ³H-thymidine was measured with a β-scintillation counter, and expressed as mean counts per minute (cpm) $\pm$ SD. The percentage of suppression was calculated by the formula: $[1 - (\text{cpm in the presence of test supernatant/cpm in the presence of control medium})] \times 100\%$.

Flow cytometric analysis of hybridoma cells. Hybridoma cells were immunostained with the following antibodies: Leu 2, Leu 3, Leu 4, Leu 8 and Leu 11 (Becton Dickinson, Mountainview, Calif.). Monoclonal antibodies were directly conjugated with fluorescein isothiocyate (FITC) or phycoerythin (PE). After staining, cell samples were analyzed using a FACscan (Becton Dickinson).

Preparation of PHA-activated hybridoma supernatant. Hybridoma cells were cultured at a density of 2×10^5/ml in the presence of PHA-P (10 μg/ml) for 3 days. Cells were then harvested, washed 3 times and resuspended with RPMI 1640 HEPES medium plus bovine albumin (10 mg/ml) (Sigma, Chemical Company, St. Louis, Mo.) at a density of 5×10^5/ml. After 48 h incubation at 37°C in 5% CO₂, cell free supernatants were filter-sterilized and stored at -37°C until use. The suppressive activity of PHA-activated hybridoma supernatant was also tested as described above.

The effect of PHA-activated hybridoma supernatants on spontaneous cytolysis. PHA-induced lymphoblasts were labeled with ⁵¹Cr, suspended in culture medium, and distributed in 96-well, round-bottomed microculture plates (1×10^4/well). We added 100 μl PHA-activated hybridoma supernatant or control medium to the plates. Triplicate 100 μl aliquots of supernatant were harvested at the indicated times and ⁵¹Cr release was determined using an auto-well gamma system. Maximum release was determined from ⁵¹Cr labeled lymphoblasts exposed to 1 *N* NaOH. Percentage cytolysis was calculated using the following formula: (experimental release/maximum release) $\times 100\%$.

Statistical analysis. Statistical analysis was performed by the paired *t*-test and $P < 0.05$ was considered significant.

Results

Establishment of a human T-cell hybridoma

Following 3 weeks of culture, macroscopic evidence of hybridoma growth was observed in approximately 30% of the wells. After cloning, one clone producing MLR inhibiting factors was established (designated C524). This hybridoma has been stable in culture and has continuously produced MLR inhibiting factors for more than 6 months. As shown in Table 1, the addition of C524 culture supernatant (C524, CS) to donor-specific primary MLR resulted in a significantly reduced response (26.5% sup-

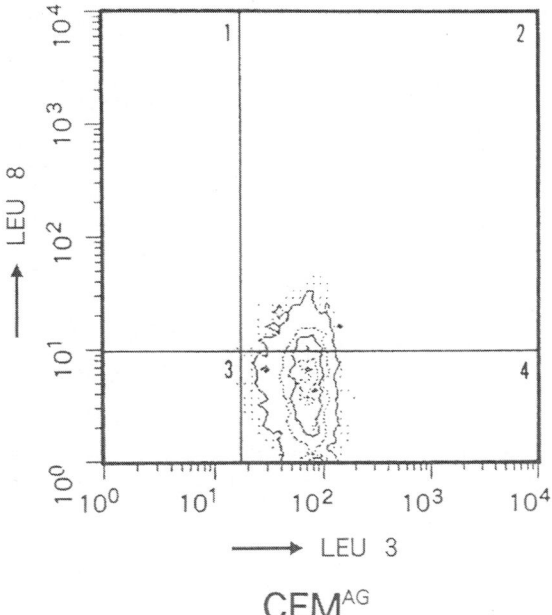

CEM^AG

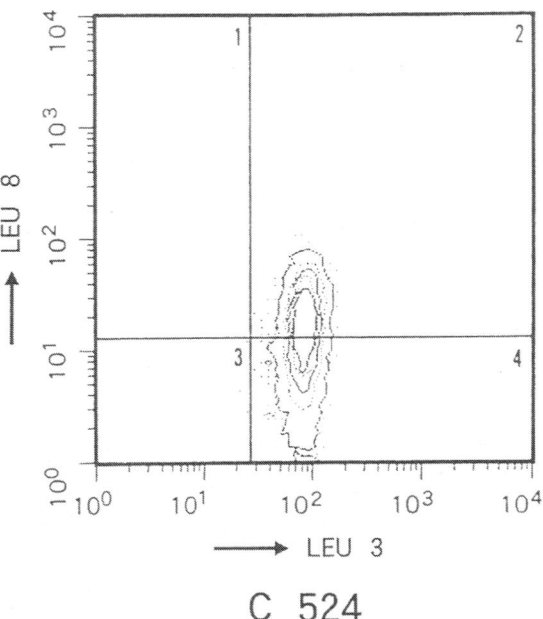

C 524

Fig. 1. Flow cytometric analysis of C524 clones: C524 and CCRF-CEM^AG cells were stained with FITC-conjugated Leu 3 antibody and PE-conjugated Leu 8 antibody and analyzed using a FACScan. Dot plots with markers set for control stained cells are shown

pression, $P < 0.001$) relative to control cultures. Furthermore, C524, CS was able to inhibit significantly not only antigen-nonspecific MLR but also MLR between controls. Supernatant of CCRF-CEM^AG showed no inhibitory effect on any MLR.

Phenotypic analysis of C524 clone

C524 cells expressed Leu 4 and Leu 3 antigen on their cell surface, but were not stained with Leu 2 or Leu 11 antibodies (data not shown). The same findings were ob-

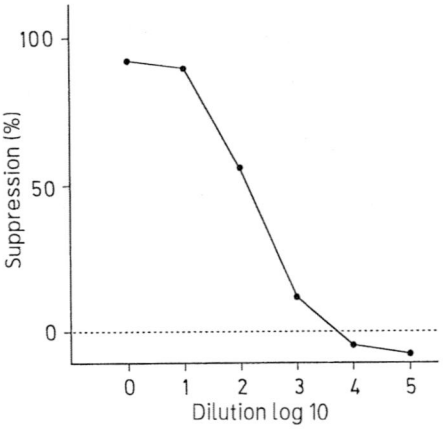

Fig. 2. Dose response of PHA-activated C524, CS to the percentage MLR suppression: Undiluted or 1:10 dilutions of PHA-activated C524, CS were added at 25% by volume to MLR culture (5×10^4 of TF-PBL and MMC-treated MU-PBL)

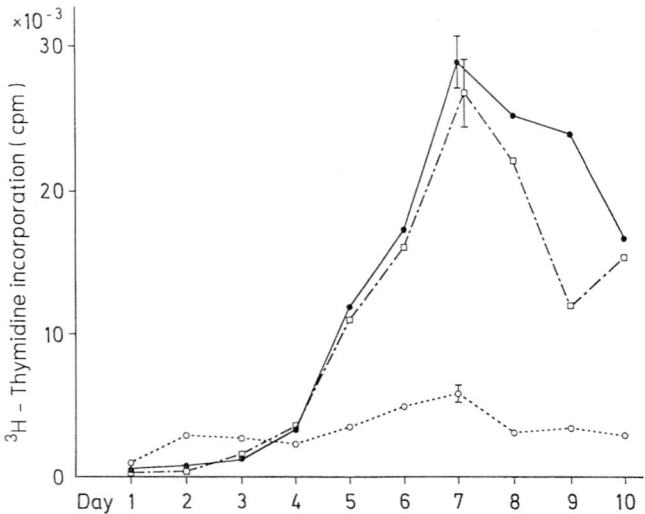

Fig. 3. Effect of PHA-activated C524, CS on the kinetics of MLR: 5×10^4 TF-PBL were cocultured with equal numbers of MU-PBL. Cells were harvested on the day indicated in medium only (●—●), with PHA-activated C524, CS (○---○) or with PHA-activated CCRF-CEM^{AG} (□---□). For graphical representation each point represents the mean of a quadruplicate sample. The standard deviation was calculated for each point. However, only the values on the day of maximal proliferation (day 7) are indicated for the sake of clarity

served on CCFR-CEM^{AG} cells. However, two-color analysis using FITC-conjugated Leu 3 and PE-conjugated Leu 8 showed that a higher expression of Leu 8 on C534 cells occurred compared with expression on CCRF-CEM^{AG} cells (Fig. 1).

Inhibition of MLR by PHA-activated C524 supernatant

To determine whether the suppressive activity of C524 was augmented after activation of mitogen, PHA-activated C524 culture supernatant (PHA-activated C524, CS) was prepared as described in Materials and methods section, and tested in MLR. Interestingly, a maked sup-

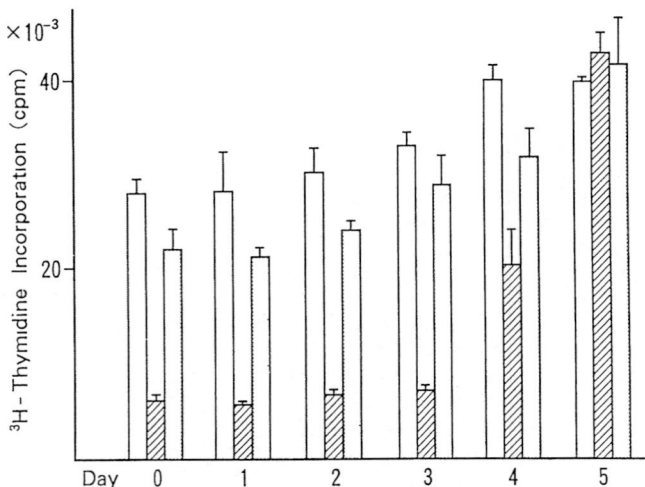

Fig. 4. Kinetics of the inhibitory effect of PHA-activated C524, CS on MLR: 5×10^4 TF-PBL was cocultured with MMC-treated MU-PBL for 6 days. On the days indicated, 50 μl medium (☐), PHA-activated C524, CS (▨), or PHA-activated CCRF-CEM^{AG}, CS (☐) were added to MLR

pression of MLR was observed when PHA-activated C524, CS was added to MLR (64–88% suppression, $P < 0.001$). Suppression by PHA-activated C524, CS was nonspecific for stimulator alloantigens and was not HLA-restricted (Table 2). Therefore, MLR between controls (TF-PBL as responder and MU-PBL as stimulator cells) was performed in the following assay. The supernatant of PHA-activated CCRF-CEM^{AG} had little effect on MLR.

Serial 1:10 dilutions of PHA-activated C524, CS were added at 25% by volume to MLR. Figure 2 shows that suppressive activity of PHA-activated C524, CS was dose-dependent, with no suppression seen at dilutions greater than 1:100.

To determine whether PHA-activated C524, CS affected the kinetics of MLR, supernatants of PHA-activated C524, CCRF-CEM^{AG}, and control medium were added at the beginning to replicate MLR cultures which were harvested serially at 1–10 days. As shown in Fig. 3, PHA-activated C524, CS significantly inhibited MLR but failed to alter its kinetics.

Furthermore, MLR was suppressed when PHA-activated C524, CS was added between days 0–3, but its addition after day 4 resulted in little or no suppression (Fig. 4).

The effect of PHA-activated C524, CS on spontaneous cytolysis

To examine the cytotoxicity of PHA-activated C524, CS, it was added at 50% by volume to the incubation of PHA-induced lymphoblasts labeled with ^{51}Cr. Figure 5 shows that PHA-activated C524, CS did not affect spontaneous cytolysis of lymphoblasts during the observation period. Therefore, the suppression by PHA-activated C524, CS was not considered to be due to cytotoxic effects.

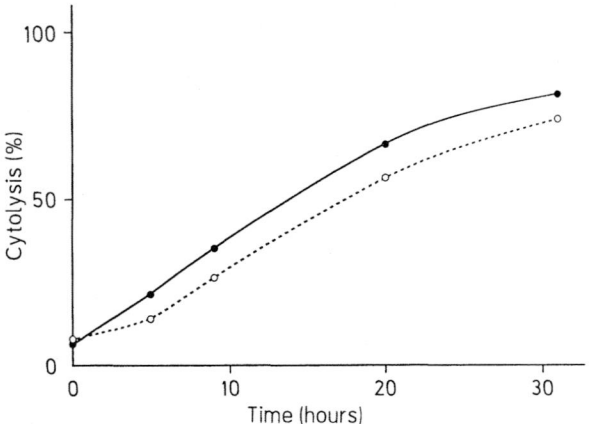

Fig. 5. The effect of PHA-activated C524, CS on spontaneous cytolysis: ^{51}Cr release of ^{51}Cr labeled lymphoblasts was measured at the indicated times in the absence (●—●) or the presence (○---○) of PHA-activated C524, CS (50% by volume). Percentage cytolysis was calculated using the formula described in Material and methods section

Discussion

DST has been used extensively prior to transplantation to improve the results of one-haplotype-identical living-related donor transplants. Recently Grailer et al. have reported the development of donor-specific cytotoxic T lymphocyte hyporesponsiveness obtained up to 2 years post-transplant in patients preconditioned with DST plus azathioprine and withdrawn from steroids 14 days following transplantation [3]. They also state that the DST effect might be most significant in the context of a reduction of immunosuppressive drug therapy.

Although several hypotheses have been proposed to explain the beneficial effect of DST, the exact mechanisms behind this effect is as yet unknown. In this study, we established a human T cell hybridoma, termed C524, producing MLR inhibiting factors by the fusion of post-DST PBL with an azaguanine-resistant mutant of a human leukemic T-cell line. The suppressive activity of the supernatant obtained from C524 was highly augmented after activation by PHA (PHA-activated C524, CS). This factor inhibited MLR dose-dependently in an antigen-nonspecific and HLA non-restricted manner. Furthermore, PHA-activated C524, CS did not affect the kinetics of MLR and showed its suppressive effect only when added early in the culture. Suppression by PHA-activated C524, CS was not considered to be due to cytotoxic effects since it did not influence spontaneous cytolysis of ^{51}Cr-labeled lymphoblasts. These results indicated that Ts clones could be induced by DST and that the immunoregulatory factors produced by activated clones may play a role in the DST effect.

Flow-cytometric analysis showed that C524 cells expressed Leu 3 and Leu 8 antigen on their cell surface. The subpopulation of T cells bearing Leu 3^+, 8^+ phenotype is reported by Mohagheghpour et al. to have suppressor inducer function [10]. They have demonstrated that the activation of Leu 2^+ suppressor effector cells generated in vitro is dependent on Leu 3^+, 8^+ cells. It is possible that suppressor effector cells are generated and inhibit proliterative responses to alloantigen when PHA-activated C524, CS is added early during the culture period.

Various antigen-nonspecific suppressor factors have been reported to inhibit the proliterative response of T cells [1, 2, 8, 14]. For example, Maki et al. have demonstrated that a murine T cell hybridoma produced "contra-IL 2", a suppressor lymphokine that inhibited interleukin 2 (IL-2) activity [8]. However, we did not observe that PHA-activated C524, CS directly inhibited IL-2 activity in the bioassay using IL-2 dependent cytotoxic T lymphocyte cell line (CTLL-2) (data not shown). In addition, PHA-activated C524, CS was thought to have the chemical properties of a protein since its suppressive activity was abolished after heat treatment or filtration, with a limiting core size of 10000 m.w. (data not shown), and thus was not likely to represent a low molecular-weight immunoregulatory substance such as prostaglandin [2, 14]. Emara and Sanfilippo have recently reported the soluble factor produced by suppressor cell line derived from a renal transplant recipient (TsEEF) [1]. TsEEF inhibited the generation of MLR and cytotoxic T cell responses, as well as mitogen-induced proliferative responses to PHA and PWM. The way in which TsEEF inhibited MLR seems to be the same as that of PHA-activated C524, CS. The other suppressive effects on the immune system of PHA-activated C524, CS and the mechanisms by which it exerts suppression are now being investigated.

Finally, although biochemical characterization and purification of the factor was not performed in this study, we consider that these approaches might be useful in explaining the mechanism of DST effect, and may also be helpful for in vivo preconditioning or immunosuppression for organ transplantation. More details and precise analysis of immunoregulatory factors produced by human suppressor clones will provide a means of applying these factors to clinical transplantation.

References

1. Emara M, Sanfilippo F (1989) Human suppressor T cells induced in vitro with an autologous renal allograft-derived T cell line II. activity and specificity of a soluble suppressor factor. Transplantation 47: 364–371
2. Fischer A, Durandy A, Griscelli C (1981) Role of prostaglandin E_2 in the induction of nonspecific T lymphocyte suppressor activity. J Immunol 126: 1452–1455
3. Gralier AP, Sollinger HW, Kawamura T, Burlingham WJ (1991) Donor-specific cytotoxic lymphocyte hyporesponsiveness following renal transplantation in patients pretreated with donor-specific transfusion. Transplantation 51: 320–324
4. Haisa M, Sakagami K, Matsumoto T, Kawamura T, Uchida S, Fujiware T, Shiozaki S, Inagaki M, Orita K (1989) Donor-specific transfusion (DST) with intermittent administration of azathioprine induces suppressor T cells and MLR-inhibiting factors without sensitization. Transplant Proc 21: 1814–1817
5. Haisa M, Sakagami K, Orita K (1990) Establishment of a human T-cell hybridoma producing an MLR suppressing factor: relationship to the mechanism of action of donor-specific transfusion. Transplant Proc 22: 1977–1980
6. Haisa M, Sakagami K, Kawamura T, Niguma T, Fujiware T, Kusaka S, Matsuoka J, Shiozaki S, Fujiware T, Onoda T, Orita K (1991) Induction of suppressor T cells by donor-specific blood

transfusions: establishment of a human T-cell hybridoma producing an MLR suppressant factor. Transplant Proc 23: 196–199

7. Kawamura T, Sakagami K, Haisa M, Morisaki F, Takasu S, Inagaki M, Oiwa T, Orita K (1989) Induction of antiidiotypic antibodies by donor-specific blood transfusions: establishment of a human-mouse hybridoma sectreting the MLR-inhibiting factor. Transplantation 48: 459–463

8. Maki T, Satomi S, Gotoh M, Monaco AP (1986) Contra-IL2: a suppressor lymphokine that inhibits IL-2 activity. J Immunol 136: 3298–3303

9. Matsumoto T, Sakagami K, Orita K (1987) Role of donor specific blood transfusions in prolongation of kidney graft survival. Transplant Proc 19: 2264–2267

10. Mohagheghpour N, Benike CJ, Kansas G, Bieber C, Engleman EG (1983) Activation of antigen-specific suppressor T cells in the presence of cyclosporin requires interactions between T cells of inducer and suppressor lineage. J Clin Invest 72: 2092–2100

11. Okada M, Yoshimura N, Kaieda T, Yamamura Y, Kishimoto T (1981) Establishment and characterization of human T hybrid cells secreting immunoregulatory molecules. Proc Natl Acad Sci USA 78: 7717–7721

12. Salvatierra O, Vincent F, Amend W, Potter D, Iwaki Y, Opelz G, Terasaki P, Duca R, Cochrum K, Hanes D, Stoney RJ, Feduska NJ (1980) Deliberate donor-specific blood transfusion prior to living related renal transplantation: a new approach. Ann Surg 192: 543–552

13. Takeuchi T, Sakagami K, Seki Y, Tsuboi K, Matsumoto M, Miyazaki M, Orita K (1985) Antiidiotypic antibodies and suppressor cells induced by donor-specific transfusion in potential kidney transplant recipients. Transplant Proc 17: 1059–1061

14. Walker C, Kristensen F, Bettens F, De Weck AL (1983) Lymphokine regulation of activated (G_1) lymphocytes 1. prostaglandin E_2-induced inhibition of interleukin 2 production. J Immunol 130: 1770–1773

Transplant Int (1992) 5 [Suppl 1]: S 659–S 660

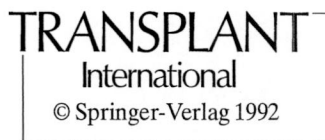

TRANSPLANT
International
© Springer-Verlag 1992

Role of leukotrienes B4 and C4 in liver allograft rejection

J. González, J. A. Cienfuegos, F. Pardo, J. Sola, J. L. Hernández, C. Rodríguez-Ortigosa, C. Benito, E. Balén, F. J. Pardo, and J. Quiroga

The Departments of Surgery, Medicine and Pathology, Clínica Universitaria, University of Navarra, Navarra, Spain

Abstract. Previous studies have shown that eicosanoids may act in vitro as immunoregulatory substances. In this study, the concentrations of leukotriene B4 (LTB4) and leukotriene C4 (LTC4) were measured in a model of allograft rejection. Six orthotopic allotransplants of the liver were performed in dogs without the administration of immunosuppressives. LTB4 levels showed an increase coinciding with the start of rejection, significant differences being present between the basal levels and those measured 24 h post-revascularization ($P < 0.05$), and every day from the 3rd postoperative day ($P < 0.01$). LTB4 rose before the parameters generally used in evaluating rejection. LTC4 levels increased significantly ($P < 0.001$) in the first 24 h, and experienced no further variations. LTB4 may play an important role in the mechanisms which bring about the response to the allograft. This substance could be a specific and early marker for rejection.

Key words: Leukotrienes – Leukotriene B4 – Leukotriene C4 – Rejection – Liver rejection – Liver transplantation

Leukotrienes (LTS) are a group of compounds derived from the metabolism of arachidonic acid which, together with the prostaglandins and the tromboxanes, are given the collective name of eicosanoids. It has previously been shown that some of these metabolites, originating via the cycloxygenase or lipoxygenase routes, potentially act as immunoregulators [1], but experience in their clinical application is very limited [2]. Various in vitro experiments [3, 4] have demonstrated that leukotriene B4 (LTB4), as well as sharing the pro-inflammatory actions of the cysteinyl leukotrienes (LTC4, LTD4, LTE4), participates in the mechanisms producing tissue lesions in response to the allograft by means of an increase in leucocyte aggregation, in the proliferation of T lymphocytes, in the secretion of

interleucine 1 and 2, and in the development of "natural killer" cell subpopulations. In this study we investigated the behaviour of LTB4 and LTC4 in the rejection of a hepatic allograft.

Materials and methods

We performed orthotopic liver transplants on six mongrel dogs weighing between 20 and 30 kgs. We used the technique described by Starzl [5–7], with some modifications. For preservation, we used, Eurocollins at 4°C, the cold ischemia time being 85 min ± 26 min. During the anhepatic phase, a femoro-porto-jugular bypass was performed with spontaneous flow. Afterwards, the venous anastomoses were performed in the following order: suprahepatic cava, infrahepatic cava, porta. After the portal venous system had been revascularized, an end to end arterial anastomosis was performed between the celiac axis of the donor and recipient. In two out of six animals the anastomosis was performed end to side between the hepatic artery of the donor and the origin of the celiac axis in the recipient. Biliary reconstruction was carried out by means of cholecystoduodenostomy. In all cases, the animals were given an autotransfusion of blood extracted a week before the operation. None of the animals was given immunosuppressives. Percutaneous liver biopsy was performed systematically on the 3rd and 5th postoperative days.

Blood samples were taken at the following stages during the study: 1 week before surgery (basal), prior to laparotomy, 8 h after revascularization of the graft through the portal vein, and every day during the postoperative period. At each stage the levels of the following were noted: aspartate aminotransferase (AST), alkaline phosphatase (ALP), bilirubin, prothombin time (PT), LTC4 and LTB4. Levels of LTB4 and LTC4 were calculated by radioimmu-

Offprint requests to: J. González M. D., Department of Surgery, Clínica Universitaria, Apartado 192. 31080, Pamplona, Navarra, Spain

Table 1.

	Basal ($n = 6$)	Day 1 ($n = 6$)	Day 3 ($n = 6$)	Day 5 ($n = 5$)	Day 7 ($n = 4$)
AST	14 ± 5	801 ± 181	170 ± 56	190 ± 83	493 ± 199
ALP	55 ± 7	223 ± 80	525 ± 267	2285 ± 414	6691 ± 392
PT	7.5 ± 0.5	11.4 ± 5.7	8.1 ± 0.6	10.4 ± 2.2	13.1 ± 3.4
Bil	0.22 ± 0.08	0.32 ± 0.16	0.61 ± 0.24	1.44 ± 1.17	2.24 ± 1.32

AST = Aspartate aminotransferase; ALP = alkaline phosphatase; PT = prothombin time; Bil = bilirubin

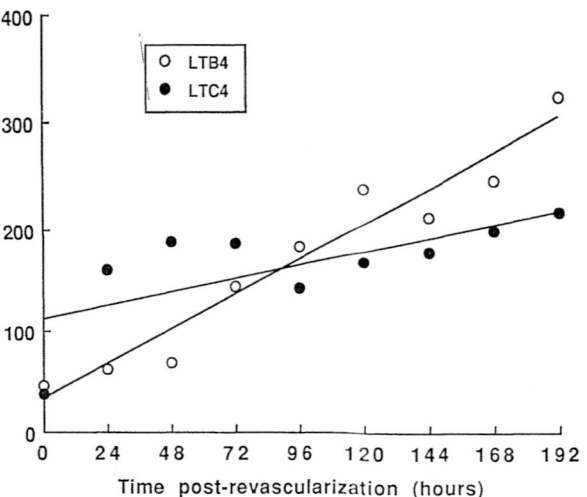

Fig. 1. Mean levels of LTB4 and LTC4

noassay. The antibody, anti-LTC4 was provided by Merck Frosst (Montreal, Canada). The antibody, anti-LTB4 was obtained from Advanced Magnetic Inc. (Cambridge, Mass. USA).

The results were expressed as mean ± SEM. The mean of the six basal dogs were used as control parameters. Observations were compared using Student's t-test for paired samples. The level of significance was set up at $P < 0.05$.

Results

The mean survival time of the six animals was 6.5 days (range 4–8 days). In all cases, pathology studies conducted after the animal's death demonstrated the presence of severe acute rejection. In two animals there were moderate pathological signs of rejection on the 3rd postoperative day. Both animals died before the 6th day.

LTB4 levels in the six dogs showed a variable development pattern. None the less, our findings showed a tendency for the mean levels of this parameter to increase as the postoperative period progressed (Fig. 1). A significant difference existed between the base level and the reading at 24 h ($P < 0.05$), and every day from the 3rd postoperative day ($P < 0.01$).

Figure 1 shows LTC4 levels rising significantly with respect to basal levels ($P < 0.001$) in the first 24 h, and then stabilizing for the rest of the postoperative period. The other parameters determined are shown in Table 1.

Discussion

This study analyzes the behaviour of LTB4 and LTC4 in a model of a hepatic allograft rejection without immunosuppression. Our results confirmed the findings of Post et al. [8], who have observed, in a similar model of allotransplant without immunosuppression, an increase in the activity of the enzymes of the 5-lipoxygenase route ocurring in the first 24 h after revascularization. These enzymes regulate the synthesis of LTB4 and LTC4.

The observation of the progressive rise in LTB4 levels as rejection becomes established constitutes a step forward in our understanding of the intimate mechanisms of the tissue lesion in response to allografts. The LTC4 levels rose in the first 24 h and showed no variations for the rest of the postoperative period. This initial increase has been reported as a parameter of good early functioning of the graft [9]. Further research is necessary in order to clarify its role in the pathology of rejection.

LTB4 levels rose earlier than the other parameters generally used to evaluate rejection (Table 1), which means that it could be used as a specific and early marker for rejection. The inhibition of the synthesis of this compound by blocking the metabolism of arachidonic acid via 5-lipoxygenase has been the subject of previous studies [10–12], and may well offer new therapeutic alternatives in the prevention and treatment of rejection.

References

1. Hagmann W, Keppler D (1988) Leukotrienes and other eicosanoids in liver pathophysiology. In: Arias IM, Jakoby WB, Popper H, Schachter D, Shafritz DA (eds) The liver: Biology and pathobiology. Raven Press Ltd, New York, pp 793–806
2. Moran M, Mozes MF, Maddux MS, Veremis S, Bartkus C, Ketel B, Pollak R, Wallemark C, Jonasson O (1990) Prevention of acute graft rejection by the prostaglandin E1 analogue misoprostol in renal-transplant recipients treated with cyclosporine and prednisone. N Engl J Med 322: 1183–1188
3. Rola-Pleszczynski M, Gagnon L, Chavaillaz PA (1988) Immune regulation by leukotriene B4. In: Levi R, Krell RD (eds) Biology of the leukotrienes. Annals of the New York academy of sciences, New York, pp 218–226
4. Rola-Pleszczynski M (1985) Immunoregulation by leukotrienes and other lipoxygenase metabolites. Immunol Today 6: 302–307
5. Starzl TE, Kaupp HA, Brock DR, Lazarus RE, Johnson RU (1960) Reconstructive problems in canine liver homotransplantation with special reference to the postoperative role of hepatic venous flow. Surg Gynecol Obstet 111: 733–743
6. Starzl TE, Marchioro TL, Porter KA, Taylor PD, Faris TD, Herrman TJ, Hlad CJ, Wadell WR (1965) Factors determining short and long term survival after orthotopic liver homotransplantation in the dog. Surgery 58: 131–155
7. Todo S, Kam I, Lynch S, Starzl TE (1985) Animal research in liver transplantation with special reference to the dog. Semin Liver Dis 5: 309–317
8. Post S, Goerig M, Otto G, Manner M, Foltis C, Hofmann W, Herfarth C (1991) Rapid increase in the activity of enzymes of eicosanoid synthesis in hepatic and extrahepatic tissues after experimental liver transplantation. Transplantation 51: 1058–1064
9. González J, Cienfuegos JA, Pardo F, Hernández JL, Benito C, Balén E, Ortigosa CR, Pardo FJ, Quiroga J (1991) Leukotriene C4 detection as an early graft function marker in liver transplantation. Transplant Proc (in press)
10. Anderson CB, Mangino MJ (1991) Arachidonate 5-lipoxygenase inhibition and acute renal allograft rejection. Transplant Proc 23: 640–642
11. Horichi H, Izumi R, Shimizu K, Konishi K, Kitabayashi K, Watanabe T, Miyazaki I (1991) Effect of 5-lipoxygenase inhibitor on canine pancreatic allotransplantation. Transplant Proc 23: 1679–1680
12. Konishi K, Watanabe T, Yabushita K, Hirosawa H, Izumi R, Miyazaki I (1991) Effect of lipoxygenase inhibitor (nordihydroguaiaretic acid, NDGA) on canine pancreatic allografts. Transplant Proc 23: 1681–1682

Transplant Int (1992) 5 [Suppl 1]: S 661–S 664

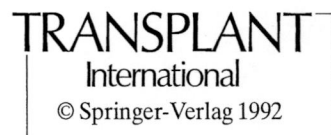

© Springer-Verlag 1992

Suppression of human lymphocyte proliferation and cytotoxic T lymphocyte generation by a soluble factor derived from K562 cells

K. Hayamizu, H. Yahata, Y. Fukuda, and K. Dohi

The Second Department of Surgery, Hiroshima University School of Medicine, Hiroshima, Japan

Abstract. The human myeloid leukemia cell line, K562, secrets a lymphocyte growth-suppressive factor (LGSF). We report our investigation of the immunological and chemical features of this factor. LGSF showed no cytolytic effect on human peripheral blood mononuclear cells (PBMC). Nevertheless, LGSF adequately suppressed in vitro alloantigen- or mitogen (PHA, ConA, PWM)-stimulated human PBMC proliferation and alloantigen-induced cytotoxic T lymphocyte generation, in antigen-nonspecific and LGSF concentration-related manners. LGSF retained activity after filtration through a 0.22 μm filter membrane and storage at – 80 °C for 6 months. Ultrafiltration experiments indicated that suppressive activity was retained in the higher molecular weight fraction (MW > 100000) and that the activity was heat-labile at 56 °C for 30 min. These results strongly suggested that LGSF is a noncytotoxically immunosuppressive substance with a high molecular weight.

Key words: Immunosuppression – Cytokine – Human leukemia cell line – Lymphocyte growth-suppressive factor – Cytotoxic T lymphocyte

---

The continuous cell line K562 was originally established by Lozzio et al. in 1975 from the pleural effusion of a patient with chronic myeloid leukemia [4]. The K562 cells are so sensitive to the direct tumoricidal activity of NK cells, K cells, and macrophages that they have been used as the standard target cells in such assays [3]. Some investigators have shown that K562 cells are able to diminish immunological reactions in vitro [1, 2, 5]. Olofsson et al. have reported that K562 cells produce a potent inhibitor of PHA-activated T-cell proliferation [5]. We confirmed the existence of lymphocyte growth-suppressive factor (LGSF) in the supernatant of cultured K562 cells which had been subcultured in our laboratory. In the present

study we investigated further the immunosuppressive activities of the factor against mitogen-stimulated lymphocyte growth, mixed lymphocyte reactions, and cytotoxic T lymphocyte generation.

Materials and methods

Cell culture. K562 cells, a gift from the Japanese Cancer Research Resources Bank, were maintained in RPMI 1640 (Gibco, Grand Island, N. Y.) containing 2 mM glutamine, 25 mM HEPES, 100 U/ml penicillin (Gibco), 100 μg/ml streptomycin (Gibco), supplemented with 10 % fetal calf serum [(FCS) Gibco] in 25 mm² tissue culture flasks (3013; Falcon, Oxnard, Calif.) at 37 °C in 5 % CO_2 humidified atmosphere. They were maintained thus in our laboratory for more than 2 years.

Preparation of LGSF. For the production of effective LGSF, exponentially growing K562 cells were cultured at 5×10^5 cells/ml in RPMI 1640, supplemented with 10 % heat-inactivated pooled human AB serum [complete medium (CM)] or without serum for 2 days, then centrifuged at 3000 rpm for 20 min. The supernatant harvested was passed through a 0.22 μm filter (Sterivex-GV; Millipore, Bedford, Mass.) and stored in conical tubes (2097; Falcon) at – 80 °C until used in the suppressor assays described below. Concentrations of LGSF presented in this paper are the final volume/volume ratio or its percentage expressions.

Preparation of lymphocytes. Human peripheral blood mononuclear cells (PBMC) were isolated from heparinized venous blood from healthy donors by using standard Ficoll-Hypaque density gradient centrifugation (Lymphoprep 1077; Nycomed, Oslo, Norway).

Mitogen-stimulated PBMC growth. Human PBMC (2×10^5) were cultured with serial dilutions of LGSF in 200 μl of CM, supplemented with 0.1 % PHA-P (Difco, Detroit, Mich.) or 64 μg/ml ConA (Miles Yedaltd) for 3 days, or with 1 % PWM (Gibco) for 5 days respectively, in each well of a flat-bottom 96-well microtiter plate (3072; Falcon). Triticated thymidine (^{3}H-TdR; Amersham, Buckinghamshire, England) (0.5 μCi/well) was added for the last 12 h of the culture period. The cells were subsequently harvested and assayed for ^{3}H-TdR uptake. The resultant suppression of the response is expressed by the percentage suppression calculated according to the formula:

% Suppression = (1 – cpm of LGSF-treated cultures/cpm of control cultures) × 100

Offprint requests to: Keisuke Hayamizu M. D., 1-2-3, Kasumi, Minami-ku, Hiroshima, 734, Japan

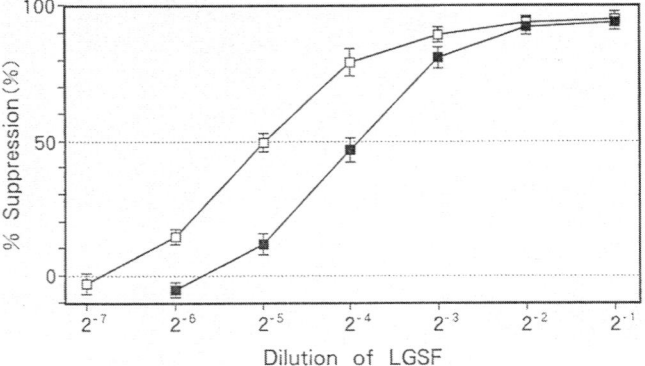

Fig. 1. Titration of suppressive activity of LGSF against PHA-stimulated lymphocyte growth. PBMC (2×10^5/culture) were cultured with 0.1% PHA and serial dilutions of LGSF prepared from the supernatant of K562 cell cultures with ($-\square-$) or without ($-\blacksquare-$) 10% pooled human AB serum in triplicate for 3 days. Cultures were assayed for ^{3}H-TdR uptake and the percentage suppression was calculated. ^{3}H-TdR uptake by the culture containing no LGSF was $69\,730 \pm 1\,642$ cpm. Data presented are the mean $\pm$ SD

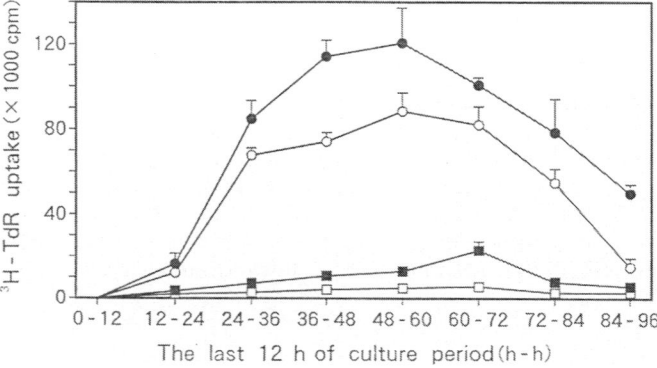

Fig. 2. Effect of LGSF on the kinetics of PHA-stimulated lymphocyte growth. PBMC (2×10^5/culture) were cultured with 2^{-1} (50%, $-\square-$), 2^{-3} (12.5%, $-\blacksquare-$), 2^{-5} (3.125%, $-\bigcirc-$) LGSF or without it (0%, $-\bullet-$), in the presence of 0.1% PHA. Three cultures were harvested every 12 h, pulsed with 0.5 µCi ^{3}H-TdR for the last 12 h of each culture period. Subsequently, the cultures were assayed for ^{3}H-TdR uptake. Data presented are the mean $\pm$ SD of the velocity of ^{3}H-TdR uptake (cpm/12 h)

The LGSF titers were expressed as the reciprocal dilutions causing 50% suppression.

One-way mixed lymphocyte reaction (MLR). Responder PBMC (1×10^5) and 2000 rad-irradiated stimulator allogeneic or autologous PBMC (1×10^5) were cultured together with 25% LGSF in 200 µl of CM in each well of the microtiter plate for 6 days. ^{3}H-TdR was added for the last 18 h of the culture period. The percentage suppression was calculated as described above.

^{51}*Cr release assay.* For the generation of cytotoxic T lymphocytes (CTL), PBMC (1×10^6/ml) were cultured with 2000 rad-irradiated PBMC (1×10^6/ml) and various dilutions of LGSF in a culture tube for 5 days. For the CTL assay, 3-day PHA-pretreated and ^{51}Cr (Na$_2$^{51}CrO$_4$; New England Nuclear, Boston, Mass.)-labeled target PBMC (1×10^4) and effector cells (5×10^5, 2.5×10^5, 1.25×10^5) in 200 µl of CM were put into each well of a U-bottom microtiter plate (Nunclon, Denmark). For the direct LGSF cytotoxicity assays, 50%

LGSF was used instead of the effector cells. After 4 h of incubation at 37°C, 100 µl of supernatant was collected and counted in a gamma counter. The percentage cytotoxicity was calculated using the following equation:

% Cytotoxicity = (experimental ^{51}Cr release – spontaneous ^{51}Cr release)/(maximum ^{51}Cr release – spontaneous ^{51}Cr release) $\times$ 100

Ultrafiltration experiment. LGSF was filtrated under high pressure using a Molcut-L (Millipore), incorporating the 100 000 nominal molecular weight limit (NMWL) membrane, and was separated into 2 fractions: the 10-fold-condensed fraction and the membrane breakthrough fraction with a lower molecular weight than 100 000 daltons. Subsequently each fraction was tested for PHA-stimulated PBMC growth-suppression assay.

Results

Effect of LGSF on mitogen-induced lymphocyte growth (Table 1). LGSF at a concentration of 25% (volume/volume) inhibited significantly the lymphocyte growth activated by the mitogens PHA, ConA and PWM. The mean percentage suppression for the 3 donors was 88% $\pm$ 3%, 89% $\pm$ 3% and 92% $\pm$ 2% respectively.

Titration of LGSF (Fig. 1). In the PHA-stimulated lymphocyte growth-suppression assay, the dose-response curve for LGSF was sigmoid shaped. The percentage suppression ranged between – 5% and 95%, over a 32-fold dilution of LGSF. The presence of serum did not affect the shape of the curve, but the LGSF titer required to produce the same effect without serum was 2.1-fold lower than that with 10% human serum.

Effect of LGSF on the kinetics of PHA-stimulated lymphocyte growth (Fig. 2). LGSF suppressed ^{3}H-TdR uptake throughout the entire culture period. The peak of ^{3}H-TdR uptake under various LGSF dilutions decreased in a LGSF dose-dependent way, but the culture time corresponding to peak uptake was almost constant.

Effect of LGSF on one-way MLR (Table 2). The 25% LGSF suppressed the proliferative response of lymphocytes stimulated by alloantigen. In six stimulator-respon-

Table 1. Effect of LGSF on mitogen-stimulated lymphocyte growth

Human PBMC	^{3}H-TdR uptake (cpm) Mitogen		
	PHA	ConA	PWM
KH	$5\,369 \pm 311$[a] $69\,515 \pm 1\,642$ (92.3)[b]	$4\,361 \pm 109$ $29\,451 \pm 1\,424$ (85.2)	$3\,383 \pm 803$ $25\,329 \pm 1\,629$ (86.6)
HY	$8\,092 \pm 230$ $60\,613 \pm 648$ (86.7)	$2\,774 \pm 145$ $33\,840 \pm 795$ (91.8)	$2\,437 \pm 34$ $29\,523 \pm 3\,056$ (91.7)
HW	$6\,313 \pm 187$ $44\,086 \pm 1\,335$ (85.7)	$5\,337 \pm 910$ $48\,857 \pm 3\,892$ (89.1)	$2\,782 \pm 405$ $30\,668 \pm 900$ (90.9)

[a] Data presented are the mean cpm of triplicates $\pm$ SD. Upper data are ^{3}H-TdR uptake of the culture with 25% LGSF and lower data are that of control

[b] Values in brackets indicate percentage suppression

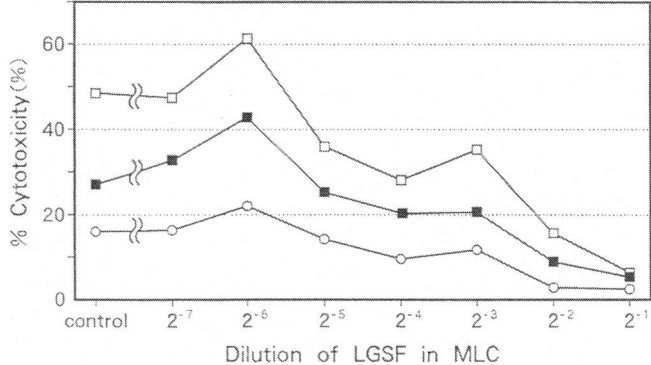

Fig. 3. Effects of LGSF concentration in the MLC on CTL generation. One-way MLCs were performed with serial dilutions of LGSF for 5 days and washed to remove the factor. Thereafter CTL activity of each MLC to stimulator (10^4/culture) as target was tested for ^{51}Cr release assay in duplicate. Effector/target cell ratios were 50/1 ($-\square-$), 25/1 ($-\blacksquare-$) and 12.5/1 ($-\bigcirc-$) respectively. Maximum ^{51}Cr released by lysed target cells per well was 5572 ± 73 cpm, and ^{51}Cr released spontaneously was 558 ± 11 cpm. The percentage cytotoxity of each test was calculated and the mean are presented

der allogeneic combinations among three donors (KH, MI, HW) expressing different HLA types, the mean percentage suppression was 85 % ± 4 %.

Effect of LGSF on alloantigen-induced CTL generation (Fig. 3). The addition of LGSF to MLC caused a decrease in the percentage cytotoxicity of the CTL generated against the allogeneic target PBMC. The percentage cytotoxicity was suppressed from 48 % to 7 % (E/T = 50), and the amount of decrease was dependent on the LGSF concentration in the MLC.

Direct cytotoxicity of LGSF. The percentage cytotoxicity of 50 % LGSF against PBMC in direct ^{51}Cr release assays was only 0.3 %. The cell viability for trypan blue exclusion of the 2-day PHA-stimulated cultures with or without

Table 2. Effect of LGSF on one-way mixed lymphocyte reaction

Responder	^{3}H-TdR uptake (cpm) Stimulator		
	KH	MI	HW
KH	$1639 \pm 532^{a, NS}$ 470 ± 993 $(-248.7)^b$	7044 ± 437 29258 ± 3148 (75.9)	5027 ± 1005 31030 ± 4018 (83.8)
MI	4471 ± 838 32050 ± 1762 (86.0)	1152 ± 147^{NS} 335 ± 283 (-243.4)	3334 ± 415 26550 ± 876 (87.4)
HW	2607 ± 156 23119 ± 1557 (88.7)	2313 ± 304 18698 ± 2165 (87.6)	1460 ± 88^{NS} 848 ± 609 (-72.3)

[a] Data presented are the mean cpm of triplicates ± SD. Upper data are ^{3}H-TdR uptake of the culture with 25 % LGSF and lower data are that of control
[b] Values in brackets indicate percent suppression
[NS] The difference between the data of LGSF-containing cultures and control are not significant ($P > 0.05$) for Student's t-test. Other data are significant ($P < 0.01$)

50 % LGSF was 95 % ± 11 % and 93 % ± 15 % respectively, and the difference was not significant using Student's t-test. Therefore, these data suggested that the inhibition occurs via a noncytotoxic mechanism.

Chemical features of LGSF. LGSF was stored at $-80\,^\circ$C in a stable condition for more than 6 months. Ultrafiltration experiments showed a 5.3 times increase in the LGSF titer of a 10-fold condensed fraction of the initial filtered supernatant using a membrane with a 100000 dalton NMWL, and the fraction that passed through the membrane revealed no suppressive activity. The fraction with the higher titer completely lost activity after incubation at $56\,^\circ$C for 30 min.

Discussion

We investigated the possibility that established human hematopoietic cell lines produce active suppressive factors against normal human lymphocyte proliferation. We found that the supernatant of K562 cell cultures showed detectable suppressive activity, and called the factor LGSF. Lozzio et al. have determined in full the character of original K562 cells, and found them to produce neither immunoglobulins nor interferons, to be free of Epstein-Barr virus and herpes-like virus particles, and to show no reverse transcriptase activity [3]. Olofsson et al. have already reported that K562 cells produce an inhibitor of cell growth. The factor is restricted to activity against hematopoietic cells. It is most active against PHA-activated T cells and myeloid stem cells, less active against erythroid precursors, and does not inhibit fibroblasts or established lines of epithelioid cells or B cells [5]. These facts gave us hope for the possibility of a clinical application for LGSF as an immunosuppressive agent with few side effects.

In this study, further immunological features were examined, and LGSF produced by K562 cells was found to suppress mitogen-stimulated lymphocyte growth not only by PHA but also by ConA and PWM in a dose-dependent manner, and to inhibit alloantigen-stimulated lymphocyte growth and CTL generation alloantigen-nonspecifically, via a noncytotoxic mechanism.

Because of their high sensitivity K562 cells are used as the standard targets in NK assays, and also in macrophage tumoricidal assays [3]. The NK sensitivity of K562 cells is diminished by a differentiating agent, sodium butyrate [1] and the anti-K562 cytotoxicity of monocytes is inhibited by the supernatant of K562 cell cultures [2]. Although the precise mechanism of this sensitivity modulation is unknown, it is interesting that our subcultured K562 cells displayed potent lymphocyte growth-suppressive activity, despite retaining NK sensitivity.

As for the chemical features of LGSF, the suspision that LGSF was an altered serum protein was ruled out by the fact that K562 cells produced this factor in a serum-free medium. In addition, LGSF was secreted only during the log-growth phase of K562 cells, and filtered through 0.22 μm pores, so the possibility that LGSF represented the influence of contaminating organisms in the supernatant was also excluded.

This study provided evidence for the production of an efficient immunosuppressive substance with a high molecular weight by the leukemic cell line K562, which showed cytostatic effects on human lymphocytes. Studies on the application of condensed LGSF for the prevention of graft rejection in vivo in animals, and the biochemical purification of LGSF are in progress.

References

1. Dokhelar M, Testa U, Vainchenker W, Finale Y, Tetaud C, Salem P, Tursz T (1982) NK cell sensitivity of the leukemic K562 cells; Effect of sodium butyrate and hemin induction. J Immunol 128: 211–216
2. Kiczka W, Szkaradkiewicz A (1986) Suppression of monocyte mediated anti K562 cytotoxicity by soluble factors in the serum of cancer patients and in the supernatant of K562 cell culture. Immunol Lett 13: 127–131
3. Lozzio BB, Lozzio CB (1979) Properties and usefulness of the original K-562 human myelogenous leukemia cell line. Leuk Res 3: 363–370
4. Lozzio CB, Lozzio BB (1975) Human chronic myelogenous leukemia cell-line with positive Philadelphia chromosome. Blood 45: 321–334
5. Olofsson T, Cline MJ (1978) Inhibitor of hematopoietic cell proliferation derived from a human leukemic cell line. Blood 52: 143–152

Transplant Int (1992) 5 [Suppl 1]: S 665–S 669

TRANSPLANT
International
© Springer-Verlag 1992

FK 506 ameliorates normothermic liver ischemia in rats by suppressing production of tumor necrosis factor

Katsunori Kawano[1], **Yang Il Kim**[1], **Shigeru Goto**[1], **Tetsuji Kai**[1], **Tatsuo Shimada**[2], **Naoshi Kamada**[3], and **Michio Kobayashi**[1]

Departments of [1] Surgery I and [2] Anatomy, Oita Medical College, Oita, Japan
[3] Department of Experimental Surgery, National Children's Medical Research Center, Tokyo, 154, Japan

Abstract. In recent years, there has been growing evidence that tumor necrosis factor-α (TNF) plays an important role in the development of hepatic injury after ischemia-reperfusion. We have previously demonstrated that the immunosuppressants, cyclosporine, azathioprine and FK 506 (FK), have a protective effect on warm ischemic injury of the rat liver. In the present study, we attempted to elucidate the mechanism for the beneficial effect of FK on liver ischemia, with special reference to the suppression of TNF production. After 60 min and 90 min of warm liver ischemia, the survival rates were significantly improved by FK pretherapy. This was associated with amelioration of hepatic injury, as assessed by histological examinations and determinations of serum AST and lipid peroxide levels in the liver. After 60 min of liver ischemia, TNF was measurable during the reperfusion period in the sera of the control animals, peaking of 6 h after reperfusion (123 ± 15.8 pg/ml, mean SEM). In contrast, pretreatment with FK significantly suppressed the elevation of serum TNF levels at the same time point (75.8 ± 13.1 pg/ml, $P < 0.05$). The present data showed that liver ischemia-reperfusion resulted in TNF production, and that FK could protect the liver from reperfusion injury by suppressing this production of TNF.

Key words: Liver ischemia – FK 506 – Lipid peroxidation – Tumor necrosis factor

Primary graft nonfunction, which has been reported to be associated with ischemic injury, is a major indication for retransplantation following liver transplantation [1]. Furthermore, there is evidence that severe preservation injury to endothelial cells results in an increased incidence of allograft rejection [2]. Recently, there has been great interest in methods for protecting the liver from ischemia-reperfusion injury. Although the precise mechanism has not been elucidated, we have recently reported that cyclosporine (CsA) and azathioprine (AZA) ameliorate both warm and cold ischemic injury of the liver in rats and pigs [3–6]. More recently, FK 506 (FK), a potent new immunosuppressive

agent, has been shown to possess a similar protective effect [7, 8], suggesting a possible linkage between the immune system and ischemic injury of the liver.

The purpose of this study was to clarify the mechanism by which FK exerts its beneficial effect on warm ischemia in the rat liver, with special reference to the suppression of lipid peroxides and of tumor necrosis factor-α (TNF) production.

Materials and methods

Female Sprague-Dawley rats weighing 200–300 g were used throughout this study. A temporary normothermic liver ischemia was induced as decribed by us in previous study [3]. Briefly, the abdomen was opened through a midline incision under light ether anesthesia. Liver ischemia was produced by occluding the hepatic artery and the portal vein to the left lateral and median lobes with a small vascular clip. The remaining hepatic lobes were excised at reperfusion, leaving only the ischemic lobes behind. The antibiotic, cefamandole sodium (100 mg/kg), was administered intramuscularly just prior to laparotomy.

The rats were assigned to two groups. In the control group (group I), the animals underwent warm liver ischemia with saline vehicle pretherapy. Group II rats received FK (1 mg/kg/day p.o.) for 4 days prior to the induction of liver ischemia. The FK 506 (Fujisawa Pharmaceutical Co., Ltd., Osaka, Japan) was suspended in a physiologic saline solution.

For the survival study, a total of 96 rats were subjected to 60 min or 90 min of liver ischemia. Autopsy was performed in all animals that died during the observation period, and survivors were sacrificed 7 days after surgery.

In a second experiment, four to nine rats were sacrificed before, during and 1, 6 and 12 h after reperfusion. Immediately before sacrifice, blood samples were taken from the inferior vena cava for measuring serum levels of aspartate aminotransferase (S-AST). They were determined by an ultraviolet method using an autoanalyzer (Jeol JCA-MS24, Japan). Serum activities of TNF were measured using an ELISA kit (Otsuka, Tokyo, Japan). At the same time, a portion of the ischemic median hepatic lobe was taken for determination of lipid perioxide content and for histological examination. Lipid peroxide was estimated as levels of malondialdehyde (MDA), using a colorimetric reaction with thiobarbituric acid [9]. Protein concentration was determined according to the method described by Lowry et al. [10]. Sections of the liver were examined with both a light and a transmission electron microscope.

The results were expressed as the mean and the standard error of the mean, and were statistically compared using the generalized Wilcoxon's test or the Student's t-test. Statistical significance was defined as a P value less than 0.05.

Offprint requests to: Katsunori Kawano, M.D., Department of Surgery I, Oita Medical Collge, Oita, 879-55, Japan

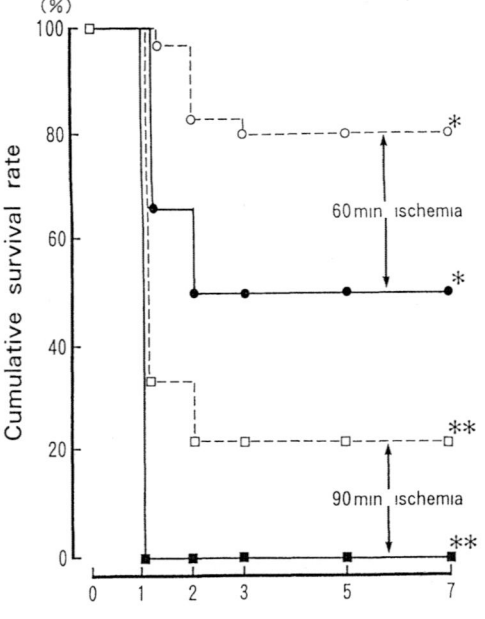

Fig. 1. Cumulative survival rates of the rats after 60 min and 90 min of liver ischemia. The differences between groups I and II were significant at * $P < 0.05$ for 60 min ischemia and * $P < 0.005$ for 90 min ischemia. (Control at 60 min –●– and at 90 min –■–; FK506 at 60 min, --○-- and at 90 min --□--)

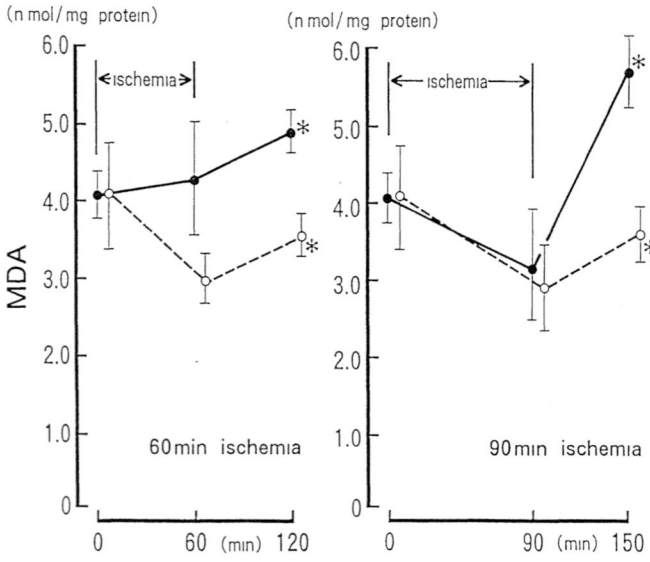

Fig. 2. The effect of FK 506 on MDA levels in an ischemic liver. MDA levels were measured before, during and 1 h after 60 min and 90 min of liver ischemia. Each point shows the mean ± SEM. The differences between groups I and II were significant at * $P < 0.01$. (control, –●–; FK 506, --○--)

Results

Cumulative survival curves after 60 min and 90 min of liver ischemia are shown in Fig. 1. Survival rates at day 7, calculated using the Kaplan-Meier method, were 50.0 % (19/38) and 80.0 % (24/30) for groups I and II respectively, after 60 min of ischemia. Those after 90 min of liver ische-

mia were 0 % (0/10) and 22.2 % (4/18) for the rats not-treated and treated with FK, respectively. The differences between the two groups after both 60 min and 90 min of liver ischemia were statistically significant ($P < 0.05$ for 60 min ischemia and $P < 0.005$ for 90 min ischemia).

Serial changes in MDA levels are depicted in Fig. 2. After 60 min of liver ischemia, the MDA levels in the control group remained steady during the ischemic period but tended to increase 1 h after reperfusion. In contrast, the MDA levels in the FK-treated group were reduced to 73.2 % of the initial value at the and of the ischemic period. At 1 h after reflow of blood, the levels in group II were significantly suppressed compared with those in group I (4.95 ± 0.30 nmol/mg protein, $n = 9$, for group I; 3.59 ± 0.29, $n = 6$, for group II; $P < 0.01$). A similar result was observed in the 90 min of liver ischemia model. At 60 min after reperfusion, the difference in the MDA levels in the two groups was statistically significant (5.72 ± 0.46, $n = 8$, for group I; 3.68 ± 0.28, $n = 5$, for group II; $P < 0.01$).

Histological alterations in representative livers taken at 1 h after reperfusion of ischemic livers are shown in Figs. 3 and 4. On light microscopic examination, parenchymal cells with eosinophilic changes and spotty necrosis of the hepatocytes were seen in the control group (Fig. 3 a). In contrast, in the FK-treated group some eosinophilic changes were seen in the hepatocytes associated with swelling, but to a lesser degree (Fig. 3 b). In group I electron microscopy showed detachment of endothelial cells from hepatocytes, thus allowing blood cells to infiltrate into Disse's space (Fig. 4 a). In contrast, the structures of the hepatic sinusoid and Disse's space were relatively well preserved in the liveer treated with FK (Fig. 4 b).

Serial changes of serum TNF levels are illustrated in Fig. 5. In the control group, the levels rose sharply at 6 h following reperfusion and declined thereafter. A similar pattern was observed in group II. When the peak values were compared, however, FK-treated animals (75.8 ± 13.1 pg/ml, $n = 7$) had significantly lower levels than those in the control group (123.2 ± 15.8, $n = 7$; $P < 0.05$). Serum levels of AST showed a parallel change with that of TNF (Fig. 6). A substantial difference between the two groups was seen at 6 h after reperfusion (10942 ± 802 IU/l, $n = 8$, for group I; $7637 P < 807$, $n = 8$, for group II, $P < 0.02$).

Discussion

As has been reported previously for CsA and AZA [3–5], we demonstrated in the present study that pretherapy with FK 506 improved the survival of rats following warm liver ischemia. This was reflected by amelioration of hepatic injury which was estimated by histological examination and quantified by measuring serum AST. We hypothesize that suppression of lipid perixodative damage and of TNF production might be the main mechanisms by which FK protects the liver from an ischemic insult.

Deleterious chemical reactions involving oxygen-derived free radicals have been shown to be the causes of

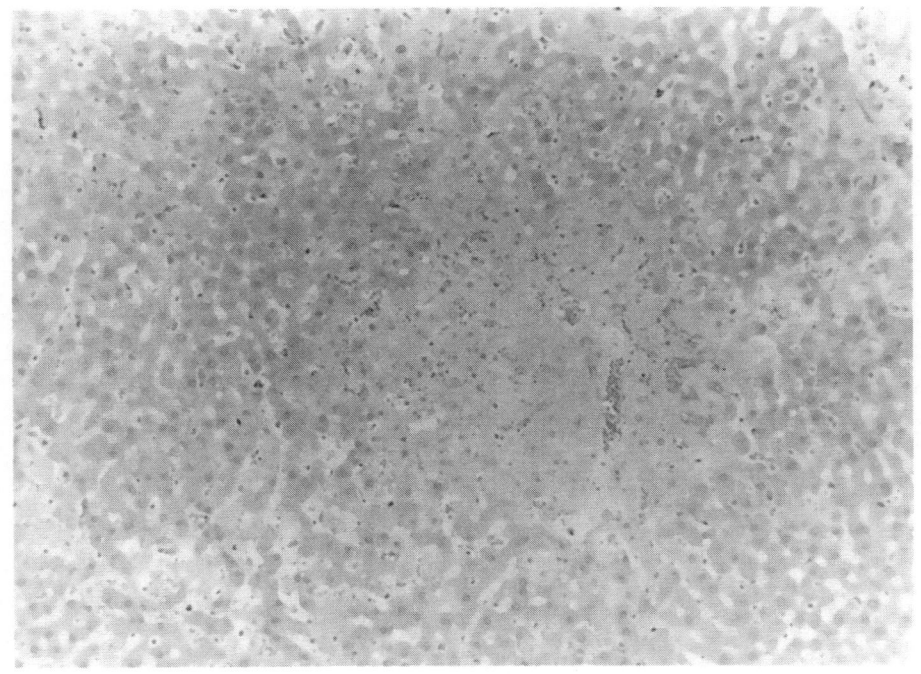

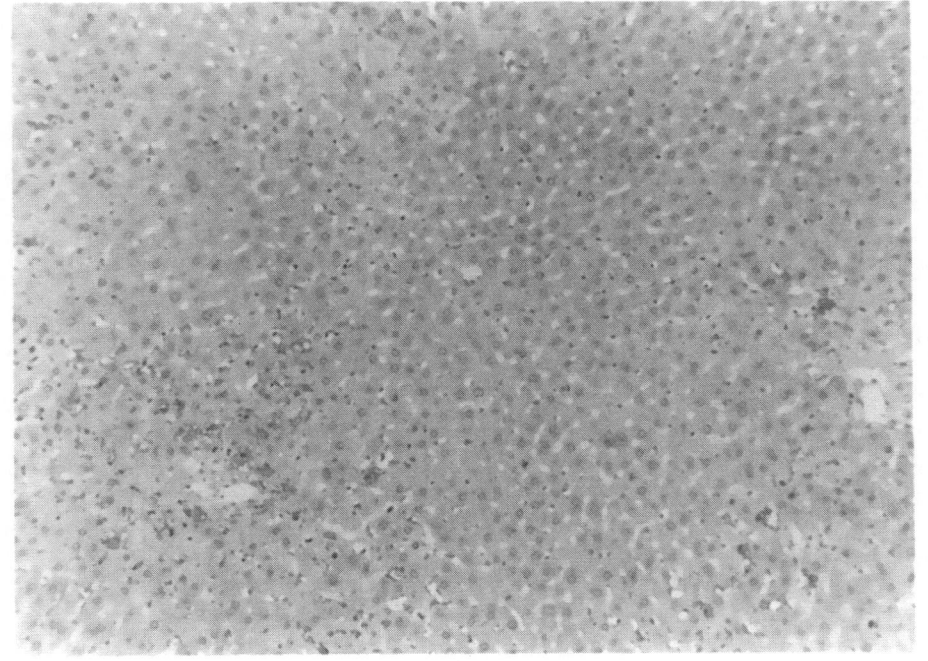

Fig. 3 a, b. Light microscopic examination of the liver **a** not treated and **b** treated with FK 506. Specimens were taken 1 h after reperfusion following 60 min of liver ischemia, H&E (× 190)

ischemia-reperfusion injury which occur immediately following reperfusion [11–13]. In the present study, it was observed that pretherapy with FK suppressed the tissue levels of MDA which is one of the stable end-products of lipid peroxides. Although there are some possible sources for the production of the free radicals, it has been suggested that reactive oxygen intermediates are released by activated hepatic macrophages [14, 15] and by circulating neutrophils [16]. In this regard, it has been reported that CsA reduces the capacity of macrophages to produce hydrogen peroxide (H_2O_2) and the superoxide anion ($Osup-_2$ [17], although whether FK suppresses such production of oxygen radicals is unknown. Thus, we postulated that FK suppressed lipid peroxide reactions, which

might initiate hepatic reperfusion injury, by inhibiting the activation of macrophages and/or neutrophils.

Cytokines are increasingly being recognized as critical mediators of ischemic injury to the liver [18]. Among the inflammatory cytokines, TNF, which is produced primarily by cells of the monocyte/macrophage lineage including the liver Kupffer cells, has been shown to exert profound effects on both neutrophils and endothelial cells. It has been reported that TNF stimulates neutrophil adhesion to rat liver sinusoidal endothelial cells and increases respiratory burst activity [16, 19]. Moreover, TNF may activate endothelial cells to initiate coagulation [20, 21], and render these cells more susceptible to neutrophil-mediated damage [22]. Taking into consideration the fact that FK

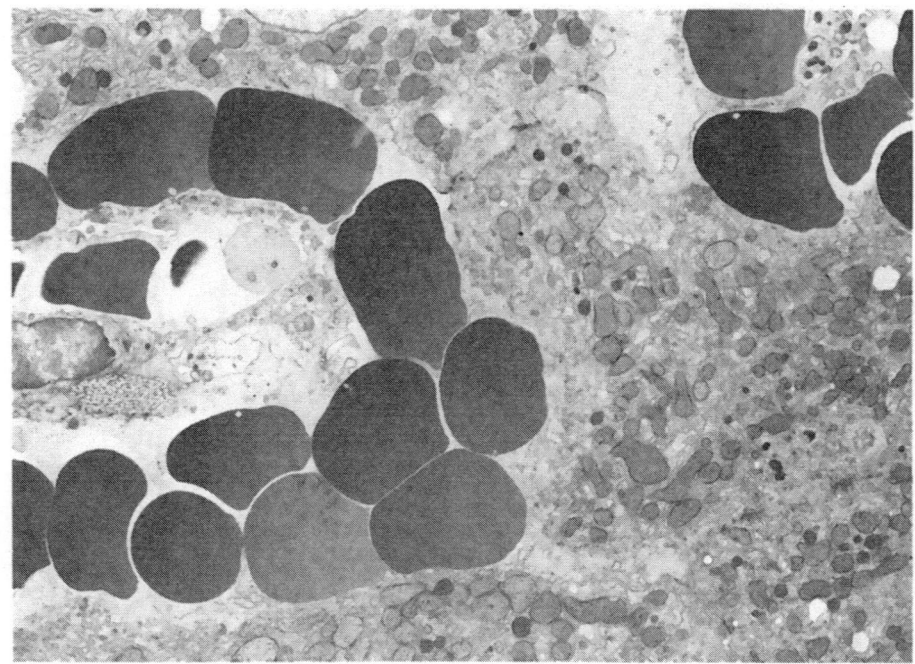

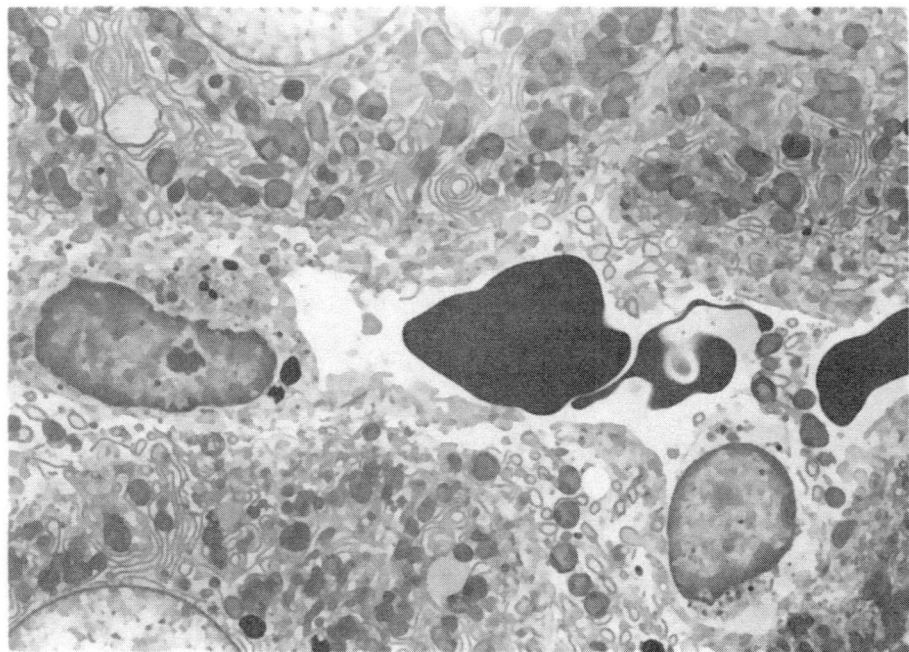

Fig. 4 a, b. Electron microscopic examination of the liver taken 1 h after reperfusion following 60 min of liver ischemia. **a** Liver of the control rats; **b** liver of the animals treated with FK 506 (× 5200)

inhibits the expression of TNF genes [23] we propose that FK exerts its protective effect against liver ischemia by suppressing the production of TNF which might accelerate hepatic injury after reperfusion.

Whether the hepatotrophic effect of FK is dependent on or independent of its immunosuppressive properties remains controversial [24]. However, it is equally conceivable that the hepatotrophic quality of this fungal agent affects the ability to recover from the ischemic injury [25]. We are testing the effect of the pretreatment of the donor or the liver graft liver FK or other immunosuppressants for a possible use in liver transplantation. Moreover, we are pursuing further experiments to observe whether this agent ameliorates pulmonary pathologic changes which are often associated with hepatic injury.

In conclusion, we confirmed the protective effect of FK 506 on warm liver ischemia in the rat. We suggested that suppressed production of lipid peroxides and TNF might account for its beneficial effect on liver ischemia.

Acknowledgements. The authors wish to thank Professor M. Ito and Mr. Y. Magari, Department of Laboratory Medicine, Oita Medical College, Oita, Japan, for assistance. This work was supported by a grant for paediatric research (63-A-05) from the Ministry of Health and Welfare and by a grant for scientific research (A-10440054) from the Ministry of Education, Science and Culture, Japan.

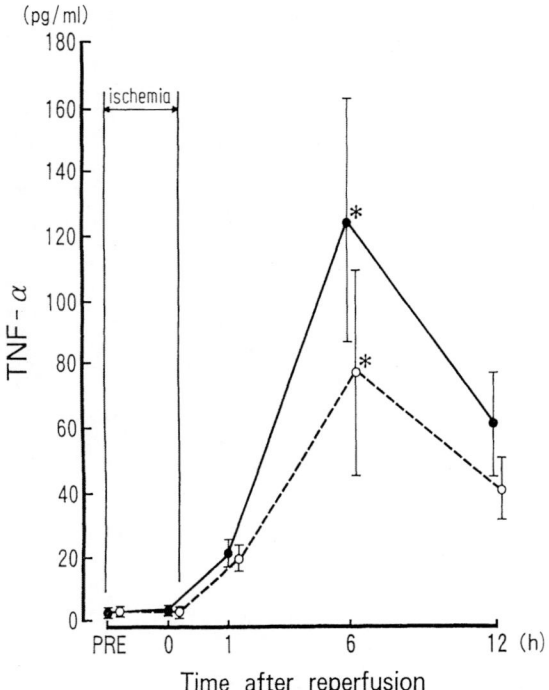

Fig. 5. Serial changes of serum TNF levels after 60 min of liver ischemia in the rats treated or not treated with FK 506. Each point shows the mean ± SEM. The differences between groups I and II were significant *$P < 0.05$ 6 h after reperfusion (control, – ● –; FK 506, -- ○ --)

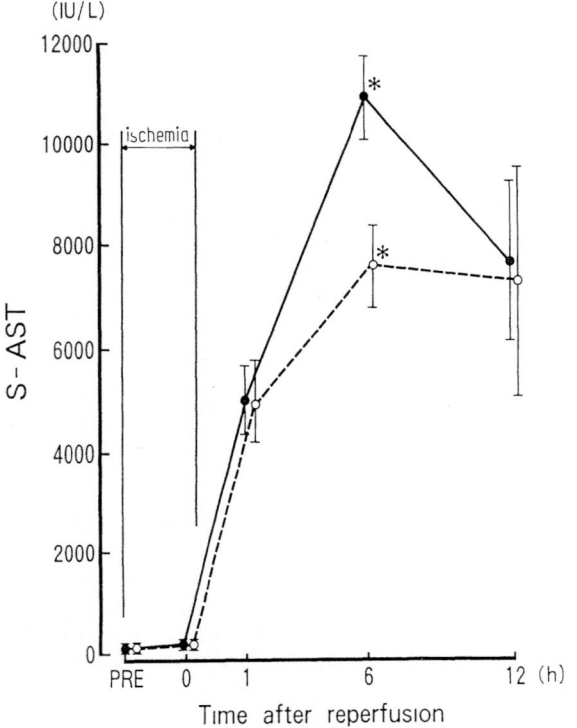

Fig. 6. Serum levels of AST following 60 min of warm liver ischemia. Each point shows the mean ± SEM. The difference between groups I and II 6 h after reperfusion was *$P < 0.02$. (control, – ● –; FK 506, -- ○ --)

References

1. Shaw BW, Wood RP (1989) Improved results with retransplantation of the liver. Transplant Proc 21: 2407–2408
2. Howard TK, Klintmalm GBG, Cofer JB, Husberg BS, Goldstein RM, Gonwa TA (1990) The influence of preservation injury on rejection in the hepatic transplant recipient. Transplantation 49: 103–107
3. Kawano K, Kim YI, Katetani K, Kobayashi M (1989) The beneficial effect of cyclosporine on liver ischemia in rats. Transplantation 48: 759–764
4. Kawano K, Kim YI, Goto S, et al (1990) Evidence that azathioprine, as well as cyclosporine, ameliorates warm ischemia in the rat liver. Transplantation 49: 1002–1003
5. Kim YI, Kawano K, Goto S, et al (1991) Beneficial effect of pretreatment with azathioprine on warm and cold ischemia of the swine liver. Transplant Proc 23: 2201–2203
6. Goto S, Kim YI, Kamada N, Kawano K, Kobayashi M (1990) The beneficial effect of pretransplant cyclosporine therapy on recipient rats grafted with a 12-hour cold-stored liver. Transplantation 49: 1003–1004
7. Kawano K, Kim YI, Goto S, Ono M, Kabayashi M (1991) A protective effect of FK 506 in ischemically injured rat livers. Transplantation 52: 143–145
8. Sakr MF, Zetti GM, Farghali H, et al (1991) Protective effect of FK 506 against hepatic ischemia in rats. Transplant Proc 23: 340–341
9. Ohkawa H, Ohishi N, Yagi K (1979) Assay for lipid peroxides in animal tissue by thiobarbituric acid reaction. Anal Biochem 95: 351–358
10. Lowry OH, Rosebrough NJ, Lewis Farr AL, Randall RJ (1951) Protein measurement with the folin phenol reagent. J Biol Chem 193: 265–275
11. McCord JM (1985) Oxygen derived free radicals in post-ischemic tissue injury. N Engl J Med 312: 159–163
12. Marubayashi S, Dohi K, Ochi K, Kawasaki T (1986) Role of free radicals in ischemic rat liver cell injury: prevention of damage by α-tocopherol administration. Surgery 99: 184–192
13. Southard JH, Marsh DC, McAnulty JF, Belzer FO (1987) Oxygen-derived free radical damage in organ preservation: activity of superoxide dismutase and xanthine oxidase. Surgery 101: 566–570
14. Shiratori Y, Kawase T, Shiina S, et al (1988) Modulation of hepatotoxicity by macrophages in the liver. Hepatology 8: 815–821
15. Arthur MJP, Kowalski-Saunders P, Wright R (1988) Effect of endotoxin on release of reactive oxygen intermediates by rat hepatic macrophages. Gastroenterology 95: 1588–1594
16. Nathan CF (1987) Neutrophil activation on biological surfaces: massive secretion of hydrogen peroxide in response to products of macrophages and lymphocytes. J Clin Invest 80: 1550–1560
17. Goldin H, Keisari Y (1989) The effect of cyclosporine on macrophage oxidative burst potential during graft-versus-host reactions in mice. Transplantation 47: 548–552
18. Colletti LM, Remick DG, Burtch GD, Kunkel SL, Strieter RM, Campbell DA (1990) Role of tumor necrosis factor in the pathophysiologic alterations after hepatic ischemia/reperfusion injury in the rat. J Clin Invest 85: 1936–1943
19. Schlayer HJ, Laaff H, Peters T, et al (1988) Involvement of tumor necrosis factor in endotoxin-triggered neutrophil adherence to sinusoidal endothelial cells of mouse liver and its modulation in acute phase. J Hepatol 7: 239–249
20. Bevilacqua MP, Pober JS, Majeau GR, Fiers W, Cotran RS, Gimbrone MA (1986) Recombinant tumor necrosis factor induces procoagulant activity in cultured human vascular endothelium. Proc Natl Acad Sci USA 83: 4533–4537
21. Nawroth PP, Stern DM (1986) Modulation of endothelial-cell hemostatic properties by tumor necrosis factor. J Exp Med 163: 740–745
22. Varani J, Bendelow MJ, Sealey DE, et al (1988) Tumor necrosis factor enhances susceptibility of vascular endothelial cells to neutrophil-mediated killing. Lab Invest 59: 292–295
23. Tocci MJ, Matkovichr DA, Collier KA, et al (1989) The immunosuppressant FK 506 selectively inhibits expression of early T cell activation genes. J Immunol 143: 718–726
24. Starzl TE, Porter KA, Mazzaferro V, Todo S, Fung J, Francavilla A (1991) Hepatotrophic effects of FK 506 in dogs. Transplantation 51: 67–70
25. Francavilla A, Barone M, Starzl TE, et al (1990) FK 506 as a growth control factor. Transplant Proc 23: 90–92

Transplant Int (1992) 5 [Suppl 1]: S670–S672

TRANSPLANT
International
© Springer-Verlag 1992

Donor directed cytotoxicity of cardiac graft infiltrating cells during cytomegalovirus infection

A. J. Ouwehand[1], **A. H. M. M. Balk**[2], **C. C. Baan**[3], **C. R. Daane**[3], **H. J. Metselaar**[4], **K. Groeneveld**[3], **N. H. P. M. Jutte**[3], **E. Bos**[1], and **W. Weimar**[3]

[1] Departments of Thoracic Surgery, [2] Cardiology, [3] Internal Medicine I and [4] II, Erasmus University Rotterdam, University Hospital Rotterdam-Dijkzigt, Rotterdam, The Netherlands

Abstract. We investigated whether cytomegalovirus (CMV) infection had an effect on donor directed cytotoxicity of cardiac graft infiltrating cells. The group we studied comprised 89 heart transplant recipients. Thirtyeight showed signs of CMV infection, and in 27 of them cytolytic activity of biopsy-derived cultures could be tested during the infection. Fity-one patients had never had CMV infection, and they were used as the control group. Eight patients had a primary, and 19 a secondary infection. We found that during CMV infection, both primary and secondary, a significantly higher proportion of the biopsy-derived cultures showed cytotoxicity against donor antigens ($P < 0.01$ when compared to the control group). In secondary infections, this was only due to an increase in donor class I directed cytotoxicity, while in primary infections a significant increase of class II directed cytotoxicity was also found ($P < 0.005$ when compared to secondary infection).

Key words: Cytomegalovirus – Alloreactivity – Graft infiltrating cells – Heart transplantation

Cytomegalovirus (CMV) infection is the most common problem due to infectious disease in immunosuppressed allograft recipients, and is a major cause of morbidity and mortality. The virus can induce viral disease, superinfections with other micro-organisms and immunomodulation. Furthermore, there may be a relationship between CMV infection and graft rejection. In the present study, we investigated the effect of CMV infection on donor directed cytotoxicity of graft infiltrating cells, and this was compared with a control group without infection.

Materials and methods

Patients. We studied CML reactivity of biopsy-derived lymphocytes from 89 heart transplant recipients. The immunosuppressive regimen consisted of cyclosporin A (CsA) and low dose prednisone.

Offprint requests to: A. J. Ouwehand, Dept. Internal Medicine I, Bd 299, Erasmus University, P. O. Box 1738, 3000 DR Rotterdam, The Netherlands

The CMV serostatus of the transplant recipients was screened for anti-CMV IgG by an ELISA. All CMV seronegative recipients received anti-CMV Immunoglobulins (Cytotect, Biotest Pharma GmbH, Dreieich, FRG), irrespective of the CMV serostatus of the allograft donor [4]. Samples of urine, throat wash, and blood were collected for virus isolation or a CMV early antigen test every 14 days for 3 months [6]. Specific anti-CMV immunofluorescence studies were done on all cultures. Routine monitoring included serology using an indirect immunofluorescence assay for IgM antibodies and an ELISA for IgG antibodies. A patient was considered to have CMV infection when a rise of CMV IgM antibodies and/or a positive CMV early antigen test was found.

All 89 patients were followed from the day of transplantation. Thirty-eight of them had CMV infection, and in 27 out of the 38 patients cytolytic activity of graft infiltrating cells could be tested during the infection. Of the 27 patients tested, 10 had clinical symptoms. Fifty-one patients had never and CMV infection, and they were used as the control group. In the patients without infection, we analyzed the biopsy-derived cells over a comparable period to the patients with infection, which was the first 228 days after transplantation (the median follow up in the patients with infection).

Culture method. Lymphocyte cultures were established from endomyocardial biopsies (EMB) as described by us in an earlier study [5]. In brief, each biopsy was cultured in a 96 well roundbottom tissue culture plate (Costar 3799, Cambridge, Mass.) with 200 µl culture medium per well, in the presence of 10^5 irradiated (40 Gy) autologous peripheral blood mononuclear leukocytes (PBMC) as feeders. Culture medium consisted of RPMI-1640-Dutch modification (Gibco, Paisley, Scotland) supplemented with 10 % v/v lectin-free lymphocult-T-LF (Biotest GmbH, Dreieich, FRG) as an exogenous source of interleukin 2 (IL-2), 10 % pooled human serum, 4 mM L-glutamine, 100 IU/ml penicillin and 100 µgg/ml streptomycin.

Cell-mediated cytotoxicity assays. A 4-h ^{51}Cr release assay was used to measure the cytotoxic capacity of the cultures against donor cells and a panel of unrelated target cells (EBV transformed B-cell lines or PHA blasts) sharing one or more HLA antigens with the donor. Serial double dilutions with E:T ratios varying from 1.25:1 up to 80:1 were used.

Results

Eighty-four EMB-derived cultures from 27 patients could be tested during CMV infection (1–7 per patient, median 2). From the individual patients without infection, one to ten biopsies (median four) yielded sufficient

Table 1. Donor directed cytotoxicity of EMB-derived cultures before, during and after infection with CMV. This is compared with the control group without infection. All patient groups were analyzed over a comparable period after transplantation

	CML specificity		
	donor n^a (%)	class I n^a (%)	DR n^a (%)
< 41 days[b]			
Before infection	62 (79)	57 (73)	43 (55)
Control group	101 (71)	92 (65)	54 (41)
≤ 228 days[c]			
During infection	74* (88)	71** (85)	37 (47)
Control group	173 (74)	157 (67)	106 (48)
229–365 days			
After infection	11 (65)	11 (65)	6 (35)
Control group	17 (65)	15 (58)	9 (38)

[a] n = number of reactive cultures
[b] median follow up before the first clinical evidence of infection (a rise of CMV-IgM and/or a positive CMV-EA test)
[c] median follow up in the patients with infection
* $P = 0.01$ when compared to the control group (X^2 test)
** $P < 0.005$ when compared to the control group (X^2 test)

Table 2. Donor directed cytotoxicity of EMB-derived cultures during primary and secondary CMV infection

	CML specificity		
≤ 228 days	donor n (%)	class I n (%)	DR n (%)
Primary infection	27 (90)	26 (87)	21* (70)
Secondary infection	47 (87)	45 (83)	16 (33)

* $P < 0.005$ when compared to cultures from secondary infected patients, and $P < 0.05$ when compared to the control group (X^2 test)

CLASS I DIRECTED CYTOTOXICITY

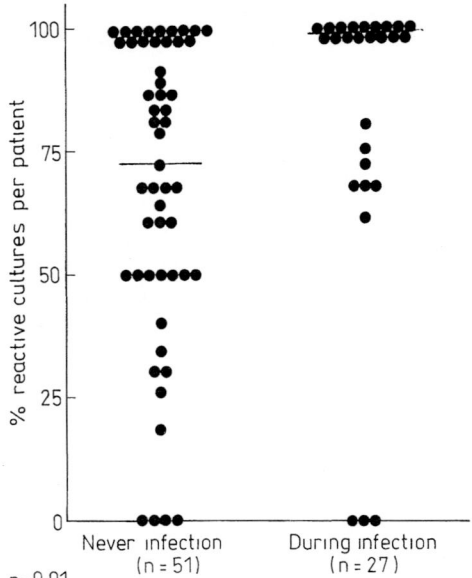

p = 0.01

Fig. 1. The percentage of cultures reactive against HLA class I mismatches for each individual patient (each *not* represents one patient). During CMV infection significantly more patients yielded a high number of reactive cultures compared to the control group who never had CMV infection ($P = 0.01$, Wilcoxon test)

Discussion

Many reports describe a relationship between CMV infection and an increased incidence of acute rejection. This relationship with rejection suggests that during infection, donor directed cytotoxic reactivity is increased. Indeed, in the present study we found an increased donor reactivity of graft infiltrating cells during infection. This proved to be due mainly to an increased cytolytic activity directed against HLA class I mismatches. Before the first clinical signs of infection could be demonstrated, we found that the cytolytic activity was comparable to the control group. This was in contrast to data described by Grundy et al. [2], who found a depression of in vitro CML responses against alloantigens early after inoculation of the virus in susceptible mice. This was followed by a phase of enhanced alloreactivity. This may have been due to other characteristics of the mouse-CMV. Our finding of increased class I directed cytotoxicity during CMV infection was consistent with the findings of others [1, 3], who have shown that the virus could directly enhance MHC class I and ICAM-1 expression on graft tissue. Grundy has shown that the virus not only increases MHC class I expression, but it also has a direct enhancing effect on the alloreactive CTL response. Von Willebrand et al. [7] have described an increased expression of HLA class II antigens on tubulus cells and endothelial cells directly after the onset of clinical symptoms, and they suggested that this was an indirect (lymphokines) consequence of the virus infection. We found that in patients with primary infection, of whom the majority had clinical symptoms, not only class I, but also class II directed cytotoxicity of graft infiltrating cells was increased. In conclusion, during

cells for cell mediated lympholysis. During CMV infection, a significantly higher percentage of donor reactive cultures was found compared to the control group ($P = 0.01$, Table 1). This proved to be due to an increase in HLA class I directed cytotoxicity ($P < 0.005$). Before signs of infection could be demonstrated, the percentage of donor (class I) reactive cultures was comparable to that in the control group over a similar period after transplantation. The highest values were measured during the infection (Table 1). After the period of the highest CMV infection incidence, CML reactivity returned to the level of the control group (Table 1). To ascertain that the increased cytolytic reactivity during CMV infection was not caused by a few patients who had provided the majority of the biopsies, we also calculated the percentage reactive cultures for each individual patient. Figure 1 shows that the increased number of HLA class I directed cytolytic biopsies during infection were derived from 24 of the 27 patients tested, and that in each of these 24 patients, the majority of the biopsies were reactive against class I antigens. In our group of 27 patients, 8 had a primary and 19 a secondary infection of whom respectively 6 (75%) and 7 (37%) had clinical symptoms. Both during primary and secondary infection, a significantly higher proportion of the EMB-derived lymphocyte cultures showed cytotoxicity against donor class I antigens compared to the control group, but in primary infected patients the percentage of class II reactive cultures was also increased (Table 2).

CMV infection we found an increased incidence of cytotoxic graft infiltrating cells directed against HLA class I mismatches. We found no evidence for an early immunosuppressive phase. In primary infections, which were often symptomatic, both class I and class II directed cytotoxicity were increased.

References

1. van Dorp, WT, Jonges E, Bruggeman CA, Daha MR, van Es LA, van der Woude F (1989) Cytomegalovirus infection directly induces MHC class I but not class II expression on endothelial cells. Transplantation 48: 469–472
2. Grundy JE, Shearer GM (1984) The effect of cytomegalovirus infection on the host response to foreign and hapten-modified self histocompatibility antigens. Transplantation 37: 484–490
3. Grundy JE, Ayles HM, McKeating JA, Butcher RG, Griffiths PD, Poulter LW (1988) Enhancement of class I HLA antigen expression by cytomegalovirus: role in amplification of virus infection. J Med Virol 25: 483–495
4. Metselaar HJ, Balk AHMM, Mochtar B, Rothbart PhH, Weimar W (1990) Prophylactic use of anti-CMV immunoglobulin in CMV seronegative heart transplant recipients. Chest 97: 396–399
5. Ouwehand AJ, Vaessen LMB, Baan CC, Jutte NHPM, Balk AHMM, Essed CE, Bos E, Class FHJ, Weimar W (1991) Alloreactive lymphoid infiltrates in human heart transplants. Loss of class II directed cytotoxicity more than three months after transplantation. Hum Immunol 30: 50–59
6. Rothbarth PhH, Diepersloot RJA, Metselaar HJ, Nooyen Y, Velzing J, Weimar W (1987) Rapid demonstration of Cytomegalovirus in clinical specimens. Infection 15: 228–231
7. Von Willebrand E, Pettersson E, Ahonen J, Hayry P (1986) CMV infection, class II antigen expression and human kidney allograft rejection. Transplantation 42: 364–367

Transplant Int (1992) 5 [Suppl 1]: S673–S675

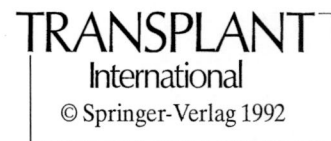

TRANSPLANT
International
© Springer-Verlag 1992

The influence of HLA-mismatches on phenotypic and functional characteristics of graft infiltrating lymphocytes after heart transplantation

A. J. Ouwehand[1], C. C. Baan[2], L. M. B. Vaessen[2], N. H. P. M. Jutte[2], A. H. M. M. Balk[3], E. Bos[1], F. H. J. Claas[4], and W. Weimar[2]

Departments of Thoracic Surgery[1], Internal Medicine I[2], Cardiology[3], Erasmus University Rotterdam, University Hospital Rotterdam-Dijkzigt, Rotterdam and Department of Immunohaematology and Blood Bank[4], University Hospital Leiden, The Netherlands

Abstract. We studied the influence of HLA mismatches on T lymphocyte cultures that were derived from endomyocardial biopsies (EMB) from 118 heart transplant recipients. From patients with DR mismatches, the majority of the EMB-derived cultures were dominated by CD4, while in patients without DR mismatches, CD8 was the predominant T cell subset. The majority (75 %) of the cultures were cytotoxic against donor antigens. A significantly ($P < 0.005$) lower proportion of the cultures showed cytotoxicity (36 %) against HLA-A antigens when compared to HLA-B (53 %) or HLA-DR (49 %). A dose effect phenomenon was detected for all HLA antigens, including HLA-A: a higher number of A, B or DR mismatches resulted in a higher number of cytotoxic cultures directed against these antigens. B and DR matching had the greatest influence on 6 month freedom from rejection. Both our experimental and clinical data indicated that HLA matching played a role in the immune response against a transplanted heart.

Key words: HLA matching – Graft infiltrating cells – Heart transplantation – Alloreactivity, Predominant phenotype

Several studies among kidney transplant recipients have shown a positive effect of HLA matching on graft outcome, especially for B and DR antigens [4, 8, 14]. The beneficial effect of DR matching has been found to be most evident in the first 5 post operative months, while the effect of matching for HLA-B antigens lasts longer [14]. In heart transplantation, the importance of HLA matching for graft survival is still debated, because in many studies numbers of patients are limited and, more importantly, numbers of well matched grafts are low, as donor hearts are randomly allocated to the recipients without reference to their HLA status. However, up to now the results indicate that HLA matching has a beneficial effect on graft survival [6, 9] or on the incidence of steroid resistant rejection [3].

The influence of HLA mismatches between donor and recipient on phenotypes and function of graft infiltrating cells has never been systematically studied. Therefore, we analyzed the effect of HLA-A, B and DR mismatches on the functional and phenotypic characteristics of these cells in a large series of endomyocardial biopsies (EMB) from 118 heart transplant recipients.

Materials and methods

Patients. We studied 1285 biopsies from 118 heart transplant recipients transplanted between September 1984 and January 1990. All patients had received preoperative blood transfusions and all received cyclosporine and low dose prednisone as maintenance immunosuppression. The actuarial patient survival was 89 % at 4 years. The mean number of HLA-mismatches between donor and recipient was 1.25, 1.62 and 1.40 for A, B, and DR, respectively. Three patients who died within 3 weeks after transplantation were excluded from this study. Endomyocardial biopsies (EMB) were taken at regular intervals. We received 4–22 biopsies from each patient (median 10).

Biopsies were cultured in interleukin 2 (IL-2) containing culture median. Phenotypes were analyzed by two-colour flow cytometry after staining with anti-Leu 4, WT31, Leu 2 and Leu 3 (Becton Dickinson, Mountain View, Calif). A more extensive phenotypic characterisation of the cultured cells is described by us in a previous study [10]. A 4-h ^{51}Cr release assay was used to measure the cytotoxic capacity against donor cells and a panel of unrelated target cells (EBV transformed B cell lines or PHA blasts) sharing one or more HLA antigens with the donor.

HLA typing. Spleen cells or peripheral blood mononuclear cells (obtained by Ficoll separation of heparinized blood) were typed for HLA class I antigens according to the standard NIH lymphocytotoxicity assay, and typed for HLA-DR by the two-colour fluorescence assay with a set of highly selected antisera [11].

Results

DR mismatches and CD4/CD8 phenotypes

In the first 180 days, the number of DR mismatches had a pronounced influence on the phenotypic composition of the EMB-derived lymphocytes (Fig. 1). Cultures from pa-

Offprint requests to: A. J. Ouwehand, Dept. Internal Medicine I, Bd 299, Erasmus University, P.O. Box 1738, 3000 DR Rotterdam, The Netherlands

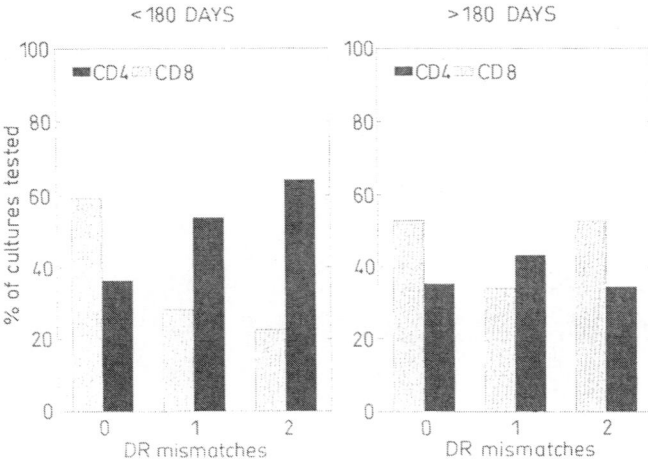

Fig. 1. Predominant phenotype of EMB-derived lymphocyte cultures in relation to the number of HLA-DR mismatches between donor and recipient

Table 1. CML specificity of EMB-derived cultures against panel cells sharing mismatched HLA A, B or DR antigens with the donor. Relation with time after transplantation. In the first 6 months, the incidence of HLA-A directed cytotoxicity was significantly lower than that against B or DR antigens ($P < 0.001$)

CML specificity	Numbers of reactive cultures		
	< 180 days n (%[1])	> 180 days n (%)	P value[2]
HLA-A	79 (38)	28 (33)	n.s.
HLA-B	127 (57)	38 (40)	< 0.01
HLA-DR	120 (55)	34 (37)	< 0.01

[1] Percentage reactive cultures
[2] X^2 test

tients without DR mismatches were most often dominated by CD8, while in cultures from patients with DR mismatches CD4 was the predominant T cell subset in the majority of cultures. After these first 6 post transplant months, no significant differences were found between the groups.

Cytotoxicity

As described by us in a previous study [10], the majority (75%) of the cultures tested (n = 324) were cytotoxic against donor antigens. In the first 6 months after transplantation a high proportion of the cultures was found to be cytotoxic against HLA-B and DR mismatches between donor and recipient, and significantly fewer were cytotoxic against HLA-A antigens (Table 1). After 6 months these differences were no longer detectable, because of a decline in the incidence of HLA-B and DR directed cytotoxicity.

HLA-mismatches and acute rejection

In the DR matched patient group 56% of patients remained free from rejection of 6 months, compared with 29% of patients with one DR mismatch and 22% with two DR mismatches. For the combination of HLA-B and DR antigens a significant effect on freedom from rejection was found: 37% in patients with two or less B and DR mismatches and 24% in patients with three or four B and DR mismatches at 6 months (P = 0.05, log rank test). No significant relationship between the number of acute rejection episodes in the 1st year and the number of mismatches on the individual A, B or DR locus was observed.

Discussion

Direct CML assays of biopsy-derived lymphocytes revealed that in the first 6 months after transplantation, HLA-B and DR antigens were important epitopes for cytotoxic lymphocytes. Cytotoxicity against B and/or DR mismatches was found significantly more often than against HLA-A antigens. This may account for the significantly lower freedom from rejection rates in the patient group with more than two B and DR mismatches. This association between the number of B and DR mismatches and freedom from rejection has also been described by others [7]. Studies on the effect of matching for HLA antigens in renal [4, 8, 14] and heart [6, 9] transplantation have shown that matching for HLA-B and DR has a significant influence on graft survival.

In the one and two DR mismatched heart allograft recipients, significantly more CD4-dominated cultures were derived from the biopsies than in the DR-matched group. CD4$^+$ cells are known to be of crucial importance in initiating rejection [1, 5]. Interaction of these cells with donor class II MHC antigens, expressed on the graft tissue and an passenger leucocytes of donor origin, results in activation of CD8$^+$ cells which recognize MHC class I antigens. Both CD4$^+$ and CD8$^+$ cells play a role in the rejection of grossly mismatched graft. Rejection of class I disparate grafts appears to be most dependent on CD8$^+$ cells, although CD4$^+$ cells can be activated as well via presentation of donor MHC class I antigens on recipient antigen presenting cells in the context of HLA class II molecules. Our data were compatible with this theory. A decline in the number of the CD4 dominated cultures was found after 180 days post transplant. Also the the incidence of DR directed cytotoxicity showed a significant decline in this period. This may be due to a lower expression of donor type class II antigens on graft tissue, and the replacement of donor dendritic cells by the patient's antigen presenting cells after such a long period following transplantation [12, 13]. As a consequence, fewer class II specific CD4$^+$ lymphocytes may be attracted to the graft.

In conclusion, we showed that in the first 6 months after transplantation, the number of DR mismatches between donor and recipient had a pronounced influence on CD4 predominance in EMB-derived cultures. Furthermore, in this period a significantly higher percentage of cytotoxic cultures was directed against HLA-B and DR mismatches than against HLA-A. This was in keeping with results of graft survival studies in renal and heart transplantation. A higher incidence of freedom from rejection was associated with a lower number of HLA-B and DR mismatches. This study showed that HLA matching between donor and recipient played a role in the immune response against a transplanted heart.

References

1. Bach FH, Sachs DH (1987) Transplantation Immunology. N Engl J Med 317: 489–492
2. Billingham ME (1982) Diagnosis of cardiac rejection by endomyocardial biopsy. J Heart Transplant 1: 25–30
3. DiSesa VJ, Kuo PC, Horvath KA, Mudge GH, Collins JJ, Cohn LH (1990) HLA histocompatibility affects cardiac transplant rejection and may provide one basis for organ allocation. Ann Thorac Surg 49: 220–224
4. Gilks WR, Gore SM, Bradley BA (1990) Renal transplant rejection. Transient immunodominance of HLA mismatches. Transplantation 50: 141–146
5. Häyry P (1989) Mechanisms of rejection. Curr Opin Immunol 1: 1230–1235
6. Khagani A, Yacoub M, McCloskey D, Awad J, Burden M, Fitzgeral M, Hawes R, Holmes J, Smith J, Banner N, Festenstein H (1989) The influence of HLA matching, donor/recipient sex, and incidence of acute rejection on survival in cardiac allograft recipients receiving cyclosporin A and azathioprine. Transplant Proc 21: 799–800
7. Laufer G, Miholic J, Laczkovics A, Wollenek G, Holzinger C, Hajek-Rosenmeier A, Wuzl G, Schreiner W, Buxbaum P, Wolner E (1989) Independent risk factors predicting acute graft rejection in cardiac transplant recipients treated by triple drug immunosuppression. J Thorac Cardiovasc Surg 98: 1113–1121
8. Opelz G (1987) Effect of HLA matching in 10.000 cyclosporine-treated cadaver kidney transplants. Transplant Proc 19: 641–646
9. Opelz G (1989) Effect of HLA matching in heart transplantation. Transplant Proc 21: 794–789
10. Ouwehand AJ, Vaessen LMB, Baan CC, Jutte NHPM, Balk AHMM, Essed CE, Bos E, Claas FHJ, Weimar W (1991) Alloreactive lymphoid infiltrates in human heart transplants. Loss of class II directed cytotoxicity more than three months after transplantation. Hum Immunol 30: 50–59
11. van Rood JJ, van Leeuwen A, Ploem JS (1976) Simultaneous detection of two cell populations by two-colour fluorescence and application to the recognition of B-cell determinants. Nature 262: 795–797
12. Steinhoff G, Wonigeit K, Schafers HJ, Haverich A (1989) Sequential analysis of monomorphic and polymorphic major histocompatibility complex antigen expression in human heart-tallograft biopsy specimens. J Heart Transplant 5: 360–370
13. Suitters A, Rose M, Higgins A, Yacoub MH (1987) MHC antigen expression in sequential biopsies from cardiac transplant patients - correlation with rejection. Clin Exp Immunol 69: 575–583
14. Thorogood J, Persijn GG, Schreuder GMTh, D'Amaro J, Zantvoort FA, van Houwelingen JC, van Rood JJ (1990) The effect of HLA matching on kidney graft survival in separate posttransplantation intervals. Transplantation 50: 146–150

Transplant Int (1992) 5 [Suppl 1]: S 676–S 678

TRANSPLANT
International
© Springer-Verlag 1992

Kidney transplant monitoring by anti donor specific antibodies

N. Torlone[1], A. Piazza[2], M. Valeri[1], P. I. Monaco[2], L. Provenzani[1], E. Poggi[1], D. Adorno[1] and C. U. Casciani[1]

[1] Clinica Chirurgica – II University of Rome, Rome, Italy
[2] CNR – Ist. Tipizzazione Tissutale e Problemi della Dialisi of L'Aquila, Italy

Summary. Donor-specific anti-HLA antibodies were studied by cytotoxicity crossmatching (CTXM) and flow cytometry crossmatching (FCXM) in 117 kidney transplant candidates; the same study was carried out in 33 cadaver-donor kidney recipients, during the first 3 post-transplant months, for which donor cells were available. Pre-transport evaluation showed that 82.9% of subjects were CTXM negative/FCXM negative, 6.8% of patients were positive in both tests, and 10.3% were CTXM negative/FCCM positive. Post-transplant monitoring for donor-specific antibodies (Abs-DS) showed that nine recipients (27.3%) were FCXM positive; six of them were IgG + and three IgM +. In comparing these results with the clinical course, a significant association between FCXM IgG + and rejection episodes was observed ($P < 0.01$).

Key words: Cytotoxicity crossmatching – Flow cytometry crossmatching – Donor-specific antibodies – Kidney transplantation

Specific anti-HLA antibodies (directed against "non-self" HLA antigens present on transplanted allograft cells) are an important element for the success of kidney transplantation. The presence of these antibodies is inevitably associated with acute or early rejection episodes; positive crossmatching, performed with the standard NIH technique – cytotoxicity crossmatching (CTXM) – is a definite contraindication to kidney transplantation. In various transplant centers, however, cases of acute or early rejection episodes have been observed in CTXM negative subjects as well [1]. These results have stimulated the study of pre-transplant anti-HLA antibody screening, which has led to the development of techniques that are more sensitive and reliable than CTXM. Among these, the flow cytometry technique (FCXM) has been proven to be one of

the most interesting [2]. Donor-specific antibodies (Abs-DS) can be directed against T and B lymphocytes, they may or not be complement fixing, they can recognize class I or II antigens and, finally, they may belong to IgG or IgM classes. The CTXM does not allow for easy and rapid antibody characterization and does not provide a full picture of the recipient's pre-transplant immune state. The FCXM, however, has proven to be a more sensitive technique for pre-transplant Abs-DS screening; it has been shown that those transplanted subjects with a negative CTXM, but a positive FCXM, have a higher incidence of acute rejection episodes during the post-transplant period [3, 4]. Furthermore, after transplantation, the FCXM allows the monitoring of specific humoral immunoreactivity directed against the transplanted organ.

The present study reports our experience in the employment of FCXM, both in the screening of kidney transplant candidates and in the monitoring of post-transplant Abs-DS.

Materials and methods

Pre-transplant screening. From June 1988 to June 1991, 117 kidney transplant candidates were studied, both by CTXM and FCXM. The organ assignement was based on a high degree of HLA-A, B, DR compatibility and on a negative result using CTXM; a positive FCXM did not contraindicate transplantation. We performed 60 transplants from cadaver-donors and all recipients were on their first transplant.

Abs-DS post-transplant monitoring. Of the 60 transplanted patients, 33, whose donor's lymphocytes were available, were studied for Abs-DS appearance during the first 3 post-transplant months. All patients had undergone an immunosuppressive protocol consisting of azathioprine, cyclosporine and prednisone; rejection episodes were treated with 1 g methylprednisolone/day for 3 days.

Complement-mediated cytotoxicity cross-matching. All sera were incubated with donor lymphocites for 60 min at room temperature. After the addition of complement, the sera were again incubated for 60 min at room temperature [5].

Flow cytometry cross-matching. This was performed by double staining, using an anti-CD3 and anti-CD20 phycoerytrin monoclonal

Offprint requests to: Nicola Torlone, Clinica Chirurgica – Osp S. Eugenio, Piazzale dell'Umanesimo, 10, 00144 Roma – Italy

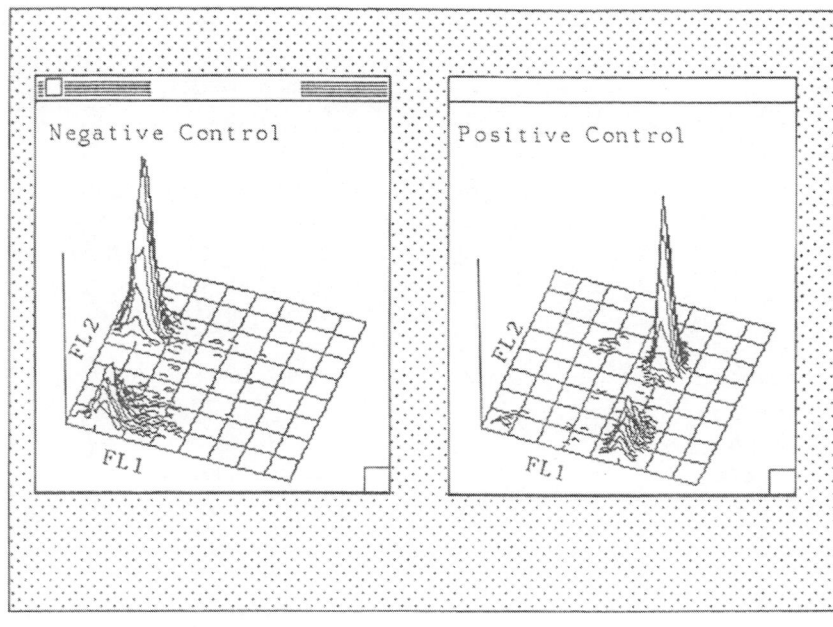

Fig. 1. FCXM. Fl1 = anti IgG o IgM; Fl2 = anti CD3 o CD20

Table 1. CTXM and FCXM results obtained from 117 patients selected for cadaver-donor kidney transplant

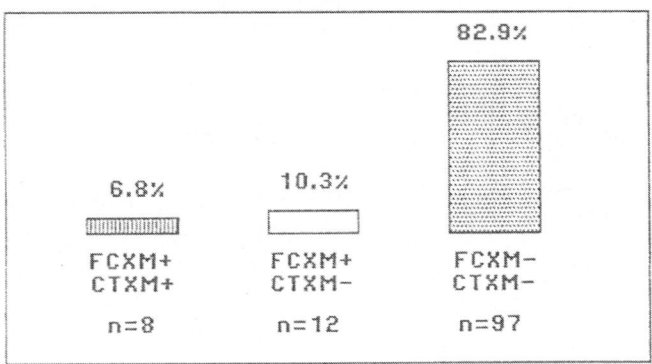

Table 2. Pre- and Post-Transplant FCXM in 33 cadaver-donor kidney transplants

antibody to identify T and B lymphocytes and using fluorescein stained anti-human IgG or IgM F(ab')2 antibodies to identify anti-lymphocyte antibodies present in the serum [6]. Positive and negative control sera were obtained, respectively, from a serum pool with a high reactivity to a cell panel (> 90%) and from a negative serum pool obtained from nontransfused male subjects. Samples were analyzed on a FACScan flow cytometer (Becton-Dickinson) and data were collected using "Lysis" software (Becton-Dickinson) (Fig. 1). The sera that presented a shift greater than 10 channels from the fluorescence 1 (fluorescein) mean curve were considered positive.

Results

Pre-transplant screening

Of the patients selected for transplantation 82.9% were CTXM negative/FCXM negative; 6.8% were positive on both tests, and 10.3% were CTXm negative/FCXM positive (Table 1).

Post-transplant monitoring

We studied 33 transplanted patients of whom 6.1% were FCXM positive before the transplant, while, at 3-month follow-up, 27.3% were positive for FCXM IgG or IgM (Table 2). During our study, 11 rejection episodes occurred and one graft was lost due to irreversible rejection. The relationship between acute rejection and the presence of Abs-DS demonstrated a significant association between these two factors ($P < 0.05$); moreover, we observed a significant association between FCXM IgG + and acute rejection ($P < 0.01$) (Table 3).

Discussion

Compared to the CTXM the FCXM has been proven to have a higher sensitivity in identifying transplant patients with Abs-DS. If the concentration of Abs-DS is lower than is required for a complement-metiated cytotoxic reaction, or if they do not fix complement, the CTXM gives

Table 3. Relationship between donor-specific antibody class and rejection episodes in 33 cadaver-donor transplants

	FCXM −	FCXM +	
		IgG	IgM
No patients	24	6	3
No rejections	5	5	1

$P < 0.01$

a negative or dubious result. The detection of Abs-DS by FCXM suggests the presence of a low titer sensitization state, which does not necessarily lead to a secondary immune response after transplantation. The clinical value of detecting these antibodies before transplantation must be correlated both to the donor-recipient HLA compatibility level and to the immunosuppressive protocol [3, 7].

In our study, monitoring in FCXM-positive recipients showed a constant decrease in the Abs-DS titer during the first post-transplant months. However, the post-transplant detection of Abs-DS by FCXM represented specific sensitization against the transplanted organ. The significant relationship, which we found between rejection episodes and post-transplant positive FCXM, confirmed the negative prognostic value of the appearance of Abs-DS. The cell immune response occurring during a rejection episode is undoubtedly accompanied by a humoral immune response. The appearance of Abs-DS is an expression of the patient's immune state, and their persistence may have a negative prognostic value in the long-term success of the transplant. Furthermore, of extreme importance is the Abs-DS class, since IgM antibodies (unlike IgG antibodies) do not seem related to the risk of acute rejection episodes.

In conclusion, compared to the CTXM technique, the FCXM technique had great advantages both before the transplant, providing a better and more exhaustive immunologic evaluation of the patient, and after the transplant, for identifying those subjects at a higher risk of rejection. In our experience, Abs-DS monitoring by FCXM was an important immunological test, providing useful information for a more effective immunosuppression.

References

1. Iwaki Y, Iguro T, Terasaki PI (1985) Nonfunctional kidneys in immunized patients. Transplant Proc 17: 2449
2. Garavoy MR, Rheinschmidt MA, Bigos M, et al (1983) Flow cytometry analysis. A high technology crossmatch technique faciliting transplantation. Transplant Proc 15: 1939–42
3. Cook DJ, Terasaki PI, Iwaki Y, Terashita GY, Lau M (1987) An approach to reducing early kidney transplant failure by flow cytometry crossmatching. Clin Transplant 1: 253–6
4. Lazda VA, Pollak R, Mazes MF, Jonasson O (1988) The relationship between flow cytometer crossmatch results and subsequent rejection episodes in cadaver renal allograft recipients. Transplantation 3: 562–5
5. Ray JG (1979) Staff Transplantation and Immunology Branch NIH. Lymphocyte microlymphocytotoxicity technique. US DHEW publication
6. Bray RA, Lebeck LK, Gebel HM (1989) The flow cytometric crossmatch. Transplantation 5: 834-40
7. Mahoney RJ, Ault KA, Given SR, Adams RJ, Breggia AC, Paris PA, Palomaki GE, Hitchcox SA, et al (1990) The flow cytometric crossmatch and early renal transplant loss. Transplantation 3: 527–35

Transplant Int (1992) 5 [Suppl 1]: S 679–S 680

TRANSPLANT
International
© Springer-Verlag 1992

Cytokines in lethal graft-versus-host disease

A. C. Knulst, C. Bril-Bazuin, G. J. M. Tibbe, A. van Oudenaren, H. F. J. Savelkoul, and R. Benner

Department of Immunology, Erasmus University, Rotterdam, The Netherlands

Graft-versus-host disease (GVHD) is caused by donor T lymphocytes that recognize foreign antigens on host tissues. This leads to T cell activation, which involves a cascade of events including the transcription of genes for cytokines and their receptors and the production of cytokines [1, 2]. One of the first cytokines to appear is interleukin 2 (IL-2). IL-2 production enhances the IL-2 receptor expression and leads to T cell proliferation. As a further step, differentation of T cells occurs, which results in the production of a certain pattern of cytokines. These cytokines influence the expression of cell surface antigens and adhesion molecules, and are able to activate other cell types such as cytotoxic T cells, macrophages and natural killer cells, which might act as effector cells in tissue destruction [2]. Insight into the sequential expression of the various cytokines involved might enable a more effective treatment of GVHD. Therefore, we investigated the occurrence of cytokines in a murine model for acute GVHD. We addressed in particular the period early after allogeneic reconstitution.

Key words: Graft-versus-host disease – Cytokines

Materials and methods

Mice. (C57BL/Ka × CBA/Rij)F1 (H-$2^{b/q}$) and BALB/c (H-2^d) mice were bred at the Department of Immunology of Erasmus University. The mice were 12–18 weeks old at the start of the experiments. Mice were kept two per cage in light-cycled rooms with access to acidified water and pelleted food ad libitum.

This study was supported by a grant from the Interuniversitary Institute for Radiation Pathology and Radiation Protection (IRS), Leiden, The Netherlands

Offprint requests to: A. C. Knulst, M. D., Dept. of Immunology, Erasmus University, P. O. Box 1738, 3000 DR Rotterdam, The Netherlands

Determination of cytokines. Serum samples and supernatants from spleen cells cultured for 24 h with Con A (1 µg/ml) [3] were assayed for cytokine activity. IL-2 was determined by a proliferative assay using an IL-2 dependent CTLL cell line, maintained in vitro in medium supplemented with rhIL-2; we used rhIL-2 as a standard (gift from Sandoz Forschungsinstitut, Wien, Austria). For the detection of interleukin 6 (IL-6), the B9 cell line was used [4]; we used rmuIL-6 as a standard (British Biotechnology, Abingdon, UK). Tumor necrosis factor (TNF)-α levels were determined by a cytotoxicity assay on WEHI 164 cells [5]; we used rmuTNF-α as a standard (gift from BASF/Knoll, Ludwigshafen, Germany). The proliferative or cytotoxic activity was measured with the MTT assay [6]. Interferon (IFN)-γ was determined in a sandwich ELISA, using a rat-anti-mouse IFN-γ mAb (XMG1.2) as a catching antibody and a polyclonal rabbit-anti-mouse IFN-γ Ab as a second step. We used rmuIFN-γ purified from CHO cells transfected with the muIFN-γ gene as a standard (kind gift from Dr. R. L. Coffman, DNAX Research Institute, Palo Alto, Calif).

Other procedures. Preparation of cell suspensions, induction of GVHD, collection of serum samples and data analysis were performed as described by us in earlier studies [7, 8].

Results and discussion

Serum samples obtained from lethally irradiated (C57BL × CBA)F1 mice, in which a lethal graft-versus-host reaction was induced by injection of 10^7 allogeneic BALB/c spleen cells, were analyzed for cytokine activity. As a control, serum samples from similarly treated mice injected with 10^7 syngeneic spleen cells were used. The results are summarized in Table 1. Since mortality occurred at day 8, from that day on the number of mice in each group became too small for statistic analysis. Therefore, no data are presented after day 8. It appeared that IL-6 levels increased from day 4 in the allogeneically reconstituted mice with a peak level at day 8, in contrast to syngeneically reconstituted mice in which no rise was found. Serum IFN-γ levels increased strongly in the allogeneically reconstituted mice between day 4 and 5, reaching a peak level at day 6. No rise was seen in the syngeneically reconstituted mice. We further determined the TNF-α activity in sera from both groups of mice. Signi-

Table 1. Symptoms of GVHD in relation to serum cytokine levels after allogeneic and syngeneic reconstitution of lethally irradiated mice. (C57BL × CBA)F1 mice were lethally irradiated and reconstituted either with 10^7 allogeneic BALB/c spleen cells or with 10^7 syngeneic spleen cells. At various days after reconstitution, serum samples were obtained from mice of each group, and analyzed for cytokine activity. Furthermore clinical symptoms were evaluated in both groups of mice

	Days after reconstitution					
	3	4	5	6	7	8
Symptoms of disease[a]	−	−	−	+	+ +	+ + +
IL-2	−	−	−	−	−	−
L-6	−	+	+	+ +	+ +	+ + +
IFN-γ	−	−	+ +	+ + +	+ +	+ +
TNF-α	−	n.d.	−	n.d.	+ + +	n.d.
Symptoms of disease[b]	−	−	−	−	−	−
IL-2	−	−	−	−	−	−
IL-6	−	−	−	−	−	−
IFN-γ	−	−	−	−	−	−
TNF-α	−	n.d.	−	n.d.	+	n.d.

[a] after allogeneic reconstution
[b] after syngeneic reconstitution
− not detectable; + low/light; + + moderate; + + + high/severe;
n.d. not determined

ficantly increased TNF-α levels were found at day 7 after allogeneic reconstitution. Serum IL-2 levels were below the detection limit (0.1 U/ml).

Since the detection of cytokines in the serum might be hampered by inhibitory or binding factors, e. g. soluble receptors, we further analyzed tissue culture supernatants of spleen cells 24 h after culture in the presence of Con A. A significantly higher activity of both IL-6 and IFN-γ was found in spleen cell supernatants from allogeneically reconstituted mice as compared to syngeneically reconstituted mice, showing a similar time-dependence as the serum levels. The TNF-α activity in spleen cell cultures was very low in both groups. IL-2 levels were below the detection limit.

Evaluation of clinical symptoms in both groups revealed that in the allogeneically reconstituted mice symptoms of acute GVHD were present at about day 6. Mortality in these mice occurred between 8 and 24 days after reconstitution, with a mean survival time of 12.5 ± 4.9 days. In the syngeneically reconstituted mice no signs of disease were found (Table 1).

Taken together, the above data indicated that a rise in IFN-γ and IL-6 levels, detectable both in serum and culture supernatants preceded the clinical symptoms and mortaility in acute GVHD. The clinical symptoms of GVHD seemed to be most closely associated with a rise in serum TNF-α activity. It is likely that the expression of these cytokines was preceded by cytokines the appeared earlier, especially IL-2. Although we could not detect IL-2 activity, possibly due to the fact that IL-2 is rapidly consumed, an important role for IL-2 was suggested by preliminary data showing decreased morbidity and mortality in acute GVHD after the in vivo administration of anti-IL-2 or anti-IL-2 receptor mAb. This stresses the importance of the use of complementary assay systems to determine the role of cytokines. Studies are underway to determine whether other cytokines also play a role in this complex disease.

References

1. Krensky AM, Weiss A, Crabtree G, Davis MM, Parham P (1990) N Engl J Med 322: 510
2. Ferrara JLM, Deeg JH (1991) N Engl J Med 324: 667
3. Cleveland MG, Annable CR, Klimpel GR (1988) J Immunol 141: 3349
4. Aarden LA, Groot de ER, Schaap OL, Lansdorp PM (1987) Eur J Immunol 17: 1411
5. Meager A, Leung H, Woolley J (1989) J Immunol Methods 116: 1
6. Mosmann T (1983) J Immunol Methods 65: 55
7. Knulst AC, Bril-Bazuin C, Benner R (1991) Eur J Immunol 21: 103
8. Knulst AC, Bazuin C, Benner R (1989) Transplantation 48: 829

Transplant Int (1992) 5 [Suppl 1]: S 681–S 683

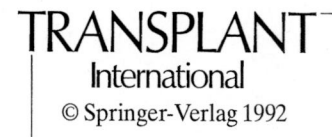

© Springer-Verlag 1992

Absence of correlation between graft-versus-host associated immunosuppression and cytotoxic T cell activity in response to major histocompatibility antigens

Ph. Lang, V. Bierre, C. Baron, S. Cholin, G. Rostoker, and B. Weil

Department of Nephrology and INSERM U. 139, Hôpital Henri Mondor, Créteil, France

Abstract. Studies in mice suggest that the T cell subset involved in graft-versus-host-reaction (GvHR) across the major histocompatibility complex (MHC) depends on the class of MHC antigens recognized by the donor cells. However, the correlation between phenotype and function is not absolute. Using a functional approach, we investigated in a parent →F_1 hybrid model differing at the whole MHC, whether graft-versus-host (GvH) associated immunosuppression was correlated with donor cytotoxic T cell activity. The immunodeficiency was tested by the ability of the F_1 mice to generate a cytotoxic T cell response against trinitrophenyl-modified syngeic cells (TNF-self) or an alloantigen. F_1 specific parental cytotoxic T cells, generated in vitro, induced less immunosuppression than naive parental cells. Specific in vivo priming increased the cytotoxicity of parental spleen cells, but decreased their capacity to induce GvH-associated immunosuppression. In contrast, nonspecific priming resulted in the usual immunodeficiency. In conclusion, there was no correlation between GvH-associated immunosuppression and cytotoxic T cell activity of the parental cells.

Key words: Graft-versus-host – Cytotoxic T cell – Immunodeficiency

On transfer of parental T cells into non irradiated, adult F_1 recipient mice, the recognition of allogenic class I plus class II major histocompatibility complex (MHC) antigens on host cells can result in a graft-vs-host (GvH) reaction characterised by a profound immunodeficiency [6, 11, 15, 17]. It has been reported that in this model, both CD4[+] and CD8[+] parental T cells are necessary to induce GvH-associated immunosuppression [5, 14]. However, the correlation between phenotype and function or phenotype and MHC class specificity is not absolute and CD8[+] lymphocytes define both cytotoxic and suppressor cells.

Using a functional rather than a phenotypic approach, we investigated whether GvH associated immunosuppression was correlated with the cytotoxic T-cell activity of parental cells.

Materials and methods

Mice. Male mice 6 to 8 weeks of age were used in all experiments. C57BL/10 (B10), B 10.BR (BR) mice were used as the donors and (C57 BL 10 × B 10.A) F_1 [(B10 × B10A) F_1] (C57 BL 10 × B10.BR) F_1 [(B10 × BR) F_1] and (B 10.BR × B 10.D2) F_1 [(BR × D2) F_1] were used as the GvH recipients.

Sensitization. Sensitization of parental cells against the F_1 hybrids was performed in vitro and in vivo. In vitro generation of cytotoxic T lymphocytes (CTL) was performed as previously described [10]. Briefly, CTL were generated in 2 ml macrocultures consisting of 4×10^6 B10 spleen cells and 1×10^6 irradiated (B10 × B10 A) F_1 spleen cells. The effectors were tested 5 days later in a 4-h ^{51}Cr release assay on Con A-stimulated spleen cells blasts. In vivo immmununization was performed by 3 intraperitoneal (i. p.) injections of BR mice with 10^7 B10 spleen cells. The spleen was removed 1 week following the last injection, and the CTL activity was tested as previously mentioned.

Injection of F_1 mice with parental spleen cells. F_1 mice were injected intravenously (i. v.) with either 4×10^7 normal parental spleen cells or 4×10^7 alloreactive T cells generated in vitro or in vivo.

GvH-associated immunosuppression. Immunosuppression was assessed 2 weeks following the induction of the GvH reaction by the ability of spleen cells to generate CTL against trinitro-phenyl-modified syngeneic cells (TNP-self) or allogeneic cells as previously described [10].

Results

Failure of in vitro generated CTL to induce GvH-associated immunodeficiency

We injected 4×10^7 B10 spleen cells obtained after in vitro culture with (B10 × B10A) F_1 cells i. v. into non-irradiated (B10 × B10A) F_1 mice. Spleen cells from these F_1 hybrid

---

Offprint requests to: Ph. Lang, Department of Nephrology, Hôpital Henri Mondor, Créteil, 94010, France

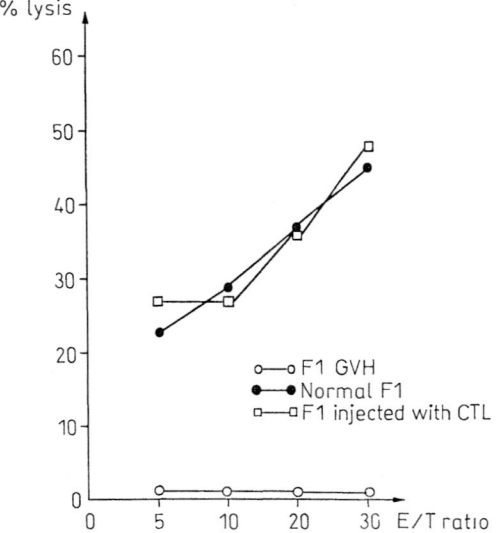

Fig.1. Inability of in vitro generated CTL to induce GVH-associated CTL suppression. B10 CTL generated against B10A were injected into (B10×B10A) F₁ and CTL assays were performed 2 weeks later against (B10×B10A) F₁ TNP-self

mice were tested 2 weeks later for their potential to generate a CTL response in vitro to irradiated TNP-self or allogeneic cells. The data in Fig.1 show that the CTL reactivity against TNP-self was not reduced. In contrast, no anti-TNP-self CTL was detected in the F₁ recipients that had been injected with 4×10^7 normal parental spleen cells. Similar results were obtanied when F₁ injected mice were tested against an allogeneic target (data not shown).

Failure of in vivo primed parental cells to induce GvH-associated immunodeficiency

BR mice were injected weekly i.p. with 10^7 B10 spleen cells. One week following the third injection, 4×10^7 BR spleen cells were injected i.v. into (B10×BR) F₁ or (BR×D2) F₁ mice and the F₁ CTL response was tested 2 weeks later against TNP-self or allogeneic cells. The CTL response of in vivo primed BR spleen cells was specifically increased (data not shown), but these cells were unable to induce a GvH-associated CTL suppression in (B10×BR) F₁ (Fig.2A). In contrast, CTL suppression was induced when immunized BR spleen cells were injected into (BR×D2) F₁ (Fig.2B) demonstrating the specificity of this finding.

Discussion

Numerous experimental models of GvH reactions giving rise to a variety of pathological symptoms have been described and it is not surprising that various effector cells have been reported to mediate the reaction. There is general agreement that mature T cells [9] are the main cause of the disease, but which particular T cells, in terms of phenotype and function, account for the various symptoms is unclear. It was assumed for a number of years that the surface antigen phenotype of lymphocytes defined

their functional activity [1, 2]. However, more recently it has been proposed that these phenotypes define the MHC antigen class for which the relevant T cell is specific or restricted, regardless of function [18]. Finally there are several reports supporting the view that there is not an absolute correlation between the phenotype and MHC antigen class specificity [12]. These findings may in part explain the controversy concerning the effector cells when using negative selection of donor T cells in various MHC disparate combinations.

A more direct approach to the question of the effector cells is to use T cell clones known to be CD4⁺ or CD8⁺ [13, 19]. However, this alternative method runs the risk that isolated cells no longer represent their ancestor, and the culture itself can select some parental T cell subsets. The functional properties of T cell clones can also be altered compared with those of their ancestor. For example, T cell clones rarely function following an i.v. injection, perhaps because they are no longer able to circulate or can only do so for a limited period of time [14]. Homing studies have shown that the majority of the injected T cell clones reside in lung and liver [19]. Furthermore, GvH disease induced by T cell clones differs in several respects form the disease caused by parental cells [19].

Because of these conceptual and technical pitfalls, we chose a functional approach to determine whether GvH-associated immunosuppression observed across a whole H-2 difference was correlated with parental cytotoxic T cell activity. Parental CTL generated in vitro were unable to induce GvH-associated CTL suppression. Although these cells had been cultured for only 5 days, the validity of this approach could be criticized; we used in vivo priming to confirm the absence of correlation between CTL activity of parental spleen cells and GvH-associated immunodeficiency. Suppressive GvH reaction across a whole H-2 difference is induced by unseparated

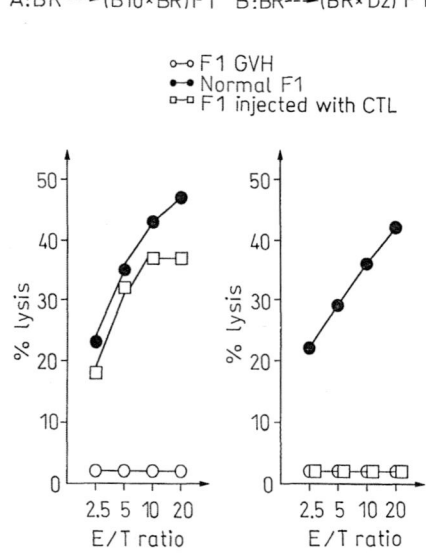

Fig.2. Inability of in vivo generated CTL to induce GVH-associated immunosuppression. BR CTL were generated by repeated i.p. immunization with B10 spleen cells and injected into **A** (B10×BR) F₁ or **B** (BR×D2) F₁. CTL assays were performed 2 weeks later against TNP-self

donor T cells, and it seems that CD4$^+$ and CD8$^+$ cells are both necessary in non-irradiated animals [14, 15]. Opinion is divided, however, on the cytotoxic or suppressor function of the CD8$^+$ cells [14, 15]. There are no convincing reports supporting the theory that CTL could easily could detectable in non-irradiated F$_1$ hybrid recipients undergoing a GvH reaction, and lethal GvH disease can develop in response to MHC antigens in the absence of CTL activity [5, 7]. In irradiated F$_1$ animals, the role of CD8$^+$ cells remains controversial and the relative contribution of various T cell subsets is determined by the particular strain combination and conditioning regimen [3, 8, 16]. In our model, the functional data which we reported, seemed to confirm the finding that parental CTL are probably not involved in GvH-associated CTL suppression. The GvH-associated CTL suppression observed in a third-party hybrid suggested that the inability of alloactivated T cells to induce immunodeficiency was not merely related to the release of various cytokines.

Acknowledgements. This study was supported by grants from A.U.R.A.

References

1. Cantor H, Boyse EA (1975) Functional subclasses of T lymphocytes bearing different Ly antigens. I. The generation of functionally distinct T cell subclasses is a differantiative process independent of antigen. J Exp Med 141: 1376–1389
2. Cantor H, Boyse EA (1975) Functional subclasses of T lymphocytes bearing different Ly antigens. II. Cooperation between subclasses of Ly cells in the generation of killer activity. J Exp Med 141: 1390–1402
3. Cobbold S, Martin G, Waldmann H (1986) Monoclonal antibodies for the prevention of graft-versus-host disease and marrow graft rejection. Transplantation 42: 239–247
4. Dailey MO, Gallatin WM, Weissman IJ, Butcher E (1983) Surface phenotype and migration properties of activated lymphocytes and T cell clones. In Parker JW, O'Brien RL (eds): Intercellular Communication in Leucocyte Culture Conference, Asilomar, Pacific Grove, California, December 1982. John Wiley and Sons Ltd, Chichester, pp 641–644
5. Elven E, Rolink AG, van der Veen F, Gleichmann E (1981) Capacity of genetically different T lymphocytes to induce lethal graft-versus-host disease correlates with their capacity to generate suppression but not with their capacity to generate anti-F$_1$ killer cells. A non-H-2 locus determines the inability to induce lethal graft-versus-host disease. J Exp Med 153: 1474–1488
6. Gleichmann ES, Pals T, Roling AG, Radasziewicz T, Gleichmann H (1984) Graft-versus-host reactions: clues to the etiopathology of a spectrum of immunological diseases. Immunol Today 5: 324–332
7. Jadus MR, Peck AB (1983) Lethal urine graft-versus-host disease in the absence of detectable cytotoxic T lymphocytes. Transplantation 36: 281–289
8. Korngold R, Sprent J (1985) Surface markers of T cells causing lethal graft-vs-host disease to class I vs class II H-2 differences. J Immunol 135: 3004–3010
9. Korngold R, Sprent J (1987) T cell subsets and graft-versus-host disease. Transplantation 44: 335–339
10. Lang Ph, Miller MW, Shearer GM (1985) Failure of bone marrow cells to reconstitute T cell immunity in graft-vs-host mice. J Immunol 134: 2052–2052
11. Lapp WS, Moller G (1969) Prolonged survival of H-2 incompatible skin allografts on F$_1$ animals treated with parental lymphoid cells. Immunology 17: 339–345
12. Macphail S, Stutman O (1987) L3T4 + cytotoxic T lymphocytes specific for class I H-2 antigens are activated in primary mixed lymphocyte reactions. J Immunol 139: 4007–4015
13. Miconnet I, Huchet R, Bonardelle D, Motta R, Canon C, Garay-Rojac E, Kress M, Reynes M, Halle-Pannenko O, Bruley-Rosset M (1990) Graft-versus-host mortality induced by noncytolytic CD4$^+$ T cell clones specific for non-H-2 antigens. J Immunol 145: 2123–2131
14. Moser M, Sharrow SO, Shearer GM (1988) Role of L3T4$^+$ and Lyt-2$^+$ donor cells in graft-versus-host immune deficiency induced across a class I, class II, or whole H-2 difference. J Immunol 140: 2600–2608
15. Pals ST, Gleichmann H, Gleichmann E (1984) Allosuppressor and allohelper T cells in acute and chronic graft-vs-host disease. V F$_1$ mice with secondary chronic GVHD contain F$_1$-reactive allohelper but no allosuppressor T cells. J Exp Med 159: 508–523
16. Pietryga DW, Blazar BR, Soderling CCB, Vallera DA (1987) The effect of T cell subset depletion on the incidence of lethal graft-versus-host disease in a murine major-histocompatibility complex mismatched transplantation system. Transplantation 43: 442–445
17. Shearer GM, Polisson RP (1980) Mutual recognition of parental and F$_1$ lymphocytes. Selective abrogation of cytotoxic potential of F$_1$ lymphocytes by parental lymphocytes. J Exp Med 151: 20–26
18. Swain S (1983) T cell subsets and the recognition of MHC class. Immunol Rev 74: 129–146
19. Tary-Lehmann M, Rolink AG, Lehmann PV, Nagy ZA, Hurtenbach U (1990) Induction of graft versus host-associated immunodeficiency by CD4$^+$ T cell clones. J Immunol 145: 2092–2098

Transplant Int (1992) 5 [Suppl 1]: S 684–S 687

TRANSPLANT
International
© Springer-Verlag 1992

Rejection prophylaxis with interleukin-2 receptor antibody BT 563: mechanisms of action on human cells

C. Herwartz[1], J. Steinmann[1], U. Bethke[4], R. Engemann[3], J. Gassel[3], S. Hoffmann[2], G. Leimenstoll[2], W. Timmermann[3], and W. Müller-Ruchholtz[1]

[1] Institute for Immunology, [2] Department of Nephrology, Kiel University, Kiel, Germany
[3] Department of Surgery, Würzburg University, Würzburg, Germany
[4] Biotest Pharma, Dreieich, Germany

Abstract. We investigated the in vitro immunosuppressive effect of BT 563, a monoclonal antibody, against the α-chain of the human interleukin-2 (IL-2) receptor (p 55), which has been used to prevent transplant rejection in several clinical trials. We also measured the proliferative T cell alloresponse and pCTL frequencies of BT 563-treated kidney transplant patients. In mixed lymphocyte cultures BT 563 caused a reduction of T cell proliferation to about 50 %. This could not be reversed by the addition of exogenous IL-2. A more effective reduction (80 %) was seen in the generation of cytotoxic T cells from CML cultures and at the clonal level. The specific T cell response after preincubation with antigen and BT 563 was not reduced so that BT 563 did not induce tolerance. The in vitro findings indicated that BT 563 had a significant but incomplete immunosuppressive effect. This correlated with the clinical course and ex vivo analysis of PBL from BT 563-treated patients after kidney transplantation.

Key words: Human IL-2 receptor – Monoclonal antibody – Graft-rejection

The human interleukin-2 (IL-2) receptor consists of two glycoproteins, p55 and p75, which by themselves display low and intermediate affinity for IL-2 and combine to form a high affinity receptor complex.

BT 563 is an IgG1 mouse monoclonal antibody, developed by Wijdenes [6], which is directed against the p55 chain of the IL-2 receptor. It blocks ligand binding to both low and high affinity receptors. Since only activated T lymphocytes express p55 following organ transplantation, the suppressive effect should concentrate on transplant reactive cells. In several clinical trials BT 563 has been used to prevent rejection after solid organ transplantation and to treat graft-versus-host disease after bone marrow transplantation.

Initial experiments have revealed that BT 563 does not deplete target cells and that the blocking of IL-2 binding is noncompetitive. To increase our understanding of the clinically observed immunosuppressive effect, we investigated the mode of action of BT 563 in various T cell assays in vitro. Additionally, anti-donor T cell reactivity in kidney transplant patients was measured before, during and after BT 563 rejection prophylaxis.

Materials and methods

BT 563. BT 563 is a mouse IgG1 monoclonal antibody against the human IL-2 receptor. It is produced and purified by Biotext Pharma according to the guidelines of the European Communities: "On the production and quality control of monoclonal antibodies of murine origin intended for use in man".

Cells. Peripheral blood lymphocytes (PBL) from healthy donors were obtained by density gradient centrifugation of heparinized blood.

MLR. One-way mixed lymphocyte reactions (MLR) were carried out with PBL from different donors. We seeded 5×10^4 responder cells and 5×10^4 irradiated stimulator cells per well into 96-well round-bottomed microculture plates in 200 µl RPMI 1640, supplemented with 15 % AB serum, glutamine and penicillin/streptomycin. After 96 h the microcultures were pulsed with 37 kBq/well ^{3}H-methylthymidine for 24 h and harvested onto glass fiber filters. Tritium incorporation was measured by liquid scintillation spectroscopy.

CML. CML assays were performed in a manner similar to MLR but evaluated for cytotoxicity by ^{51}chromium release on day 7.

Limiting dilution assays. Limiting dilution assays for donor-reactive CTL precursors were performed according to the consensus protocol of the European pCTL Workshop [12]. Briefly, graded numbers of PBL were cocultured with 5×10^4 irradiated kidney donor spleen cells in round-bottomed microtiter plates as described above. We added 10 U/ml recombinant IL-2 in fresh medium on days 3 and 6. On day 12 ^{51}Cr-labelled target cells were added directly to the microcultures. The supernatant was removed after 4 h and the amount of ^{51}Cr released was determined by gamma counting. Microcultures were defined as positive when counts were higher than those of con-

Offprint requests to: Jörg Steinmann, Inst. f. Immunology, Kiel University, Michaelisstr. 5, D-2300 Kiel 1, Germany

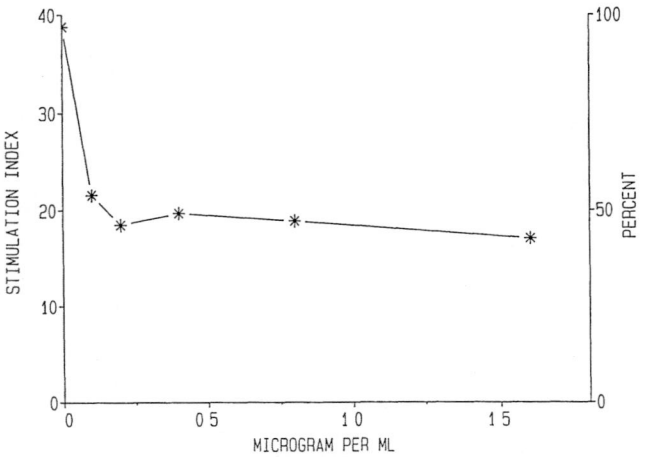

Fig. 1. Reduction of the stimulation index in mixed lymphocyte cultures by increasing concentrations of BT 563

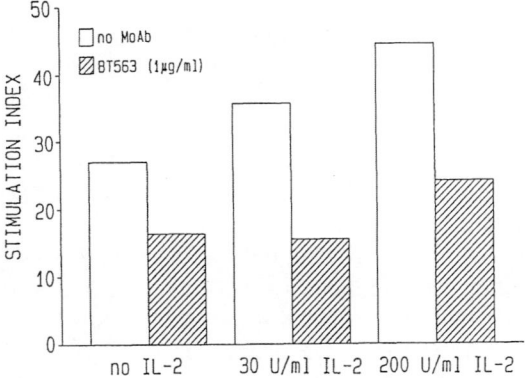

Fig. 2. Influence of exogenous IL-2 on the suppressive effect of BT 563 in mixed lymphocyte cultures

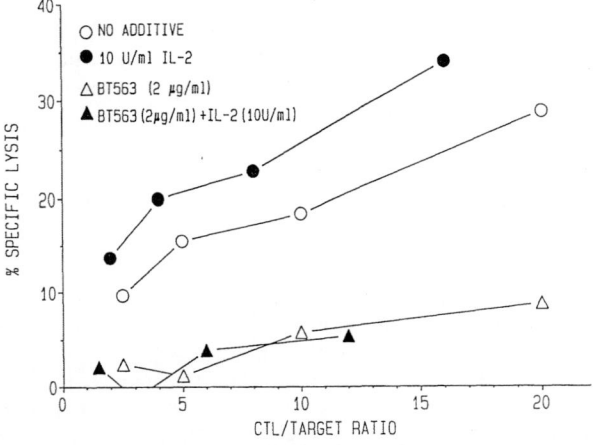

Fig. 3. Inhibition of cell-mediated lysis by BT 563 with and without exogenous IL-2

trols (spontaneous release, irradiated stimulators alone) plus 3-fold standard deviation. Due to the assay setup, pCTL anti-donor frequencies lower than 3 per million were not signfiicantly different than zero. Frequencies were calculated according to Taswell (Lausanne) using the Strijbosch computer program distributed by F. Claas, Eurotransplant, Leiden (Netherlands). By measuring the proliferative response of the sequentially diluted PBL on day 10, expressed as ^{3}H-thymidine uptake, it was possible to calculate the frequency of clonable T-cells.

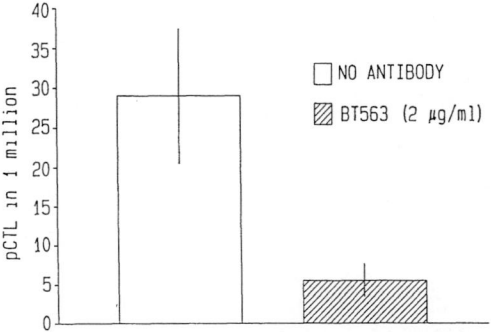

Fig. 4. Reduction of pCTL frequencues by BT 563, measured in limiting dilution cultures

Results and discussion

Effects of BT 563 in vitro

BT 563 inhibited the MLR. The clinically adjusted concentration of BT 563 was 2 µg/ml. In in vitro MLR we tested the effect of the antibody up to 5 µg/ml. As shown in Fig. 1, as little as 0.25 µg/ml BT 563 reduced the stimulation index to about 50 %. Higher concentrations did not, however, increase the suppressive effect.

IL-2 did not overcome the immunosuppressive effect. Figure 2 showed that IL-2 enhanced proliferation in MLR, but that the proportional suppressive effect of pretreatment with saturating concentrations of BT 563 was not influenced. This finding indicated that IL-2 and BT 563 do not share the same epitope on the α-chain of the receptor and that the inhibitory effect of BT 563 was not due to competition.

BT 563 reduced the generation of cytotoxic T cells. The IL-2 dependent differentiation of cytotoxic T cells was more effectively influenced by BT 563. Figure 3 demonstrates that 2 µg/ml BT 563 strongly reduced the in vitro development of alloreactive T cells in the standard CML assay. Also this suppressive effect could not be overcome by the addition of exogenous IL-2. This finding could also be demonstrated at the clonal level by performing limiting dilution analysis. As shown in Fig. 4, the frequency of clonable alloreactive cells from the peripheral blood was reduced to 20 %. This appeared to indicate that the antibody treatment left out a T cell population which proliferates and differentiates in the presence of BT 563.

BT 563 did not anergize antigen-specific T cells. To determine whether BT 563 was able to induce anergy, we investigated the antigen-specific response of PBL after 1 week of preincubation with antigen and BT 563. Compared to fresh PBL, we could not detect a significant reduction of the pCTL-frequency as shown in Fig. 5.

Concerning the proliferative response, similar results were seen in secondary MLR (data not shown). These findings indicated that BT 563 did not induce tolerance in alloreactive T cells. Taken together, our in vitro data demonstrated that BT 563 had a significant but limited immunosuppressive effect on the alloreactive T cell response. To investigate the clinical effect of BT 563, we analysed

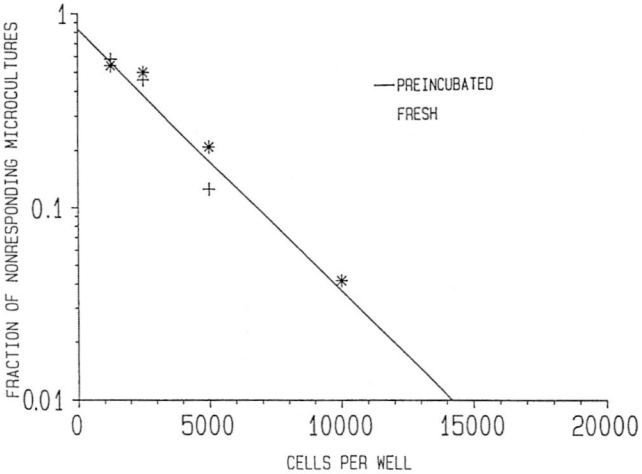

Fig. 5. pCTL frequencies of preincubated PBL compared to fresh cells

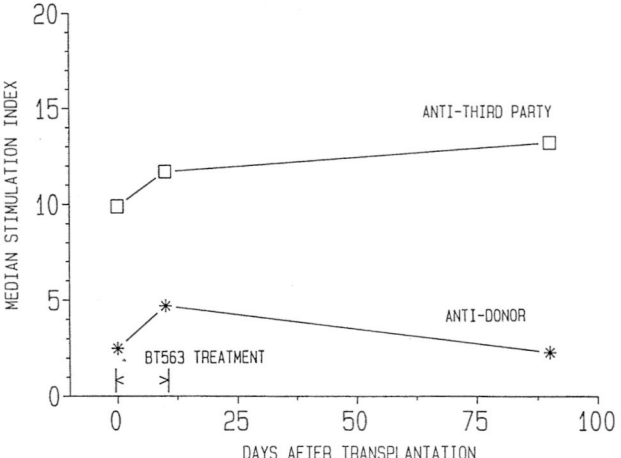

Fig. 6. Mean stimulation index in MLR of nine kidney transplant patients before, during and after BT 563 treatment

PBL from kidney transplant patients before, during and after BT 563 rejection prophylaxis.

Effects of BT 563 in vivo in a phase II clinical trial

Nine kidney transplant patients were treated with BT 563, 10 mg per day, from day 0 until day 9 after transplantation, in addition to cyclosporin A (CsA) and prednisolone. One patient rejected the kidney in association with CMV infection on day 28, four patients had stable graft function after episodes of rejection and four patients showed no signs of rejection.

BT 563 treatment did not reduce MLC-reactivity and pCTL frequency. PBL from the kidney transplant patients were prepared from day 0, 10 and 90 after transplantation and both proliferative activity and pCTL frequencies were measured. The general allogeneic reactivity was determined by coculturing with HLA-mismatched third-party cells and compared to the specific reactivity against HLA-matched donor cells, which is generally lower due to pretransplant typing. As shown in Fig. 6 the mean stimula-

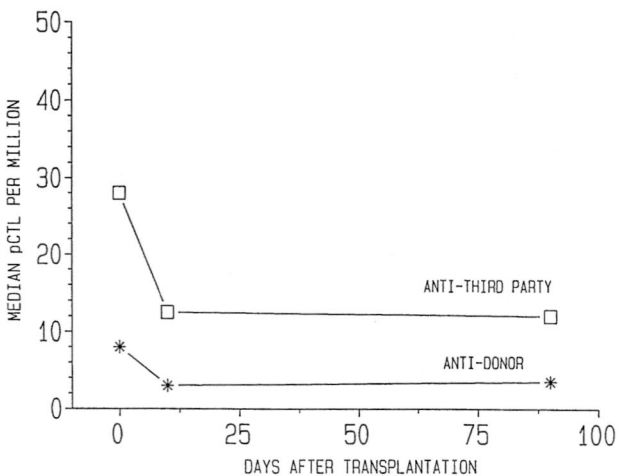

Fig. 7. Mean pCTL frequencies of BT 563-treated kidney transplant patients

tion index increased slightly between day 0 and day 10. This correlated with an increase in the percentage of IL-2 receptor α-chains expressing T cells and the serum levels of interleukin-6 IL-6 (Data not shown). On day 90 the mean MLR stimulation index was at the pretransplant level again, whereas the anti-third-party index was further but not significantly increased.

In contrast to the MLR stimulation index, the mean pCTL frequency was significantly reduced against donor and third-party on day 10 and remained on this low level until day 90 as shown in Fig. 7. Since Kosugi et al. [8] have demonstrated that CsA abrogates the development of mature T cells, we interpreted this target-independent effect as CsA determined, rather than due to BT 563. However, a controlled clinical study is necessary to clarify this important point.

In summary, in vitro, ex vivo and clinical data in kidney transplantation indicated that BT 563 has an immunosuppressive effect. So far we are not able to support the hypothesis that the antibody induces donor-specific nonreactivity.

References

1. Audrain M, Boeffard F, Soulillou JP, Jacques Y (1991) Synergistic action of monoclonal antibodies directed at p55 and p75 chains of the human IL-2 receptor. J Immunol 146:884
2. Blaise D, Olive D, Hirn M, et al (1991) Prevention of acute GVHD by in vivo use of anti-interleukin-2 receptor monoclonal antibody (33B3.1) a feasibility trial in 15 patients. Bone Marrow Transplant
3. Brown PS, Parenteau GL, Dirbas FM, et al (1991) Anti-Tac-H, a humanized antibody to the interleukin 2 receptor, prolongs primate cardiac allograft survival. Proc Natl Acad Sci USA 88:2663
4. Carpenter CB, Kirkman RL, Shapiro ME, et al (1989) Prophylactic use of monoclonal anti-IL-2 receptor antibody in cadaveric kidney transplantation. Am J Kidney Dis 14:54
5. Chabannes D, Mauff BL, Hallet MM, Jacques Y, Soulillou JP (1988) Effect of cyclosporine on interleukin 2 receptor expression in a human alloreactive T cell clone. Transplantation 46:97
6. Hervé P, Wijdenes J, Bergerat JP, Milpied N, Gaud C, Bordigoni P (1988) Treatment of acute graft-versus-host disease with monoclonal antibody to IL-2 receptor. Lancet II:1072

7. Jacques Y, Audrain M, Boeffard F, Soulillou JP (1991) Concerted action of monoclonal antibodies directed at the p55 and p75 chains of the human interleukin-2 receptor. Transplant Proc 23:1068

8. Kosugi A, Sharrow SO, Shearer GM (1989) Effect of Cyclosporin A on Lymphocytes. I. Absence of mature T cells in thymus and periphery of bone marrow transplanted mice treated with cyclosporin A. J Immunol 142:3026

9. Kupiec-Weglinski JW, Mariani G, Tanaka K et al (1989) Biodistribution of anti interleukin 2 receptor monoclonal antibodies correlates with their therapeutic efficacy following transplantation. Cell Immunol 123:148

10. Plaetinck G, Come MC, Corthesy P et al (1990) Control of IL-2 receptor-α expression by IL-1, tumor necrosis factor and IL-2. J Immunol 145:3340

11. Read MH, Shapiro ME, Strom TB et al (1989) Prolongation of primate renal allograft survival by anti-Tac, an anti-human IL-2 receptor monoclonal antibody. Transplantation 47:55

12. Sharrock CEM, Kaminski E, Man S (1990) Limiting dilution analysis of human T cells: a usefull clinical tool. Immunol Today 11:281

13. Turka LA, Carpenter CB, Yunis EJ, Milford EL (1989) Selective sparing of suppressor cells generated in mixed lymphocyte response by an anti interleukin-2 receptor antibody. Transplantation 47:182

14. Zola H, Weedon H, Thompson GR, Fung MC, Ingley E, Hapel AJ (1991) Expression of IL-2 receptor p55 and p75 chains by human B lymphocytes: effects of activation and differentiation. Immunology 72:167

Transplant Int (1992) 5 [Suppl 1]: S 688–S 689

TRANSPLANT
International
© Springer-Verlag 1992

Hyaluronic acid accumulation; the mechanism behind graft rejection edema

G. Tufveson, B. Gerdin, E. Larsson, T. Laurent, J. Wallander, A. Wells, and R. Hällgren

The Departments of Surgery, Medical and Physiological Chemistry, Pathology and Internal Medicine, University of Uppsala, Uppsala, Sweden

Abstract. Hyaluronic acid (HA) is an important stabilizing consistuent of the loose connective tissue and regulates water homeostasis. Thus, excessive accumulation of HA in interstitial tissue immobilizes water and may thereby contribute to interstitial tissue edema. By the use of biotin labelled core protein and an avidin-enzyme system, we visualized HA in grafted rat kidney, rat heart, rat small bowel and also in human kidneys. By an extraction procedure the tissue amounts of HA were measured in the experimental grafts. Simple techniques for measuring water content were also employed. The extracellular amounts of HA increased between 100 % and 350 % in rejecting tissues as compared to syngeneic controls. The relative water content also increased and correlated well with the HA accumulation. The clinical value of these experimental observations was confirmed in human transplantation where rejecting kidney allografts demonstrated a highly significant increase in HA staining in the interstitium as compared to non-rejecting biopsy specimens. We therefore concluded that transplantation edema – a key features of graft rejection – is regulated by the accumulation of HA not only under experimental conditions but also in the clinical setting.

Key words: Hyaluronic acid – Transplantation edema – Rejection

We have shown in two recent studies that HA – an important stabilizing constituent of the loose connective tissue and regulator of water homeostasis – accumulates during graft rejection in rat renal and cardiac grafts [2, 3]. In those studies we also found a correlation between the accumulation of HA and the water content of the tissue. We drew the tentative conclusion that the HA accumulation is the major mechanism behind graft rejection edema. The aim of the present communication was to review our findings regarding rat heart and rat kidney allografts and compare those with new findings emerging from the present studies of rejecting rat small bowel and human kidney allografts.

Materials and methods

Animals. Lewis rats and DA rats or Lewis × DA F1-hybrid rats (originally obtained from Bantin & Kingman, N Humberside, UK and Möllegaard, Skensved, Denmark) were bred in our own animal quarters. Parental strain animal transplants were performed for obtaining rejection in kidney and heart allografts, whereas F1 hybrids were transplanted into Lewis rats for small bowel transplants.

Patients. The records of 153 patients were retrospectively analyzed and biopsy reports were studied. Only biopsies where the graft status was classified as denfitely rejecting ($n = 39$) or definitely stable ($n = 38$) were selected for the present investigation ($n = 77$). All patients received base line immunosuppression with triple drug therapy as outlined elsewhere [1]. These biopsy specimens were restained for HA according to a protocol shown elsewhere [7].

Transplant procedures. Heterotopic cardiac [4], orthotopic renal [3], and heterotopic small bowel transplants [6] were performed as described elsewhere.

Tissue preparation: extraction of tissue hyaluronan and calculation of water content. All experimental animals mentioned in this paper were sacrificed 2, 4 or 6 days after transplantation. Only the data for animals harvested 6 days posttransplantation are shown. Tissue handling and processing is describe in detail elsewhere [3]. Briefly, one part of the specimens obtained were analyzed for HA and water content and were weighed immediately on filter paper at room temperature (wet weight, ww) and later after lyophilization at $-80\,°C$ for 4 days (dry weight, dw). The relative water content of the specimens was calculated according to the formula: $100 × /(ww - dw)/(ww)/$. The HA was extracted from pulverized dried tissue with 0.5 M NaCl. The material was extracted with 2 ml of the buffer for 16 h with constant shaking at $4\,°C$. The samples were then centrifuged for 15 min at $2,000\ g$. The supernatants were recovered and the HA concentrations were analyzed in duplicate with a radiometric assay (Pharmacia Diagnostics, Uppsala, Sweden), according to the principles previously outlined [5].

Data presentation. All data are presented as mean $\pm$ SEM. For the human tissues the intensity and the amount of HA stain in the inter-

Offprint requests to: Gunnar Tufveson, Transplantation Unit, University Hospital, S-751 85 Uppsala, Sweden

Table 1. Amounts of hyaluronan extracted and relative water content (mean ± SEM)

Organ	Type	n	HA (μg/g dw)	Water (%)
Kidney	Syngeneic	5	180 ± 10	75.2 ± 1
	Allogeneic	5	350 ± 20	84.3 ± 1
Heart	Syngeneic	3	465 ± 42	79.6 ± 0.3
	Allogeneic	4	930 ± 13	82.9 ± 0.7
Small bowel	Syngeneic	3	80 ± 35	74.0 ± 1.0
	Semi allogenric	4	280 ± 25	83.0 ± 1.0

stitium was given as intensity, graded into an abritary scale from 0–3 where zero denotes no or absence of stain and 3 represents intense staining. Due to lack of sufficient material for further sectioning only 32 of the stable grafts and 35 of the acute rejecting grafts were available for the final evaluation.

Statistical differences between group means were carried out by means the Student's t-test for the experimental animals and with the Mann-Whitney U-test for the clinical material.

Results

The results for the animal experiments are summarized in Table 1. Table 1 depicts the HA concentrations in kidney, heart, and small bowel grafts when performed in either allogeneic or syngeneic conditions. Table 1 also depicts the water content of the tissues. The HA concentration on the 6th day after allografting increased 100–350% as compared to the syngeneic situation. The water concentration also increased significantly. There was a significant correlation between the relative water content and HA content of the allogeneic grafts ($r = 0.51$, $P < 0.01$ for kidneys; $r = 0.62$, $P < 0.05$ for hearts and $r = 0.72$, $P < 0.01$ for small bowels).

Non rejecting human kidney grafts were scored to have an interstitial HA content of $1.031 ± 0.08$ and acutely rejecting kidney grafts were arbitrarily scored to have a mean of $1.9 ± 0.13$.

Discussion

In this communication we showed that the HA content increased in three different experimental settings; that is, non-immunosuppressed rejection of cardiac, renal and small bowel allografts. We also found a good correlation between HA and the increased water content in the tissues. We were also able to confirm these findings of increased HA content in a clinical setting. These findings have been extensively discussed elsewhere [2, 3]. The finding of a good clinical correlation to the experimental findings strengthens the validity of the interpretation put forward that HA binds water and thereby immobilizes water in the interstitial tissue. Two clinical implications are clear: (1) HA staining, may in certain instances, add to the diagnostic potency of routine histology, and (2) it explains why the edema of grafted tissue undergoing rejection is resistent to diuretics and calls for other procedures, e. g. HA degradation in a connective tissue to decrease the edema and thereby improve graft function.

Acknowledgements. These research investigations were carried out with the support of Njursjukas Förening i C, U, W, X län, the Elof Eriksson Fund and the Maud and Birger Gustavsson Fund and the Swedish Medical Research Council.

References

1. Brynger H, Persson H, Flatmark A, Albrechtsen D, Frödin L, Tufveson G, Gäbel H, Weibull H, Möller E, Lundgren G, Groth CG (1988) No effect of blood transfusions or HLA matching on renal graft success rate in recipients treated with cyclosporine-prednisolone or cyclosporine-azathioprine-prednisolone; the Scandinavian experience. Transplant Proc 20 [Suppl 3]:261–263
2. Hällgren R, Gerdin B, Tengblad B, Tufveson G (1990) Accumulation of Hyaluronan (Hyaluronic acid) in myocardial interstitial tissue parallels development of transplantation edema in heart allografts in rats. J Clin Invest 85:668–673
3. Hällgren R, Gerdin B, Tufveson G (1990) Hyaluronic acid accumulation and redistribution in rejecting rat kidney graft: Relationship to the transplantation edema. J Exp Med 171:2063–2076
4. Olausson M, Mjörnstedt L, Lindholm L, Brynger H (1984) Nonsuture organ grafting to the neck vessels in rats. Acta Chir Scand 150:463–467
5. Tengblad A (1980) Quantitative analysis of hyaluronate in nanogram amounts. Biochem J 185:101–105
6. Wallander J, Holtz A, Larsson E, Gerdin B, Läckgren G, Tufveson G (1988) Small-bowel transplantation in the rat with a non suture cuff technique: Technical and immunological considerations. Transplant Int 1:135–139
7. Wells AF, Larsson E, Tengblad A, Fellström B, Tufveson G, Klareskog L, Laurent TC (1990) The localization of hyaluronan in normal and rejected human kidneys. Transplantation 50:240–243

Transplant Int (1992) 5 [Suppl 1]: S690–S691

TRANSPLANT
International
© Springer-Verlag 1992

Expression of activation markers, HLA class II and IL-2R in acute vascular rejection of human renal allografts

E. von Willebrand, K. Salmela, H. Isoniemi, E. Taskinen, L. Krogerus, and P. Häyry

Transplantation Laboratory and Fourth Department of Surgery, University of Helsinki, Helsinki, Finland

Abstract. We analyzed the expression of class II antigens on graft tubular cells and the expression of IL-2R on lymphoid cells in 314 prospective aspiration biopsies taken from 30 consecutive patients with histologically verified acute vascular rejection (AVR). Based on histology, two main groups were seen: 11 grafts had features of AVR only and 19 grafts had a combination of AVR and acute cellular rejection (ACR). The AVR findings were also predominant in the latter group. In the grafts with a combination of AVR and ACR, patterns similar to ordinary ACR were seen in class II and IL-2R expression. On the contrary, no class II or IL-2R induction could be seen in the grafts with pure AVR and irreversible rejection. This pattern, demonstrated by immunocytology, suggested that AVR is a heterogenous group of rejections, where different cellular and molecular mechanisms are operating. Humoral mechanisms might be involved in these rejections.

Key words: Class II antigens – IL-2R – Acute vascular rejection – Acute cellular rejection

The association between tubular cell class II induction and renal allograft rejection has been confirmed in several studies [1–3]. We have demonstrated previously that class II induction is associated only with blastogenic inflammation (acute cellular rejection) in the graft [2] but not with nonblastogenic patterns of inflammatory infiltrates. The induction of interleukin-2 (IL-2) receptors on activated lymphoid cells of the inflammatory infiltrate has been demonstrated during acute cellular rejection (ACR) of human kidney transplants [4–5], where it follows closely the pattern of blastogenic inflammation [5]. The induction of these activation markers, class II expression on the tubular cells and IL-2R expression on activated lymphoid

cells is thus well established in acute ACR. In acute vascular rejection (AVR), very little is known about the induction of activation markers. To elucidate this question, we have recently analyzed the expression of class II antigens on the graft tubular cells, and the expression of IL-2 receptors on lymphoid cells in serial renal aspiration biopsies taken from 20 consecutive patients with AVR before, during and after acute vascular rejection episodes that were verified histologically [6]. We have now extended the study to 30 consecutive patients with histologically verified acute vascular rejection.

Materials and methods

A total of 314 aspiration biopsies were obtained from 30 consecutive patients with histologically verified AVR during the first posttransplant month. Altogether 571 renal transplants were performed between 1987 and 1990, at our center. The acute vascular rejections usually occurred early, on days 2 to 31 posttransplant (mean, day 10). The patients were monitored with frequent fine needle aspiration biopsies (FNABs) at 1–3 day intervals, from days 3–30 after transplantation. Altogether 314 aspiration biopsies were performed, mean, 10.4 per patient. Evaluation of class II and IL-2R expression was done by indirect immunoperoxidase staining using monoclonal antibodies. Class II determination was done from 235 biopsies, on average from 8 biopsies per patient and IL-2R determination from 135 biopsies, on average 5 biopsies per patient. Histological biopsies were taken from all 30 patients with AVR throughout the rejection period and after the rejection. Altogether 63 histological biopsies were taken and investigated.

Results

Based on histological findings, the grafts were categorized into four groups: group I ($n = 12$), combination of AVR and ACR, with reversible rejections (REV). Group II ($n = 7$), AVR and ACR with irreversible rejections (IRR). Group III ($n = 3$), pure AVR with REV and group IV ($n = 8$), pure AVR with IRR.

Tables 1 and 2 demonstrate the sequences in tubular cell class II expression and in lymphoid IL-2R expression

Offprint requests to: Eeva von Willebrand, M.D., Transplantation Laboratory, University of Helsinki, Haartmaninkatu 3, SF 00290 Helsinki, Finland

Table 1. Sequence of class II expression on tubular cells in the different groups

	Group I (n = 12)	Group II (n = 7)	Group III (n = 3)	Group IV (n = 8)
Day 5	4 ± 2	14 ± 7	15 ± 5	4 ± 1
Day 0–2	$36 \pm 6^*$	39 ± 5	41 ± 9	$7 \pm 2^*$
Day 5–7	$49 \pm 7^*$	28 ± 7	31 ± 10	7 ± 1
Day 10–15	$37 \pm 4^*$	34 ± 9	33 ± 5	$5 \pm 0^*$
Day 22–25	12 ± 5	$43 \pm 3^{**}$	24 ± 7	6 ± 1

Percentage of positive tubular cells ± SEM in the aspiration biopsies during the course of AVR

* indicates significant differences ($P < 0.001$) between the groups I and IV

** indicates significant differences ($P < 0.001$) between the groups I and II

Table 2. Sequence of IL-2 receptor expression in the different groups

	Group I (n = 12)	Group II (n = 7)	Group III (n = 3)	Group IV (n = 8)
Day 5	0 ± 0	0 ± 0	0 ± 0	0 ± 0
Day 0–2	4 ± 1	4 ± 2	7 ± 2	0.1 ± 0.1
Day 5–7	4 ± 1	6 ± 2	0 ± 0	0.4 ± 0.2
Day 10–15	2 ± 1	3 ± 1	0 ± 0	0 ± 0
Day 22–25	0.4 ± 0.3	4 ± 2	0 ± 0	0.3 ± 0.3

Total number of IL-2R positive cells ± SEM in the aspiration biopsies during AVR

of all 30 grafts in the study. All 19 grafts with a combination of AVR and ACR displayed class II induction and IL-2R expression, closely correlating the blast response of the rejection, with 40–50% positive tubular cells during the 1st week after the onset of rejection, and declining thereafter to prerejection levels in grafts with reversible rejection (group I). In grafts with irreversible rejection (group II), tubular cell class II expression and lymphoid IL-2R expression remained elevated. The same pattern of class II and IL-2R expression was observed in grafts with pure AVR and reversible rejections (group III). On the contrary, a completely different finding was seen in grafts with pure AVR and irreversible rejections (group IV): there was neither class II induction on tubular cells nor IL-2R expression on lymphoid cells. The persistant inflammation was dominated by mononuclear phagocytes, and no blast response could be detected.

Discussion

This study confirmed our earlier observations that in AVR, a close relationship exists between IL-2R and tubular cell class II induction, when AVR is associated with ACR. Furthermore, the study demonstrated that in histologically pure AVR, i.e. without features of interstitial blastogenic cellular rejection, two different patterns of IL-2R and class II expression exist.

All 19 grafts with a combination of AVR and ACR on histology displayed class II upregulation, which was closely associated with IL-2R expression on lymphoid cells and also closely associated with blast cell infiltration in the graft. The local release of gamma interferon and/or other cytokines by the activated lymphocytes and lymphoid blast cells, could be the mechanism responsible for this induction. Also the profile of class II expression would support this concept; in the reversible rejections the blast cells and IL-2R expressing cells disappeared and the tubular cell class II expression returned to pre-rejection level. On the other hand, in the irreversible rejections the blast response and the IL-2R expressing cells persisted as did also the tubular cell class II upregulation. Treatment had no permanent effect on the upregulation in the irreversible rejections.

Completely different findings were seen in the grafts with a pure AVR pattern of histology and irreversible rejection. On immunocytology, none of these grafts demonstrated upregulation of class II antigens on tubular cells or expression of IL-2R on lymphoid cells; also the cytological pattern of inflammation was clearly different. The inflammation was dominated by mononuclear phagocytes, which appeared in these grafts shortly after transplantation. This pattern of inflammation, demonstrated by immunocytology, may represent an entirely different inflammatory cascade, not dominated by the usual T cell driven mechanisms. Humoral mechanisms might be involved in these reactions.

References

1. Fuggle SV, McWhinnie DL, Chapman JR, Taylor HM, Morris PJ (1986) Sequential analysis of HLA-Class II antigen expression in human renal allografts. Induction of tubular Class II antigens and correlation with clinical parameters. Transplantation 42:144–150
2. Hall B, Duggin GG, Philips J, Bishop GA, Horvath JS, Tiller DJ (1984) Increased expression of HLA-DR antigens on renal tubular cells in renal transplants: relevance to the rejection response. Lancet II:247–251
3. Hancock WW, Gee D, De Moerloose P, Rickles FR, Ewan VA, Atkins RC (1985) Immunohistological analysis of serial biopsies taken during human renal allograft rejection Changing profile of infiltrating cells and activation of the coagulation system. Transplantation 39:430–438
4. Häyry P, von Willebrand E (1986) The influence of the pattern of inflammation and administration of seroids on Class II MHC antigen expression in renal transplants. Transplantation 42: 358–363
5. von Willebrand E, Häyry P (1987) Relationship between cellular and molecular markers of inflammation in human kidney allograft rejection. Transplant Proc 19: 1644–1645
6. von Willebrand E, Salmela K, Isoniemi H, Krogerus L, Taskinen E, Häyry P (1991) Induction of HLA Class II antigen and IL-2 receptor expression in acute vascular rejection of human kidney allografts. Transplantation, in press

Cytokines

Transplant Int (1992) 5 [Suppl 1]: S 695–S 697

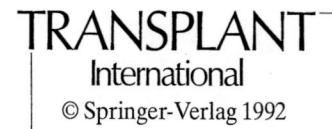

© Springer-Verlag 1992

T-cell receptor Vβ gene usage by lymphocytes infiltrating human renal allografts

I. E. Gecim[1], S. E. Christmas[2], R. Brew[2], B. F. Flanagan[2], N. J. Wheatcroft[2], A. Bakran[1], and R. A. Sells[1]

[1] Renal Transplant Unit and [2] Department of Immunology, Royal Liverpool University Hospital, Liverpool, United Kingdom

Abstract. T cell lines have been derived from human kidney allograft biopsies using mitogenic stimulation. Southern blotting using a T-cell receptor (TCR) Cβ probe revealed an oligoclonal pattern of rearranged bands in all 12 samples analysed. In some cases, differences in band patterns were noted between independent cultures from the same biopsy. Most T-cell clones derived from 2 biopsies showed different patterns of rearranged bands. The polymerase chain reaction (PCR) was used to study TCR Vβ gene usage in allograft-derived T-cell cultures. This was more sensitive and more informative than Southern blotting and revealed that most TCR Vβ genes were expressed in T cells from biopsies showing cellular rejection. The potential usefulness of this technique to quantify TCR V gene usage in allospecific T-cell populations is discussed.

Key words: Renal transplantation – T-cell receptor – Lymphocytes

The human T-cell repertoire for antigen is generated by somatic rearrangement of the T-cell receptor (TCR), variable diversity, and adjoining gene segments [1]. There are over 50 distinct TCR Vβ gene segments which can be assigned to around 20 subgroups on the basis of sequence homology and a similar diversity of TCR Vα segments which together contribute to the high degree of combinatorial diversity of the TCR αβ heterodimer [2]. In the mouse, T cells expressing certain Vβ genes predominantly recognise particular alloantigens [3] and are consequently deleted during thymic ontogeny in strains bearing that particular alloantigen [4, 5]. However, in man it is not clear whether T cells expressing particular Vβ genes are predominantly reactive with distinct alloantigenic determinants. If this is the case, a more specific form of immuno-

suppression might be possible in transplant patients using reagents against TCR gene products which are predominantly reactive towards the relevant mismatched HLA antigen(s).

Studies of small numbers of alloreactive T-cell clones have revealed a bias in TCR Vβ gene usage [6–8], but it is not known whether this is a general phenomenon and whether individual alloantigens preferentially stimulate selected T-cell subsets. Previous studies of rejecting human renal transplants have shown that infiltrating T cells stimulated either with donor alloantigen [9] or with interleukin 2 (IL-2) [10] have an oligoclonal pattern of TCR β gene rearrangements. We have used mitogenically stimulated T cells from renal allograft biopsies to estimate the degree of oligoclonality of the total cellular infiltrate. These studies have been extended by using the polymerase chain reaction (PCR) to identify TCR Vβ gene expression in these T-cell cultures. This has revealed that although T cells from rejecting allografts show oligoclonal patterns of TCR β gene rearrangement using Southern blotting, expression of most TCR Vβ genes can be detected in these infiltrates using the PCR.

Materials and methods

T-cell culture. Needle biopsies ca. 10×1 mm in diameter were taken from kidneys of transplant patients with deteriorating renal function. Biopsies were gently disaggregated in a small volume of phosphate buffered saline (PBS) using opposing 21 G needles and filtered through fine gauze. Cells were washed with PBS and resuspended in 3 ml RPMI 1640 plus 10 % heat-inactivated fetal calf serum + antibiotics (RPMI-CS). They were then plated in 100-μl aliquots into 96-well, round-bottomed plates containing feeder mixture comprising RPMI-CS plus 2×10^5 allogeneic peripheral blood mononuclear cells/ml and 10^5 B lymphoblastoid cells/ml (both given 5000 rads γ-irradiation), 100 U/ml IL-2 (Biotest), 1 μg/ml phytohaemagglutinin (PHA; Wellcome), 1 μg/ml indomethacin (100 μl feeder mixture/well). This culture system results in clonal proliferation of almost 100 % of peripheral blood αβ T cells [11]. Plates were examined after incubating for 10–16 days at 37 °C in an atmosphere of 5 % CO_2, and in those samples in which almost all wells were positive for T-cell growth, cells from rows of 8 wells were pooled and

Offprint requests to: Dr. S. E. Christmas, Department of Immunology, Royal Liverpool University Hospital, P. O. Box 147, Liverpool L69 3BX, United Kingdom

PATIENT JML

Eco RI   **Cβ probe**

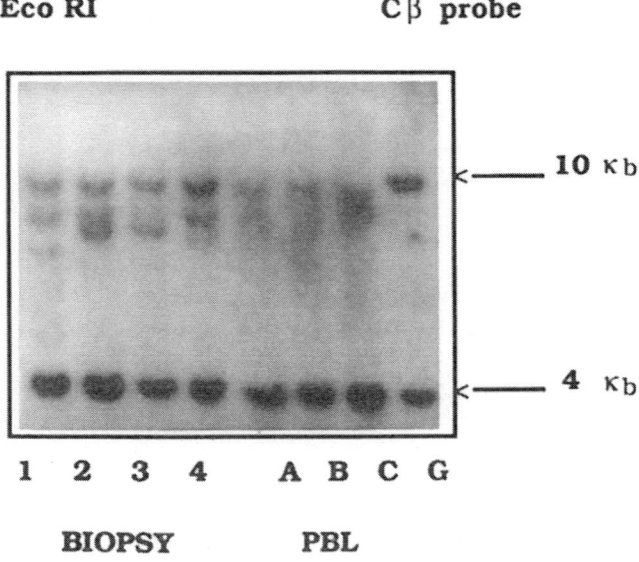

← 10 κb

← 4 κb

1   2   3   4   A   B   C   G

BIOPSY   **PBL**

Fig. 1. Southern blot analysis of DNA from 4 independent T-cell populations *(1–4)* derived from the same kidney transplant biopsy from patient JML compared with PBL samples *(A–C)* from the same patient. *G,* germ-line DNA

PATIENT EL

Eco RI   **Cβ probe**

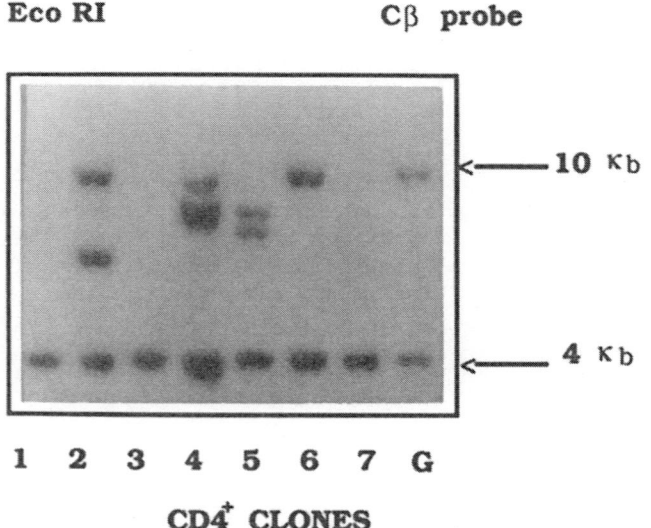

← 10 κb

← 4 κb

1   2   3   4   5   6   7   G

CD4⁺ CLONES

Fig. 2. Southern blot analysis of DNA from CD4$^+$ T-cell clones obtained from a kidney transplant biopsy from patient EL

grown for a further 4–10 days in the same feeder mixture but without PHA. For most biopsies, 10^6–10^7 T cells were obtained from at least three independent aliquots of the same biopsy. In some experiments, T cells were cloned directly from the biopsy extract by plating out at limiting dilution as above and growing clones for 3–4 weeks prior to phenotypic analysis with monoclonal antibodies against CD3, CD4, and CD8 (Dako).
TCR β gene analysis. RNA was prepared from aliquots of 1–5×10^5 T cells from each biopsy using a micro-method [7]. The remainder of the cells were lysed in the presence of sodium dodecylsulphate (SDS) and proteinase K, and the DNA was extracted with phenol

and chloroform and precipitated with ammonium acetate and ethanol [12]. The DNA was then dried and redissolved in TE buffer, pH 7.6. For Southern blotting, 10–15 μg aliquots were digested with *Eco*RI and electrophoresed in a 0.7% agarose gel. The DNA was transferred to a nylon membrane (Hybond N, Amersham) and hybridised with a ^{32}P-labelled TCR C probe (pB400, Dr. M. J. Owen, ICRF, London) [13]. For PCR analysis, the RNA was converted to cDNA with reverse transcriptase using a Cβ oligonucleotide primer [7]. The cDNA was divided into 20 aliquots and the PCR performed using unique primers for human TCR Vβ subgroups 1–20 together with a Cβ primer [7]. The PCR was carried out using 12 cycles of 1 min denaturation at 94 °C, 2 min annealing at 55 °C and 2 min extension at 72 °C followed by 20 similar cycles but with a 3 min extension time. The reaction was terminated with single cycles with extension times of 4.2 min and 5.2 min at 72 °C. The PCR products were then run on a 2% agarose gel and visualised in the presence of ethidium bromide. In some experiments, the PCR products were then blotted onto Hybond N and hybridised with an internal Cβ oligonucleotide end-labelled with γ-^{32}P-dATP. The relative intensities of bands obtained by ethidium bromide staining or autoradiography were estimated visually on a scale of 0–3 where 0 = band absent and 3 = strong band. Sensitivity and specificity controls were performed using cDNA from the T-cell line Jurkat, which expresses Vβ 8, and from normal peripheral blood lymphocytes (PBL). The former gave only a single band with the Vβ 8 primer and the latter gave bands with all 20 TCR Vβ primers as expected.

Results

Southern blot analysis

Of 60 biopsies studies, T-cell growth was noted in almost all wells in 26 (43%), most of which were diagnosed histologically as having cellular rejection. In all 12 cases in which multiple samples were analysed using Southern blotting, discrete rearranged bands were observed with DNA digested with *Eco*RI and hybridised with the Cβ probe (Fig. 1). In some cases, independent T-cell DNA samples from the same biopsy showed similar patterns of rearranged bands, but in others the rearranged bands sizes were clearly different in separate samples from the same biopsy. In contrast, PBL DNA from all samples showed a smear around the 7–10kb region in which no discrete bands were discernible (Fig. 1). T-cell clones were generated from biopsies from 2 patients with cellular rejection, and these comprised roughly equal numbers of CD4$^+$ and CD8$^+$ clones. When analysed using Southern blotting, most CD4$^+$ clones had differently sized rearranged bands (Fig. 2), as did most CD8$^+$ clones (data not shown).

Polymerase chain reaction experiments

Biopsy T-cell cDNA from 4 patients with cellular rejection and 1 with pyelonephritis was amplified by the PCR using TCR Vβ and Cβ primers. In the former 4 cases, the majority of the TCR Vβ genes were being expressed in the biopsy T-cell infiltrate. In 3 independent T-cell populations from the same biopsy (patient GC), a similar but not identical pattern of Vβ gene usage was found (Table 1). When biopsy T-cell populations were compared with PBL from the same patient, there was again a similar but not identical pattern of TCR Vβ gene usage (Table 2). A more

Table 1. Polymerase chain reaction (PCR) analysis of T-cell receptor (TCR) Vβ gene usage in 3 independent T-cell lines from the same biopsy from patient G. C. who was showing cellular rejection. The intensity of the bands stained with ethidium bromide was estimated according to the following scale: 3 = strong band, 2 = intermediate band, 1 = weak band, – = nothing visible

Biopsy	TCR Vβ Gene																			
	1	2	3	4	5	6	7	8	9	10	11	12	13	14	15	16	17	18	19	20
1	3	1	2	2	3	–	–	2	1	–	1	2	2	2	–	–	–	1	–	–
2	2	2	3	1	1	1	2	2	1	–	–	1	3	2	–	–	–	2	–	–
3	2	2	3	2	2	–	2	3	1	–	1	1	2	2	1	1	2	–	–	1

Table 2. PCR analysis of TCR Vβ gene usage by biopsy T cells and PBL from patient B. G. who was showing cellular rejection. Band intensities were scored as in Table 1

	TCR Vβ Gene																			
	1	2	3	4	5	6	7	8	9	10	11	12	13	14	15	16	17	18	19	20
Biopsy	2	2	3	–	2	–	–	1	1	–	–	2	3	2	1	1	2	1	–	–
PBL	1	2	3	1	2	–	–	1	1	–	1	1	2	2	1	2	2	3	1	–

Table 3. PCR analysis of TCR Vβ gene usage in 2 biopsy T-cell lines from patient H. W. suffering from pyelonephritis as assessed by visualisation of an ethidium bromide-stained gel (EtBr) or by hybridisation with an internal Cβ probe (Probe). Band intensities were scored as in Table 1

	TCR Vβ Gene																			
	1	2	3	4	5	6	7	8	9	10	11	12	13	14	15	16	17	18	19	20
1. EtBr	–	1	1	–	–	–	–	–	–	–	–	–	1	–	–	–	2	–	–	–
1. Probe	1	2	3	–	1	–	–	–	–	–	–	–	1	1	–	–	3	1	–	–
2. EtBr	–	–	1	–	–	–	–	–	–	–	–	–	1	–	–	–	2	–	–	1
2. Probe	2	1	2	–	1	–	–	1	–	–	–	–	3	2	–	–	3	1	–	2

visible, as has been reported previously [10]. However, results with the PCR showed that in all samples evidencing cellular rejection, the majority of the TCR Vβ subgroups was represented, indicating that Southern blotting is a relatively insensitive way of detecting T-cell polyclonality.

The PCR analysis of independent T-cell populations derived from the same biopsy showed similar patterns of TCR Vβ gene usage, indicating that the technique is reproducible. The similar pattern of TCR Vβ gene usage between the biopsy and peripheral T cells suggests either that there was a predominance of 'innocent bystanders' in the infiltrates studied or that T cells expressing a wide range of TCR Vβ genes can recognise a small number of alloantigens. The use of donor stimulator cells in in vitro culture experiments with allograft-derived T cells may reveal which of these is the case. A more accurate method of quantifying the PCR products would be needed to detect any relative increases or decreases in the proportions of T cells expressing different TCR Vβ genes following stimulation with alloantigen. Although the PCR products could readily be visualised in ethidium bromide-stained gels, the sensitivity of detection was increased by hybridisation with an internal Cβ oligonucleotide probe. This revealed bands which were not visible in the gel. The subjective method used for quantifying PCR products by estimating band intensities can undoubtedly be improved upon by using densitometry or by serially diluting PCR products [14] followed by probing with a Cβ probe, and future work will address this.

Acknowledgements. This work was supported by a grant to I. E. G. from the British Council. N. J. W. was the recipient of a Wellcome Trust Vacation Scholarship.

sensitive method of detecting PCR products not visible by ethidium bromide staining was to hybridise then with an internal Cβ oligonucleotide probe (Table 3). This also showed that there was a considerably more restricted pattern of TCR Vβ gene usage in a biopsy from a patient subsequently diagnosed histologically as suffering from pyelonephritis rather than cellular rejection.

Discussion

We have used mitogenic stimulation to study TCR Vβ gene usage by the total T-cell population infiltrating renal allografts during a rejection episode. Although this does not take into account the specificity of T cells for donor alloantigen, in the absence of donor material this is a convenient way of analysing both donor-specific and nonspecific T cells within allograft biopsies. All 12 biopsies studied in detail had oligoclonal patterns of TCR β gene rearrangement as detected by Southern blotting. Statistically spealcing, each independent sample from a single biopsy contained the progeny of at least 30 T-cell clones, but in such samples only a few rearranged bands were

References

1. Siu G, Clark S, Yoshikai Y, Malissem M, Yanagi Y, Strauss E, Mak T, Hood L (1984) Cell 37: 393
2. Wilson RK, Lai E, Concannon P, Barth RK, Hood LE (1988) Immunol Rev 101: 149
3. Kappler J, Wade T, White J, Kushnir E, Blackman M, Bill J, Roehm N, Marrack P (1987) Cell 49: 263
4. Kappler J, Roehm N, Marrack P (1987) Cell 49: 273
5. Bill J, Kanagawa O, Woodland DL, Palmer E (1989) J Exp Med 169: 1405
6. Beall SS, Lawrence JV, Bradley DA, Mattson DH, Singer DS, Biddison WE (1987) J Immunol 139: 1320
7. Bragado R, Lauzurica P, Lopez D, Lopez de Castro JA (1990) J Exp Med 171: 1189
8. Wilson KE, Ball E, Stasny P, Capra JD (1991) Scand J Immunol 33: 131
9. Miceli MC, Finn OJ (1989) J Immunol 142: 81
10. Frisman DM, Hurwitz AA, Bennett WT, Boyle LA, Fallon JT, Dec GW, Colvin RB, Kurnick JT (1990) Hum Immunol 28: 208
11. Christmas SE (1989) Eur J Immunol 19: 741
12. Sambrook J, Fritsch EF, Maniatis T (1989) Molecular cloning: a laboratory manual, 2nd edn. Cold Spring Harbor, New York
13. Collins MKL, Kissonerghis AM, Dunne MJ, Watson CJ, Rigby PWJ, Owen MJ (1985) EMBO J 4: 1211
14. Dallman MJ, Larsen CP, Morris PJ (1991) J Exp Med 174: 493

Transplant Int (1992) 5 [Suppl 1]: S 698–S 702

TRANSPLANT
International
© Springer-Verlag 1992
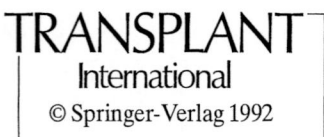

Effects of interleukin 2 receptor b chain (P75)-specific monoclonal antibody on the generation of cytotoxic T lymphocytes and suppressor T cells in mixid lymphocyte culture

S. Kusaka, K. Sakagami, T. Fujiwara, M. Uda, and K. Orita

First Department of Surgery, Okayama University Medical School, Okayama, Japan

Abstract. The interaction of interleukin 2 (IL-2) with its receptor (IL-2R) plays an essential role in the proliferation and differentiation of T cells. The IL-2R β-chain is considered to function directly in the intracellular signal transduction. In this study, we investigated using a newly established IL-2R β-chain-specific monoclonal antibody (MAb) (TU-25) and an IL-2R α-chain-specific MAb (H-31). The IL-2-induced proliferation of concanavalin blasts and the mixed lymphocyte reaction (MLR) were suppressed by TU-25 in combination with H-31. This combination had a greater suppressive effect than each of them alone. The generation of cytotoxic T lymphocytes (CTL) using a cell-mediated lympholysis (CML) assay, was not inhibited by TU-25 alone. TU-25 in combination with H-31 suppressed the generation of CTL completely in this assay even if recombinant IL-2 (rIL-2) was added. Although the CTL generation was inhibited, cells that suppressed a fresh MLR were preserved. Our study suggests that the combination of TU-25 with H-31 completely blocks the functional high-affinity binding site of IL-2 but does not inhibit the generation of suppressor cells. This may lead to immunosuppressive therapy using an IL-2R β-chain-specific MAb in combination with an IL-2R α-chain-specific MAb in clinical organ transplantation.

Key words: Interleukin 2 (IL-2) – IL-2 receptor – Monoclonal antibody – Suppressor cell

Interleukin 2 (IL-2) is produced by allostimulated T cells and acts via its receptor (IL-2R) on the surface of T cells. The binding of IL-2 to the IL-2R leads to the proliferation and the differentiation of T cells. There are three forms of receptor, which have three different affinities to IL-2. The high-affinity one has been shown to be composed of at least two distinct subunits, IL-2R α-chain (p55) and IL-2R β-chain (p75), each of which exhibits low-affinity and in-

termediate-affinity to IL-2 [13, 21, 22]. The IL-2R β-chain has a larger intracellular domain than the IL-2R α-chain. The interaction between IL-2 and the intermediate- or high-affinity receptor can induce intracellular signal transduction, indicating that the IL-2R β-chain directly functions in the signal transduction pathway [3, 4, 14].

Recently, monoclonal antibodies (MAb) directed against the IL-2R β-chain have been produced [9, 17, 21]. In this study, we used a newly established IL-2R β-chain-specific MAb (TU-25) and an IL-2R α-chain-specific MAb (H-31) and observed their effects on the proliferation of T cells by allostimulation or IL-2 and the generation of cytotoxic T lymphocytes (CTL) or suppressor T cells.

Materials and methods

Antibodies. The H-31 and TU-25 are IgG$_1$ MAb directed against the IL-2R α- and β-chains, respectively, and were kindly given by Dr. Sugamura (Tohoku University, Sendai, Japan). The 2-3D1, which was used as a control MAb, is also an IgG$_1$ MAb directed against *Escherichia coli*.

IL-2-induced proliferation of ConA blasts. Peripheral blood lymphocytes (PBL) were isolated by Ficoll-Hypaque gradient density centrifugation. Concanavalin A (ConA) blasts were obtained by stimulating PBL with 5 µg/ml ConA (Gibco Laboratories, Grand Island, N. Y.) for 3 days in RPMI 1640 medium containing 25 mM HEPES (Difco Laboratories, Detroit, Mich.) and 10% fetal calf serum (FCS; Difco Laboratories) at 37 °C, 5% CO$_2$. The ConA blasts were washed twice and plated out at a concentration of 1×10^4 cells/well in 200 µl of culture medium in 96-well, flat-bottomed plates (Falcon tissue culture plate, 3072). The H-31 and TU-25 were tested in the presence of different concentrations of recombinant IL-2 (rIL-2). After 48 h incubation (37 °C, 5% CO$_2$), the cultures were pulsed with 1.0 µCi/well of tritiated thymidine (TdR) for 18 h, harvested, and then counted for radioactivity.

Inhibition of the MLR. Equal numbers (5×10^4) of responder cells and MMC-treated stimulator cells were plated in 96-well, round-bottomed plates (FALCON tissue culture plate, 3077). In the presence or absence of MAb, the cells were cultured for 6 days, harvested, and pulsed with 1 µCi/well of ^{3}H-TdR 18 h before harvesting.

Induction of CTL and the CML assay. The induction of CTL was carried out in mixed lymphocyte culture (MLC). Equal numbers (1×10^7) of responder cells and MMC-treated stimulator cells were

Offprint requests to: S. Kusaka, M. D., First Department of Surgery, Okayama University Medical School, 2-5-1 Shikata-cho, Okayama 700, Japan

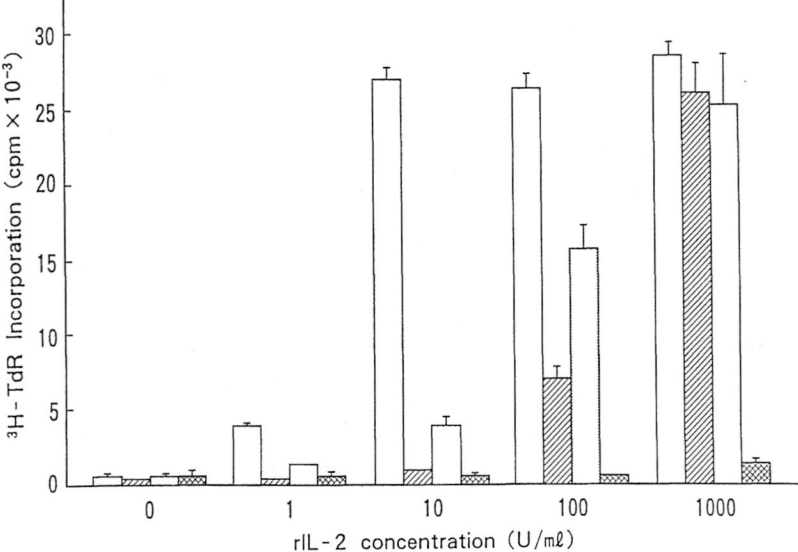

Fig. 1. Inhibitory effect of H-31 and TU-25 on interleukin 2 (IL-2)-induced proliferation. Concanavalin A (ConA) blasts were cultured without monoclonal antibody, MAb (□) or with H-31 (50 μg/ml; ▨), TU-25 (50 μg/ml; ▢), or H-31 (50 μg/ml) + TU-25 (50 μg/ml) (▨) in the presence of rIL-2

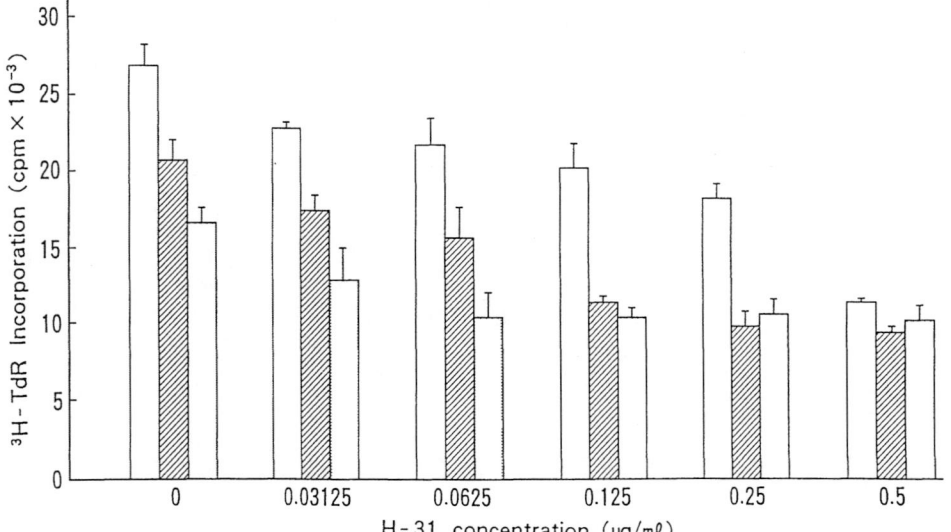

Fig. 2. Inhibitory effect of H-31 and TU-25 on the mixed lymphocyte reaction (MLR) which was performed in the presence of H-31 without TU-25 (□) or with TU-25 (1.25 μg/ml) (▨) or TU-25 (2.5 μg/ml) (□)

cocultured for 7 days in a total volume of 20 ml in the presence or absence of MAb. These induced cells were used as effector cells in a cell-mediated lympholysis (CML) assay. Target cells, fresh stimulator PBL, or third-party PBL were cultured for 3 days in culture medium containing 50 μg/ml phytohemagglutinin (PHA-P; Difco Laboratories) and labeled with ^{51}Cr. Target cells (1×10^4/well) were added to effector cells in 96-well, round-bottomed plates. After 6 h incubation, the supernatant from each well was harvested using a supernatant collection system (Skatron, Lier, Norway), and ^{51}Cr release was determined using an autowell gamma-system. Spontaneous release was determined by incubating the target cells in medium alone, while maximum release was determined by target cells exposed to 1 N NaOH. The percentage lysis of target cells was calculated according to the formula: % Cytotoxicity = (Experimental release − Spontaneous release) × 100 (Maximum release − Spontaneous release)

CTL generation in the presence of exogeneous rIL-2. Various concentrations of rIL-2 were added at the initiation of the MLC in the presence of H-31 (1.0 μg/ml) or H-31 (1.0 μg/ml) and TU-25 (2.0 μg/ml) or in the absence of MAb. The percentage lysis of target cells was determined and calculated as described above.

Generation of suppressor cells. Equal numbers (1×10^7) of responder cells and MMC-treated stimulator cells were cocultured for 10 days in a total volume of 20 ml in the presence of 1.0 μg/ml of H-31 and 2.0 μg/ml of TU-25 or in the absence of MAb. After 10 days, the cells were harvested, washed twice, and restimulated using the same al-

logeneic stimulator cells for 4 days in the absence of MAb. After 14 days from the initiation of culture, the induced cells were harvested, MMC-treated, and added as regulators in a primary MLR. Regulator cells were mixed with 5×10^4 fresh autologous PBL and 5×10^4 MMC-treated PBL (as specific stimulators or third-party stimulators). To measure the control response, autologous fresh PBL were MMC-treated and added as regulators. Cells were cultured for 6 days and pulsed with 1 μCi/well of ^{3}H-TdR 18 h before harvesting. The percentage suppression was calculated by the formula: % Suppression = 1 − cpm (responder + stimulator + induced regulator) × 100 cpm (responder + stimulator + fresh autologous regulator)

Results

As shown in Fig. 1, the rIL-2-induced proliferation of ConA blasts was suppressed by either H-31 or TU-25 alone at low concentrations of rIL-2. H-31 showed a stronger suppression action than TU-25. Proliferation was completely inhibited in the presence of both H-31 and TU-25 despite a high concentration of rIL-2 (1000 U/ml).

Figure 2 indicates that both H-31 and TU-25 showed suppressive effects on the MLR in a dose-dependent manner. Inhibition of the MLR by H-31 was stronger than that by TU-25 at the same concentration. H-31 brought about

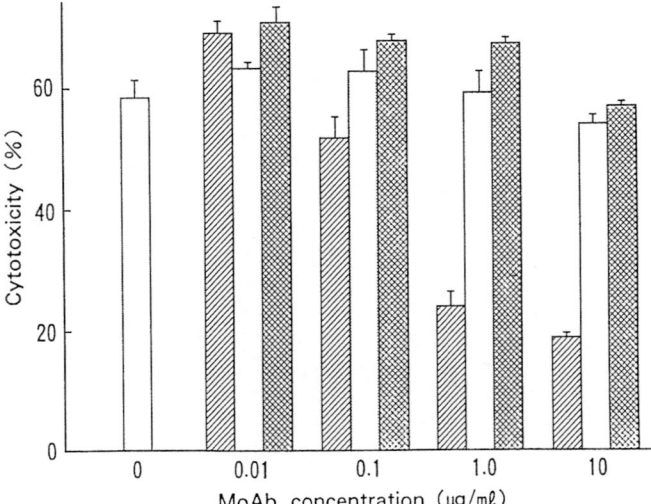

Fig. 3. Inhibitory effect of H-31 and TU-25 on cytotoxic T lymphocyte (CTL) generation. Induction of CTL was performed without MAb (☐) or in the presence of H-31 (▨), TU-25 (☐), or control MAb (2-3D1) (▩). Cell-mediated lympholysis (CML) assay was performed at 50:1 of effector-to-target ratio

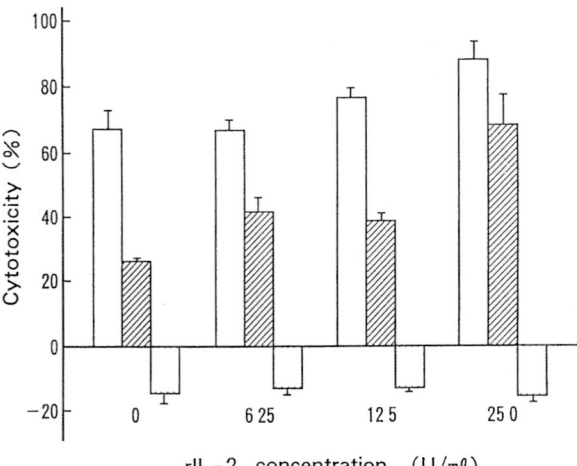

Fig. 5. Effect of H-31 and TU-25 on CTL generation in the presence of exogenous recombinant IL-2 (rIL-2). Induction of CTL was carried out without MAb (☐) or with H-31 (1.0 μg/ml; ▨) or H-31 (1.0 μg/ml) + TU-25 (2.0 μg/ml) (☐) in the presence of rIL-2. CML assay was performed at 50:1 of effector-to-target ratio

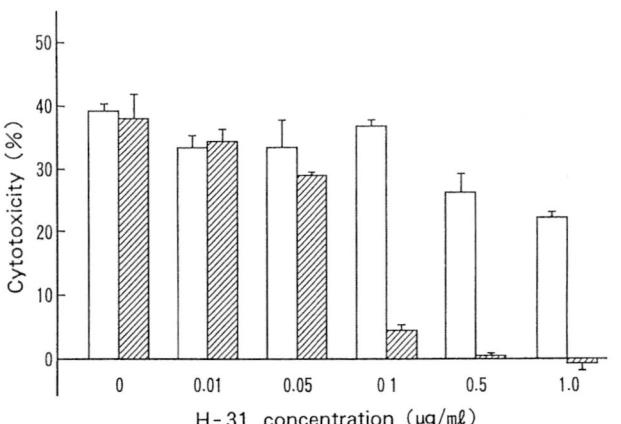

Fig. 4. Combined effect of TU-25 with H-31 on CTL generation. Induction of CTL was performed in the presence of H-31 without TU-25 (☐) or with TU-25 (2.0 μg/ml; ▨). CML assay was performed at 50:1 of effector-to-target ratio

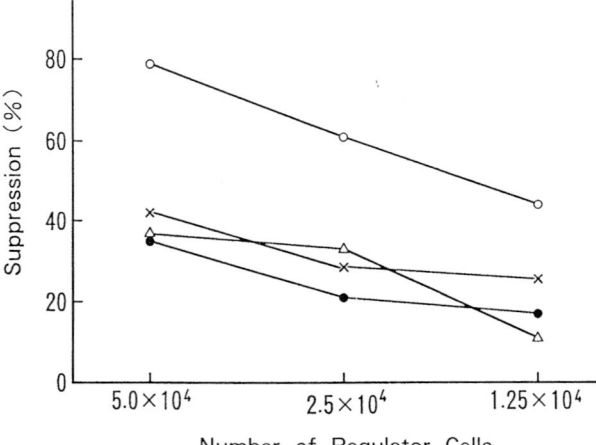

Fig. 6. Suppression of MLR by autologous cells primed in the presence of H-31 and TU-25. Control regulator cells, primed in the absence of MAb, were MMC-treated and added to fresh specific MLR (o—o) or third-party MLR (x—x). Modified primed cells, cultured in the presence of H-31 (1.0 μg/ml) + TU-25 (2.0 μg/ml), were MMC-treated and added to fresh specific MLR (●—●) or third-party MLR (△—△)

24% inhibition at a concentration of 0.125 μg/ml; in combination with TU-25 (1.25 μg/ml) it showed 57% inhibition, which was equal to the inhibition at a concentration of 0.5 μg/ml of H-31 alone.

To determine whether H-31 or TU-25 alone could inhibit the generation of CTL, they were added at the initiation of the MLC. As shown in Fig. 3, 2–3D1, a control MAb, did not affect the percentage cytotoxicity. H-31 alone inhibited CTL generation in a dose-dependent manner, and 59% inhibition was observed at a concentration of 1.0 μg/ml. In contrast, TU-25 alone had no inhibitory effect on CTL generation at any concentration.

To test the combined effect of TU-25 with H-31, they were added at various concentrations at the initiation of cultures. Figure 4 reveals that in the presence of various concentrations of H-31, the addition of TU-25 (2.0 μg/ml) reduced CTL generation much more effectively than the same concentration of H-31 alone. H-31 at a concentra-

tion of 0.5 μg/ml showed 43% inhibition of CTL generation, but 99% inhibition was observed in combination with TU-25 (2.0 μg/ml). Furthermore, TU-25 inhibited CTL generation in a dose-dependent manner in the presence of H-31 at a concentration of 0.1 μg/ml.

As shown in Fig. 5, when rIL-2 was added in the controls, the percentage cytotoxicity was augmented in a dose-dependent manner. The inhibitory effect of H-31 on CTL generation was reduced when rIL-2 was added. The percentage cytotoxicity was returned to the level of the control at a concentration of 25 U/ml. In the combination of H-31 (1.0 μg/ml) with TU-25 (2.0 μg/ml), the inhibitory effect on CTL generation was preserved despite the presence of rIL-2.

As shown in Fig. 6, the control regulator cells (R') showed 79% inhibition of fresh specific MLR (regulator cells 5 × 10⁴). However, at the same time (as shown in

Table 1. Cytotoxicity 2 weeks after the initiation of culture

Effector	Target	% Cytotoxicity (Mean ± SD)			
		Effector to target ratio			
		50:1	25:1	12.5:1	6.25:1
R' (Control)	D (Specific)	78.4 ± 4.9	67.4 ± 1.3	53.9 ± 1.8	39.7 ± 1.6
R" (H-31 1.0 µg/ml + TU-25 2.0 µg/ml)	D	3.6 ± 0.5	4.0 ± 1.2	1.9 ± 0.9	0.5 ± 1.5
R'	C (Third party)	11.4 ± 0.8	3.3 ± 0.6	0.7 ± 0.8	− 1.0 ± 0.7
R"	C	− 5.4 ± 0.6	− 2.2 ± 0.7	− 0.5 ± 0.5	− 1.7 ± 1.0

Table 1), 78% cytotoxicity was observed for the specific stimulator cells (effector-to-target ratio was 50:1). Modified cells primed in the presence of H-31 and TU-25 (R") also showed an inhibition of specific MLR and third-party MLR (35% and 37% inhibition, respectively). This inhibition was weaker than the control regulator cells (R") showed no cytotoxicity to both stimulator cells, although they were restimulated without MAb.

Discussion

MAbs directed against the IL-2R α-chain have been shown to inhibit the proliferation of allostimulated T cells and the generation of CTL by allogeneic stimulation in vitro [2]. In this study, we tested the effect of TU-25, a newly established IL-2R β-chain-specific MAb, on the proliferation of T cells and on the generation of CTL or suppressor cells.

H-31, an IL-2R α-chain-specific MAb, showed some inhibitory effects on the proliferation of T cells or the generation of CTL. Moreover, H-31 and TU-25 together showed synergistic effects in a dose-dependent manner. Interestingly, although the IL-2R β-chain is considered to be responsible for signal transduction, little inhibitory effect was observed with the addition of TU-25 alone. However, TU-25 showed inhibitory effects in the presence of H-31 in a dose-dependent manner which were synergistic.

These effects may be explained by several IL-2 binding studies [8, 24]. It was reported that when lymphocytes were stimulated in allogeneic cultures at 37 °C, new β-chains were synthesized on the lymphocytes to form high-affinity receptors in cooperation with free α-chains. Once high-affinity receptors have formed, IL-2 can interact very rapidly with them, since the affinity of the receptors is much higher than that of the IL-2R β-chain-specific MAb.

Kamio et al. showed that an IL-2R β-chain-specific MAb completely inhibited the binding of the IL-2R β-chain with IL-2 at 4 °C, but at 37 °C the high-affinity IL-2R reappeared [5]. This was considered to be due to the replacement of the IL-2R β-chain-specific MAb by α-chain-mediated IL-2. They suggested that the IL-2R α-chain functions as a dimension converter of IL-2.

Treatment with antibodies against the IL-2R α-chain has been demonstrated to prolong graft survival or prevent allograft rejection in mice, rats, and monkeys [6, 10–12]. Recently, pilot studies and randomized trials have been performed in clinical human kidney transplantation [1, 7, 15]. The treatment was effective in preventing early rejection in combination with cyclosporin A or corticosteroids. An IL-2R α-chain-specific MAb was effective in acute rejection, but as shown in this study, the addition of exogenous rIL-2 to ConA blasts or CML assay reversed its inhibitory effect. Single therapy may not be sufficient to block the high-affinity IL-2R.

It has been shown that the IL-2R α-chain-specific MAb did not inhibit MLC-generated suppressor cells in vivo and in vitro [20]. Tan et al. reported that activation of antigen-specific T suppressor-inducer and T suppressor-effector cells appeared to be relatively IL-2 independent in their study using α-chain-specific MAb [19]. As shown above, primed cells in the presence of H-31 and TU-25 did not show such a strong and antigen-specific effect. Also, during stimulation without MAb they did not show any cytotoxicity. It was reported that in immunofluorescence analysis, the IL-2R α-chain and β-chain were preferentially expressed on CD4+ and CD8+ T cells with CD45RO+ (memory) phenotypes, respectively [16]. These CD45RO+ CD4+ and CD8+ T cells, unlike CD45RO− cells, proliferate in response to exogenous IL-2. This may explain why suppressor cells were not inhibited by IL-2R-specific MAbs.

When T cells are exposed to alloantigens, high-affinity receptors are synthesized, and the interaction of IL-2 with them stimulates mitosis and clonal expansion of the progenitors. Immunosuppressive therapy against the high-affinity IL-2R may be relatively specific and a target in the alloantigen-specific T-cell repertoire. Recently, the existence of the third component of IL-2R, the γ-chain (p64), was demonstrated [18]. This receptor is thought to be associated with the β-chain and to be concerned with intracellular signal transduction. The inhibition of this new receptor (γ-chain receptor) will be necessary for complete blockade of the high-affinity receptor.

Thus, our study suggests that immunosuppressive therapy using an IL-2R β-chain-specific MAb in combination with an IL-2R α-chain-specific MAb may be a new therapeutic strategy in clinical organ transplantation.

References

1. Cantarovich D, Le Mauff B, Hourmant M, Giral M, Denis M, Jacques Y, Soulillou JP (1989) Anti-IL2 receptor monoclonal antibody (33B3.1) in prophylaxis of early kidney rejection in humans: a randomized trial versus rabbit antithymocyte globulin. Transplant Proc 21: 1769–1771

S702

2. Depper JM, Leonard WJ, Robb RJ, Waldmann TA, Greene WC (1983) Blockade of the interleukin 2 receptor by anti Tac antibody: inhibition of human lymphocyte activation. J Immunol 131: 690–696

3. Hatakeyama M, Tsudo M, Minamoto S, Kono T, Doi T, Miyata T, Miyasaka M, Taniguchi T (1989) Interleukin 2 receptor β chain gene: generation of three receptor forms by cloned human and β chain cDNA's. Science 244: 551–556

4. Hatakeyama M, Mori H, Doi T, Taniguchi T (1989) A restricted cytoplasmic region of IL-2 receptor β chain is essential for growth signal transduction but not for ligand binding and internalization. Cell 59: 837–845

5. Kamio M, Uchiyama T, Arima N, Itoh K, Ishikawa T, Hori T, Uchino H (1990) Role of α chain-IL-2 complex in the formation of the ternary complex of IL-2 and high-affinity IL-2 receptor. Int Immunol 2: 521–530

6. Kirkmann RL, Barrett LV, Storm TB, Gaulton GN, Kelley VE, Kolton WA, Schoen FJ, Ytheier A, Strom TB (1985) The effect of anti interleukin-2 receptor monoclonal antibody on allograft rejection. Transplantation 40: 719–722

7. Kirkmann RL, Shapiro ME, Carpenter CB, McKay DB, Milford EL, Ramos EL, Tilney NL, Waldmann TA, Zimmerman CE, Storm TB (1991) A randmized prospective trial of anti-Tac monoclonal antibody in human renal transplantation. Transplant Proc 23: 1066–1067

8. Lowenthal JW, Greene WC (1987) Contrasting interleukin 2 binding properties of the α (p55) and β (p70) protein subunits of the human high-affinity interleukin 2 receptor. J Exp Med 166: 1156–1161

9. Ohbo K, Takeshita T, Asao H, Kurahayashi Y, Tada K, Mori H, Hatakeyama M, Taniguchi T, Sugamura K (1991) Monoclonal antibodies defining distinct epitopes of the human IL-2 receptor β chain and their differential effects on IL-2 response. J Exp Med (in press)

10. Reed MH, Shapiro ME, Strom TB, Milford EL, Carpenter CB, Weinberg DS, Reimann KA, Letvin NL, Waldmann TA, Kirkmann RL (1989) Prolongation of primate renal allograft survival by anti-TAC, an anti-human IL-2 receptor monoclonal antibody. Transplantation 47: 55–59

11. Sakagami K, Ohsaki T, Ohnishi T, Saito S, Matsuoka J, Orita K (1988) The effect of anti-interleukin 2 monoclonal antibody treatment of the survival of rat cardiac allograft. J Surg Res 46: 262–266

12. Shapiro ME, Kirkman RL, Reed MH, Puskas JD, Mazoujian G, Letvin NL, Carpenter CB, Milford EL, Waldmann TA, Strom TB, Schlossman SF (1987) Monoclonal anti-IL2 receptor anti-

body in primate renal transplantation. Transplant Proc 19: 594–598

13. Sharon M, Klausner RD, Cullen BR, Chizzonite R, Leonard WJ (1986) Novel interleukin-2 receptor subunit detected by cross-linking under high-affinity conditions. Science 234: 859–863

14. Siegel JP, Sharon M, Smith PL, Leonard WJ (1987) The IL-2 receptor β chain (p70): role in mediating signals for LAK, NK, and proliferative activities. Science 238: 75–78

15. Solillou JP, Peyronnet P, Le Mauff B, Hourmant M, Olive D, Mawas C, Delaage M, Hirn M, Jacques Y (1987) Prevention of rejection of kidney transplants by monoclonal antibody directed against interleukin 2. Lancet I: 1339–1342

16. Taga K, Kasahara Y, Yachie A, Miyawaki T, Taniguchi N (1991) Preferential expression of IL-2 receptor subunits on memory populations within CD4+ and CD8+ T cells. Immunology 72: 15–19

17. Takeshita T, Goto Y, Tada K, Nagata K, Asao H, Sugamura K (1989) Monoclonal antiboy defining a molecule possibly identical to the p75 subunit of interleukin 2 receptor. J Exp Med 169: 1323–1332

18. Takeshita T, Asao H, Suzuki J, Sugamura K (1990) An associated molecule, p64, with high-affinity interleukin 2 receptor. Int Immunol 2: 477–480

19. Tan P, Anasetti C, Martin PJ, Hansen JA (1990) Alloantigen-specific T suppressor-inducer and T suppressor-effector cells can be activated despite blocking the IL-2 receptor. J Immunol 145: 485–488

20. Tanaka K, Turka LA, Kupiec-Weglinski JW, Milford EL, Ueda H, Diamantstein T, Carpenter CB, Tilney NL (1990) Evidence that monoclonal antibodies against the 55kD subunit of the rat IL-2 receptor do not inhibit the development of suppressor cells generated in mixed lymphocyte culture. Transplantation 50: 125–131

21. Teshigawara K, Wang HM, Kato K, Smith KA (1987) Interleukin 2 high-affinity receptor expression requires two distinct binding proteins. J Exp Med 165: 223–238

22. Tsudo M, Kozak RW, Goldman CK, Waldmann TA (1986) Demonstration of a non-Tac peptide that binds interleukin 2: a potential participant in a multichain interleukin 2 receptor complex. Proc Natl Acad Sci USA 83: 9694–9698

23. Tsudo M, Kitamura F, Miyasaka M (1989) Characterization of the interleukin 2 receptor β chain using three distinct monoclonal antibodies. Proc Natl Acad Sci USA 86: 1982–1986

24. Wang HM, Smith KA (1987) The interleukin 2 receptor: functional consequences of its bimolecular structure. J Exp Med 166: 1055–1169

Quality of Life

Transplant Int (1992) 5 [Suppl 1]: S 705–S 707

TRANSPLANT
International
© Springer-Verlag 1992

Quality of life before and after liver transplantation: experiences with 7 patients with primary biliary cirrhosis in a 2-year follow-up

A. Lähteenmäki[1], K. Höckerstedt[2], S. Kajaste[2], and M. Huttunen[1]

[1] Department of Psychiatry and [2] Fourth Department of Surgery, Helsinki University Hospital, Helsinki, Finland

Abstract. Seven patients with end-stage primary biliary cirrhosis were evaluated both before and 1 and 2 years after liver transplantation using a clinical psychiatric interview and the self-rating questionaire SCL-90. Neuropsychological tests were done before and 1 year after operation. Preoperatively, all patients had a poor general condition and overall quality of life. Flattening of emotions and reactions, regression, disturbances of verbal memory and cognitive function, and dependence on close relatives were observed. One year after transplantation, 6 patients had a much better overall quality of life, and with five patients it improved still further during the 2nd year, but only 2 patients felt that their life situation had fully stabilised. However, nearly all of them experienced phases of moderate or even severe depression or anxiety during those 2 years. On neuropsychological tests patients appeared to be near their normal level. The only patient who died during this follow-up (some months after transplantation) had in her life history a prominent sense of insecurity and mistrust. It seems to take more than a year for the majority of patients to give up the regressive mode of experience and turn to adult interests in life again, as well as psychologically experience the new liver as part of oneself.

Key words: Liver transplantation – Quality of life

The number of liver transplantations has increased and the long-term results have improved considerably in the past few years [9]. There is a growing need to know more of the patients' quality of life and about the long-term recovery process also from the psychological point of view. There are some studies dealing with psychiatric diagnosis [13] or neuropsychological complications [1]

before or after liver transplantation and a few studies with a follow-up from before transplantation to some time after it [5, 11, 12] and only one with a multidimensional perspective to the recovery process including the quality of life [6, 7].

We describe in this study different aspects of the quality of life before and after liver transplantation on three main levels of human life: internal (both somatic and psychic), interpersonal, and functional level, which are all related to each other (Fig. 1).

Materials and methods

We examined 7 adult patients with primary biliary cirrhosis (PBC) who were undergoing liver transplantation in Helsinki. There were 6 women and 1 man. Their mean age was 53 years, (range 45–64). They were evaluated both before and 1 and 2 years after liver transplantation by using a clinical psychiatric interview and a self-rating questionare. Neuropsychological evaluations were done before and 1 year after transplantation. Preoperative evaluations were performed just after the decision of transplantation had been made and the patients put on the waiting list.

The psychiatric interview was semistructured so that the same topics were discussed with every patient, starting from the present life situation and the course of their illness to the coming operation and the future, with special interest in their fears, hopes, and fantasies and their relationship to their family and other people near them. The basic sense of security or insecurity and the ways with which they had reacted to stressful situations or big losses in the past were estimated from their life history.

As a self-rating questionare we used the SCL-90 [3]. It is a 90-item symptom checklist with 9 primary symptom dimensions and 3 global indices of distress. Each item is rated on a 5-point scsale ranging from Not-at-all at one pole to Extremely at the other.

The neuropsychological evaluation was done before and 1 year after transplantation using the following methods [8]: Wechsler Adult Intelligence Scale (WAIS), Wechsler Memory Scale (WMS), trail making test for visuomotor tracking, Stroop test for capacity to resist mental interference.

The neuropsychological findings were compared with a reference group of 53 healthy Finnish males aged 41–50 years. Two patients were retransplanted some months after the first transplantation and their follow-up evaluations were done 1 and 2 years after the second transplantation.

Offprint requests to: K. Höckerstedt, M. D., IV Department of Surgery, Helsinki University Hospital, Kasarminkatu 11, SF-00130 Helsinki, Finland

Functional
level

Interpersonal
level

Internal
level

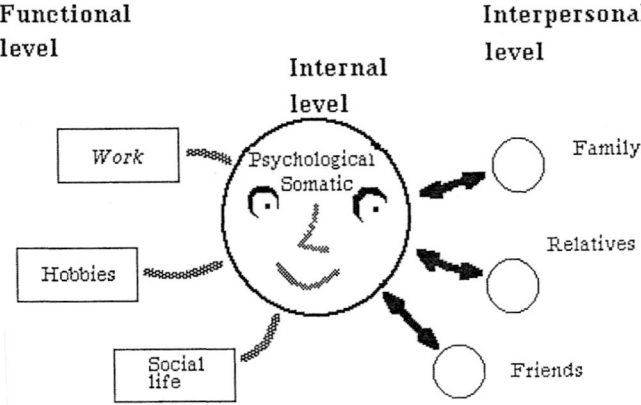

Fig. 1. Different levels of quality of life

Results

Before transplantation all patients were in a poor general somatic condition; they were tired, muscle wasting was evident, most of them had ascites and had had variceal bleedings. None of them was able to work anymore, and they had all moderate to severe difficulties in daily functioning. General flattening of emotions and reactions was evident with every patient when compared with the way they reacted and described their feelings and life situations in the follow-up evaluations. They needed a lot of help and felt dependent on either their family and close relatives or hospital staff. Two of the patients felt insecure, and they did not receive much support or understanding at home. One of them was the only patient who died during this follow-up (some months after transplantation). The rest of the patients found support from family and relatives very important and helpful.

One year after transplantation, all 6 patients had a clearly better somatic condition, although they all experienced various somatic complications during that year. Also, every patient had a much better general functional ability. Four patients were able to work somehow in or outside home and had picked up some hobby. Two patients still seemed to need quite a lot of help at home. All patients felt that their functional ability became even better during the 2nd year; they were all able to do duties at home almost normally, they felt more independent and had interests and hobbies of their own. Two patients had a cataract that somewhat restricted their functioning.

The neuropsychological tests showed some impairment in intelligence (WAIS) and in memory (WMS) before transplantation in every patient (Table 1). These impairments improved to the expected level 1 year after transplantation. Visuoconstructive apraxia was more marked in all these patients before transplantation, and some impairment still remained in the mental flexibility of 5 patients 1 year after it.

The results of SCL-90 (Table 2) showed as a general tendency that all successfully transplanted patients were feeling better 1 year after transplantation; they had fewer somatic complaints, they were less depressed and anxious and less sensitive in their relationships with other people than before transplantation. After 2 years the scores were even better. During the 1st year, the interviews revealed

phases of moderate or even severe depression in 5 patients and general anxiety or anxiety attacks in 4 patients. During the 2nd year 2 patients had a phase of depression, and 3 still felt anxiety, although less severely than during the 1st year. With 1 patient the depression was long lasting, and her condition worsened during the 2nd year. These difficulties were often related to somatic complications, occasionally to a family problem, but also to inner psychic conflicts and fears.

Discussion

Different organ transplantations have common features from the psychological point of view [10]. Liver transplantation has though its specific features, with hepatic encephalopathy and neurological symptoms [1, 12] that influence all levels of the quality of life.

On the functional level there was much improvement from the preoperative situation in which all patients needed help in everyday life to the point where they all managed quite well in normal daily duties and interests in adult life. Nevertheless, most of these patients felt after 2 years that some of their life energy was still missing.

On the interpersonal level, support from family and other relatives seemed to be most important as has been noticed in several studies before [2, 7]. The general sense of security and ability to be helpless without shame seemed to support the recovery from transplantation. In this study, insecurity and lack of family support were related to a poor outcome. This could be a risk factor, and an extra effort should be made to offer such patients more support.

In this group of patients there was less impairment in intelligence and memory tests and more visuomotor apraxia than was found in another group of patients ($n = 8$) tested with the same methods [5].

On the psychological level, varying degrees of depression and anxiety were observed in every patient sometime during these 2 years. A self-rating questionnaire did not

Table 1. Neuropsychological test results before and after transplantation

	Before transplant ($n = 7$)	After transplant ($n = 6$)	Controls ($n = 53$)
Wechsler Adult Intelligence Scale			
VS	106 ± 12.3	111 ± 10.7	110 ± 13.3
PS	98 ± 14.3	108 ± 10.0	109 ± 12.9
Wechsler Memory	106 ± 20.1	120 ± 20.2	118 ± 15.6
Stroop C Scale	172 ± 28.7	115 ± 20.3	110 ± 24.6
Trail B	157 ± 52.1	132 ± 54.0	101 ± 46.0

Mean ± SD

Table 2. SCL-90 results before and after transplantation

	Before Transplant	1 year after	2 years after
Somatization	64 ± 3.6	58 ± 9.8	54 ± 10.8
Depression	64 ± 7.3	54 ± 9.8	52 ± 4.3
Anxiety	61 ± 6.0	56 ± 8.2	48 ± 7.4
Interpersonal sensitivity	61 ± 8.2	53 ± 9.7	48 ± 8.9
Global severity index	65 ± 4.2	58 ± 6.1	52 ± 6.5

reveal these individual variations well. There seemed to be a general tendency of denying symptoms and difficulties in the questionnaire, compared with what these patients said in the interviews. The same observation was made by Heyink et al. in their study [4]. Many of these patients seemed to need denial before transplantation as a psychological defence mechanism. Under such extreme circumstances, denial can be helpful in dealing with overwhelming emotions. Also, the drowsiness and flattening of emotions caused by hepatic encephalopathy could be a shelter from overly strong emotions. Several patients found their sense of humor to be important in this recovery process.

We describe in this study different aspects of the quality of life from the experience of 7 patients before and after liver transplantation. There is a great individual variation in the psychological recovery process. Although all successfully transplanted patients already feel much better 1 year after transplantation, it seems to take about 2 years for them to stabilise the new life situation.

References

1. Adams DH, Gunson B, Honigsberger L, et al (1987) Neurological complications following liver transplantation. Lancet I: 949–951

2. Christopherson LK (1986) Quality of life; organ transplantation and artificial organs. Intl J Techn Assist Health Care 2: 553–562

3. Derogatis LR (1983) SCL-90. Clinical Psychometric Research, MD, Thomson

4. Heyink J, Tymstra T, Slooff MJH, et al (1989) Liver transplantation–psychosocial problems following the operation. Transplantation 49: 1018–1019

5. Höckerstedt K, Kajaste S, Isoniemi H, et al (1990) Tests for encephalopathy before and after liver transplantation. Transplant Proc 22: 1576–1578

6. Küchler T, Kober B, Brölsch C, et al (1991) Quality of life after liver transplantation: can a psychosocial support program contribute? Transplant Proc 23: 1541–1544

7. Küchler T, Kober B, Broelsch C, et al (1991) Quality of life after liver transplantation. Clin Transplant 5: 94–101

8. Lezak MD (1983) In: Neuropsychological assessment, 2nd edn. Oxford University Press, New York

9. Markus BH, Dickson ER, Grambsch PM, et al (1989) Efficacy of liver transplantation in patients with primary biliary cirrhosis. N Engl J Med 320: 1709–1713

10. Surman OS (1989) Psychiatric aspects of organ transplantation. Am J Psychiatry 146: 972–982

11. Surman OS, Dienstag JL, Cosimi AB, et al (1987) Psychosomatic aspects of liver transplantation. Psychother Psychosom 48: 26–39

12. Tarter RE, Switala J, Arria A, et al (1990) Subclinical hepatic encephalopathy. Transplantation 50: 632–637

13. Trzepacz PT, Brenner R, Thiel DH Van (1989) A psychiatric study of 247 liver transplantation candidates. Psychosomatics 30: 147–153

Transplant Int (1992) 5 [Suppl 1]: S 708–S 710

TRANSPLANT
International
© Springer-Verlag 1992

Effect of kidney transplantation on quality of life measures*

A. Pietrabissa[1], A. Ciaramella[2], M. Carmellini[1], G. Massimetti[2], P. C. Giulianotti[1], M. Ferrari[1], I. Corradi[2], and F. Mosca[1]

[1] Istituto di Chirurgia Generale e Sperimentale, [2] Istituto di Clinica Psichiatrica, Universita' di Pisa, Italy

Abstract. Assessing the quality of life should be an essential part of the long-term results of surgery, particularly for those procedures that may influence a patient's lifestyle and body image. Eliminating the need for dependence on chronic hemodialysis, kidney transplantation improves the patient's autonomy but exposes them to the side-effects of immunosuppression and the constant threat of rejection. The purpose of this study was to compare the quality of life of patients on the waiting list for a kidney transplantation to that of those already transplanted at our Center to quantify carefully the impact of this therapy on the patient's physical, emotional, and social well-being. Computer analysis of the data collected from self-administered questionnaires revealed that the vast majority of successfully transplanted patients experience a significant improvement in almost all the areas investigated compared with the pretransplant group. In addition, we tried to use the questionnaire to predict which type of patient will adjust more fully to the impact of a kidney transplantation and which will probably need posttransplant psychological care and social support. Aside from clinical factors such as the time spent on hemodialysis before transplantation, the gender, the age, as well as the source of the organ (living vs. cadaver donor) seem to play a role in the final outcome of a successful kidney transplantation.

Key words: Quality of life – Kidney transplantation – Health status measurement

Over the past 10 years the results of kidney transplantation have improved dramatically. However, even when kidney function is excellent and the patient is discharged from the hospital in a few weeks, the posttransplant medical regimen can be stressful, and patients may report side-effects attributable to the immunosuppression that have the potential to compromise their quality of life. Patients with a successful transplant may also experience difficulty in resuming their role in society, particularly after many years of dialysis. Although other studies have documented that patients adapted to the impact of a kidney transplantation such that lifestyles, although altered, were not impaired [1, 2, 7], it has been suggested that behavioral and cultural differences between the patient populations of different countries can considerably affect the results of the quality of life surveys [4]. Our purpose, therefore, was to compare the quality of the lives of patients on chronic hemodialysis with that of patients after a successful transplant performed at our Center. The need for such a study was felt since this is to our knowledge the first on this subject conducted in our country.

Patients and methods

Data were collected by sending self-administered questionnaires with multiple-choice questions to 81 patients who had undergone a kidney transplantation at our Center between 1982 and 1990 and to 271 patients maintained on hemodialysis while on the waiting list for a donor. The questionnaire was a transcultural version of that designed by Simmons and others at the University of Minnesota to assess the quality of life in uremic and transplant patients [8]. Items in the questionnaire were categorised into three major dimensions: physical well-being, emotional well-being, and social well-being. Within each dimension, particular subdimensions were measured with multiple-choice questions and with scales and scores constructed from the multiple-choice questions. These measures were chosen because they had been used in similar research projects [9] where they proved to be reliable and valid health tests for chronically ill patients and therefore could provide a basis for future comparisons. The exact instrument along with its reliability and validity information has been previously reported [8]. As an additional investigation, we tried to use the questionnaire to detect which patients will adjust more fully to the kidney transplant and, which is perhaps the most crucial point, which ones will need greater posttransplant psychological care and social support. For this purpose, the relationship between age, sex, education, time spent on dialysis, and type of donor (living vs. cadaver), and the emotional and social well-being scores was analyzed.

The Student's t-test was used to test for significant differences between the groups. For data that did not fit the assumption required for a t-test, χ^2 analysis was performed. P values less than 0.05 were chosen for statistical significance.

* Supported by a grant from AIDO (Associazione Italiana Donatori Organi) and APRIC (Associazione Pisana Per le Ricerche In Chirurgia)

Offprint requests to: Dr. A. Pietrabissa, M.D., Istituto di Chirurgia Generale e Sperimentale, Universita' di Pisa, Ospedale Cisanello, Via Paradisa, 2-56124 Pisa, Italy

Results

Out of 352 sent by post, 243 questionnaires returned to the Center for analysis: 172 from patients on dialysis (63% answer rate) and 71 from transplant patients (88% answer rate). There was no significant difference between the two groups in regard to the following variables used to check for comparability: age, sex, education, marital status, and time spent on dialysis.

The physical well-being dimension was designed to assess the level of health improvement and refers to the patients' evaluation of their health and to the level of physical activity possible given their physical condition [3]. Not surprisingly, posttransplant patients have fewer physical problems than patients on chronic hemodialysis (Table 1). In addition, patients were asked how often they encountered problems with symptoms of uremia and whether all uremic symptoms had been considerably reduced, or if they had any difficulty with a list of ordinary life activities. Some patients still have difficulty with walking, climbing stairs, and lifting things. In general, the posttransplant patient showed an important health improvement, to the point that 42% could say their health was not a problem, in comparison with only 9% of the pretransplant group, and 53% classified themselves as, "I am well and doing the same things I did before my illness" compared with 18% in the pretransplant group.

More than with physical well-being, a successful transplant leads to a dramatic improvement in the patients' self-esteem, as well as in all the other subdimensions of emotional well-being, including a reduction in anxiety and feelings of depression (Table 2).

The last dimension, social well-being, refers to a general satisfaction and participation in social activities and life roles such as job, friends, and family adjustment. There was evidence of a statistically significant improvement in 2 subdimensions out of 4 (Table 3). Our data indicate that the patient after transplant appears to be socializing more with people outside the family. However, only 18% of patients classified themselves as very satisfied with their job, compared with 9% of those on chronic hemodialysis. A lack of suitable job opportunities in our country could be responsible for the low numbers in both cases: It indicates that transplant patients tend to remain unemployed even when they are able to work again.

Male patients showed some tendency to be better adjusted after transplant, the low anxiety score achieving statistical significance (Fig. 1). However, it should be noticed that considering the general population, women are more likely to score lower than men in this area [8]. Among the other possible explanations, is the impact of body-image upon these areas: More than one-third of patients reported having a "fuller face" and abnormal hair growth, characteristic of immunosuppression. As expected, these problems of unattractive appearance were reported by about 50% of women and by less than 20% of men. Considering age, although with no statistical significance, there seems to be a tendency for younger patients to be less accepting of health problems after transplant. Education might be expected to make a difference, too, meaning that higher education could be associated

Table 1. Physical well-being analysis results

Subdimensions	Mean scores	
	Pretransplant	Posttransplant
Health satisfaction	2.76	4.22*
Physical well-being summary[a]	12.38	11.81
General well-being[a]	7.45	5.56*
Domosthings	4.74	5.33

[a] Lower scores reflected better well-being
* two way analysis of variance: $P \leq 0.05$

Table 2. Emotional well-being analysis results

Subdimensions	Mean scores	
	Pretransplant	Posttransplant
Self-esteem scale	3.18	5.14*
Index of depression	1.39	2.84*
Index of anxiety	1.47	2.47*
Independence	2.04	2.47*
Control over destiny	1.75	2.58*
Positive affect scale	5.30	7.42*

* Two-way analysis of variance: $P \leq 0.05$

Table 3. Social well-being analysis results

Subdimensions	Mean scores	
	Pretransplant	Posttransplant
Social well-being summary	10.79	11.87*
Family well-being summary[a]	10.24	11.07
Social role satisfaction[a]	4.32	4.29
General satisfaction	11.76	8.60*

[a] Lower scores reflect better well-being
* Two-way analysis of variance: $P \leq 0.05$

with fewer rehabilitation problems. Our data, however, showed no consistent differences considering patients after transplant with less or more than 8 years of school. Looking at the time spent on dialysis before transplant, there is some evidence that patients who have been on dialysis for less than 1 year, with a higher level of emotional well-being pretransplant, are more likely to remain better adjusted after transplant if compared with longstanding dialyzed patients, reaching statistical significance on the self-esteem score. Finally, our data suggest that recipients of cadaver kidneys show a greater emotional adjustment after transplant, probably because of fewer problems in the relationship with the donor as compared with living related donors (11 patients in this study) [6].

Discussion

Quality of life variables are rarely considered as outcome measures in controlled trials of surgical treatment [5, 10, 11]. The purpose of this study was to document the quality of life of kidney transplant patients versus dialysis patients in our geographical area. Our results provide further evidence that patients receiving a successful kidney transplant have a higher quality of life as measured subjectively by physical, emotional, and social well-being. It is known that the quality of life may also vary depending on the immunosuppression therapy; however, most of the patients in-

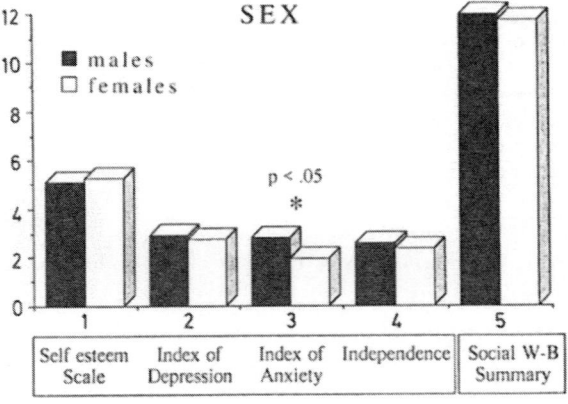

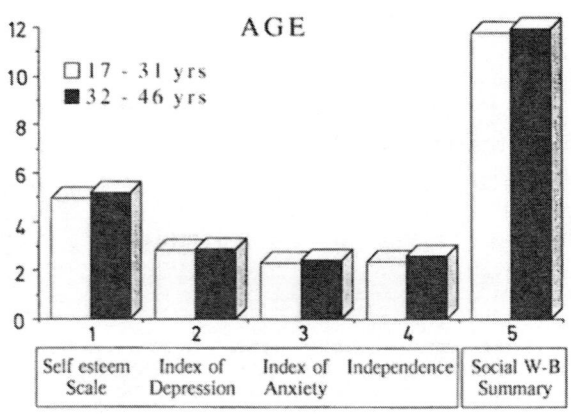

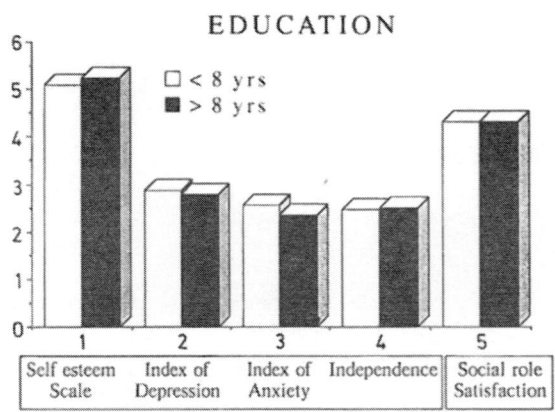

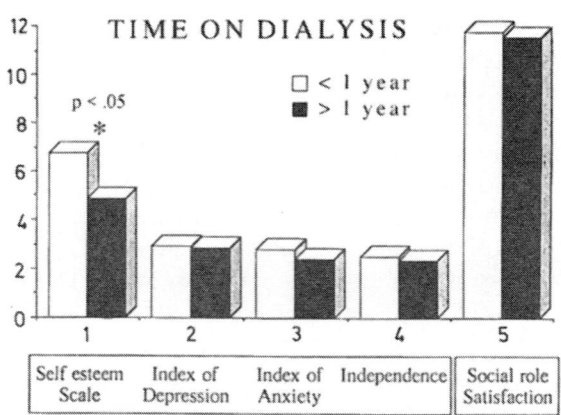

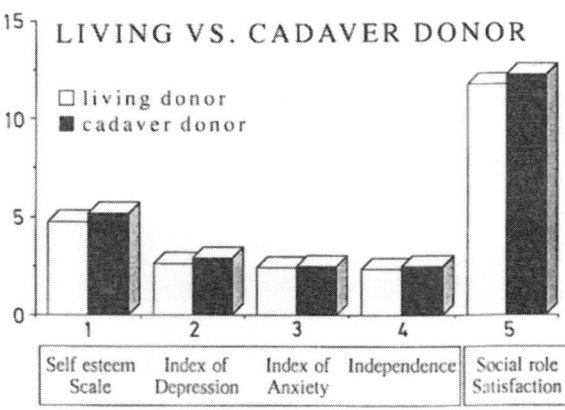

Fig. 1. Relationship of transplant patients' variables to emotional and social well-being scores

References

1. Evans RW, Manninen DL, Garrison JP Jr (1985) The quality of life of patients with end-stage renal disease. N Engl J Med 312: 553
2. Johnson RG, McCauley CR, Copley JB (1982) The quality of life of hemodialysis and transplant patients. Kidney Int 22: 286
3. Jones BM, Taylor FJ, Wright OM (1990) Quality of life after heart transplantation in patients assigned to double- or triple-drug therapy. J Heart Transplant 9: 392–396
4. Katz S (1987) The science of quality of life. J Chron Dis 40: 459–463
5. O'Young J, McPeek B (1987) Quality of life variables in surgical trials. J Chronic Dis 40: 513–522
6. Simmons RG, Anderson CR (1982) Related donors and recipients five to nine years posttransplant. Transplant Proc 13: 40
7. Simmons RG, Anderson C, Kamstra L (1984) Comparison of quality of life of patients on continous ambulatory peritoneal dialysis, hemodialysis, and after transplantation. Am J Kidney Dis 4: 253
8. Simmons RG, Klein SD, Simmons RL (1987) Gift of life: the effect of organ transplantation on individual, family, and societal dynamics. Transaction, New Brunswick
9. Simmons RG, Abress L, Anderson CR (1988) Quality of life after kidney transplantation. Transplantation 45: 415–421
10. Troidl H, Kusche J, Vestweber KH (1987) Quality of life: an important endpoint both in surgical practice and research. J Chronic Dis 40: 523–528
11. Ware JE Jr (1987) Standards for validating health measures: definition and content. J Chronic Dis 40: 473–480

cluded in this study received triple-drug therapy, and it was therefore impossible to distinguish separate subgroups.

Our analysis suggests that some patients are more likely to benefit from psychological support in the posttransplant period: women, young people, those who spent a long time on dialysis, and living related recipients.

Although clinical considerations will always be the main determinant of the decision-making process in surgery, we believe that quality of life information is also needed by both surgeons and patients in selecting the most appropriate therapy for each case and to guide health policy decisions [10].

Transplant Int (1992) 5 [Suppl 1]: S711–S715

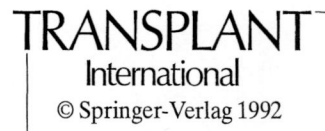

© Springer-Verlag 1992

Cognitive and behavioural status of paediatric patients 1 year after cardiac or cardiopulmonary transplantation

J. Wray, R. Radley-Smith, and M. Yacoub

Cardiothoracic Unit, Harefield Hospital, Harefield, United Kingdom

Abstract. Cardiac and cardiopulmonary transplantation are being increasingly used as methods of treatment for children with end-stage heart or lung disease, but little is documented about their psychological adjustment to such procedures. In all, 45 children who had undergone heart or heart-lung transplantation were studied 1 year after operation and compared with 39 children who had undergone bone marrow transplantation, 49 children who had undergone conventional cardiac surgery and 46 normal healthy children. None of the 3 treatment groups differed significantly with respect to developmental, cognitive or behavioural measures, but there were significant differences between the transplant and normal groups in the areas of developmental and cognitive functioning. The initial diagnosis of the transplant patients was found to be an important factor in the postoperative psychological functioning.

Key words: Behaviour – Cognition – Heart Transplantation – Heart-lung transplantation – Children

---

With the increasing use of cardiac and cardiopulmonary transplantation for the treatment of children with end-stage heart or lung disease, attention is now being given to the psychological adjustment of children following these procedures. Although it is accepted that children with chronic illness are more likely to experience major psychological and social difficulties than their healthy peers [18], there are still very few published data on the psychological aspects of paediatric heart and heart-lung transplantation. Studies of children 1–5 years after heart transplantation suggested that in most cases the children had returned to age-appropriate activities, including school, and that few were experiencing cardiac-related symptoms [4, 10, 16, 17]. Whilst the side effects of immunosuppressive therapy are still not clear, poor growth has been found in many children taking steroids [24], which may have significant psychological repercussions. The effects

of transplantation on the parents have also been assessed, but these studies, together with those on the children themselves, tend to be based on very small sample sizes. The focus has been on heart, rather than heart-lung, recipients in the school-age group, with little attention being given to preschoolers.

In order to address some of these issues with the Harefield patients, a systematic evaluation of paediatric patients and their families is carried out before and at regular intervals after transplantation. This paper reports some of the findings of patients seen 1 year after heart or heart-lung transplantation.

Methods

Patient selection. Between January 1984 and August 1991, 201 heart and heart-lung transplants were performed at the Harefield Hospital on children and adolescents under the age of 17 years. Of the 63 patients eligible for inclusion in the study (criteria for inclusion were that the child and family spoke English, that they were domiciled in the UK or Eire, that the child was under 17 years of age and that they attended the Harefield Hospital for follow-up), 45 patients have been assessed 1 year after transplantation. (The remaining 18 patients were less than 1 year post-transplant).

There were 19 boys and 26 girls, and 37 (82%) came from intact, 2-parent families. The mean age at assessment was 9.6 years (range 1.3–16.0). Of the 45 patients seen, 29 had undergone heart transplantation, of whom 25 had an original diagnosis of cardiomyopathy, 3 had congenital heart disease, and 1 had Kawasaki disease. Sixteen children had had a heart-lung transplant, 8 of whom had pulmonary vascular disease, and 8 had cystic fibrosis. Twelve (27%) of the patients had undergone previous cardiothoracic surgery related to their disease – primarily those with an initial diagnosis of congenital heart disease. One heart-lung recipient had undergone a second transplant for chronic rejection, and a further 2 patients were awaiting retransplantation. At the time of the assessment, 2 children were hospitalised, and a further 6 patients were experiencing problems with repeated infection and/or rejection episodes. Seven of these 8 patients were heart-lung recipients.

Reference group selection. For comparison, 3 reference groups were assessed with the same measures. The first group consisted of 39 children who had undergone bone marrow transplantation (BMT) for a variety of congenital and acquired disorders (mean age at assessment 8.6 years). The second group consisted of 49 patients

---

Offprint requests to: J. Wray Cardiothoracic Unit, Harefield Hospital, Harefield, Middlesex UB9 6JH, United Kingdom

who had undergone conventional cardiac surgery (mean age at assessment 6.8 years) for correction ($n = 46$) or palliation ($n = 3$) of congenital heart disease. The BMT and cardiac surgery groups were seen 1 year after treatment. The third group was a group of 46 normal healthy children (mean age at assessment 8.2 years). The four groups did not differ significantly with respect to sex and social class, but they differed significantly with respect to age – the cardiac surgery group were significantly younger than the transplant group. The reference groups were selected from a prospective study undertaken at the Westminster Children's Hospital between 1984 and 1988. At the time of assessment a similar proportion of children in the transplant, BMT, and cardiac surgery groups were experiencing medical problems.

Measures used

Cognitive development was assessed using either the Ruth Griffiths Mental Development Scales for children of 0–3.5 years [6] or the short form IQ estimate of the British Ability Scales (BAS) for children of 3.6–17.0 years [3]. Two children in the transplant group could not be tested due to neurological damage following transplantation, which was sustained as a result of cardiac arrest prior to establishing cardiopulmonary bypass. These two children were assessed as being in the severely mentally handicapped range. Two children in the cardiac surgery group also could not be tested due to neurological damage following open heart surgery. Although no measure of cognition or behaviour in these neurologically impaired patients is included in the final analysis, they are mentioned so that the groups studied are representative of the status of patients after transplantation or open heart surgery. School attainment tests covering arithmetic (BAS), reading (BAS) and spelling (Schonell graded spelling test) [23] skills were administered to the children aged 5.0–14.4 years. With the exception of the children with impaired neurological status, all of the children in each of the 3 groups were assessed with the appropriate measures of developmental or cognitive ability.

The behaviour of the children was assessed by questionnaires completed by the parents and teachers. Questionnaire assessment of the behaviour of children under 3 years of age was not undertaken because of the lack of suitable measures. The behaviour at home of children of 3.0–5.0 years was assessed with the Richman BCL [20] and for children of 5.0–17.0 years with the Rutter A scales [22]. The behaviour at school was assessed with the Rutter B scales [22], completed by the teachers. The recommended cut-off scores were used in order to identify those children with a significant degree of problem behaviour. Compliance rates for the completion of the questionnaires were 93% for the transplant group, 82% for the BMT group, 96% for the cardiac surgery group and 93% for the normal group.

In addition to assessing the child, the parents were seen for a semistructured interview during which information was collected on demographic, social and medical variables. Specific questions were asked regarding the amount of schooling missed and the child's previous medical history. The cardiologists at the Harefield Hospital and the hospitals at which the cardiac surgery group were patients were also asked to rate the child's medical condition at the time of the assessment.

Statistical analysis. The developmental and cognitive measures were compared using analysis of variance. The Richman and Rutter scores were analysed using the Kruskal-Wallis analysis of variance for nonparametric data.

Results

Development: 0–3.5 years

Ten children in the transplant group, all of whom had an initial diagnosis of cardiomyopathy, were assessed with the Ruth Griffiths Scales. All of the mean subtest scores

and overall IQ score were within the normal range. Comparison with the children in the BMT ($n = 8$), cardiac surgery ($n = 14$) and normal ($n = 11$) groups indicated that the transplant group obtained significantly lower scores in all areas of development compared with the normal group, but none of the groups of children who had undergone medical treatment differed from one another (Fig. 1).

Cognitive ability: 3.6–17.0 years

The performance on all of the subtests and the overall IQ of the transplant patients fell within the normal range. The IQ score for the group ($n = 31$) was $99.94 + 16.77$ (SD), and the mean scores on the attainments were arithmetic $92.21 + 18.94$, reading $94.42 + 18.13$ and spelling $84.37 + 18.55$. The initial diagnosis of the transplant patients was categorised into cardiomyopathy ($n = 15$), cystic fibrosis ($n = 8$) and congenital heart disease ($n = 8$). In terms of overall IQ and attainment scores with the initial diagnosis as the dependent variable, children with an initial diagnosis of congenital heart disease performed at a lower level on all of the cognitive parameters. The difference reached significance on the overall IQ score, with both the cardiomyopathy and cystic fibrosis groups obtaining a significantly higher score than the congenital heart disease group (Fig. 2).

Comparison with the reference groups indicated that the transplant group performed at a lower level on all parameters, although the differences only reached statistical significance on the spelling test (Fig. 3).

Behaviour at home

Six of the 27 transplant patients (22.2%) on whom Rutter A data were available obtained scores indicative of a significant degree of problem behaviour at home, and the majority of the behaviour problems were of a neurotic nature. There were again marked differences in the prevalence of problem behaviour between the subgroups.

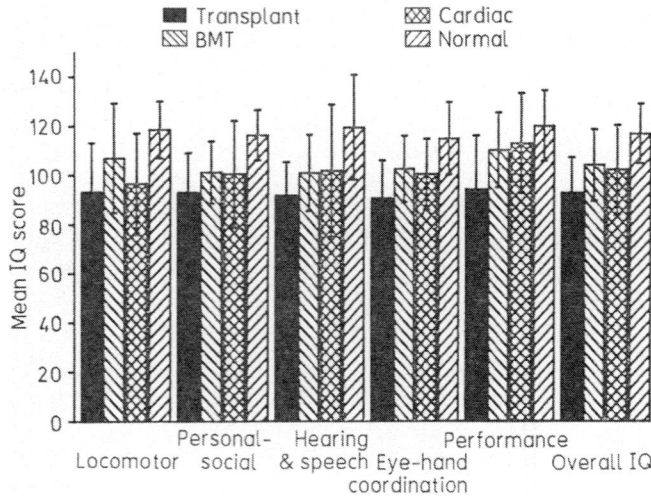

Fig. 1. Developmental ability: comparison of the transplant and reference groups

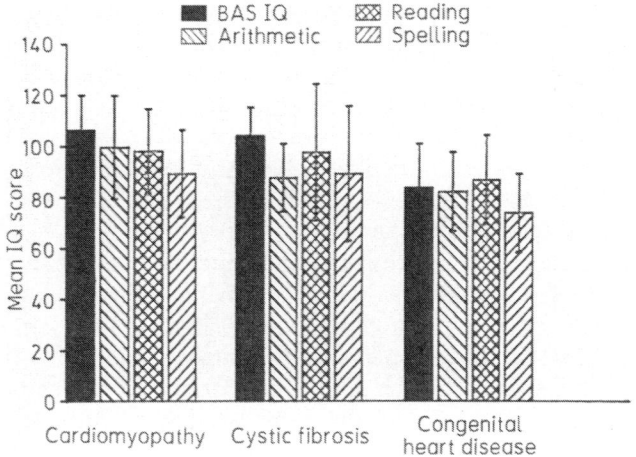

Fig. 2. Cognitive ability of the transplant group according to initial diagnosis

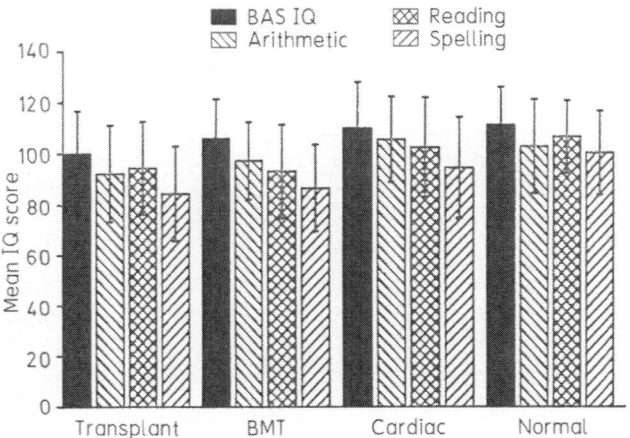

Fig. 3. Comparison of the transplant group with the reference groups: cognitive ability 5–17 years

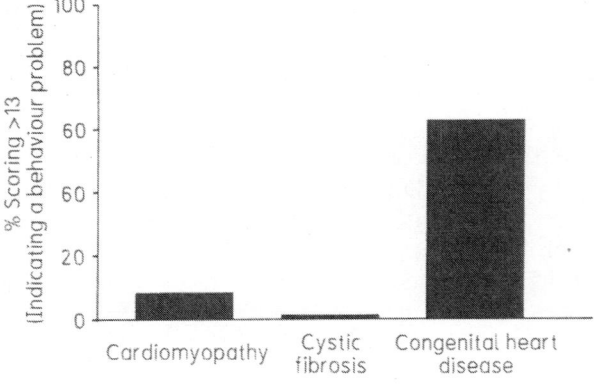

Fig. 4. Prevalence of a significant degree of problem behaviour at home as a function of the initial diagnosis

The group with an initial diagnosis of congenital heart disease obtained a significantly higher score on the Rutter A scale and had a significantly higher proportion of children with scores indicative of problem behaviour than the children originally diagnosed with cardiomyopathy or cystic fibrosis (Fig. 4).

Comparison with the reference groups yielded no statistically significant differences in the prevalence of be-

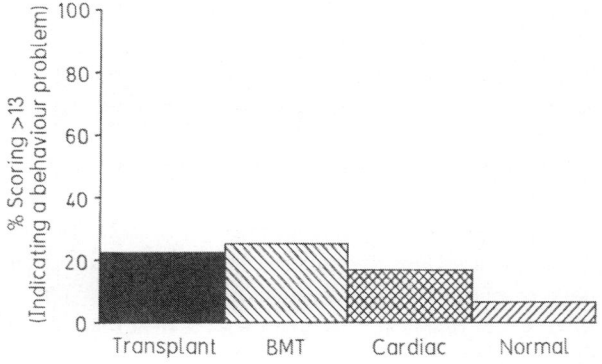

Fig. 5. Comparison of the transplant group with the reference groups: behaviour at home

haviour problems, although the proportion of children with problem behaviour was higher in the 3 treatment groups than in the normal group (Fig. 5).

Behaviour at school

Thirty-two children were eligible for school, 19 of whom were at full-time normal school, 2 were at school part-time, and 3 were at a special school. The reason for non-attendance at school was ongoing medical problems in all 8 cases. One child attending scholl on a part-time basis was able to attend full-time but for psychological reasons was not doing so. This child had had a good medical outcome from the transplantation but had experienced severe adjustment problems posttransplant.

Four of the 18 patients on whom Rutter B data were available were rated as having a significant degree of problem behaviour, of whom 3 children had an original diagnosis of congenital heart disease. Comparison with the reference groups indicated that the prevalence of problem behaviour was similar in all of the groups of children who had undergone medical treatment but was higher than that seen in the normal group.

Discussion

Heart and heart-lung transplantation are major surgical procedures necessitating intensive medical support and follow-up. The risks involved in the treatment are such that transplantation is only undertaken when there is no alternative form of treatment available. The patients are often chronically ill prior to surgery, with a very poor quality of life and life expectancy. Although there is a dramatic improvement in the clinical condition of most patients after transplantation, regular clinic visits are necessary, and uncertainty about the future remains. Both the patient and family have to adjust to the fact that the child is no longer chronically sick and in many cases is able to lead a completely normal life, sometimes for the first time.

The results of this study indicate that the cognitive and behavioural status of transplant patients 1 year after transplantation is similar to that of other groups of children who have, or have had, a chronic illness. The limitations of the data with respect to sample size are acknowledged, but in the context of the paucity of documented research on the psychological adjustment of paediatric heart and heart-lung transplant patients, these findings do address some of the deficits in the existing literature.

The findings in the younger age group suggest that children undergoing cardiac transplantation before the age of 3 years are developing within the normal range, according to the standardised means for the tests, although their development is significantly behind that of a group of normal healthy children. The lower scores obtained by all 3 groups of children who had undergone medical treatment compared with the normal group correspond with findings in the literature that young children suffering from chronic illness, and particularly cardiac-related problems, are at risk for exhibiting developmental delay [11–13, 21].

In the absence of neurological damage, cognitive development in school-age children who have undergone heart or heart-lung transplantation is within the normal range, although the performance was at a lower level compared with the reference groups, particularly on the short-term memory test. Whilst the heart/heart-lung, BMT and cardiac surgery groups were comparable in terms of the level of medical disability at the time of assessment, the initial diagnosis appeared to be an important factor in the postoperative cognitive status, which would explain the trend for lower scores in the transplant group compared with the reference groups. Whilst it is recognised that congenital heart disease can have a deleterious effect on cognitive function, impairment is more frequently associated with the presence of a cyanotic lesion [1, 9, 14, 15]. The cardiac surgery group predominantly consisted of children with acyanotic lesions, whereas the transplant group consisted of a higher proportion of children with cyanotic heart disease. Cystic fibrosis and cardiomyopathy, together with the conditions for which bone marrow transplantation was the chosen treatment, are not known to have any deleterious effect on brain development, and this is substantiated by the performance of the subgroups of the transplant group. In this paper no preoperative measures to indicate whether the IQ score was lower prior to transplantation are available, but other studies of chronically ill children have found this to be the case [19]. The transplant and BMT patients had also missed more schooling than the children in the cardiac surgery and normal groups, which is likely to have contributed to the lower scores obtained by the transplant and BMT groups on the academic attainments.

In terms of the behaviour at home, the number of children on whom Richman BCL data were available was too small for statistical analysis to be valid, but behaviour problems were reported in the preschool age group following transplantation. Temper tantrums, eating and sleeping difficulties and anxieties were areas of specific concern to the parents of all 3 groups of hospitalised children, and the frequency of reporting of such problems was higher than in the normal group.

For the children of 5 years and older, the Rutter A data indicated that a higher proportion of children had a significant degree of problem behaviour than the expected rate of 10 % for the normal population [22]. The types of problems were predominantly of a neurotic nature and included misery, irritabilty, sleeping and eating difficulties and anxieties. The initial diagnosis was again a significant factor in the prevalence of problem behaviour, with children transplanted for congenital heart disease manifesting the greatest degree of problem behaviour. The majority of children obtaining a score indicative of a significant degree of problem behaviour were well at the time of the assessment but were having difficulties in adapting to the transplant and to the changes in their lifestyle now that they were no longer chronically ill. For 3 of the patients in particular, all of whom originally had congenital heart disease, their problems in behaviour were related to a poor body image and a low self-esteem.

The results of the transplant and reference groups, whilst not demonstrating any significant differences between the groups, are relevant in terms of chronic illness/hospitalisation per se. All 3 groups of patients who had undergone medical treatment had a higher prevalence of problem behaviour than their healthy peers, and this corresponds to the level of emotional and behavioural disorder found in other studies of chronically ill children [5, 7]. Increased levels of depression, anxiety and aggression have also been reported in paediatric kidney and bone marrow transplant recipients [2, 8, 19].

The pattern of behaviour at school was very similar to that reported at home, with the children initially diagnosed with congenital heart disease manifesting the highest proportion of problem behaviour. Comparison with the reference groups indicated similar patterns of problem behaviour in the 3 groups of children who had undergone medical treatment, and a higher proportion of children in these 3 groups manifested a significant degree of problem behaviour at school compared with the normal group. The types of problems included poor concentration, lack of motivation and overly anxious behaviour.

This paper reports a single, retrospective assessment of 45 patients 1 year after heart or heart-lung transplantation and clearly indicates that there are important psychological effects associated with such procedures in children. A similar conclusion has also been reached by Uzark and Crowley [25]. The findings indicate the importance of conducting a controlled, prospective study involving all family members, thereby enabling changes over time in psychosocial functioning to be monitored and comparisons to be made with other groups of chronically ill children and also with normal healthy children. Ultimately, therapeutic interventions will be planned to reduce psychiatric morbidity in this group of paediatric patients and families.

References

1. Aram DM, Ekelman BL, Ben-Shachar G, Levinsohn MW (1985) Intelligence and hypoxemia in children with congenital heart disease: fact or artifact? J Am Coll Cardiol 6: 889–893
2. Bernstein DM (1977) Psychiatric assessment of the adjustment of transplanted children. In: Simmons RG, Klein S, Simmons RL (eds) Gift of life. The social and psychological impact of organ transplantation. John Wiley & Sons, New York, pp 119–147

3. Elliot CD (1983) The British ability scales. Introductory handbook, technical handbook and manual for administration and scoring. NFER-Nelson, Windsor
4. Fricker FJ, Griffith BP, Hardesty RL, Trento A, Gold LM, Schmeltz K, Beerman LB, Fischer DR, Matthews RA, Neches WH, Park SC, Zuberbuhler JR, Lennox CC, Bahnson HT (1987) Experience with heart transplantation in children. Pediatrics 79: 138–146
5. Garralda ME, Jameson RA, Reynolds JM, Postlethwaite RJ (1988) Psychiatric adjustment in children with chronic renal failure. J Child Psychol Psychiatry 29: 79–91
6. Griffiths R (1970) The abilities of young children. A comprehensive system of mental measurement for the first eight years of life. Child Development Research Centre, London
7. Heller A, Rafman S, Zvagulis I, Pless IB (1985) Birth defects and psychosocial adjustment. Am J Dis Child 139: 257–263
8. Korsch BM, Negrete VP, Gardner JE (1973) Kidney transplantation in children: psychosocial follow-up study on child and family. J Pediatr 83: 399–408
9. Kramer HH, Awiszus D, Sterzel U, van Halteren A, Classen R (1989) Development of personality and intelligence in children with congenital heart disease. J Child Psychol Psychiat 30: 299–308
10. Lawrence KS, Fricker FJ (1987) Pediatric heart transplantation: quality of life. J Heart Transplant 6: 329–333
11. Linde LM, Rasof B, Dunn OJ (1967) Mental development in congenital heart disease. J Pediatr 71: 198–203
12. Linde LM, Rasof B, Dunn OJ (1970) Longitudinal studies of intellectual and behavioural development in children with congenital heart disease. Acta Paediatr Scand 59: 169–176
13. Newburger JW, Silbert AR, Buckley LP, Fyler DC (1984) Cognitive function and age at repair of transposition of the great arteries in children. N Engl J Med 310: 1495–1499
14. O'Dougherty MM, Wright F, Garmezy N, Loewenson R, Torres F (1983) Later competence and adaptation in infants who survive severe heart defects. Child Dev 54: 1129–1142
15. O'Dougherty M, Wright FS, Loewenson RB, Torres F (1985) Cerebral dysfunction after chronic hypoxia in children. Neurology 35: 42–46
16. Pahl E, Fricker FJ, Trento A, Griffith B, Hardesty R, Gold L, Lawrence K, Beerman L, Fischer D, Neches W (1988) Late follow-up of children after heart transplantation. Transplant Proc 20: 743–746
17. Pennington DG, Sarafian J, Swartz M (1985) Heart transplantation in children. Heart Transplant 4: 441–445
18. Pless IB, Satterwhite BB (1975) Family functioning and family problems. In: Haggerty RJ, Roghman KJ, Pless IB (eds) Child, health and the community. John Wiley & Sons, New York, pp 41–54
19. Pot-Mees C (1989) The psychosocial effects of bone marrow transplantation in children. Eburon, Delft
20. Richman N, Graham PJ (1971) A behavioural screening questionnaire for use with three-year-old children. Preliminary findings. J Child Psychol Psychiatry 12: 5–33
21. Rosenthal A, Castaneda AR (1975) Growth and development after cardiovascular surgery in infants and children. Prog Cardiovasc Dis XVIII: 27–37
22. Rutter M, Tizard J, Whitmore K (1970) Education, health and behaviour. Longman, London
23. Schonell FJ, Schonell FE (1949) Diagnostic and attainment testing. Oliver & Boyd, Edinburgh
24. Starnes VA, Bernstein D, Oyer PE, Gamberg PL, Miller JL, Baum D, Shumway NE (1989) Heart transplantation in children. J Heart Transplant 8: 20–26
25. Uzark K, Crowley D (1989) Family stresses after pediatric heart transplantation. Prog Cardiovasc Nurs 46: 382:388

The Donor Problem

Transplant Int (1992) 5 [Suppl 1]: S719–S721

TRANSPLANT
International
© Springer-Verlag 1992

Perioperative hemodynamic heterogeneity of brain dead organ donors

P. K. Duke, M. A. B. Ramsay, T. C. Gunning, A. W. Paulsen and L. C. Roberts

Baylor University Medical Center, Dallas, Texas, USA

Brain death is accompanied by a loss of homeostatic mechanisms leading to physiologic changes which have been shown to be detrimental to donor organs prior to procurement [2,4]. The management of the brain dead organ donor (BDOD) is frequently left to transplant coordinators, often registered nurses, who follow standardized protocols for that management. The use of a standardized protocol assumes that these donors display homogeneity. To investigate this assumption, the anesthesiology fellows and faculty involved in multiorgan transplantation at the Baylor University Medical Center/UTSWMC conducted a study into the perioperative hemodynamics of the BDOD.

Key words: Brain dead – Hemodynamics

Methods

To demonstrate perioperative hemodynamic changes over time in this population, the investigators placed an arterial pressure line and pulmonary artery thermodilution catheter into each of 13 brain dead patients scheduled for organ donation surgery. These patients ranged in age from 16 to 58 years. All patients received dopamine infusions of 3–5 µg/kg · min throughout the perioperative period. Data were collected up until the time of aortic cross-clamping on the following parameters: cardiac index (CI), heart rate (HR), mean arterial pressure (MAP), systemic vascular resistance (SVR), central venous pressure (CVP), mean pulmonary artery pressure (MPAP), and blood temperature (BT).

Results

Looking at the ranges of each parameter for each patient, one may observe that not only were the patients disparate from one another, but each individual donor displayed variability in all parameters throughout the perioperative period (Table 1). Overall, the CI ranged from 1.0 to 8.8 l, HR from 70 to 176 cpm, MAP from 48 to 118 mmHg, SVR from 188 to 2782 PZU, CVP from 1 to 28 mmHg, MPAP from 9 to 36 mmHg, and BT from 31.5° to 39.2°C. Graphs were generated for CI, HR, MAP, and MPAP (Fig. 1). These were plotted over time with t_0 being the time of aortic cross-clamp application. All four graphs show a scattering of data points, demonstrating hemodynamic heterogeneity among this group of BDOD.

A further investigation followed the transplant recipients into the postoperative period looking for evidence

Table 1. Data for 13 brain dead organ donors

Patient	CI (l)	HR (bpm)	MAP (mmHg)	SVR (PRU)	CVP (mmHg)	MPAP (mmHg)	BT (°C)
1	1.4–3.6	109–129	64–105	751–2782	1–10	12–33	32.9–36.1
2	3.4–7.6	101–109	61–76	259–924	2–15	15–34	35.2–35.9
3	3.5–7.2	147–157	44–60	188–492	10–17	22–36	37.9–39.2
4	1.4–1.8	87–99	78–100	2189–2269	12–15	9–12	31.5–31.7
5	1.2–2.6	70–114	50–65	583–1911	10–15	11–14	31.6–32.4
6	2.9–4.2	84–101	65–91	724–1453	4–11	21–32	35.3–35.9
7	4.3–4.8	90–109	68–118	499–863	6–10	16–21	35.2–35.7
8	2.5–3.3	99–106	61–75	716–1053	7–18	19–31	33.0–33.2
9	3.2–4.8	118–140	57–88	375–871	5–14	10–26	33.5–35.6
10	1.3–2.6	124–147	73–105	1687–2537	6–10	11–21	32.9–36.3
11	1.0–4.2	101–120	48–88	580–1680	6–10	14–25	31.9–33.2
12	2.3–8.8	147–176	51–114	548–594	20–28	26–31	33.7–35.3
13	3.8–4.8	115–130	64–75	647–716	10–12	15–19	33.9–35.0

CI, cardiac index; HR, heart rate; MAP, mean arterial pressure; SVR, systemic vascular resistance; CVP, central versus pressure; MPAP, mean pulmonary artery pressure; BT, blood temperature

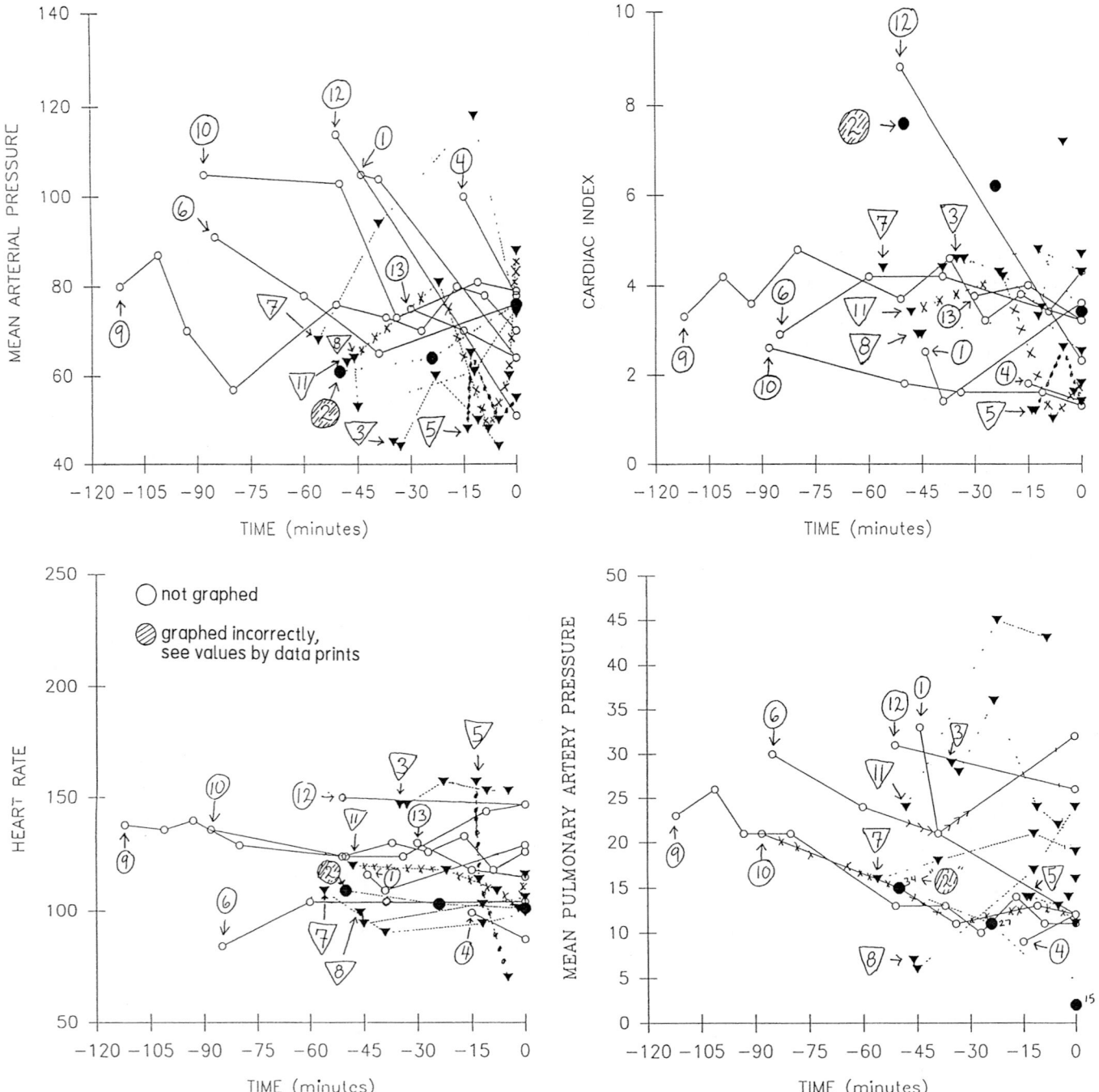

Fig. 1. Data from 13 brain dead organ donors (nos.): ○ successful transplant, ▼ limited harvest due to instability, ● primary graft failure

of primary graft failure. Of 41 organs transplanted, only 1 patient, a heart recipient, experienced primary graft failure. In this instance, the perioperative hemodynamic course of the heart donor, donor 2, included a period of circulatory instability and cardiopulmonary resuscitation. Two transplanted livers failed during the course of the study but were not considered primary failures. The liver from donor 9 failed 10 days after transplantation and the liver from donor 10 failed at 30 days. The perioperative hemodynamic course of these two donors was not clinically significantly different from the other donors in the study.

Five of the donors were considered by the transplant surgeons to have had perioperative periods of hemodynamic instability that may have compromised some or-

gans, making them unsuitable for transplantation. These were patients who experienced transient periods of MAP readings below 60 mm Hg. In these cases a limited harvest, excluding heart, liver, or both, occurred. Other than experiencing MAP < 60 mm Hg, these patients were not hemodynamically clinically significantly different from the other donors in the study.

Discussion

BDOD is frequently the subject of less than meticulous management after the declaration of brain death [2]. This is unfortunate in light of the fact that a single donor can benefit as many as 5–15 recipients [1, 2]. The care of these patients is often left to persons who follow standardized protocols in their management. We have demonstrated that BDOD are not a homogeneous group but are heterogeneous in their hemodynamic picture. This does not fit the profile of a group that can be well managed by following a standardized protocol.

According to Odom in a recent article, minimal monitoring for the BDOD should include hourly measurement of temperature, pulse, blood pressure, and urine output. He suggests that an arterial line would be useful for continuous blood pressure monitoring and blood sampling. A CVP line is not recommended unless inotropc drugs are administered. Use of a pulmonary artery (PA) catheter is not mentioned [3].

In our experience, transplant surgeons have refused to harvest certain organs from donors who have displayed hemodynamic instability, because they feel the organs may have been compromised. Organs are being wasted that could have potentially been used for transplantation because the donor suffered detrimental hemodynamic changes while awaiting surgery [2]. Use of a pulmonary artery thermodilution catheter in the perioperative care of BDOD may lead to better management through directed, rather than standardized, care, thus decreasing the loss of donor organs prior to procurement.

References

1. Frist WH, Fanning WJ (1990) Donor management and matching. Cardiol Clin 8:1 55–71
2. Ghosh S, Hardy I, Kneeshaw J, Latimer D, Oduro A (1990) Management of donors for heart and heart-lung transplantation. Anaesthesia 45: 672–675
3. Odom NJ (1990) Organ donation. Br Med J 300: 1571–1575
4. Wicomb WN, Cooper DKC, Novitzky D (1986) Impairment of renal slice function following brain death, with reversibility of injury by hormonal therapy. Transplantation 41: 29–32

Transplant Int (1992) 5 [Suppl 1]: S 722–S 724

TRANSPLANT
International
© Springer-Verlag 1992

A reliable and safe way of shortening cadaver kidney ischemia time: prenephrectomy tissue typing using donor lymph node cells

M. F. X. Gnant[1], T. Sautner[1], A. Rosenmayr[2], C. Banhegyi[1], P. Wamser[1], P. Goetzinger[1], and F. Muehlbacher[1]

[1] 1st Department of Surgery and [2] Institut für Blutgruppenserologie, University of Vienna, Vienna, Austria

Abstract. The purpose of this study was to investigate the impact of prenephrectomy donor tissue typing on tissue typing quality and transplantation outcome in human kidney transplantation. We report on 680 consecutive kidney transplantations performed at the Vienna Transplantation Center from 1986 to June 1991. In 343 of them, HLA typing was performed using donor lymph node cells obtained in a small surgical procedure several hours before organ retrieval. The mean cold ischemia time (CIT) could be reduced to 17.7 h in these patients compared with 21.9 h in the control group ($n = 337$, conventional tissue typing using spleen lymphocytes obtained during the organ removal, $P = 0.0001$). There was a trend towards better initial and long-term function in the lymph node group; however, this did not reach statistical significance. The clarity of tissue typing results was significantly better when lymph nodes were used as the lymphocyte source. We conclude that prenephrectomy tissue typing is a feasable and inexpensive method of shortening CIT in renal transplantation and favors HLA typing, both likely to benefit transplantation outcome particularly within organ exchange programs.

Key words: Renal transplantation – Organ donor – HLA typing – Prenephrectomy tissue typing – Cold ischemia time

Despite the introduction of new storage solutions, cold ischemia time (CIT) remains of crucial importance to the functioning of a cadaveric renal graft, at least for the organ function in the immediate postoperative period. Some studies have been published showing an effect of CIT on long-term function, too. Furthermore, there is evidence that graft function depends mainly on the number of HLA antigens shared between the recipient and the respective donor. Organ exchange organizations such as Eurotransplant intend to minimize HLA-mismatches by selecting the optimal recipient for an organ available, based on the stored data of the thousands of patients on the multinational waiting list. The benefit of organ sharing in achieving the greatest possible HLA-matching between donor and recipient may be impaired by the additional time necessary for transportation of the organ from the donor center to the recipient center [2].

The aim of our study was to investigate the effects of prenephrectomy donor tissue typing on CIT and its impact on the quality of HLA type determination. Furthermore, we investigated the effects of CIT shortening on primary and long-term graft function.

Materials and methods

Since 1982, in Austria organ donation has been based on a law of the so-called presumed consent. This means that, if no declaration of dissent is found with a potential organ donor, he or she is considered as agreeing with organ donation [6]. The regulation is comparable with those of Belgium or France [10] and follows the guidelines of the European Council [3].

We report on 683 consecutive cadaveric kidney transplantations performed at our center using kidneys procured within our own catchment area from January 1986 to June 1991. Details about procurement strategies and logistics are described elsewhere [4, 5]. The remainder of the 1048 kidneys available (368, 35.1 %) were shipped to other centers of the Eurotransplant community. In 3 of the 683 consecutive cases (0.4 %), neither lymph nodes nor spleen could be obtained from the donor for various reasons. Tissue typing was performed using donor blood in these cases. The following analyses are confined to the 680 transplantations with HLA typing based on donor spleen or lymph nodes.

The 680 transplantations were divided into 2 groups: In group A ($n = 343$, 50.4 %) inguinal donor lymph nodes were obtained in a small surgical procedure after the first brain death determination hours before organ removal. After a short incision of the skin, the inguinal lymph nodes near the femoral vein were prepared, dissected, and stored in cold saline. The procedure was performed under sterile conditions by a transplant coordinator at the donor ICU, without the need for an operation theatre or nurse. In the first cases, the operation was done on both donor sides, but it quickly turned out that enough material could be obtained with one or two lymph nodes

Offprint requests to: Dr. M. Gnant, 1st Department of Surgery, University of Vienna, General Hospital, Alser Straße 4, A-1097 Vienna, Austria

Table 1. Donor parameters

	Group A ($n = 343$)	Group B ($n = 337$)	P value
Age (years)	35.2 ± 14.7	37.5 ± 15.4	0.04
Sex (% male)	68.4	66.5	0.3
Blood group (O-A-B-AB)	129-149-51-14	126-150-45-16	0.7
Cause of death (% trauma)	60.2	55.3	0.7
Traffic accident (%)	36.2	29.8	0.06
Stay in ICU (days)	2.79 ± 0.16	2.69 ± 0.17	0.8
Circulation (% stable)	58.2	65.2	0.1
Reversible cardiac arrest (%)	8.72	9.29	0.6

ICU, intensive care unit

Table 2. Recipient characteristics

	Group A ($n = 343$)	Group B ($n = 337$)	P value
Age (years)	45.9 ± 13.6	46.3 ± 13.3	0.7
Sex (% male)	63.9	56.4	0.05
Days on dialysis	826.1 ± 58.0	935.2 ± 56.1	0.7
Duration of kidney disease (years)	8.85 ± 0.8	8.34 ± 0.6	0.8
Mismatches HLA-A + B	1.87 ± 0.06	1.92 ± 0.06	0.8
Mismatches HLA-DR	0.41 ± 0.04	0.48 ± 0.03	0.1
Retransplants (%)	16.9	14.9	0.8
Patients with PRAs (%)	29.2	33.6	0.5
Patients with PRAs > 40%	11.1	12.5	0.7
(%)	31.6	29.6	0.4
Anatomical variations (%)	38.5 ± 13.2	37.9 ± 12.7	0.9
Anastomosis procedure (min)			
Perioperative (30 days) mortality (%)	2.2	2.9	0.6
Immunosuppression (% including ATG)	33.1	34.0	0.9
	81.2	80.5	0.9
Immediate graft function (%)	17.7 ± 6.8	21.9 ± 5.6	0.0001
Cold ischemia time (h)			
One year graft survival, all patients (%)	87.7	84.6	0.09
One year graft survival, without PRNF (%)	92.4	87.2	0.05
Four year graft survival, all patients (%)	80.1	73.2	0.06

PRA, panel reactive antibodies; PRNF, primary nonfunction; ATG, antithymocyte globulin

from one side. Usually the complete procedure was finished within 30 min. Appropriate HLA tissue typing started immediately afterwards. This procedure was approved by the ethics committee of our institution. In group B ($n = 337$, 49.6%) tissue typing was performed using cells from the donor spleen removed at the time of organ retrieval.

The quality of the tissue typing results was assessed according to a score by doctors and technicians without knowledge about the way the lymphatic material had been retrieved from the donor. After determination of the donor's HLA type and crossmatching, recipients were selected in the same way in both groups, namely be HLA-matching, preimmunization, and waiting time as ranked selection criteria. Results of tissue typing were checked in the Eurotransplant laboratory. For organ perfusion and storage we used Euro-Collins and UW solution [7]. Transplantations were performed in a standardized surgical procedure, the immunosuppressive regimen consisted of cyclosporine and prednisone or was given as sequential immunosuppression with antithynocyte globulin (ATG) for the first 10 days and cyclosporine thereafter, as described elsewhere [1]. For stastical analysis we used Student's t-test and χ^2 test whenever appropriate. Survival curves were calculated according to the Kaplan Meier method [8]. Differences between groups with respect to survival were tested using Mantel's test [9].

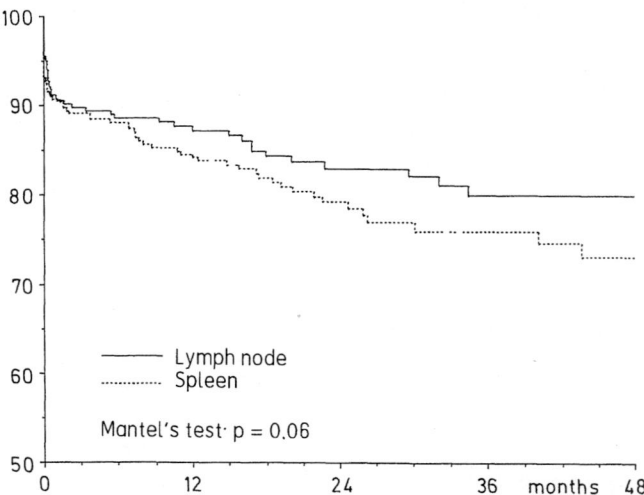

Fig. 1. Graft survival for lymph node ($n = 343$) vs. spleen ($n = 337$) tissue typing, no cases excluded

Results

The two groups were comparable with respect to all donor parameters (Table 1). Donor age, however, was slightly higher in group B (35.2 vs 37.5 years, $P = 0.04$). Cold ischemia time was significantly shorter in group A ($17.7 ± 6.8$ h) than in group B ($21.9 ± 5.6$ h) (mean ± standard deviation, $P < 0.0001$).

Recipient data and outcome of transplantations are summarized in Table 2. The primary nonfunction rate in group A was 4.2% compared with 7.1% in group B ($P = 0.06$). The actuarial 1-year graft survival was 87.7% in group A as compared with 84.6% in group B (no cases excluded, $P = 0.09$). If graft with PRNF were excluded, the figures are 92.4% and 87.2%, respectively ($P = 0.05$). After 4 years, 80.1% of grafts were functioning in group A and 73.2% in group B (no cases excluded, $P = 0.06$). The graft function curves for both groups are given in Fig. 1.

The quality of tissue typing remained unchanged, with virtually no discrepancies between the methods. However, in group A only 5.1% of reactions were difficult to interpret as compared with 16.7% ambiguous serological reactions in group B ($P < 0.0001$).

Discussion

We have shown the consequences of prenephrectomy tissue typing using donor inguinal lymph nodes. There is a significant impact on the CIT and clarity of tissue typing results. There is a trend towards fewer grafts with PRNF, most likely due to the shortened CIT. The 1-year and 4-year actuarial survival, too, show a trend in favor of lymph node typing. To statistically detect the effects of a 4-h difference in CIT, however, obviously requires very large data samples, with respect to the 1-year graft survival. The additional costs of the prenephrectomy lymph node sampling are minimal.

From these results, we conclude that tissue typing from donor lymph node cells obtained before nephrectomy provides two major advantages, shortening of the CIT and facilitation of clearer typing results, without reducing the quality of HLA determination; both factors are likely to benefit organ sharing and the outcome of transplantations.

References

1. Banhegyi C, Rockenschaub S, Muehlbacher F, Balcke P, Kovarik J (1991) Preliminary results of a prospective randomized clinical trial comparing cyclosporine A to antithymocyte-globulin immunosuppressive induction therapy in kidney transplantation. Transplant Proc 4: 197–199
2. Banhegyi C, Sautner T, Gnant M, Goetzinger P, Wamser P, Muehlbacher F (1991) Transplantation of shipped full-house kidneys versus local poorly matched grafts–does a shorter cold ischemic time outweigh a worse match? Transplant Proc (in press)
3. Council of Europe (1978) Harmonisation of legislations of member states relating to removal, grafting and transplantation of human substances. Legal Affairs, Resolution 29
4. Gnant M, Muehlbacher F (1990) Kidney transplantation: getting the numbers right. Lancet I: 479
5. Gnant M, Sautner T, Muehlbacher F, Steininger R, Laengle F, Piza F (1989) Professionelle Organgewinnung als Vorraussetzung zum Erreichen der notwendigen Transplantationsfrequenz: Erfahrungen mit der Organspende am Transplantationszentrum Wien. Wien Klin Wochenschr 23: 824–828
6. Gnant M, Wamser P, Goetzinger P, Sautner T, Steininger R, Muehlbacher F (1991) The impact of presumed consent law and decentralized organ procurement system on organ donation: quadruplication of number of organ donors. Transplant Proc (in press)
7. Jamieson NV, Sundberg R, Lindell S, et al (1988) Preservation of the canine liver for 24–48 hours using simple cold storage with UW solution. Transplantation 46: 517–522
8. Kaplan EL, Meier P (1958) Nonparametric estimation from incomplete observations. J Am Stat Assoc 53: 457–481
9. Mantel N (1966) Evaluation of survival data and two new rank order statistic avising in its consideration. Cancer Chemother Rep 50: 163–165
10. Stuart FP, Veith FJ, Cranford RE (1981) Brain death laws and patterns of consent to remove organs for transplantation from cadavers in the United States and 28 other countries. Transplantation 31: 238–244

Transplant Int (1992) 5 [Suppl 1]: S 725–S 726

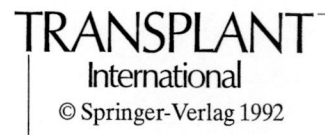

© Springer-Verlag 1992

Assessment of costs to donor hospitals for organ transplantation

C. Wight, M. G. M. Rowland, A. Morris, and P. J. F. Friend

Department of Surgery, Addenbrooke's Hospital, Cambridge, United Kingdom

In 1987, die Department of Health in the UK set up a working party to identify reasons contributing to a shortfall in donor organs. One recommendation was reimbursement to the District Health Authorities for costs incurred in providing the donor organs. The figure chosen was not to be seen as an incentive to donate organs, merely as an appropriate compensation for the costs incurred. There would be no direct payment to doctors, trustees or relatives of the donor. With the development of the competitive health care environment in the United Kingdom, the reimbursement of donating hospital costs is being considered with these data.

Key words: Costs – Donor hospitals

Method

The study started on May 1st, 1989. Prospective information on resource use was sought by questionnaire for all potential donors in 5 Health Regions during a 7-month period. The period of care for which data were collected was from the time of the second brain stem death tests to the closure of the operating theatre. The information was obtained and recorded by Transplant Coordinators or by the key ward or operating theatre staff concerned. Costs directly attributable to the management of a potential donor included staff, consumables, capital costs, general services and capital charging.

Staff costs. Medical and nursing costs were based on recorded time spent with the donor, and on behalf of the donor but away from the bedside. For nursing staff the midpoint of the relevant salary scale was used, plus 30% for extra duty allowance and cover and a further 15% on costs (employers' contributions for pensions, etc.). For medical staff the midpoint of the salary scale for each grade of staff was taken. Gross costs were used which included average merit awards for consultants and UMT for junior staff. Ancillary staff costs were based on time spent from the opening to closure of the operating theatre and in transporting the donor between the ward, operating theatre and mortuary. The midpoint of the relevant salary scale was used. Gross costs were used plus an additional 30% for overtime.

Offprint requests to: C. Wight, Department of Surgery, Addenbrooke's Hospital, Hills Road, Cambridge CB2 200, United Kingdom

Consumables. Drugs were costed at the East Anglian contract price. Tests and disposables were based on the Addenbrooke's Hospital costs. Blood products were costed at standard Blood Transfusion Service costs.

Capital costs. All items of capital equipment were attributed to individual donors according to use, based on estimates of present values, using a discount rate of 6%. Ward equipment costs were attributed on a daily basis, theatre equipment on a session basis. Indirect hospital costs were apportioned to the donor on a daily rate.

General services. Such items as administration, medical records, training, catering, cleaning, laundry, transport, etc. were also included. The Addenbrooke's Hospital mid-1989 prices were used and were based on the length of time between confirmation of brain stem death and the onset of organ retrieval.

Capital charging. It is estimated that this will add 20% to current revenue costs. The cost of the donors' use of resources was therefore increased by 20%. The only exception to this was for charges attributed specifically to items of capital equipment priced at £1,000 or more.

Data analysis was carried out using the Statistical Package for the Social Sciences (SPSS Inc.) and Supercalc 5 (Computer Associates).

Results

Clinical information was obtained on 112 potential donors. This comprised data on 38 kidney donors, 70 multi-organ donors, and 4 potential donors from whom organs

Table 1. Consolidated costs by category of cost (£)

Cost category	Mean	Minimum	Maximum	Total (%)
A. Staff consulting	16	0	103	1820 (3)
B. Blood products	26	0	386	2910 (5)
C. Investigations	28	0	192	3105 (7)
D. Drugs maintenance	21	0	193	2392 (4)
E. Drugs operation	10	0	158	1111 (2)
F. Equipment and theatre	76	0	94	8552 (15)
G. Ward staff	166	0	758	18636 (34)
H. Theatre staff	131	0	524	14704 (27)
I. General services	17	0	93	1831 (3)
Total	492	0	1396	55061 (100)

Table 2. Consolidated costs by category of donor (£)

	Number	Mean	Median	Minimum	Maximum	Total
Kidney	38	410	375	134	887	15566
Multi-organ	70	559	482	151	1396	39123
Abandoned	4	93	82	0	208	373
All donors	112	492		0	1396	55062

were not retrieved. Costs consolidated by category cost are shown in Table 1. Costs consolidated by category of donor are shown in Table 2.

Discussion

It is clear that staff salaries contribute substantially (>60%) to the estimate of overall costs.

The actual mean duration of the interval between the diagnosis of brain stem death and the start of the donor operation was 5.4 h, with a median of 4.0 h for kidney donors and 5.5 h for multi-organ donors. The interval between the first and second tests for brain stem death varied from 0 to 64 h with a mean of 9 h.

The mean duration of the donor operation was 1.5 h for kidney donation (median 1.25) but longer at 3.2 h for multi-organ retrieval (median 3). To be added to this is the recorded time spent opening, preparing and closing the theatre. This time difference between the two categories of donor will be reflected in the overall costs.

Proposing a single figure estimate of costs incurred in relation to potential donors not coming to organ retrieval is problematical. The stage at which plans may be abandoned is variable. The main component of the costs will be directly related to the number of staff and the time spent in caring for the donor. Looking at the relative cost contributions of the maintenance period and of organ retrieval, the split was approximately 55:45 in our study for all categories combined.

In conclusion, a median cost of £375 for a kidney donor and £482 for a multi-organ donor should be taken as minimum estimates. Though less correct statistically, the mean values obtained may be more realistic and are most unlikely to be overestimates. A value of around 45% of the mean might well be a reasonable estimate of the cost incurred in the care of potential donors not coming to successful donor operation, though clearly overcompensating in the situation where plans for organ retrieval were abandoned at an early stage.

Transplant Int (1992) 5 [Suppl 1]: S 727–S 729

TRANSPLANT
International
© Springer-Verlag 1992

Impact of donor age on living related donor kidney transplantation

M. Sobh, A. El-Salam Yousif, A. Shokeir, A. Shaaban, M. Kenawy, A. El-Sherif, and M. Ghoneim

Urology and Nephrology Center, University of Mansoura, Mansoura, Egypt

Abstract. Two comparable groups of kidney transplant recipients were identified according to the age of their kidney donors. The first group (A) comprised 42 recipients of donors aged < 40 years, and the second group (B) comprised 48 recipients of donors aged > 50 years. The patients were followed for a mean period of 26 months (range 13–50 months). Post-transplant renal function and graft survival were assessed together with the frequency of post-transplant proteinuria and hypertension. Moreover, the functional reserve of the grafts was determined by comparing the clearance values, obtained by both isotope and chemical means, before and after a combined infusion of dopamine and an amino acids preparation. The graft function was significantly better in group A according to the serum creatinine levels (μmol/l) at 1 month (107 ± 4.5 vs. 134 ± 10.7, $P < 0.01$), 12 months (119 ± 5.3 vs. 181 ± 88, $P < 0.05$) and at last follow-up visit (118 ± 6.2 vs. 223 ± 63, $P < 0.03$) for groups A and B, respectively. The graft survival in group A was significantly higher than that in group B (100 % vs. 87 % at 1 year, $P < 0.05$). The graft functional reserve was significantly better in group A than in group B. Post-transplant proteinuria was significantly more frequent in group B recipients (70 % vs. 40 %, $P < 0.03$). The age of the donors had no impact on the incidence of post-transplant hypertension. These observations suggest that the transplantation of a kidney from an older live kidney donor is associated with an inferior post-transplant outcome.

Key words: Donor age – Kidney transplantation

In many countries, living related donors are still the main source of kidneys for transplantation in view of the poor legal definition and deficient organization of cadaveric donor work-up. The excessive demand for donor kidneys has necessitated the continued use of those available as ef-

ficiently as possible. In many cases these donors are more than 50 years old. The impact of kidney age on graft survival is contradictory; Matas et al. [1] showed no difference in graft survival of kidneys from living donors older or younger than 45 years. Similarly, Wetzels et al. [2] found that donor age did not affect the outcome of renal transplantation. On the other hand, Rao et al. [3] reported that graft survival and renal function in recipients of older donor kidneys (> 50 years) were significantly lower than in a control group who received kidneys from donors between 11 and 50 years of age.

With a view to clarifying the impact of kidney age on the outcome of kidney transplantation, we evaluated 90 consecutive patients who received kidneys from young and older living related donors. Evaluation involved estimation of the graft functional reserve and the trends of decline in graft function over time.

Materials and methods

In this analysis we studied 90 consecutive renal transplants performed in our centre between 1987 and 1989. All patients received kidneys from living related donors (24 from fathers, 26 from mothers and 40 from siblings). The recipients were stratified into two groups according to the age of the donors. The first group (A) comprised 42 recipients of donors aged < 40 years (31.2 ± 6.1 years), and the second group (B) comprised 48 recipients of donors aged > 50 years (56 ± 8.0 years).

Both groups of recipients were comparable with respect to age, sex, duration of pretransplant dialysis, frequency of blood transfusions prior to transplantation and mean time since transplantation. Table 1 summarizes the characteristics of the recipients in both groups. In addition, the HLA-A, B and DR tissue antigens were similarly distributed in both groups, with the majority having an one-haplotype HLA match. Furthermore, the surgical technique employed was similar in the two groups. Retransplantation and children below the age of 16 years were excluded.

The protocol of immunosuppression was identical for both groups of recipients and included simultaneous administration of prednisolone and azathioprine (AZA). In selected cases, cyclosporine (CsA) was used with variable doses of prednisolone. The initial dose of CsA was 12.5 mg/kg daily, and it was decreased thereafter to maintain the whole blood trough levels at 100–200 ng/ml

Offprint requests to: Dr. M. Sobh, Urology and Nephrology Center, University of Mansoura, Egypt

Table 1. Characterestics of patients

Factors analysed	Group A (n = 42)	Group B (n = 48)
Age (years)	26.9 ± 7	30.6 ± 8
Sex (male/female)	31/11	35/13
Duration of pretransplant dialysis (months)	42.2 ± 4	41.5 ± 5
Prior transfusions (units)	3.2 ± 2	3.1 ± 2.5
Mean time since transplantation (months)	23 ± 4	25 ± 5
Tissue matching		
One haplotype	39	38
Full match	2	9
Complete mismatch	1	1
Type of primary immunosuppression		
Prednisone + azathioprine	25	19
Prednisone + cyclosporine	9	8
Triple	8	21

Table 2. Post-transplant serum creatinine level (μmol/l; mean ± SD)

Time of measurement after transplantation	Serum creatinine Group A	Group B	P value
At 1 month	107 ± 4.5	134 ± 10.7	0.015
At 3 months	107 ± 4.5	151 ± 13.4	0.03
At 6 months	116 ± 4.5	160 ± 16	0.02
At 12 months	119 ± 5.3	181 ± 88	0.05
At the most recent follow-up visit	118 ± 6.2	223 ± 63	0.03

(Sandoz, radioimmunoassay, RIA kits). AZA in an initial dose of 2–3 mg/kg daily, was adjusted according to the white blood cell counts, and prednisolone was slowly tapered from a dose of 90 mg/day to 10 mg/day over a period of 6 months.

Acute rejection episodes were diagnosed on a clinical basis and confirmed by fine needle aspiration cytology (FNAC) [4]. Tru-cut biopsy was performed when FNAC result was inconclusive. Rejection episodes were treated by 750 mg methylprednisolone given intravenously on 5 consecutive days.

The patients were followed for a mean period of 26 months (range 13–50 months). Patient and graft survival were assessed together with the frequency of post-transplant proteinuria and hypertension. Chronic rejection was diagnosed on a clinical basis and confirmed in all cases by the examination of a core biopsy. The serum creatinine level was measured at 1, 3, 6 and 12 months and at the most recent follow-up visit. The graft glomerular filtration rate (GFR) was measured by technetium-99m diethylene triamine peuta-acetic acid (^{99m}Tc-DTPA) scans [5] and by the determination of the endogenous creatinine clearance. Moreover, the functional reserve of the graft was assessed by the simultaneous infusion of dopamine (2.5 μg/kg·min) and a 10% solution of an amino acid preparation, Vamin N (80 ml/h) for 12 h. During the procedure, a diuresis of at least 100 ml/h was maintained by orally administered fluids. At 6 h after combined dopamine and amino acids infusion, when the GFR reaches its maximum level, the isotope clearance was measured using ^{99m}Tc-DTPA scans. Furthermore, an urine sample was collected, and the endogenous creatinine clearance was measured at the end of the 12 h. The functional reserve of the graft was determined by comparing the clearance values obtained by both isotope and chemical means with the corresponding values obtained before the infusion of dopamine and amino acids.

For statistical analysis we used Student's t-tests for paired and unpaired comparisons, χ^2 test of proportions and Fisher's exact test.

Results

Patient and graft survival

At 1 year, the patient survival rate was not significantly different among the 2 groups (100% vs. 96% for groups A and B, respectively). However, the 1-year graft survival in recipients of group A was significantly higher than that of group B (100% vs. 87%, $P = 0.05$). Six patients from group B lost their grafts; 2 of them had died of uraemia by 1 year post-transplant.

Graft function, functional reserve and post-transplant complications

The serum creatinine values at 1, 3, 6 and 12 months and at the last follow-up visit were significantly lower in group A recipients compared with those of group B (Table 2). The response of the graft to the infusion of dopamine and the amino acids preparation is depicted in Table 3. The graft functional reserve, measured by both chemical and isotope means, was significantly higher in the recipients of group A than in those of group B. Acute rejection episodes were documented equally in both groups (in 35 out of 42 patients in group A, and in 40 out of 48 patients in group B). Although the incidence of post-transplant hypertension was higher in group B recipients, the difference was not statistically significant (36% in group A vs. 49% in group B, $P = 0.5$). Furthermore, post-transplant proteinuria was significantly more frequent in group B (70%) than in group A (40%) recipients ($P = 0.03$).

Discussion

The results of our analysis showed that the recipients of kidneys from living related donors older than 50 years have a lower graft survival and reduced post-transplant renal function compared with recipients whose donors were younger than 40 years of age. These observations are in agreement with the clinical data reported by other in-

Table 3. Effect of infusion of dopamine (D) and amino acids preparation (A) on the glomerular filtration rate (GFR; ml/min)

	GFR estimated by creatinine clearance			Isotope GFR		
	Value before D&A	Value after D&A	Graft reserve	Value before D&A	Value after D&A	Graft reserve
Group A	72.05 ± 13.43	89.54 ± 10.79	15.9 ± 9.43*	63.7 ± 8.07	75 ± 10.09	11.24 ± 7.5**
Group B	51.18 ± 18.5	66.5 ± 16.5	7.7 ± 5.06*	64.75 ± 7.8	70 ± 11.29	5.2 ± 6.15**

Mean ± SD
* $P = 0.0001$, ** $P = 0.0002$

vestigators [3, 6, 7]. Moreover, our study draws attention to the fact that kidneys from older donors have less functional reserve capacity as reflected by a smaller increase in GFR after the infusion of a dopamine and amino acids preparation. The decline in graft function observed in kidneys obtained from older age donors could be explained by the anatomical and functional changes known to occur in human kidneys with aging. The aged kidney is a seat of progressive glomerular sclerosis, atherosclerotic occlusion of renal vessels and hyalinization, causing a reduction in the number of functioning nephrons [3, 8]. Rao and associates [3] summarized the factors that may shorten the survival of aged kidneys when transplanted into a uraemic patient as the combined effects of compensatory renal haemodynamic injury (pre-existing aging effect) and the post-transplant exposure to noxious events such as acute tubular necrosis, graft rejection, sepsis and nephrotoxic drugs.

This study showed that the development of hypertension in allograft recipients is not dependent on the age of donation. This result is supported by Torres et al. [9], who concluded that neither the age of the donors nor their predisposition to developing hypertension significantly influences the blood pressure status of the recipients. Darmady [6], however, reported a higher risk of post-transplant hypertension in recipients of older grafts compared with younger ones. Differences among authors may reflect the multiplicity of risk factors associatied with the development of hypertension in renal transplant patients.

A significant association between post-transplant proteinuria and the age of the kidney donors is evident in our study. Indeed, post-transplant proteinuria may be attributed to several causes, including recurrence of the original kidney disease, the appearance of de novo nephropathy, chronic rejection or ligation of one of the long veins draining the graft [10]. Since the age of a kidney graft is unlikely to affect all the causes of proteinuria equally, the demonstrated association may reflect variation in the relative frequency of each of these causes among different populations of kidney recipients. Indeed, an earlier report by Talseth and associates [11] stated that donor age is not related to an increase in blood pressure or protein excretion at follow-up.

In conclusion, the levels of renal function and the renal functional reserve of kidneys obtained from older live donors are significantly inferior to those of younger live donors when measured at corresponding time points following renal transplantation. The clinical significance of these findings, however, should await longer follow-up studies, particularly in view of the continuous shortage of organs for renal transplantation.

Acknowledgement. We thank Miss Ghada Abdallah for her secretarial work during the preparation of the manuscript.

References

1. Matas AJ, Simmons RL, Kjellstrand CM, et al (1976) Transplantation of the aging kidney. Transplantation 21: 160–161
2. Wetzels JFM, Hoitsma AJ, Koene RA (1986) Influence of cadaver donor age on renal graft survival. Clin Nephrol 25: 256–259
3. Rao KV, Kasiske BL, Odlund MD, et al (1990) Influence of cadaver donor age on post-transplant renal function and graft outcome. Transplantation 49: 91–95
4. Sobh MA, Moustafa FE, Ghoneim MA (1987) Fine-needle aspiration biopsy: a reproducibility study and a correlation with the tru-cut biopsy in the evaluation of renal allotransplants. Nephrol Dial Transplant 2: 562–567
5. Jackson JH, Blue PW, Ghaed N (1985) Glomerular filtration rate determination with routine renal scanning. Radiology 154: 203–205
6. Darmady EM (1974) Transplantation and the aging kidney. Lancet 2: 1046–1047
7. Morling N, Ladefoged J, Lange P, et al (1975) Kidney transplantation and donor age. Tissue Antigens 6: 163–166
8. Ljungqvist A, Lagergren C (1962) Normal intrarenal arterial pattern in adult and aging human kidneys. J Anat 96: 285–300
9. Torres VE, Offord KP, Anderson CF, et al (1987) Blood pressure determinants in living related renal allograft donors and their recipients. Kidney Int 31: 1383–1390
10. Abouna GM, Kogure H, Porter KA, Sobel RE (1973) Homotransplantation. JAMA 226: 631
11. Talseth T, Fauchald P, Skrede S, et al (1986) Long-term blood pressure and renal function in kidney donors. Kidney Int 29: 1072–1076

Worldwide distribution ● Rapid publication

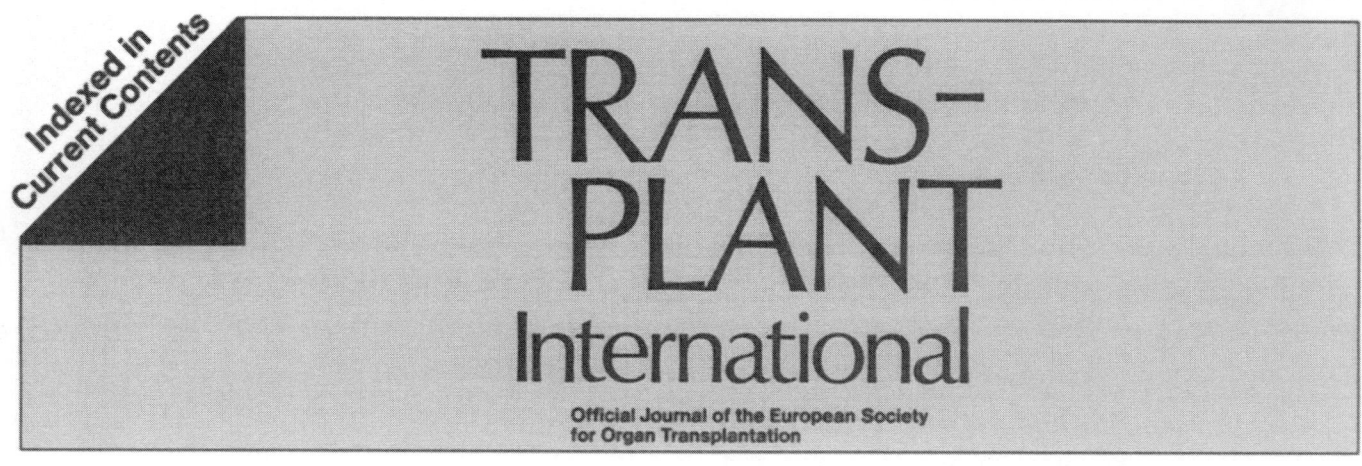

Indexed in Current Contents

TRANS-PLANT International

Official Journal of the European Society for Organ Transplantation

ISSN 0934-0874   Title No. 147

Contents of Volume 4, Number 2

Send now for your free sample copy or subscription!

Editor-in-Chief

G. Kootstra
Department of Surgery,
University Hospital,
P. Debyelaan 25,
P. O. Box 5800,
6202 AZ Maastricht,
The Netherlands

Editorial Board

H. Brynger, Göteborg
W. A. Buurman, Maastricht
P. Häyry, Helsinki
R. A. P. Koene, Nijmegen
W. Land, Munich
P. McMaster, Birmingham
M. J. Mihatsch, Basel
G. Opelz, Heidelberg
B. Ringe, Hannover
R. van Schilfgaarde, Groningen
G. Sirchia, Milan
J. P. Soulillou, Nantes
J. P. Squifflet, Brussels
J. Wallwork, Cambridge

in cooperation with
a distinguished
International Advisory Board

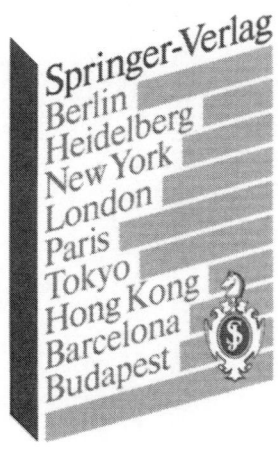

Springer-Verlag
Berlin
Heidelberg
New York
London
Paris
Tokyo
Hong Kong
Barcelona
Budapest

**D. K. C. Cooper, E. Kemp, K. Reemtsma,
D. J. G. White (Eds.)**

Xenotransplantation

The Transplantation of Organs and Tissues Between Species

1991. XXIX, 583 pp. 153 figs. 68 tabs. Hardcover
ISBN 3-540-53875-5

The possibility of transplanting organs and tissues between animal species – a field known as xenotransplantation – has captured the imagination of a handful of scientists for decades. In recent years, however, advances in immunology and immunosuppressive therapy, together with the chronic shortage of organ donors, have stimulated widespread interest in xenotransplantation in the international scientific community. The greatly increasing number of experimental efforts during the past few years is clear evidence of the upsurge in interest in this topic.

The work of the world's leading researchers is documented in this book – the first comprehensive volume to be published on the subject. It gives a detailed overview of the present status of xenotransplantation and is essential reading for anyone interested in the medical, scientific or ethical aspects of this rapidly developing field. The wide range of information presented will help the reader pinpoint advances of great potential and evaluate prospects for clinical application in the near future.

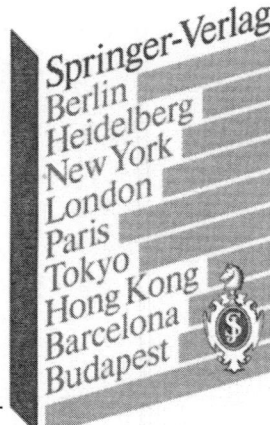

Springer-Verlag
Berlin
Heidelberg
New York
London
Paris
Tokyo
Hong Kong
Barcelona
Budapest